125.00

D1460385

125.00

Multiple Sclerosis Therapeutics

Fourth Edition

Multiple Sclerosis Therapeutics

Fourth Edition

Edited by

Jeffrey A. Cohen, MD
Director, Experimental Therapeutics Program, Mellen Center for Multiple Sclerosis Treatment and Research, Neurological Institute, Cleveland Clinic, Cleveland, OH, USA

Richard A. Rudick, MD
Director, Mellen Center for Multiple Sclerosis Treatment and Research, Neurological Institute, Cleveland Clinic, Cleveland, OH, USA

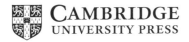

CAMBRIDGE
UNIVERSITY PRESS

CAMBRIDGE UNIVERSITY PRESS
Cambridge, New York, Melbourne, Madrid, Cape Town,
Singapore, São Paulo, Delhi, Tokyo, Mexico City

Cambridge University Press
The Edinburg Building, Cambridge CB2 8RU, UK

Published in the United States of America by Cambridge University
Press, New York

www.cambridge.org
Information on this title: www.cambridge.org/
9780521766272

First published 2011

Printed in the United Kingdom at the University Press, Cambridge

A catalog record for this publication is available from the British Library

Library of Congress Cataloging in Publication data
Multiple sclerosis therapeutics / edited by Jeffrey A. Cohen,
Richard A. Rudick. – 4th ed.
    p.   ;   cm.
Includes bibliographical references and index.
ISBN 978-0-521-76627-2 (hardback)
I. Cohen, Jeffrey A. (Jeffrey Alan), 1954–   II. Rudick, Richard A.
III. Title.
[DNLM: 1. Multiple Sclerosis – therapy.   2. Clinical Trials as Topic –
methods.   3. Magnetic Resonance Imaging.   4. Multiple Sclerosis –
pathology.   5. Outcome Assessment (Health Care) WL 360]
LC classification not assigned
616.8′34 – dc23   2011030483

ISBN 978-0-521-76627-2 Hardback

Contents

Section IV – Therapy in clinical practice

Contributors

Douglas L. Arnold, MD
James McGill Professor of Neurology; Director, Magnetic Resonance Spectroscopy Unit, Montreal Neurological Institute, McGill University, Montreal, Quebec, Canada

Laura J. Balcer, MD, MSCE
Department of Neurology, University of Pennsylvania School of Medicine, Philadelphia, PA, USA

Amit Bar-Or, MD, FRCPC
Associate Professor, Neurology & Neurosurgery and Associate Professor, Microbiology & Immunology, McGill University; Director, Experimental Therapeutics Program, Montreal Neurological Institute; Staff Neurologist, Montreal Neurological Hospital, McGill University Hospital Center, Montreal, Quebec, Canada

Sergio E. Baranzini, PhD
Department of Neurology, University of California at San Francisco, San Francisco, CA, USA

Frederik Barkhof, MD, PhD
Professor, Department of Diagnostic Radiology, VU University Medical Center, Amsterdam, The Netherlands

Robert A. Bermel, MD
Mellen Center for Multiple Sclerosis Treatment and Research, Neurological Institute, Cleveland Clinic, Cleveland, OH, USA

Francois A. Bethoux, MD
Mellen Center for Multiple Sclerosis Treatment and Research, Neurological Institute, Cleveland Clinic, Cleveland, OH, USA

Dennis N. Bourdette, MD
Chair and Roy and Eulalia Swank Family Research Professor, Department of Neurology, Oregon Health Sciences University, Portland, OR, USA

Richard K. Burt, MD
Division of Immunotherapy, Department of Medicine, Northwestern University, Feinberg School of Medicine, Chicago, Il, USA

Peter A. Calabresi, MD
Professor of Neurology, Director, The John Hopkins Multiple Sclerosis Center, Director, Division of Neuroimmunology and Neuroinfectious Diseases, Department of Neurology, John Hopkins University, Baltimore, MD, USA

Zografos Caramanos, MA
Magnetic Resonance Spectroscopy Unit, Montreal Neurological Institute, McGill University, Montreal, Quebec, Canada

Tanuja Chitnis, MD
Department of Neurology, Brigham and Women's Hospital, Center for Neurologic Disease, Partners MS Center, Harvard Medical School, Boston, MA, USA

Stacey S. Cofield, PhD
Department of Biostatistics, University of Alabama at Birmingham, Birmingham, AL, USA

Jeffrey A. Cohen, MD
Director, Experimental Therapeutics Program, Mellen Center for Multiple Sclerosis Treatment and Research, Neurological Institute, Cleveland Clinic, Cleveland, OH, USA

Nadine Cohen, PhD
Senior Vice President, Regulatory Affairs, Biogen Idec Inc., Cambridge, MA, USA

Alasdair J. Coles, PhD, FRCP
Department of Clinical Neurosciences, University of Cambridge, Addenbrooke's Hospital, Cambridge, UK

Devon Conway, MD, MSC
Mellen Center for Multiple Sclerosis Treatment and Research, Neurological Institute, Cleveland Clinic Foundation, Cleveland, OH, USA

Stuart D. Cook, MD
University of Medicine and Dentistry, New Jersey Medical School, Newark, NJ, USA

Gary R. Cutter, PhD
Department of Biostatistics, University of Alabama at Birmingham, Birmingham, AL, USA

Peter J. Darlington, PhD
Research Associate, Montreal Neurological Institute, Neuroimmunology Unit, McGill University, Montreal, Quebec, Canada

Ann Dodds-Frerichs, MBA
Senior Director, Regulatory Affairs, Biogen Idec Inc., Cambridge, MA, USA

Ranjan Dutta, PhD
Project Staff, Department of Neurosciences, Cleveland Clinic, Cleveland, OH, USA

Gilles Edan, MD
Chef de Service de Neurolosie Clinique Neurologie, CHU Pontchaillou, Rennes, France

Michelle Fabian, MD
Assistant Professor of Neurology, Corinne Goldsmith Dickinson Center for Multiple Selerosis, Department of Neurology, Mount Sinai School of Medicine, New York, NY, USA

Franz Fazekas, MD
Department of Neurology, Medical University of Graz, Graz, Austria

Massimo Filippi, MD
Neuroimaging Research Unit, Institute of Experimental Neurology, Division of Neuroscience, San Raffaele Scientific Institute, Vita-Salute, San Raffaele University, Milan, Italy

Elizabeth Fisher, PhD
Department of Biomedical Engineering, Lerner Research Institute, Cleveland Clinic, Cleveland, OH, USA

Paulo Fontoura, MD, PhD
Department of Immunology, Faculty of Medical Sciences, New University of Lisbon, Lisbon, Portugal

Corey C. Ford, MD, PhD
Department of Neurology, University of New Mexico, Albuquerque, NM, USA

Robert J. Fox, MD
Medical Director, Mellen Center for Multiple Sclerosis Treatment and Research, Neurological Institute, Cleveland Clinic, Cleveland, OH, USA

Natasha Frost, MD, MSC
Dean Health System, Madison, WI, USA

Alex Z. Fu, PhD
Department of Quantitative Health Sciences, Cleveland Clinic, Cleveland, OH USA

Siegrid Fuchs, MD
Department of Neurology, Medical University of Graz, Graz, Austria

Kazuo Fujihara, MD
Dept of Multiple Sclerosis Therapeutics and Neurology, Tohoku University, Sendai, Japan

Kristin M. Galetta, MS
Department of Neurology, University of Pennsylvania School of Medicine, Philadelphia, PA, USA

Jeroen J.G. Geurts, PhD
MR Center for MS Research, VU University Medical Center, Amsterdam, The Netherlands

Gavin Giovannoni, MBBCh, PhD
Blizard Institute of Cell and Molecular Science, Barts and The London School of Medicine and Dentistry, Queen Mary University of London, London, UK

Nada Gligorov, PhD
Assistant Professor of Medical Education, Mount Sinai School of Medicine, New York, NY, USA

Ralf Gold, MD
Department of Neurology, St. Josef-Hospital and Ruhr-University Bochum, Bochum, Germany

Andrew D. Goodman, MD
Department of Neurology, University of Rochester School of Medicine and Dentistry, Rochester, NY, USA

Myla D. Goldman, MD, MSc
Department of Neurology, University of Virginia, Charlottesville, VA, USA

Jenny Guerre, MD
Department of Neurology, University of New Mexico, Albuquerque, NM, USA

Stephen L. Hauser, MD
Professor and Chair, Department of Neurology, University of California at San Francisco, San Francisco, CA, USA

Peter B. Imrey, PhD
Professor of Medicine, Department of Quantitative Health Sciences, Cleveland Clinic, Cleveland, OH, USA

Douglas R. Jeffery, MD, PhD
The Multiple Sclerosis Center at Advance Neurology, Advance, NC, USA

Stephen E. Jones, MD, PhD
Department of Diagnostic Radiology, Imaging Institute, Cleveland Clinic, Cleveland, OH, USA

Adam I. Kaplin, MD, PhD
Assistant Professor of Psychiatry and Neurology, Departments of Psychiatry and Behavioral Sciences and Neurology, John

Hopkins University School of Medicine, Baltimore, MD, USA

Michael W. Kattan, PhD
Chair, Department of Quantitative Health Sciences, Cleveland Clinic, Cleveland, OH, USA

B. Mark Keegan, MD
Associate Professor and Consultant of Neurology, Department of Neurology, School of Medicine, Mayo Clinic, Rochester, MN, USA

Kyle C. Kern, MS
Staff Research Associate, Department of Neurology, David Geffen School of Medicine, UCLA, Los Angeles, CA, USA

Zhaleh Khaleeli, PhD
Specialist Registrar in Neurology, Institute of Neurology, University College London, Queen Square, London, UK

Samia J. Khoury, MD
Department of Neurology, Brigham and Women's Hospital, Center for Neurologic Disease, Partners MS Center, Harvard Medical School, Boston, MA, USA

Joep Killestein, MD, PhD
Department of Neurology, VU Medical Center, Amsterdam, The Netherlands

Soo Hyun Kim, MD
Cardiovascular Medicine, Section of Vascular Medicine, Cleveland Clinic, Cleveland, OH, USA

R. Philip Kinkel, MD
Director, Multiple Sclerosis Program, Beth Israel Deaconess Medical Center; Associate Professor of Neurology, Harvard Medical School, Boston, MA, USA

Stephen C. Krieger, MD
Assistant Professor of Neurology, Corinne Goldsmith Dickinson Center for Multiple Sclerosis, Department of Neurology, Mount Sinai School of Medicine, New York, NY, USA

Lauren B. Krupp, MD
Stony Brook University Medical Center, Department of Neurology, Stony Brook, NY, USA

Emmanuelle Le Page, MD
Service de Neurologie, Hôpital Pontchaillou, Rennes, France

David Leppert, MD
Associate Professor, Department of Neurology, University Hospital Basel, Switzerland

Scott Litwiller, MD
Urologic Associates of Oklahoma, Tulsa, OK, USA

Fred D. Lublin, MD
Saunders Family Professor of Neurology, Corinne Goldsmith Dickinson Center for Multiple Sclerosis, Department of Neurology, Mount Sinai School of Medicine, New York, NY, USA

Henry F. McFarland, MD
Chief, Neuroimmunology Branch, National Institute of Neurological Disorders and Stroke, National Institutes of Health, Bethesda, MD USA

Joseph C. McGowan, PhD
Exponent Inc. Philadelphia, PA, USA

Don Mahad, MD, PhD
Mellen Center for MS Treatment and Research, Neurological Institute, Cleveland Clinic, Cleveland, OH, USA

Jahangir Maleki, MD, PhD
Neurological Center for Pain, Neurological Institute, Cleveland Clinic, Cleveland, OH, USA

Ruth Ann Marrie, MD, PhD
Associate Professor of Medicine, Departments of Internal Medicine and Community Health Sciences, University of Manitoba, Winnipeg, Manitoba, Canada

Paul M. Matthews, MD, DPhil
Centre for Neurosciences, Division of Experimental Medicine and Toxicology, Imperial College, London; GlaxoSmithKline Clinical Imaging Centre, Hammersmith Hospital, London, UK

Francesca Milanetti, MD
Division of Immunotherapy, Department of Medicine, Northwestern University, Feinberg School of Medicine, Chicago, IL, USA; Division of Clinical Immunology and Rheumatology, S. Andrea University Hospital, "Sapienza" University of Rome, II School of Medicine, Rome, Italy

Aaron E. Miller, MD, FAAN
Professor of Neurology, Corinne Goldsmith Dickinson Center for Multiple Sclerosis, Department of Neurology, Mount Sinai School of Medicine, New York, NY, USA

Deborah M. Miller, PhD
Director, Comprehensive Care, Mellen Center for Multiple Sclerosis Treatment and Research, Cleveland Clinic, Neurological Institute, Cleveland, OH, USA

Xavier Montalban, MD
Unitat de Neuroimmunologia Clínica, Multiple Sclerosis Centre of Catalonia (CEM-Cat), Vall d'Hebron University Hospital, Barcelona, Spain

Charity J. Morgan, PhD
Food and Drug Administration, Silver Spring, MD, USA

Ichiro Nakashima, MD
Department of Multiple Sclerosis Therapeutics and Neurology, Tohoku University, Sendai, Japan

Sridar Narayanan, PhD
Department of Neurology and Neurosurgery, Magnetic Resonance Spectroscopy Unit, Montreal Neurological Institute, McGill University, Montreal, Quebec, Canada

Avindra Nath, MD
The John Hopkins Multiple Sclerosis Center, Department of Neurology, John Hopkins University, Baltimore, MD, USA

Paul W. O'Connor, MD, MSc
Waugh Family Chair in Multiple Sclerosis Research; Professor, Department of Health Policy, Management and Evaluation, University of Toronto, Toronto, Ontario, Canada

Jorge R. Oksenberg, PhD
Department of Neurology, University of California at San Francisco, San Francisco, CA, USA

A. John Petkau, PhD
Professor, Department of Statistics, University of British Columbia, Vancouver, British Columbia, Canada

Michael D. Phillips, MD
Department of Diagnostic Radiology, Imaging Institute, Cleveland Clinic, Cleveland, OH, USA

J. Theodore Phillips, MD, PhD
Director, Multiple Sclerosis Program, Baylor Institute for Immunology Research, Baylor University Medical Center, Dallas, TX, USA

Tammy Phinney, MSC
Director, Regulatory Affairs, Biogen Idec Inc., Cambridge, MA, USA

Sean J. Pittock, MB, BAO, BCh, MMedSci, MD
Associate Professor of Neurology, Department of Neurology, College of Medicine, Mayo Clinic, Rochester, MN, USA

Sarah M. Planchon, PhD
Mellen Center for MS Treatment and Research, Neurological Institute, Cleveland Clinic, Cleveland, OH, USA

Chris H. Polman, MD, FRCP, FRCPI
Professor and Chair, Department of Neurology, VU Medical Center, Amsterdam, The Netherlands

Alexander Rae-Grant, MD
Mellen Center for Multiple Sclerosis Treatment and Research, Neurological Institute, Cleveland Clinic Foundation, Cleveland, OH, USA

Stephen M. Rao, PhD
Director, Schey Center for Cognitive Neuroimaging, Lov Ruvo Center for Brain Health, Neurological Institute, Cleveland Clinic, Cleveland, OH, USA

Stephen C. Reingold, PhD
President, Scientific and Clinical Review Associates, LLC Salisbury, Connecticut and New York City, NY, USA

Maria A. Rocca, MD
Neuroimaging Research Unit, Institute of Experimental Neurology, Division of Neuroscience, San Raffaele Scientific Institute, Vita-Salute, San Raffaele University, Milan, Italy

Richard A. Rudick, MD
Director, Mellen Center for Multiple Sclerosis Treatment and Research, Neurological Institute, Cleveland Clinic, Cleveland, OH, USA

Amber R. Salter, MPH
Department of Biostatistics, University of Alabama at Birmingham, Birmingham, AL, USA

Paula Sandler, PhD
Vice President, Regulatory Affairs, Biogen Idec Inc., Cambridge, MA, USA

Jaume Sastre-Garriga, MD
Unitat de Neuroimmunologia Clínica, Multiple Sclerosis Centre of Catalonia (CEM-Cat), Vall d'Hebron University Hospital, Barcelona, Spain

John R. Scagnelli, MD
Department of Neurology, University of Virginia, Charlottesville, VA, USA

Dana J. Serafin, BA
Stony Brook University Medical Center, Department of Neurology, Stony Brook, NY, USA

Lynne Shinto, ND, MPH
Associate Professor, Deparmtent of Neurology, Oregon Health and Science University, Portland, OR, USA

Nancy L. Sicotte, MD
Department of Neurology, Cedars-Sinai Medical Center, Los Angeles, CA, USA

Jack H. Simon, MD, PhD
Professor, Department of Diagnostic Radiology, Oregon Health and Science University; Chief, Imaging, Portland VA Medical Center, Portland, OR, USA

Per Soelberg Sørensen, MD, DMSc
Danish Multiple Sclerosis Center, Department of Neurology, Copenhagen University Hospital Rigshospitalet, Copenhagen, Denmark

Ryan E. Stagg, MD
Department of Psychiatry and Behavioral, Sciences, John Hopkins University School of Medicine, Baltimore, MD, USA

James M. Stankiewicz, MD
Department of Neurology, Brigham and Women's Hospital, Center for Neurologic Disease, Partners MS Center, Harvard Medical School, Boston, MA, USA

Lael A. Stone, MD
Mellen Center for Multiple Sclerosis Treatment and Research, Neurological Institute, Cleveland Clinic, Cleveland, OH, USA

Amy Sullivan, PsyD
Mellen Center for Multiple Sclerosis Treatment and Research, Neurological Institute, Cleveland Clinic, Cleveland, OH, USA

Matthew Sutliff, PT
Mellen Center for Multiple Sclerosis Treatment and Research, Neurological Institute, Cleveland Clinic, Cleveland, OH, USA

Jessica Szpak
Dean Health System, Madison, WI, USA

Alan J. Thompson, MD, FRCP, FRCPI, FAAN
Dean, University College London, Faculty of Brain Sciences, London, UK

Bruce D. Trapp, PhD
Chairman, Department of Neuroscience, Lerner Research Institute, Cleveland Clinic, Cleveland, OH, USA

Helen Tremlett, BPharm, MRPharmS, PhD
Faculty of Medicine, Division of Neurology, Brain Research Centre, Faculty of Medicine University of British Columbia, Vancouver, British Columbia, Canada

Maria Trojano, MD
Professor of Neurology, Department of Neurological and Psychiatric Sciences, University of Bari, Bari Italy

Orla Tuohy, MB
Department of Clinical Neurosciences, University of Cambridge, Addenbrooke's Hospital, Cambridge, UK

Rhonda R. Voskuhl, MD
Professor, Department of Neurology; Director, Multiple Sclerosis Program, UCLA, Los Angeles, USA

Marc K. Walton, MD, PhD
Associate Director for Translational Medicine, Office of Translational Sciences, Center for Drug Evaluation and Research, FDA, Silver Spring, MD, USA

Mike P. Wattjes, MD
MS Center Amsterdam, Department of Radiology, VU University Medical Center, Amsterdam, The Netherlands

Emmanuelle Waubant, MD, PhD
Department of Neurology, University of California at San Francisco, San Francisco, CA, USA

Martin S. Weber
Department of Neurology, Technische Universität München, Munich, Germany

Howard L Weiner, MD
Department of Neurology, Brigham and Women's Hospital, Center for Neurologic Disease, Partners MS Center, Harvard Medical School, Boston, MA, USA

Brian G. Weinshenker, MD
Professor of Neurology, Department of Neurology, College of Medicine, Mayo Clinic, Rochester, MN, USA

Bianca Weinstock-Guttman, MD
Department of Neurology, State University of New York, Buffalo; Buffalo General Hospital, Buffalo, NY, USA

Jeffrey L. Winters, MD,
Department of Laboratory Medicine and Pathology, Mayo Clinic, Rochester, MN, USA

Jerry S. Wolinsky, MD
Professor, Department of Neurology; Bartels Family Professorship; Opal C. Rankin Professorship, The University of Texas Health Science Center at Houston, Houston, TX, USA

Vijayshree Yadav, MD, MCR
Assistant Professor, Department of Neurology, Oregon Health and Science University, Portland, OR, USA

E. Ann Yeh, MD
Pediatric MS and Demyelinating Disorders Center of the JNI, Women and Children's Hospital of Buffalo, Buffalo, NY, USA

Scott S. Zamvil, MD
Department of Neurology, University of California at San Francisco, San Francisco, CA, USA

Abbreviations list

This list includes abbreviations that were utilized in multiple chapters.

Abbreviation	Full name
9HPT	Nine-Hole Peg Test
AA	African American
AE	adverse event
APC	antigen presenting cell
AQP4	aquaporin-4
ARR	annualized relapse rate
B-cell	B lymphocyte
BBB	blood–brain barrier
BDNF	brain-derived neurotrophic factor
BPF	brain parenchymal fraction
CD	clinically definite
CDMS	clinically definite multiple sclerosis
CI	confidence interval
CIS	clinically isolated syndrome
cMRI	conventional magetic resonance imaging
CNS	central nervous system
CSF	cerebrospinal fluid
DMT	disease-modifying therapy
DTI	diffusion tensor imaging
EAE	experimental autoimmune encephalomyelitis
EBV	Epstein Barr virus
EDSS	Expanded Disability Status Scale
ELISA	enzyme-linked immunosorbent assay
EMA	European Medicines Agency
FDA	Food and Drug Administration
FSS	Functional System Score
GA	glatiramer acetate, Copaxone
GABA	gamma-aminobutyric acid
Gd-enhancing	gadolinium-enhancing
GM	gray matter
HLA	human leukocyte antigen
HR	hazard ratio
HRQoL	health-related quality of life
IFNβ	interferon beta
IFNβ-1b	interferon beta-1b
IFNβ-1a(IM)	interferon beta-1a by intramuscular injection
IFNβ-1a(SC)	interferon beta-1a by subcutaneous injection

Abbreviation	Full name
Ig	immunoglobulin
IL-#	interleukin, e.g. IL-2
IM	intramuscular
IMD	immunomodulatory drug
IRIS	immune reconstitution inflammatory syndrome
i.v.	intravenous
IVIg	intravenous immunoglobulin
MBP	myelin basic protein
MHC	major histocompatibility complex
MMP	matrix metalloproteinase
MOG	myelin oligodendrocytes glycoprotein
MP	methylprednisolone
MRI	magnetic resonance imaging
MRS	magnetic resonance spectroscopy
MS	multiple sclerosis
MSFC	Multiple Sclerosis Functional Composite
MSQLI	Multiple Sclerosis Quality of Life Inventory
MSSS	Multiple Sclerosis Severity Scale
MxA	Myxovirus resistance protein A
NAA	N-acetyl aspartate
NAb	neutralizing antibody
NABT	normal-appearing brain tissue
NAWM	normal-appearing white matter
NMO	neuromyelitis optica
NP	neuropsychological
OCBs	oligoclonal bands
OCT	optical coherence tomography
ON	optic neuritis
OR	odds ratio
PASAT	Paced Auditory Serial Addition Test
PLEX	plasma exhange
PLP	proteolipid protein
PML	progressive multifocal leukoencephalopathy
PP	primary progressive
PPMS	primary progressive multiple sclerosis
QoL	quality of life
RCT	randomized controlled trial

RNFL	retinal nerve fiber layer	SP	secondary progressive
ROC	receiver operating characteristic	SPMS	secondary progressive multiple sclerosis
RR	relapsing–remitting	T25FW	Timed 25-Foot Walk
RRMS	relapsing–remitting multiple sclerosis	T-cell	T lymphocyte
SAE	serious adverse event	TCR	T-cell receptor
s.c.	subcutaneous	TGFβ	transforming growth factor-beta
SDMT	Symbol Digits Modalities Test	TNFα	tumor necrosis factor-alpha
SNP	single nucleotide polymorphism	WM	white matter

Foreword

Multiple Sclerosis Therapeutics is now in its fourth edition and remains the definitive source of information about the theory and art of clinical trials for this complex disorder. The first edition of the book appeared in 1999, only a few years after regulatory approval of the first agents to modify the multiple sclerosis (MS) disease course. Subsequent editions have appeared every 3 to 5 years, attesting to the rapid progress that has been made over the past decade. However, this fourth edition serves as a reminder that we still have only partially effective therapies for only some forms of the disease, that available therapies have problematic side effects and remain extremely expensive, and that there remains a strong demand for safer, more effective, more tolerable, and more affordable therapeutic agents for all forms of MS. An interesting irony to the progress that has been made is that our past success has created new problems in clinical trial theory, design, and conduct. The availability of multiple relatively safe and effective immunomodulatory therapies stresses the need to identify new biological modes of action that might be useful for MS, thus underscoring the problem that we still do not know entirely what causes the disease. And, with many patients worldwide having access to available therapy, the practical and ethical challenges of testing the next generation(s) of therapies require entirely new ways of thinking about trial design and interpretation.

Compared with prior editions, the current volume contains expansive chapters on the biology and demographics of MS, including separate chapters on disease pathology, immunology, genetics, and epidemiology. New MS treatments will require our ability to better target the etiopathology of the disease. Thus, this emphasis on the fundamentals of the disease process helps to chart progress in disease pathology that will surely result in new therapeutic modalities.

An extensive treatment of clinical trial methodology is provided in 19 chapters, providing updated information on clinical assessment, imaging outcomes, biological markers, and evolving developments in regulatory review. New information about cortical lesions in MS – previously a relatively underappreciated locus of disease pathology – points to modalities such as double inversion recovery imaging and other measures of cortical pathology that should be in the "mix" of assessments done to track changes in the brain by MRI. A review of data on neutralizing antibodies that often develop in subjects using interferon therapy has been moved from the prior edition's section on specific therapeutic modalities to the current section on trial design considerations, a reflection perhaps of the need to pay attention to the complexities of evaluating long-term efficacy and of combining new experimental therapies with available therapies which may no longer be effective in some subjects.

The fourth edition contains 27 separate chapters devoted to specific available or experimental therapies for MS, a significant increase over the prior edition. Significantly, there are new chapters on therapies that were not particularly visible at the time of the prior edition 5 years ago: cladribine, fingolimod, fumarate, laquinimod, and teriflunomide, all represent a new era of oral therapy for MS; and alemtuzumab and daclizumab may represent the next steps for monoclonal antibody therapy. A new chapter on mesenchymal and neural stem cell transplantation represents a "brave new world" for MS therapeutics and would not have been possible to include previously. Finally, no discussion of MS therapies today would be complete without a review of the current knowledge and controversy about chronic cerebrospinal venous insufficiency, its detection, prevalence, relevance, and treatment.

Of highly practical impact is the final section of the volume, on "Therapy in Clinical Practice." Recent therapeutic achievements dictate the need for practical advice to practitioners around the world and the expansion of treatment-focus fellowship programs for MS physicians and allied health professionals is an indication of the need for "texts" like Multiple Sclerosis Therapeutics. Diagnosis and treatment of neuromyelitis optica (NMO) is given a new chapter, emphasizing both the recent development of a biological marker for the disease (the aquaporin 4 autoantibody assay) and the prominent role that NMO and NMO spectrum disorders play in the differential diagnosis for MS. Many clinicians are newly focused on diagnosis, treatment, and management of pediatric-onset MS and this topic as well is given a new chapter in the present edition. Also previously not addressed is the topic of comorbidities in patients with MS, which highlights the need to consider and treat non-MS pathologies as well as MS itself, whether these be associated with the underlying autoimmune nature of the disease, a symptomatic consequence of the disease or its treatments, or are simply coincidental.

This will not be the final edition of Multiple Sclerosis Therapeutics. Fundamental and applied research related to MS is burgeoning and will result in new, especially non-immunomodulatory, interventions with novel modes of action that may be used to combine with, or replace, current therapies. Ongoing clinical studies described in this fourth edition will be completed in the next few years and some, at least, will be added to our mix of available therapies with the consequent need for new perspectives on patient management for relapsing and likely progressive forms of MS. Increased focus on biomarkers – cellular, biochemical and imaging – and their potential as valid clinical surrogates will alter the outcomes that we monitor in MS trials. A better understanding of the genetic basis for MS and its subtypes and a better, biologically based definition of MS phenotypes and more efficient and accurate diagnostic procedures will result in more targeted clinical trial recruitment based on rational objective data and might well usher in an era of "personalized medicine." Regulatory agencies worldwide have already begun to stress the importance of head-to-head comparisons of new agents against available agents to provide a sense of relative safety and efficacy to guide physicians, patients, and third-party payers. And regulators are on the cusp of providing formal guidance for adaptive trial design in an effort to streamline current trial and statistical protocols and guidelines for the development of biosimilar agents, creating the possibility of "generic" products for MS with all of their challenges.

For any practitioner, clinical investigator, or fundamental or applied scientist who hopes his or her work will have an impact on new treatments for MS, *Multiple Sclerosis Therapeutics* is an invaluable resource. Its regular updating has provided an ongoing MS history for more than a decade and will serve to guide and prepare us all for the exciting developments to come.

Stephen C. Reingold, PhD
President, Scientific and Clinical Review Associates,
LLC Salisbury, Connecticut and New York City, NY, USA

Preface

The field of multiple sclerosis therapeutics is rapidly changing. Understanding of the disease is improving, leading to new concepts with major diagnostic and therapeutic implications. Clinical trial methodology is evolving, and there are numerous ongoing or recently completed clinical trials for novel therapeutic strategies in all categories of the disease. As a result, a variety of new therapeutic options are emerging. Multiple sclerosis therapy is now proactive – there is general consensus that early diagnosis and initiation of disease-modifying drug therapy, and active monitoring of patients during therapy are essential to delay or prevent neurological disability. For all these reasons, we felt a single text, providing a comprehensive summary of the dynamic field of multiple sclerosis therapeutics, would be valuable.

This book has been substantially updated from the prior edition: over 50% of the material is new, including new chapters on pathology, epidemiology, gray matter imaging, neuromyelitis optica, pediatric multiple sclerosis, medical comorbidities, chronic cerebrospinal venous insufficiency, and a wide range of emerging therapies. All chapters have been substantially revised to provide current information, particularly on rapidly evolving topics such as genetics, magnetic resonance imaging and other endpoints, drug mechanism of action and potential adverse effects, and neuroprotection and repair strategies. The current status of recently approved disease-modifying and symptomatic drugs for multiple sclerosis is summarized. Experts provide overviews on disease and symptom management. This book will be an essential reference for practitioners caring for patients with multiple sclerosis, investigators planning or conducting clinical trials, clinical and research trainees, and clinical trial sponsors.

We thank the authors and co-authors who provided current and comprehensive chapters. We also gratefully acknowledge Cassandra Talerico, PhD for expert assistance in compiling the book. Finally, we dedicate this book to our wives and families for their patience and support.

J. A. Cohen and R. A. Rudick

Aspects of multiple sclerosis that relate to experimental therapeutics

Richard A. Rudick and Jeffrey A. Cohen

The purpose of this chapter is to discuss key features of multiple sclerosis (MS) that relate to clinical trial design or treatment. The emphasis will be on aspects of the disease that create challenges for developing effective therapies, and for using them in practice. These include the subclinical nature of early-stage MS, phenotypic and disease heterogeneity, and complexities related to measuring disease severity. Many of these topics are covered in greater detail throughout the book. This chapter will end with a brief discussion about current controversies in the MS experimental therapeutics field.

Disease features relevant to clinical trials
MS pathology is largely subclinical in early MS

Relapsing remitting MS (RRMS) patients have periodic relapses occurring at variable rates, but generally less than one per year. Serial MRI demonstrates many more new lesions than clinical relapses, with most studies demonstrating a rate of new MRI lesions about 10–20-fold higher than clinical relapses.[1,2] In some patients, MRI shows active disease for years with no clinical relapses, indicating that MS disease activity may be entirely subclinical in some patients during the early stage of the disease. New inflammatory lesions in white matter begin with gadolinium (Gd) enhancement, marking sites of inflammatory lesions (Chapter 9).[3–5] Approximately 50% of untreated RRMS patients have Gd-enhancing lesions on a cranial MRI scan obtained when the disease is inactive clinically.[6,7] Even the number of Gd-positive lesions drastically underestimates disease activity, however. First, gray matter pathology is present in MS patients, even early in the disease (Chapters 2, 11, and 13), and Gd-enhancement rarely occurs in gray matter lesions. Second, disease in normal appearing white matter is well recognized, and correlates with progressive atrophy. Therefore, Gd-enhancing lesions, themselves mostly asymptomatic, are just the "tip of the iceberg" with respect to MS pathology.

There are several implications of this for clinical trials. First, relapse counts are meaningful clinical outcomes in RRMS, but inherently insensitive, and it is difficult to measure clinical disability in RRMS patient groups, because RRMS patients don't generally get disabled during the time-frame of a clinical trial. Second, insensitivity of clinical outcomes in RRMS drives up sample sizes, which become prohibitive in active arm designs (Chapter 21). Third, the subclinical nature of disease activity in RRMS forms the basis for screening putative therapies using MRI outcomes, including MRI parameters as secondary outcomes, and potentially using MRI as a primary outcome measure in RRMS trials. In that regard, Sormani and colleagues conducted a pooled analysis of 23 clinical trials that included MRI lesion measurements, to test the effect of interventions on lesions and relapse rate.[8] The effect of the intervention on MRI lesions was strongly correlated with the effect of the intervention on relapses, accounting for over 80% of the total variance. This indicates that formation of new lesions in RRMS is clinically relevant, and supports the argument that MRI disease activity could be used as a primary outcome for RRMS trials. While many have advocated for this, use of MRI as a primary outcome measure has not achieved regulatory agency acceptance (Chapter 18).

Progressive destructive pathology starts early in the disease

The rationale for early intervention in MS is the presence of widespread tissue damage at the earliest stages of the disease.[9–11] Once RRMS is established, residual clinical disability is usually minimal or absent early in the disease, yet there is ongoing tissue damage, as evidenced by accumulation of T2-bright MRI lesions,[1] T1-hypointense lesions,[12] and brain atrophy (Chapter 11).[13–16] Gray matter lesions are frequent in MS autopsy material.[17] Although these lesions are not visualized with standard MRI methods, gray matter atrophy has been documented early in the disease.[18,19] It is widely believed that the ongoing destructive pathology sets the stage for later conversion to secondary progressive MS (SPMS), in which disability accumulates. According to this model, tissue destruction proceeds without frank neurological disability progression until a threshold is surpassed. Beyond that stage, progressive neurological disability ensues. The threshold hypothesis was supported by studies correlating retinal nerve fiber layer (RNFL) thickness with visual acuity.[20] Visual acuity was maintained until RNFL thickness declined to about 75 microns, and then fell off rapidly with further loss of RNFL thickness. The implication of this for clinical trials is that disease-modifying drug therapy should be viewed as providing secondary neuroprotection, i.e. treatment prevents neurodegeneration by inhibiting inflammation, and thereby decreases the amount of brain injury and delays or prevents SPMS.

Disease manifestations are heterogeneous

Another factor complicating MS clinical trials is disease heterogeneity, which is one of the hallmarks of MS. Patients manifest varying patterns of clinical features, variable clinical course, and variable disease severity. This creates hurdles for clinical trials, as heterogeneity complicates outcomes assessment, and increases required sample sizes. The myriad clinical manifestations include neuropsychological impairment (itself multifaceted), visual loss, eye movement abnormalities, weakness, spasticity, incoordination, imbalance, sensory loss, paresthesias, gait impairment, bowel and bladder dysfunction, sexual dysfunction, fatigue, and paroxysmal phenomena. Individuals manifest these features in varying combinations, and the symptoms change over time. Even within multiply affected families, there is striking clinical heterogeneity between affected family members. Disease heterogeneity is poorly understood in MS, as genome-wide association studies have mostly focused on disease susceptibility genes, rather than disease modifying genes (Chapter 4).

Managing the wide variety of MS symptoms is crucially important for patient well-being, but is increasingly challenging with increasing complexity and emphasis on disease modifying drug therapy. Heterogeneity in clinical manifestations also presents significant challenges for the design of clinical trials. Subjects in separate trials and treatment arms within a given trial exhibit variable admixtures of clinical manifestations that are not necessarily evenly matched between study groups. Multidimensional clinical outcome measures are needed to capture the range of ways in which MS affects patients (Chapter 6). The traditional clinical outcome measure – Expanded Disability Status Scale (EDSS) – is heavily weighted to motor impairment, particularly gait dysfunction. Common symptoms such as cognitive dysfunction, sphincter disturbances, pain, and fatigue have significant effects on functional status and quality of life (QOL), but may not correlate well with measures of physical impairment and disability. This forms a strong rationale for including patient-reported outcomes in clinical trials as a measure of the impact of intervention on disease-related symptoms (Chapter 8). It is possible that therapies may have different effects on specific disease manifestations, i.e. benefit for some with no effect or deleterious effects on others. This is an under-explored area.

Evolution of the MS disease process – the "MS categories"

Because the clinical course of MS evolves over decades, there has been interest in subcategorizing MS into discrete groupings.

The current classification system was based on clinical phenomenology of the clinical disease course,[21] not on the underlying biological mechanisms. According to this classification, MS begins with a clinically isolated syndrome (CIS), defined as an initial clinical episode with features typical for inflammatory demyelination (e.g. optic neuritis, partial transverse myelitis). With additional clinical episodes, CIS evolves to clinically definite RRMS. Even in the absence of a second relapse, a patient meets criteria for clinically definite MS when new MRI lesions are observed during follow-up.[22] RRMS then evolves to SPMS in many but not all patients. About 15% of patients have primary progressive MS (PPMS), meaning that progressive disability ensues without prior relapses. In RRMS patients, periodic relapses occur at irregular and unpredictable intervals, averaging approximately one per year, but declining with disease duration. Episodic attacks of neurological dysfunction are followed by partial or complete recovery, separated by clinically stable intervals. Relapses become less conspicuous over the years, and over 60% of RRMS patients transition to SPMS. During this stage physical and cognitive disability gradually worsens, and disease worsening is refractory to known treatment.

RRMS and SPMS present different challenges in study design. In RRMS, relapses are infrequent, occur at irregular intervals, and pose significant measurement challenges, and disability progression tends to be minimal during the course of a clinical trial. There seems to be some "drift" in MS severity in the direction of more benign disease. This may be driven by increased awareness of MS and widespread use of MRI scanning for patients with non-specific symptoms such as fatigue, paresthesias, or headache.[23] The SPMS stage of the disease is also difficult to study, but for different reasons. Deterioration occurs slowly over the course of years, and there is significant within-patient and between-patient variability. Further, while trials tend to restrict patients by disease category, transition from RRMS to SPMS does not occur at a precise point in time. Clinical relapses become less distinct, recovery becomes less complete, and gradual worsening in the absence of relapses eventually becomes apparent. Transition to the SPMS stage, which commonly occurs during the fourth and fifth decade of life, can be estimated only in retrospect, once it is clear that the patient has gradually worsened in the absence of acute relapses. Because of the indistinct boundary between RR and SPMS, many patients could be entered into either a RRMS or a SPMS clinical trial, depending on how the clinician chooses to classify the individual patient.

A consensus has emerged that PPMS (Chapter 52) should be considered separately for clinical trials. This is based on the uncertainty about the etiological relationship between PPMS and SPMS. Prototypical PPMS patients have symptom onset at a later age, typically between ages 40 and 60, and the female preponderance seen with relapsing forms of MS is not evident. These patients commonly present with insidiously progressive spastic weakness, imbalance, and sphincter dysfunction; diffuse and less nodular T2-hyperintense lesions on cranial MRI; few if any Gd-enhancing lesions; and less indication of inflammation in cerebrospinal fluid (CSF).[24] PPMS may be less dependent on inflammation, and neurodegenerative mechanisms may underlie the disease. Some PPMS patients have clinical, MRI, and CSF findings similar to SPMS. These patients may be similar to SPMS, but without clinically distinct relapses during the early disease stage. This is probably also true of another clinical category – progressive relapsing MS (PRMS) – in which there is gradual neurological progression from onset but with subsequent superimposed relapses. Thus, studies in PPMS are problematic for two reasons. These cases are relatively uncommon, and clinical trial groups contain admixtures of disease etiologies. It is unknown whether "SPMS-like PPMS" and "pure PPMS" patients have similar pathogenic mechanisms driving disease progression, or whether they would respond similarly to treatment intervention.

Common practice has been to select relatively homogeneous patient groups for inclusion in clinical trials by entering patients with a specified disease category, and creating disability limits based on the EDSS.[25] As a result of widespread acceptance of the disease categories, separate trials have been conducted for patients with CIS, RRMS, SPMS, and PPMS. This strategy aims to reduce between-patient variability and to increase the power to show therapeutic effects with a given sample size. However, there are some drawbacks. Narrow entry criteria impede recruitment; it may not be clear whether the results of a trial enrolling a highly selected cohort of patients can be extrapolated to other groups of MS patients; and the distinction between clinical disease categories is imprecise and based on clinical features that are disconnected from underlying disease mechanisms. Conversely, different clinical trials that nominally studied the same patient population almost certainly contain different mixes of patients. This point is well illustrated by the European and North American trials of interferon beta-1b (IFNβ-1b) in SPMS. These two trials used similar entry criteria, but enrolled distinct patient populations that yielded different results with the same therapeutic agent.[26] The problem of classifying patients is most problematic at the interface between RRMS and SPMS, as discussed above. Biological markers for the different MS categories would be valuable, but are not currently available.

Disease severity can not be accurately predicted in individuals or groups

Because of the highly variable future course for newly diagnosed MS patients, there is a compelling need for prognostic markers for treatment decision-making at the individual patient level. Prognostic markers would not only serve the need for better clinical decision-making, but also would help with informative enrollment into clinical trials. Data from the pre-therapeutic era suggested that 50% of MS patients were unable to carry out household and employment responsibilities 10 years after disease onset, 50% required an assistive device to walk after 15–20 years, and 50% were unable to walk at all after

25 years.[27] About 10% of patients have an unusually severe disease course, deteriorating to severe disability in only a few years, while 10%–20% exhibit mild disease with minimal disability decades after symptom onset. Distinguishing these severe and mild cases early after symptom onset has proved difficult.

Selective enrollment has been attempted in clinical trials. The approach has been to enroll patients at risk for disease activity, excluding patients not likely to change during the trial. In groups of patients, milder disease has been associated with sensory symptoms or optic neuritis at onset, good recovery from relapses and infrequent relapses early in the disease course.[13–15] Conversely, symptom onset at an older age, progressive disease from onset, and poor relapse recovery mark a relatively worse prognosis. Clinical features have not been useful for informative enrollment, however. The presence of multiple white matter lesions at the time of first MS symptom has proven very useful, as it is associated with much higher risk of disease activity in the next 5 years.[28] Also, the amount of T2 lesion accrual during the initial 5 years after onset is a modest predictor of EDSS 20 years later.[29] Despite this, T2 lesion load has not been used for informative enrollment strategies in clinical trials.

Most trials employ relapses or progression during a specified time period prior to the trial, or Gd-enhancing lesions on screening MRIs to identify patients with increased likelihood of disease activity during the trial. This is supported by a study showing that relapse rate prior to the trial and disease duration were the best predictors of on-study relapse rate.[30] In that study, disease course and Gd-enhancement status did not provide additional information. That study used a pooled data set from natural history studies and the placebo groups of randomized clinical trials, with a substantially larger sample size compared with previous analyses. A second study examined factors that predicted on-study Gd-enhancement, a common efficacy end-point in Phase 2 studies.[31] A combination of younger age at onset, shorter disease duration, recent relapses, and T2 lesion volume predicted Gd-enhancement. In other studies, the presence of Gd-enhancing lesions at baseline predicted frequency of clinical relapses, as well as increased T2 lesion volume and brain atrophy progression over the subsequent two years.[13,32] However, all of the identified predictors, alone or in combination, are only modestly predictive of disease activity during a trial. The advantages of informative enrollment need to be balanced against the difficulty of finding eligible patients, and the problem of generalizing results when the entry criteria are restrictive.

Heterogeneity in pathological mechanisms

Studies of a large number of biopsy and autopsy specimens suggested that the mechanisms leading to tissue damage differ from patient to patient.[33–36] Four distinct patterns of pathology were proposed. Analogous to experimental autoimmune encephalomyelitis, in patterns I and II the myelin sheath appears to be the target of the destructive process, mediated by macrophages in pattern I and antibody and complement deposition in pattern II. Pattern III is characterized by an ill-defined lesion border with early loss of adaxonal myelin-associated glycoprotein. This pattern is similar to that seen in some viral encephalitides and in cerebral ischemia. In pattern IV, there is a sparse inflammatory reaction, with prominent non-apoptotic degeneration of oligodendrocytes in the periplaque white matter. At present, pathologically distinct MS subgroups cannot be defined on the basis of biomarkers, or functional assays. However, most now recognize neuromyelitis optica (NMO) as a distinct disorder (Chapter 53). It has long been known that NMO differs from typical MS clinically, by imaging features, pathology,[37] and response to MS disease-modifying drugs. But the watershed event was the observation that NMO is associated with antibodies to aquaporin-4, an astrocyte water channel.[38,39] Presumably, better understanding of MS pathological heterogeneity will lead to more rationale approaches to personalized use of disease-modifying drugs.

Complexities related to measurement tools that impact clinical trials

Clinical measures: relapses, physical function, neuropsychological performance (Chapters 6–8)

The annualized relapse rate or the number of relapses are the most common primary outcome measure for RRMS clinical trials. Relapse frequency was the primary outcome measure in pivotal trials of two of the three IFNβ products,[40,41] the glatiramer acetate trial,[42] and the natalizumab trials.[43,44] These studies led to world-wide approval by regulatory agencies, and marketing of the products. Relapses are considered clinically relevant by regulatory agencies, because they are defined by new neurological symptoms and signs and are therefore assumed to have clinical impact. The relationship between relapse number and future disability is weak, however.[45] Relapses may be subjective, and influenced by bias, over- or under-reporting, and treatment unmasking. There are no accepted methods to quantify relapse severity or recovery from relapse. Lastly, the amount of relapse rate reduction considered "clinically important" has never been defined. The rate of relapse in MS clinical trial populations has fallen over time. This indicates that more recent trials have enrolled patients with less active disease, lowering the power of recent trials to show treatment arm differences, and making comparison across trials completely impractical.

The EDSS is an ordinal scale ranging from 0 to 10 that classifies disability severity according to 19 steps.[25] A score of 0 means a normal neurological examination; a score of 3.5 is computed when there is moderate disability in more than one functional system (e.g. visual, motor, cerebellar, sensory, bowel, bladder, etc.), but the patient is able to walk an unlimited distance without assistance. A score between 4.0 and 6.0 indicates limited distance walking. Level 6.0 indicates the need for unilateral assistance to walk, 6.5 bilateral assistance, and ≥7.0 measures severity in non-ambulatory patients. There is debate whether the EDSS measures disability accurately at the low end, because it

has been very difficult to standardize the scoring for the functional system scales and small changes within the functional systems have unclear clinical relevance; and the middle and high ranges are insensitive to change, and so lower the power of clinical trials. Despite criticism, the EDSS has been the standard measure of neurologic disability in nearly all MS clinical trials.

Since the mid-1990s, the EDSS has been used to determine "disability progression," by identifying patients with confirmed worsening from the baseline score. The proportion of patients in different treatment arms are compared directly, or using survival curves. The most common definition of "disability progression" in RRMS trials is worsening from baseline by at least 1.0 EDSS point, confirmed at the next three-month study visit. A minority of trials have required six-month confirmation. The EDSS may revert to baseline more commonly if the three-month definition is used,[46] probably because of residual effects of relapses still present at three-months. The relevance of confirmed EDSS worsening in the early stages of MS remains controversial. One study showed a strong observed correlation between six-month confirmed EDSS worsening and clinical outcome eight years later.[47] There are no similar studies using three-month confirmation. A pooled analysis of multiple clinical trials demonstrated a strong association between treatment effect on relapse rate, and treatment effect on confirmed EDSS worsening, suggesting these two measures are inter-related in RRMS patients.[48] Despite continued criticism of EDSS as a clinical outcome measure, confirmed EDSS worsening has been accepted by regulatory agencies as a primary "disability progression" end-point for RRMS trials.

Because of perceived limitations of the EDSS, a National MS Society task force recommended the MS Functional Composite (MSFC), a three-part composite consisting of timed measures of ambulation, upper extremity function, and cognition.[49] The MSFC has been extensively tested and validated but has yet to achieve its intended purpose – to replace the EDSS as a primary clinical measure of MS-related disability. A substantial part of the problem lies in difficulty interpreting the clinical relevance of the results. As originally recommended, the three MSFC measures are transformed to a single Z score, defined as the average of the Z scores from the ambulation, upper extremity, and cognitive tests. Not only is the clinically relevant Z-score difference not defined, but also the choice of reference population influences the weighting of the different components within the MSFC,[50] so the optimal population used to normalize clinical trial test scores is debatable. Recently, a group analyzed MSFC data collected during the natalizumab placebo-controlled trial, and proposed using the MSFC to identify a disability progression event, analogous to how the EDSS is used.[51] Disability progression defined using MSFC scores correlated with traditional measures of disease activity and progression, and demonstrated treatment effects similar to EDSS. It is hoped that the addition of a sensitive visual function measure (e.g. low contrast visual acuity), and perhaps substituting a cognitive measure with less learning effect than PASAT, will improve

MSFC performance characteristics and may promote use of the MSFC as a more sensitive primary outcome measure.

Neuropsychological impairment, particularly changes in processing speed, complex attention, and verbal learning, has been noted in approximately 50% of MS cases in population-based studies, and has been associated with significant vocational and social disability.[52,53] The effects of treatment on neuropsychological test performance have been reported, although the popularity of neuropsychological testing in MS clinical trials has declined because of research subject burden, and cost considerations. Only six published randomized MS clinical trials included measures of neuropsychological outcome.[54] Results were mixed. Neuropsychological testing is obviously critical for studies specifically targeting neurocognitive deficits, but these tests have not achieved widespread use in clinical trials. Efforts are under way to develop and validate more brief neuropsychological test batteries that might be more practical for MS trials.[55]

Patient-reported quality of life measures (Chapter 8)[56]

Generic health related (HR)-QOL measures include the Symptom Impact Profile and the Medical Outcomes Study 36-Item Short-Form Survey (SF-36). Hybrid measures are the MS Quality of Life Index and MSQOL-54; MS-specific instruments include the Functional Assessment of MS and MS Impact Scale-29. No consensus exists concerning the optimal patient self-report HR-QOL instrument for MS clinical trials. At least eight clinical trials have reported the effects of IFNβ or glatiramer acetate on HR-QOL in MS. The AFFIRM study of natalizumab found a strong association between the physical component score of the SF-36 and the EDSS score, relapse rate, and treatment effects.[57] Patient-reported HR-QOL measures are appealing in that they capture the overall burden of MS, but they are insensitive because clinical changes may occur while HR-QOL remains the same. In addition, many HR-QOL measures are non-specific, affected by non-disease factors, and are therefore are considered most appropriate as secondary outcome measures.

Conventional MRI measures (Chapters 9,11)

All contemporary MS trials include lesion and brain atrophy measures. Gd-enhancing lesions, T2-bright lesions, and lesions that appear dark on T1-weighted scans – the so-called "black holes" – comprise the standard lesion assessment, although image acquisition parameters and the lesion analysis methods have not been standardized. Consequently, lesion "numbers" can not be compared directly across studies. Lesions that enhance after intravenous Gd infusion indicate blood–brain barrier disruption and inflammatory activity. Enhancement lasts 1–4 weeks, so frequent MRI scans are required to capture all Gd-enhancing lesions. During and following enhancement, lesions appear bright on T2-weighted scans, and once formed, T2 hyperintense lesions persist indefinitely. The typical clinical trial includes counts of both Gd-enhancing

lesions and new or newly enlarging T2 lesions. Both are considered measures of new inflammatory activity. All currently approved MS disease-modifying therapies have been shown to reduce enhancing lesions.

The volume of T2 lesions is an estimate of overall MS disease burden. Reductions in the accumulation of T2 lesion volume have been reported in active treatment arms compared to placebo for most MS trials. The significance of this is not clear because the rate of accumulation of T2 lesions correlates weakly with disability progression over the short term.[58] This may be due to non-specificity of T2 lesions – only about half of all T2 bright lesions are associated with demyelination demonstrated pathologically.[59] However, T2 lesion volume correlates modestly with future brain atrophy,[60] and accumulation of T2 volume in the five years following MS onset is predictive of the clinical status 20 years later.[61] Also, the T2 lesion volume is one of the best measures for confirming that clinical trial treatment arms are well matched at baseline.

Lesions appearing dark on T1-weighted scans not related to current or recent Gd-enhancement ("black holes") correspond to regions with axonal loss.[62] Black hole volume correlates strongly with T2 volume, however, and has not been very useful as a clinical trial outcome measure. A newer use of black hole data is to determine the proportion of Gd-enhancing lesions that develop into chronic black holes. It has been proposed that this metric may be a useful indicator of neuroprotection.[63]

Brain atrophy is used as a marker of severe tissue destruction. The techniques vary for quantifying brain atrophy, but generally break into two categories. One is to measure normalized brain volume at two points in time, and subtract the two measures;[14] the other is a more direct measure of brain volume change, in which the two MRI studies are co-registered, and the software measures the changes in brain edges from the MRI pairs.[64] Both of these methods have been applied in MS clinical trials to estimate whole brain atrophy. Atrophy measures have some advantages over lesion measurements. Most significantly, brain atrophy reflects the net effect of the CNS pathology in MS. Furthermore, brain atrophy correlates more strongly with disability than do lesion measures, and also predicts subsequent disability.[60] However, interpretation of brain atrophy results is complicated. First, in the initial period after starting anti-inflammatory therapies, loss of brain volume accelerates, presumably because of inflammation and associated edema resolves. This has been termed pseudoatrophy.[65] Pseudoatrophy has been observed in the initial year with nearly all drugs that strongly inhibit new lesion formation; an interesting exception to this was reported for fingolimod,[66,67] which significantly reduced new lesion formation, but which slowed brain volume loss in the first year compared with placebo. Generally, however, treatment effects on brain atrophy of anti-inflammatory drugs are observed in the second year of treatment. An additional problem with brain atrophy measures is the extremely low rate of change – brain volumes decline about 0.2% per year in healthy controls, and about 0.5% to 1% per year in

MS patients. Because the changes are very small, highly reproducible methods and studies of adequate duration are required.

Current controversies in MS trials

Relapse rate

Relapses are subjective. Because symptoms fluctuate, and are influenced by many factors – fever, high ambient temperature, anxiety, intercurrent illness, and sleep deprivation, among others – it is often not clear whether an individual MS patient has experienced a relapse or not. Also, the required duration beyond which symptoms must persist has not been standardized. Some studies use 24 hours, others 48 hours. The precise methodology to evaluate possible relapses is not standardized either. Some studies use an examining neurologist who is blinded to the treatment arm. In some cases, the examining neurologist is instructed to "not talk to the patient," but then how does the neurologist determine some of the functional system scores, e.g. bladder / bowel? All definitions require an objective change on neurological examination, but practice is variable in allowing examining neurologists access to prior neurological examination data vs. conducting an unbiased new examination without reference to prior scores. Also, recovery is rarely quantified, and no studies require a neurological exam to establish a new baseline after an initial relapse. This makes the finding of "new neurological signs" very difficult for relapses that occur after an initial on-study relapse. For all these reasons and others, relapses remain quite subjective, and differences in relapse ascertainment almost certainly exist between examiners, sites, and studies. A recent practice has been to use an "objective" adjudication committee to review case report forms and confirm relapses. While this approach helps standardize relapse scoring, it does not make relapse assessment more consistent, still allowing potential ascertainment biases. The impact of adjudication committees to quantify relapses in MS trials has not been studied.

Another major issue with relapse as an outcome measure is its uncertain relationship to long-term clinical outcome. Natural history studies have shown only a weak relationship between relapse frequency and subsequent disability, or conversion to SPMS. While IFNβ and glatiramer acetate were approved based on an approximate one-third reduction in relapse rate, no studies have documented whether a one-third reduction in relapse rate correlates with a significant benefit in later disability progression.

EDSS

The EDSS has been criticized vociferously, and for decades. Some of the more significant concerns relate to the ordinal nature of the scale, which essentially means that simple statistical analysis of EDSS change can not be done. The significance of a patient worsening from a 1.0 to a 2.0 is vastly different than for a patient worsening from a 6.0 to a 7.0, yet the difference is 1.0 EDSS units. Therefore, magnitude of EDSS change should be avoided as a clinical trial metric. Another very significant problem is that MS patients remain at particular levels of the EDSS for variable amounts of time. Therefore, the proportion of patients at each EDSS level in the treatment arms of a clinical trial becomes relevant when a metric based on frequency of EDSS worsening is the primary outcome. This detail is not always reported. The EDSS score itself is difficult to derive, particularly at the lower end of the scale. Standardized training is important, and has been implemented in many, but not all MS trials. However, the impact of EDSS training is not clear.

Confirmed EDSS worsening is now a standard metric, but the details are still somewhat variable. Also, most studies require a ≥ 1.0 point change from baseline at EDSS levels below 5.5, and a ≥ 0.5 point change at EDSS 5.5 and above. Most studies require the EDSS change to persist at least three months. What happens when the three-month sustained change reverts back below the threshold at a subsequent visit, or at the final visit? This has been documented to occur in clinical trials,[46] presumably because of noise in the measurement tool, and because of the residual effects of relapses. The latter problem may be reduced by requiring EDSS worsening to persist for at least six months.

Another common criticism of the EDSS is that it fails to capture information about major dimensions of MS. In particular, the EDSS is relatively insensitive to visual impairment, and even more insensitive to neuropsychological impairment. Most studies indicate that EDSS correlates, even in RRMS patients, with walking ability.

As with relapse reduction, the clinical significance of confirmed EDSS worsening vis-à-vis long-term clinically meaningful disability is not clear. An analysis of disability progression in the Phase 3 IM IFNβ-1a study[47] demonstrated strong correlation between disability progression in the clinical trial (defined with six-month confirmation of EDSS worsening) and clinical status eight years later. This is reassuring, and suggests that confirmed EDSS worsening in RRMS is meaningfully related to disability progression, at least as used in that particular trial.

Relevance of MRI lesions

At the time MRI was developed and applied to the study of MS patients, there was great hope that MRI visible lesions represented a window into disease pathology, and that MRI visible lesions would suffice as a sensitive, specific, and predictive imaging marker useful for patient care and clinical trials. Complexities and uncertainties soon became apparent, and continue to this day. The main problem has been the limited predictive value of MRI lesions early in the disease, and the low-modest correlations between lesions and MS-related disability. There are many potential reasons for the so-called "MRI-clinical paradox." First, MRI-detectable lesions represent only a small portion of MS pathology. Standard MRI does not detect lesions in the gray matter, which constitutes about 65% of brain parenchyma. MRI visible lesions are restricted to white matter, and hence demonstrate pathology in about

35% of the target end-organ. Gray matter atrophy has been shown to more strongly correlate with disability than white matter atrophy.[18,61,68] Finally, even within white matter, there are many reports of diffuse abnormalities in the tissue distant from lesions. Lesion size fluctuates over time, which introduces sampling noise when MRI scans are done infrequently, as in most clinical trials. Finally, there is almost certainly temporal dissociation between development of lesions and clinical events such as relapses or progression. This degrades the magnitude of cross-sectional correlations.

Despite these limitations, MRI lesions are included as primary outcome measures in Phase 2 proof-of-concept trials, and as important secondary outcome measures in registration trials. The effect of subcutaneous IFNβ-1b on T2 bright lesions was an important consideration in the approval of subcutaneous IFNβ-1b in 1993 by the USA FDA, a watershed event in the field of MS therapeutics. The recent pooled analysis showing a strong relationship between therapeutic effects on lesions and relapses strongly supports the measurement of MRI lesions in MS clinical trials.

The role of brain atrophy measures in MS trials

A National error MS Society-supported workshop on MRI measures for neuroprotection concluded that brain atrophy measures are currently a logical metric for studies of possible neuroprotective interventions.[69] However, many caveats were discussed at the meeting, and some were listed in the publication. First, brain atrophy measures are non-specific – loss of myelin and axons, gliosis, edema, and state of hydration all affect brain volumes. Second, there are various techniques used to measure brain atrophy, and results may not necessarily correlate strongly. There are very few studies in which multiple techniques were compared using the same patient sample and imaging set. Third, there are many published reports documenting pseudoatrophy – accelerated brain volume loss in the 4–6 months after initiating anti-inflammatory therapy, presumably due to resolution of edema. The kinetics of Wallerian degeneration within the central nervous system also complicate the use of brain atrophy measures in clinical trials. Assuming a treatment is instantaneously effective in stopping neuronal injury, the impact of tissue injury occurring prior to treatment will play out over an undefined length of time. Use of brain atrophy methods in clinical trials probably requires establishing a stable baseline months after starting intervention because of pseudoatrophy and the kinetics of Wallerian degeneration. The optimal trial design using brain atrophy has not been defined at present. Regional measures of brain atrophy, e.g. gray matter atrophy, cortical atrophy, or specific structures such as the thalamus, may be more useful, but development of techniques, including their validation and comparison between techniques is at an early stage. Application to multicenter trials is only beginning. Despite the caveats, brain atrophy measures are standard secondary outcomes in MS trials, and will likely play an increasingly important role.

Gray matter pathology

It is now clear that gray matter pathology is prominent in MS, and more closely relates to disability than white matter pathology, but measuring gray matter pathology using imaging techniques within clinical trials is at an early stage. There are no specific, sensitive measures of gray matter or cortical lesions, although work in this area is rapidly accelerating and there are promising methods.[70,71] Because sensitive imaging methods are lacking, fundamental questions about gray matter pathology remain, e.g. is gray matter affected before, simultaneously, or after white matter injury? What is the mechanistic relationship between gray matter and white matter pathology?

Contemporary issues in MS trials

Optimal study designs for primary neuroprotection

There are no demonstrably effective therapies for primary neuroprotection, though it appears possible to slow the neurodegerative process in early-stage MS with immunomodulatory or immunosuppressive drugs. Presumably, this form of neuroprotection is secondary to the anti-inflammatory effect. How can we best measure primary neuroprotection? What is the optimal patient population? What is the optimal study design? What are the optical outcome measures? A recent trial of lamotrigine used multiple measures of CNS atrophy, and multiple clinical measures to test the hypothesis that sodium channel blockade in progressive MS would be neuroprotective.[71] The results were largely negative for this pioneering study.

Declining disease severity in contemporary MS trials

As discussed in Chapter 21, there is an urgent need for more sensitive and predictive outcome measures. This need is driven by the widespread availability of partially effective therapies, which has two consequences. First, placebo-controlled studies have become controversial, supplanted in many cases by active arm comparison studies. Active arm comparison studies require many more patients. The more important impact of available disease-modifying therapy is the selection of more benign patients for clinical trials of unproven agents. Neurologists are naturally reluctant to enroll highly active patients in clinical trials where one or more arms entails an unproven therapy, opting to treat highly active patients with established treatment. This results in a selection bias in the direction of enrolling less severe patients for current clinical trials. This was thought to explain the low event rate in a recent study comparing s.c. IFNβ-1a with glatiramer acetate.[72] In addition, the move toward early diagnosis and treatment, combined with widespread use of MRI has led to the diagnosis of MS in a large number of patients who in a prior era would not have gotten a diagnosis. Some of these patients have mild MS, and some may not have MS at all.

Personalized medicine – from trials to patient care

Results from clinical trials rarely provide insights into individual treatment response. But in an era of multiple disease-modifying drugs, it becomes desirable to select the proper drug for the proper patient at the proper time. Therefore, methods for rational selection of disease modifying drugs, and techniques to rationally monitoring treatment effectiveness are badly needed (Chapter 23). Presently, there are no validated biological markers that predict individual responsiveness to available drugs, though efforts are under way to correlate genotype, gene expression, proteomics, and pathways with effects of disease modifying drugs. There is emerging literature on the use of MRI to monitor patients treated with IFNβ, for the purposes of predicting long-term benefits,[73–75] but no current MRI markers that predict treatment response at the time therapy is initiated.

Observational and follow-up studies

Clinical trial durations of 2–3 years are feasible, notwithstanding the increasing difficulty of maintaining a placebo arm, but the impact of MS evolves over the course of a decade or longer, and rare serious adverse effects of immunomodulatory or immunosuppressive drugs may emerge only years after use of the treatment, as with natalizumab.[76] Consequently, long-term follow-up studies for efficacy and toxicity are much needed. But long-term follow-up studies cannot definitively determine causality, i.e. between intervention and outcome, because there is no concurrent comparison group.

This has lead to newer approaches, such as propensity matching to allow comparison of more similar groups.[77] There have been published long-term follow-up studies for all the IFNβ products,[78–80] and for glatiramer acetate.[81] These studies have suggested a beneficial effect of disease-modifying drug therapy in delaying the onset of SPMS, or in lowering progression to EDSS milestones. As noted,[82] causal inferences about the therapeutic effectiveness of disease-modifying drugs in long-term follow-up studies are difficult due to design constraints. Long-term follow-up studies are very useful for determining long-term tolerability and emergence of rare adverse effects.

Post-approval monitoring

As discussed in Chapter 18, there has been an expanded emphasis on adverse event monitoring, and risk minimization procedures for approved MS drugs. The natalizumab progressive multifocal leukoencephalopathy experience, and occurrence of leukemia and cardiotoxicity with mitoxantrone have ushered in a new era in MS therapeutics, with more effective but more toxic therapies. This has occurred at a time of heightened awareness of risk with marketed pharmaceuticals (e.g. rofecoxib;[83] rosiglitazone.[84]) Clearly, efficacy needs to be balanced with risk, and risk needs to be defined over the long duration of MS. Availability of more effective, riskier drugs further drives the need for accurate prognostic markers for disease severity, and rational methods to personalize the use of disease-modifying drugs.

References

1. Paty DW, Li DK, UBC MS/MRI Study Group, The IFNB Multiple Sclerosis Study Group. Interferon beta-1b is effective in relapsing–remitting multiple sclerosis. II. MRI analysis results of a multicenter, randomized, double-blind, placebo-controlled trial. *Neurology* 1993;43:662–7.

2. McFarland HF, Frank JA, Albert PS, *et al.* Using gadolinium-enhanced magnetic resonance imaging lesions to monitor disease activity in multiple sclerosis. *Ann Neurol* 1992;32(6): 758–66.

3. Miller DH, Rudge P, Johnson G, *et al.* Serial gadolinium enhanced magnetic resonance imaging in multiple sclerosis. *Brain* 1988;111(4):927–39.

4. Katz D, Taubenberger JK, Cannella B, McFarlin DE, Raine CS, McFarland HF. Correlation between magnetic resonance imaging findings and lesion development in chronic, active multiple sclerosis. *Ann Neurol* 1993;34(5): 661–9.

5. Bruck W, Bitsch A, Kolenda H, Bruck Y, Stiefel M, Lassmann H. Inflammatory central nervous system demyelination: correlation of magnetic resonance imaging findings with lesion pathology. *Ann Neurol* 1997;42(5): 783–93.

6. Harris JO, Frank JA, Patronas N, McFarlin DE, McFarland HF. Serial gadolinium-enhanced magnetic resonance imaging scans in patients with early, relapsing–remitting multiple sclerosis: implications for clinical trials and natural history. *Ann Neurol* 1991;29(5):548–55.

7. Thompson AJ, Miller D, Youl B, *et al.* Serial gadolinium-enhanced MRI in relapsing/remitting multiple sclerosis of varying disease duration. *Neurology* 1992;42(1):60–3.

8. Sormani MP, Bonzano L, Roccatagliata L, Cutter GR, Mancardi GL, Bruzzi P. Magnetic resonance imaging as a potential surrogate for relapses in multiple sclerosis: a meta-analytic approach. *Ann Neurol* 2009;65(3): 268–75.

9. Ge Y, Gonen O, Inglese M, Babb JS, Markowitz CE, Grossman RI. Neuronal cell injury precedes brain atrophy in multiple sclerosis. *Neurology* 2004;62(4):624–7.

10. Gallo A, Rovaris M, Riva R, *et al.* Diffusion-tensor magnetic resonance imaging detects normal-appearing white matter damage unrelated to short-term disease activity in patients at the earliest clinical stage of multiple sclerosis. *Arch Neurol* 2005;62(5): 803–8.

11. Rovaris M, Gambini A, Gallo A, *et al.* Axonal injury in early multiple sclerosis is irreversible and independent of the short-term disease evolution. *Neurology* 2005;65(10):1626–30.

12. Van Den Elskamp IJ, Lembcke J, Dattola V, *et al.* Persistent T1 hypointensity as an MRI marker for treatment efficacy in multiple sclerosis. *Mult Scler* 2008;14(6):764–9.

13. Simon JH, Jacobs LD, Campion MK, *et al.* A longitudinal study of brain atrophy in relapsing multiple sclerosis. The Multiple Sclerosis Collaborative Research Group (MSCRG). *Neurology* 1999;53(1):139–48.

14. Rudick RA, Fisher E, Lee JC, Simon J, Jacobs L. Use of the brain parenchymal fraction to measure whole brain atrophy in relapsing–remitting MS. Multiple Sclerosis Collaborative Research Group. *Neurology* 1999;53(8):1698–704.

15. Brex PA, Jenkins R, Fox NC, *et al.* Detection of ventricular enlargement in patients at the earliest clinical stage of MS. *Neurology* 2000;54(8):1689–91.

16. Chard DT, Griffin CM, Parker GJ, Kapoor R, Thompson AJ, Miller DH. Brain atrophy in clinically early relapsing–remitting multiple sclerosis. *Brain* 2002;125(2):327–37.

17. Geurts JJ, Bo L, Pouwels PJ, Castelijns JA, Polman CH, Barkhof F. Cortical lesions in multiple sclerosis: combined postmortem MR imaging and histopathology. *Am J Neuroradiol* 2005;26(3):572–7.

18. Fisher E, Lee JC, Nakamura K, Rudick RA. Gray matter atrophy in multiple sclerosis: a longitudinal study. *Ann Neurol* 2008;64:255–265.

19. Chard DT, Griffin CM, Rashid W, *et al.* Progressive grey matter atrophy in clinically early relapsing–remitting multiple sclerosis. *Mult Scler* 2004;10(4):387–91.

20. Costello F, Coupland S, Hodge W, *et al.* Quantifying axonal loss after optic neuritis with optical coherence tomography. *Ann Neurol* 2006;59(6):963–9.

21. Lublin FD, Reingold SC. Defining the clinical course of multiple sclerosis: results of an international survey. *Neurology* 1996;46, 907–11.

22. Polman CH, Reingold SC, Edan G, *et al.* Diagnostic criteria for multiple sclerosis: 2005 revisions to the "McDonald Criteria." *Ann Neurol* 2005;58(6):840–6.

23. Marrie RA, Cutter G, Tyry T, Hadjimichael O, Campagnolo D, Vollmer T. Changes in the ascertainment of multiple sclerosis. *Neurology* 2005;65(7):1066–70.

24. Thompson AJ, Kermode AG, Wicks D, *et al.* Major differences in the dynamics of primary and secondary progressive multiple sclerosis. *Ann Neurol* 1991;29(1):53–62.

25. Kurtzke JF. Rating neurologic impairment in multiple sclerosis: an expanded disability status scale (EDSS). *Neurology* 1983;33(11):1444–52.

26. Bagnato F, Butman JA, Gupta S, *et al.* In vivo detection of cortical plaques by MR imaging in patients with multiple sclerosis. *Am J Neuroradiol* 2006;27(10):2161–7.

27. Weinshenker B. The natural history of multiple sclerosis. *Neurol Clin* 1995;13:119–46.

28. Filippi M, Horsfield MA, Morrissey SP, *et al.* Quantitative brain MRI lesion load predicts the course of clinically isolated syndromes suggestive of multiple sclerosis. *Neurology* 1994;44: 635–641.

29. Fisniku LK, Chard DT, Jackson JS, *et al.* Gray matter atrophy is related to long-term disability in multiple sclerosis. *Ann Neurol* 2008;64(3):247–54.

30. Held U, Heigenhauser L, Shang C, Kappos L, Polman C. Predictors of relapse rate in MS clinical trials. *Neurology* 2005;65(11):1769–73.

31. Barkhof F, Held U, Simon JH, *et al.* Predicting gadolinium enhancement status in MS patients eligible for randomized clinical trials. *Neurology* 2005;65(9):1447–54.

32. Simon JH, Jacobs LD, Campion M, *et al.* Magnetic resonance studies of intramuscular interferon beta-1a for relapsing multiple sclerosis. The Multiple Sclerosis Collaborative Research Group. *Ann Neurol* 1998;43(1):79–87.

33. Lucchinetti C, Bruck W, Rodriquez M, Lassmann H. Distinct pattern of multiple sclerosis pathology indicates heterogeneity in pathogenesis. *Brain Pathol* 1996;6(3):259.

34. Lucchinetti C, Bruck W, Parisi J, Scheithauer B, Rodriguez M, Lassmann H. Heterogeneity of multiple sclerosis lesions: implications for the pathogenesis of demyelination. *Ann Neurol* 2000;47(6):707–17.

35. Lassmann H, Bruck W, Lucchinetti CF. The immunopathology of multiple sclerosis: an overview. *Brain Pathol* 2007;17(2):210–18.

36. Lucchinetti CF, Bruck W, Lassmann H. Evidence for pathogenic heterogeneity in multiple sclerosis. *Ann Neurol* 2004;56(2):308.

37. Lucchinetti CF, Mandler RN, McGavern D, *et al.* A role for humoral mechanisms in the pathogenesis of Devic's neuromyelitis optica. *Brain* 2002;125(7):1450–61.

38. Weinshenker BG, Wingerchuk DM, Pittock SJ, Lucchinetti CF, Lennon VA. NMO-IgG: a specific biomarker for neuromyelitis optica. *Dis Markers* 2006;22(4):197–206.

39. Lennon VA, Wingerchuk DM, Kryzer TJ, *et al.* A serum autoantibody marker of neuromyelitis optica: distinction from multiple sclerosis. *Lancet* 2004;364(9451):2106–12.

40. PRISMS Study Group. Randomised double-blind placebo-controlled study of interferon beta-1a in relapsing/remitting multiple sclerosis. PRISMS (Prevention of Relapses and Disability by Interferon beta-1a Subcutaneously in Multiple Sclerosis) Study Group [see comments]. *Lancet* 1998;352(9139):1498–504.

41. The IFN-b Multiple Sclerosis Study Group. Interferon beta-1b is effective in relapsing–remitting multiple sclerosis. I. Clinical results of a multicenter, randomized, double-blind, placebo-controlled trial. *Neurology* 1993;43:656–61.

42. Johnson KP, Brooks BR, Cohen JA, *et al.* Copolymer 1 reduces relapse rate and improves disability in relapsing–remitting multiple sclerosis: results of a phase III multicenter, double-blind placebo-controlled trial. *Neurology* 1995;45(7):1268–76.

43. Rudick RA, Stuart WH, Calabresi PA, *et al.* Natalizumab plus interferon beta-1a for relapsing multiple sclerosis. *N Engl J Med* 2006;354(9):911–23.

44. Polman CH, O'Connor PW, Havrdova E, *et al.* A randomized, placebo-controlled trial of natalizumab for relapsing multiple sclerosis. *N Engl J Med* 2006;354(9):899–910.

45. Kremenchutzky M, Cottrell D, Rice G, *et al.* The natural history of multiple sclerosis: a geographically based study. 7. Progressive-relapsing and relapsing-progressive multiple sclerosis: a re-evaluation. *Brain* 1999;122 (10):1941–50.

46. Ebers GC, Heigenhauser L, Daumer M, Lederer C, Noseworthy JH. Disability as an outcome in MS clinical trials. *Neurology* 2008;71(9):624–31.

47. Rudick RA, Lee JC, Cutter GR, *et al.* Disability progression in a clinical trial of relapsing–remitting multiple sclerosis: eight-year follow-up. *Arch Neurol* 2010;87:1329–35.

48. Sormani MP, Bonzano L, Roccatagliata L, Mancardi GL, Uccelli A, Bruzzi P. Surrogate endpoints for EDSS worsening in multiple sclerosis. A meta-analytic approach. *Neurology* 2010;75(4):302–9.

49. Rudick R, Antel J, Confavreux C, *et al.* Recommendations from the National Multiple Sclerosis Society Clinical Outcomes Assessment Task Force. *Ann Neurol* 1997;42(3):379–82.

50. Fox RJ, Lee JC, Rudick RA. Optimal reference population for the multiple sclerosis functional composite. *Mult Scler* 2007;13(7):909–14.

51. Rudick RA, Polman CH, Cohen JA, *et al.* Assessing disability progression with the multiple sclerosis functional composite. *Mult Scler* 2009;15(8):984–97.

52. Rao SM, Leo GJ, Bernardin L, Unverzagt F. Cognitive dysfunction in multiple sclerosis. I. Frequency, patterns, and prediction. *Neurology* 1991;41(5):685–91.

53. Rao SM, Leo GJ, Ellington L, Nauertz T, Bernardin L, Unverzagt F. Cognitive dysfunction in multiple sclerosis. II. Impact on employment and social functioning. *Neurology* 1991;41(5):692–6.

54. Cohen JA, Rudick RA (eds.) *Multiple Sclerosis Therapeutics*. 3rd ed. United Kingdom: Informa Healthcare, 2007.

55. Benedict RH, Cookfair D, Gavett R, *et al.* Validity of the minimal assessment of cognitive function in multiple sclerosis (MACFIMS). *J Int Neuropsychol Soc* 2006;12(4):549–58.

56. Rudick RA, Miller DM. Health-related quality of life in multiple sclerosis: current evidence, measurement and effects of disease severity and treatment. *CNS Drugs* 2008;22(10):827–39.

57. Rudick RA, Miller D, Hass S, *et al.* Health-related quality of life in multiple sclerosis: effects of natalizumab. *Ann Neurol* 2007;62(4):335–46.

58. Barkhof F. MRI in multiple sclerosis: correlation with expanded disability status scale (EDSS). *Mult Scler* 1999;5(4):283–6.

59. Fisher E, Chang A, Fox RJ, *et al.* Imaging correlates of axonal swelling in chronic multiple sclerosis brains. *Ann Neurol* 2007;62(3):219–28.

60. Fisher E, Rudick RA, Cutter G, *et al.* Relationship between brain atrophy and disability: an 8-year follow-up study of multiple sclerosis patients. *Mult Scler* 2000;6(6):373–7.

61. Fisniku LK, Chard DT, Jackson JS, *et al.* Gray matter atrophy is related to long-term disability in multiple sclerosis. *Ann Neurol* 2008;64(3):247–54.

62. van Walderveen MA, Kamphorst W, Scheltens P, *et al.* Histopathologic correlate of hypointense lesions on T1-weighted spin-echo MRI in multiple sclerosis. *Neurology* 1998;50(5):1282–8.

63. van dE, I, Lembcke J, Dattola V, *et al.* Persistent T1 hypointensity as an MRI marker for treatment efficacy in multiple sclerosis. *Mult Scler* 2008;14(6):764–9.

64. Smith SM, Zhang Y, Jenkinson M, *et al.* Accurate, robust, and automated longitudinal and cross-sectional brain change analysis. *Neuroimage* 2002;17(1):479–89.

65. Zivadinov R, Reder AT, Filippi M, *et al.* Mechanisms of action of disease-modifying agents and brain volume changes in multiple sclerosis. *Neurology* 2008;71(2):136–44.

66. Cohen JA, Barkhof F, Comi G, *et al.* Oral fingolimod or intramuscular interferon for relapsing multiple sclerosis. *N Engl J Med* 2010;362(5):402–15.

67. Kappos L, Radue EW, O'Connor P, *et al.* A placebo-controlled trial of oral fingolimod in relapsing multiple sclerosis. *N Engl J Med* 2010;362(5):387–401.

68. Rudick RA, Nakamura K, Lee J-C, Fisher E. Gray matter atrophy correlates with MS disability progression measured with MSFC but not EDSS. *J Neurol Sci* 2009;282:106–11.

69. Barkhof F, Calabresi PA, Miller DH, Reingold SC. Imaging outcomes for neuroprotection and repair in multiple sclerosis trials. *Nat Rev Neurol* 2009;5(5):256–66.

70. Calabrese M, Filippi M, Gallo P. Cortical lesions in multiple sclerosis. *Nat Rev Neurol* 2010;6(8):438–44.

71. Chard DT, Miller DH. What you see depends on how you look: Gray matter lesions in multiple sclerosis. *Neurology* 2009;73(12):918–19.

72. Mikol DD, Barkhof F, Chang P, *et al.* Comparison of subcutaneous interferon beta-1a with glatiramer acetate in patients with relapsing multiple sclerosis (the REbif vs Glatiramer Acetate in Relapsing MS Disease [REGARD] study): a multicentre, randomised, parallel, open-label trial. *Lancet Neurol* 2008;7(10):903–14.

73. Rudick RA, Lee JC, Simon J, Ransohoff RM, Fisher E. Defining interferon beta response status in multiple sclerosis patients. *Ann Neurol* 2004;56(4):548–55.

74. Durelli L, Barbero P, Bergui M, *et al.* MRI activity and neutralising antibody as predictors of response to interferon beta treatment in multiple sclerosis. *J Neurol Neurosurg Psychiatry* 2008;79(6):646–51.

75. Prosperini L, Gallo V, Petsas N, Borriello G, Pozzilli C. One-year MRI scan predicts clinical response to interferon beta in multiple sclerosis. *Eur J Neurol* 2009;16(11):1202–9.

76. Yousry TA, Major EO, Ryschkewitsch C, *et al.* Evaluation of patients treated with natalizumab for progressive multifocal leukoencephalopathy. *N Engl J Med* 2006;354(9):924–33.

77. Trojano M, Pellegrini F, Fuiani A, *et al.* New natural history of interferon-beta-treated relapsing multiple sclerosis. *Ann Neurol* 2007;61(4):300–6.

78. Rudick RA, Cutter GR, Baier M, *et al.* Estimating long-term effects of disease-modifying drug therapy in multiple sclerosis patients. *Mult Scler* 2005;11(6):626–34.

79. Ebers GC, Traboulsee A, Li D, *et al.* Analysis of clinical outcomes according to original treatment groups 16 years after the pivotal IFNB-1b trial. *J Neurol Neurosurg Psychiatry* 2010;81(8):907–12.

80. Kappos L, Traboulsee A, Constantinescu C, *et al.* Long-term subcutaneous interferon beta-1a therapy in patients with relapsing–remitting MS. *Neurology* 2006;67(6):944–53.

81. Ford C, Goodman AD, Johnson K, *et al.* Continuous long-term immunomodulatory therapy in relapsing multiple sclerosis: results from the 15-year analysis of the US prospective open-label study of glatiramer acetate. *Mult Scler* 2010;16(3):342–50.

82. Marriott JJ, O'Connor PW. Lessons learned from long-term multiple sclerosis treatment trials. *Mult Scler* 2010;16(9):1028–30.

83. Dabu-Bondoc S, Franco S. Risk-benefit perspectives in COX-2 blockade. *Curr Drug Saf* 2008;3(1):14–23.

84. Woodcock J, Sharfstein JM, Hamburg M. Regulatory action on rosiglitazone by the U.S. Food and Drug Administration. *N Engl J Med* 2010;363(16):1489–91.

Chapter 2

The pathology of multiple sclerosis

Ranjan Dutta and Bruce D. Trapp

Introduction

Descriptions of putative MS date back as early as the Middle Ages, but it was in the nineteenth century when MS was definitively recognized as a distinct disease. The first pathological report was published by Jean-Martin Charcot, Professor of Neurology at the University of Paris in 1868 in the *Leçons du mardi*.[1] He examined a young woman who presented with tremor, slurred speech, and abnormal eye movements. When she died, Charcot had the chance to study her brain and document the characteristic scars he termed "plaques" coining the definition of "*la sclerose en plaques*." Pathologically, the diagnosis of MS is therefore confirmed by the presence of multifocal inflammatory demyelinated plaques distributed over time and space within the CNS.

Typically, MS lesions involve breakdown of the blood–brain barrier, multifocal inflammation, demyelination, oligodendrocyte loss, reactive gliosis, and axonal degeneration.[2,3] While immune-mediated destruction of CNS myelin and oligodendrocytes is considered the primary pathology in MS, it is well established that progressive axonal loss is the major cause of neurological disability in MS.[2,4] Various approaches including magnetic resonance imaging (MRI),[5] magnetic resonance spectroscopy (MRS)[6,7] functional magnetic resonance imaging (fMRI),[5,7,8] and morphological analysis of MS tissue[2,4] provide evidence for axonal loss as the major cause of irreversible neurological disability in MS.

Axonal loss in MS

Although often a controversial subject, axonal pathology was mentioned in early reports that included descriptions of axonal swellings, axonal transection, Wallerian degeneration, as well as discussions regarding the functional consequences of such pathology (see review by Kornek *et al.*).[9]

Inflammatory demyelination as a cause of axonal loss

A series of papers in the late 1990s described a variety of axonal changes in actively demyelinating lesions present in postmortem MS brains. These studies concentrated mainly on alterations in the axonal cytoskeleton or the accumulation of proteins that are transported down the axon. Axonal accumulation of the amyloid precursor protein (APP) was reported in acutely demyelinated axons.[10] APP is present at undetectable levels in normally myelinated axons, but can accumulate to detectable levels following demyelination. There were also reports of accumulation of the pore-forming subunit of N-type calcium channel[11] and metabotropic glutamate receptors[12] in acutely demyelinated axons.[13] Cytoskeletal alterations in acutely demyelinated axons are not unexpected, as one of the functions of myelin is to stabilize the axonal cytoskeleton to maximize transport to pre-synaptic terminals. Phosphorylation increases the extension of sidearms from the neurofilaments and this in turn increases interfilament spacing and axonal diameter. One of the best characterized myelin-induced axonal changes is therefore to study the phosphorylation of axonal neurofilaments.[14] As expected, many demyelinated axons contained a dramatic increase in non-phosphorylated neurofilament epitopes.[15] In addition, a striking number of non-phosphorylated neurofilament-positive ovoids were present in acute MS lesions.[15] Many of the ovoids were transected ends of axons. Upon transection of a CNS axon, the axonal segment distal to the transection will degenerate (Fig. 2.1(a)). The part of the axon still connected to the neuronal cell body can survive and mend the cut. Axonal transport continues in this axon, but the mended end cannot handle the transported material which accumulates and forms an ovoid (Fig. 2.1(a)). Three-dimensional reconstruction of the ovoids established that most were connected to a single axon and thus represented the cut end of transected axons (Fig. 2.1(b)). This observation is important for two reasons. First, once a CNS axon is cut, the function of that axon is lost permanently. Second, the number of transected axons in acute MS lesions exceeds 11 000 per mm^3 of lesion area. Transected axons were identified and quantified in MS lesions from patients with disease durations ranging from 2 weeks to 27 years.[15] The identification of significant axonal transection in patients with short disease duration and prominent inflammatory demyelination established that axonal loss occurs at disease onset in MS. Positive correlations between inflammatory activity of MS lesions

Multiple Sclerosis Therapeutics, Fourth Edition, ed. Jeffrey A. Cohen and Richard A. Rudick. Published by Cambridge University Press.
© Cambridge University Press 2011.

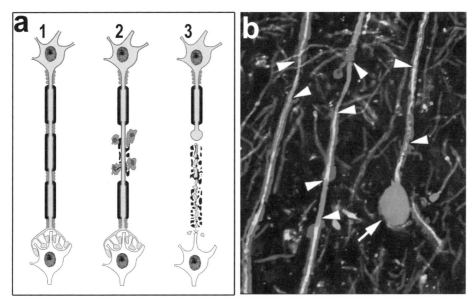

Fig. 2.1. Axons are transected during inflammatory demyelination. (*a*) Schematic summary of axonal response during and following transection. 1. Normal appearing myelinated axon. 2. Demyelination is an immune-mediated or immune cell-assisted process. 3. As many as 11 000 axons/mm³ of lesion area are transected during the demyelinating process. The distal end of the transected axon rapidly degenerates while the proximal end connected to the neuronal cell body survives. Following transection, the neuron continues to transport molecules and organelles down the axon, and they accumulate at the proximal site of the transection. These axon retraction bulbs are transient structures that eventually "die back" to the neuronal perikarya or degenerate. Transected axons were detected in confocal images of an actively demyelinating MS lesion stained for myelin protein (*red*) and axons (*green*). The three vertically oriented axons have areas of demyelination (*arrowheads*), which is mediated by microglia and hematogenous monocytes. The axon on the right ends in a large swelling (*arrowhead*), or axonal retraction bulb, which is the hallmark of the proximal end of a transected axon. Quantification of axonal retraction bulbs has established significant axonal transection in demyelinating lesions of MS. Reproduced from Trapp and Nave, 2008,[2] (Panel a), and Trapp *et al.*, 1998.[15] (Panel b) with permission (see also color plate section).

and axonal damage suggests inflammation modulates axonal pathology in MS patients.[10–13,15,16]

Despite all this axonal loss occurring in acute MS lesions, relapses are reversible because of the remarkable ability of the human brain to compensate for neuronal loss. For example, it has been estimated that Parkinson's patients lose over 70% of dopaminergic neurons before they show clinical signs.[17] In MS brain tissue, approximately 22% axonal loss at sites distal to a fatal brain stem lesion[18] was reported. An acute demyelinated lesion is therefore unlikely to generate enough axonal loss to produce irreversible neurological disability. Axonal loss, therefore, does not have an immediate clinical readout during early stages of RRMS. With time and additional lesions, however, axonal loss can drive the clinical aspects of MS. In a chronic model of EAE neurological impairment correlated with axon loss.[19] Axonal loss in MS patients is supported by a variety of analyses including whole brain atrophy[20] and reductions in the neuronal specific amino acid *N*-acetyl aspartate acid (NAA).[21] The conversion of RR-MS to SP-MS is therefore thought to occur when the brain exhausts its capacity to compensate for further axonal loss.[22]

Loss of axons by immune-mediated mechanisms

In acute MS lesions, axonal pathology and the number of transected axons correlate with the number of immune cells and therefore with inflammatory activity.[10,13,15] Demyelinated

axons are therefore vulnerable to inflammation surrounding an actively demyelinating white matter lesion. Activated immune and glial cells release proteolytic enzymes, matrix metalloproteases, cytokines, oxidative products, and free radicals, all of which can damage axons. For example, inducible nitric oxide synthetase (iNOS), a key enzyme required for synthesis of nitric oxide (NO), is significantly increased in acute MS lesions.[23] NO and its derivative, peroxynitrite, reduce axonal survival by inhibiting mitochondrial respiration and modifying activity of ion channels. Demyelinated axons are also vulnerable to excitotoxic damage by glutamate. Activated immune cells, axons, and astrocytes are potential sources for excessive levels of glutamate in acute MS lesions.[24] MRS studies of MS brains have detected elevated glutamate levels in acute MS lesions.[25]

Another possible mechanism of axonal degeneration in MS is a specific immunologic attack on the axon. Immune-mediated axonal transection is suggested by the strong correlation between inflammation and axonal transection. The terminal axonal ovoids are often surrounded by macrophages and activated microglia in acute MS lesions.[15] Whether these cells are directly attacking axons, protecting axons, or removing debris remains to be determined. Direct immunologic targeting of axons is not without precedence. Primary immune-mediated attack against gangliosides on peripheral nervous system (PNS) axons has been identified as a cause of axonal degeneration in the autoimmune disease acute motor axonal neuropathy (AMAN), a variant of Guillain–Barré syndrome

(GBS).[26] Unlike AMAN, antibodies to axonal components in the CNS have not been localized to MS lesions.[26] Additionally, since most axons survive the acute demyelinating process it seems unlikely that there is a specific immunologic attack against axons. Cytotoxic $CD8^+$ T-cells have been identified as possible mediators of axonal transection in MS lesions, in EAE mice and in vitro.[2] Furthermore, some reports indicate that axonal subpopulations may be targeted by immune-mediated mechanisms.[27] Despite the current paucity of direct evidence supporting a specific immunologic attack on axons in MS, the possibility remains of cell-mediated mechanisms of axon loss.

Loss of myelin-derived trophic support as a cause of axonal loss

"Proof-of-principle" that chronic demyelinated axons degenerate is derived from mice that lack individual myelin proteins. The myelin-associated glycoprotein (MAG), $2',3'$ cyclic nucleotide $3'$-phosphodiesterase (CNP), and proteolipid protein (PLP) can be removed from oligodendrocytes without major effects on the process of myelination.[28] All three lines of mice, however, developed a late onset, slowly progressing axonopathy and axonal degeneration. These studies established that in addition to axonal insulation, myelin/oligodendrocytes provide trophic support that is essential for long-term axonal survival. The axonal pathology that precedes axonal degeneration is different in the MAG-null mice when compared to the PLP- and CNP-null mice. Axonal atrophy precedes axonal degeneration in MAG-deficient mice. The reduction in axonal caliber is most prominent in paranodal regions of the myelin internodes and is due in part to reduced phosphorylation on neurofilaments.[29] In PLP- and CNP-null mice, axonal swelling precedes axonal degeneration. These swellings occur most often at distal paranodes, suggesting a defect in retrograde axonal transport at nodes of Ranvier.[30,31] Compared to the PLP-null mice, CNP-null mice have a more severe axonal phenotype.[32] PLP-null mice also have alterations in compact myelin membrane spacing. In addition, axonal degeneration was prominent in PLP-null mice when their compact myelin phenotype was rescued by the peripheral myelin protein, P0.[33] While the MAG- and CNP-null mice segregate the role of oligodendrocytes in myelin formation and axonal survival, the mechanisms by which these proteins provide this support are currently unknown.

If removal of single myelin proteins can cause axonal degeneration without affecting the structure of myelin, it should not be surprising that loss of myelin in MS can cause axonal degeneration. Several findings support axonal loss during the latter stages of MS. The MS brain undergoes continuous atrophy when new inflammatory demyelinating lesions are rare.[17] Pathological studies have identified transected axons and axoplasmic changes that render the axon dysfunctional and at risk to degenerate. Postmortem studies have identified axonal retraction bulbs, the histological hallmark of transected axons, in chronic inactive lesions.[16] While numbers are small, these ovoids are transient structures and the accumulative degeneration of chronically demyelinated axons over decades would be substantial. Estimates of total axonal loss in spinal cord, corpus callosum, and optic nerve lesions approach 70%.[2] As discussed in detail below, the 30% of demyelinated axons which remain in these chronic lesions have significant structural and molecular changes that are detrimental to normal function and survival.[2] These observations implicate axonal degeneration as a cause of irreversible neurological impairment during chronic progressive stages of MS.

Degeneration of chronically demyelinated axons

Due to the paucity of animal models where demyelinated axons persist for extended periods of time, it is difficult to directly test mechanisms by which chronically demyelinated axons degenerate. The central hypotheses revolve around an imbalance between energy demand and energy supply.[2] In normal myelinated fibers, Na^+ channels are concentrated at nodes of Ranvier, allowing the action potential to rapidly "jump" from node to node. When Na^+ enters nodal axoplasm, it is rapidly exchanged for extracellular K^+ by the Na^+/K^+ ATPase. This continuous energy-dependent ion exchange is required for maintenance of axonal polarization to support the repetitive axonal firing essential for many neuronal functions. Thus, myelination not only promotes rapid nerve conduction but also conserves energy. While loss of myelin *per se* may not kill axons, it renders them more vulnerable to physiological stress and degeneration by substantially increasing the energy requirements for nerve conduction. Following demyelination, Na^+ channels become diffusely distributed along the denuded axolemma. This supports depolarization of the demyelinated axonal segment and permits less efficient non-saltatory action potential propagation at the cost of increased energy required to restore trans-axolemmal Na^+ and K^+ gradients. If axonal Na^+ rises above its nominal concentration of ≈ 20 mM,[34] the Na^+/Ca^{2+} exchanger, which exchanges axoplasmic Ca^{2+} for extracellular Na^+, will operate in the reverse Ca^{2+}-import mode. With increasing electrical traffic, axoplasmic Ca^{2+} will rise and eventually a Ca^{2+}-mediated degenerative response will be initiated. An underlying mechanism of Ca^{2+}-mediated axonal degeneration is reduced axoplasmic ATP production. This impairs Na^+/K^+ ATPase function which causes axoplasmic ionic imbalances and leads to Ca^{2+}-mediated injury. Excessive axoplasmic Ca^{2+} accumulation will cause a vicious cycle of impaired mitochondrial operation, reduced energy production and compromised axonal transport. This vulnerability to degeneration is compounded by several additional factors. The mitochondria that reach chronically demyelinated axoplasm are likely to be compromised and have a reduced capacity for ATP production caused by decreased neuronal transcription of nuclear encoded mitochondrial genes.[35] Additional support for degeneration of chronically demyelinated axons comes from ultrastructural studies of chronically demyelinated spinal cord lesions.[35] In the same lesions which averaged 70% axonal loss, 50% of the remaining demyelinated axons contained fragmented neuro-filaments and dramatically reduced numbers of mitochondria and microtubules. Another feature of the chronic MS lesions is axonal swelling. Histological comparison of axons in normal appearing white matter, acute MS lesions, and chronic MS lesions detected a statistically significant increase in axonal diameters in chronic MS lesions.[36] In addition, axonal swelling correlated with T1 and MTR changes on MRI (but not T2 only MRI changes).[36] Altered T1 and MTR sequences identify chronic lesions with severe axonal loss and swelling whereas T2-only changes correlated with breakdown of the blood–brain barrier, with or without acute demyelination. Axoplasmic swelling is therefore a pathological hallmark of chronically demyelinated CNS axons that is likely to reflect, in part, increased axoplasmic Ca^{2+}.

Recent studies also support the notion that chronically demyelinated axolemma eventually loose critical molecules that are essential for propagation of action potential.[37] Thus, many chronically demyelinated axons may be dysfunctional prior to degeneration because they lack voltage-gated Na channels and/or Na^+/K^+ ATPase.[37] In addition, a linear correlation was reported between the percentages of demyelinated axons with and without Na^+/K^+ ATPase and both T1 contrast ratio ($P < 0.0006$) and MTR ($P < 0.0001$).[37] In acutely demyelinated lesions, Na^+/K^+ ATPase was detectable on demyelinated axolemma while 58% of chronic lesions contained less than 50% Na^+/K^+ ATPase-positive demyelinated axons. Chronically demyelinated axons that lack Na^+/K^+ ATPase therefore cannot exchange axoplasmic Na^+ for K^+ and are incapable of nerve transmission. Reduced exchange of axonal Na^+ for extracellular K^+ will also increase axonal Na^+ concentrations, which will, in turn, reverse the Na^+/Ca^{2+} exchanger and lead to an increase in axonal Ca^{2+} and contribute to Ca^{2+}-mediated axonal degeneration. These data support the concept that many chronically demyelinated axons are non-functional before degeneration. Loss of axonal Na channels and/or Na^+/K^+ ATPase is likely to be a contributor to continuous neurological decline in chronic stages of MS and quantitative MRI may provide a valuable predictor of this process in longitudinal studies of MS patients.

Can axonal degeneration in MS be prevented?

Persistent demyelinated axonal Na^+ accumulation that increases with depolarization[37] is thought to contribute to Ca^{2+}-mediated axonal degeneration in MS brain. Inhibition of Na^+ channel and Ca^{2+}-mediated activators are thus logical therapeutic targets that may delay axonal degeneration and permanent neurological disability in MS patients. In animal models of MS, systemic administration of the class I anti-arrhythmic flecainide[38] or Na^+ channel-blocking anticonvulsants (lamotrigine, phenytoin, carbamazepine)[37] reduced neurological disability and have prompted Phase 1 trials of Na^+ channel blocking agents in MS patients. Two of these drugs, phenytoin and carbamazepine, although being protective in EAE, also show acute exacerbation of disease and

an increase in inflammatory markers following withdrawal of these agents after disease induction.[39] In a Phase 2 clinical trial, lamotrigine did not have significant effects between placebo and SPMS patients.[40] One of the other axon protective mechanisms in myelin disease is remyelination as repair of myelin restores conduction and prevents axonal degeneration. Current remyelination therapies focus on transplantation of oligodendrocyte producing cells and manipulation of endogenous remyelination.[41] Studies are also beginning to unravel the molecular mechanisms by which myelin-forming cells provide trophic support to axons (for review, see[28]). A small molecule therapy which mimics the axonal trophic support of myelin could delay axonal degeneration independent of immunosuppressive and/or regenerative strategies.

Pathology of cortical lesions

In addition to the commonly described white matter locations, demyelination also occurs in the gray matter of MS patients.[2] This can be quite extensive and may exceed white matter demyelination in some cases. The full extent of gray matter demyelination, however, is unknown because gray matter lesions are not detected by standard MRI analyses. Current knowledge is derived from histological analysis of postmortem brains. Three patterns of demyelination (Types I, II, and III) (Fig. 2.2(a)–(c)) have been described. Type I lesions occur at the leukocortical junction, resulting in demyelination affecting white matter and contiguous cortex. Type II lesions are small, perivascular demyelinated lesions that are restricted to the cortex. Type III lesions are strips of demyelination that extend into the cortex from the pial surface. They can traverse several gyri and often stop at cortical layers 4 or 5. They can extend to the white matter, but at present there is no indication that they demyelinate axons in the white matter. All three cortical lesion types are detected in the same MS brain. Type II lesions do not significantly contribute to the cortical lesion load and it appears from limited analysis that Type III lesions are the major contributor to cortical lesion load. However, it is unknown whether sub-grouping patients with variable pathogenesis[42] will identify patients with dominant cortical lesion subtypes. Mechanisms of demyelination and characteristics of the immune response or demyelinating inflammatory environment may differ for each cortical lesion subtype. In a prospective study analyzing cingulate gyrus and frontal, parietal, and temporal cortices from 20 post-mortem MS brains, approximately 27% of the cortical area was found to be demyelinated.[43] A key question is how cortical lesions are formed. There are some trends that prove important in elucidating the underlying mechanisms of cortical demyelination. For example, Type III lesions appear to be more prominent in brain regions with deep sulci, which usually contain large vessels and expanded Virchow–Robin spaces. These expanded CSF compartments often harbor foci of immune cells which may contribute to subpial demyelination. Cortical demyelination is prominent in most, but not all, MS brains.

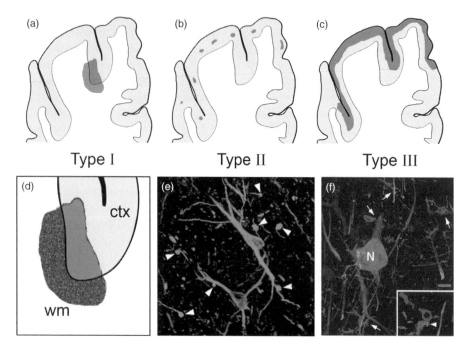

Fig. 2.2. Cortical pathology in multiple sclerosis: Three types of cortical lesions were identified in MS. Type I lesions affect subcortical white matter and cortex (a). Type II lesions are small, circular intracortical lesions, often centered on vessels (b). Type III lesions extend from the pial surface into the cortex and often involve multiple gyri (c). Cortex is light gray, white matter is white, and orange represent areas of demyelination. (d) Cortical demyelination occurs without significant infiltration of hematogenous leukocytes, which is schematically depicted in a Type I lesion (ctx, cortex; wm, white matter). (e) Axons and dendrites are transected (white arrowheads) during cortical demyelination. (f) Stellate-shaped microglia were identified in close apposition to neuronal perikarya and extending processes to and around neurofilament-positive neurites (arrows). (Inset) High-magnification image of microglial process (red, arrowhead) ensheathing a branch of an apical dendrite (green). N, neuron. (Adapted from Trapp and Nave, 2008,[2] Peterson et al., 2001,[44] with permission (see also color plate section).

Decreased inflammation in cortical lesions

The number of inflammatory cells in the white matter of Type I cortical lesions is significantly less than the gray matter component of the same lesion (Fig. 2.2(d)).[44] The cortical part of Type I lesions contain 6 times fewer CD68-positive microglia/macrophages and 13 times fewer CD3-positive lymphocytes than the white matter. In cortical lesions, perivascular cuffing was rare and when present contained few cells.[44,45] Regulation of leukocyte migration in the cortex appears to be different from the white matter. One possibility for the lack of cortical leukocytic infiltration may be due to the differential regulation and expression of cell adhesion molecules by cortical endothelial cells. Antigen-specific lymphocytes produce pro-inflammatory cytokines, inducing a cascade of cytokine and chemokine expression by resident astrocytes and microglia.[46] Thus endothelial cells, astrocytes, and microglia all help modulate the inflammatory signals in cortex and white matter lesions, which influence the inflammatory cell character of the immune response.

The paucity of leukocytes in cortical MS lesions indicates that demyelination can occur without extensive leukocytic infiltration. This implies induction of demyelination may not require a large influx of leukocytes and that the trafficking of leukocytes into white matter lesions is related to phagocytosis of myelin debris rather than the destruction of myelin. Type III lesions, which accounted for ∼50% of the total cortical lesions identified, have the most interesting pattern of demyelination.[44] Many Type III lesions extend from the pial surface to cortical layers three or four, often affecting multiple gyri. This pattern of demyelination suggests factors in CSF may cause demyelination or loss of oligodendrocytes in Type III lesions compared to Type I and II cortical lesions.

Neuronal damage in cortical lesions

Transected axons, transected dendrites, and neuronal apoptosis were identified in cortical lesions from MS patients with clinical disease ranging from 2 weeks to 27 years.[44] Substantial neuronal injury occurs in cortical lesions despite reduced cortical inflammation. Neurofilament-positive swellings were detected along dendrites and axons, suggesting disruption of normal cellular transport. Confocal analysis identified many of these swellings as the terminal ends of axons and dendrites (Fig. 2.2(e)). Neuritic (axons and dendrites) transection in cortical lesions correlated with microglial activation. The correlation between neuritic transection and microglial activation of the lesion suggests that dendrites and demyelinated axons may be vulnerable to microglial activation associated with cortical demyelination.

The destruction of dendrites is a previously unidentified pathological change in MS that can contribute to neurological disability by decreasing synaptic input into the cortex. The functional deficit induced by axonal transection will vary depending upon which axons are transected. If transection of efferent axonal inputs occurs close to their targets, they may have the ability to sprout and reinnervate post-synaptic densities. However, proximal transection of afferent axonal outputs of cortical neurons will result in the irreversible functional loss of the neuron since reinnervation of the target is not possible. Axonal transection may result in apoptosis or atrophy of the affected neuron, depending on the amount of remaining target-derived support.[47] As cortical neurons die or atrophy this will reduce the trophic support for their afferent neurons and eventually these target-deprived neurons may die or atrophy.[47] Neuronal or axonal damage unrelated to axonal transection may also result in apoptotic neuronal death. A recent study reported CSF collected from a primary progressive MS patient during ongoing inflammatory activity induced apoptosis of neurons in vitro.[48] This implies a diffusible factor in the CSF mediates neuronal damage and death. If demyelination, deafferentation, or inflammatory mediators secreted by activated microglia cause neuronal apoptosis, then therapeutic intervention may help preserve the neuron and maintain the neuronal circuitry. Detection of substantial neuronal apoptosis in chronic active and chronic inactive lesions suggests that neuronal death may result from chronic insults to neurons, dendrites, or axons in addition to direct immune attack during the demyelinating process.[44]

Microglial targeting of neurons in cortical MS lesions

Microglia are the resident macrophages of the CNS responsible for monitoring pathological changes and in cortical MS lesions they were detected closely associated with neurons.[44] Elongated microglia were oriented perpendicular to the pial surface, closely apposed, and ensheathing apical dendrites and axons in active and chronic active cortical lesions. In addition, other highly ramified stellate-shaped microglia often extended processes to neuronal perikarya and ensheathed dendrites or axons (Fig. 2.2(f)). Unlike microglia/macrophages in white matter lesions which often surrounded the transected ends of axons[15] microglia in cortical lesions did not appear to target the transected ends of neurites. The targeting of neurons by microglia in cortical lesions is suggestive of synaptic stripping.[37] It remains to be determined whether microglia in cortical lesions are actively targeting synaptic terminals and whether the association of microglia with neurons is destructive or protective. It is probable that the microglia are targeting neurons already damaged. For example, activated microglia target damaged neurites and neurons in Alzheimer's disease (AD).[49] Some of the most promising AD therapeutics are anti-inflammatory drugs that target activated microglia.[50] Similar anti-inflammatory drugs, which reduce microglial activation in the cerebral cortex, may also benefit MS patients.

Contribution of cortical lesions to neurological disability and neuronal compensation

Neuronal damage in motor and sensory cortex would exacerbate ambulatory decline in MS patients. In addition to motor and sensory deficits, gray matter lesions may provide the pathological correlate for the cognitive and executive dysfunction that arises in 40%–70% of MS patients.[2] Recent studies have also suggested that there may be a global cortical pathology in MS patients, possibly independent of demyelination. Studies utilizing brain imaging techniques to measure cortical thickness raised the possibility that cortical thinning is an early event in MS pathogenesis, is independent of white matter lesion load, and is different from brain atrophy patterns in normal aging.[51] Cortical regions with cortico–cortical connections were reported to have more thinning than primary sensory or motor

cortices. If these conclusions are verified by larger prospective studies using more sensitive imaging techniques, it could establish that cortical pathology precedes white matter lesions in MS.

A number of adaptive and neuroprotective mechanisms repress or delay the neuronal degeneration and neurological decline in MS patients. Functional MRI studies have identified the activation of cortical areas that compensate for functional loss caused by new MS lesions. Other mechanisms of neuronal compensation operate at the cellular level and include alterations in neuronal gene expression. These gene changes were first identified by unbiased comparisons of 33 000 mRNA transcripts in motor cortices from control and MS patients. Among the 555 significantly altered transcripts, 488 were decreased and 67 were increased in MS cortex.[35,52] Of the 67 genes increased in MS cortex, nine were members of the ciliary neurotrophic factor (CNTF) family. CNTF is a neurotrophic factor that enhances neuronal survival during development and in disease. An active and functionally significant role of CNTF in MS patients is supported by the report that MS patients with CNTF-null mutations have an earlier disease onset and a more aggressive disease course.[53] These gene changes were present in myelinated motor cortices, where they represent part of the endogenous defense mechanism mounted by the MS brain to maintain neurons and combat progressive neurological decline.

Functional consequences

The concept of MS as an inflammatory demyelinating and neurodegenerative disease provides a framework to help explain disease progression and development of permanent neurological disability in MS patients. The time from clinical disease onset of MS to a score of 4 on the Expanded Disability Status Scale (EDSS) ranges from 1 to 33 years; however once patients reach EDSS 4, the time to EDSS 7 was less variable.[54] These observations suggest the initiation of a cascade of neuronal degeneration occurs once a pathological threshold is reached. The progression of neurological disability from EDSS 4 to EDSS 7 occurs by neurodegenerative mechanisms other than inflammatory-mediated axonal transection.[54,55] The identification of neuronal pathology in MS, specifically the destruction of axons and dendrites along with neuronal apoptosis, provides a pathological substrate for the progressive disability many MS patients experience, and suggests early inflammatory activity may initiate a state of pre-programmed neuronal degeneration.

Prevention of persistent neurological disability is the main goal when treating neurological diseases. Since inflammatory-mediated tissue destruction begins at disease onset and may occur in the absence of clinical symptoms during RR-MS, early continuous proactive application of disease-modifying therapeutics is warranted to prevent and delay accumulating neuronal damage. Thus, inflammation remains a major therapeutic target. Other mechanisms also contribute to neuronal damage during different stages of MS; therefore clarification of the pathophysiology of neurodegeneration in MS is crucial. In contrast to most neurodegenerative diseases, patients with MS can be identified early before the occurrence of extensive neurodegeneration by the presentation of symptoms mediated by inflammatory demyelination. Therefore, neuroprotective therapeutics may have a greater probability of clinical efficacy in MS patients since treatment can be initiated before extensive axonal loss. Additionally, MS patients may benefit from the combination of neuroprotective therapies along with current anti-inflammatory and immunomodulatory treatments. The development of neuroprotective drugs applicable to MS is an urgent goal for MS researchers.

Future challenges

The major challenge for MS researchers is to develop therapies that stop or prevent MS. Understanding the cause of the disease is necessary for this goal. Since MS is not inherited, gene linkage studies will not identify a causative gene or altered cellular pathway. It is fundamentally important to determine whether inflammatory demyelination is primary or secondary in the MS disease process. Are RRMS and PPMS the same disease with different clinical presentations? One can argue that the concept of MS as an autoimmune disease induced by molecular mimicry has little direct support despite decades of searching for the initiating environmental agent. The past decade has seen renewed interest in the role of the axon and in axon-myelin interactions in the pathogenesis of MS. It is possible that this interaction is the key to understanding the cause of MS and it also remains possible that MS is a primary neurodegenerative disease with secondary inflammatory demyelination. Regardless of the cause of MS, axons and neurons are important therapeutic targets.

Acknowledgments

The work is in part by supported by NMSS RG-4280 (RD), NIH NS38667 and NIH NS35058 (BDT). The authors would like to thank Dr. Christopher Nelson for assisting with the editing.

References

1. Charcot M. Histologie de la sclerose en plaques. *Gaz Hosp* 1868; 141: 554–5, 557–8.

2. Trapp BD, Nave KA. Multiple sclerosis: an immune or neurodegenerative disorder? *Annu Rev Neurosci* 2008; 31: 247–69.

3. Prineas J. Pathology of Multiple Sclerosis. In Cook S, eds. *Handbook of Multiple Sclerosis*. Marcel Dekker, 2001; 289–324.

4. Stadelmann C, Albert M, Wegner C, Bruck W. Cortical pathology in multiple sclerosis. *Curr Opin Neurol* 2008; 21: 229–34.

5. Bakshi R, Thompson AJ, Rocca MA, *et al.* MRI in multiple sclerosis: current status and future prospects. *Lancet Neurol* 2008; 7: 615–25. S1474-

6. De SN, Filippi M. MR spectroscopy in multiple sclerosis. *J Neuroimaging* 2007; 17 Suppl 1: 31S–5S.

7. Tartaglia MC, Arnold DL. The role of MRS and fMRI in multiple sclerosis. *Adv Neurol* 2006; 98: 185–202.

8. Filippi M, Bozzali M, Rovaris M, *et al.* Evidence for widespread axonal damage at the earliest clinical stage of multiple sclerosis. *Brain* 2003; 126: 433–7.

9. Kornek B, Lassmann H. Axonal pathology in multiple sclerosis. A historical note. *Brain Pathol* 1999; 9: 651–6.

10. Ferguson B, Matyszak MK, Esiri MM, Perry VH. Axonal damage in acute multiple sclerosis lesions. *Brain* 1997; 120: 393–9.

11. Kornek B, Storch MK, Bauer J, *et al.* Distribution of a calcium channel subunit in dystrophic axons in multiple sclerosis and experimental autoimmune encephalomyelitis. *Brain* 2001; 124: 1114–24.

12. Geurts JJ, Wolswijk G, Bo L, *et al.* Altered expression patterns of group I and II metabotropic glutamate receptors in multiple sclerosis. *Brain* 2003; 126: 1755–66.

13. Bitsch A, Schuchardt J, Bunkowski S, Kuhlmann T, Bruck W. Acute axonal injury in multiple sclerosis. Correlation with demyelination and inflammation. *Brain* 2000; 123: 1174–83.

14. Sanchez I, Hassinger L, Paskevich PA, Shine HD, Nixon RA. Oligodendroglia regulate the regional expansion of axon caliber and local accumulation of neurofilaments during development independently of myelin formation. *J Neurosci* 1996; 16: 5095–105.

15. Trapp BD, Peterson J, Ransohoff RM, Rudick R, Mork S, Bo L. Axonal transection in the lesions of multiple sclerosis. *N Engl J Med* 1998; 338: 278–85.

16. Kornek B, Storch MK, Weissert R, *et al.* Multiple sclerosis and chronic autoimmune encephalomyelitis: a comparative quantitative study of axonal injury in active, inactive, and remyelinated lesions. *Am J Pathol* 2000; 157: 267–76.

17. Trapp BD, Ransohoff RM, Fisher E, Rudick RA. Neurodegeneration in multiple sclerosis: Relationship to neurological disability. *The Neuroscientist* 1999; 5: 48–57.

18. Bjartmar C, Kinkel RP, Kidd G, Rudick RA, Trapp BD. Axonal loss in normal-appearing white matter in a patient with acute MS. *Neurology* 2001; 57: 1248–52.

19. Wujek JR, Bjartmar C, Richer E, *et al.* Axon loss in the spinal cord determines permanent neurological disability in an animal model of multiple sclerosis. *J Neuropathol Exp Neurol* 2002; 61: 23–32.

20. De Stefano N, Guidi L, Stromillo ML, Bartolozzi ML, Federico A. Imaging neuronal and axonal degeneration in multiple sclerosis. *Neurol Sci* 2003; 24 Suppl 5: S283–6.

21. Arnold DL. Magnetic resonance spectroscopy: imaging axonal damage in MS. *J Neuroimmunol* 1999; 98: 2–6.

22. Trapp BD, Ransohoff R, Rudick R. Axonal pathology in multiple sclerosis: relationship to neurologic disability. *Curr Opin Neurol* 1999; 12: 295–302.

23. Bo L, Dawson TM, Wesselingh S, *et al.* Induction of nitric oxide synthase in demyelinating regions of multiple sclerosis brains. *Ann Neurol* 1994; 36: 778–86.

24. Steinman L. Multiple sclerosis: a two-stage disease. *Nat Immunol* 2001; 2: 762–4.

25. Srinivasan R, Sailasuta N, Hurd R, Nelson S, Pelletier D. Evidence of elevated glutamate in multiple sclerosis using magnetic resonance spectroscopy at 3 T. *Brain* 2005; 128: 1016–25.

26. Ho TW, McKhann GM, Griffin JW. Human autoimmune neuropathies. *Annu Rev Neurosci* 1998; 21: 187–226.

27. Evangelou N, Konz D, Esiri MM, Smith S, Palace J, Matthews PM. Size-selective neuronal changes in the anterior optic pathways suggest a differential susceptibility to injury in multiple sclerosis. *Brain* 2001; 124: 1813–20.

28. Nave KA, Trapp BD. Axon-glial signaling and the glial support of axon function. *Annu Rev Neurosci* 2008; 31: 535–61.

29. Yin X, Crawford TO, Griffin JW, *et al.* Myelin-associated glycoprotein is a myelin signal that modulates the caliber of myelinated axons. *J Neurosci* 1998; 18: 1953–62.

30. Klugmann M, Schwab MH, Puhlhofer A, *et al.* Assembly of CNS myelin in the absence of proteolipid protein. *Neuron* 1997; 18: 59–70.

31. Griffiths I, Klugmann M, Anderson T, *et al.* Axonal swellings and degeneration in mice lacking the major proteolipid of myelin. *Science* 1998; 280: 1610–13.

32. Lappe-Siefke C, Goebbels S, Gravel M, *et al.* Disruption of Cnp1 uncouples oligodendroglial functions in axonal support and myelination. *Nat Genet* 2003; 33: 366–74.

33. Yin X, Baek RC, Kirschner DA, *et al.* Evolution of a neuroprotective function of central nervous system myelin. *J Cell Biol* 2006; 172: 469–78.

34. Stys PK, Lehning E, Saubermann AJ, Lopachin RM, Jr. Intracellular concentrations of major ions in rat myelinated axons and glia: calculations based on electron probe X-ray microanalyses. *J Neurochem* 1997; 68: 1920–8.

35. Dutta R, McDonough J, Yin X, *et al.* Mitochondrial dysfunction as a cause of axonal degeneration in multiple sclerosis patients. *Ann Neurol* 2006; 59: 478–89.

36. Fisher E, Chang A, Fox R, *et al.* Imaging correlates of axonal swelling in chronic multiple sclerosis brains. *Ann Neurol* 2007; 62: 219–28.

37. Trapp BD, Stys PK. Virtual hypoxia and chronic necrosis of demyelinated axons in multiple sclerosis. *Lancet Neurol* 2009; 8(3): 280–91.

38. Bechtold DA, Kapoor R, Smith KJ. Axonal protection using flecainide in experimental autoimmune encephalomyelitis. *Ann Neurol* 2004; 55: 607–16.

39. Black JA, Liu S, Carrithers M, Carrithers LM, Waxman SG. Exacerbation of experimental autoimmune encephalomyelitis after withdrawal of phenytoin and carbamazepine. *Ann Neurol* 2007; 62: 21–33.

40. Kapoor R, Furby J, Hayton T, *et al.* Lamotrigine for neuroprotection in secondary progressive multiple sclerosis: a randomised, double-blind, placebo-controlled, parallel-group trial. *Lancet Neurol* 2010; 9: 681–8.

41. Gallo V, Armstrong RC. Myelin repair strategies: a cellular view. *Curr Opin Neurol* 2008; 21: 278–83.

42. Lucchinetti C, Bruck W, Parisi J, Scheithauer B, Rodriguez M, Lassmann H. Heterogeneity of multiple sclerosis lesions: implications for the pathogenesis of demyelination. *Ann Neurol* 2000; 47: 707–17.

43. Bo L, Vedeler CA, Nyland HI, Trapp BD, Mork SJ. Subpial demyelination n the cerebral cortex of multiple sclerosis patients. *J Neuropath Exp Neurol* 2003; 62: 723–32.

44. Peterson JW, Bo L, Mork S, Chang A, Trapp BD. Transected neurites, apoptotic neurons and reduced inflammation in cortical MS lesions. *Ann Neurol* 2001; 50: 389–400.

45. Bo L, Vedeler CA, Nyland H, Trapp BD, Mork SJ. Intracortical multiple sclerosis lesions are not associated with increased lymphocyte infiltration. *Mult Scler* 2003; 9: 323–31.

46. Lo D, Feng L, Li L, *et al.* Integrating innate and adaptive immunity in the whole animal. *Immunol Rev* 1999; 169: 225–39.

47. al Abdulla NA, Martin LJ. Projection neurons and interneurons in the lateral geniculate nucleus undergo distinct forms of degeneration ranging from retrograde and transsynaptic apoptosis to transient atrophy after cortical ablation in rat. *Neuroscience* 2002; 115: 7–14.

48. Alcazar A, Regidor I, Masjuan J, Salinas M, Alvarez-Cermeno JC. Axonal damage induced by cerebrospinal fluid from patients with relapsing–remitting multiple sclerosis. *J Neuroimmunol* 2000; 104: 58–67.

49. Mochizuki A, Peterson JW, Mufson EJ, Trapp BD. Amyloid load and neural elements in Alzheimer's disease and nondemented individuals with high amyloid plaque density. *Exp Neurol* 1996; 142: 89–102.

50. Combs CK, Johnson DE, Karlo JC, Cannady SB, Landreth GE. Inflammatory mechanisms in Alzheimer's disease: inhibition of beta-amyloid-stimulated proinflammatory responses and neurotoxicity by PPARgamma agonists. *J Neurosci* 2000; 20: 558–67.

51. Charil A, Dagher A, Lerch JP, Zijdenbos AP, Worsley KJ, Evans AC. Focal cortical atrophy in multiple sclerosis: relation to lesion load and disability. *Neuroimage* 2007; 34: 509–17.

52. Dutta R, McDonough J, Chang A, *et al.* Activation of the ciliary neurotrophic factor (CNTF) signalling pathway in cortical neurons of multiple sclerosis patients. *Brain* 2007; 130: 2566–76.

53. Giess R, Maurer M, Linker R, *et al.* Association of a null mutation in the CNTF gene with early onset of multiple sclerosis. *Arch Neurol* 2002; 59: 407–9.

54. Confavreux C, Vukusic S, Moreau T, Adeleine P. Relapses and progression of disability in multiple sclerosis. *N Engl J Med* 2000; 343: 1430–8.

55. Noseworthy JH, Lucchinetti C, Rodriguez M, Weinshenker BG. Multiple sclerosis. *N Engl J Med* 2000; 343: 938–52.

Chapter

3

The immunology of multiple sclerosis

Amit Bar-Or and Peter J. Darlington

Introduction

Understanding the immunology of multiple sclerosis (MS) and how it contributes to different clinical features poses a number of challenges, including an ever-growing body of animal and human studies that may, at times, appear to be in conflict. Still widely considered to be an autoimmune disease, the risk of developing MS is influenced by complex genetic-environmental interactions (Fig. 3.1). The clinical presentation and course of MS can exhibit considerable heterogeneity between patients – and even within a given patient at different times during his illness. The more typical course manifests with patients initially experiencing a period of relapsing remitting symptoms and signs, which may resolve completely or only partially, thereby contributing to "relapse-related" progressive disability. Subsequently, a progressive course of neurological deterioration may occur, which seems independent of further relapses and remissions (Fig. 3.2). What initiates an aberrant immune response in MS is not established. Disease relapses are generally thought to be caused by episodes of inadequately controlled peripheral activation of central nervous system(CNS)-directed pro-inflammatory immune cells, with resultant peri-vascular inflammation in the brain and spinal cord. Neurological dysfunction that develops during a relapse is thought to reflect consequences of focal inflammatory injury involving peri-vascular demyelination and axonal injury. During remission, early functional recovery likely reflects primarily resolution of focal inflammation and edema, and re-establishment of conduction at sites of focal inflammatory demyelination, with potential for some remyelination and network redistribution to contribute to further recovery. Axonal injury, which can be quite substantial at sites of acute focal inflammation, is likely less forgiving and is considered to be the major cause of persistent relapse-related disability that does not improve over time. The underlying biological mechanisms that contribute to the "percolating" progression of disability that evolves in apparent absence of relapses and remissions are less well understood but likely represent a combination of processes within the CNS involving both inflammation and degeneration. Whether the biological processes underlying such "progressive disease" are shared in patients described as having secondary progressive

MS (SPMS) and primary progressive MS (PPMS) has not been established. In this chapter, we will focus on how the immune system is thought to contribute to the MS process through the different disease phases, including initiation and propagation, and in different anatomical compartments.

How firm is the autoimmune hypothesis in MS?

While many accept that MS is both initiated and propagated as an "autoimmune disease," it is worth considering how well MS fits this definition. Several criteria must be met for a disease to have a frank autoimmune etiology. These include: (i) the presence of immune mediators within sites of pathology in patients who have the illness; (ii) the absence of such mediators in persons or tissues without the illness; (iii) the ability of the putative immune mediators to adoptively transfer the disease; and (iv) demonstration that removal of these mediators has therapeutic effects. While MS fulfills the first requirement quite well, relatively few features of MS lesions have been established as specific to the MS pathologic state. Although CNS inflammatory disease can be transferred by autoreactive CD4 T-cells in animal models, this criterion has not been met in efforts to transfer disease to animals using implicated immune factors or cells of MS patients, unlike passive-transfer experiments in myasthenia gravis in which patient serum can induce disease in recipient animals. The fourth criterion: "removal of the mediators," has been achieved to variable degrees using a variety of immune modulators and immunosuppressive strategies (described in other chapters), mostly targeting the peripheral immune system. While these strategies have been effective in limiting relapses, none to date have been particularly effective in slowing disease progression that is not relapse related. While the above highlights the difficulty in conclusively establishing MS as an autoimmune disease, it does not preclude key roles of immune-mediated responses in either disease initiation or propagation. The failure of currently approved therapies to halt disease progression, particularly later in disease course, underscores the presence of important CNS-compartmentalized aspects of MS pathophysiology (local

Multiple Sclerosis Therapeutics, Fourth Edition, ed. Jeffrey A. Cohen and Richard A. Rudick. Published by Cambridge University Press.
© Cambridge University Press 2011.

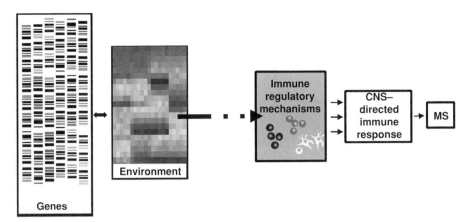

Fig. 3.1. Immune pathogenesis of multiple sclerosis. Interplay exists between different environmental exposures and multiple genes that influence susceptibility at the levels of both the immune system and the target organ. These complex gene–environment interactions, occurring in early life, ultimately converge and lead to insufficient function of immune regulatory mechanisms, with subsequent loss of tolerance to self-antigens and the development or propagation of target-directed autoimmune disease (AID), such as MS.

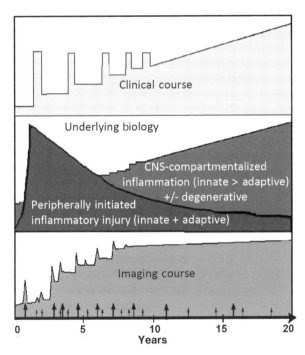

Fig. 3.2. Peripherally mediated and CNS-compartmentalized immune responses: relationship to MS disease course. The common clinical course in MS (top) involves relapses and remissions in the earlier stages of illness, and subsequently progressive worsening without clinically evident relapses and remissions. Imaging parameters applied during the clinical course (bottom), can track the accumulation of T2 hyperintense lesion volume (shaded) as a marker of disease burden, as well as identify time points (arrows) when gadolinium enhancing lesions are present, reflecting local breach of the blood–brain barrier, a measure of active inflammation. However, an imaging:clinical dissociation exists since, later in disease course, progression of disability occurs without further accumulation of T2 lesion burden and in the absence of gadolinium enhancing lesions. This points to the presence of at least two distinct biological mechanisms underlying CNS tissue injury in MS (middle). Earlier in disease course, peripherally-mediated waves of inflammation prevail, corresponding to some clinically manifest relapses and remissions. Later in disease, ongoing injury predominantly relates to CNS-compartmentalized processes that likely include local (CNS-compartmentalized) inflammatory responses, as well as CNS degeneration.

inflammation and/or degeneration) that can be relatively resistant to peripheral immune intervention and may be particularly dominant later in the disease process (Fig. 3.2). These putative CNS events may also relate to the initial abnormalities in MS which trigger the immune response. A "smoldering" degenerative process in the CNS may trigger subsequent rounds of immune cell activation and recruitment. While it is not straightforward to ascertain definitively whether faulty immune regulation is the primary initiating event or a secondary response in MS, various observations, in aggregate, provide strong presumptive evidence that immune responses play important roles in MS pathophysiology and are not merely epiphenomena of CNS tissue injury. These include: (i) the implication of immune-related risk alleles in genetic studies; (ii) identification of environmental risk factors that can impact immune responses; (iii) the presence of inflammatory mediators at sites of CNS pathology in patients; and (iv) the observations that immune manipulations diminish (and sometime aggravate) disease activity.

A framework to describe the immunology of MS

Through a combination of animal and human data, an overall framework has emerged to describe how immune responses in MS may begin, and how they may lead to CNS damage and subsequent clinical disability (Fig. 3.3). Each step within this broad framework of MS immune-pathophysiology also provides an opportunity for therapeutic intervention. The prevailing view, in large part driven by data derived from animal models, most prominently experimental autoimmune encephalomyelitis (EAE), has been that triggering of MS relapses is initiated by peripheral activation of CD4 helper T-cells with the potential to react against self-tissue antigens of the CNS. The source of antigen during such peripheral activation may come from pathogen-associated (e.g. viruses) antigens that can share similarities with CNS antigens and may thus be recognized by CNS autoreactive T-cells, a process called molecular mimicry (Step 1a of Fig. 3.3). Alternatively, peripheral activation of CNS autoreactive T-cells may occur if CNS antigens leak out of the

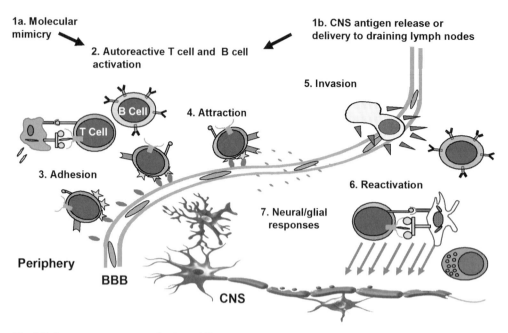

Fig. 3.3. Immune responses contributing to MS propagation. Autoreactive T-cells are activated in the periphery by either molecular mimicry (1a), or by endogenous CNS antigen leaking or carried out of the CNS (1b). Immune cells activated in the periphery including T-cells, myeloid cells and B-cells (2) upregulate surface molecules that enable them to more efficiently adhere (3) to the endothelial cells of the blood–brain barrier (BBB) and respond to local chemokine gradients (4). Active secretion of matrix proteases (5) facilitates immune cell invasion into the CNS where they may become reactivated (6) and impact on the biology of CNS elements (7). These steps also represent rational therapeutic targets for MS immune-therapies. Disease-relevant immune responses are also propagated within the CNS by both infiltrating cells that can become chronically activated in situ, and/or by chronically activated CNS resident cells such as microglia. These processes of CNS-compartmentalized inflammation may take place independent of ongoing peripheral events. Successful immune therapy in MS ultimately requires treatments that result in beneficially modulating inflammation both in the periphery and within the CNS.

CNS or are carried by antigen presenting cells (APC) to peripheral lymph nodes (Step 1b). These processes need not be mutually exclusive. In the case of the latter, there is a presumption of some unknown insult in the CNS that allows CNS antigens, normally compartmentalized, to leak out. Once the CD4 T-cells recognize the antigen and are activated in the periphery (Step 2), this pool of helper T-cells facilitates activation of other immune cells such as CD8 cytotoxic T-cells, B-cells, myeloid cells and NK cells. The activated immune cells can then more efficiently enter the CNS through a series of interactions with the endothelial cells of the blood–brain barrier (BBB), involving adhesion (Step 3), chemo-attraction (Step 4), and subsequent invasion (Step 5) by extravasation between BBB cells or through transendothelial migration. Once in the CNS, further activation occurs in response to the local inflammatory environment and by activated APC carrying self-antigens (Step 6). The activated immune cells may then damage myelin/oligodendrocytes and axons, either through direct mechanisms involving cell–cell contact or secretion of toxic molecules, or by indirectly activating other cells in the brain (e.g. resident microglia), which contribute to tissue injury (Step 7). In addition to adaptive immune responses mediated by T-cells and B-cells, innate immune cells – myeloid cells, gamma-delta T-cells, NK cells, and possibly neutrophils, and mast cells – have been implicated, though neutrophils and mast cells are rarely seen within MS lesions. The innate immune system likely participates throughout the various steps of the disease process, directly or through innate-adaptive "bridges," and may also importantly integrate environmental cues, such as through toll-like receptor signaling by pathogen-associated molecules. Of note, immune cells may also contribute to protection and repair mechanisms, which perhaps should not be surprising considering that response to injury and tissue-repair represent key roles of the normal immune system.

Peripheral immune activation and MS attacks
Evidence for involvement of auto-reactive T-cells in MS

Normally, the adaptive immune system repertoire is generated to efficiently react against foreign antigens, while avoiding strong responses to self-antigens. Despite "central tolerance" mechanisms, which delete the majority of self-reactive T-cell precursors during the process of "thymic education," a significant pool of naive (antigen inexperienced) but potentially autoreactive T-cells can be found in the circulation of normal individuals. These include T-cells with a capacity to recognize CNS antigens. Thus, the mere presence of CNS-reactive T-cells is not sufficient to cause CNS disease, and there is considerable overlap in the frequencies and functional response profiles of CNS autoreactive T-cells of MS patients and healthy controls. On the average, it appears that circulating myelin-reactive T-cells from MS patients exhibit a higher state of activation, require less co-stimulation, tend to be of higher avidity, and preferentially belong to the memory T-cell pool, as compared to myelin-reactive T-cells derived from adult healthy controls.[1] Establishing the role of such cells in disease initiation is difficult given the long duration between sampling for immune studies and the biological disease onset. Studies in pediatric-onset MS may be more revealing, since the lag between disease onset and immune assessment may be shorter.[2] In adults with established MS, correlation between myelin reactive T-cell responses and disease activity/relapses has been reported by some, but not all investigators. This may reflect the substantial biological variability across individuals, the difficulty determining whether MS is "active," the extent to which peripheral measures can inform us about CNS-relevant immune responses, and challenges inherent to studies of human immunology, such as low signal-to-noise characteristics of auto-antigen responses, and added variability related to different assays and approaches to sample handling.[1]

Pasteur's introduction of a neural-tissue containing vaccine as a therapy for rabies resulted in episodes of acute disseminated encephalomyelitis (ADEM). This provided proof-of-principle that peripheral activation of target-specific immune responses could be directed to CNS tissue in humans. The peripheral immunization of animals with myelin components (typically MBP, MOG, PLP) resulting in development of inflammatory demyelination of the CNS established the EAE paradigm as the animal model most extensively used to dissect mechanisms of peripherally triggered CNS inflammation. While EAE is not MS, it continues to provide insights important to our understanding of the human disease. In EAE, transfer of activated CNS-reactive T-cells from affected animals to healthy animals does transfer the illness, which establishes EAE as an auto-immune T-cell-mediated disease.

Genetic and environmental risk factors implicated in MS immunology

There is debate over the event(s) that trigger the first MS attack and subsequent relapses. In the case of Pasteur's vaccine, or in the EAE model, the immunization protocols typically contain adjuvants, which are capable of strongly stimulating the adaptive immune response. But in the case of MS, the disease arises spontaneously, with no common, singular triggering mechanism discovered to date. The spontaneous nature of MS underscores one key difference between the human disease and experimental models. Moreover, humans are genetically heterogeneous and live in "dirty" environments, while animal models typically examine genetically inbred strains, studied under specific pathogen-free conditions.

In the context of human autoimmune diseases including MS, the prevailing view is that disease is triggered when certain environmental exposure, such as common viruses, triggers immune dysregulation in genetically a susceptible host. Recent genome-wide association studies (Chapter 4) have identified several additional genetic risk factors for MS, most of which

appear related to the immune system. The strongest risk factor continues to be linked to particular major histocompatibility complex (MHC) alleles, with minor contributions from genes encoding the interleukin (IL)-7 receptor, IL-2 receptor, and a number of other immune-related genes that encode cell-surface and intracellular signaling proteins.[3] These genetic studies support the concept that immune pathways are involved in disease risk, but even the most strongly implicated genes – the MHC alleles – individually contribute relatively little risk, underscoring the "multi-gene" nature of MS. It is likely that differences in particular combinations of risk/protection alleles present across patients with MS, as well as epi-genetic phenomena, contribute to these observations. Certain immune-related genes may also influence disease severity.[4,5] Genes unrelated to the immune system may also confer risk as pathways relating to glutamate metabolism and axon guidance have been implicated.[3]

The overall genetic background of MS patients appears insufficient to account for the development of disease. Concordance rates in identical twins is approximately 30% and a recent study in MS discordant identical twins revealed no differences in either single nucleotide polymorphisms, or in epigenetic modifications evaluated (e.g. methylation of genes).[6] Lifestyle and environmental factors that have been proposed to influence risk of developing MS include gut flora, EBV exposure, and vitamin D levels. Vitamin D is particularly interesting, as there is not only epidemiological evidence, but a biological link that may relate to modulation of HLA risk-conferring haplotypes.

Autoreactive T-cells may be activated by auto-antigens or by foreign antigens through molecular mimicry

A key unresolved question is where putative autoantigens first come from. One theory is that CNS antigens pass from the brain into draining regional lymph nodes. It has been demonstrated that myelin proteins injected into the brain or CSF can be found in the cervical lymph nodes of animals, and can in turn induce humoral and cellular immune responses in the periphery.[7] Although the brain was traditionally considered to be immune-privileged due to the BBB and lack of a draining lymphatic system, it is now appreciated that immune cells percolate through the CNS as part of normal immune surveillance and that at least two distinct pathways may exist for drainage of antigen into cervical lymph nodes. One such route for antigen drainage is via the interstitial fluid (ISF) along the basement membranes of blood vessels, and another via the CSF, thought to be principally through the cribriform plate and nasal lymphatics.[8] Another route may involve APC carrying antigen from the CNS to regional lymph nodes. Elegant studies of cervical lymph nodes identified APC containing myelin antigens, and significantly more of these cells were found in EAE-induced animals, as well as in MS patients compared to controls.[9]

The other main theory of how peripheral naive T-cells may be primed into CNS antigen-reactive effectors invokes the concept of molecular mimicry between self- and foreign peptide/MHC complexes. This theory is based on the appreciation that any given T-cell receptor (TCR), while considered to recognize a "specific" cognate antigen, in fact has an inherent polyspecificity, and can recognize a range of potential peptide/MHC ligands, a few with higher affinity, and perhaps even more with lower affinity.[10] Peptide screening experiments have proven the concept of polyspecificity (also referred to as degeneracy or cross-reactivity), and yielded new candidate antigens in MS and other autoimmune diseases. Peptides derived from herpes simplex, Epstein–Barr (EBV) or influenza viruses, when presented in the context of MHC molecules, may trigger responses of T-cells that can also react to myelin.[11] An extension of this molecular mimicry concept is "structural equivalence," whereby two different MHC molecules, encoded by the individual's two MHC alleles, bind two distinct antigens, e.g. epitopes of the self-antigen MBP and the foreign antigen EBV, creating two antigen-MHC complexes that may result in triggering CNS-reactive T-cells as part of the immune response to the virus antigen.[12] This implies that the foreign peptide sequences that may have little similarity with the autoreactive peptide can nonetheless be relevant, making it more challenging to discover new pathogen antigens capable of triggering autoreactive immune responses.

Many of the proposed auto-antigens in MS derive from EAE experiments, most commonly myelin proteins including MBP, PLP as well as MOG. Since no single antigen has been established as the major MS target, it is possible that the predominant auto-antigen targets differ across patients and, indeed, may change within the same individual over time (for example from one relapse to another), in keeping with the concept of "epitope spread." This is a well-established phenomenon in EAE, where, for example, disease induction with PLP139–151 leads initially to a PLP139–151 restricted T-cell response which, over time, switches to other PLP peptides (intra-molecular spread), and eventually to other myelin protein peptides (inter-molecular spread) such as MOG.[13]

Perhaps the most direct indication that peripheral activation of autoreactive T-cells can contribute to MS disease activity came from studies of patients treated with an altered peptide ligand (APL) of MBP.[14] APLs were developed as synthetic peptides with minor alterations in amino acid sequence compared to cognate autoantigens. Certain APLs were identified that, while still able to engage the autoreactive TCR in the context of MHC presentation, induced a different outcome of T-cell activation. A particular APL of the encephalitogenic peptide MBP83–99 peptide led to an anti-inflammatory (Th2) shift in MBP reactivity in the EAE model, and was associated with improved outcomes. While Th2 shifts were found in one APL clinical trial that also suggested clinical benefits in MS patients, another trial, employing a higher dose of the same APL, was associated with significant increases in brain MRI activity in several patients. In the latter study, induction of MBP-reactive pro-inflammatory (Th1) responses were documented in blood, providing strong evidence that antigen-specific modulation

of CNS-reactive T-cells in the periphery of MS patients can impact disease activity within the CNS. Newer antigen-specific approaches are being pursued including DNA-vaccine technology, that may enable presentation of myelin antigens to the immune system of patients in such a way as to down-regulate myelin-specific reactivity.[14,15]

T-cell co-stimulation as a therapeutic target (Chapter 41)

T-cell stimulation through TCR engagement alone, often referred to as signal 1, is insufficient to activate a naive T-cell, and could instead lead to a state of functional unresponsiveness called anergy. TCRs such as CD28, which binds B7.1 (CD80) and B7.2 (CD86) molecules on professional APCs, as well as a host of other receptor-ligand interactions between T-cells and APCs, contribute to the overall "co-stimulatory" environment a T-cell encounters. The integration of such co-stimulatory signaling influences the threshold of T-cell activation and can also impact cell survival and differentiation. In addition to co-stimulation, negative (co-inhibitory) signals are essential for maintaining T-cell homeostasis. The classical example is the T-cell CTLA-4 receptor which, when knocked out in animals, manifests in multi-organ autoimmunity. CTLA-4 binds strongly to B7 molecules thus competing for binding with CD28, and can also deliver negative signals that oppose T-cell receptor signaling, which together serve to inhibit TCR-mediated stimulation. An Ig-fusion protein of CTLA-4 (CTLA-4-Ig), which potently blocks B7-mediated co-stimulation of T-cells, was recently introduced into early-phase clinical trials in MS.[16] A number of other co-stimulators as well as co-inhibitors such as ICOS, PD1/2 and HLA-G, have been implicated in modulating disease in both EAE and MS, and represent potentially attractive therapeutic targets.[1]

T-cell differentiation into functionally distinct subsets influences autoimmune disease outcome

Naive T-cells can differentiate into functionally distinct effector/memory subsets upon activation. Three "effector" CD4 T-cell subsets that have been relatively well characterized include Th1, Th2, and Th17 cells, named based on the cytokine profiles they produce. The cytokine environment during activation, which is modified by the local APCs or other neighboring immune cells, influences the outcome of T-cell differentiation. For example, Th1 differentiation can be driven by IL-12; Th2 by IL-4; while Th17 differentiation is influenced by IL-1β, IL-6, and TGFβ.[17,18] IL-23 appears important in helping to maintain memory Th17 cells. Unique transcription factors have been associated with each subset, Tbet for Th1, GATA-3 for Th2, and RORγ (RORC) for Th17,[19] though the biology of these transcription factors is not mutually exclusive as, for example, Tbet has been described as essential for CNS inflammation mediated by both Th1 and Th17 cells.[20] The Th17 associated transcription factor RORγ and the regulatory T-cell (Treg) associated transcription factor FOXP3 may oppose each other, and the outcome of T-cell polarization is further influenced by a combination of TCR signaling strength and cytokine-driven STAT signaling.[19] This complex transcriptional control of Th17 is also regulated upstream by a class of small RNA molecules called microRNA. In particular, elevated microRNA-326 is reportedly associated with Th17 responses in MS patients; in EAE up- or down-modulating microRNA-326 has a corresponding effect on disease activity.[21]

Adoptive transfer of either Th1 or Th17 can cause EAE, albeit with notable differences in the resulting disease.[22,23] Th17 responses have been implicated as pathogenic in EAE as well as patients with MS. Cells that make IL-17 and no IFNγ, and cells that make both IL-17 and IFNγ (referred to as Th1/17) may act in the periphery, at the blood–brain barrier, or within the CNS.[24–26] MS therapies that are variably effective in controlling new CNS lesion activity are known to diminish not only Th1 responses, but also Th17 responses. This has been documented with IFNβ,[27] glatiramer acetate,[28,29] fingolimod,[30] and rituximab.[31] A recent study indicated that IFNβ treatment response was correlated to the pre-treatment level of serum IL-17F, suggesting that Th17 responses should be studied further as a potential biomarker for clinical responses to IFNβ.[32] The impact of experimental therapy on Th17 responses is of considerable interest. In EAE, for example, disease amelioration by mesenchymal stem cells (MSCs) is mediated by inhibition of both Th1 and Th17 responses.[33] Interestingly, recent studies suggest a reciprocal effect may occur in humans, with MSC inducing increased responses of Th17 cells, despite concomitant decreases in Th1 and Th1/17 responses.[34] This highlights the importance of careful immune monitoring of T-cell differentiation in future clinical trials using MSCR. The precise mechanisms by which Th17 responses contribute to pathogenesis are unknown. One report showed that IL-17 and IL-22, another cytokine made by Th17 cells, can increase permeability of human BBB endothelial cells,[24] and it has been suggested that Th17 cells contribute to an initial breach of the BBB which may then facilitate recruitment and participation of Th1 effector cells.[35] While the precise mechanisms and relative importance of Th1 and Th17 continue to be debated, additional subsets have been discovered including a subset defined by IL-9 production (referred to as Th9), and a T-cell population expressing GM-CSF, and their relevance to MS is being explored.[22,26,36–39]

In contrast to Th1 and Th17 responses, Th2 responses are considered "anti-inflammatory" in the context of MS and most EAE models. Possible mechanisms include the capacity of Th2 cells to oppose Th1 and Th17 differentiation, in part thought to be through IL-4 production. Several established MS therapies including IFNβ and glatiramer acetate are thought to shift immune responses towards a Th2 profile. Such "Th2 immune deviation" continues to represent one attractive strategy for novel MS therapeutics. It should be kept in mind that, under certain situations, unchecked Th2 responses may contribute to exacerbation of CNS inflammation, however.[40,41]

Regulatory T-cells and control of autoimmunity

Several subsets of regulatory T-cells are capable of potently inhibiting activation of other T-cells, including suppression of autoimmune responses.[42] Best studied are the natural Tregs (nTreg) that are generated in the thymus, as well as inducible T regs (iTreg) that arise from activated T-cells in the periphery. Resting nTregs exhibit high surface levels of the CD25 subunit of the IL-2 receptor and nuclear expression of FoxP3, as well as surface expression of CD62-ligand and lack of CD127 (IL-7 receptor). The latter two criteria help distinguish Tregs from activated T-cells, which upregulate CD25 and can express low/intermediate levels of FoxP3 in human samples. It is presumed that cell–cell contact between T regs and effector T-cells for some Treg subsets while other Treg subsets appear capable of suppressing neighboring T-cell responses through secretion of cytokines including IL-10.[43,44] In MS, reduced suppressor function in ex vivo assays,[42] as well as diminished migratory capacity of nTreg cells[45] have been described. Some but not all groups have suggested that the number of Tregs may also be lower in MS patients vs. healthy controls. In a recent report, the frequency and function of a subset of Tregs expressing CD39, a cell surface ATPase that mediates part of the suppressive function of T regs, was decreased in MS patients suggesting a link between phenotype and function.[46] This study also demonstrated that CD39 expressing Tregs inhibited Th17 T-cells, further linking MS disease development with insufficiently controlled Th17 T-cell responses. A unique interplay between Tregs and Th17 T-cells has now been recognized. Functional interactions between these two cell types may be important for treatment of MS and other immune-mediated conditions in the future.

In contrast to nTreg, iTreg (such as Tr1) cells arise from activated T-cells in the periphery, and are defined by lack of or transient expression of FOXP3, an intermediate level of CD25 expression and typically the secretion of IL-10, a cytokine with a wide range of immuno-regulatory properties. In MS, the ability of Tr1 cells to produce IL-10 is impaired in ex vivo assays,[47] indicating that defects in regulatory T-cells may apply to both the natural and induced compartments. It is not known whether stimulation of Tr1 cells will successfully impact already differentiated auto-aggressive cells, or needs to be applied before the autoreactive T-cells are induced.[48]

B-cells as important regulators of T-cell responses in MS (Chapter 42)

Clinical trials of B-cell depletion with rituximab and more recently ocrelizumab, which efficiently eliminate circulating B-cells, have demonstrated substantial reductions in new brain lesions, and relapses in MS patients, underscoring an important contribution of B-cells to the development of disease activity (see Chapter 42). B-cell depletion in these studies was not accompanied by decreased CSF oligoclonal bands or CSF levels of immunoglobulins. This indicates that the benefit of B-cell removal reflects non-antibody dependent B-cell function. In addition to secretion of antibodies, human B-cells are known to serve as APC to T-cells, regulate local immune responses through elaboration of pro-inflammatory (e.g. LT, TNFα) or anti-inflammatory (IL-10) cytokines, contribute to formation of lymph tissue architecture, and act as transducers at the innate-adaptive immune interface. Abnormalities in one or more of these B-cell functions could contribute to MS disease activity. Circulating B-cells from MS patients expressed increased levels of the B7.1 (CD80) costimulatory molecule,[49,50] and were deficient in producing the immunosuppressive cytokine IL-10[51–53] possibly leading to excessive T-cell responses.

More recently, B-cells of MS patients were also found to secrete abnormally increased levels of LT and lower levels of IL-10 compared with B-cells of healthy controls when activated in the presence of viral-associated molecules. This indicates that common infections may induce B-cells of MS patients to respond with an exaggerated pro-inflammatory effector cytokine profile.[31] These abnormalities in peripheral MS B-cells may underlie their capacity to contribute to new MS disease activity through activation of abnormal T-cell responses in the periphery, a premise supported by the recent demonstration that circulating T-cells in MS patients treated with rituximab exhibit significantly decreased Th1 and Th17 responses[31] and may be relevant to targeting CNS antigens.[54] Studies of B-cell depletion in EAE have also pointed to important influences of peripheral B-cells on T-cell-mediated CNS inflammation.[55,56] Of note, these animal studies further underscore the emerging appreciation that the B-cell pool includes both pro-inflammatory B-cells as well as anti-inflammatory B-cells (Bregs) which may have opposing roles on disease activity. Thus, while targeting B-cell responses in the periphery of patients with MS represents an attractive therapeutic strategy for limiting relapsing disease activity, elucidating both the normal roles and the disease implications of particular B-cell subsets will help to define the optimal approach and achieve the risk/benefit balance necessary for long-term intervention.

Involvement of the innate immune system in peripheral immune responses

The innate immune system rapidly senses foreign pathogen-associated structures without the need for adaptive antigen-specific recognition or memory responses. Recently, a number of "innate-adaptive bridges" have been identified, which can be considered new therapeutic targets for MS and other autoimmune diseases. For example, killer NK cells, normally involved in tumor and pathogen clearance, are also capable of regulating autoreactive T-cells, a property that is be enhanced

by daclizumab, an anti-CD25 (high affinity IL-2 receptor) antibody under investigation in ongoing MS trials (Chapter 33).[57] Initially designed to block IL-2 signaling in CD4 T-cells, a major effect of daclizumab in vivo is the induction of an increased frequency of circulating NK cells with cytotoxic function towards activated T-cells, which may compensate for decreased Tregs seen in the same patients. In a similar fashion, innate γδ T-cells may have a protective role involving control of autoreactive T-cells, though the overall contribution of this subset in MS has been difficult to establish given its potential to also contribute to CNS damage (see next section). Myeloid cells are also viewed as members of the innate immune response and, as indicated above, play an integral role in controlling T-cell responses both in the periphery and within the CNS where they are abundant in the typical inflammatory MS lesions. Myeloid cells can also differentiate into pro- or anti-inflammatory APCs, for example Type-1 myeloid cells can induce activation of Th1 responses, which may be pathogenic, whereas modulation of myeloid cells towards a Type-2 APC phenotype can promote anti-inflammatory Th2 responses.[58,59] An abnormal balance between functionally distinct subsets of plasmacytoid dendritic cells has been recently implicated in MS.[60]

An emerging field of study in MS relates to the contribution of the innate toll-like receptors (TLRs), a family of receptors expressed by many cell types that are designed to recognize an array of structural features derived from pathogens. While the relevance of TLR signals in MS remains to be determined, studies show that certain TLR signals can exacerbate chronic inflammation in EAE, and that the adjuvants sometimes used to induce EAE contain multiple toll ligands that impact on the disease development.[61] Another innate-adaptive bridge may be represented by the recent observation that, compared to normal B-cells, B-cells of MS patients exhibit exaggerated pro-inflammatory cytokine profiles when TLR9 on their surface is ligated during activation, which could contribute to exaggerated Th1 and Th17 T-cell responses.[31]

Immune cell invasion into the CNS: more than one route

Once thought to be immune-privileged, it is now accepted that the normal CNS is subjected to immune surveillance. In the context of MS, the perivascular immune cell infiltration typical of deep white matter lesions has been thought to reflect abnormal immune cell transmigration across BBB endothelial cells. The BBB represents a boundary that separates the circulating blood from the CNS and is composed of tightly bound endothelial cells surrounded by a continuous basement membrane and a supporting layer of astrocyte footpads. While the BBB is relatively impermeable, in part due to the presence of tight junction molecules between endothelial cells, the presence of inflammatory signals results in up-regulated surface expression of adhesion molecules on BBB endothelial cells, that promotes entry of immune cells through a multi-step process referred to as extravasation or transmigration (Fig. 3.3).

Extravasation begins with the immune cell rolling and tethering/arresting, which is mediated by selectins and integrins, as well as the involvement of chemoattraction. The production of tissue lytic enzymes (Fig. 3.3), such as the matrix metalloproteinases (MMP), results in breakdown of the basement membrane, further facilitating invasion into the CNS.

In MS, endothelial cells display elevated levels of cell adhesion molecules including ICAM-1, VCAM-1, and ALCAM, some of which appear to correlate with the extent of immune cell infiltration.[62] Perivascular inflammatory cells within MS lesions have the capacity to express relevant ligands for these adhesion molecules. The clinical trial program of the anti-VLA-4 antibody, natalizumab, confirmed impressive efficacy using this strategy, though enthusiasm was tempered by the emergence progressive multifocal leukoencephalopathy (PML). More selective strategies of targeting trafficking may be viable as emerging findings indicate that different immune cell subsets preferentially use distinct adhesion molecules when interacting with brain endothelial cells.[63,64]

In addition to trafficking from the blood into the CNS parenchyma across endothelial vessel walls, it is now recognized that immune cells can also traffic from the blood into the CSF across the choroid plexus, as well as from the blood into the subarachnoid space, across post-capillary venules at the pial surface.[35,65] Additional considerations may apply to leukocyte entry into the spinal cord where EAE lesions primarily occur and can also occur in MS. The comparative effects of VLA-4 blockade at different anatomical sites of the CNS have been most thoroughly characterized. VLA-4 blockade diminishes lymphocyte adhesion to choroid plexus cells (in vitro), while at the pial surface it inhibits rolling/arrest, and at the spinal cord the main effect was on the adhesion and capture steps of extravasation.[66]

Several chemokine receptors and ligands are emerging as key regulators of immune cell trafficking along the different routes of CNS entry described above.[67] In a recent study, the choroid plexus was shown in mouse and human settings to express the chemokine CCL20 which facilitated entry of Th17 T-cells that express CCR6 (the CCL20 chemokine receptor).[35] Another chemokine receptor, CXCR3, is over expressed by lymphocytes in the CSF of MS patients, suggesting an involvement in migration from blood to CSF.[67]

Impact of immune responses within the CNS
(Re)activation of T-cells within the CNS

The presence of clonally expanded CD4 and CD8 T-cells persisting in the CNS,[68] suggests that T-cells can be activated or re-activated within the CNS compartment (Fig. 3.3). Infiltrating myeloid cells as well as brain resident cells such as microglia, can function as APCs given their capacity to express MHC class I and II and costimulatory molecules, and thereby contribute to local re-activation of T-cells.[69] Blood-derived macrophages are abundant in typical perivascular inflammatory lesions and crossing the BBB may alter the properties of myeloid cells such

Table 3.1. *Immune mechanisms that could contribute to CNS injury in MS*

Cellular-mediated cytotoxicity, including:
o Antigen-specific CNS-reactive CD8 T-cells and CD4 T-cells
o Non-antigen-specific CD8 and CD4 T-cells (bystander injury)
o Infiltrating macrophage; reactive resident microglia
o Innate effectors: natural killer (NK) cells, NK T-cells, γδ T-cells
o Failure to downregulate the immune response (prolonged retention, limited apoptosis of pro-inflammatory cells)
o Deficient regulatory cell function
o Apoptotic signals (leading to neural and/or glial cell death)

Injury by soluble (humoral) immune mediators, including:
o Antigen-specific CNS-reactive antibodies; injury through complement fixation and/or antibody dependent cytotoxicity (ADCC)
o Pro-inflammatory cytokines (including Th1 cytokines, IL-17, osteopontin TNFα, IL-1β)
o Nitric oxide and reactive oxygen species
o Leukotrienes, plasminogen activators
o Matrix metalloproteinases (MMP)
o Glutamate-mediated cytotoxicity

that they acquire dendritic cell (DC) properties that can in turn promote expansion of Th17 T-cells in the CNS perivascular spaces and parenchyma.[25] Microglia, like peripheral myeloid cells, can activate T-cells and produce cytokines that polarize T-cell responses. For example, IL-23 (known to sustain Th17 responses), can be expressed by microglia within MS lesions.[70] Subsets of microglia may also adopt Type 2 APC functions that are able, in turn, to drive anti-inflammatory Th2 T-cell differentiation.[58] This function may represent an attractive target for immune modulatory therapy.[71,72] Astrocytes in an inflammatory state can also produce cytokines that impact on T-cell polarization, including IL-23 and IL-12.[73]

Several hypotheses have been proposed to explain how T-cells mediate CNS injury, including direct T-cell : target cell interactions, indirect damage to myelin or axons through activation of local microglia, or production of toxic molecules (Fig. 3.3, and Tables 3.1 and 3.2). In vitro studies have not supported a major role for CD4 myelin-reactive T-cells in direct killing of adult oligodendrocytes. However, neurons cultured in vitro are susceptible to activated CD4 and CD8 T-cells; both MHC-dependent and MHC-independent mechanisms have been proposed.[74,75] In MS lesions, neurons express MHC I, and in vitro studies show that electrical silencing and additional pro-inflammatory signals can induce MHC I expression on neurons and subsequent sensitivity to antigen-dependent effects of CD8 T-cells.[75] Several mechanisms have been proposed to explain CD8 T-cell-mediated damage to neurons and oligodendrocytes.[76,77] In contrast to neuromyelitis optica, and possibly Rasmussen's encephalitis, astrocytes do not appear to be directly targeted in MS, although fragmentation of the astrocyte cytoskeletal protein GFAP has been recognized.[78]

Relative importance of CD4 vs. CD8 T-cells

CD4 T-cells are more frequently found in the perivascular infiltrate, but are less common in brain parenchyma, where CD8 T-cells predominate.[79,80] With cellular and molecular approaches, it has been demonstrated that populations of

Table 3.2. *Immune mechanisms that could contribute to CNS recovery, protection and repair*

Mediators that could serve to decrease pro-inflammatory responses, including:
○ Anti-inflammatory cytokines (including Th2 cytokines, IL-10, TGFβ)
○ Anti-inflammatory (Type 2) antigen-presenting cells
○ Regulatory/suppressive T-cell subsets (Tr1, Th2, Th3, CD4+CD25hi nTreg; CD8 HLA-E, other)
○ NK and γδ T-cells (by killing activated auto-reactive T-cells)
○ Pro-apoptotic signals (leading to death of pro-inflammatory immune cells)
○ Tissue inhibitors of matrix metalloproteinases (TIMPs)

Mechanisms that could promote CNS protection and repair, including:
○ Release of neurotrophic factors (BDNF, NGF, others)
○ Clearance of inhibitory myelin molecules (Nogo, MAG) by macrophage/microglia
○ Cytokines promoting CNS progenitor cells (e.g. TNFα via TNFR2) and remyelination (IL-1β inducing IGF-1)
○ Protective autoimmunity
○ Pro-myelinating antibodies
○ Some prostaglandins, lipoxins, antithrombin

CD8 T-cells within the CNS compartment of patients can share the same TCR, and may persist there long term.[79,81] Increased frequencies of CNS-specific auto-reactive CD8 T-cells have also been reported in the circulation of MS patients compared to controls,[82-84] though it is not clear in what compartment disease-relevant CD8 T-cells undergo clonal expansion. Nor is it clear whether clonal expansion of CD8 T-cells is in response to peripheral or CNS stimulation. Though considerably less well studied in EAE compared with CD4 T-cells, studies of CD8 T-cell-mediated disease have implicated pro- and anti-inflammatory roles for different CD8 T-cell subsets and have identified novel mechanisms by which CD8-cells contribute to CNS inflammation.[85] Elucidating the roles of functionally distinct CD8 T-cell subsets in the human disease and their potential as therapeutic targets is of considerable interest.[85,86]

B-cell responses within the CNS

Abnormally increased levels of CSF Ig have long been recognized and several lines of evidence indicate intra-clonal expansion of B-cells and plasma cells within the CSF and lesions of MS patients, observations that have been taken as evidence for antigen-driven expansion and antibody production within the CNS.[87-92] Numerous observations implicate antibodies in the pathogenesis of white matter lesions: co-deposition of IgG with activated complement fragments and complexes at the borders of active MS lesions; presence of anti-myelin antibody in lesions; capping of surface IgG on microglia/macrophages engaged in myelin breakdown; and the presence of Ig and myelin fragments within phagocytic macrophage or microglia in lesions.[90-95] Some studies correlated higher levels of CSF IgG and IgM with worse MS disease prognosis,[96-98] while lack of CSF oligoclonal bands (OCBs) has been associated with a more benign MS course.[99] It is noteworthy that adoptive transfer of anti-myelin antibodies does not induce EAE in absence of CNS directed T-cell responses, suggesting that these antibodies do not initiate the immune-mediated CNS injury, but rather influence its severity. A recent study of anti-myelin antibodies in pediatric-onset MS supports this interpretation.[100]

Elucidating the antigen(s) specificity for CNS antibodies of MS patients has proven elusive, and it remains unclear the extent to which intrathecal antibodies in MS patients are pathogenic.[1] CSF antibodies recognizing myelin, neuronal, and viral antigens have been reported by some but not all groups.[90-92] Of the putative myelin antigens in MS, myelin oligodendrocyte glycoprotein (MOG) is a leading contender. MOG is located on the surface of intact myelin, and is known to be encephalitogenic in EAE.[94,101] Furthermore, anti-MOG antibodies have been identified within EAE lesions as well as within lesions and CSF from MS patients.[94,95,102] Studies of myelin antibodies in serum as an MS biomarkers for diagnosis or prognosis have yielded conflicting results.[1] In the case of anti-MOG antibodies, immunoassays that retain the naturally occurring three-dimensional conformation of MOG epitopes are crucial, and this presents a significant technical challenge.[103-107] While proteins derived from compact myelin have been traditionally considered the main disease targets in MS – a concept largely driven by studies in EAE – of renewed interest is recent work revisiting the possibility that relevant immune responses by both T-cells and B-cells/antibodies may target non compact myelin structures such as neuronal/axoglial epitopes,[108] or non-protein antigens such as lipids.[98,109-111] It should be kept in mind that antibodies within the CNS could also have beneficial effects during the course of MS. In certain contexts, Igs can have a down regulatory effect on inflammation by binding to inhibitory Fc receptors.[112] There is also evidence suggesting that antibodies binding oligodendrocytes promote remyelination.[113] In EAE, remyelination can be promoted by antibodies against Lingo-1, a protein expressed both in neurons and oligodendrocytes, which acts as a negative regulator of myelination.[114] Antibodies targeting Nogo A, which have been described in MS serum and CSF,[115] can promote axonal extension,[116,117] consistent with the observation that silencing Nogo A can promote functional recovery in demyelinating disease.[118]

B-cells within the MS CNS may also contribute to disease independent of antibody production via any of the multiple antibody-independent functions of B-cells described earlier. While CNS inflammation is known to trigger several molecular mechanisms that down-regulate local immune responses – such as HLA-G and B7-H1 mediated down-regulation of T-cell activation[119,120] or CD200-CD200R mediated down-regulation of myeloid cells[121] – the inflamed CNS environment in MS patients may provide a supportive milieu to B-cells. Activated astrocytes in MS lesions exhibit up-regulated expression of B-cell activating factor (BAFF), a potent B-cell survival and growth factor.[122] Corcione *et al.* described that CSF of MS patients was enriched for B-cell subsets typical of lymph node tissue and also harbored elevated levels of lymphogenic mediators including LTα, CXCL12, and CXCL13, a known B-cell chemotactic factor. The authors suggested that these factors may provide a favorable environment for B-cells within the MS CNS, where they may recapitulate the stages of B-cell differentiation typically observed in secondary lymphoid organs.[123] While B-cells and plasma cells represent a minor fraction of the typical perivascular inflammatory lesions in MS, they are considerably more abundant in immune cell aggregates identified in the meninges.[123–126] These lymphoid aggregates recapitulate features of lymphoid germinal centers. Such structures, reportedly composed of chronically activated B-cells, plasma cells, T-cells and cells with follicular dendritic cell (DC) features expressing CXCL13, have been referred to as "tertiary" or "ectopic" follicles, and have been described within the target organs of several other autoimmune diseases, typically evolving later in the disease process.[127] Magliozzi et al. reported that in MS brains these follicle-like structures could be found adjacent to subpial cortical demyelinating lesions, raising the intriguing possibility that immune–immune interactions within follicle-like structures may contribute, potentially through soluble factors, to the subpial cortical pathology in MS patients (Chapter 2).[126] B-cells are known to play important roles in the formation and maintenance of normal lymphoid germinal centers and follicle architecture, with particular roles attributed to B-cell LT-alpha and LT-beta. It is intriguing to speculate that B-cells present in meningeal follicle-like structures within the inflamed MS CNS, can express LT and inflammatory chemokines that may contribute to the maintenance of such structures, as well as to other MS-relevant immune responses. The recent discovery that activated B-cells of MS patients exhibit an over propensity to produce LT (as well as TNFα) in the face of diminished induction of IL-10[31] may be relevant in this regard, as are reports that peripheral B-cell depletion using rituximab results in diminished CSF levels of chemokines including CXCL13,[128] as well as decreased T-cell numbers within the CSF of patients.[129]

Innate-immune-mediated injury in the CNS

Several types of innate immune cells have been implicated in MS tissue injury. Innate γδ T-cells differ from adaptive αβ T-cell in several respects including usage of the γ and δ TCR chains which produce an invariant TCR recognizing primarily phospholipids, and the apparent lack of a traditional memory pool. The CSF and lesions of MS patients have been shown to contain γδ T-cells, and in vitro experiments show that γδ T-cells have the capacity to kill human oligodendrocytes and astrocytes through cytotoxic mechanisms.[78,130] Dissecting the contribution of γδ T-cells using animal models has been challenging; variable effects on EAE disease activity upon depletion of these cells may reflect their potential for both pro- and

anti-inflammatory roles.[131] NK cells, which can also contribute to both induction and down-regulation of immune responses, may play different roles in different tissue compartments. They have been implicated in bystander neuronal injury,[78] though they are present in relatively small numbers in typical MS lesions. Microglia, important innate immune effectors that are resident to the brain, can contribute to tissue injury in several ways beyond activation of T-cells, including production of injurious (and potentially protective) cytokines, glutamate, matrix proteases, nitric oxide, oxygen radicals, and pro-apoptotic signals, all of which may participate at sites of injury in non-antigen-dependent ways; the capacity of microglia to respond to (both internal and external) cues, and transduce environmental signals continues to be an area of active investigation.[69,132,133]

Protective and reparative potential of immune responses in MS

Immune responses within the CNS need not always be detrimental. Both cellular immune responses as well as soluble factors can have protective and potentially growth permissive influences capable of limiting injury, as well as promoting survival and repair of neural elements.[134,135] Microglia may play a key role in regenerative therapies through clearing myelin debris thus facilitating remyelination and preventing axon degeneration.[69,136] Relevant soluble factors are thought to include neurotrophic molecules, reparative cytokines, as well as particular antibodies, as indicated above, that may support clearance of debris, remyelination, and neurite outgrowth.[137] Mechanisms by which individual cytokines (such as IL-1β, TNFα), matrix metalloproteinases, and apoptotic molecules may contribute locally to either tissue injury or neural protection/repair are complex and may, in part, explain why therapies such as anti-TNFα agents appear to be detrimental in MS. Modulating the immune system to harness its neuroprotective/reparative potential is of considerable therapeutic interest. For example, in addition to mediating Th2 and Type 2 APC immune deviation, treatment with glatiramer acetate has also been implicated in supporting a growth permissive CNS environment.[138,139] Other emerging therapies that may favorably impact both the immunology and neurobiology of MS may include fingolimod[140] (Chapter 30) and fumarate/BG00012 (Chapter 31).[141] The future challenge for harnessing neuroprotective and reparative immune responses will be to find the balance between promoting the potentially beneficial effects of the immune system within the CNS while avoiding the detrimental ones, as underscored by the dual roles of microglia.[69]

References

1. Bar-Or A. The immunology of multiple sclerosis. *Semin Neurol* 2008;28(1): 29–45.

2. Banwell B, Bar-Or A, Cheung R, et al. Abnormal T-cell reactivities in childhood inflammatory demyelinating disease and type 1 diabetes. *Ann Neurol* 2008;63(1):98–111.

3. Oksenberg JR, Baranzini SE. Multiple sclerosis genetics–is the glass half full, or half empty? *Nat Rev Neurol*; 6(8):429–37.

4. Okuda DT, Srinivasan R, Oksenberg JR, et al. Genotype–phenotype correlations in multiple sclerosis: HLA

genes influence disease severity inferred by 1HMR spectroscopy and MRI measures. *Brain*, 2009;132(1):250–9.

5. O'Brien M, Lonergan R, Costelloe L, *et al*. OAS1: a multiple sclerosis susceptibility gene that influences disease severity. *Neurology* 2010;75(5):411–18.

6. Baranzini SE, Mudge J, van Velkinburgh JC, *et al*. Genome, epigenome and RNA sequences of monozygotic twins discordant for multiple sclerosis. *Nature*; 464(7293):1351–6.

7. Cserr HF, Harling-Berg CJ, Knopf PM. Drainage of brain extracellular fluid into blood and deep cervical lymph and its immunological significance. *Brain Pathol*; 2:269–76.

8. Weller RO, Galea I, Carare RO, Minagar A. Pathophysiology of the lymphatic drainage of the central nervous system: Implications for pathogenesis and therapy of multiple sclerosis. *Pathophysiology* 2010;17(4):295–306.

9. de Vos AF, van Meurs M, Brok HP, *et al*. Transfer of central nervous system autoantigens and presentation in secondary lymphoid organs. *J Immunol* 2002;169(10):5415–23.

10. Wucherpfennig KW, Allen PM, Celada F, *et al*. Polyspecificity of T cell and B cell receptor recognition. *Semin Immunol* 2007;19(4):216–24.

11. Wucherpfennig KW, Strominger JL. Molecular mimicry in T cell-mediated autoimmunity: viral peptides activate human T cell clones specific for myelin basic protein. *Cell* 1995 10; 80(5):695–705.

12. Lang HL, Jacobsen H, Ikemizu S, *et al*. A functional and structural basis for TCR cross-reactivity in multiple sclerosis. *Nat Immunol* 2002;3(10):940–3.

13. Vanderlugt CL, Miller SD. Epitope spreading in immune-mediated diseases: implications for immunotherapy. *Nat Rev Immunol* 2002;2(2):85–95.

14. Giacomini PS, Bar-Or A. Antigen-specific therapies in multiple sclerosis. *Expert Opin Emerg Drugs* 2009;14(3):551–60.

15. Bar-Or A, Vollmer T, Antel J, *et al*. Induction of antigen-specific tolerance in multiple sclerosis after immunization with DNA encoding myelin basic protein in a randomized, placebo-controlled phase 1/2 trial. *Arch Neurol* 2007;64(10):1407–15.

16. Viglietta V, Bourcier K, Buckle GJ, *et al*. CTLA4Ig treatment in patients with multiple sclerosis: an open-label, phase 1 clinical trial. *Neurology* 2008;71(12):917–24.

17. Korn T, Oukka M, Kuchroo V, Bettelli E. Th17 cells: effector T cells with inflammatory properties. *Semin Immunol* 2007;19(6):362–71.

18. Bettelli E, Oukka M, Kuchroo VK. T(H)-17 cells in the circle of immunity and autoimmunity. *Nat Immunol* 2007;8(4):345–50.

19. Zhu J, Paul WE. Peripheral CD4+ T-cell differentiation regulated by networks of cytokines and transcription factors. *Immunol Rev*; 238(1): 247–62.

20. Yang Y, Weiner J, Liu Y, *et al*. T-bet is essential for encephalitogenicity of both Th1 and Th17 cells. *J Exp Med* 2009;206(7):1549–64.

21. Du C, Liu C, Kang J, *et al*. MicroRNA miR-326 regulates TH-17 differentiation and is associated with the pathogenesis of multiple sclerosis. *Nat Immunol* 2009;10(12):1252–9.

22. Jager A, Dardalhon V, Sobel RA, Bettelli E, Kuchroo VK. Th1, Th17, and Th9 effector cells induce experimental autoimmune encephalomyelitis with different pathological phenotypes. *J Immunol* 2009;183(11): 7169–77.

23. Kroenke MA, Carlson TJ, Andjelkovic AV, Segal BM. IL-12- and IL-23-modulated T cells induce distinct types of EAE based on histology, CNS chemokine profile, and response to cytokine inhibition. *J Exp Med* 2008;205(7):1535–41.

24. Kebir H, Kreymborg K, Ifergan I, *et al*. Human TH17 lymphocytes promote blood–brain barrier disruption and central nervous system inflammation. *Nat Med*. 2007;13(10):1173–5.

25. Ifergan I, Kebir H, Bernard M, *et al*. The blood-brain barrier induces differentiation of migrating monocytes into Th17-polarizing dendritic cells. *Brain* 2008;131(Pt 3):785–99.

26. Kebir H, Ifergan I, Alvarez JI, *et al*. Preferential recruitment of interferon-gamma-expressing TH17 cells in multiple sclerosis. *Ann Neurol* 2009;66(3):390–402.

27. Prinz M, Kalinke U. New lessons about old molecules: how type I interferons shape Th1/Th17-mediated autoimmunity in the CNS. *Trends Mol Med*; 16(8):379–86.

28. Aharoni R, Eilam R, Stock A, *et al*. Glatiramer acetate reduces Th-17 inflammation and induces regulatory T-cells in the CNS of mice with relapsing–remitting or chronic EAE. *J Neuroimmunol* 2010;225(1–2):100–11.

29. Begum-Haque S, Sharma A, Kasper IR, *et al*. Downregulation of IL-17 and IL-6 in the central nervous system by glatiramer acetate in experimental autoimmune encephalomyelitis. *J Neuroimmunol* 2008;204(1–2):58–65.

30. Mehling M, Lindberg R, Raulf F, *et al*. Th17 central memory T cells are reduced by FTY720 in patients with multiple sclerosis. *Neurology*; 75(5):403–10.

31. Bar-Or A, Fawaz L, Fan B, *et al*. Abnormal B-cell cytokine responses a trigger of T-cell-mediated disease in MS? *Ann Neurol* 2010;67(4):452–61.

32. Axtell RC, de Jong BA, Boniface K, *et al*. T helper type 1 and 17 cells determine efficacy of interferon-beta in multiple sclerosis and experimental encephalomyelitis. *Nat Med* 2010;16(4):406–12.

33. Rafei M, Campeau PM, Aguilar-Mahecha A, *et al*. Mesenchymal stromal cells ameliorate experimental autoimmune encephalomyelitis by inhibiting CD4 Th17 T cells in a CC chemokine ligand 2-dependent manner. *J Immunol* 2009;182(10):5994–6002.

34. Darlington PJ, Boivin MN, Renoux C, *et al*. Reciprocal Th1 and Th17 regulation by mesenchymal stem cells: Implication for multiple sclerosis. *Ann Neurol* 2010;68(4):540–5.

35. Reboldi A, Coisne C, Baumjohann D, *et al*. C-C chemokine receptor 6-regulated entry of TH-17 cells into the CNS through the choroid plexus is required for the initiation of EAE. *Nat Immunol* 2009;10(5):514–23.

36. Ponomarev ED, Shriver LP, Maresz K, Pedras-Vasconcelos J, Verthelyi D, Dittel BN. GM-CSF production by autoreactive T cells is required for the activation of microglial cells and the onset of experimental autoimmune encephalomyelitis. *J Immunol* 2007;178(1):39–48.

37. Nowak EC, Weaver CT, Turner H, *et al.* IL-9 as a mediator of Th17-driven inflammatory disease. *J Exp Med* 2009;206(8):1653–60.

38. Elyaman W, Bradshaw EM, Uyttenhove C, *et al.* IL-9 induces differentiation of TH17 cells and enhances function of FoxP3+ natural regulatory T cells. *Proc Natl Acad Sci USA* 2009;106(31): 12885–90.

39. Beriou G, Bradshaw EM, Lozano E, *et al.* TGF-beta induces IL-9 production from human Th17 cells. *J Immunol* 2010;185(1):46–54.

40. Genain CP, Abel K, Belmar N, *et al.* Late complications of immune deviation therapy in a nonhuman primate. *Science* 1996;274(5295): 2054–7.

41. Pedotti R, Mitchell D, Wedemeyer J, *et al.* An unexpected version of horror autotoxicus: anaphylactic shock to a self-peptide. *Nat Immunol* 2001;2(3):216–22.

42. Cvetanovich GL, Hafler DA. Human regulatory T cells in autoimmune diseases. *Curr Opin Immunol* 2010;22(6):753–60.

43. Huang YH, Zozulya AL, Weidenfeller C, Schwab N, Wiendl H. T cell suppression by naturally occurring HLA-G-expressing regulatory CD4+ T cells is IL-10-dependent and reversible. *J Leukoc Biol* 2009;86(2):273–81.

44. Gandhi R, Farez MF, Wang Y, Kozoriz D, Quintana FJ, Weiner HL. Cutting edge: human latency-associated peptide+ T cells: a novel regulatory T cell subset. *J Immunol* 2010;184(9): 4620–4.

45. Schneider-Hohendorf T, Stenner MP, Weidenfeller C, *et al.* Regulatory T cells exhibit enhanced migratory characteristics, a feature impaired in patients with multiple sclerosis. *Eur J Immunol* 2010;40(12):3581–90.

46. Fletcher JM, Lonergan R, Costelloe L, *et al.* CD39+Foxp3 +regulatory T Cells suppress pathogenic Th17 cells and are impaired in multiple sclerosis. *J Immunol* 2009;183(11):7602–10.

47. Astier AL, Meiffren G, Freeman S, Hafler DA. Alterations in CD46-mediated Tr1 regulatory T cells in patients with multiple sclerosis. *J Clin Invest* 2006;116(12):3252–7.

48. Korn T, Reddy J, Gao W, *et al.* Myelin-specific regulatory T cells accumulate in the CNS but fail to control autoimmune inflammation. *Nat Med* 2007;13(4):423–31.

49. Genc K, Dona DL, Reder AT. Increased CD80(+) B cells in active multiple sclerosis and reversal by interferon beta-1b therapy. *J Clin Invest* 1997;99(11):2664–71.

50. Bar-Or A, Oliveira EM, Anderson DE, *et al.* Immunological memory: contribution of memory B cells expressing costimulatory molecules in the resting state. *J Immunol* 2001;167(10):5669–77.

51. Duddy ME, Alter A, Bar-Or A. Distinct profiles of human B cell effector cytokines: a role in immune regulation? *J Immunol* 2004;172(6):3422–7.

52. Duddy M, Niino M, Adatia F, *et al.* Distinct effector cytokine profiles of memory and naive human B cell subsets and implication in multiple sclerosis. *J Immunol* 2007;178(10):6092–9.

53. Correale J, Farez M, Razzitte G. Helminth infections associated with multiple sclerosis induce regulatory B cells. *Ann Neurol* 2008;64(2):187–99.

54. Harp CT, Ireland S, Davis LS, *et al.* Memory B cells from a subset of treatment-naive relapsing–remitting multiple sclerosis patients elicit CD4(+) T-cell proliferation and IFN-gamma production in response to myelin basic protein and myelin oligodendrocyte glycoprotein. *Eur J Immunol* 2010;40(10):2942–56.

55. Matsushita T, Yanaba K, Bouaziz JD, Fujimoto M, Tedder TF. Regulatory B cells inhibit EAE initiation in mice while other B cells promote disease progression. *J Clin Invest* 2008;118(10):3420–30.

56. Weber MS, Prod'homme T, Patarroyo JC, *et al.* B-cell activation influences T-cell polarization and outcome of anti-CD20 B-cell depletion in central nervous system autoimmunity. *Ann Neurol* 2010;68(3):369–83.

57. Martin JF, Perry JS, Jakhete NR, Wang X, Bielekova B. An IL-2 paradox: blocking CD25 on T cells induces IL-2-driven activation of CD56(bright) NK cells. *J Immunol* 2010;185(2): 1311–20.

58. Kim HJ, Ifergan I, Antel JP, *et al.* Type 2 monocyte and microglia differentiation mediated by glatiramer acetate therapy in patients with multiple sclerosis. *J Immunol* 2004;172(11):7144–53.

59. Weber MS, Starck M, Wagenpfeil S, Meinl E, Hohlfeld R, Farina C. Multiple sclerosis: glatiramer acetate inhibits monocyte reactivity in vitro and in vivo. *Brain* 2004;127(Pt 6):1370–8.

60. Schwab N, Zozulya AL, Kieseier BC, Toyka KV, Wiendl H. An imbalance of two functionally and phenotypically different subsets of plasmacytoid dendritic cells characterizes the dysfunctional immune regulation in multiple sclerosis. *J Immunol* 2010;184(9):5368–74.

61. Racke MK, Drew PD. Toll-like receptors in multiple sclerosis. *Curr Top Microbiol Immunol* 2009;336:155–68.

62. Ransohoff RM. Mechanisms of inflammation in MS tissue: adhesion molecules and chemokines. *J Neuroimmunol* 1999;98(1):57–68.

63. Cayrol R, Wosik K, Berard JL, *et al.* Activated leukocyte cell adhesion molecule promotes leukocyte trafficking into the central nervous system. *Nat Immunol* 2008;9(2):137–45.

64. Ifergan I, Kebir H, Terouz S, *et al.* Role of Ninjurin-1 in the migration of myeloid cells to CNS inflammatory lesions. *Ann Neurol.* 2011; in press.

65. Bartholomaus I, Kawakami N, Odoardi F, *et al.* Effector T cell interactions with meningeal vascular structures in nascent autoimmune CNS lesions. *Nature* 2009;462(7269):94–8.

66. Ransohoff RM, Kivisakk P, Kidd G. Three or more routes for leukocyte migration into the central nervous system. *Nat Rev Immunol* 2003;3(7):569–81.

67. Holman DW, Klein RS, Ransohoff RM. The blood–brain barrier, chemokines and multiple sclerosis. *Biochim Biophys Acta* 2011;1812(2):220–30.

68. Hohlfeld R, Meinl E, Dornmair K. B- and T-cell responses in multiple sclerosis: novel approaches offer new insights. *J Neurol Sci* 2008;274(1–2): 5–8.

69. Ransohoff RM, Cardona AE. The myeloid cells of the central nervous system parenchyma. *Nature* 2010;468(7321):253–62.

70. Li Y, Chu N, Hu A, Gran B, Rostami A, Zhang GX. Increased IL-23p19 expression in multiple sclerosis lesions and its induction in microglia. *Brain* 2007;130(Pt 2):490–501.

71. Durafourt BA, Lambert C, Johnson TA, Blain M, Bar-Or A, Antel JP.

Differential responses of human microglia and blood-derived myeloid cells to FTY720. *J Neuroimmunol* 2011;230 (1–2):10–16.

72. Lambert C, Desbarats J, Arbour N, *et al.* Dendritic cell differentiation signals induce anti-inflammatory properties in human adult microglia. *J Immunol* 2008;181(12):8288–97.

73. Constantinescu CS, Tani M, Ransohoff RM, *et al.* Astrocytes as antigen-presenting cells: expression of IL-12/IL-23. *J Neurochem* 2005;95(2):331–40.

74. Giuliani F, Goodyer CG, Antel JP, Yong VW. Vulnerability of human neurons to T cell-mediated cytotoxicity. *J Immunol* 2003;171(1):368–79.

75. Neumann H, Medana IM, Bauer J, Lassmann H. Cytotoxic T lymphocytes in autoimmune and degenerative CNS diseases. *Trends Neurosci* 2002;25(6):313–19.

76. Melzer N, Meuth SG, Wiendl H. CD8+ T cells and neuronal damage: direct and collateral mechanisms of cytotoxicity and impaired electrical excitability. *FASEB J* 2009;23(11):3659–73.

77. Wang T, Lee MH, Johnson T, *et al.* Activated T-cells inhibit neurogenesis by releasing granzyme B: rescue by Kv1.3 blockers. *J Neurosci* 2010;30(14):5020–7.

78. Darlington PJ, Podjaski C, Horn KE, *et al.* Innate immune-mediated neuronal injury consequent to loss of astrocytes. *J Neuropathol Exp Neurol* 2008;67(6):590–9.

79. Babbe H, Roers A, Waisman A, *et al.* Clonal expansions of CD8(+) T cells dominate the T cell infiltrate in active multiple sclerosis lesions as shown by micromanipulation and single cell polymerase chain reaction. *J Exp Med* 2000;192(3):393–404.

80. Hoftberger R, Aboul-Enein F, Brueck W, *et al.* Expression of major histocompatibility complex class I molecules on the different cell types in multiple sclerosis lesions. *Brain Pathol* 2004;14(1):43–50.

81. Skulina C, Schmidt S, Dornmair K, *et al.* Multiple sclerosis: brain-infiltrating CD8+ T cells persist as clonal expansions in the cerebrospinal fluid and blood. *Proc Natl Acad Sci USA* 2004;101(8):2428–33.

82. Tsuchida T, Parker KC, Turner RV, McFarland HF, Coligan JE, Biddison WE. Autoreactive CD8+ T-cell responses to human myelin protein-derived peptides. *Proc Natl Acad Sci USA* 1994;91(23):10859–63.

83. Buckle GJ, Hollsberg P, Hafler DA. Activated CD8+ T cells in secondary progressive MS secrete lymphotoxin. *Neurology* 2003;60(4):702–5.

84. Crawford MP, Yan SX, Ortega SB, *et al.* High prevalence of autoreactive, neuroantigen-specific CD8+ T cells in multiple sclerosis revealed by novel flow cytometric assay. *Blood* 2004;103(11):4222–31.

85. Goverman J. Autoimmune T cell responses in the central nervous system. *Nat Rev Immunol* 2009;9(6): 393–407.

86. York NR, Mendoza JP, Ortega SB, *et al.* Immune regulatory CNS-reactive CD8+T cells in experimental autoimmune encephalomyelitis. *J Autoimmun.* 2010;35(1):33–44.

87. Harp C, Lee J, Lambracht-Washington D, *et al.* Cerebrospinal fluid B cells from multiple sclerosis patients are subject to normal germinal center selection. *J Neuroimmunol* 2007;183(1–2):189–99.

88. Obermeier B, Mentele R, Malotka J, *et al.* Matching of oligoclonal immunoglobulin transcriptomes and proteomes of cerebrospinal fluid in multiple sclerosis. *Nat Med* 2008;14(6):688–93.

89. von Budingen HC, Gulati M, Kuenzle S, Fischer K, Rupprecht TA, Goebels N. Clonally expanded plasma cells in the cerebrospinal fluid of patients with central nervous system autoimmune demyelination produce "oligoclonal bands." *J Neuroimmunol* 2010;218(1–2):134–9.

90. Archelos JJ, Storch MK, Hartung HP. The role of B cells and autoantibodies in multiple sclerosis. *Ann Neurol* 2000;47(6):694–706.

91. Cross AH, Trotter JL, Lyons J. B cells and antibodies in CNS demyelinating disease. *J Neuroimmunol* 2001;112(1–2):1–14.

92. Fraussen J, Vrolix K, Martinez Martinez P, *et al.* B cell characterization and reactivity analysis in multiple sclerosis. *Autoimmun Rev* 2009;8(8):654–8.

93. Storch MK, Piddlesden S, Haltia M, Iivanainen M, Morgan P, Lassmann H. Multiple sclerosis: in situ evidence for antibody- and complement-mediated demyelination. *Ann Neurol* 1998;43(4):465–71.

94. Genain CP, Cannella B, Hauser SL, Raine CS. Identification of autoantibodies associated with myelin damage in multiple sclerosis. *Nat Med* 1999;5(2):170–5.

95. O'Connor KC, Appel H, Bregoli L, *et al.* Antibodies from inflamed central nervous system tissue recognize myelin oligodendrocyte glycoprotein. *J Immunol* 2005;175(3):1974–82.

96. Izquierdo G, Angulo S, Garcia-Moreno JM, *et al.* Intrathecal IgG synthesis: marker of progression in multiple sclerosis patients. *Acta Neurol Scand* 2002;105(3):158–63.

97. Villar LM, Masjuan J, Gonzalez-Porque P, *et al.* Intrathecal IgM synthesis predicts the onset of new relapses and a worse disease course in MS. *Neurology* 2002;59(4):555–9.

98. Villar LM, Sadaba MC, Roldan E, *et al.* Intrathecal synthesis of oligoclonal IgM against myelin lipids predicts an aggressive disease course in MS. *J Clin Invest.* 2005;115(1):187–94.

99. Zeman AZ, Kidd D, McLean BN, *et al.* A study of oligoclonal band negative multiple sclerosis. *J Neurol Neurosurg Psychiatry.* 1996;60(1):27–30.

100. O'Connor KC, Lopez-Amaya C, Gagne D, *et al.* Anti-myelin antibodies modulate clinical expression of childhood multiple sclerosis. *J Neuroimmunol* 2010;223(1–2):92–9.

101. Genain CP, Nguyen MH, Letvin NL, *et al.* Antibody facilitation of multiple sclerosis-like lesions in a nonhuman primate. *J Clin Invest* 1995;96(6): 2966–74.

102. Klawiter EC, Piccio L, Lyons JA, Mikesell R, O'Connor KC, Cross AH. Elevated intrathecal myelin oligodendrocyte glycoprotein antibodies in multiple sclerosis. *Arch Neurol* 2010;67(9):1102–8.

103. Zhou D, Srivastava R, Nessler S, *et al.* Identification of a pathogenic antibody response to native myelin oligodendrocyte glycoprotein in multiple sclerosis. *Proc Natl Acad Sci USA* 2006;103(50):19057–62.

104. Lalive PH, Menge T, Delarasse C, *et al.* Antibodies to native myelin oligodendrocyte glycoprotein are serologic markers of early inflammation in multiple sclerosis. *Proc Natl Acad Sci USA* 2006;103(7):2280–5.

105. O'Connor KC, McLaughlin KA, De Jager PL, *et al.* Self-antigen tetramers discriminate between myelin autoantibodies to native or denatured protein. *Nat Med* 2007;13(2): 211–17.

106. Chan A, Decard BF, Franke C, *et al.* Serum antibodies to conformational and linear epitopes of myelin oligodendrocyte glycoprotein are not elevated in the preclinical phase of multiple sclerosis. *Mult Scler* 2010;16(10):1189–92.

107. Selter RC, Brilot F, Grummel V, *et al.* Antibody responses to EBV and native MOG in pediatric inflammatory demyelinating CNS diseases. *Neurology* 2010;74(21):1711–15.

108. Derfuss T, Linington C, Hohlfeld R, Meinl E. Axo-glial antigens as targets in multiple sclerosis: implications for axonal and grey matter injury. *J Mol Med* 2010;88(8):753–61.

109. Kanter JL, Narayana S, Ho PP, *et al.* Lipid microarrays identify key mediators of autoimmune brain inflammation. *Nat Med* 2006;12(1):138–43.

110. Garcia-Barragan N, Villar LM, Espino M, Sadaba MC, Gonzalez-Porque P, Alvarez-Cermeno JC. Multiple sclerosis patients with anti-lipid oligoclonal IgM show early favourable response to immunomodulatory treatment. *Eur J Neurol* 2009;16(3):380–5.

111. Podbielska M, Dasgupta S, Levery SB, *et al.* Novel myelin penta- and hexa-acetyl-galactosyl-ceramides: structural characterization and immunoreactivity in cerebrospinal fluid. *J Lipid Res* 2010;51(6):1394–406.

112. Ravetch JV, Bolland S. IgG Fc receptors. *Annu Rev Immunol* 2001;19:275–90.

113. Warrington AE, Asakura K, Bieber AJ, *et al.* Human monoclonal antibodies reactive to oligodendrocytes promote remyelination in a model of multiple sclerosis. *Proc Natl Acad Sci USA* 2000;97(12):6820–5.

114. Mi S, Miller RH, Tang W, *et al.* Promotion of central nervous system remyelination by induced differentiation of oligodendrocyte precursor cells. *Ann Neurol* 2009;65(3):304–15.

115. Reindl M, Khantane S, Ehling R, *et al.* Serum and cerebrospinal fluid antibodies to Nogo-A in patients with multiple sclerosis and acute neurological disorders. *J Neuroimmunol* 2003;145(1–2):139–47.

116. Karnezis T, Mandemakers W, McQualter JL, *et al.* The neurite outgrowth inhibitor Nogo A is involved in autoimmune-mediated demyelination. *Nat Neurosci* 2004;7(7):736–44.

117. Li W, Walus L, Rabacchi SA, *et al.* A neutralizing anti-Nogo66 receptor monoclonal antibody reverses inhibition of neurite outgrowth by central nervous system myelin. *J Biol Chem* 2004;279(42):43780–8.

118. Yang Y, Liu Y, Wei P, *et al.* Silencing Nogo-A promotes functional recovery in demyelinating disease. *Ann Neurol* 2010;67(4):498–507.

119. Magnus T, Schreiner B, Korn T, *et al.* Microglial expression of the B7 family member B7 homolog 1 confers strong immune inhibition: implications for immune responses and autoimmunity in the CNS. *J Neurosci* 2005;25(10): 2537–46.

120. Wiendl H, Feger U, Mittelbronn M, *et al.* Expression of the immune-tolerogenic major histocompatibility molecule HLA-G in multiple sclerosis: implications for CNS immunity. *Brain* 2005;128(Pt 11):2689–704.

121. Liu Y, Bando Y, Vargas-Lowy D, *et al.* CD200R1 agonist attenuates mechanisms of chronic disease in a murine model of multiple sclerosis. *J Neurosci* 2010;30(6):2025–38.

122. Krumbholz M, Theil D, Derfuss T, *et al.* BAFF is produced by astrocytes and up-regulated in multiple sclerosis lesions and primary central nervous system lymphoma. *J Exp Med* 2005;201(2):195–200.

123. Corcione A, Casazza S, Ferretti E, *et al.* Recapitulation of B cell differentiation in the central nervous system of patients with multiple sclerosis. *Proc Natl Acad Sci USA* 2004;101(30): 11064–9.

124. Prineas JW. Multiple sclerosis: presence of lymphatic capillaries and lymphoid tissue in the brain and spinal cord. *Science.* 1979;203(4385):1123–5.

125. Serafini B, Rosicarelli B, Magliozzi R, Stigliano E, Aloisi F. Detection of ectopic B-cell follicles with germinal centers in the meninges of patients with secondary progressive multiple sclerosis. *Brain Pathol* 2004;14(2):164–74.

126. Magliozzi R, Howell O, Vora A, *et al.* Meningeal B-cell follicles in secondary progressive multiple sclerosis associate with early onset of disease and severe cortical pathology. *Brain* 2007;130 (Pt 4):1089–104.

127. Vinuesa CG, Sanz I, Cook MC. Dysregulation of germinal centres in autoimmune disease. *Nat Rev Immunol* 2009;9(12):845–57.

128. Piccio L, Naismith RT, Trinkaus K, *et al.* Changes in B- and T-lymphocyte and chemokine levels with rituximab treatment in multiple sclerosis. *Arch Neurol* 2010;67(6):707–14.

129. Cross AH, Stark JL, Lauber J, Ramsbottom MJ, Lyons JA. Rituximab reduces B cells and T cells in cerebrospinal fluid of multiple sclerosis patients. *J Neuroimmunol* 2006;180(1–2):63–70.

130. Freedman MS, Ruijs TC, Selin LK, Antel JP. Peripheral blood gamma-delta T cells lyse fresh human brain-derived oligodendrocytes. *Ann Neurol* 1991;30(6):794–800.

131. Petermann F, Rothhammer V, Claussen MC, *et al.* gammadelta T cells enhance autoimmunity by restraining regulatory T-cell responses via an interleukin-23-dependent mechanism. *Immunity* 2010;33(3):351–63.

132. Antel J, Owens T. Multiple sclerosis and immune regulatory cells. *Brain* 2004;127(Pt 9):1915–16.

133. DeBoy CA, Rus H, Tegla C, *et al.* FLT-3 expression and function on microglia in multiple sclerosis. *Exp Mol Pathol* 2010;89(2):109–16.

134. Martino G, Adorini L, Rieckmann P, *et al.* Inflammation in multiple sclerosis: the good, the bad, and the complex. *Lancet Neurol* 2002;1(8):499–509.

135. Yong VW, Rivest S. Taking advantage of the systemic immune system to cure brain diseases. *Neuron* 2009;64(1):55–60.

136. Villoslada P, Moreno B, Melero I, *et al.* Immunotherapy for neurological diseases. *Clin Immunol* 2008;128(3):294–305.

137. Rodriguez M, Warrington AE, Pease LR. Invited article: human natural autoantibodies in the treatment of neurologic disease. *Neurology* 2009;72(14):1269–76.

138. Skihar V, Silva C, Chojnacki A, *et al.* Promoting oligodendrogenesis

and myelin repair using the multiple sclerosis medication glatiramer acetate. *Proc Natl Acad Sci USA*. 2009;106(42):17992–7.

139. Arnon R, Aharoni R. Neuroprotection and neurogeneration in MS and its animal model EAE effected by glatiramer acetate. *J Neural Transm* 2009;116(11):1443–9.

140. Miron VE, Ludwin SK, Darlington PJ, *et al*. Fingolimod (FTY720) enhances remyelination following demyelination of organotypic cerebellar slices. *Am J Pathol* 2010;176(6):2682–94.

141. Gold R. Oral therapies for multiple sclerosis: a review of agents in phase III development or recently approved. *CNS Drugs* 2011;25(1):37–52.

Chapter

4

The genetics of multiple sclerosis

Jorge R. Oksenberg, Sergio E. Baranzini, and Stephen L. Hauser

The likelihood that an individual will develop MS is strongly influenced by her or his ethnic background and family history, suggesting that genetic susceptibility is a key determinant of the risk. For example, high prevalence rates are found in Scandinavia, Iceland, the British Isles, and North America (~1 to 2 in 1000) whereas, with the notable exception of Sardinia, lower frequencies are characteristic of southern European populations.[1] The disease is uncommon among Asians, Amerindians, African Blacks, and native populations of New Zealand and Australia. Within families, monozygotic twins have a higher concordance rate (20%–30%) compared to dizygotic twins of the same sex (2%–5%),[2–4] and after adjusting for age, non-twin siblings of an affected individual are 10–15 times more likely to develop MS than the general population.[5–10] Second and third degree relatives are also at an increased risk,[8,11] and studies in Canadian half-siblings,[12] spouses,[13] and adoptees[14] further support the conclusion that genetic, rather than environmental, risk factors underlie familial clustering.

This body of compelling epidemiological data fueled a longstanding search, spanning the last 50 years, to identify and characterize the genetic underpinnings of MS in order to gain insights into the fundamental etiology of the disease (Fig. 4.1). The available data, including the results from recent genome-wide association studies (GWAS),[15] have clarified the role of genetic factors in MS pathogenesis and provided strong empirical support for a polygenic model of inheritance driven primarily by allelic variants relatively common in the general population.[1] GWAS examine single nucleotide variation across genomes to identify genetic factors that are associated with a quantifiable trait. Commercially available "SNP chips or arrays" typically used in GWAS contain probes for polymorphisms selected on the basis of frequency and linkage disequilibrium parameters to efficiently capture large portions of common variation across the genome. Thus, the selected polymorphisms acts as surrogate markers of the broad genomic loci putatively associated with the trait of interest. Rapid rises have been observed in the density of the tested polymorphisms (currently $>10^6$) per study and in the number of published GWAS. Given the very large number of simultaneous tests in each study, various P

value cut-off points have been used to assess the statistical significance of associations (from $P < 5 \times 10^{-7}$ to $P < 1 \times 10^{-10}$), and a number of replication strategies have been employed to confirm the screening results. The Wellcome Trust Case Control Consortium has proposed that GWAS for complex diseases should involve at least 2000 cases and 2000 controls, and that P values of $< 5 \times 10^{-7}$ would be needed to ensure that results are most likely true. Naturally, larger sample sizes would be needed to detect smaller effect sizes to ensure the validity of this proposed threshold. Despite being a very young experimental approach, GWAS have already identified hundreds of polymorphisms associated with several diseases and traits, providing new knowledge and important biological insights. Most of these associated variants confer small increments to risk (1.2-fold–1.5-fold).

MS is also characterized by only modest heritability, a characteristic that is shared with many other common diseases. Although the effect of any given predisposing variant is modest, the possibility exists that multifaceted gene–gene (epistatic) and/or gene–environment interactions could substantially increase the contribution of some variants to the overall genetic risk (Fig. 4.2). Susceptibility genes may be subject to epigenetic modifications, which greatly increase the complexity of MS inheritance.[25–28]

The incidence of MS seems to have increased considerably over the last century – notwithstanding improved surveillance – and this increase may have occurred primarily in women.[16] Since it is unlikely that the distribution and frequency of genetic risk factors have changed over such a short period of time, this increasing frequency points in the direction of environmental factors. The influence of migration, latitude, and month of birth on disease prevalence is also consistent with a role for the environment adding substantially to the risk burden.[17,18] A large number of environmental exposures have been proposed as MS triggers, but robust evidence for a role of Epstein–Barr virus (EBV) in particular, has been shown by both epidemiologic[19] and laboratory studies.[20–22] However, since EBV is a ubiquitous herpesvirus with a world-wide distribution, this factor alone is insufficient to explain the uneven incidence of MS across

Multiple Sclerosis Therapeutics, Fourth Edition, ed. Jeffrey A. Cohen and Richard A. Rudick. Published by Cambridge University Press.
© Cambridge University Press 2011.

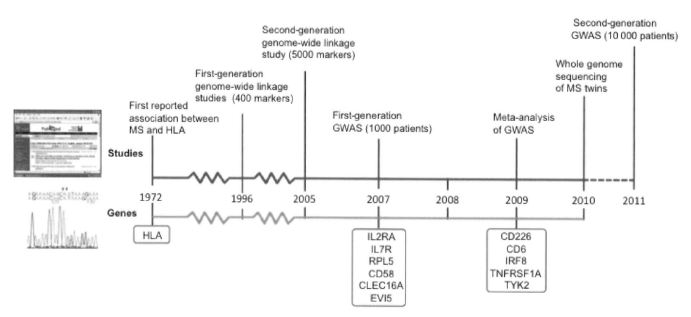

Fig. 4.1. Timeline of MS genetic research. Early success in identifying the role of *HLA* was immediately followed by intense, yet mostly unproductive efforts in the search of additional susceptibility genes. The recent publication of genome-wide association studies and identification of novel true disease genes has ignited the field with considerable drive. With the aid of high-powered laboratory technologies, we are now in a position to define the full array of genes, molecules, and pathways operating in MS. This goal can only be achieved if sufficient knowledge exists to distinguish disease variants, reliably classify therapeutic outcomes, and capture key individual molecular profiling variables.

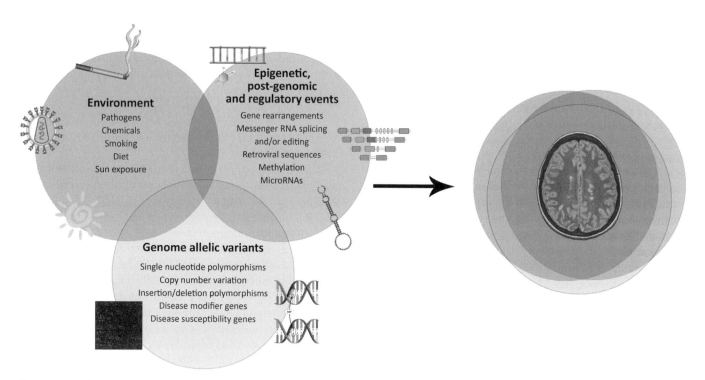

Fig. 4.2. Multiple sclerosis as a complex disease. MS is a complex genetic disease, characterized by a polygenic heritable component, epigenetic changes, and multifaceted interactions with environmental factors. The full roster of disease genes (susceptibility and modifiers) and environmental triggers in MS remains incomplete, whereas the study of epigenetic and other regulatory mechanisms linked to MS susceptibility is only beginning to emerge (see also color plate section).

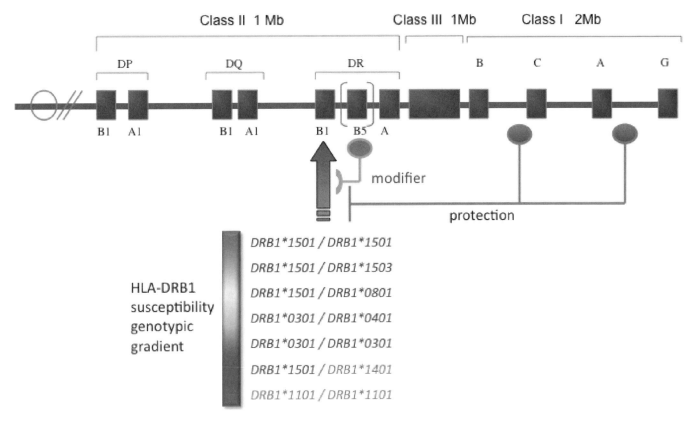

Fig. 4.3. The HLA system in MS. The human leukocyte antigen (*HLA*) gene complex is located on the short arm of chromosome 6 at p21.3, spanning almost 4000 KB of DNA. The full sequence of the region was completed and reported in 1999. From 224 identified loci, 128 are predicted to be expressed and about 40% to have immune-response functions. There are two major classes of HLA-encoding genes involved in antigen presentation. The telomeric stretch contains the *class I* genes, whereas the centromere proximal region encodes *HLA-class II* genes. The *HLA-class II* gene *DRB5* (in brackets) is only present in the DR51 haplotypic group (*DRB1*15* and *16* alleles). HLA class I and class II encoded molecules are cell surface glycoproteins whose primary role in an immune response is to display and present short antigenic peptide fragments to peptide/MHC-specific T cells, which can then become activated by a second stimulatory signal and initiate an immune response. In addition, HLA molecules are present on stromal cells on the thymus during development helping to determine the specificity of the mature T cell repertoire. A third group of genes collectively known as *class III*, cluster between the *class I* and *II* regions and include genes coding for complement proteins, 21a-hydroxylase, tumor necrosis factor, and heat shock proteins. This super-locus contains at least one gene (*HLA-DRB1*) that strongly influences susceptibility to MS. *HLA-DRB1* allelic copy number and *cis/trans* effects have been detected, and suggest a disease association gradient, ranging from high vulnerability (*DRB1*15* homozygotes and *DRB1*15/08* heterozygotes) to moderate susceptibility (*DRB1*03* homozygotes and heterozygotes) and resistance (*DRB1*15/*14* heterozygotes; in this genotypic configuration, the presence of *DRB1*14:01* neutralizes the susceptibility effect of *DRB1*15:01*). Modified from Figure 1, Oksenberg JR et al. Nature Reviews Genetics 9:516–526, 2008 (see also color plate section).

different populations. An attractive explanation for the latitude effect on MS is that sun exposure protects against MS by raising blood levels of vitamin D.[23] It is noteworthy that the disease concordance rate in monozygotic twins appears to vary by latitude of birthplace: latitudes with higher MS prevalence also show a higher concordance rate in twins.[24] This pattern is consistent with the hypothesis that gene–environment interactions importantly shape an individual's risk for MS.

The HLA locus and MS susceptibility

The human leukocyte antigen (*HLA*) gene cluster in chromosome 6p21.3 (Fig. 4.3) represents by far the strongest MS susceptibility locus genome-wide, explaining approximately 7%–10% of the total (genetic and non-genetic) variance. The association with this locus was observed across virtually all populations, and in both primary progressive and

relapsing-remitting patients, suggesting that *HLA*-related mechanisms contribute to both phenotypes.[29] The primary signal arises from the *HLA-DRB1* gene in the class II segment of the locus; individuals who are *HLA-DRB1*15:01* homozygous or *HLA-DRB1*15:01/*08:01* heterozygous carry a high-risk genotype (independent of family history, odds ratios – OR = 9.8 and 7.7 were observed, respectively, compared with a range between 3.5 and 5.0 for *HLA-DRB1*15:01/X*).[30] Individuals with *HLA-DRB1*03:01/*03:01* genotypes carry a moderate risk genotype (OR = 1.8), and individuals with *HLA-DRB1*15:01/*14:01* appear to carry a protective genotype (OR = 0.2).[30–33] Finally, the class I genes *HLA-A*, *HLA-B*, *HLA-C* and/or *HLA-G* have been proposed each to exert a protective effect on MS susceptibility, although the mutual independence of these signals remains to be resolved.[34–36]

Additional genetic interactions within the MHC region have also been identified. Perhaps the most interesting relates to *HLA-DRB5*, a class II gene immediately telomeric of *HLA-DRB1*; *HLA-DRB5* is a productive gene on the MS-associated *HLA-DRB1*15:01* haplotype, but is a pseudogene on most other *HLA* haplotypes. *HLA-DRβ5DRα* heterodimers appear to be effective myelin antigen-presenting molecules,[37] and elegant experiments using triple *DRB1-DRB5-hTCR* transgenic mice support functional epistasis (interaction) between *HLA-DRB1* and *HLA-DRB5* genes whereby DRβ5 modifies the T-cell response activated by DRβ1 through activation-induced cell death, resulting in a milder and relapsing form of autoimmune demyelinating experimental disease.[26] Similarly, in African Americans with MS, carriers of the *HLA-DRB1*15* with *HLA-DRB5*null* haplotypes have a more severe disease course than with *HLA-DRB5* wild types.[38] Although based on a small number of individuals with the rare *DRB5*null* mutation, the convergence of findings obtained from HLA-humanized EAE mice with human MS genetic data supports a modulatory role of *HLA-DRB5* gene products on the progression of autoimmune demyelinating disease.

The exact mechanism by which *HLA-DRB1* contributes to MS risk is unknown; however, multiple theories have been proposed, including binding of a specific peptide antigen to this *HLA* molecule; modulating a response to vitamin D via promoters that have vitamin D response elements; and influencing central T-cell tolerance. Despite the remarkable molecular dissection of the *HLA* region in MS in recent years, it is evident that further studies are needed to determine the mechanism or mechanisms by which *HLA* genes contribute to MS susceptibility.

Genome-wide association studies in MS

Two main biological issues contributed to thwart gene-discovery efforts in MS. First, the effect attributable to each individual allelic variant is modest. Second, the true signals need to be isolated from the abundant genetic variation that characterizes the human population as a whole, leading to the inescapable conclusion that the discovery of genes influencing MS risk must rely primarily on very large patient datasets and well-matched controls. By the mid 2000s, large, multicenter DNA collections had been established and the development of new laboratory and analytical approaches matured to a stage that permitted exploration of the human genome with remarkable coverage and precision. In 2007, the International Multiple Sclerosis Genetics Consortium (IMSGC) completed and reported a trio-based study assaying 500 000 single nucleotide polymorphisms (SNPs) in 931 MS families.[39] The classic *HLA-DRB1* risk locus stood out with remarkably strong statistical significance ($P < 1 \times 10^{-81}$). Extending the analysis of the 110 most promising non-*HLA* SNPs identified in the screen into additional trios, cases and controls enabled a combined replication analysis involving more than 12 000 samples, and confirmed a subset of SNPs associated with disease susceptibility, including the interleukin 2 receptor alpha chain (*IL2RA* also known as CD25) on chromosome 10p15, *CD58 (LFA3)* on chromosome 1p13,

and *IL7R* (CD127) on chromosome 5p13. Subsequently, other groups independently replicated these hits. Additional follow-up experiments refined some of the association signals, identified additional risk loci, and revealed early mechanistic insights into the functional consequences of the identified gene variants, such as an increase in the soluble to membrane-bound ratio for the IL2 and IL7 receptors.[40–44] To date, eight GWAS have been reported for MS susceptibility, all in populations of European descent (Table 4.1), including recent scans of a high-risk isolate from Finland and a Sardinian cohort.[39,45–51] A summary of the top candidate susceptibility genes is presented in Table 4.2. Interestingly, some of the allelic variants associated with MS have also emerged in GWAS of several other autoimmune diseases, suggesting that common underlying mechanisms might exist for various autoimmune conditions (Fig. 4.4).[52,53]

Taken together, the data from GWAS appear to support the long-held view that MS susceptibility rests on the action of common sequence allelic variants (that is, risk alleles with a population frequency of >5%) in multiple genes. It is important to note, however, that the associated SNPs do not necessarily represent the causative variants. Extremely fine mapping of each locus associated with MS risk using highly saturated customized SNPs arrays or direct sequencing of the entire coding and non-coding regions is likely to further refine the associated candidate regions and may lead to the identification of the true causative variant or variants for each MS risk locus. Despite the expanding roster of risk loci, our understanding of MS genetics remains incomplete. Some models estimate that the available non-HLA data from GWAS only explain approximately 3% of the total variance in MS risk.[54] Thus, the missing heritability of MS must reside in additional very low-effect common variants, in rare causative alleles, and/or in gene–gene interactions. A GWAS comprising 10 000 cases and high-density SNP–CNV platforms is near completion by the IMSGC. This study is adequately powered to identify common risk alleles with odds ratios as modest as 1.2.[55] In addition, multiple efforts to identify rare variants are underway through the use of second-generation sequencing methods and whole exome and whole genome sequencing approaches.

Genotype–phenotype associations

Concordance in families for some clinical metrics such as severity or age-of-onset suggests that, in addition to susceptibility, genes modestly influence disease trajectory and course.[56–59] The availability of GWAS datasets allowed the pursuit of agnostic genome-wide screens to characterize the genetic component of disease expression, including the response to immunomodulatory drugs (see also Chapter 23).[46,60,61] A GWAS in 372 MS patients using brain glutamate concentration as a quantitative trait, measured using two-dimensional echo time-averaged proton spectroscopic imaging, identified a variant within the gene sulfatase modifying factor 1 (*SUMF1*) affecting variation in MS brain glutamate concentrations.[62] DNA variants in this

Table 4.1. *Genome-wide association screens in MS*

Study	Design	Population origin	Number of screened samples	Number of SNPs	Featured loci/genes
Wellcome Trust CCC (2007)	Cases-shared controls	UK	1000 cases 1500 controls	14 436 (non-synonymous)	*IL7R*
IMSGC (2007)	Family and case control	US, UK	931 family trios	334 923	*HLA, IL2R, IL7R, CLEC16, CD58, EVI5, TYK2*
Comabella *et al.* (2008)	Pooled case-control	Spain	242 cases 242 controls	500 000	*HLA, 13q31.3*
GeneMSA C. (2009)	Case-control	US, The Netherlands, Switzerland	978 cases 8883 controls	551 642	*HLA, GPC5, PDZRNA4, CSMD1*
ANZ C. (2009)	Case-shared controls	Australia and New Zealand	1618 cases 3413 controls	303 431	*HLA, METTL1, CD40*
De Jager *et al.* (2009)	Meta-analysis and case-control	US, UK, The Netherlands, Switzerland	2624 case 7220 controls	2 557 248 (imputed)	*TNFRSF1A, IRF8, CD6, RGS1*
Jakkula *et al.* (2010)	Isolated case-control	Finland	68 cases 136 controls	297 343	*STAT3*
Sanna *et al.* (2010)	Case-control	Sardinia	882 cases 872 controls	6 600 000 (imputed)	*HLA, CBLB*
Nischwitz *et al.* (2010)	Case-control	Germany	590 cases 825 controls	300 000	*HLA, VAV2, ZNF433*

Table 4.2. *Multiple sclerosis susceptibility loci (2010)*

Gene	Associated SNP	Location	Risk allele	Estimated OR	Protein function/process
CD58	rs2300747	1p13	A	1.18	Cell adhesion, co-stimulation
EVI5	rs10735781	1p22.1	G	1.23	Rab GTPase activator, cell cycle
KIF21B	rs12122721	1pter-q31	G	1.22	Transport along axonal microtubules
RGS1	rs2760524	1q31	G	1.13	GTPase activator
CBLB	rs9657904	3q13	A	1.40	Calcium ion binding
TMEM39A	rs1132200	3q13	C	1.24	Membrane component
IL12A	rs4680534	3q25	C	1.11	Interleukin
IL7R	rs6897932	5p13	C	1.04	Cytokine receptor
HLA	DRB1*15:01	6p21	–	3.0	Immune response
IL2R	rs2104286	10p15	T	1.18	Cytokine receptor
CD6	rs17824933	11q13	G	1.16	Cell adhesion
MTTL1	rs703842	12q13	A	1.23	tRNA modification
TNFRSF1	rs1800693	12p13.2	C	1.23	Cytokine receptor
MPHOSPH9	rs1790100	12q24	G	1.10	Cell cycle
CLEC16A	rs12708716	16p13.3	A	1.17	Not determined
IRF8	rs17445836	16q24.1	G	1.33	Transcription
STAT3	rs744166	17q21	G	1.15	Transcription activator
CD226	rs763361	18q22.3	T	1.04	Cell adhesion
TYK2	rs34536443	19p13.2	G	1.30	Signaling
CD40	rs6074022	20q12	G	1.22	Co-stimulation

Top allelic variants identified in MS GWAS. Listed are genes with robust genome-wide evidence of association ($P < 5 \times 10^{-8}$) or that have been identified in more than two independent studies. In addition, suggestive evidence of association ($5 \times 10^{-8} < P < 5 \times 10^{-6}$) has been reported for *IL7, MMEL1, GPC5, PTGER4 CXCR4, ZMIZ1, OLIG3,* and *CD40*.

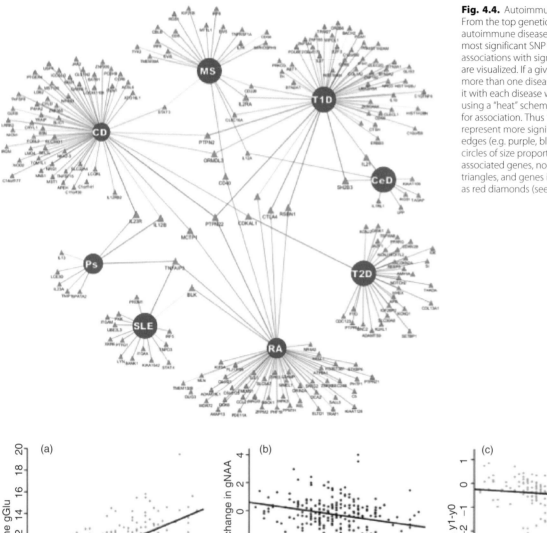

Fig. 4.4. Autoimmune disease-gene network. From the top genetic associations in 7 autoimmune diseases and Type 2 diabetes, the most significant SNP per gene was selected. Only associations with significance of at least $P < 10^{-7}$ are visualized. If a given gene was identified in more than one disease, multiple lines connecting it with each disease were drawn. Lines are colored using a "heat" scheme according to the evidence for association. Thus "hot" edges (e.g. red, orange) represent more significant associations than "cold" edges (e.g. purple, blue). Diseases are depicted by circles of size proportional to the number of associated genes, non-MHC genes by gray triangles, and genes in the MHC region are shown as red diamonds (see also color plate section).

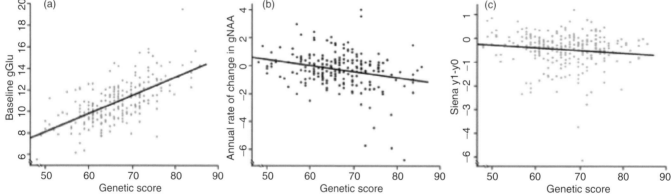

Fig. 4.5. Correlation between glutamate genetic score and phenotypic variables. (a) For a module of N genes, each patient was assigned a genetic score (GS) (from 0 to 2*N) corresponding to the total number of risk alleles carried at the N loci. (b) Correlation of glutamate genetic scores with grey matter glutamate concentration. (c) Correlation of genetic scores with NAA change over 1 year. Genetic scores explain more variance in NAA decline than expected given the a priori correlation between glutamate level and NAA decline. Similarly, correlation between genetic scores and brain atrophy was significant and higher than that expected from a priori correlation between glutamate level and brain atrophy. *Modified from Fig. 4, Baranzini SE et al. Brain 133:2603–2611, 2010[62].*

gene may indirectly regulate extracellular glutamate by altering the activity of steroid sulfatases. A network-based pathway analysis based on established protein–protein interactions to define the biological relationships among genes complemented the mining of the data, and a module composed of 70 genes associated with glutamate biology was identified; individuals carrying a higher number of associated alleles from genes in this module showed the highest levels of glutamate, and show greater decreases in N-acetylaspartate and in brain volume over

one year of follow-up (Fig. 4.5). Results from these analyses indicated that variance in the activity of neurochemical pathways implicated in neurodegeneration is explained, at least in part, by the inheritance of definable genetic variants. These data also validate the concept that spectroscopy and other emerging high-resolution imaging techniques provide valid quantitative endophenotypes for genetic association studies directed towards identifying factors that contribute to the heterogeneity of clinical expression of MS.

Full genome sequencing in MS

The ultimate goal of genetic studies in MS is to identify all of the genetic variants that contribute to disease susceptibility and/or clinical phenotypes. With the advent of next-generation sequencing, the ability to efficiently sequence an entire human genome and directly assay for all genetic variations has become a reality. In an initial experiment, the entire genomes of a female MS-discordant monozygotic (MZ) twin pair were sequenced from CD4+ T-cells, generating over one billion, high-quality, whole-genome sequences, corresponding to approximately 22-fold coverage of each genome, i.e. each position in the genome was sequence on average 22 times.[63] These are the first female, twin, and autoimmune genome sequences reported. The twin genomes contained ten of thirteen previously identified MS susceptibility SNPs. Approximately ~3.6 million single nucleotide polymorphisms (SNPs), ~200 000 insertion-deletion polymorphisms (indels), 27 copy number variations (CNVs), and 1.1 million mCpG dinucleotides (methylation sites) were detected, but no SNPs, indels, or CNVs differed between the twins. The study also reported the mRNA transcriptome and epigenome sequences of CD4+ T-cells from three MS discordant MZ twin pairs. Of ~29 000 expressed genes, 8214 differed in level of transcription between twins and tantalizing allelic differences in the levels of mRNA expression between twins were observed. Two hundred and sixty eight heterozygous cSNPs were associated with allelic imbalance in cis at 188 loci in the twins' transcriptomes, as determined by significant deviation of aligned genomic and mRNA read counts. Interestingly, 115 (43%) of these cSNPs differed between twins (i.e. differential allelic expression), suggesting that some gene expression differences between twins represent chromatid-specific alterations in transcription. This study inaugurated the era of whole-genome sequencing in MS and highlighted the importance of understanding epigenetic regulation of expression in the genetic architecture of MS. As the costs of sequencing continue to fall, large-scale whole genome sequencing studies in MS may become the norm. Future whole genome studies that examine a greater number of individuals from the same family with a multi-case family history of MS may provide greater power to detect genetic differences that are associated with MS.

Extracting translational applications from genetic data

Using GWAS data to predict individual risk for developing MS through genetic testing is a tempting scenario. However, the modest familial recurrence risk of the disease, the low prior risk of disease in the population, the fact that most individuals in the population carry common MS risk alleles and never develop the disease, and the determining role of non-genomic factors make the ability to generate a diagnostic test that can differentiate individuals at a high risk for developing MS from those at low risk, not feasible at the present time.

A weighted log-additive integrative approach was recently used to collectively account for 17 established genetic variants and their transmission in 1213 independent MS families encompassing both sporadic and multi-case pedigrees.[64] Interestingly, the analysis demonstrated a higher aggregation of susceptibility variants in multi-case, compared to sporadic MS families (Fig. 4.6). Furthermore, a greater burden of susceptibility variants in siblings of MS patients was associated with two-fold increased risk of MS (Fig. 4.7). However, the cumulative score of common genetic variants only captures part of the variance, suggesting that attempts to extend the paradigm of monogenic genetic counseling with instruments integrating GWAS identified SNPs is, at the least, immature. This may radically change if highly penetrant (rare) variants and/or high-impact environmental triggers are discovered. Molecular diagnostics may then become a reality to identify those at a high risk of developing MS as well as to predict individual clinical courses.

Biomarkers of disease progression

High throughput methods of analysis have enabled the characterization of gene expression signatures characteristic of the disease[65] and multiple efforts are underway to identify biomarkers of therapeutic response (see also Chapter 23).[66] We recently reported the expression of genes involved in the CD4+ T-cell cycle to be correlated with progression from an early stage (CIS) to clinically definite disease. Among these genes, the expression of TOB1 (transducer of ERBB2–1) was particularly illuminating as individuals with low expression of this gene at diagnosis of CIS were more likely to progress to full blown MS.[67] A Kaplan–Meyer survival curve showed that 100% of patients with low TOB1 expression at baseline had converted to CDMS 9 months later, while only 20% of patients with normal TOB1 expression had converted in the same period of time. In vitro T-cell stimulation and immunization of C57Bl/6 mice with MOG35–55 also resulted in downregulation of TOB1, suggesting this gene is involved in a central process that controls T-cell cycle and when its expression decreases, cells proliferate more thus advancing the pathogenic process.

In conclusion, extensive epidemiological and laboratory results confirm that genetic variation is an important determinant of susceptibility to MS and suggests that such variation also influences when symptoms develop, how the disease progresses, and perhaps how well individuals respond to treatment. Although the association of *HLA* and MS susceptibility has been known for almost four decades, the identification of additional disease variants has been made feasible only recently with the introduction of large capacity fixed SNPs arrays, capable to interrogate individual genomes with remarkable fidelity and coverage, and the assembly of large DNA collections thorough multicenter collaborations. Ultimately, the goal of MS genetic studies is to provide a better understanding of MS in order to improve patient care in the clinic. For the first time

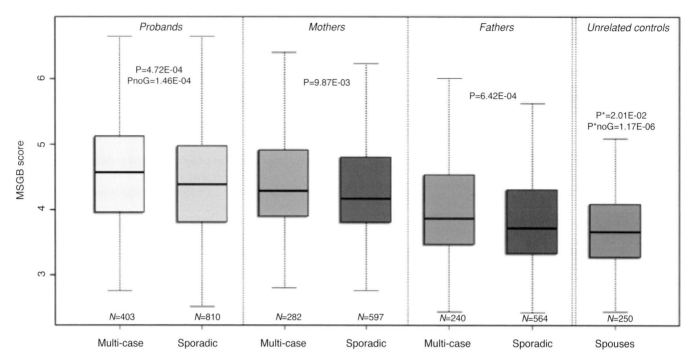

Fig. 4.6. MSGB differentiates multi-case from sporadic MS families. A weighted log-additive integrative approach termed MS Genetic Burden (MSGB) was used to account for the well-established genetic variants from previous association studies and meta-analyses. The MSGB scoring algorithm includes one SNP per MS-associated genomic locus: CLEC16A, EVI5, IL2RA, CD58, TYK2, IRF8, CD226, CD6, GPC5, IL7R, HLA-DRB1, TNFRSF1A, IL12A, MPHOSPH9, RGS1, KIF21B, TMEM39A. The corresponding genetic burden and its transmission was analyzed in 1213 independent MS families encompassing both sporadic and multi-case families. The MSGB distribution is presented using box-plots and shows a higher aggregation of susceptibility variants in multi-case, compared to sporadic MS families. In addition, the MSGB of both mothers and fathers are higher in multi-case families than in sporadic MS families. The MSGB values of all patients and parents are significantly greater than genetically unrelated controls. Modified from Figure 1, Gourraud P-A *et al. Annals Neurology* 69:65–74, 2010.[64]

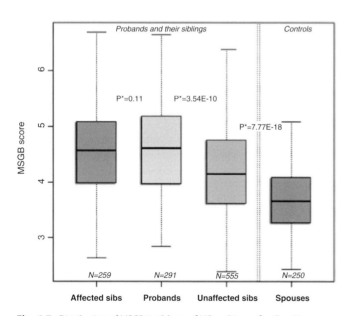

Fig. 4.7. Distribution of MSGB in siblings of MS multi-case families. No difference in MSGB can be detected between the probands and the affected siblings of the same pedigree. Unaffected siblings, on the other hand, have lower MSGB than the probands but still carry greater MSGB than controls. A greater MSGB in siblings of MS patients was associated with an increased risk of MS (OR = 2.1, P = 0.001). Modified from Figure 3, Gourraud P-A *et al. Annals Neurology* 69:65–74, 2010.[64]

in history the MS genetics community is within reach of identifying the full array of genes, pathways, and networks operating in MS. In addition to gene identification, these studies will drive a forceful paradigm shift in the study of MS by allowing a more refined representation of the genetic contributions to disease pathogenesis. Equally important, understanding the genetic and molecular events that underlie MS pathogenesis will be of paramount importance in the development of more effective strategies for disease management, prevention, and repair.

In a recently completed multicenter collaborative GWAS involving 9772 cases, nearly all of the previously suggested associations were Replicated, and at least 29 novel susceptibility loci were identified.[68]

Key terms

Copy number variations (CNVs) represent polymorphic alterations (duplications or deletions) of genomic DNA sequence consisting of between ten thousand and five million bases.

Endophenotypes are heritable and measurable components of a disease along the pathway between the genotype and the symptoms.

Epigenetics is the study of heritable changes in the expression of a gene or the phenotype caused by mechanisms other than changes in the corresponding DNA sequence.

Epistasis was originally defied as the masking of the expression of a gene at one position by one or more genes at other positions. It is the statistical description of the interaction phenomenon where the effects of one gene are modified by one or several other genes.

Genome wide association studies (GWAS) examine single nucleotide variation across genomes to identify DNA variants unevenly distributed between a group of unrelated individual carriers of a quantifiable trait and an unrelated group of unrelated controls. Commercially available single nucleotide polymorphism chips or arrays typically used in GWAS contain probes for polymorphisms selected on the basis of frequency and linkage disequilibrium parameters to efficiently capture large portions of common variation across the genome. Thus, the selected polymorphisms acts as surrogate markers of the broad genomic loci putatively associated with the trait of interest.

Haplotype refers to the combination of alleles at different genes on the same chromosome that are transmitted together as a block.

Heritability is the proportion of the total phenotypic variation for a given characteristic in a population that can be attributed to genetic variance among individuals.

Indel (insertion–deletion polymorphism) represents a specific mutation class resulting in an insertion or deletion and a net gain or loss in nucleotides (typically one or two base pairs).

Linkage disequilibrium (LD) describes and quantifies the condition in which the frequency of a particular haplotype in the population is significantly different from that expected if the loci were assorting independently.

Single nucleotide polymorphisms (SNPs) are single nucleotide (A, T, C, G) DNA variation occurring among individuals. By consensus, for a variation to be considered a SNP, it must occur in at least 1% of the population.

References

1. Rosati G. The prevalence of multiple sclerosis in the world: an update. *Neurol Sci* 2001; 22:117–39.

2. Willer CJ, Dyment DA, Risch NJ, Sadovnick AD, Ebers GC. Twin concordance and sibling recurrence rates in multiple sclerosis. *Proc Natl Acad Sci USA* 2003; 100:12877–82.

3. Hansen T, Skytthe A, Stenager E, Petersen HC, Bronnum-Hansen H, Kyvik KO. Concordance for multiple sclerosis in Danish twins: an update of a nationwide study. *Mult Scler* 2005; 11:504–10.

4. Hawkes CH, Macgregor AJ. Twin studies and the heritability of MS: a conclusion. *Mult Scler* 2009; 15: 661–7.

5. Mackay RP. Familial occurrence of multiple sclerosis and its implications. *Arch Neurol Psychiatry* 1950; 64: 155–7.

6. Schapira K, Poskanzer DC, Miller H. Familial and conjugal multiple sclerosis. *Brain* 1963; 86:315–32.

7. Doolittle TH, Myers RH, Lehrich JR, *et al.* Multiple sclerosis sibling pairs: clustered onset and familial predisposition. *Neurology* 1990; 40:1546–52.

8. Robertson NP, Fraser M, Deans J, Clayton D, Walker N, Compston DA. Age-adjusted recurrence risks for relatives of patients with multiple sclerosis. *Brain* 1996; 119:449–55.

9. Hemminki K, Li X, Sundquist J, Hillert J, Sundquist K. Risk for multiple sclerosis in relatives and spouses of patients diagnosed with autoimmune and related conditions. *Neurogenetics* 2009; 10:5–11.

10. Sawcer S, Ban M, Wason J, Dudbridge F. What role for genetics in the prediction of multiple sclerosis? *Ann Neurol* 2010; 67:3–10.

11. Carton H, Vlietinck R, Debruyne J, *et al.* Risks of multiple sclerosis in relatives of patients in Flanders, Belgium. *J Neurol Neurosurg Psychiatry* 1997; 62:329–33.

12. Sadovnick AD, Ebers GC, Dyment DA, Risch NJ, Group. Evidence for genetic basis of multiple sclerosis. *Lancet* 1996; 347:1728–30.

13. Ebers GC, Yee IM, Sadovnick AD, Duquette P. Conjugal multiple sclerosis: population-based prevalence and recurrence risks in offspring. *Ann Neurol* 2000; 48:927–31.

14. Ebers GC, Sadovnick AD, Risch NJ. A genetic basis for familial aggregation in multiple sclerosis. *Nature* 1995; 377:150–1.

15. Johnson BA, Oksenberg JR. The role of genetics in multiple sclerosis. In D Valle *et al.* (eds): *Scriver's OMMBID*, New York: McGraw-Hill, http://wwwommbidcom, 2010.

16. Orton SM, Herrera BM, Yee IM, *et al.* Sex ratio of multiple sclerosis in Canada: a longitudinal study. *Lancet Neurol* 2006; 5:932–6.

17. Ascherio A, Munger KL. Environmental risk factors for multiple sclerosis. Part I: the role of infection. *Ann Neurol* 2007; 61:288–99.

18. Ascherio A, Munger KL. Environmental risk factors for multiple sclerosis. Part II: Noninfectious factors. *Ann Neurol* 2007; 61:504–13.

19. Ascherio A, Munger KL, Lennette ET, *et al.* Epstein–Barr virus antibodies and risk of multiple sclerosis: a prospective study. *J Am Med Assoc* 2001; 286:3083–8.

20. Cepok S, Zhou D, Srivastava R, *et al.* Identification of Epstein–Barr virus proteins as putative targets of the immune response in multiple sclerosis. *J Clin Invest* 2005; 115(5):1352–60.

21. Serafini B, Rosicarelli B, Franciotta D, *et al.* Dysregulated Epstein–Barr virus infection in the multiple sclerosis brain. *J Exp Med* 2007; 204:2899–912.

22. Salvetti M, Giovannoni G, Aloisi F. Epstein–Barr virus and multiple sclerosis. *Curr Opin Neurol* 2009; 22:201–6.

23. Raghuwanshi A, Joshi SS, Christakos S. Vitamin D and multiple sclerosis. *J Cell Biochem* 2008; 105:338–43.

24. Islam T, Gauderman WJ, Cozen W, Hamilton AS, Burnett ME, Mack TM. Differential twin concordance for

multiple sclerosis by latitude of birthplace. *Ann Neurol* 2006; 60: 56–64.

25. Brassat D, Motsinger AA, Caillier SJ, *et al.* Multifactor dimensionality reduction reveals gene–gene interactions associated with multiple sclerosis susceptibility in African Americans. *Genes Immun* 2006; 7:310–15.

26. Gregersen JW, Kranc KR, Ke X, *et al.* Functional epistasis on a common MHC haplotype associated with multiple sclerosis. *Nature* 2006; 443:574–7.

27. Casaccia-Bonnefil P, Pandozy G, Mastronardi F. Evaluating epigenetic landmarks in the brain of multiple sclerosis patients: a contribution to the current debate on disease pathogenesis. *Prog Neurobiol* 2008; 86:368–78.

28. Otaegui D, Baranzini SE, Armananzas R, *et al.* Differential micro RNA expression in PBMC from multiple sclerosis patients. *PLoS ONE* 2009; 4:e6309.

29. Barcellos LF, Oksenberg JR, Begovich AB, *et al.* HLA-DR2 dose effect on susceptibility to multiple sclerosis and influence on disease course. *Am J Hum Genet* 2003; 72:710–6.

30. Barcellos LF, Sawcer S, Ramsay PP, *et al.* Heterogeneity at the HLA-DRB1 locus and risk for multiple sclerosis. *Hum Mol Genet* 2006; 15:2813–24.

31. Oksenberg JR, Barcellos LF, Cree BA, *et al.* Mapping multiple sclerosis susceptibility to the HLA-DR locus in African Americans. *Am J Hum Genet* 2004; 74:160–7.

32. Dyment DA, Herrera BM, Cader MZ, *et al.* Complex interactions among MHC haplotypes in multiple sclerosis: susceptibility and resistance. *Hum Mol Genet* 2005; 14:2019–26.

33. Lincoln MR, Ramagopalan SV, Chao MJ, *et al.* Epistasis among HLA-DRB1, HLA-DQA1, and HLA-DQB1 loci determines multiple sclerosis susceptibility. *Proc Natl Acad Sci USA* 2009; 106:7542–7.

34. Yeo TW, De Jager PL, Gregory SG, *et al.* A second major histocompatibility complex susceptibility locus for multiple sclerosis. *Ann Neurol* 2007; 61:228–36.

35. Rioux JD, Goyette P, Vyse TJ, *et al.* Mapping of multiple susceptibility variants within the MHC region for 7 immune-mediated diseases. *Proc Natl Acad Sci USA* 2009; 106:18680–5.

36. Cree BA, Rioux JD, McCauley JL, *et al.* A major histocompatibility Class I locus contributes to multiple sclerosis susceptibility independently from HLA-DRB1*15:01. *PLoS ONE* 2010; 5:e11296.

37. Prat E, Tomaru U, Sabater L, *et al.* HLA-DRB5*0101 and -DRB1*1501 expression in the multiple sclerosis-associated HLA-DR15 haplotype. *J Neuroimmunol* 2005; 167:108–19.

38. Caillier SJ, Briggs F, Cree BA, *et al.* Uncoupling the roles of HLA-DRB1 and HLA-DRB5 genes in multiple sclerosis. *J Immunol* 2008; 181: 5473–80.

39. The International Multiple Sclerosis Genetics Consortium. Risk alleles for multiple sclerosis identified by a genomewide study. *N Engl J Med* 2007; 357:851–62.

40. Gregory SG, Schmidt S, Seth P, *et al.* Interleukin 7 receptor alpha chain (IL7R) shows allelic and functional association with multiple sclerosis. *Nat Genet* 2007; 39:1083–91.

41. The International Multiple Sclerosis Genetics Consortium. Refining genetic associations in multiple sclerosis. *Lancet Neurol* 2008; 7:567–9.

42. The International Multiple Sclerosis Genetics Consortium. Comprehensive follow-up of the first genome-wide association study of multiple sclerosis identifies KIF21B and TMEM39A as susceptibility loci. *Hum Mol Genet* 2010; 19:953–62.

43. De Jager PL, Jia X, Wang J, *et al.* Meta-analysis of genome scans and replication identify CD6, IRF8 and TNFRSF1A as new multiple sclerosis susceptibility loci. *Nat Genet* 2009; 41(7):776–82.

44. Maier LM, Anderson DE, Severson CA, *et al.* Soluble IL-2RA levels in multiple sclerosis subjects and the effect of soluble IL-2RA on immune responses. *J Immunol* 2009; 182:1541–7.

45. Burton PR, Clayton DG, Cardon LR, *et al.* Association scan of 14,500 nonsynonymous SNPs in four diseases identifies autoimmunity variants. *Nat Genet* 2007; 39:1329–37.

46. Baranzini SE, Wang J, Gibson RA, *et al.* Genome-wide association analysis of susceptibility and clinical phenotype in multiple sclerosis. *Hum Mol Genet* 2009; 18:767–78.

47. Comabella M, Craig DW, Morcillo-Suarez C, *et al.* Genome-wide scan of 500,000 single-nucleotide polymorphisms among responders and nonresponders to interferon beta therapy in multiple sclerosis. *Arch Neurol* 2009; 66:972–8.

48. Australia and New Zealand Genetics Consortium. Genome-wide association study identifies new multiple sclerosis susceptibility loci on chromosomes 12 and 20. *Nat Genet* 2009; 41:824–8.

49. Nischwitz S, Cepok S, Kroner A, *et al.* Evidence for VAV2 and ZNF433 as susceptibility genes for multiple sclerosis. *J Neuroimmunol* 2010; 227:162–6.

50. Jakkula E, Leppa V, Sulonen AM, *et al.* Genome-wide association study in a high-risk isolate for multiple sclerosis reveals associated variants in STAT3 gene. *Am J Hum Genet* 2010; 86:285–91.

51. Sanna S, Pitzalis M, Zoledziewska M, *et al.* Variants within the immunoregulatory CBLB gene are associated with multiple sclerosis. *Nat Genet* 2010; 42:495–7.

52. Baranzini SE. The genetics of autoimmune diseases: a networked perspective. *Curr Opin Immunol* 2009; 21:596–605.

53. The International Multiple Sclerosis Genetics Consortium. The expanding genetic overlap between multiple sclerosis and type I diabetes. *Genes Immun* 2009; 10:11–14.

54. Bush WS, Sawcer SJ, de Jager PL, *et al.* Evidence for polygenic susceptibility to multiple sclerosis – the shape of things to come. *Am J Hum Genet* 2010; 86:621–5.

55. Oksenberg JR, Baranzini SE, Sawcer S, Hauser SL. The genetics of multiple sclerosis: SNPs to pathways to pathogenesis. *Nat Rev Genet* 2008; 9:516–26.

56. Brassat D, Azais-Vuillemin C, Yaouanq J, *et al.* Familial factors influence disability in MS multiplex families. *Neurology* 1999; 52:1632–6.

57. Barcellos LF, Oksenberg JR, Green AJ, *et al.* Genetic basis for clinical expression in multiple sclerosis. *Brain* 2002; 125:150–8.

58. Hensiek AE, Seaman SR, Barcellos LF, *et al.* Familial effects on the clinical

course of multiple sclerosis. *Neurology* 2007; 68:376–83.

59. DeLuca GC, Ramagopalan SV, Herrera BM, *et al.* An extremes of outcome strategy provides evidence that multiple sclerosis severity is determined by alleles at the HLA-DRB1 locus. *Proc Natl Acad Sci USA* 2007; 104:20896–901.

60. Byun E, Caillier SJ, Montalban X, *et al.* Genome-wide pharmacogenomic analysis of the response to interferon beta therapy in multiple sclerosis. *Arch Neurol* 2008; 65:337–44.

61. Brynedal B, Wojcik J, Esposito F, *et al.* MGAT5 alters the severity of multiple sclerosis. *J Neuroimmunol* 2010; 220:120–4.

62. Baranzini SE, Srinivasan R, Khankhanian P, *et al.* Genetic variation influences glutamate concentrations in brains of patients with multiple sclerosis. *Brain* 2010; 133:2603–11.

63. Baranzini SE, Mudge J, van Velkinburgh JC, *et al.* Genome, epigenome and RNA sequences of monozygotic twins discordant for multiple sclerosis. *Nature* 2010; 464:1351–6.

64. Gourraud P-A, McElroy J, Caillier S, *et al.* Aggregation of multiple sclerosis genetic variants in multiple and single affected families. *Ann Neurol* 2010; 69:65–74.

65. Achiron A, Gurevich M. Peripheral blood gene expression signature mirrors central nervous system disease:

the model of multiple sclerosis. *Autoimmun Rev* 2006; 5:517–22.

66. Goertsches RH, Hecker M, Zettl UK. Monitoring of multiple sclerosis immunotherapy: from single candidates to biomarker networks. *J Neurol* 2008; 255 (Suppl 6):48–57.

67. Corvol JC, Pelletier D, Henry RG, *et al.* Abrogation of T cell quiescence characterizes patients at high risk for multiple sclerosis after the initial neurological event. *Proc Natl Acad Sci USA* 2008; 105:11839–44.

68. International Multiple Sclerosis Genetics Consortium and the Welcome Trust Case-Control Consortium. Genetic risk and a primary role for cell-mediated immune mechanisms in multiple sclerosis. *Nature* in press.

Chapter

5

The epidemiology of multiple sclerosis

Ruth Ann Marrie and Helen Tremlett

Introduction

Multiple sclerosis (MS) is well recognized for geographic and temporal variation in disease risk.[1] Despite many studies exploring this variation in disease risk and putative etiologic factors, the etiology of MS remains unknown; it is thought that multiple environmental factors act together in a genetically susceptible individual to cause disease. Heterogeneity in disease outcomes is also well recognized in MS, but poorly understood; as with the etiology of the disease it is likely that multiple genetic and environmental factors influence outcome. This heterogeneity of etiology and outcome poses challenges for the design and interpretation of clinical trials.

Most MS patients present with a relapsing–remitting (RR) course, characterized by a fluctuating course of relapses and remissions.[2] Clinical manifestations are stable between relapses, but most patients will ultimately develop gradual disability progression with or without superimposed relapses, termed secondary progressive MS (SPMS).[2,3] Approximately 10%–15% of MS patients present with primary progressive MS (PPMS) in which patients exhibit gradual worsening from disease onset without relapses.[2] Initial manifestations of MS vary widely, but most individuals with RRMS present with optic neuritis or sensory symptoms.[4] Most patients ultimately will experience a constellation of symptoms including weakness, sensory symptoms, bowel and bladder dysfunction, fatigue, spasticity, pain, and cognitive impairment.

Changing face of multiple sclerosis

Recent studies suggest that the demographic characteristics of MS are changing. Specifically, several studies suggest that the female to male sex ratio is rising, and that this change is too great to be accounted for entirely by changes in ascertainment, although it is difficult to completely assess this issue.[5] While evidence exists of an increased risk of MS in certain racial (Caucasian) and ethnic (Scandinavian and Scottish) groups, as well as resistance among other racial and ethnic groups, including black Africans, Asians, Hutterites, Aborigines, Maori, and Native Americans,[1] findings among the pediatric MS population suggest this is also changing. Two North American centers

reported a higher than expected frequency of pediatric patients with non-Caucasian ancestry.[6]

The clinical characteristics of MS populations may also be changing. In Sardinia, a region with a relatively stable, ethnically homogeneous population, the mean age of onset is becoming progressively earlier in successive generations.[7] Unlike the age of diagnosis, age of onset should not be influenced substantially by changes in diagnostic criteria or techniques. In Norway, the mean age of onset is also becoming progressively earlier, and the ratio of persons diagnosed with relapsing remitting vs. primary progressive MS at onset is increasing – from 1.93 in the 1910–1929 birth cohort to 16.0 in the 1970–1979 birth cohort.[8] These observations raise the question of whether other aspects of the disease, such as relapse rates and disability progression, may also be changing along with sex ratios, but some studies do not concur with these observations.[9] Possible explanations for these observations include (i) the typically later ages of onset and diagnosis of PPMS compared with RRMS such that in more recent birth cohorts some persons may still be diagnosed with PPMS in the future, reducing the observed ratio between RRMS and PPMS; (ii) decreasing delays between symptom onset and diagnosis might lead to more accurate characterization of disease subtype; or (iii) increased identification of mild cases due to increased awareness and more sensitive diagnostic tests (e.g. MRI), favoring RRMS.

In an examination of more than 16 000 participants in the North American Research Committee on Multiple Sclerosis (NARCOMS) Registry, the diagnostic delay between initial symptom onset and diagnosis decreased steadily with later year of symptom onset ($r = -0.43$, $P < 0.0001$).[10] In a subset of 5548 participants who enrolled in NARCOMS at or near the time of MS diagnosis, the proportion with mild disability at diagnosis increased with later calendar year of symptom onset, even after accounting for the diagnostic delay.[10] It is uncertain whether these findings are due to changes in the ascertainment of disease, that is, the identification of persons with mild disease who would not have been diagnosed in an earlier era; or due to true changes in disease severity. This distinction is very important from the perspective of the etiology of MS and pathogenesis, but the observation also has important implications for clinical research, regardless of the underlying explanation. If

Multiple Sclerosis Therapeutics, Fourth Edition, ed. Jeffrey A. Cohen and Richard A. Rudick. Published by Cambridge University Press.
© Cambridge University Press 2011.

sample size calculations for clinical trials are based on the behavior of more severely affected historical cohorts of MS patients, they may be inadequate. For example, the PROMiSE trial tested glatiramer acetate in primary progressive MS but was halted early because of the rate of progression of disability was substantially lower than expected.[11]

Natural history of multiple sclerosis and prognostic factors

"Natural history" refers to the progression of disease independent of drugs or other exogenous factors known to alter the disease course. Advances in statistical analyses, access to powerful software, and acceptance of "survival analyses" have moved the field of MS natural history forward. Herein we will focus on studies applying these modern approaches in, where possible, a population-based setting with long-term follow-up data. The Expanded Disability Status Scale (EDSS) represents the most widely accepted measure of disease progression in MS, and is used in many natural history studies. Developed by Kurtzke, it is an ordinal scale, ranging from 0 (no neurological symptoms) to 10 (death due to MS).[12] It was first introduced as the 11-point "Disability Status Scale" and later as the 20-point Expanded Disability Status Scale, incorporating a Functional Systems Scale (FSS), and allowing half-point increases.[12] The heavy reliance of the EDSS on a patient's ability to walk especially after a score of 5.0; its inability to fully capture the range of symptoms associated with MS, such as fatigue or cognitive impairment; and inter-rater variability, especially with the lower scores, are well-recognized limitations of the EDSS, which should be considered as we review the findings of these studies.[13]

Natural history of relapsing onset MS

Relapsing onset MS (R-MS) encompasses RR and SPMS. The increasing use of immunomodulatory drugs (IMDs) in relapsing forms of MS means that our chance to describe the true natural history in these patients may be drawing to a close. Considerable variation in disease progression has been reported between studies for those with R-MS, ranging from a median of 18 to 35 years to reach EDSS 6 ("requires a cane to walk") from MS onset (see Table 5.1). Similar variation is also observed between studies when other disability outcomes based on the DSS/EDSS are examined. Substantial heterogeneity also exists within studies; for instance, while it might take 50% of a relapsing at onset cohort 30 years to reach EDSS 6.0, one-quarter of patients did so within an estimated 19 years and another one-quarter took over 40 years.[21] Generally, a trend exists for a slower disease progression to be reported in later studies; these findings appear largely independent of any IMD treatments. However, differences in study design (e.g. prospective vs. retrospective), definition of outcome (e.g. use of "sustained" or "confirmed" EDSS outcome or both) or geographical location (hence different medical facilities, environment or latitude) might all contribute to heterogeneity between cohorts

and outcomes. Intriguingly, the median time to SPMS appears reasonably consistent between studies, being around 20 years from MS onset, although fewer studies have contributed to this finding (Table 5.1).[29,33]

Relapses are the hallmark of relapsing onset MS. Most natural history studies show that relapses naturally decrease over time,[22,34,35] although not all do so.[36,37] Accurately measuring relapse rates in clinical practice is challenging. The more frequently patients are followed up, the more relapses are recalled and recorded; patients seen every 3 months report more relapses than those seen yearly. Nonetheless, a decrease in relapses by 17% for every five years' disease duration was recently reported.[22] This decrease varied according to the patient's age at onset of MS, with the largest decreases seen in those older at onset. Clinically, these findings imply that if a drug reduces relapse rates, its greatest potential for a population impact would be when relapses are at or near their peak, in patients under 40 years old and within the first five to ten years of disease onset.[22]

Natural history of primary progressive MS

As with R-MS, considerable variation exists between PPMS studies, with time to reach EDSS 6 taking from six to 21 years from onset of PPMS symptoms (Table 5.1). Intriguingly, the proportion of patients with PPMS also differs between studies, ranging from 6% to 20% of the overall cohort; the more recent studies seem to report proportionally fewer PPMS patients, although this temporal trend is not consistent (Table 5.1). Whether these differences reflect a real change in the presenting disease course, or a shift in the recognition of PPMS vs. R-MS possibly driven by the licensing of IMDs approved only for the use of those with R-MS, remains to be investigated. The study setting might also influence the types of patients included in these natural history series, raising the possibility of referral bias.

Changes in natural history and impact on clinical trial design

The differences in disease progression as observed in contemporary vs. older natural history studies have already impacted MS clinical trials, as mentioned above with the early termination of the PROMiSe trial. Also, the natural decrease in relapses over time and low relapse rates observed in natural history studies have been mirrored in recent clinical trials,[38] compromising statistical power. The design of future clinical trials will need to consider the disease activity levels reported in contemporary natural history studies, as these represent the types of patients available for recruitment into today's clinical trials.

Traditional prognostic factors

Clearly, MS is a heterogeneous disease and the desire to predict an individual's disease course is strong. Unfortunately, existing prognostic factors are primarily applicable at the population

Table 5.1. *Characteristics and select findings of the main longitudinal natural history studies published over the last decade*

Location/ group	Setting	Data collection period	Diagnostic criteria	Cohort size (n)	Cohort characteristics	Median time to EDSS[a] 6 (95% CI)	Median time to SPMS (95% CI)
London, Ontario, Canada[3,14,15]	An out-patient MS specialist clinic with a population-based sub-group, Middlesex County ~90% captured[3,14]	1972–1984[3,14] (Updates: 1984–1991; 1992–1997)	Definite, probable or possible MS (Poser)[3,14]	1099[3,14] (1972–1984 cohort)	R-MS: 722 (66%)[3,14] PPMS: 216 (20%)[15] Female: 722 (66%)[3,14] Mean onset age: 30.5 years[3,14] (1972–1984 cohort)	All: 15 years[3] R-MS: 18 years[15] PPMS: 8 years[15] (1972–1984 cohort)	-
Lyon, France[c,16,17,18]	Clinic-based, serving as the referral center for the city of Lyons and the Rhône–Alpes region since 1976, but "representative of the general population,"[16] Out-patient clinic	1976–1997[16,17]	Definite or probable MS (Poser)[16]	1844[16]	R-MS: 1562 (85%)[16] PPMS: 282 (15%)[16] Female: 1187 (64%)[16] Mean onset age: 31 years (SD10)[16]	All: 20.1 years (18.1–22.5)[17] R-MS: 23.1 years (20.1–26.1)[17] PPMS: 7.1 years (6.3–7.9)[17]	All: 19.1 years[18] Females: NA Males: NA
Olmsted county, USA[19,20]	Patients seen at either the Mayo Clinic, the Olmsted Medical Group or the Olmsted Community Hospital, resulting in a population-based cohort[19,20]	1991–2000	Definite MS (Poser)[19,20]	201[19,20]	R-MS: 190 (94%)[19,20] PPMS: 11 (6%)[19,20] Female: 140 (70%)[19,20] Median onset age: 31.2 years[19,20]	All: 28.6 years§[19] R-MS:- PPMS: 6.3 years[b,19]	-
British Columbia, Canada[21,22,23,24,25,26]	All four out-patient MS specialist clinics in the province of British Columbia; 80% of the MS population captured[21]	1980–2003[21] *Cohort 1:* Select criteria *Cohort 2:* all patients[23]	Definite MS (Poser)[21,23]	*Cohort 1:* 2837[21] *Cohort 2:* 5779	*Cohort 1:* R-MS: 2485 (88%)[21] PPMS: 352 (12%)[21,26] Female: 1997 (70%)[21] Mean onset age: 30.6 years (SD:10.0)[21] *Cohort 2:* R-MS: 5277 (90%)[23] PPMS: 552 (10%)[23]	*Cohort 1:* All: 27.9 years (26.5–29.3)[21] R-MS: 30.3 years (28.6–32.0)[21] PPMS: 13.3 years (11.0–15.5)[21,26] *Cohort 2: PPMS:* 14.0 years (11.3–16.7)[23]	*Cohort 1:* All: 18.9 years (18.2–19.7)[22,25] Females: 20.0 years (19.1–21.0)[22,25] Males: 15.6 years (14.2–17.0)[22,25] *Cohort 2:* 21.4 years (20.6–22.2)
Nova Scotia, Dalhousie MS Research Unit Canada[24,27,28]	Clinic-based, being Nova Scotia's only specialized referral service for MS, but "representative of the general population"[27,28]	1979–2004[27,28]	Definite MS, (Poser or MacDonald)[27,28]	1607[27]	R-MS: 1333 (83%)[27] PPMS: 274 (17%)[27] Female: 1194 (74%)[27] Mean onset age: NA	All: 32.4 years (27.3–35.6)[27,28] R-MS:35.6 years (29.4.1–41.2)[b,27,28] PPMS: 20.9 years (15.9–23.8)[b,27,28]	-
Lorraine, France[d,29,30]	Population-based; the Lorraine MS Regional Network; comprising neurologists (office-based practice and hospitals), MS centers, radiologists, biologists, nurses, physiotherapists, and the MS Association[30]	1996–2003[30]	Definite or probable MS (Poser)[19]	2871[29]	R-MS: 2518 (87%)[29] PPMS: 353 (13%)[29] Female: 794 (28%)[29] Mean onset age: 33 years (SD:10)[29]	All: 23.3 years (21.7–24.3)[29] R-MS: 24.5 years (22.7–26.5)[29] PPMS: 10.3 years (6.0–15.2)[29]	All: 20.0 years (18.6–21.0)[29] Females: 21.1 years (11.4–31.1)[29] Males: 15.7 years (8.2–31.3)[29]

Key:

NA = Not available; R-MS = relapsing onset MS; PPMS = primary progressive MS; SPMS = secondary progressive MS; DSS = Disability Status Scale Score; EDSS = Expanded Disability Status Scale Score (EDSS 6 = "requires a cane to walk")

[a] = EDMUS Impairment scale (DSS adapted) was used by Lyon, France[16,17]

[b] = Not explicitly published, figures derived from the authors (personal communications: Pittock S, 2009 and Brown M, 2009). For Nova Scotia, once treatment with an immunomodulatory drug was commenced, subsequent data for that patient were truncated.

[c] = Approximately half of the R-MS patients received immunosuppressants, predominantly azathioprine. However, as none to date have been shown to convincingly impact long-term irreversible disability, the authors argue that reported findings should be unaffected.

[d] = Use of immunomodulatory drugs was not reported in the Lorraine cohort, which was formed in the post-IMD era. Findings could be impacted by immunomodulatory drug use. However, no IMD to date has been shown to have an impact in PPMS and consensus has not been reached as to whether IMDs favorably alter long-term disease progression in those with relapsing-onset MS or not.

Where cohorts/studies have had updates, the focus of the table has been the defining cohort in which the main disease progression finding(s) were reported.

Other studies worthy of note:

Newcastle, Australia (n = 159)[31] reported a median time to DSS 6 of 24 years (95%CI:19–27) (95%CI gratefully obtained by personal communications: Macaskill P and McLeod J, 2009) and median age at DSS 6 of 52 years (95%CI unavailable). Findings were from a cross-sectional study which can provide some useful information, albeit with less robust estimates. Older longitudinal population-based natural history databases, such as Göteborg, Sweden (n = 308) have been reviewed elsewhere.[32]

level (Table 5.2). From onset of MS to fixed disability milestones, most studies concur that women as compared to men, those with a younger rather than older age at MS onset, and those with a relapsing rather than progressive onset have a better outcome, that is, slower disability progression (Table 5.2). Perceptions regarding age of onset, however, change somewhat when a patient's age when reaching a fixed disability milestone is examined, that is, time from birth is considered rather than time from onset of MS symptoms. Then, an older age at onset is considered favorable, as patients with a younger onset age will, on average, still reach disability milestones at a younger age compared to their older counterparts. This has also been observed in patients with childhood onset MS.[43] Regardless of whether one considers time from onset or birth, a relapsing onset course still appears advantageous (Table 5.2), but findings conflict for sex.

Onset symptoms have been examined as possible predictors of disease progression with inconsistent findings, hampered by the lack of consensus on the classification and grouping of onset symptoms (Table 5.2).

The impact of relapses on disease progression in MS is an area of particular interest, partly driven by the modest clinical effect of the current IMDs for MS, which reduce relapses.[4] Generally, it was assumed that this reduction in relapse rates would result in a beneficial long-term impact on disease progression, but a convincing long-term impact of the IMDs has not been shown yet,[4] and some natural history studies suggest a possible dissociation between relapses and long-term disability. Incomplete recovery from the first attack has been associated with more rapid progression to fixed disability milestones, as have early relapses within the first two to five years from MS onset,[16,29,39,41] although this is not an entirely consistent finding.[40] One study examined the impact of later relapses occurring more than five years from MS onset and found little evidence of an association with long-term disability, except in patients with an age of onset under 25 years.[41] Some of these analyses pose significant challenges, however; such as immortal time bias.[42] In studies examining the impact of the time between attacks on long-term disease progression, the time interval is immortal because the outcome of interest by definition cannot occur during this interval, leading to misclassification of the exposure period which is now typically artificially lengthened as it contains the "immortal time period" and hence results are biased. The bias is always in favor of a positive association, regardless of the true association. That is, using this approach, a longer time between attacks (time interval = a) will invariably result in a corresponding overall longer time to disease progression (time interval = a + p), irrespective of whether this is true or not.

Some studies have examined the impact of relapses indirectly by comparing disease progression between specific groups of patients.[16,17,44] Generally, most of these studies showed the early inflammatory phase of the disease is dissociated from the subsequent progressive phase.[16,17,44] For instance, once a certain disability level or the progressive phase is reached, progression thereafter to higher fixed disability

milestones appears similar for most sub-groups examined, although not all.[16,17,44] One study found that progression to DSS 6, 8, or 10 was similar across different phases or forms of progressive MS once the actual progressive phase had begun, including PP MS and patients with "single attack progression," where only a single attack occurs before the onset of progression.[44]

Other factors which may influence prognosis

Although many studies have focused on the prognostic significance of initial relapse location and severity, age of symptom onset and other characteristics of disease,[45] a growing body of literature examines the influence of other patient-related characteristics on prognosis such as race, comorbid diseases, and health behaviors.

Non-Whites have a lower risk of MS than Whites, and are more likely to present with variant forms of demyelinating disease, such as neuromyelitis optica.[46] Although results vary across studies, race also appears to be associated with disease outcome. Phillips et al. reviewed the medical records of 33 African Americans (AA) and 56 Whites examined at two sites in Atlanta, Georgia and compared them to patients enrolled in the Optic Neuritis Treatment Trial.[47] Not only did AAs present with severe visual loss at baseline (93%) more often than non-AA patients in the Optic Neuritis Treatment Trial (36%, $P = 0.0001$), they had less recovery 12 months after onset. Investigators from the New York State Multiple Sclerosis Consortium observed that AAs in their 18-center registry had more severe cognitive disability than non-AAs participating in the registry.[48] Several studies suggest that AAs experience more ambulatory disability than Whites after accounting for disease duration and treatment status.[49,50] Cree et al. evaluated 802 patients and found that AAs had higher odds of needing a unilateral assistive device to walk (HR 1.67; 95% CI: 1.29–2.15).[50] In an examination of 21 557 participants in the NARCOMS Registry, a self-report registry for persons with MS, AA participants had increased disability in multiple domains including ambulation (OR 1.37; 95% CI: 1.11–1.67), vision (OR 1.59; 95% CI: 1.19–2.08), and hand function (OR 1.27; 95% CI: 1.00–1.61) when compared to White participants.[49]

One study investigated possible racial differences in treatment responsiveness. Cree et al. conducted a post-hoc analysis of the EVIDENCE trial, a comparative trial of two formulations of interferon-beta-1a, using data from 36 AA and 616 White participants.[51] As compared to Whites, AAs were less likely to be relapse free than Whites at 24 weeks (56% vs. 70%) or at 48 weeks (47% vs. 57%). After adjusting for the pre-treatment relapse rate and treatment status, AAs had 45% reduced odds of being relapse free, but this did not reach statistical significance. After 24 weeks AAs had a higher median number of combined unique lesions (active T2- and T1-weighted gadolinium-enhancing lesions), and more new T2 lesions at 48 weeks. Again, the findings were not statistically significant after adjustment. Although the sample size was small, the authors concluded

Table 5.2. *Characteristics associated with time to disability milestones (DSS/ EDSS or the EDMUS Impairment scale (DSS adapted))*

Clinical characteristic	From onset of MS		From birth (age of the patient at disability milestones)	
	Positively associated (better outcome)	Not associated	Positively associated (better outcome)	Not associated
Sex	*Female* British Columbia, Canada[21] London, Canada[39] Lorraine, France[29] Lyon, France[16]	Göteborg, Sweden[40]	*Female* Lyon, France[16]	British Columbia, Canada[21]
Age at MS symptom onset	*Older age* British Columbia, Canada[21] London, Canada[39] Lorraine, France[29] Lyon, France[16] Göteborg, Sweden[40]		*Older age* British Columbia, Canada[21] Lyon, France[16]	
Disease course (typically RR vs. PPMS)	*RR disease course* British Columbia Canada[21] London, Canada[39] Lorraine, France[29] Lyon, France[16] Göteborg, Sweden[40]		*RR disease course* British Columbia Canada[21] Lyon, France[16]	
Onset symptoms Balance/ataxia	*Absence of symptom* London, Canada[39]	Lorraine, France[29]		
Brain stem		Göteborg, Sweden[29] Lyon, France[16]		Lyon, France[16]
Cerebellar, ataxia or brain stem		British Columbia, Canada[21]		British Columbia, Canada[21]
Diplopia and/or vertigo		London, Ontario, Canada[39]		
Long-tract involvement	*Absence of symptom* Lyon, France[16]	Lorraine, France[29]		Lyon, France[16]
Motor (insidious)	*Absence of symptom* London, Canada[39]			
Motor (acute)		London, Ontario, Canada[39]		
Motor (not specified)		British Columbia, Canada[21]		British Columbia, Canada[21]
Optic neuritis/optic nerve involvement	*Presence of symptom* London, Canada[39] Lyon, France[16]	British Columbia, Canada[21]		British Columbia, Canada[21] Lyon, France[16]
Spinal symptoms		Göteborg, Sweden[40]		
Sensory		British Columbia, Canada[21] London, Canada[39]		British Columbia, Canada[21]
Monoregional onset symptoms	Göteborg, Sweden[40] Lorraine, France[29]			
Relapses Complete recovery from first attack	Göteborg, Sweden[40] Lorraine, France[29] Lyon, France[16]			
Longer time between the first two attacks	*London, Ontario, Canada[39] *Lorraine, France[29] *Lyon, France[16]	Göteborg, Sweden[40]		
Relapse rate or total number of relapses in the first 2 to 5-years	*Lower rate/fewer relapses* British Columbia, Canada (short-term impact only)[41] London, Canada[39] Lorraine, France[29] Lyon, France[16]	British Columbia, Canada (minimal long-term impact)[41] Göteborg, Sweden[40]		
Relapse occurring later in the disease course (>5–10 or 10-years from onset)		British Columbia, Canada (minimal long-term impact)[41]		

Findings from multivariate analysis reported where possible.
Key for Table 5.2:
*These findings could be subject to immortal time bias as the time to end-point was measured from onset of MS rather than from the second attack.[42]
RRMS = relapsing–remitting MS; SPMS = secondary progressive MS; PPMS = primary progressive MS
DSS = Disability Status Scale Score; EDSS = Expanded Disability Status Scale Score EDMUS = European Database for Multiple Sclerosis, the Lyon, France group uses the "EDMUS Impairment scale", which is DSS adapted.

that AAs appeared to respond less to treatment. An alternative explanation is that AAs responded to treatment similarly to non-AA participants, but had more severe disease at baseline.

In studies of racial differences in disease severity or treatment response, race is really being used as a proxy for ancestry and the associated underlying biologic differences. While this approach has some limitations because race does not completely capture ancestry, and other important social and cultural factors may covary with race, these findings highlight the potential impact of different underlying biologies in influencing clinical phenotype, severity and response to treatment. As knowledge of these differences grows, planned subgroup analyses to determine whether treatment responses apply equally to all subgroups will be important. These differences also increase the problems inherent in comparing treatment findings from one population to another, depending on the underlying population substructure.

Comorbid diseases

A growing literature suggests that comorbid conditions influence central nervous system disease. Vascular risk factors and stroke may accelerate the progression of Alzheimer's disease.[52] Comorbid diabetes, congestive heart failure, and vision impairment are associated with increased mortality in Parkinson's disease.[53] Stroke recovery may be delayed by comorbidity.[54] Comorbidity also appears to influence several aspects of MS, including disability progression and quality of life.

Comorbid diseases are common in MS. In the NARCOMS population, the most common comorbidities reported were hypercholesterolemia (37%), hypertension (30%), arthritis (16%), irritable bowel syndrome (13%), and chronic lung disease (13%).[55] In the Canadian Community Health Survey, respondents with MS reported multiple comorbidities including back problems (35%), non-food allergies (29%), arthritis (26%), hypertension (17%), depression (16%), and migraine (14%).[56] Mental comorbidities are also common in MS. Depression has a lifetime prevalence of 50%, and anxiety may affect up to 30% of patients.[57,58] In some series, autoimmune thyroid disease affects up to 10% of the MS population.[59-61] Although persons with MS typically present for the first time between the ages of 20 and 40 years, up to one-third may have comorbidities at the time of diagnosis,[62] with the proportion of affected persons increasing with age at presentation.[55]

As compared with the general population and chronic disease populations such as inflammatory bowel disease and rheumatoid arthritis, persons with MS report lower health-related quality of life (HRQOL).[63] Several studies suggest that comorbidity influences HRQOL,[56,64] a common end-point in clinical trials. A study of 262 MS patients found poorer physical HRQOL in relapsing remitting MS patients with comorbid musculoskeletal and respiratory conditions,[64] but the study was cross-sectional. In the Canadian Community Health Survey, 335 persons with MS completed the Health Utilities Mark 3 as a measure of HRQOL.[56] The mean overall HRQOL score of

participants with no comorbidity (0.64) was 0.12 points higher than that of respondents with one or more comorbidities (0.52).

Given the reported increased frequency of comorbid autoimmune disease in MS as compared to the general population,[61,65] the earliest studies of the influence of comorbidity on disease progression examined autoimmune disease. Tourbah et al. conducted a five-year prospective study of 64 patients with definite or probable MS.[66] No difference in the type of clinical course, age at symptom onset or presenting symptoms was observed according to the presence or absence of antinuclear antibodies. Investigators in Nova Scotia, Canada reviewed the medical records of 1709 of 1730 persons followed at the provincial MS Clinic and found that patients with relapsing remitting MS and comorbid autoimmune disease had more rapid disability progression than patients without those comorbidities.[67]

As discussed previously, both respiratory and musculoskeletal comorbidities negatively influence HRQOL; other findings suggest they adversely affect disability also. In another multivariable analysis of the Nova Scotia MS population, patients with asthma experienced more rapid disability progression to an EDSS of 3 as compared to patients without asthma ($P = 0.027$).[68] Dallmeijer et al. followed 146 patients with newly diagnosed MS for 3 years, of whom 65 (44%) had one or more comorbidities at baseline.[69] Twenty (14%) had musculoskeletal comorbidities – those affected experienced a 5-point decline in the motor scale of the Functional Independence Measure while those without such comorbidities experienced only a two-point decline.

Participants in the NARCOMS Registry who reported having vascular comorbidities, including hypertension, hypercholesterolemia, diabetes, heart disease, and peripheral vascular disease, experienced more rapid progression of ambulatory disability than those without comorbidities. The median time from MS diagnosis to needing a unilateral assistive device to walk was 18.8 (95 % CI: 18.4, 19.3) years in participants without vascular comorbidities, but was 6.0 years earlier in participants with vascular comorbidities at diagnosis (12.8; 95%: 12.3, 13.4).[70] This difference corresponded to a hazard ratio of 2.03 (95% CI: 1.86, 2.23), which decreased slightly to 1.68 (95% CI: 1.51, 1.87) after adjusting for sex, year of symptom onset, age of symptom onset, income, health insurance status, race, and region of residence. While most of these studies have focused their attention on the impact of physical comorbidities, the impact of comorbid mental illness is relevant also. Again investigators in Nova Scotia found that the presence of psychiatric syndromes was associated with more rapid progression of disability.[71] The mechanism underlying these findings is unknown. Comorbidities could influence the pathophysiology of MS or adherence to treatment; or these findings could reflect the impact of multiple diseases additively influencing a common outcome, such as mobility.

All studies examining the impact of comorbidity on disability have focused on ambulation. While this is clearly important, it is also relevant to know whether comorbid diseases or health behaviors influence disability in domains such as cognition, upper extremity function, and vision. The magnitude of the impact and how this differs across domains is also important. Where treatment benefits may not be uniform across domains, the presence of comorbidities that may further modify disability and treatment response complicates the interpretation of treatment benefit. We do not know how comorbidities influence treatment decisions, or treatment responses in MS.

Health behaviors

The risk and outcomes of many chronic diseases are influenced by health behaviors, such as smoking, alcohol consumption, and level of physical activity. Because these behaviors also influence health outcomes independent of their effects on the risk of chronic disease,[72] and are potentially modifiable, they deserve attention. Smoking has received more attention than other health behaviors in MS, both as an etiologic factor and as a prognostic factor. The first study of smoking as a prognostic factor used the General Practice Research Database (United Kingdom) to examine the association between smoking and the time to developing secondary progressive MS.[73] As compared to never smokers, smokers with relapsing remitting MS had an increased risk of SPMS (HR 3.6; 95% CI 1.3–9.9).

Findings from subsequent studies have been inconsistent, possibly reflecting differences in the outcomes used, and methods of ascertainment. For three years, Di Pauli et al. followed 129 patients with a clinically isolated syndrome at high risk for developing MS, and found that smokers were more likely to develop definite MS (HR 1.8; 95% CI: 1.2–2.8).[74] Two studies found no association between smoking and disability progression, while four confirmed the findings of the British study.[75–80] Two of the studies examining the effects of smoking on MS found that smokers had a greater T2-lesion burden and greater brain atrophy when compared to non-smokers.[79,80] Strikingly, in 205 Portuguese women with definite MS smoking had a protective effect in women carrying the ApoE–e4 isoform, such that smokers had lower scores on the Expanded Disability Status Scale ($P = 0.033$) and Multiple Sclerosis Severity Score ($P = 0.023$) as compared with non-smokers.[81] The study was restricted to women from a clinic-based population and needs to be replicated, but highlights the potential difficulty of examining prognostic factors when multiple interacting factors may be relevant. Common to all of but one these studies was the failure to account for potential confounding effects due to alcohol intake, obesity or comorbid diseases associated with smoking.[75]

Immunomodulatory drug treatments for MS

Prior to the 1990s the mainstay of MS treatment was symptomatic support and short courses of corticosteroids for relapses. The first IMDs for MS were licensed in the mid-1990s. Since then, their uptake world-wide has been rapid, despite the modest effects shown in short-term clinical trials. Given the chronic lifelong nature of MS, there is a real need to determine the long-term impact of these drugs, but a long-term clinical trial with a suitable untreated control group is ethically questionable. Pharmacoepidemiological studies using "real world" data derived from clinical practice represent a cost-effective means of evaluating the long-term effectiveness of IMDs. Typically, these are retrospective studies which require sophisticated statistical modeling to account for the lack of randomization that would normally take place in a (randomized) clinical trial. Issues such as switching drugs, lack of adherence, irregular follow-up, loss to follow-up, presence of comorbid diseases, and health behaviors which might impact outcome add to the complexity. Nonetheless, these studies represent an important contribution to our understanding of IMDs for MS and the conduct of pharmacoepidemiological and post-marketing effectiveness studies in MS. These issues will be discussed further in Chapter 20.

Novel treatment targets and epidemiological studies

Rational drug targeting in MS is challenging, particularly in a disease where the cause is unknown and the mechanisms surrounding progression are poorly understood. Along with evidence from the basic sciences, epidemiological studies can provide insights into potentially novel treatments, as well as the rationale and hypotheses for testing these treatments in clinical trials. For example, vitamin D and estrogen are being evaluated in clinical trials based partly on epidemiological observations. With vitamin D, for example, the observation of an increased frequency of MS with increasing distance from the equator led to ecological and case control studies showing an inverse association between higher levels of exposure to sunlight and the risk of developing MS. Given the relationship between sunlight exposure and vitamin D production, much work has focused on the relationship between vitamin D and MS. A growing body of evidence suggests that vitamin D may influence gene expression, immunological function, and disease risk in MS.[82] Further, the results of the first clinical trials of vitamin D supplementation in MS support further research in this area.[83]

Other novel treatment approaches which could be considered based on emerging epidemiological observations include modification of comorbid diseases or health behaviors (smoking, exercise, (safe) sunlight exposure, diet, body weight), or preventing infectious exposures. Epstein–Barr virus (EBV) is an infectious agent of particular interest. Antibodies to EBV are more common in persons with MS than the general population.[84] Case control and cohort studies suggest an increased risk of MS in persons with a history of infectious mononucleosis.[85] Further, some studies also suggest that the risk of MS is nine-fold higher among persons with elevated anti-EBNA-1 titers who are HLA-DR15 positive when compared with persons who do not have elevated titers and are HLA-DR15 negative.[86]

Other untapped applications of natural history studies include the possible identification of commonly used drugs (e.g. antidepressants or statins) which might influence the MS disease course, by linkage of MS natural history data with drug exposure on a large scale. Findings from these studies would be hypothesis generating, but could pave the way for novel uses of existing, inexpensive medications.

Conclusions

Heterogeneity remains the hallmark of MS. While reasons for this diversity remain incompletely understood, efforts at understanding sources of variation should include examination of a broader range of factors beyond the oft-studied clinical parameters such as race/ethnicity, social factors, environmental factors, comorbid diseases and health behaviors. More detailed characterization of MS cohorts and MS individuals according to these factors could help us understand differences in disease behavior that have relevance to prognostication, clinical trial design, and individualized therapy, thereby maximizing treatment adherence and effectiveness while minimizing adverse events related to treatment, and optimizing outcomes.

References

1. Pugliatti M, Sotgiu S, Rosati G. The worldwide prevalence of multiple sclerosis. *Clin Neurol Neurosurg* 2002;104:182–91.

2. Lublin FD, Reingold SC. Defining the clinical course of multiple sclerosis: Results of an international survey. *Neurology* 1996;46:907–11.

3. Weinshenker BG, Bass B, Rice PA, *et al.* The natural history of multiple sclerosis: A geographically based study. 1. Clinical course and disability. *Brain* 1989;112:133–46.

4. Compston A, McDonald I, Noseworthy J, *et al. McAlpine's Multiple Sclerosis.* 4th edn. London: Churchill Livingstone Elsevier, 2006.

5. Koch-Henriksen N, Sorensen PS. The changing demographic pattern of multiple sclerosis epidemiology. *Lancet Neurology* 2010;9:520–32.

6. Ness JM, Chabas D, Sadovnick AD, *et al.* Clinical features of children and adolescents with multiple sclerosis. *Neurology* 2007;68:S37–45.

7. Cocco E, Sardu C, Lai M, Spinicci G, Contu P, Marrosu MG. Anticipation of age at onset in multiple sclerosis: a Sardinian cohort study. *Neurology* 2004;62:1794–8.

8. Celius EG, Smestad C. Change in sex ratio, disease course and age at diagnosis in Oslo MS patients through seven decades. *Acta Neurol Scand* 2009;120:27–9.

9. Barnett MH, Williams DB, Day S, Macaskill P, McLeod JG. Progressive increase in incidence and prevalence of multiple sclerosis in Newcastle, Australia: a 35-year study. *J Neurol Sci* 2003;213:1–6.

10. Marrie RA, Cutter G, Tyry T, Hadjimichael O, Campagnolo D, Vollmer T. Changes in the ascertainment of multiple sclerosis. *Neurology* 2005;65:1066–70.

11. Wolinsky JS, Narayana PA, O'Connor P, *et al.* Glatiramer acetate in primary progressive multiple sclerosis: Results of a multinational, multicenter, double-blind, placebo-controlled trial. *Ann Neurol* 2007;61:14–24.

12. Kurtzke JF. Rating neurologic impairment in multiple sclerosis: an expanded disability status scale (EDSS). *Neurology* 1983;33:1444–52.

13. Noseworthy JH, Vandervoort MK, Wong CJ, Ebers GC. Interrater variability with the Expanded Disability Status Scale (EDSS) and Functional Systems (FS) in a multiple sclerosis clinical trial. *Neurology* 1990;40:971–5.

14. Weinshenker BG, Bass B, Rice GP, *et al.* The natural history of multiple sclerosis: A geographically based study. 2. Predictive value of the early clinical course. *Brain* 1989;112:1419–28.

15. Cottrell DA, Kremenchutzky M, Rice GPA, *et al.* The natural history of multiple sclerosis: a geographically based study. 5. The clinical features and natural history of primary progressive multiple sclerosis. *Brain* 1999;122:625–39.

16. Confavreux C, Vukusic S, Adeleine P. Early clinical predictors and progression of irreversible disability in multiple sclerosis: an amnesic process. *Brain* 2003;126:770–82.

17. Confavreux C, Vukusic S, Moreau T, Adeleine P. Relapses and progression of disability in multiple sclerosis. *N Engl J Med* 2000;343:1430–8.

18. Confavreux C, Vukusic S. Age at disability milestones in multiple sclerosis. *Brain* 2006;129:595–605.

19. Pittock SJ, Mayr WT, McClelland RL, *et al.* Disability profile of MS did not change over 10 years in a population-based prevalence cohort. *Neurology* 2004;62:601–6.

20. Pittock SJ, Mayr WT, McClelland RL, *et al.* Change in MS-related disability in a population-based cohort: a 10-year follow-up study. *Neurology* 2004;62:51–9.

21. Tremlett H, Paty D, Devonshire V. Disability progression in multiple sclerosis is slower than previously reported. *Neurology* 2006;66:172–7.

22. Tremlett H, Zhao Y, Joseph J, Devonshire V. Relapses in multiple sclerosis are age- and time-dependent. *J Neurol, Neurosurg Psychiatry* 2008;79:1368–74.

23. Koch M, Kingwell E, Rieckmann P, Tremlett H. The natural history of primary progressive multiple sclerosis. *Neurology* 2009;73:1996–2002.

24. Koch M, Kingwell E, Rieckmann P, Tremlett H. The natural history of secondary progressive MS. *J Neurol, Neurosurg Psychiatry* 2010;81:1039–43.

25. Tremlett H, Yinshan Zhao, Devonshire V. Natural history of secondary-progressive multiple sclerosis. *Mult Scler* 2008;14:314–24.

26. Tremlett H, Paty D, Devonshire V. The natural history of primary progressive MS in British Columbia, Canada. *Neurology* 2005;65:1919–23.

27. Brown M, Andreou P, Kirby S, Murray J. EDSS natural history atlas: MS disability progression in Nova Scotia 1979–2004. *Mult Scler* 2008;14:P540.

28. Brown MG, Kirby S, Skedgel C, *et al.* How effective are disease-modifying drugs in delaying progression in relapsing-onset MS? *Neurology* 2007;69:1498–507.

29. Debouverie M, Pittion-Vouyovitch S, Louis S, Guillemin F. Natural history of multiple sclerosis in a population-based cohort. *Eur J Neurol* 2008;15:916–21.

30. Debouverie M, Louis S, Pittion-Vouyovitch S, Roederer T,

Vespignani H. Multiple sclerosis with a progressive course from onset in Lorraine-Eastern France. *J Neurol* 2007;254:1370–5.

31. McLeod JG, Barnett MH, Macaskill P, Williams DB. Long-term prognosis of multiple sclerosis in Australia. *J Neurol Sci* 2007;256:35–8.

32. Confavreux C, Compston A. The natural history of Multiple Sclerosis. In: Compston A, McDonald I, Noseworthy J, *et al.*, eds. *McAlpine's Multiple Sclerosis.* 4th edn. London: Churchill Livingstone Elsevier, 2006.

33. Confavreux C, Vukusic S. Natural history of multiple sclerosis: a unifying concept. *Brain* 2006;129: 606–16.

34. Broman T, Andersen O, Bergmann L. Clinical studies on multiple sclerosis. I. Presentation of an incidence material from Gothenburg. *Acta Neurol Scandinavica* 1981;63:6–33.

35. Patzold U, Pocklington PR. Course of multiple sclerosis. First results of a prospective study carried out of 102 MS patients from 1976–1980. *Acta Neurol Scand* 1982;65:248–66.

36. Goodkin DE, Hertsgaard D, Rudick RA. Exacerbation rates and adherence to disease type in a prospectively followed-up population with multiple sclerosis. Implications for clinical trials. *Arch Neurol* 1989;46:1107–12.

37. Confavreux C, Aimard G, Devic M. Course and prognosis of multiple sclerosis assessed by the computerized data processing of 349 patients. *Brain* 1980;103:281–300.

38. Mikol DD, Barkhof F, Chang P, *et al.* Comparison of subcutaneous interferon beta-1a with glatiramer acetate in patients with relapsing multiple sclerosis (the REbif vs Glatiramer Acetate in Relapsing MS Disease [REGARD] study): a multicentre, randomised, parallel, open-label trial. *Lancet Neurol* 2008;7:903–14.

39. Weinshenker BG, Rice GP, Noseworthy JH, Carriere W, Baskerville J, Ebers GC. The natural history of multiple sclerosis: A geographically based study. 3. Multivariate analysis of predictive factors and models of outcome. *Brain* 1991;114:1045–56.

40. Runmarker B, Andersen O. Prognostic factors in a multiple sclerosis incidence cohort with twenty-five years of follow-up. *Brain* 1993;116:117–34.

41. Tremlett H, Yousefi M, Devonshire V, Rieckmann P, Zhao Y, and the UBC Neurologists. The impact of multiple sclerosis relapses on progression diminishes with time. *Neurology* 2009;17:1616–23.

42. Suissa S. Immortal Time Bias in Pharmacoepidemiology. *Am J Epidemiol* 2008;167:492–9.

43. Renoux C, Vukusic S, Mikaeloff Y, *et al.* Natural history of multiple sclerosis with childhood onset. *N Engl J Med* 2007;356:2603–13.

44. Kremenchutzky M, Rice GPA, Baskerville J, Wingerchuk DM, Ebers GC. The natural history of multiple sclerosis: a geographically based study 9: Observations on the progressive phase of the disease. *Brain* 2006;129: 584–94.

45. Langer-Gould A, Popat RA, Huang SM, *et al.* Clinical and demographic predictors of long-term disability in patients with relapsing–remitting multiple sclerosis: a systematic review. *Arch Neurol* 2006;63: 1686–91.

46. Argyriou AA, Makris N. Neuromyelitis optica: a distinct demyelinating disease of the central nervous system. *Acta Neurol Scand* 2008;118:209–17.

47. Phillips PH, Newman NJ, Lynn MJ. Optic neuritis in African Americans. *Arch Neurol* 1998;55:186–92.

48. Weinstock-Guttman B, Jacobs LD, Brownscheidle CM, *et al.* Multiple sclerosis characteristics in African American patients in the New York State Multiple Sclerosis Consortium. *Mult Scler* 2003;9:293–8.

49. Marrie RA, Cutter G, Tyry T, Vollmer T, Campagnolo D. Does multiple sclerosis-associated disability differ between races? *Neurology* 2006;66:1235–40.

50. Cree BA, Khan O, Bourdette D, *et al.* Clinical characteristics of African Americans vs. Caucasian Americans with multiple sclerosis. *Neurology* 2004;63:2039–45.

51. Cree BA, Al-Sabbagh A, Bennett R, Goodin D. Response to interferon beta-1a treatment in African American multiple sclerosis patients. *Arch Neurol* 2005;62:1681–3.

52. Mielke MM, Rosenberg PB, Tschanz J, *et al.* Vascular factors predict rate of progression in Alzheimer disease. *Neurology* 2007;69:1850–8.

53. Fernandez HH, Lapane KL. Predictors of mortality among nursing home residents with a diagnosis of Parkinson's disease. *Med Sci Monitor* 2002;8:CR241–6.

54. Studenski SA, Lai SM, Duncan PW, Rigler SK. The impact of self-reported cumulative comorbidity on stroke recovery. *Age Ageing* 2004;33:195–8.

55. Marrie RA, Horwitz R, Cutter G, Tyry T, Campagnolo D, Vollmer T. Comorbidity, socioeconomic status, and multiple sclerosis. *Mult Scler* 2008;14:1091–8.

56. Warren SA, Turpin KV, Pohar SL, Jones CA, Warren KG. Comorbidity and health-related quality of life in people with multiple sclerosis. *Int J MS Care* 2009;11:6–16.

57. Goldman Consensus Group. The Goldman Consensus statement on depression in multiple sclerosis. *Mult Scler* 2005; 11:328–37.

58. Korostil M, Feinstein A. Anxiety disorders and their clinical correlates in multiple sclerosis patients. *Mult Scler* 2007;13:67–72.

59. Niederwieser G, Buchinger W, Bonelli RM, *et al.* Prevalence of autoimmune thyroiditis and non-immune thyroid disease in multiple sclerosis. *J Neurol* 2003;250:672–5.

60. Barcellos LF, Kamdar BB, Ramsay PP, *et al.* Clustering of autoimmune diseases in families with a high-risk for multiple sclerosis: a descriptive study. *Lancet Neurol* 2006;5:924–31.

61. Sloka JS, Pryse-Phillips WEM, Stefanelli M, Joyce C. Co-occurrence of autoimmune thyroid disease in a multiple sclerosis cohort. *J Autoimmune Dis* 2005;2:9.

62. Marrie RA, Horwitz RI, Cutter G, Tyry T, Campagnolo D, Vollmer T. Comorbidity delays diagnosis and increases disability at diagnosis in MS. *Neurology* 2009;72:117–24.

63. Rudick RA, Miller DM, Clough JD, Gragg LA, Farmer RG. Quality of life in multiple sclerosis: Comparison with inflammatory bowel disease and rheumatoid arthritis. *Arch Neurol* 1992;49:1237–42.

64. Turpin KV, Carroll LJ, Cassidy JD, Hader WJ. Deterioration in the health-related quality of life of persons with multiple sclerosis: the possible warning signs. *Mult Scler* 2007;13:1038–45.

65. Bernstein CN, Wajda A, Blanchard JF. The clustering of other chronic inflammatory diseases in inflammatory bowel disease: a population-based study. *Gastroenterology* 2005;129: 827–36.

66. Tourbah A, Clapin A, Gout O, *et al.* Systemic autoimmune features and multiple sclerosis: a 5-year follow-up study. *Arch Neurol* 1998;55:517–21.

67. Kirby S, Brown MG, Andreou P, *et al.* Progression of multiple sclerosis in patients with other autoimmune diseases. *Can J Neurol Sci* 2009;36: S-29.

68. Kirby S, Brown MG, Murray TJ, *et al.* Progression of multiple sclerosis in patients with other autoimmune diseases. *Mult Scler* 2005;11:S28–9.

69. Dallmeijer AJ, Beckerman H, de Groot V, van de Port IGL, Lankhorst GJ, Dekker J. Long-term effect of comorbidity on the course of physical functioning in patients after stroke and with multiple sclerosis. *J Rehab Med* 2009;41:322–6.

70. Marrie RA, Rudick R, Horwitz R, *et al.* Vascular comorbidity is associated with more rapid disability progression in multiple sclerosis. *Neurology* 2010;74:1041–7.

71. Kirby S, Fisk JD, Brown MG, *et al.* Progression of multiple sclerosis in patients with psychiatric syndromes. *Mult Scler* 2005;11:S28–9.

72. Tammemagi CM, Neslund-Dudas C, Simoff M, Kvale P. Smoking and lung cancer survival. The role of comorbidity and treatment. *Chest* 2004;125:27–37.

73. Hernan MA, Jick SS, Logroscino G, Olek MJ, Ascherio A, Jick H. Cigarette smoking and the progression of multiple sclerosis. *Brain* 2005;128: 1461–5.

74. Di Pauli F, Reindl M, Ehling R, *et al.* Smoking is a risk factor for early conversion to clinically definite multiple sclerosis. *Mult Scler* 2008;14:1026–30.

75. Pittas F, Ponsonby AL, Van Der Mei IA, *et al.* Smoking is associated with progressive disease course and increased progression in clinical disability in a prospective cohort of people with multiple sclerosis. *J Neurol* 2009;256:577–85.

76. Sundstrom P, Nystrom L. Smoking worsens the prognosis in multiple sclerosis. *Mult Scler* 2008;14:1031–5.

77. Koch M, van Harten A, Uyttenboogaart M, De Keyser J. Cigarette smoking and progression in multiple sclerosis. *Neurology* 2007;69:1515–20.

78. D'hooghe MB, Nagels G. Smoking behavior and multiple sclerosis severity. *Mult Scler* 2005;11:S27.

79. Healy BC, Ali EN, Guttmann CRG, *et al.* Smoking and disease progression in multiple sclerosis. *Arch Neurol* 2009;66:858–64.

80. Zivadinov R, Weinstock-Guttman B, Hashmi K, *et al.* Smoking is associated with increased lesion volumes and brain atrophy in multiple sclerosis. *Neurology* 2009;73:504–10.

81. Sena A, Couderc R, Ferret-Sena V, *et al.* Apolipoprotein E polymorphism interacts with cigarette smoking in progression of multiple sclerosis. *Eur J Neurol* 2009;16:832–7.

82. Cantorna MT. Vitamin D and multiple sclerosis: an update. *Nutr Rev* 2008;66: S135–8.

83. Burton JM, Kimball S, Vieth R, *et al.* A phase I/II dose-escalation trial of vitamin D3 and calcium in multiple sclerosis. *Neurology* 2010;74:1852–9.

84. Ascherio A, Munch M. Epstein–Barr virus and multiple sclerosis. *Epidemiology* 2000;11:220–4.

85. Marrie RA, Wolfson C. Multiple sclerosis and Epstein–Barr virus: a review. *Canadian Journal of Infectious Diseases* 2002;13:111–18.

86. Jager PLD, Simon KC, Munger KL, Rioux JD, Hafler DA, Ascherio A. Integrating risk factors: HLA-DRB1* 1501 and Epstein–Barr virus in multiple sclerosis. *Neurology* 2008;70:1113–18.

Measures of neurological impairment and disability in multiple sclerosis

Gary R. Cutter, Charity J. Morgan, Amber R. Salter, Stacey S. Cofield, and Laura J. Balcer

Introduction

This chapter describes the measurement of impairment and disability for use in MS clinical trials, rather than from a patient care perspective. Measuring impairment and disability for individual patients differs from evaluating the impact of therapies on impairment and disability. For patient care, we focus on the individual in order to alleviate suffering, prevent problems, and lessen the impact of the disease. In the latter, we assess evidence in favor of a therapy in order to determine whether that therapy is beneficial to patients in general. For patient care, clinical assessments identify problems, document the course of disease, provide etiological clues, prevent consequences of the disease, and guide therapeutic interventions. Because of the complexity of the multiple sclerosis (MS) disease process and the variety of clinical features, clinical tools are most effectively applied by skilled clinicians. Good clinical care could be viewed as a series of informal clinical trials, in which the clinician uses each patient as a study, in which the patient serves as his own control. Individualizing treatment is central to patient care, and successful response at the level of the individual patient is the goal. This ongoing "n of 1" trial is appropriate for patients, and results in many anecdotes, but is neither appropriate nor accepted for experimental studies. To evaluate the impact of treatment on impairment and disability, clinical measurements are needed that derive from a population of patients under a predefined, common protocol. Many concepts discussed in this chapter are relevant at the patient care level, but the reader should realize that optimal measures for clinical trials may differ significantly from evaluative methods for individualized patient care.

Impairment and disability differ somewhat based on the specific classification system (e.g. WHO,[1] the Nagi model,[2] AMA,[3] Social Security Administration (SSA)),[4] but impairment and disability may become quite dissociated at the individual patient level. For example, a wheelchair-bound paraplegic may be working full-time, and would therefore not meet the SSA's definition of disability, while a surgeon might have a relatively minor injury to a digital nerve that limits his ability to perform critical neurosurgical techniques. Thus, definitions that seem clear, and in general can be applied to groups of impacted individuals, nevertheless fail to meet our expectations in certain cases. Thus, we often accept outcomes at the group level that suffer deficiencies at the individual level and vice versa. This compromise occurs as well with clinical trial outcomes.

The value of any one outcome measure of disability in MS is often debated. For example, some believe that detailed cognitive testing is essential to characterize a patient's disability, while others are content with a more global assessment. Part of this divide stems from the perspective of the observer. Two general perspectives of disability drive measurement approaches. The *medical model* of disability focuses on the individual, specifically their impairment and its precise definition. The goal of treatment is to alleviate consequences of the impairment, to return the individual to normal functioning or as close to normal functioning as possible. This model requires accurate diagnosis of the impairment and its pathology. It relies on detailed understanding of normal function in order to develop the goals of intervention. In this model, patients are commonly labeled in terms of disability (e.g. wheelchair-bound) rather than by level of impairment. The second perspective is the *health psychology* perspective. This vantage point focuses heavily on coping behaviors and developing strategies to minimize the effects of impairment. The view is that a person is disabled not only by their impairment, but also by how they respond to it. From this perspective, an assessment of daily living activities and how a patient plans to accomplish certain tasks make up the tools for assessing that patient. Both approaches are valid, and both can lead to valid outcome measures for clinical trials. Interventions that seek to effect cure are best measured from the medical model perspective. Interventions designed to ameliorate symptoms can often be approached using the health psychology perspective.

This chapter deals primarily with the measurement of impairment or disability from a medical model perspective, in part because of Food and Drug Administration (FDA) demands for clinical relevance for therapeutic findings warranting approval. While there is a wide range of measurement tools for application in MS, encompassing everything from fatigue to bowel and bladder functioning, this chapter focuses on global clinical trial outcome measures rather than specific symptomatic therapy outcomes.

Multiple Sclerosis Therapeutics, Fourth Edition, ed. Jeffrey A. Cohen and Richard A. Rudick. Published by Cambridge University Press.
© Cambridge University Press 2011.

Methodological issues in measuring impairment and disability

Measures can be grouped into four classes:[5] (1) biological assays use laboratory methods, such as the presence and amount of neutralizing antibodies, serum glutamic pyruvic transaminase (SGPT) to evaluate liver function, etc.; (2) performance measures are standardized procedures for testing human function, such as the Timed 25-Foot Walk[6] or the 9-Hole Peg Test[7]; (3) rating scales are ordered (ordinal) scales requiring human assessment, the most common in MS being Kurtzke's Expanded Disability Status Scale (EDSS);[8] and (4) self-report measures require the individual patient to provide information about his condition from his own perspective. The Incapacity Status Scale[9] and the MS Quality of Life Inventory[10] are examples of such self-report measures, also called patient reported outcomes or PROs.

These four classes of measurement provide an assessment framework. The uses of the measurements are, however, not restricted amongst the differing classes. In other words, a particular research question could be addressed: by a laboratory test, a measure of patient function, a clinical rating scale, or a self-report. In clinical medicine, more than one measure is often used to evaluate patient status, check progress, alter the course of therapy or make other recommendations. In a clinical trial, it is generally preferred to identify a single measure as the primary outcome, but in addition use other secondary dimensions of the patient's well-being. There is a natural conflict between a complete clinical assessment of a patient from a physician's perspective and the index measure used in a clinical trial. The primary end-point by itself is often inadequate at the individual level. This is because a single measure nearly always aggregates information to an average or otherwise representative value, and is usually seen as inadequate for individual patients. Clinicians feel an obligation to understand their patient in as detailed a manner as possible, while the trial outcome measure may ignore entirely important factors of a specific patient's condition. The conflict may not show in the choice of instruments, but can and does influence the interpretation of the results.

Some instruments measure disease-specific functions or conditions. Examples are ambulation, bladder infections, or cognitive function. Other instruments aim to measure disease dysfunction in a non-specific manner, thus enabling comparison across diagnostic conditions. The adult Functional Independence Measure (FIM)[11] is a generic instrument used to measure impairment in a number of diseases or conditions. There are benefits and disadvantages to both disease-specific and generic instruments. They must be weighed and related to the primary research question. These considerations of perspective are especially true with quality of life instruments because of the personal nature of the perspective. Clinicians generally prefer disease-specific instruments. In areas of psychosocial evaluation, disease-specific approaches are too narrow. Broad-based assessments tend to be too cumbersome or

time-consuming, leading to a proliferation of choices and often a lack of consensus on the best measurement techniques. As can be seen from the SSA[4] definition for disability ("the inability to engage in any substantial, gainful activity by reason of any medically determinable physical or mental impairment(s), which can be expected to result in death or which has lasted or can be expected to last for a continuous period of not less than 12 months"), vested interests invalidate the patient's perspective as the sole determinant of disability. In the context of a clinical trial, disease-specific approaches often have more merit with respect to the illness under investigation, while generic measures provide more generalizability and the normative context for the results.

Another measurement issue is whether to choose an instrument that explores a single dimension of impairment vs. one that addresses a broader spectrum. For certain clinical trials, a more specific outcome measure is preferred, while in other trials, multiple responses may be important. Ambulation may be a key outcome measure in a trial of 4-aminopyridine, where the mechanism of action is thought to improve nerve conduction in demyelinated fiber. An outcome such as Guy's Neurological Disability Scale[12] may not offer the specificity desired. In a trial of disease-modifying therapy, e.g. an interferon trial, a more global measure such as the EDSS may be preferable because the principal question relates to the overall condition of the patient. Thus, while no single measure is ever likely to be completely adequate to characterize an MS patient, investigators must choose the end-point that most appropriately addresses the question being asked in a given clinical trial.

Because it is difficult to characterize impairments and disability associated with the multiple clinical manifestations of MS, optimal outcome measures in MS clinical trials may evolve to a narrow question of treatment. Composite clinical measures for assessing the impact of treatment on a group of patients, or surrogate measures shown to correlate, predict and be tantamount to other clinical outcomes, may evolve, but unfortunately, what the key primary outcome is or should be is unclear. In cardiovascular disease, it might be death, a subsequent myocardial infarction, or percentage stenosis. In cancer, it can be mortality, disease-free survival, or even tumor size. However, in MS, we do not have a particular outcome that can reliably stated to be the outcome of choice. A patient presenting with optic neuritis may believe that vision is their primary outcome, but in the long term, this may not in fact be the outcome of choice. While impairment-free survival or disease activity free survival may be the desire, the outcome most commonly used is the EDSS. When a gold-standard outcome that all agree upon is the important clinically meaningful outcome, a search for surrogate outcomes ensues. Surrogates shorten the development time of new drugs. If there is no gold-standard from which to gauge MS progression and/or disability, then surrogates are still sought after, but it requires much more effort to demonstrate that these outcomes are tantamount to longer-term outcomes. We must first understand just what a surrogate outcome is.

Surrogate outcomes

Surrogate outcome measures have been studied in a variety of diseases (cancer, heart disease, human immunodeficiency virus (HIV), etc.) and have been hoped for within the MS community. Surrogate outcomes are variables that have specific properties. When used to establish the effectiveness of a treatment, criteria for the validation of surrogates are stringent.[13] First, the surrogate must predict future clinical disease. Second, the effect of treatment on clinical disease must be explained by the effect of the treatment on the surrogate; that is, the treatment needs to impact the clinical outcome by working through the surrogate. Third, the surrogate must work over various classes of treatment in the same manner.

A surrogate end-point is one that is measured instead of the biologically definitive or most relevant clinical end-point. Fleming[14] defines a surrogate end-point as "a response variable for which a test of the null hypothesis of no relationship to the treatment groups under comparison is also a valid test of the corresponding null hypothesis based on the true end-point". Alternatively, the FDA defines a surrogate marker as any non-clinical measure that can reliably predict clinical changes "within a reasonable amount of time", and also as "a laboratory measurement or physical sign used as a substitute for a clinically meaningful endpoint that measures directly how a patient feels, functions, or survives".[15]

A surrogate end-point needs to be convincingly associated with a definitive clinical outcome so that it can be used as a reliable replacement. A good surrogate should yield the same inference about the disease as the definitive end-point and also be responsive to treatments. A good surrogate can shorten clinical trials because of its short latency with respect to the natural history of the disease. It is advantageous to use it in cases where the definitive end-point is inaccessible due to time constraints, difficulty of measurement or cost. There are disadvantages to surrogate end-points. For example, eligibility criteria for a clinical trial may depend on the surrogate measurement truncating a population, which reduces both the predictive validity of a measure and the correlation with other variables. Furthermore, a weak association between the surrogate and the true outcome may not reflect the effects of treatment, as when the treatment affects the true outcome through a mechanism not involving the surrogate, and thus does not predict treatment effects on the definitive end-points accurately.

The EDSS is not tantamount to the MS disease outcome. Many clinical practices never measure this composite scoring of the patient. Nevertheless, the EDSS is the gestalt that most agree is the clinical condition of the patient. The EDSS tends to predict future status over reasonable time domains, and has grown to become the outcome measure of choice in clinical trials. However, in terms of the formal definitions of surrogate outcomes, the EDSS has not been validated to fulfill the characteristics required for a surrogate. It has long been known that the EDSS is somewhat unreliable from visit to visit, varying in general by one point or more and yielding slightly more than 50%

agreement from visit to visit. MS clinical trialists introduced the concept of sustained change in part to avoid the unreliability of the EDSS. While this approach provides better properties for the EDSS, few data are available to show that the predictive validity of the EDSS and the treatment effects observed are sufficiently high to warrant the label as a surrogate. However, the EDSS remains the unchallenged standard outcome for trials. Thus, the field of MS lacks a definitive outcome measure, making all the more important a keen understanding of this classic MS outcome as well as other measures of impairment and disability.

The EDSS is thought of as an ordinal scale. An ordinal scale represents a series that orders the possible outcomes into a rank order. While in general the EDSS orders patients in terms of MS disability severity, the true requirements of an ordinal scale may not be technically met. A patient, who is terribly debilitated by cognitive dysfunction as a result of their MS, may not be rated at the highest levels of the EDSS as the focus is mostly on physical disability. Nevertheless, the EDSS is almost always considered as an ordinal scale rather than nominal (a scale that assigns values for classes or names, such as Male $= 0$ and Female $= 1$). If we accept the EDSS as ordinal, we have to consider the implications. Results from running a marathon can be seen as an ordinal scale with the winner having the lowest "score" or rank and the last finisher, the highest rank. The actual times of finishing would be the underlying numerical outcome, but we can use the ranks to examine the data. That is, the first person with finishing position 1 has the fastest time and just by knowing the finishing position we have no idea whether the second finisher was 1 second behind or 1 minute behind, we just know that the first person was faster than the second. Would we add these together? Does the first person plus the second person equal the third person – of course not! Adding ordinal data points as if they were numerical measures may not make sense. However, thinking about two people and averaging their finishing position $(1 + 2)/2 = 1.5$, while somewhat inappropriate from the ordinal scale perspective, does seem to tell us something about where these two participants finished the race.

Why? Because we do associate the underlying scale with something we feel is meaningful: the rank of the finish. Could we average the Transportation Safety Administrations color-coded ordinal scale of alert status: low, guarded, elevated, high, severe? Yesterday it was yellow (third level), today it was orange (fourth level), so on average the color is light orange; or is the level 3.5? Clearly, discussing what we think the mixture of orange and yellow will look like does not really convey interesting results – but arbitrarily calling yellow a 3 and orange a 4, the average of 3.5 is not totally meaningless, although it violates mathematical principles. This incongruity between mathematical no-nos and some intuitive meaning is what continues to support the use of averaging of ordinal variables, especially the EDSS. Many journal articles report the average EDSS in trial participants. The authors usually are well aware that you should not use ordinal data as numerical, but it has become commonplace and as with the TSA alert codes, the average suggests a meaning despite violating the assumptions. Averaging the EDSS is used merely to describe the comparability of the treated populations. More appropriate to the form of the EDSS data are non-parametric statistics such as the median as a measure of central tendency and the inter-quartile range (25th and 75th percentiles) as a measure of variability.

While we use and tolerate some parametric statistics on the EDSS, there are limitations to applying mathematics and statistics to ordinal data. One common statistical test applied somewhat inappropriately to the EDSS is the t-test to demonstrate baseline comparability. Just as adding the first and second place runners does not yield the third place runner, so too adding and then averaging the EDSS values is not a meaningful number to compute or test. However, for testing the differences between two groups based on this "metric," we can see what happens. Purists will argue that one should use non-parametric statistics to compare the two sets of EDSS scores. If we replace the EDSS values of each participant with the rank of that person's EDSS score and apply the Wilcoxon Rank Sum test for comparing two groups, the results will be actually quite close in terms of P-values. The t-test will often show a lower P-value than the non-parametric rank test, because the EDSS is like a rank with ties, which tends to underestimate the variance slightly. Thus, while one should keep in mind that the EDSS is an ordinal variable, the EDSS can, in some instances, be used as a numerical summary measure if one is willing to assume it truly measures disability on a single scale and one is careful about the manner in which the data are summarized and tested.

This discussion is a prerequisite to a discussion of another outcome measure that has been discussed as an improvement for the EDSS. The Multiple Sclerosis Severity Scale (MSSS), devised by Roxburgh et al.,[16] purports to improve on the EDSS by providing a score that is indexed by the EDSS and time since the onset of original symptoms. The underlying premise is that patients who have reached a particular EDSS level with a shorter disease duration are progressing faster than those who took longer to reach that disability level. The score assigned is in effect a number that represents the percentage of MS patients reaching a particular EDSS score given time since the onset of the disease divided by 10. For example, an MSSS score of 5.0 means that a patient appears to be progressing at the median rate and a 9.0 means that 90% of patients progress at a slower rate. This appealing approach can arguably be used to compare a population at a single cross-section of time. On the other hand, one needs to keep in mind that ascertaining when symptoms began is subject to a variety of errors and thus, we are trading one variable, the EDSS, which is known to be precise to within plus or minus one step, for two variables (EDSS and disease duration) measured with error. Values can be obtained from the table provided in the Roxburgh et al. paper.[16] Some researchers want to use MSSS values to determine change in disease progression over time. The use of the MSSS is quite problematic as each row of the MSSS table is in effect the ranks of 1000 patients for that duration of disease (taking into account ties at the same EDSS levels). As was noted above with the marathon race

example, measuring the difference between two ranks does not really provide any information about the change.

The poor meaning of the changes can be further illustrated by considering a normal distribution. In a normal distribution characterized by "z-scores" which range from negative to positive symmetrically about zero, percentiles or ranks of 1000 observations could be obtained from the cumulative distribution of these z-scores. If we assume the value of the z-score is a measure of the underlying disease (as we do for the EDSS) then a z-score of -3.0 would correspond to having only four people with this z-score or lower. There would be 500 patients at or below a z-score of zero, etc. From this example we might see how difficult it is to interpret changes change in the MSSS. A change of 50 points from a rank of 9166 to 9866 takes you from a z-score of -2.1 to -2.2, indicating progression or worsening of the patient, but when the z-score is -0.30, a change in ranks by 50 in either direction effectively does not change your z-score substantively. Thus the mere measure of change on the rank scale is not always associated with a change in the z-score or the underlying disease score.

Thus on the disability scale, a change of one point on the MSSS may be important (if in the "tails" of the distribution), but may be absolutely inconsequential if in the mid-range. Because of the different meanings of the changes in some portions of the MSSS range, the resulting changes lack consistency and are hard to interpret.

Outcomes and the Multiple Sclerosis Functional Composite

In 1994, a meeting, "Outcomes assessment in multiple sclerosis clinical trials", was held in Charleston, SC, USA. Participants of this meeting[17] recommended the development of an improved clinical outcome measure for MS clinical trials that met several criteria: (1) the measure should be multidimensional to reflect the varied clinical expression of MS across patients and over time; (2) the individual dimensions should change relatively independently over time; and (3) measures of cognitive function should be included, in addition to those clinical dimensions already incorporated into the Kurtzke EDSS.[8,18] These recommendations led the National Multiple Sclerosis Society's (NMSS) Advisory Committee on Clinical Trials to appoint the Task Force on Clinical Outcomes Assessment. The development of the Multiple Sclerosis Functional Composite (MSFC) resulted from the analysis of a pooled data set of placebo control groups and natural history study databases.[19] The Task Force developed six guiding principles for the composite development and analyses that are reported in this paper, and which still apply to the development of any purported outcome measure: (1) to use measures that reflect the major clinical dimensions of MS; (2) to avoid redundancy; (3) to use simple rather than complex measures; (4) to improve on the valuable characteristics of the EDSS; (5) to emphasize measures sensitive to change; and (6) to develop an outcome measure that will be useful in clinical trials (and may or may not be directly useful for clinical care).

The Task Force identified the major clinical dimensions of MS – arm, leg, cognitive, and visual function – and specified criteria by which to evaluate candidate measures of these dimensions.[20]

The criteria established to select candidate component measures included: good correlation with the biologically relevant clinical dimensions; good reliability of the measurement (the ability to obtain the same result on repeat testing when no change occurred); the ability to show change over time; and the availability of a minimum of two data points one year apart in time in the pooled data set. Construct validity (the extent to which the measure of interest correlates with other measures in predicted ways, but for which no true criterion exists) was used to reduce the number of candidate measures. This was based on the logic that individual measures within the same clinical dimension should correlate with each other (convergent validity) and not with measures of different clinical dimensions (discriminant validity). Applying these criteria, a subset of candidate measures was selected. Reliability estimates were observed from the literature and means and standard deviations of change and the relationship between changes in these candidate variables and in the EDSS were assessed. Both the concurrent and predictive validity of each composite measure were evaluated. Concurrent validity was defined as change in the composite measure compared with concurrent change in the EDSS over a one-year period. Predictive validity was defined as change in the composite occurring over the first year of follow-up compared with subsequent change in EDSS among those patients with no change in EDSS during the first year. Predictive validity was felt to illustrate and best validate the composite construction. Detailed discussion of this process is given by Cutter et al.[21]

The MSFC is a unified score representing the combination of results from three performance tests: the 9-Hole Peg Test (9HPT), the Timed 25-Foot Walk (T25FW), and the 3-Second Paced Auditory Serial Addition Test (PASAT-3). These performance tests are combined to form a single score.[22] The MSFC score incorporates three clinical dimensions representing arm, leg, and cognitive function to create a single score that can be used to detect change over time in a group of MS patients. No measure of visual function was found at the time that could be used in the MSFC. Recent developments in other measures (discussed below) provide a potential important addition to the MSFC in the visual domain.

The concept of the MSFC is rather simple. The results of three functional tests are combined into a single number that represents the relative impairment of an individual compared with the group or an external reference group. Since the underlying units of measurement differ between these tests (time in seconds for the 9HPT and T25FW, and the number of correct answers for the PASAT-3), it is necessary to identify a sensible way in which to combine variables that evaluate different dimensions. A z-score was selected as a common metric for this purpose. The z-score is a standardized number representing how close a test result is to the mean of the standard or reference population to which the result is compared on one functional domain. The z-score is expressed in units of standard deviation, and when the underlying distribution of assessments is normally distributed the values will generally range from -3 to $+3$, although there are no restrictions on its values. Owing to the non-linear way in which the body fails when functions deteriorate, these z-scores are often highly skewed as a person loses functions. For example, MS patients in the early phase of the disease can walk 25 feet in 5–7 seconds, declining by a few seconds as their EDSS increases, until they begin to reach handicaps in ambulation where assistive devices are necessary. At this stage of MS, T25FW typically exceeds 25–30 seconds. The calculated z-scores score for these cases often greatly exceed three standard deviations from the mean.

The standard deviation of a measure is, on average, how far a randomly selected observation is from the mean in original units of measurement, ignoring the direction of the difference, whereas the z-score is a relative measure. A z-score of 2 implies that an observation is two standard deviation units above the mean. It is often stated that the clinical meaning of a standard deviation of 2 is too difficult to interpret, because clinical meaning depends on what is being measured: seconds, number correct, etc. Some clinicians argue that these underlying units would need to be known before the clinical interpretation and value could be considered as meaningful. This assertion is not the case, but rather one of custom and comfort with how results are reported. For example, in medicine, we define laboratory abnormalities in this way, marking them as adverse events or critical limits, when they are two or three times the upper or lower limit of normal clinical values. This concept depends on the normative values and how many standard deviation units the upper limit of normal is.

Just as twice or three times the upper limit of normal adjusts for differences in methods of laboratory assessment and internal reference values, *the z-score is a relative measure indicating how many standard deviation units the current observation is from the mean of the reference population, and the units are the same irrespective of the underlying measurement scale.* For example, the number of seconds required to perform a test can be represented on the same z-score scale as the number of correct responses on the PASAT-3 if we are willing to assume that they are both continuous measures. This allows the results from tests using different metrics (e.g. seconds and number correct) to be combined as a single overall average measure, indicating where a person falls on these combined dimensions. The three components of the MSFC are combined by creating a z-score for each individual component, then averaging the three z-scores to create the MSFC. Implicit in this approach is the idea that patients who deteriorate or improve on all three component measures will have an overall larger change than patients who change on only one of the three measures. Also, patients who deteriorate in one area but improve in another may show no change on the MSFC, because the MSFC represents the *average* change in the three domains. The MSFC has now been used in many studies and trials. It has been criticized as difficult to interpret and lacking clinical meaning.

Table 6.1. *Baseline to month-24 change in the MSFC and component z-scores from the IMPACT study*

	Placebo (n = 219)	IFNβ-1a (n = 217)	P value[a]
MSFC Mean ± SD	−0.495 ± 1.58	−0.362 ± 1.41	0.033
Median (IQR)	−0.161 (−0.417, 0.028)	−0.096 (−0.305, 0.066)	
T25FW Mean ± SD	−1.191 ± 3.13	−0.979 ± 2.62	0.378
Median (IQR)	−0.113 (−0.622, −0.006)	−0.076 (−0.402, 0.00)	
9HPT Mean ± SD	−0.290 ± 0.494	−0.202 ± 0.476	0.024
Median (IQR)	−0.305 (−0.594, 0.027)	−0.169 (−0.457, 0.105)	
PASAT-3 Mean ± SD	−0.004 ± 0.473	+0.094 ± 0.498	0.061
Median (IQR)	0.000 (−0.163, 0.244)	+ 0.081 (−0.081, 0.244)	

[a] Analysis of covariance on ranks stratified on baseline Expanded Disability Status Scale (EDSS) and Gd-enhancement on baseline magnetic resonance imaging (MRI); T25FW, Timed 25-Foot Walk; 9HPT, 9-Hole Peg Test; PASAT-3, 3-second Paced Auditory Serial Addition Test; IQR, Inter-quartile range; IFN, interferon.

Consider the International Multiple Sclerosis Secondary Progressive Avonex Controlled Trial (IMPACT).[23,24] In this study, there was a significant difference in the MSFC between the interferon-treated group and the placebo group (Table 6.1). The mean MSFC difference was 0.133 (0.065 difference in medians). The FDA did not believe that these were clinically significant differences and wanted evidence of clinical effects. But, what is an intelligence quotient (IQ) score or the college examination SAT or ACT scores? We are familiar with them and attach meaning to them. However, these scores only have meaning in that they have been used sufficiently that we all purport to understand them. Most ACT scores have at best a correlation of about 0.50 with graduation rates.[25] We know that high 20s are a good ACT score and that values below 20 are poor, but what does a difference mean? Amherst College boasts a mean ACT of 31, while Massachusetts Institute of Technology's (MIT's) mean is 32. Compare these averages with the University of Wisconsin's 26.3, the University of Missouri's 25.4 and Michigan State's score of 24. The differences correlate vaguely with our notions about these schools, but does this mean something for the individual student?

Similarly, an overall difference in scores on the MSFC tells us something, but just as a one-point difference between MIT and Amherst is insufficient to characterize what is clinically meaningful about the difference in the schools, it does give us some information. As for the widely used outcome measure in MS, the EDSS, consider the interpretation of change in the EDSS. This task is really no easier – just more accepted. For example, if a patient changes by one point on the EDSS, what does this change mean? Unless one has more detailed information (as in the components of the MSFC), all that can really be said is that he/she has worsened by one point on the EDSS, what has become conventional as a significant amount. If we say that a patient has gone from an EDSS 2 to a 3, we have a set of descriptions that enable us to envision the kind of changes the patient has experienced. But the changes that occur in going from a 2 to a 3, a one-point change, are not the same as the one-point change of a 6 to a 7; just knowing the amount of change in the EDSS does not mean clarity in the information from the change.

So what information was there in the MSFC for the IMPACT study? The absolute difference tells us that the means of the two groups are slightly more than 0.13 standard deviation units apart. But what does that imply? Is this clinically meaningful? One way to examine this difference is to consider a so-called effect size. That is, the difference observed between the groups relative to the standard deviation within the groups, similar in concept to the z-score discussed above. In the case of the IMPACT study, the effect size is about 0.08 or 0.09. Effect sizes have been characterized[26] as small, medium, and large. Values of 0.30 or below are considered small and 0.80 or above, large, and medium is somewhere in between. Thus, while the difference found in the MSFC in IMPACT is statistically significant, using these guidelines, the effect size and, thus, expected consequence from the treatment studied is small. Other information is available from the MSFC in IMPACT. Table 6.1 shows the component z-scores of the MSFC. Only the 9HPT difference is statistically significant, but computing the effect size of each component to assess the findings shows an effect size of 0.07 for T25FW, 0.18 for the 9HPT and 0.20 for the PASAT-3. This approach shows effect sizes that consistently favor treatment, all small, with the T25FW showing the smallest. Thus, we can conclude that there was a small but consistent treatment effect. While benefit was not significant for each component, the MSFC reflects the combined benefits for all three domains. This type of analysis shows consistency of the outcomes across all three components. If there were no effect, this would happen by chance 12.5% of the time (each component has a 50/50 chance of being favorable and, thus, the probability of all three being favorable is $(1/2)^3 = 1/8 = 12.5\%$).

Table 6.2 examines the magnitude of the absolute changes to discover what clinical meaning might be associated with these results. The mean times on the T25FW went from about 14.5 seconds to 32 in the placebo group and 29 seconds in the IFNβ-1a (IM) group, with a tripling of the standard deviations, indicating the presence of some excessively long times to complete the test. As noted above, when patients reach levels of impairment that are the beginnings of handicap, non-linear declines in function are often seen, producing a skewed distribution of results. When such skewness is present, using means to represent groups can be rather misleading, and comparison of the medians is often substituted. Using the shift in median times over 2 years still gives a value of 2.8 seconds for the placebo

Table 6.2. *Raw scores of MSFC component tests from the IMPACT Study (See Table 6.1 for definitions)*

	Placebo ($n = 219$)		IFNβ-1a (IM) ($n = 217$)	
T25FW	**Baseline**	**Month 24**	**Baseline**	**Month 24**
Mean ± SD	14.6 ± 15.4	32.0 ± 53.0	14.4 ± 17.4	29.0 ± 47.0
Median (IQR)	9.1 (6.5, 16.1)	11.9 (7.3, 27.1)	9.1 (6.4, 14.6)	10.4 (7.1, 22.1)
9HPT	**Baseline**	**Month 24**	**Baseline**	**Month 24**
Mean ± SD	33.2 ± 30.0	53.1 ± 90.3	31.1 ± 16.1	44.7 ± 82.8
Median (IQR)	27.5 (23.2, 34.8)	29.6 (23.8, 39.8)	26.4 (23.0, 32.8)	27.5 (23.7, 37.0)
PASAT-3	**Baseline**	**Month 24**	**Baseline**	**Month 24**
Mean ± SD	46.7 ± 12.3	46.7 ± 13.7	47.1 ± 12.3	48.3 ± 12.9
Median (IQR)	51.0 (39.0, 57.0)	52.0 (38.0, 58.0)	52.0 (39.0, 57.0)	54.0 (43.0, 58.0)

group (9.1 to 11.9), representing a change of over 30%. Similarly, in the IFNβ-1a group, the median change in the time walk went from 9.1 to 10.4 seconds, a 14% increase. However, is this an indication of a change that is clinically important, and should we believe that it is a difference in the absence of statistical significance? It has been reported by Schwid et al.[27] that changes of 20% or more could be considered thresholds for a true change in function for an individual. Thus, we are seeing group-level changes in the placebo group that might be expected to be important, but not seeing a comparable change in the treated group. For the 9HPT, the test that gave a statistically significant difference, we see only an 8% change in the median time for this test in the placebo group, compared with a 4% improvement in the IFNβ-1a group. There is also a 4% improvement in the IFNβ-1a group on the PASAT, vs. 2% in the placebo. We see that the percentage change is double for all three individual components of the MSFC in the IFNβ-1a group.

The point of the preceding paragraphs is not to say that the FDA made a mistake in its assessment about the treatment benefit of this drug, but only to suggest that the evidence was consistent with benefit not only for the 9HPT, but for all three components. The effect was small, and given the limited evidence for long-term benefits of any MS therapy currently licensed, it would seem unlikely that the benefits would translate into major advances for secondary progressive MS patients. Nevertheless, these data support the utility of the MSFC in assessing impairment and disability.

Potential improvements to the Multiple Sclerosis Functional Composite

The notion that clinically meaningful change needs to exceed 20% to be functionally significant has been advanced by Schwid et al.,[27] confirmed by Hoogervorst et al.[28] and utilized by Vaney et al.[29] Vaney uses the two motor components of the MSFC (the T25FW and 9HPT) to develop an assessment based on the number of 20% changes that occur. He points out that the MSFC is sensitive to the standard population chosen; the broader and more variable the population is at baseline, the more difficult it is to show a change. His population ranges from EDSS 1.5 to

EDSS 9, which indeed accentuates this deficiency. The MSFC was developed as a clinical trial outcome measure, whereas Vaney's goal was to develop a tracking tool for the individual clinician. Using a clever transformation, he develops a measure (closely related to the MSFC) that offers clinically meaningful results based on percentage changes. His SaGAs, the Short and Graphic Ability Score, provides counts of meaningful changes.

Additional work has been conducted to examine ways in which to make the MSFC changes more clinically meaningful. As Vaney has done, these new examinations include counting the number of 20% changes, using percentage change in the composite or using inverse changes. To date, no single approach with overall best performance has been identified. What may improve the MSFC substantively is identifying potential visual components.

Contrast sensitivity was identified as providing a significant signal in the Optic Neuritis Treatment Trial,[30] and has been explored in a number of investigations and publications. Visual dysfunction occurs in 80% of patients with MS during their disease, and is a presenting feature in 50%.[31,32] Balcer et al.[33] evaluated several tests of binocular contrast sensitivity and contrast letter acuity, concluding that Sloan charts and the Pelli–Robson contrast sensitivity measures provide useful means of distinguishing MS patients from normal controls and showing change over time within MS patients. Several papers have demonstrated key components of the use of the contrast letter acuity assessed by Sloan letter charts. Balcer et al.[33] have shown that these measurements are highly reliable (intraclass correlations exceeding 0.90), and can be simplified for use in the clinic setting. These measures also have face validity in that the average number correct declines with decreasing contrast.

Results for 224 MS patients and 153 disease-free controls from a cross-sectional study of visual outcome measures (MS Vision Prospective (MVP) cohort) showed that contrast letter acuity (Sloan charts, $P < 0.0001$, receiver operating characteristic (ROC) area under the curve 81%) and contrast sensitivity (Pelli–Robson, $P = 0.003$, ROC area under the curve 78%) best distinguished MS patients from disease-free controls. Adjusting for age, the odds of being an MS patient were nearly 2.4, based on contrast letter acuity scores. Correlations of Sloan chart scores with MSFC and EDSS scores in both studies were significant and moderate in magnitude (approximately 0.56), demonstrating that Sloan chart scores reflect visual and neurological dysfunction not entirely captured by the EDSS or MSFC.[34] Contrast letter acuity (Sloan charts) and contrast sensitivity (Pelli–Robson) demonstrate the capacity to identify binocular visual dysfunction in MS. Sloan chart testing also captures unique aspects of neurological dysfunction not captured by current EDSS or MSFC components, making it a strong candidate visual function test for the MSFC.

In a small substudy in the IMPACT trial, Baier et al.[35] showed that these measures demonstrated predictive validity. That is, a change in the Sloan letter chart scores over the first year predicted the change in the EDSS over the subsequent year. More formal evaluation of these potential additions to the MSFC awaits analyses of ongoing ancillary studies that should provide evidence for the value of the addition of a vision component to the MSFC.

The latest modification to the MSFC was published by Rudick et al.[36] using data from the AFFIRM study of natalizumab. A patient was considered to have progressed if there was a 20% change in any of the components of the MSFC persisting for at least 3 months. This was then compared to a 15% change. "Sustained MSFC worsening" was proposed as a "disability event," and compared with other measures. Rudick et al. concluded "MSFC Progression-20 and MSFC Progression-15 are sensitive measures of disability progression; correlate with EDSS, relapse rates, and SF-36 PCS; and are capable of demonstrating therapeutic effects in randomized, controlled clinical studies." This approach to use of the MSFC is appealing, because it eliminated the need to standardize MSFC scores using an external standard to create z-scores. This may make it easier to compare results across studies; further, correlation of MSFC progression with relapse rates, EDSS, and SF-36 provide criterion validation of this approach. Recently Polman et al.[37] provided an extensive discussion of the status of the MSFC as of 2010.

Other measures of impairment and disability

The majority of other measures of impairment and disability have been scales rather than functional measures. Several scales have been identified that seem to contain important information about the clinical status of the patient. These include Guy's Neurological Disability Scale, the Multiple Sclerosis Impact Scale (MSIS-29), the Scripps Neurological Rating Scale, the Functional Independence Measure, the Ambulation Index and the Patient Determined Disease Steps.

Several of these have been evaluated, each having pros and cons, proponents and detractors. The arguments that brew over the plethora of candidates may be summed up by the same questions as for quality of life. What is the question? What is the goal? Does one need a disease-specific outcome or a more generic instrument? Should one focus on symptom evaluation or disability or impairment? The field of MS has not placed much confidence to date in self-administered questionnaires. However, the Guy's Neurological Disability Scale appears to have reasonable properties. The North American Research Consortium on Multiple Sclerosis (NARCOMS) registry has made extensive use of self-assessment scales. More attention to these self-administered scales might be beneficial in reducing the complexity of trials and blinded evaluations by examiners, if such scales can be shown to be good surrogates. With both the FDA and NIH more focused on PROs, it is clear that these outcomes should not be ignored, but in chronic diseases with extensive long-term horizons for the consequences of disease, patient reported outcomes often suffer from shifts in patient perspectives some times leading to little change in PROs due to these perceptions by patients. Still, patients offer a unique personal perspective that is important, cost effective, and meaningful.

Conclusions

The measurement of impairment and disability requires a focus on the question being addressed. When the question requires a clinical trial, outcome measures of group performance are preferred. Continuous measures are preferred over ordinal scales. These measures may result in therapeutic benefits without obvious clinical benefits, but, by using such tools, benefits can be inferred from their effect sizes. The MSFC is a measure of impairment that represents a paradigm shift from ordinal outcomes to those more sensitive to change. Clinical interpretability is likely to improve as more information is collected and published. New and better measures will surely be developed.

Finally, careful consideration of sentinel events in the course of the progression of MS needs to be underlined. These events may be magnetic resonance imaging (MRI) benchmarks, achieving some level of EDSS disability that is reliably assessed or some measured functional tests. Once clear benchmarks are established as outcomes, then the search for surrogates to simplify the trials and speed the research in MS will be enhanced.

References

1. World Health Organization. *International Classification of Impairments, Disabilities, and Handicaps.* Geneva: WHO, 1980.

2. Nagi S. Disability concepts revisited: implications for prevention. In Sussman MG, ed. *Sociology and Rehabilitation.* Washington, DC: American Sociological Association, 1965: 100–13.

3. American Medical Association. *The Guides to the Evaluation of Permanent Impairment*, 5th edn. Chicago, IL: AMA, 2001: 2.

4. Social Security Administration. *Disability Evaluation under Social Security, Office of Disability, Publication No. 64–039*, Washington, DC, 2001.

5. LaRocca NG. *Statistical and Methodological Consideration in Scale*

Construction in Quantification of Neurologic Deficit. Stoneham, MA: Butterworth Publishers, 1989.

6. Schwid SR, Goodman AD, Mattson DH, *et al*. The measurement of ambulatory impairment in multiple sclerosis. *Neurology* 1997; 49: 1419–24.

7. Mathiowetz V, Weber K, Kashman N, Volland G. Adult norms for 9 Hole Peg Test of finger dexterity. *Occup Ther J Res* 1985; 5: 24–38.

8. Kurtzke JF. Rating neurologic impairment in multiple sclerosis: an Expanded Disability Status Scale (EDSS). *Neurology* 1983; 33: 1444–52.

9. National Multiple Sclerosis Society. *MRD Minimal Record of Disability for Multiple Sclerosis*. New York: NMSS, 1985.

10. Ritvo PG, Fischer JS, Miller DM, *et al*. *Multiple Sclerosis Quality of Life Inventory: A User's Manual*. New York: National Multiple Sclerosis Society, 1997.

11. Granger CV, Hamilton BB, Keith RA, *et al*. Advances in functional assessment for medical rehabilitation. *Top Geriatr Rehabil* 1986; 1: 59–74.

12. Sharrack B, Hughes RA. The Guy's Neurological Disability Scale (GNDS): a new disability measure for multiple sclerosis. *Mult Scler* 1999; 5: 223–33.

13. Prentice RL. Surrogate endpoints in clinical trials: definition and operational criteria. *Stat Med* 1989; 8: 431–40.

14. Fleming T. Surrogate markers in AIDS and cancer trials. *Stat Med* 1994: 13: 13–14.

15. www.fda.gov/ohrms/dockets/dailys/02/Jun02/060602/02D-0095_emc-000001-01.doc,06–14–2002.

16. Roxburgh RH, Seaman SR, Masterman T, *et al*. Multiple sclerosis severity score: using disability and disease duration to rate disease severity. *Neurology* 2005; 64: 1144–51.

17. Whitaker JN, McFarland HF, Rudge P, Reingold SC. Outcomes assessment in multiple sclerosis clinical trials: a critical analysis. *Mult Scler* 1995; 1: 37–47.

18. Kurtzke JF. A new scale for evaluating disability in multiple sclerosis. *Neurology* 1955; 5: 580–3.

19. Rudick R, Antel J, Confavreux C, *et al*. Clinical outcomes assessment in multiple sclerosis. *Ann Neurol* 1996; 40: 469–79.

20. Rudick R, Antel J, Confavreux C, *et al*. Recommendations from the National Multiple Sclerosis Society Clinical Outcomes Assessment Task Force. *Ann Neurol* 1997; 42: 379–82.

21. Cutter GR, Baier ML, Rudick RA, *et al*. Development of a multiple sclerosis functional composite as a clinical trial outcome measure. *Brain* 1999; 122: 871–82.

22. Fischer JS, Jak AJ, Kniker JE, *et al*. *Administration and Scoring Manual for the Multiple Sclerosis Functional Composite (MSFC)*. New York: Demos Publishing, 1999.

23. Cohen JA, Cutter GR, Fischer JS, *et al*. Use of the multiple sclerosis functional composite as an outcome measure in a phase III clinical trial. *Arch Neurol* 2001; 58: 961–7.

24. Cohen JA, Cutter GR, Fischer JS, *et al*. Benefit of interferon beta-1a on MSFC progression in secondary progressive MS. *Neurology*. 2002; 59: 679–87.

25. Allison P. *Missing Data*. Thousand Oaks, CA: Sage Publications, 2001.

26. Cohen J. *Statistical Power for the Behavioral Sciences*, 2nd edn. Hillsdale, NJ: Erlbaum, 1988.

27. Schwid SR, Goodman AD, McDermott MP, *et al*. Quantitative functional measures in MS: what is a reliable change? *Neurology* 2002; 58: 1294–6.

28. Hoogervorst EL, Kalkers NF, Cutter GR, *et al*. The patient's perception of a (reliable) change in the Multiple Sclerosis Functional Composite. *Mult Scler* 2004; 10: 55–60.

29. Vaney C, Vaney S, Wade DT. SaGAS, the Short and Graphic Ability Score: an alternative scoring method for the motor components of the Multiple Sclerosis Functional Composite. *Mult Scler* 2004: 10: 231–42.

30. The Optic Neuritis Study Group. Visual function 5 years after optic neuritis: experience of the Optic Neuritis Treatment Trial. *Arch Ophthalmol* 1997; 115: 1545–52.

31. McDonald WI, Barnes D. The ocular manifestations of multiple sclerosis. 1. Abnormalities of the afferent visual system. *J Neurol Neurosurg Psychiatry* 1992; 55: 747–52.

32. Newman NJ. Multiple sclerosis and related demyelinating diseases. In Miller NR, Newman NJ, eds. *Walsh and Hoyt's Clinical Neuro-Ophthalmology*, 5th edn. Baltimore: Williams & Wilkins, 1998: 5539–676.

33. Balcer LJ, Baier ML, Cohen JA, *et al*. Contrast letter acuity as a visual component for the Multiple Sclerosis Functional Composite. *Neurology* 2003; 61: 1367–73.

34. Balcer LJ, Baier ML, Pelak VS, *et al*. New low-contrast vision charts: reliability and test characteristics in patients with multiple sclerosis. *Mult Scler* 2000; 6: 163–71.

35. Baier ML, Cutter GR, Rudick RA, *et al*. Low-contrast letter acuity testing captures visual dysfunction in patients with multiple sclerosis. *Neurology* 2005; 64: 992–5.

36. Rudick RA, Polman CH, Cohen JA, *et al*. Assessing disability progression with the Multiple Sclerosis Functional Composite. *Mult Scler* 2009; 15(8): 984–97.

37. Polman CH, Rudick, RA. The Multiple Sclerosis Functional Composite: a clinically meaningful measure of disability. *Neurology* 2010; 74 (Suppl 3): S8–S15.

Assessment of neuropsychological function in multiple sclerosis

Stephen M. Rao

Cognitive function is often impaired in multiple sclerosis (MS) patients,[1] with nearly half of MS patients exhibiting deficits on neuropsychological (NP) testing.[2,3] The functional consequences of MS-related cognitive impairment can be devastating. Cognitive impairment has a direct impact on the ability to maintain employment,[4-6] driving skills and safety,[7,8] involvement in social activities,[4] personal and community independence,[4,6,9,10] and the likelihood of benefiting from inpatient rehabilitation.[11] Not surprisingly, it is a major source of caregiver strain.[12,13]

Cognitive impairment is correlated with brain abnormalities as visualized by various MRI techniques.[14] These studies have demonstrated that NP tests correlate with T2- and T1-weighted white matter lesions as well as lesions in gray matter visualized by inversion recovery pulse sequences; brain atrophy, as measured in whole brain volume, gray matter volume, brain parenchymal fraction, ventricular diameter, and callosal area; and microscopic pathology, as visualized by magnetization transfer, diffusion tensor, and proton spectroscopy, in both lesions and normal appearing brain tissue. Furthermore, deteriorating cognitive function has been associated in longitudinal studies with increasing cerebral lesion burden over 1-year[15] and 4-year[16] intervals, and with decreasing brain parenchymal volume over a 2-year period.[17]

Secondary progressive MS patients typically perform more poorly on NP testing than do patients with relapsing remitting or primary progressive MS.[18-20] Surprisingly, NP test scores correlate only weakly with disease duration and neurologic disability.[3,21,22] The weak cross-sectional correlations between cognitive dysfunction and disease duration may be due to the highly variable clinical presentation associated with MS; progression on NP tests is best appreciated in longitudinal, natural history studies (see below). Neurologic disability, as typically assessed by the Expanded Disability Standard Scale (EDSS), tends to emphasize disability associated with ambulation. As a consequence, lesions affecting primarily brain regions associated with higher cognitive functions will not have an impact on the EDSS; likewise, lesions of the spinal cord may impact ambulation, but have no effect on cognitive functions. Traditional clinical outcome measures,

therefore, are generally insensitive to MS-associated cognitive deficits.[23]

Not all cognitive functions are equally susceptible to disruption by MS. Deficits in learning and recall of new information ("recent memory") occur in 22%–31% of MS patients.[3] Impairment of information processing speed and working memory (i.e. the ability to simultaneously buffer and manipulate information) is also common, with 22%–25% of patients exhibiting deficits.[3] Less common, but significant deficits are observed on visuospatial abilities and executive functions (including reasoning, problem-solving, and planning/sequencing) in 12%–19% of patients.[3] In contrast, on measures of auditory attention span and language abilities, around 7–8% of patients are affected,[3] although recent natural history studies suggest that deficits in these domains become evident when cohorts are followed for longer periods of time.[6,24] It is important to recognize that the severity and pattern of cognitive deficits may vary considerably across individual MS patients.[19,25,26] This heterogeneity of NP impairment can best be appreciated when large samples of patients are administered a comprehensive NP battery.[27,28]

The natural history of MS-related cognitive impairment has been reported from studies conducted prior to the appearance of approved disease-modifying drugs (Table 7.1). Typically, the longitudinal NP performance of MS patients has been compared with that of demographically comparable healthy controls tested at the same intervals.[6,9,24,29,30] Of these, three studies used multiple follow-up intervals ranging up to 10 years.[6,9,24] These studies differed considerably in terms of disease characteristics, NP measures, and data analysis methods. Despite these interpretive problems, several conclusions may be drawn from these studies. First, cognitive impairment is not inevitable in MS: some patients appear to maintain intact cognitive function well into their disease, whereas other patients develop cognitive impairment early in their disease. Second, cognitive impairment is unlikely to remit to any significant extent, but cognitive deficits may remain stable for long periods of time before worsening. Third, progression rates vary considerably across patients and across cognitive functions, but on average,

Multiple Sclerosis Therapeutics, Fourth Edition, ed. Jeffrey A. Cohen and Richard A. Rudick. Published by Cambridge University Press.
© Cambridge University Press 2011.

Table 7.1. *Controlled natural history studies of MS-related cognitive dysfunction*

Study	Initial sample	Design and data analysis	Outcome
Dutch study (1990)[29]	39 patients (51% RR) vs. 24 HC *MS group:* Mean DSS = 3.5 (range = 1–7) Mean age = 42 (range = 17–73)	4-year follow-up (*n* = 33) Cross-sectional between-group and longitudinal within-group comparisons on individual tests	Initial deficits (choice reaction time, verbal and visual learning, reading speed and finger tapping) persisted over time; a few patients (6%–12%) deteriorated markedly, and one improved
Italian study (1995, 2001)[6,9]	50 patients (88% RR) vs. 70 HC *MS group:* Mean EDSS = 2.0 (SD = 1.5) Mean age = 29.9 (SD = 8.5) Mean education = 11.4 (SD = 3.6)	4.5-year (*n* = 49) and 10-year (*n* = 45) follow-up Cross-sectional between-group comparisons on individual tests	Initial deficits in verbal memory and executive functions persisted and new deficits emerged at 4.5 years (verbal fluency and auditory comprehension) and 10 years (attention span); 12/49 patients (24%) worsened by 4.5 years, and 19/45 (42%) deteriorated by 10 years
Finnish study (1997)[30]	45 patients (86% CP) vs. 35 HC *Intact MS group (n = 22)* Mean EDSS = 5.0 (SD = 1.8) Mean age = 43.3 (SD = 8.7) Mean education = 11.6 (SD = 3.5) *Impaired group (n = 23):* Mean EDSS = 5.5 (SD = 1.3) Mean age = 43.3 (SD = 7.2) Mean education = 11.0 (SD = 2.9)	2- to 4-year follow-up (*n* = 42) Cross-sectional between-group comparisons on individual tests Longitudinal between-group comparisons of difference scores on individual tests	Performance of intact group remained relatively stable over time (though 35% worsened slightly); impaired groups deficits in attention span, processing speed, verbal fluency, verbal memory, visual memory, and susceptibility to interference continued to worsen (only 23% of this group were stable or improved)
USA study (1998)[24]	100 patients (39% RR) vs. 100 HC *MS group:* Mean EDSS = 4.1 (SD = 2.2) Mean age = 45.7 (SD = 11.3) Mean education = 13.2 (SD = 2.4)	3-year (*n* = 84) and 8-year (*n* = 59) follow-up Cross-sectional and longitudinal between-group comparisons on individual tests (Group x Time ANOVA) Comparison of actual change with regression-based estimates derived from HCs	Deficits in most domains were evident at all time points and some of these (i.e. verbal abilities, verbal fluency, processing speed/working memory, calculation ability, and visual perception) worsened significantly over time; 21/84 patients (25%) met criteria for a significant deterioration at 3 years, whereas only 10/59 (17%) did at 8 years

Notes

The *Jennekens-Schinkel et al.*[29] test battery consisted of: confrontation naming; word generation; reading (100 words); writing to dictation; figure copy; Knox Cubes; Wechsler Memory Scale; 10-item list learning task (auditory and visual); 7/24 Spatial Recall Test; Stroop test; Wisconsin Card Sort (Nelson version); Raven's Progressive Matrices; and finger tapping.

The *Amato et al.*[6,9] test battery included: Blessed Information–Memory–Concentration Test; Token Test; Figure copy; Digit Span (forward); Corsi Blocks; Randt Repeatable Memory Battery (5 Words and Paired Words); Set Test; and Raven's Progressive Matrices.

The *Kujala et al.*[30] test battery included: Mini-Mental State Examination; 20-item object naming; verbal fluency (letters); BVRT errors; WAIS-R Digit Span, Digit Symbol, Block Design, and Similarities; Paced Auditory Serial Addition Test (PASAT); WMS Logical Memory; 20-item verbal paired associate recall; 7/24 Spatial Recall Test; 20-item object recall; and Stroop test.

The *Bobholz et al.*[24] test battery consisted of: WAIS-R Verbal subtests; oral comprehension; Boston Naming Test (abbreviated); Controlled Oral Word Association Test; Digit Span; reaction time tasks (simple and choice); PASAT; Stroop test; Sternberg Memory Scanning; Brown-Peterson task; Story Recall; Buschke Verbal Selective Reminding Test; 7/24 Spatial Recall; President's Test; Judgment of Line Orientation; Benton Visual Form Discrimination; Hooper Visual Organization Test; Benton Facial Recognition; Wisconsin Card Sorting Test; Booklet Category Test; Standard Raven's Progressive Matrices.

approximately 5%–9% of patients will experience deterioration on NP tests annually. This latter statistic is important to keep in mind when performing power analyses for clinical trials that employ cognitive measures as outcomes.

The purpose of this chapter is to provide: (1) an overview of controlled clinical trials of disease-modifying and symptomatic medications in which NP outcomes have been explicitly assessed, (2) an overview of factors complicating NP outcome assessment in MS clinical trials, and (3) a list of recommendations regarding NP outcome assessment for future MS clinical trials. More comprehensive reviews of MS-related cognitive dysfunction are also available.[1,31–33] It is beyond the scope of this chapter to provide a review of non-pharmacologic clinical trials designed to treat cognitive dysfunction in MS.[34]

Clinical trials of disease-modifying medications

As the prevalence and functional consequences of MS-related cognitive dysfunction became more widely recognized, several definitive trials of disease-modifying medications for relapsing remitting MS[35–40] and progressive MS[41–43] incorporated NP outcome measures.[43–49] Tables 7.2 (relapsing remitting MS) and 7.3 (progressive MS) provide an overview of these trials. Purposely excluded are non-randomized or open-label trials. Trials involving natalizumab[39] and oral fingolimod[40] administered the Multiple Sclerosis Functional Composite (MSFC), but were not included in the tables because they did not report separate performance on the cognitive component represented by the Paced Auditory Serial Addition Test (PASAT).

Table 7.2. *Randomized clinical trials of disease-modifying medications with NP outcome assessment: relapsing remitting MS*

Trial	Initial sample	NP measures and design	Primary NP analysis	NP outcome
Betaseron[a] (IFNβ-1b)[35,45]	372 patients EDSS = 0.0–5.5	Focused battery (WMS Logical Memory and Visual Reproduction, Trials A & B, Stroop) at 2 years and 4 years only ($n = 30$ at a single site)	2-way ANOVAs (Group x Test Time) of demographically adjusted scores from individual tests	Significant treatment effect (Group x Test Time interaction) on Delayed Visual Reproduction ($P < 0.03$), favoring high-dose group ($P < 0.003$), with a similar trend on Trials B ($P < 0.14$)
Copaxone (glatiramer acetate)[36,46]	251 patients EDSS = 0.0–5.0	Focused battery (Selective Reminding Test, 10/36 SRT, PASAT, SDMT, and Word List Generation) at Baseline, 12 months, and 24 months ($n = 248$)	2-way ANCOVAs (Group x Site x Test Time) of individual scores, with baseline score as covariate	No significant treatment effects
Avonex (IFNβ-1a(IM))[37,47]	301 patients EDSS = 0.0–3.5	Broad-spectrum battery at Baseline and 2 years, and focused battery every 6 months x 24 months ($n = 166$ with 2 years of assessment and treatment)	MANOVAs of demographically adjusted 2-year change scores on 3 sets of factor analytically derived variables, with baseline score as a covariate[b]	Significant treatment effects on memory and information processing ($P = 0.011$), with a trend on visuospatial abilities and executive functions ($P = 0.085$); secondary analyses confirmed treatment effects on briefer battery (MANOVA) and PASAT deterioration (survival analysis)
Tysabri (natalizumab) AFFIRM[38,49,50]	942 patients EDSS = 0–5.5	PASAT-3″ (as component of MS Functional Composite) at baseline, then every 3 months x 24 months ($n = 627$ received treatment)	Time to sustained worsening (0.5 standard deviation decrease in score sustained for 12 weeks)	Increases in test scores in both groups over 2 years; sustained worsening was 7% in natalizumab group and 12% in placebo group; survival analysis was significant ($P = 0.013$)

[a] Caution is urged in interpreting NP outcomes from this study because NP measures were not administered prior to initiating treatment and the groups differed on several NP measures at the first (Year 2) assessment.

[b] Memory and information processing measures included CVLT Total 1–5, Ruff Figural Fluency Test (RFFT) Error Ratio, Stroop Interference Score, and CALCAP Sequential RT; Measures of visuospatial abilities and executive functions included WCST Perseverative Errors, Tower of London Total # Moves; 20 Questions % Good Hypotheses, WMS-R Visual Span Forward, and Rennick Visual Search Trials.

Table 7.3. *Randomized clinical trials of disease-modifying medications with NP outcome assessment: progressive MS*

Trial	Initial sample	NP measures and design	Primary NP analysis	NP outcome
Methotrexate[41,44]	60 CPMS patients EDSS = 3.0–6.5	Broad-spectrum battery at Baseline, 12 months, 24 months ($n = 40$); focused NP battery every 6 weeks x 24 weeks to a subset of patients ($n = 35$)	MANCOVA of 2-year change scores on 5 variables (15-item BNT, WAIS-R Block Design, PASAT-2″, CVLT Long Delay Free Recall, and WCST Perseverative Responses), with age and education as covariates	Trend toward beneficial overall treatment effect ($P = 0.07$), due primarily to effects on PASAT-2″ ($P = 0.002$); effect on PASAT was evident early in treatment
Betaferon (IFNβ-1b)[42,48]	718 SPMS patients EDSS = 3.0–6.5	Broad-spectrum battery (Selective Reminding Test, 10/36 SRT, PASAT, SDMT, Word List Generation) at baseline, 12 months, 24 months, and 36 months. ($n = 476$ received treatment; 197 healthy controls served as controls for practice effects)	Non-parametric ANCOVAs of change from baseline to last visit on individual tests (stratified by country), with age, gender, education, and baseline score as covariates	No significant treatment effect on individual tests; secondary analyses indicated that fewer IFNβ-1b patients met criteria for "new or worsened cognitive impairment" at 24 months ($P = 0.039$)
Avonex (IFNβ-1a (IM))[43]	436 SPMS patients EDSS = 3.5–6.5	PASAT-3 (as component of MS Functional Composite) at three baseline visits, then every 3 months x 24 months ($n = 217$ received treatment)	Non-parametric ANCOVA of change from baseline to 24 months, stratified by baseline EDSS and Gd enhancement	Trend toward beneficial treatment effect on PASAT-3″ ($P = 0.061$)

The trials depicted in Tables 7.2 and 7.3 differ substantially in terms of their sample sizes, patients, disease course, level of disability at study entry, breadth, and timing of NP outcome assessment, and methods of statistical analysis. In all studies, beneficial effects were observed on primary clinical outcome measures (e.g. relapse rate, EDSS) in each of these trials. One might, therefore, expect positive NP effects as well. These trials provide unusually stringent tests of the NP effects of disease-modifying therapies, however. Cognitive impairment was not an explicit entry criterion, so trial participants varied widely in their levels of cognitive functioning. Even effective disease-modifying medications should not be expected to improve NP performance in cognitively intact patients. Not surprisingly, positive treatment effects on NP tests are undoubtedly attenuated in cognitively heterogeneous samples.

Despite these caveats, the trials listed in Tables 7.2 and 7.3 suggest that beneficial effects of disease-modifying therapies can extend to cognitive function, although these effects may be subtle. Statistically significant NP effects were most often observed on composite NP outcome measures (e.g. multivariate analyses or analyses of "number of failed tests"). In addition, significant effects were more likely to be observed when demographic factors (e.g. age, education, sex), important influences on NP test performance, were carefully controlled by converting raw scores to age- and education-corrected scores based on published norms[45] or using demographic variables as covariates in statistical analyses.[44,47,48] Considerations in the selection of NP outcome measures and the choice of statistical approaches are discussed later in this chapter.

NP studies of symptomatic medications

Table 7.4 summarizes clinical trials designed to assess the efficacy of medications as symptomatic treatment for cognitive impairment. Patients enrolling in these symptomatic trials were required to have documented cognitive deficits, or at minimum subjective cognitive complaints. The typical trial involved a relatively small number of patients ($n < 70$) and was conducted at a single site.[51–56] Recently, larger ($n > 100$) multisite trials have begun to appear in the literature.[57,58] Table 7.5 summarizes drug studies in which the NP impact of symptomatic treatments was of secondary interest and cognitive impairment was not an explicit selection criterion.[59–65] A brief perusal of Tables 7.4 and 7.5 indicates that the trials differ considerably in study design (cross-over vs. parallel groups), sample sizes, choice of NP measures, and statistical analyses.

Results from trials of symptomatic medications conducted in cognitively impaired MS patients (Table 7.4) are mixed. Medications approved for the treatment of Alzheimer's disease (donepezil, rivastigmine, memantine) show either no clinical benefit or a very modest benefit in treating MS-related cognitive dysfunction. Likewise, *Ginkgo biloba* did not appear to be effective for treatment of cognitive dysfunction.[53] Surprisingly, L-amphetamine sulfate, a stimulant, appears to have a promising effect on verbal and visuospatial episodic memory, but no effect on measures of information processing speed and attention.[57] Also promising is the effect of modafinil on measures of simple attention and working memory.[54] Trials that involve amantadine and various forms of aminopyridine, conducted with cognitively heterogeneous patients, do not seem to have a positive treatment effect on NP outcome measures (Table 7.5).

Factors complicating NP outcome assessment in MS trials

Several factors complicate the assessment of NP outcomes in MS trials, although none is insurmountable. The first methodological challenge is the inherently heterogeneous nature of cognitive impairment in MS.[18,25–28] Only about half of all MS patients develop measurable cognitive deficits, and those who do vary considerably in terms of which functions are involved and to what extent. This cognitive heterogeneity has implications for both patient selection and the choice of NP outcome measures. With the advent of the MSFC, disease modifying trials tend to rely solely on a single NP measure, the PASAT. This test is capable of identifying 45%–74% of patients diagnosed with cognitive dysfunction relative to results derived from a comprehensive NP battery.[3,66] Thus, whereas the PASAT is a sensitive measure of cognitive dysfunction in MS, a quarter to half of patients with cognitive dysfunction, primarily in other domains (e.g. episodic memory), will not be classified as impaired from this single test instrument.

A second challenge pertains not only to NP outcome measures but to all potential outcome measures in MS clinical trials: measures with good discriminative properties (i.e. ones that can detect impairment in MS patients relative to healthy controls) do not necessarily have optimal sensitivity to measuring change over time. The differential sensitivity of specific tests is undoubtedly related to several factors, including test difficulty, the potential range and distribution of scores (i.e. floor or ceiling effects), and test reliability. Guyatt and his colleagues[67] have presented a method for evaluating a measure's sensitivity to change, or "responsiveness," that has been applied to the evaluation of MS neurologic rating scales,[68–70] functional abilities scales[69,71,72] and MS quality of life instruments.[73] Responsiveness is an important factor to consider in selecting both NP outcome measures and specific variables from these measures for statistical analyses.

A third factor complicating NP outcome assessment is inherent in many (if not most) NP tests and other performance-based measures: they are often subject to practice effects, regardless of the length of the interest interval.[74–76] Practice effects may differ across populations (e.g. patient groups vs. healthy controls) and even among patients within the same population.[74,75,77] Furthermore, practice effects are not entirely eliminated by using alternate, equivalent forms.[78–80] Practice effects are likely the result of two forms of learning: episodic and procedural learning. In this context, procedural learning refers to the acquisition of knowledge about how to take a test rather than being re-exposed to previous test stimuli. Unlike episodic memory, procedural learning is highly resistant to forgetting. Practice effects can meaningfully influence the interpretation of clinical trial outcomes. For example, a highly significant ($P = 0.005$) difference was observed between natalizumab and placebo groups on the PASAT over the 2-year trial;[50] both groups, however, showed an improvement in performance. If

Table 7.4. Placebo-controlled clinical trials of symptomatic medications for cognitive dysfunction in patients with documented or subjective cognitive deficits at entry

Study	Sample/study design	NP measures	Primary analysis	Outcome
i.v. physostigmine[51]	Four patients (EDSS 3.0–6.0) with documented memory impairment 6-week placebo-controlled crossover (no washout)	Focused battery (Buschke SRT and Digit Span Forward) at baseline, then weekly × 6 weeks	Paired t-tests (1-tailed) on individual measures	Significant treatment effects ($P < 0.05$) on selected Buschke SRT variables (LTS, LTR, STR) and consistent trends ($P < 0.10$) on others; no effect on Digit Span
Donepezil hydrochloride (10 mg/day × 24 weeks)[52]	n = 69 MS patients with documented cognitive impairment 24-week randomized, double-blind, parallel group	Broad-spectrum battery (Brief Repeatable Battery, Tower of Hanoi) at baseline and 24 weeks	Independent samples t-test on pre-post change scores; ANCOVA using age, EDSS, baseline testing, and reading score	Significant treatment effect on primary outcome measure, Buschke SRT ($P < 0.05$); nonsignificant trend for PASAT ($P < 0.10$); no effect on 10/36, SDMT, Word List Generation, and Tower of Hanoi
Ginkgo biloba (240 mg/day × 12 weeks)[53]	n = 39 MS patients with documented impairment on PASAT or CVLT-II 12-week randomized, double-blind, parallel group	Broad-spectrum battery (PASAT, CVLT-II, Stroop, SDMT, Stroop, Useful Field of View Test) at baseline and 12 weeks	Independent samples t-test on pre-post change scores; correction for multiple comparisons	No significant treatment effects; a trend for improved function in the drug group on the Stroop test; more impaired patients at baseline demonstrated a stronger treatment effect
Modafinil (200 mg/day × 16 weeks)[54]	n = 49 RRMS patients with documented impairment on attention measures 6-week randomized, single-blind, parallel group	Broad-spectrum battery (PASAT, CPT, CVLT, Trials, ANAM, Digit Span, Digit Symbol, verbal and visuospatial fluency)	Independent samples t-test on pre-post change scores; no correction for multiple comparisons	Significant ($P < 0.05$) treatment effects on measures of simple attention span, working memory, and verbal fluency; non-significant trends on measures of sustained attention and episodic memory
Rivastigmine (6 mg/day × 12 weeks)[55]	n = 60 MS patients (19 RR, 31 SP, 10 PP) with documented impairment on Wechsler Memory Scales 12 week, randomized, double-blind, parallel group	Focused Battery (subtests of Wechsler Memory Scales)	Independent samples t-test on pre-post change scores	No significant treatment effects observed on the Wechsler Memory Scale General Memory score or subtest scores
Rivastigmine (9 mg/day × 16 weeks)[56]	n = 15 MS patients (12 RR and 3 SP) with subjective complaints of cognitive impairment 32-week randomized, single-blind, crossover (no washout)	Broad-spectrum battery (Brief Repeatable Battery, Stroop, N-Back) at baseline, 16 and 32 weeks	Paired t-tests on average z-scores	Non-significant trend ($P = 0.07$) on BRB for improved cognitive function on vs. off rivastigmine; no performance effects of drug on Stroop and N-Back tasks administered during functional MRI scans
L-amphetamine sulfate (30 mg/day × 29 days)[57]	n = 151 MS patients with documented impairment on SDMT or CVLT-II or PASAT 28 day, randomized, double-blind, parallel group (2:1 drug:placebo)	Broad-spectrum battery (SDMT, CVLT-II, Brief Visual Memory Test, PASAT) at baseline and at 29 days	ANCOVA with baseline scores serving as covariate	No significant effect on primary NP outcome measure (SDMT); significant treatment effects observed on memory measures (delayed recall on the CVLT, $P = 0.012$; total recall and delayed recall on Brief Visual Memory Test ($P = 0.041$ and < 0.01, respectively)
Memantine (20 mg/day × 16 weeks)[58]	n = 114 MS patients (RR, PP, and SP) with documented impairment on PASAT or CVLT-II 16-week randomized, double-blind, parallel group	Broad-spectrum battery (PASAT, CVLT-II, Stroop, SDMT, COWAT, DKEFS) at baseline and 16 weeks	Independent samples t-test on pre-post change scores	No significant treatment effects observed on the primary (PASAT, CVLT-II) and secondary NP outcome measures

Table 7.5. *Placebo-controlled clinical trials of symptomatic medications for cognitive dysfunction in patients with a range of cognitive function at entry*

Study	Sample and study design	NP measures	Primary analysis	NP outcome
Amantadine hydrochloride (100 mg bid)[59]	29 patients (55% RRMS) with mean EDSS = 4.0 (SD = 1.4) and symptomatic daily fatigue x 3 months 10-week placebo-controlled crossover (including 2-week washout)	Broad-spectrum battery at baseline; focused battery (Grooved Pegboard, Trials, SDMT, Consonant Trigram, Stroop, CPT, COWAT) at baseline, 4 weeks, and 10 weeks	Repeated measures ANOVA (Condition x Test Time) of individual tests	Significant treatment effect on Stroop Interference ($P < 0.05$) and trend on Stroop Color Naming ($P = 0.08$)
4-aminopyridine (up to 10 mg qid)[60]	20 patients (90% CPMS) with EDSS 2.5–8.0 4-week placebo-controlled cross-over (no washout)	Broad-spectrum battery (16-item verbal learning, 10/36 SRT, PASAT, SDMT, Word List Generation) at baseline, 2 weeks, 4 weeks	t-tests comparing conditions on change scores for individual measures	No significant treatment effects, but trends on PASAT-2" ($P = 0.09$) and 10/36 SRT Delayed Recall ($P = 0.06$)
3,4 diaminopyridine (up to 100 mg/day, divided)[61]	36 patients (81% CPMS) with EDSS 2.5–9.0 and leg weakness 90-day placebo-controlled crossover, including 30-day washout	Broad-spectrum battery (Buschke Selective Reminding, 10/36 SRT, PASAT, SDMT, Word List Generation) at baseline, 30 days, 60 days, 90 days	Paired Wilcoxon signed rank tests comparing scores on individual measures during placebo and DAP conditions	No significant treatment effects
Amantadine (100 mg bid) vs. pemoline (56.25 mg)[62]	45 patients with EDSS < 6.5 and documented fatigue 6-week placebo-controlled parallel groups	Broad-spectrum battery (Digit Span, SDMT, Trials, Buschke Selective Reminding, BVRT) at baseline, 6 weeks	ANOVAs (Group x Test Time) of individual measures	Significant treatment effect on written SDMT ($P < 0.03$), favoring amantidine; similar trend on oral SDMT ($P < 0.08$)
Amantadine (100 mg bid)[63]	24 patients (58% SPMS) with EDSS ≤ 6.5 and documented fatigue (FSS > 4) Placebo-controlled cross-over, including 10-day washout	Focused battery (computerized visual selective attention task administered twice, 2 weeks apart (once in each condition)	MANOVA (Condition x Test Time) on RTs	No overall treatment effect, although amantadine significantly enhanced practice effects (but attenuated initial learning) in patients with longer disease duration ($P < 0.002$)
4-aminopyridine (32 mg qd)[64]	54 progressive MS patients 12-month placebo-controlled crossover	Focused battery	Between-group change on individual tests	No significant treatment effects
Sustained release 4-aminopyridine (10–40 mg qd)[65]	36 patients (7 RR, 3 PP, 26 SP) 7-week randomized, double-blind, placebo-controlled, dose-ranging	Focused battery (PASAT as part of MSFC) administered at baseline and once per week x 7 weeks	Repeated measures ANOVA	No significant treatment effects

strictly interpreted, one might conclude from this study, probably erroneously, that natalizumab improves cognitive functioning.

A fourth challenge in assessing NP outcomes in MS trials is the definition of abnormal performance. On most NP measures, normal performance is not intuitively obvious, but instead, must be defined with respect to some normative group (i.e. demographically comparable healthy controls). A placebo control group in a randomized clinical trial can serve as a reference for evaluating treatment effects, but not for defining the presence and magnitude of cognitive impairment. Assessing NP outcomes is similar to assessing other quantifiable functional abilities (e.g. timed gait, fine motor speed, and coordination) in this respect. Development of longitudinal normative databases

for quantitative functional outcome measures (including NP tests) would greatly facilitate analysis and interpretation of clinical trial data.

Finally, as mentioned above, only about 5%–9% of patients will experience deterioration on NP tests annually in natural history studies,[6,9,24] even when practice effects are controlled using longitudinally yoked healthy control subjects as a reference. This relatively low rate suggests that most disease-modifying trials would require very large patient samples to identify a treatment effect using NP tests as outcomes.

The remainder of this chapter is intended to guide NP test selection, study design, and statistical analysis for those wishing to incorporate NP outcome assessment into their clinical trials.

Recommendations for design and analysis of NP outcome assessment in MS trials

Is a single NP measure adequate for assessing cognition in clinical trials? This question applies principally to trials of disease-modifying medications, since trials of symptomatic interventions for MS-related cognitive dysfunction will most likely include measures assessing several domains of interest. Investigators may wonder, for example, whether the cognitive component of the MS Functional Composite[81–84] (i.e. the Paced Auditory Serial Addition Test[3,85]) is sufficient for assessing NP outcomes in a clinical trial. Although the MSFC, which comprises quantitative tests of arm/hand, leg, and cognitive function, clearly represents an important advance in MS clinical outcome assessment, it was not designed to comprehensively assess either cognitive or physical function. Just as neurologic function in MS cannot be adequately captured by assessing only one functional system, no single NP test provides a comprehensive assessment of the treatment effects in a cognitively heterogeneous disease like MS.

With these caveats in mind, the PASAT has several features to recommend it for this purpose. The 3-second version can be administered in less than 5 minutes. It is multidimensional and therefore capable of detecting change in more than one domain of cognitive function. Specifically, the PASAT taps calculation ability and processing speed/working memory,[86] both of which have been shown to deteriorate over time in MS.[24] Finally, the PASAT's sensitivity to treatment effects or trends has already been demonstrated in several MS disease-modifying clinical trials.[43,44,47,50] The PASAT also have some disadvantages: it does not assess learning and memory, which are commonly impaired in MS; it is a challenging task, one that may meet with resistance from both patients and examiners; it is prone to practice effects; and patients may adopt strategies while performing the PASAT that effectively alter task demands and potentially compromise the task's sensitivity, particularly at faster stimulus presentation rates.[87]

In recent years, there has been some discussion of substituting the PASAT with the oral version of the Symbol Digit Modalities Test (SDMT) as the cognitive component of the MSFC.[88,89] Drake *et al.*[88] administered the SDMT and PASAT to 400 MS patients and 100 demographically matched controls; a subset of MS patients ($n = 115$) were retested 2.1 years later. The two tests were equally adept at discriminating MS patients from healthy controls based on a receiver operating characteristic (ROC) analysis. The test-retest correlations for the PASAT and SDMT were 0.78 and 0.74, respectively. No statistically significant differences were observed in longitudinal changes in raw test scores (39.9 ± 13.5 to 41.9 ± 14.5 for the PASAT; 49.2 ± 11.8 to 48.9 ± 12.2 for the SDMT), suggesting that practice effects are comparable in MS patients. As acknowledged by Drake *et al.*,[88] there are no available data to show that the SDMT is more or less sensitive to medication effects than the PASAT.

Which NP measures should be included in future symptomatic MS trials? Comprehensive assessment of the NP effects of symptomatic treatments will necessarily involve several measures that capture different cognitive domains. Unfortunately, faced with a plethora of available NP measures, each MS investigator group has chosen a slightly different combination of tests. Some have adopted a broad-spectrum approach (i.e. selecting measures that together assess a broad range of cognitive domains), whereas others have opted for more focused batteries that cover only one or two domains of interest. A focused battery has the advantage of narrowing the number of primary outcome measures. However, the drug demonstrated a non-significant treatment effect on the primary NP measures of attention and a positive treatment effect on the secondary measures assessing episodic memory.[57] One alternative is to use composite measures (using z-scores as done in the MSFC) or to calculate the number of statistically worsened scores in a broad-spectrum battery.

The broad-spectrum approach has the disadvantage of being time consuming, with some batteries taking over an hour to administer. Use of a broad-spectrum NP battery may also increase the risk of Type II statistical errors (i.e. failure to detect a true treatment effect) if it includes unresponsive measures or if alpha level adjustments to accommodate multiple statistical tests are too stringent. The Brief Repeatable NP Battery (BRB)[90] is a frequently used broad-spectrum battery in clinical MS trials and takes approximately 30 minutes to administer. A more comprehensive broad-spectrum battery for monitoring MS patients is the Minimal Assessment of Cognitive Function in MS (MACFIMS)[91] (see Table 7.6). The MACFIMS takes approximately 90 minutes to administer and was created on the basis of a consensus panel of neuropsychologists convened by the Consortium of MS Centers (CMSC) in 2001. To date, the MACFIMS has not been used in its entirety as part of a medication trial.

Do computerized NP test batteries offer advantages relative to traditional paper-and-pencil tests? In recent years, several computerized NP batteries have begun to appear in the MS neuropsychology literature.[92–94] Some computerized NP tests closely resemble their paper-and-pencil counterparts with some modifications needed to accommodate a manual than verbal response. Other computerized tests draw heavily from the cognitive neuroscience literature and have not been widely used clinically. Computerized testing offers several advantages: (1) test instructions and administration can be better standardized than paper-and-pencil tests, thus reducing administration errors within and across sites in a clinical trial, (2) computerized tests can measure reaction times with millisecond accuracy, and (3) test scoring is accurate and immediate. One common misconception about computerized tests is that they do not require the presence of a human test administrator. Another concern about computerized tests is the overreliance on a manual response. MS-related motor impairment due to lesions located outside the cerebral hemispheres may give the false impression of cognitive impairment on reaction time measures. In addition, MS patients are more impaired on free recall than recognition episodic memory tests;[1] computerized

Table 7.6. *Tests in the minimal assessment of cognitive function in MS (MACFIMS)*

Test	Estimated administration time	Comment
Processing speed and working memory		
Paced Auditory Serial Addition Test (PASAT)	10 minutes	Rao version, using 3.0- and 2.0-second interstimulus intervals. Two equivalent forms are available.
Symbol Digit Modalities Test (SDMT)	5 minutes	Oral administration only. Multiple forms are available, although their equivalence has not been established.
Learning and memory		
California Verbal Learning Test-II (CVLT-2)	25 minutes	There are two equivalent alternate forms.
Brief Visuospatial Memory Test-Revised (BVMT-R)	10 minutes	There are six equivalent alternate forms.
Executive functions		
California Sorting Test (CST)	25 minutes	Two equivalent forms are available. To conserve time, only free sort condition may be administered.
Visuospatial perception		
Judgment of Line Orientation Test (JLO)	10 minutes	Two forms are described in the manual but are actually the same test items administered in a different order.
Language/Other		
Controlled Oral Word Association Test (COWAT)	5 minutes	Two alternate forms are available.

Data: reproduced with permission.[91]
Note: It is recommended that the MACFIMS be supplemented by a measure of estimated premorbid abilities (e.g. National Adult Reading Test [NART]; North American Adult Reading Test [NAART]; WRAT-3 Reading, or selected WAIS-R Verbal subtests) at the baseline study visit, a measure of self-reported depression (Chicago Multiscale Depression Inventory [CMDI] at all study visits, and other measures of potential confounding factors as appropriate for the study population.

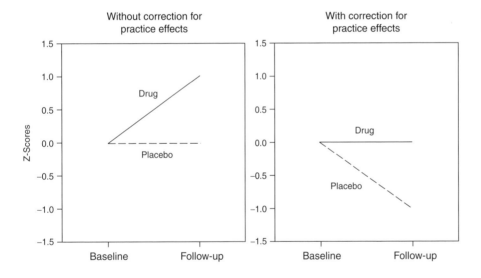

Fig. 7.1. Results of hypothetical clinical trial involving a NP outcome measure.

tests typically measure only recognition memory. Computerized tests are relatively new and typically do not have extensive normative databases. Finally, only one clinical trial[63] has used a computerized test battery to date.

Can anything be done regarding practice effects? In a randomized, placebo-controlled, parallel group clinical trial, drug effects can be identified whether or not an instrument demonstrates practice effects (see left panel of Fig. 7.1). In this hypothetical trial, the treated group demonstrates an improvement in NP test performance and the placebo group's NP performance is unchanged. As mentioned previously, one might infer from these data that the drug agent has "improved" cognitive function. While this could be the case, practice effects are a reasonable alternative explanation. One method for "correcting" practice effects would be to adjust the MS patient's NP scores based on the performance of healthy control subjects administered NP tests on the same retest schedule as used in the clinical trial. The right panel of Fig. 7.1 illustrates such an adjustment. Note that the magnitude of difference between the drug and placebo groups is unchanged. The adjustment allows for a more reasonable measurement of disease progression in the placebo group of disease-modifying trials. There are, however, two potential problems with this approach: (1) a longitudinal NP database derived from healthy control subjects demographically matched to MS patients does not currently exist, and (2) this approach assumes that practice effects are comparable in MS and healthy control subjects.

An alternative approach is to administer NP outcome measures several times prior to initiating treatment. This "run-in" approach at the outset of a trial would not only permit estimation of the natural variability in test performance in clinically stable patients but also allow test performance to be stabilized, thereby minimizing practice effects during the treatment phase. Such an approach was adopted in the clinical trial of IFNβ-1a (IM) for secondary progressive MS.[43] There are some disadvantages to this approach, however. Not only does a run-in add costs to conducting a clinical trial, but it assumes that practice effects will plateau after a fixed number of assessments. Unfortunately, learning curves may vary considerably across NP tests and test samples. In addition, massing NP test administrations may produce artificially elevated test scores at baseline and give the false impression that cognitive functions have declined after a 1- or 2-year follow-up assessment.

Given the low rate of progression of cognitive functioning in MS patients, is it possible to enrich a clinical trial by selecting patients with a higher rate of progression? As mentioned previously, natural history studies suggest that 5%–9% of patients will experience deterioration on NP tests annually in natural history studies.[6,9,24] A recent longitudinal study[95] suggests that more extensive MRI involvement at baseline can predict a more rapid decline in NP test performance over a five year retest interval. Similar findings were observed in another study.[96] Clinical trials with a focus on NP outcome measures, therefore, may wish to enrich their samples with patients having more extensive brain involvement on MRI scans at entry.

What should be done to ensure the quality of NP data collected during clinical trials? Several steps can be taken to increase the likelihood that NP data collection will be complete and accurate, thereby reducing error variance. First, the neuropsychologist responsible for this component of the clinical trial should ensure that examiners who will be administering and scoring the NP outcome measures are appropriately trained. Optimal reliability is achieved when training is centralized and when a standardized manual and training procedures are used.[97] Second, examiners should practice administering and scoring the NP outcome measures several times prior to administering them to study participants. Finally, all test protocols (including "practice protocols") should be reviewed at a central NP coordinating center, which should provide timely feedback to examiners regarding the accuracy of test administration and scoring. The NP coordinating center should also be responsible for transcribing data onto case report forms.

How should NP outcome measures be analyzed statistically? Analysis of NP outcomes in MS clinical trials has typically consisted of comparing the mean change in test performance of patients in different treatment conditions from baseline to the end of the treatment phase, using analysis of variance-based (ANOVA) methods or analogous non-parametric procedures. In most trials, NP measures have been analyzed individually for evidence of treatment effects, and demographic factors that can influence NP test performance have not been controlled. The conventional approach to NP outcome assessment has not consistently yielded statistically significant results, however, even for treatments with documented effects on other outcome measures.

Several steps can be taken to improve the sensitivity of NP outcome analyses. First, it is essential to minimize irrelevant sources of variance ("noise") in order to be able to detect treatment effects ("signal"), which are often subtle. One method for minimizing error variance is to standardize test procedures and testing conditions, as recommended earlier. Irrelevant variance can be further reduced by statistically "extracting" the effects of demographic factors that can affect test performance. Adjustment of raw test scores or covariance analysis is only appropriate when treatment groups are demographically comparable at baseline, however.

Second, subtle treatment effects may be more evident when multiple outcome measures are analyzed simultaneously.[98] If data from demographically matched healthy controls are available, analysis of aggregate NP outcomes might include counting "number of failed tests," as was done in a secondary outcome analysis for the IFNβ-1b trial in secondary progressive MS.[48] An alternative approach would be to construct a NP composite variable or to perform a multivariate analysis of variance (MANOVA). (Both yield identical results statistically if equal weightings are used in constructing the composite.) In order to maximize the sensitivity of a NP composite, its component variables must not be highly correlated and the individual measures should be sensitive to change within the time frame of the trial (cf. IFNβ-1a (IM) trial for relapsing remitting MS,[47] where treatment effects or trends were observed on composites of domains commonly compromised in MS, but not on a composite measure of attention span and overall verbal abilities).

Third, when NP outcome measures are administered several times during the treatment phase, statistical techniques that make use of all available data should be employed. One such approach is random-effects regression modeling (also known as hierarchical linear modeling, or HLM), in which slopes and intercepts are calculated for each individual patient in order to characterize different patterns of change over time.[99–102] HLM cannot only accommodate variable follow-up intervals, but it also permits interpolation of missing data. In addition, it can incorporate adjustments for demographic variables, practice effects, and regression to the mean. Applications in neurologic disease have included analysis of NP progression in Alzheimer's disease[102] and HIV infection,[103–105] treatment outcome analysis in an ALS clinical trial,[106] and secondary analyses of NP outcome data from the IFNβ-1a (IM) trial.[47]

Another statistical approach that makes use of all available data is survival analysis, which calculates the length of time it takes for patients to reach a predetermined criterion for significant deterioration.[107,108] An extension of survival analysis that incorporates both deterioration and improvement, termed multi-state analysis, is also available.[109] Survival analysis has been widely adopted as the primary method for analyzing clinical outcomes in trials of disease-modifying medications for MS.[37,41–43,110,111] It was also used in a secondary NP outcome analysis in the trial of IFNβ-1a (IM) in relapsing remitting MS.[47] In that trial, a conventional statistical cutoff was used as the criterion for significant deterioration (i.e. change of at least 0.5 SD relative to baseline), but alternatively, the reliable change index[112–115] or regression-based norms for change[76,116,117] could be used to establish the criterion for meaningful change.

Finally, variations in treatment response among patients assigned to the same treatment condition can be obscured if analyses are confined to treatment groups as a whole. Consequently, subgroup analyses should be performed. One simple method for subdividing patients neuropsychologically is to perform a median split based on patients' initial NP performance. A more sophisticated method for grouping patients would be to use cluster analysis to identify patients who differ in their baseline pattern of performance on several different NP measures.[27,28] If healthy control data are available, patients can be categorized based on whether they were neuropsychologically intact or impaired at baseline. NP subgroup membership can then serve as a between-subjects factor (or potentially a covariate) in analyses of treatment response.

Can a positive outcome involving NP outcome measures be accepted as an indication of treatment efficacy by governmental oversight agencies such as the FDA? At present, no NP test is accepted as an outcome measure by the FDA for MS clinical trials. Thus it is unlikely that a change in drug labeling is likely to occur even if the medication has a positive effect in treating cognition or preventing its progression. In part, this may be due to the traditional view that disability in MS is influenced more by sensory and motor symptoms rather than cognitive dysfunction (despite evidence to the contrary[1]). One problem is a lack of understanding of how changes in NP testing over time translate into changes in the activities of daily living in MS patients. Investigators in schizophrenia, through a partnership with the NIH, FDA, and pharmaceutical industry, have established a method for validating a NP battery (MATRICS) suitable for clinical trials.[118] Their experience may serve as a model for validating NP measures for MS trials.

Future directions

With the recent development of functional MRI, it has been possible to image MS patients while they perform cognitive tests in the scanner.[119–122] In general, these fMRI studies have demonstrated that, even when cognitive testing is comparable to healthy controls, MS patients exhibit a larger number of activated regions, an increase in MR signal change and spatial extent in regions also activated by controls, and a decrease in laterality indices (indicating more bilateral activation). These compensation brain changes often correlate with the extent of structural brain changes (T2 lesion burden).[123] Using a Stroop activation task, Parry *et al.*[124] employed fMRI as an outcome measure for assessing the efficacy of rivastigmine, a cholinesterase inhibitor, in five MS patients. All five demonstrated a normalization of the activation pattern relative to control subjects as a result of this intervention; no drug-related brain changes were observed in the control subjects. These promising results suggest that fMRI may become a useful outcome measure for assessing the neural correlates of cognitive performance in MS clinical trials involving symptomatic therapies.

Concluding remarks

The widespread prevalence of MS-related cognitive dysfunction, its direct relationship to cerebral MS lesions but weak relationship to physical disability, and its devastating functional impact are now widely recognized. There is convincing evidence from clinical trials of both disease-modifying therapies and symptomatic treatments that NP outcome measures can detect even subtle treatment effects, provided that sensitive measures are chosen and appropriate statistical techniques are applied. Furthermore, recent large-scale studies of symptomatic treatments for MS-related cognitive dysfunction show some progress in identifying medications that may be useful for treating memory and attentional dysfunction. Now that there is consensus regarding a comprehensive, yet practical, approach for assessing cognitive function in MS, attention can turn to development of a longitudinal normative database to correct for practice effects, methods for aggregating test scores, and empirically supported criteria for significant change to move NP outcome assessment forward in the next generation of MS clinical trials.

Acknowledgment

I want to thank Joshua Cohen for his assistance with the literature review.

References

1. Bobholz JA, Rao SM. Cognitive dysfunction in multiple sclerosis: a review of recent developments. *Curr Opin Neurol* 2003;16: 283–8.

2. Heaton RK, Nelson LM, Thompson DS, Burks JS, Franklin GM. Neuropsychological findings in relapsing-remitting and chronic-progressive multiple sclerosis. *J Consult Clin Psychol* 1985;53: 103–10.

3. Rao SM, Leo GJ, Bernardin L, Unverzagt F. Cognitive dysfunction in multiple sclerosis. I. Frequency, patterns, and prediction. *Neurology* 1991;41: 685–91.

4. Rao SM, Leo GJ, Ellington L, Nauertz T, Bernardin L, Unverzagt F. Cognitive dysfunction in multiple sclerosis. II.

Impact on employment and social functioning. *Neurology* 1991;41: 692–6.

5. Beatty WW, Blanco CR, Wilbanks SL, Paul RH, Hames KA. Demographic, clinical, and cognitive characteristics of multiple sclerosis patients who continue to work. *J Neurol Rehabil* 1995;9: 167–73.

6. Amato MP, Ponziani G, Siracusa G, Sorbi S. Cognitive dysfunction in early-onset multiple sclerosis: a reappraisal after 10 years. *Arch Neurol* 2001;58: 1602–6.

7. Schultheis MT, Garay E, DeLuca J. The influence of cognitive impairment on driving performance in multiple sclerosis. *Neurology* 2001;56: 1089–94.

8. Schultheis MT, Garay E, Millis SR, DeLuca J. Motor vehicle crashes and violations among drivers with multiple sclerosis. *Arch Phys Med Rehabil* 2002;83: 1175–8.

9. Amato MP, Ponziani G, Pracucci G, Bracco L, Siracusa G, Amaducci L. Cognitive impairment in early-onset multiple sclerosis. Pattern, predictors, and impact on everyday life in a 4-year follow-up. *Arch Neurol* 1995;52: 168–72.

10. Higginson CI, Arnett PA, Voss WD. The ecological validity of clinical tests of memory and attention in multiple sclerosis. *Arch Clin Neuropsychol* 2000;15: 185–204.

11. Langdon DW, Thompson AJ. Multiple sclerosis: a preliminary study of selected variables affecting rehabilitation outcome. *Mult Scler* 1999;5: 94–100.

12. Knight RG, Devereux RC, Godfrey HP. Psychosocial consequences of caring for a spouse with multiple sclerosis. *J Clin Exp Neuropsychol* 1997;19: 7–19.

13. Chipchase SY, Lincoln NB. Factors associated with carer strain in carers of people with multiple sclerosis. *Disabil Rehabil* 2001;23: 768–76.

14. Filippi M, Rocca MA, Benedict RH, *et al.* The contribution of MRI in assessing cognitive impairment in multiple sclerosis. *Neurology* 2010;75: 2121–8.

15. Hohol MJ, Guttmann CR, Orav J, *et al.* Serial neuropsychological assessment and magnetic resonance imaging analysis in multiple sclerosis. *Arch Neurol* 1997;54: 1018–25.

16. Sperling RA, Guttmann CR, Hohol MJ, *et al.* Regional magnetic resonance imaging lesion burden and cognitive function in multiple sclerosis: a longitudinal study. *Arch Neurol* 2001;58: 115–21.

17. Zivadinov R, Sepcic J, Nasuelli D, *et al.* A longitudinal study of brain atrophy and cognitive disturbances in the early phase of relapsing-remitting multiple sclerosis. *J Neurol Neurosurg Psychiatry* 2001;70: 773–80.

18. Fischer JS. Using the Wechsler Memory Scale-Revised to detect and characterize memory deficits in multiple sclerosis. *Clin Neuropsychol* 1988;2: 149–72.

19. Filippi M, Horsfield MA, Morrissey SP, *et al.* Quantitative brain MRI lesion load predicts the course of clinically isolated syndromes suggestive of multiple sclerosis. *Neurology* 1994;44: 635–41.

20. Grossman M, Armstrong C, Onishi K, *et al.* Patterns of cognitive impairment in relapsing–remitting and chronic progressive multiple sclerosis. *Neuropsychiatry Neuropsychol Behav Neurol* 1994;7: 194–210.

21. Van Den Burg W, van Zomeren AH, Minderhoud JM, Prange AJ, Meijer NS. Cognitive impairment in patients with multiple sclerosis and mild physical disability. *Arch Neurol* 1987;44: 494–501.

22. Beatty WW, Goodkin DE, Hertsgaard D, Monson N. Clinical and demographic predictors of cognitive performance in multiple sclerosis. Do diagnostic type, disease duration, and disability matter? *Arch Neurol* 1990;47: 305–8.

23. Whitaker JN, McFarland HF, Rudge P, Reingold SC. Outcomes assessment in multiple sclerosis clinical trials: a critical analysis. *Mult Scler* 1995;1: 37–47.

24. Bobholz JA, Rao SM, Sweet LH, Patterson K, Binder JR, Lobeck L. Cognitive decline in multiple sclerosis: An 8-year longitudinal investigation. *J Int Neuropsychol Soc* 1998;4: 35.

25. Rao SM, Hammeke TA, McQuillen MP, Khatri BO, Lloyd D. Memory disturbance in chronic progressive multiple sclerosis. *Arch Neurol* 1984;41: 625–31.

26. Beatty WW, Wilbanks SL, Blanco CR, Hames KA, Tivis R, Paul RH. Memory disturbance in multiple sclerosis: reconsideration of patterns of performance on the selective reminding test. *J Clin Exp Neuropsychol* 1996;18: 56–62.

27. Ryan L, Clark C, Klonoff H. Patterns of cognitive impairment in relapsing-remitting multiple sclerosis and their relationship to neuropathology on magnetic resonance images. *Neuropsychology* 1996;10: 176–93.

28. Fischer JS, Jacobs LD, Cookfair DL, *et al.* Heterogeneity of cognitive dysfunction in multiple sclerosis. *Clin Psychol* 1998;12: 286.

29. Jennekens-Schinkel A, Laboyrie PM, Lanser JB, Van Der Velde EA. Cognition in patients with multiple sclerosis after four years. *J Neurol Sci* 1990;99: 229–47.

30. Kujala P, Portin R, Ruutiainen J. The progress of cognitive decline in multiple sclerosis. A controlled 3-year follow-up. *Brain* 1997;120 (2): 289–97.

31. Fischer JS. Cognitive impairment in multiple sclerosis. In Cook SD, ed. *Handbook of Multiple Sclerosis.* New York: Marcel Dekker, 2001: 233–55.

32. Amato MP, Zipoli V, Portaccio E. Multiple sclerosis-related cognitive changes: a review of cross-sectional and longitudinal studies. *J Neurol Sci* 2006;245: 41–6.

33. Genova HM, Sumowski JF, Chiaravalloti N, Voelbel GT, DeLuca J. Cognition in multiple sclerosis: a review of neuropsychological and fMRI research. *Front Biosci* 2009;14: 1730–44.

34. O'Brien AR, Chiaravalloti N, Goverover Y, DeLuca J. Evidenced-based cognitive rehabilitation for persons with multiple sclerosis: a review of the literature. *Arch Phys Med Rehabil* 2008;89: 761–9.

35. The IFNB Multiple Sclerosis Study Group. Interferon beta-1b is effective in relapsing–remitting multiple sclerosis. I. Clinical results of a multicenter, randomized, double-blind, placebo-controlled trial. *Neurology* 1993;43: 655–61.

36. Johnson KP, Brooks BR, Cohen JA, *et al.* Copolymer 1 reduces relapse rate and improves disability in relapsing–remitting multiple sclerosis: results of a phase III multicenter, double-blind placebo-controlled trial. The Copolymer 1 Multiple Sclerosis Study Group. *Neurology* 1995;45: 1268–76.

37. Jacobs LD, Cookfair DL, Rudick RA, *et al.* Intramuscular interferon beta-1a for disease progression in relapsing multiple sclerosis. The Multiple Sclerosis Collaborative Research Group (MSCRG). *Ann Neurol* 1996;39: 285–94.

38. Polman CH, O'Connor PW, Havrdova E *et al.* A randomized, placebo-controlled trial of natalizumab for relapsing multiple sclerosis. *N Engl J Med* 2006;354: 899–910.

39. Rudick RA, Stuart WH, Calabresi PA, *et al.* Natalizumab plus interferon beta-1a for relapsing multiple sclerosis. *N Engl J Med* 2006;354: 911–23.

40. Cohen JA, Barkhof F, Comi G, *et al.* Oral fingolimod or intramuscular interferon for relapsing multiple sclerosis. *N Engl J Med* 2010;362: 402–15.

41. Goodkin DE, Rudick RA, VanderBrug MS, *et al.* Low-dose (7.5 mg) oral methotrexate reduces the rate of progression in chronic progressive multiple sclerosis. *Ann Neurol* 1995;37: 30–40.

42. European Study Group on interferon beta-1b in secondary progressive MS. Placebo-controlled multicentre randomised trial of interferon beta-1b in treatment of secondary progressive multiple sclerosis. *Lancet* 1998;352: 1491–7.

43. Cohen JA, Cutter GR, Fischer JS, *et al.* Benefit of interferon beta-1a on MSFC progression in secondary progressive MS. *Neurology* 2002;59: 679–87.

44. Goodkin DE, Fischer JS. Treatment of multiple sclerosis with methotrexate. In Goodkin DE, Rudick RA, eds. *Multiple Sclerosis: Advances in Clinical Trial Design, Treatment and Future Perspectives*. London: Springer, 1996: 251–89.

45. Pliskin NH, Hamer DP, Goldstein DS, *et al.* Improved delayed visual reproduction test performance in multiple sclerosis patients receiving interferon beta-1b. *Neurology* 1996;47: 1463–8.

46. Weinstein A, Schwid SI, Schiffer RB, McDermott MP, Giang DW, Goodman AD. Neuropsychologic status in multiple sclerosis after treatment with glatiramer acetate (Copaxone). *Arch Neurol* 1999;56: 319–24.

47. Fischer JS, Priore RL, Jacobs LD, *et al.* Neuropsychological effects of interferon beta-1a in relapsing multiple sclerosis. Multiple Sclerosis Collaborative Research Group. *Ann Neurol* 2000;48: 885–92.

48. Langdon DW, Thompson AJ, Hamalainen P, *et al.* Effect of IFNB-1b on cognition in secondary progressive multiple sclerosis. 2006 (unpublished).

49. Havrdova E. The effects of natalizumab on a test of cognitive function in patients wiuth relapsing multiple sclerosis (MS). *Eur J Neurol* 2006;13 (Suppl. 2): 307.

50. Polman CH, Rudick RA. The multiple sclerosis functional composite: a clinically meaningful measure of disability. *Neurology* 2010;74 Suppl 3: S8–15.

51. Leo GJ, Rao SM. Effects of intravenous physostigmine and lecithin on memory loss in multiple sclerosis: Report of a pilot study. *J Neurol Rehabil* 1988;2: 123–9.

52. Krupp LB, Christodoulou C, Melville P, Scherl W, Mac Allister W, Elkins LE. Donepezil improved memory in multiple sclerosis in a randomized clinical trial. *Neurology* 2004;63: 1579–85.

53. Lovera J, Bagert B, Smoot K, *et al.* Ginkgo biloba for the improvement of cognitive performance in multiple sclerosis: a randomized, placebo-controlled trial. *Mult Scler* 2007;13: 376–85.

54. Wilken JA, Sullivan C, Wallin M, *et al.* Treatment of multiple sclerosis-related cognitive problems with adjunctive modafinil: rationale and preliminary supportive data. *Int J MS Care* 2008;10: 1–10.

55. Shaygannejad V, Janghorbani M, Ashtari F, Zanjani HA, Zakizade N. Effects of rivastigmine on memory and cognition in multiple sclerosis. *Can J Neurol Sci* 2008;35: 476–81.

56. Cader S, Palace J, Matthews PM. Cholinergic agonism alters cognitive processing and enhances brain functional connectivity in patients with multiple sclerosis. *J Psychopharmacol* 2009;23: 686–96.

57. Morrow SA, Kaushik T, Zarevics P, *et al.* The effects of L-amphetamine sulfate on cognition in MS patients: results of a randomized controlled trial. *J Neurol* 2009;256: 1095–102.

58. Lovera JF, Frohman E, Brown TR, *et al.* Memantine for cognitive impairment in multiple sclerosis: a randomized placebo-controlled trial. *Mult Scler* 2010;16: 715–23.

59. Cohen RA, Fischer M. Amantadine treatment of fatigue associated with multiple sclerosis. *Arch Neurol* 1989;46: 676–80.

60. Smits RC, Emmen HH, Bertelsmann FW, Kulig BM, van Loenen AC, Polman CH. The effects of 4-aminopyridine on cognitive function in patients with multiple sclerosis: a pilot study. *Neurology* 1994;44: 1701–5.

61. Bever CT, Jr., Anderson PA, Leslie J, *et al.* Treatment with oral 3,4 diaminopyridine improves leg strength in multiple sclerosis patients: results of a randomized, double-blind, placebo-controlled, crossover trial. *Neurology* 1996;47: 1457–62.

62. Geisler MW, Sliwinski M, Coyle PK, Masur DM, Doscher C, Krupp LB. The effects of amantadine and pemoline on cognitive functioning in multiple sclerosis. *Arch Neurol* 1996;53: 185–8.

63. Sailer M, Heinze HJ, Schoenfeld MA, Hauser U, Smid HG. Amantadine influences cognitive processing in patients with multiple sclerosis. *Pharmacopsychiatry* 2000;33: 28–37.

64. Rossini PM, Pasqualetti P, Pozzilli C, *et al.* Fatigue in progressive multiple sclerosis: results of a randomized, double-blind, placebo-controlled, crossover trial of oral 4-aminopyridine. *Mult Scler* 2001;7: 354–8.

65. Goodman AD, Cohen JA, Cross A, *et al.* Fampridine-SR in multiple sclerosis: a randomized, double-blind, placebo-controlled, dose-ranging study. *Mult Scler* 2007;13: 357–68.

66. Rosti E, Hamalainen P, Koivisto K, Hokkanen L. PASAT in detecting cognitive impairment in relapsing–remitting MS. *Appl Neuropsychol* 2007;14: 101–12.

67. Guyatt G, Walter S, Norman G. Measuring change over time: assessing the usefulness of evaluative instruments. *J Chronic Dis* 1987;40: 171–8.

68. Koziol JA, Lucero A, Sipe JC, Romine JS, Beutler E. Responsiveness of the Scripps neurologic rating scale during a multiple sclerosis clinical trial. *Can J Neurol Sci* 1999;26: 283–9.

69. Sharrack B, Hughes RA, Soudain S, Dunn G. The psychometric properties of clinical rating scales used in multiple sclerosis. *Brain* 1999;122 (1): 141–59.

70. Hobart J, Freeman J, Thompson A. Kurtzke scales revisited: the application of psychometric methods to clinical intuition. *Brain* 2000;123 (5): 1027–40.

71. Van Der Putten JJ, Hobart JC, Freeman JA, Thompson AJ. Measuring change in disability after inpatient rehabilitation: comparison of the responsiveness of the Barthel index and the Functional Independence Measure. *J Neurol Neurosurg Psychiatry* 1999;66: 480–4.

72. Hobart J, Freeman J, Lamping D, Fitzpatrick R, Thompson A. The SF-36 in multiple sclerosis: why basic assumptions must be tested. *J Neurol Neurosurg Psychiatry* 2001;71: 363–70.

73. Hobart J, Lamping D, Fitzpatrick R, Riazi A, Thompson A. The Multiple Sclerosis Impact Scale (MSIS-29): a new patient-based outcome measure. *Brain* 2001;124: 962–73.

74. Dikmen SS, Heaton RK, Grant I, Temkin NR. Test-retest reliability and practice effects of expanded Halstead–Reitan Neuropsychological Test Battery. *J Int Neuropsychol Soc* 1999;5: 346–56.

75. McCaffrey RJ, Westervelt HJ. Issues associated with repeated neuropsychological assessments. *Neuropsychol Rev* 1995;5: 203–21.

76. Salinsky MC, Storzbach D, Dodrill CB, Binder LM. Test-retest bias, reliability, and regression equations for neuropsychological measures repeated over a 12–16-week period. *J Int Neuropsychol Soc* 2001;7: 597–605.

77. Frank R, Wiederholt WC, Kritz-Silverstein DK, Salmon DP, Barrett-Connor E. Effects of sequential neuropsychological testing of an elderly community-based sample. *Neuroepidemiology* 1996;15: 257–68.

78. Bever CT, Jr., Grattan L, Panitch HS, Johnson KP. The brief repeatable battery of neuropsychological tests for multiple sclerosis: a preliminary serial study. *Mult Scler* 1995;1: 165–9.

79. Hannay HJ, Levin HS. Selective reminding test: an examination of the equivalence of four forms. *J Clin Exp Neuropsychol* 1985;7: 251–63.

80. Benedict RH, Zgaljardic DJ. Practice effects during repeated administrations of memory tests with and without alternate forms. *J Clin Exp Neuropsychol* 1998;20: 339–52.

81. Rudick R, Antel J, Confavreux C, *et al.* Clinical outcomes assessment in multiple sclerosis. *Ann Neurol* 1996;40: 469–79.

82. Rudick R, Antel J, Confavreux C, *et al.* Recommendations from the National Multiple Sclerosis Society Clinical Outcomes Assessment Task Force. *Ann Neurol* 1997;42: 379–82.

83. Cutter GR, Baier ML, Rudick RA, Cookfair DL, Fischer JS, Petkau J, *et al.* Development of a multiple sclerosis functional composite as a clinical trial outcome measure. *Brain* 1999;122 (5): 871–82.

84. Fischer JS, Rudick RA, Cutter GR, Reingold SC. The Multiple Sclerosis Functional Composite Measure (MSFC): an integrated approach to MS clinical outcome assessment. National MS Society Clinical Outcomes Assessment Task Force. *Mult Scler* 1999;5: 244–50.

85. Gronwall DMA. Paced auditory serial-addition task: a measure of recovery from concussion. *Percept Mot Skills* 1977;44: 367–73.

86. Hiscock M, Caroselli JS, Kimball LE. Paced serial addition: modality-specific and arithmetic-specific factors. *J Clin Exp Neuropsychol* 1998;20: 463–72.

87. Fisk JD, Archibald CJ. Limitations of the Paced Auditory Serial Addition Test as a measure of working memory in patients with multiple sclerosis. *J Int Neuropsychol Soc* 2001;7: 363–72.

88. Drake AS, Weinstock-Guttman B, Morrow SA, Hojnacki D, Munschauer FE, Benedict RH. Psychometrics and normative data for the Multiple Sclerosis Functional Composite: replacing the PASAT with the Symbol Digit Modalities Test. *Mult Scler* 2010;16: 228–37.

89. Brochet B, Deloire MS, Bonnet M, *et al.* Should SDMT substitute for PASAT in MSFC? A 5-year longitudinal study. *Mult Scler* 2008;14: 1242–9.

90. Rao SM, NMSS Cognitive Function Study Group. *A Manual for the Brief Repeatable Battery of Neuropsychological Tests in Multiple Sclerosis.* New York: National MS Society, 1990.

91. Benedict RH, Fischer JS, Archibald CJ, *et al.* Minimal neuropsychological assessment of MS patients: a consensus approach. *Clin Neuropsychol* 2002;16: 381–97.

92. Tombaugh TN, Berrigan LI, Walker LA, Freedman MS. The Computerized Test of Information Processing (CTIP) offers an alternative to the PASAT for assessing cognitive processing speed in individuals with multiple sclerosis. *Cogn Behav Neurol* 2010;23: 192–8.

93. Wilken JA, Kane R, Sullivan CL, *et al.* The utility of computerized neuropsychological assessment of cognitive dysfunction in patients with relapsing–remitting multiple sclerosis. *Mult Scler* 2003;9: 119–27.

94. Achiron A, Doniger GM, Harel Y, ppleboim-Gavish N, Lavie M, Simon ES. Prolonged response times characterize cognitive performance in multiple sclerosis. *Eur J Neurol* 2007;14: 1102–8.

95. Penny S, Khaleeli Z, Cipolotti L, Thompson A, Ron M. Early imaging predicts later cognitive impairment in primary progressive multiple sclerosis. *Neurology* 2010;74: 545–52.

96. Summers M, Fisniku L, Anderson V, Miller D, Cipolotti L, Ron M. Cognitive impairment in relapsing–remitting multiple sclerosis can be predicted by imaging performed several years earlier. *Mult Scler* 2008;14: 197–204.

97. Cohen JA, Fischer JS, Bolibrush DM, *et al.* Intrarater and interrater reliability of the MS functional composite outcome measure. *Neurology* 2000;54: 802–6.

98. Goldsmith CH, Smythe HA, Helewa A. Interpretation and power of a pooled index. *J Rheumatol* 1993;20: 575–8.

99. Bryk AS, Raudenbush SW. Application of hierarchical linear models to assessing change. *Psychol Bull* 1987;1987: 147–58.

100. Nich C, Carroll K. Now you see it, now you don't: a comparison of traditional versus random-effects regression models in the analysis of longitudinal follow-up data from a clinical trial. *J Consult Clin Psychol* 1997;65: 252–61.

101. Krause MS, Howard KI, Lutz W. Exploring individual change. *J Consult Clin Psychol* 1998;66: 838–45.

102. Gould R, Abramson I, Galasko D, Salmon D. Rate of cognitive change in Alzheimer's disease: methodological approaches using random effects models. *J Int Neuropsychol Soc* 2001;7: 813–24.

103. Selnes OA, Galai N, Bacellar H, *et al.* Cognitive performance after progression to AIDS: a longitudinal study from the Multicenter AIDS Cohort Study. *Neurology* 1995;45: 267–75.

104. Selnes OA, Galai N, McArthur JC, *et al.* HIV infection and cognition in intravenous drug users: long-term follow-up. *Neurology* 1997;48: 223–30.

105. Stern Y, Liu X, Marder K, *et al.* Neuropsychological changes in a prospectively followed cohort of homosexual and bisexual men with and without HIV infection. *Neurology* 1995;45: 467–72.

106. Lai EC, Felice KJ, Festoff BW, *et al.* Effect of recombinant human insulin-like growth factor-I on progression of ALS. A placebo-controlled study. The North America ALS/IGF-I Study Group. *Neurology* 1997;49: 1621–30.

107. Greenhouse JB, Stangl D, Bromberg J. An introduction to survival analysis: statistical methods for analysis of clinical trial data. *J Consult Clin Psychol* 1989;57: 536–44.

108. Luke DA, Homan SM. Time and change: Using survival analysis in clinical assessment and treatment evaluation. *Psychol Assess* 1998;10: 360–78.

109. Hartmann A, Schulgen G, Olschewski M, Herzog T. Modeling psychotherapy outcome as event in time: an application of multistate analysis. *J Consult Clin Psychol* 1997;65: 262–8.

110. The Multiple Sclerosis Study Group. Efficacy and toxicity of cyclosporine in chronic progressive multiple sclerosis: a randomized, double-blinded, placebo-controlled clinical trial. *Ann Neurol* 1990;27: 591–605.

111. Secondary Progressive Efficacy Clinical Trial of Recombinant Interferon-beta-1a in MS (SPECTRIMS) Study Group. Randomized controlled trial of interferon- beta-1a in secondary progressive MS: Clinical results. *Neurology* 2001;56: 1496–504.

112. Heaton RK, Temkin N, Dikmen S, *et al.* Detecting change: a comparison of three neuropsychological methods, using normal and clinical samples. *Arch Clin Neuropsychol* 2001;16: 75–91.

113. Jacobson JS, Truax P. Clinical significance: a statistical approach to defining meaningful change in psychotherapy research. *J Consult Clin Psychol* 1991;59: 12–19.

114. Speer DC, Greenbaum PE. Five methods for computing significant individual client change and improvement rates: support for an individual growth curve approach. *J Consult Clin Psychol* 1995;63: 1044–8.

115. Sawrie SM, Chelune GJ, Naugle RI, Luders HO. Empirical methods for assessing meaningful neuropsychological change following epilepsy surgery. *J Int Neuropsychol Soc* 1996;2: 556–64.

116. Martin RC, Sawrie SM, Roth DL, *et al.* Individual memory change after anterior temporal lobectomy: a base rate analysis using regression-based outcome methodology. *Epilepsia* 1998;39: 1075–82.

117. Temkin NR, Heaton RK, Grant I, Dikmen SS. Detecting significant change in neuropsychological test performance: a comparison of four models. *J Int Neuropsychol Soc* 1999;5: 357–69.

118. Green MF, Nuechterlein KH, Gold JM, *et al.* Approaching a consensus cognitive battery for clinical trials in schizophrenia: the NIMH-MATRICS conference to select cognitive domains and test criteria. *Biol Psychiatry* 2004;56: 301–7.

119. Sweet LH, Rao SM, Primeau M, Durgerian S, Cohen RA. Functional magnetic resonance imaging response to increased verbal working memory demands among patients with multiple sclerosis. *Hum Brain Mapp* 2006;27: 28–36.

120. Wishart HA, Saykin AJ, McDonald BC, *et al.* Brain activation patterns associated with working memory in relapsing–remitting MS. *Neurology* 2004;62: 234–8.

121. Audoin B, Ibarrola D, Ranjeva JP, *et al.* Compensatory cortical activation observed by fMRI during a cognitive task at the earliest stage of MS. *Hum Brain Mapp* 2003;20: 51–8.

122. Staffen W, Mair A, Zauner H, *et al.* Cognitive function and fMRI in patients with multiple sclerosis: evidence for compensatory cortical activation during an attention task. *Brain* 2002;125: 1275–82.

123. Bobholz JA, Rao SM, Lobeck L, *et al.* fMRI study of episodic memory in relapsing–remitting MS: correlation with T2 lesion volume. *Neurology* 2006;67: 1640–5.

124. Parry AM, Scott RB, Palace J, Smith S, Matthews PM. Potentially adaptive functional changes in cognitive processing for patients with multiple sclerosis and their acute modulation by rivastigmine. *Brain* 2003;126: 2750–60.

Chapter

8

Health-related quality of life assessment in multiple sclerosis

Deborah M. Miller, Michael W. Kattan, and Alex Z. Fu

Role of health-related quality of life assessment in the conduct of evidence-based medicine

Healthcare providers are placing increasing emphasis on the practice of evidence-based medicine, "a conscientious, explicit, and judicious use of current best evidence in making decisions about the care of individual patients."[1] Evidence-based medicine refers not only to use of evidence from research studies, including clinical trials, to guide practice in general, but also to use of data from the individual patient to guide his or her therapy. Three types of evidence are generally acceptable for guiding treatment decisions in individual patients:

- Anatomical or biological evidence (e.g. magnetic resonance imaging, cerebrospinal fluid measures)
- Clinical evidence (e.g. Multiple Sclerosis Functional Composite, Expanded Disability Status Scale)
- Patient-derived evidence

An emerging area of research to guide clinical decision-making is comparative effectiveness research, designed to inform health care decisions by providing evidence about the benefits and harms of different treatment options.[2] According to the Agency for Healthcare Research and Quality, comparative effectiveness research requires the development, expansion, and use of a variety of data sources to conduct timely and relevant research and disseminate the results in a timely and usable fashion that is relevant to a range of health care stake holders.[3] Patient reports are considered an essential component of comparative effectiveness research.[4]

The patient-generated category of evidence may be evaluated at several levels of complexity, including general quality of life (QoL) and more specific health-related quality of life (HRQoL), or in terms of discrete patient-reported outcomes such as functional status, walking ability, or self-efficacy. This chapter focuses on HRQoL assessments. Patient-derived data are increasingly accepted as an important assessment domain in clinical research for most chronic conditions, including multiple sclerosis (MS) (see the Proceedings from the annual meetings of the International Society for Quality of Life Research).

Important goals of treatments for conditions that carry substantial morbidity but have minimal impact on mortality are to reduce the disease impact on patients' lives and to assure that interventions result in more good than harm. Achieving these goals can be demonstrated only with patient input. Furthermore, measures of patient perception and clinical data derived from examiners are not redundant.[5-7] Moreover, patient functioning in the somewhat artificial setting of the treatment center is not always duplicated in the home setting,[8] indicating that clinical assessments do not always reflect a person's abilities at home.

Currently, most empirical evidence available to inform evidence-based medicine in MS is anatomical, biological, or clinical. The Multiple Sclerosis Council for Clinical Practice Guidelines noted that the lack of patient perceptions and preference data about treatment options has effectively left the recipients of care removed from systematic clinical decision-making.[9] This chapter addresses these important patient perceptions in terms of HRQoL. Health-related quality of life is defined and assessment techniques are reviewed. Recommendations follow for future directions for MS HRQoL assessment.

Two approaches to HRQoL assessment are considered in this chapter. They are health profiles and utility assessment. Health profiles are based on psychometric techniques[10] and typically include several subscales that assess theoretically and empirically distinct domains of HRQoL. These subscales can be calculated into summary or global scores. The majority of HRQoL research reported in this chapter includes health profile assessments.

Utility measures are derived from economic and decision theory. They reflect patient preferences for different health states and are summarized in a single summary score. These measures incorporate preference measurements, and allow patients to assess their willingness to accept various health states in relation to death. Kaplan and Anderson[11] explain that they use this approach at the health policy level to explain the benefits of medical care, behavioral intervention, or prevention programs in terms of well-years, in order to compare outcomes across very different interventions. At the individual level, this method is useful in helping patients with life-threatening conditions to make judgments about their willingness to accept

Multiple Sclerosis Therapeutics, Fourth Edition, ed. Jeffrey A. Cohen and Richard A. Rudick. Published by Cambridge University Press.
© Cambridge University Press 2011.

potentially life-saving treatments that have profound negative cost or health status side effects.[12]

Health profile assessment of quality of life
Definition

Since the Food and Drug Administration (FDA) has offered guidance on using HRQoL measures to support labeling claims, the definition of HRQoL has become more systematized.[13] The FDA guidance describes HRQoL as a multi-domain concept that represents the patient's overall perception of the impact of an illness and its treatment. HRQoL measures capture, at a minimum, physical, psychological (including emotional and cognitive), and social functioning. Knowledge about interpreting clinically important HRQoL change is rapidly advancing through the use of quantitative and qualitative methods.[14,15] However, there is much to learn about the interactions of HRQoL components. Traugott[16] drew an analogy between HRQoL and immunological studies, noting a number of quantitative and qualitative abnormalities of the immune system associated with MS. These immunological changes are considered important, but their cause, significance, and the relationships among immunological markers and the disease are not fully understood. Similar uncertainties apply to HRQoL parameters.

Quality of life is considered to be but one domain of health, as defined by the World Health Organization,[17] and HRQoL is a discrete component of general quality of life. Guyatt et al.[6] noted that, while general quality of life can be affected by many factors beyond the scope of health care, including economic instability, civil unrest or poor environment, these general factors have only an indirect relationship with HRQoL and are not included in its definition. Schipper et al.[18] agreed that, while factors such as equal opportunity and social security are important to community health, these factors extend beyond the more immediate goal of treating the sick. These authors offer the following definition of HRQoL: "'Quality of life' in clinical medicine represents the functional effect of an illness and its consequent therapy upon a patient, as perceived by the patient." This construct includes four broad domains: physical and occupational function, psychological function, social interaction, and somatic sensation. They established several operational characteristics of HRQoL assessment that help to further define the construct. First and foremost, HRQoL is subjective. As Schipper et al.[18] explain: " … in clinical medicine the ultimate observer of the experiment is not a dispassionate third party but a most intimately involved patient." Since the goal of treatment is to minimize the manifest consequences of disease, they note, HRQoL represents "the final common pathway of all the physiological, psychological and social inputs into the therapeutic process." The second characteristic of HRQoL is that it is multi-factorial. Having operationally defined HRQoL as the integration of four domains, it is important to assure that patients' daily experiences in all these regards are explored in the questionnaire, albeit in a manner that is parsimonious

and minimizes respondent burden. The third characteristic is self-administration. Because HRQoL is subjective, there is concern that external administration would in some way influence the patient report. The final characteristic is that HRQoL is time-variable, meaning that it fluctuates with time.

Generic vs. specific approaches to health-profile HRQoL measurement

HRQoL measures look at patients' reports of their perceived health in either very general or very particular terms. Measures that assess the former are referred to as generic assessments, and those that measure the latter as disease- or symptom-specific assessments.

Generic measures assess general well-being and are intended to be broad assessments. They tap a wide range of health concepts, and are useful in making broad comparisons across general populations or persons with different conditions, or comparing the relative benefits of different treatments for the well-being of a community. In contrast, disease-specific measures focus on aspects of health that are significant to the disease or intervention under consideration. The major reason for adopting this approach is to assure that the measure is sensitive to different health states within a condition. It is especially useful in clinical trials, because it increases the ability to detect change caused by an intervention and, as important, allows intense assessment of both positive and negative impacts of the intervention. For this reason in particular, the use of disease-specific measures is especially important in MS, which can manifest a broad range of symptoms that fluctuate over time. In order to allow both the detailed assessment inherent in disease-specific measures and a more general comparison of a study sample with the general population or with other disease groups, it is commonly recommended that short generic measures be combined with disease-specific ones.

Utility assessment of health-related quality of life
Definition

It is common practice to measure quality of life using comprehensive instruments with multiple domains. However, when trying to decide which treatment has better outcomes, interpretation of multiple domains becomes complicated. Suppose a study involves a comparison of two treatments for MS. One treatment might be found to have a better effect on MRI endpoints but a worse side-effect profile. Which treatment, on average, has the better health outcome? The problem is obviously more difficult when several domains (i.e. quality of life aspects) are involved,[19] which is the more typical scenario. When looking at multiple domains, the decision of which treatment is preferable is obvious only when all the quality of life domains favor one treatment over the other. When domains disagree, or when quality of life disagrees with quantity of life,[20] it becomes difficult to judge between treatments.

Assessing the utility for current health provides a theoretically attractive solution to this issue.[21] Utility, in this context is a number that measures, under conditions of uncertainty, an individual's preference for a state of health. It is measured using the von Neumann–Morgenstern utility theory.[22] A patient's utility is assessed on a scale from 0 to 1, where 0 represents a state of health which the patient perceives to be as bad as death, and 1 represents perfect health. The principal value of a utility measure arises from the ability to compute quality-adjusted survival, measured in quality-adjusted life years (QALY).[23] We achieve this by multiplying quantity of life by quality of life, as measured by the patient's utility.[19,24–27] For example, if a patient lives 1 year of life with utility 0.9, this amounts to $1 \times 0.9 = 0.9$ QALYs. If we were to measure the patient's utility routinely, until death, we could compute his or her quality-adjusted survival. If all patients were followed until death, we would sum the products of these quantity/quality of life values. Conceptually, determining QALY[1] allows us to compare treatment outcomes comprehensively by simultaneously analyzing quality and quantity of life; and[2] resolves conflicts when one treatment gives a better quality of life for some end-points, but not all. As a summary, the global utility assessment is irreplaceable when QALY is the outcome of interest, but it is by no means a replacement for disease- or symptom-specific quality of life measurements.

Approaches to utility assessment of HRQoL

Utility assessment is an increasingly active area of research in MS.[28] Depending on whether the research purpose is operating at the individual or population patient level, utility can be elicited with different approaches. At the individual patient level, an investigator can elicit the patient's own utilities for different possible outcome states. This is referred to as direct utility elicitation. Among the various methods for directly eliciting utilities, the three most popular ones are the visual analog scale, time trade-off, and standard gamble. At the patient population level, there are many pre-scored multi-attribute health status classification systems available. They provide preference-based index scores pre-defined from a large group of people in the population. With a ready-made questionnaire and a set of weights, these methods are also referred to as indirect utility elicitation. The most commonly seen include the European Quality of Life-5D, Health Utility Index Mark 2 and 3, the Quality of Well Being (QWB) scale, and the Short Form -6D. Both direct and indirect utility elicitations are commonly used with their well-understood properties, and they are valuable research tools for quantifying the impact of treatment on the quality of life of patients.

Visual analog scale

The easiest and probably most common method is the visual analog scale, also called the rating scale or feeling thermometer. With this method, patients are usually shown a line or thermometer-like drawing, scaled from 0 to 100, where 0 represents death and 100 represents perfect health. Patients are asked to indicate where on the line they feel their current health is located. Utility is then computed by dividing the corresponding number by 100. Clearly, this is an easy method to administer. However, it has a considerable drawback: the 0 to 100 scale has no real external meaning. In other words, one patient's belief of what an "80" is may be very different from another's.[23]

Time trade-off

The time trade-off is another popular utility assessment method. This approach presents the patient with a choice between some fixed period of time in the patient's current health and a shorter period of time in perfect health. The time trade-off utility is computed as the minimum period of time in perfect health that the patient is willing to accept, divided by the fixed period of time offered in current health. For example, if the patient has no preference between 3 years in perfect health and 5 years in present health, the time trade-off utility is 3/5 = 0.6. This approach has limitations. In particular, guaranteeing a minimum duration of time in current health may produce a highly unrealistic scenario when the patient has a degenerative or life-threatening condition.[29] Furthermore, utility scores measured by time trade-off are affected by the patients' time preference, and not in any uniform or proportionate way. It is problematic for discounting future time-trade-off derived QALY, which is a typical way of calculating long-term accumulative QALY or quality-adjusted survivals.

Standard gamble

Perhaps the most accepted utility assessment method is the standard gamble, because it is based directly on the fundamental axioms of utility theory.[30–35] In its most typical form, the standard gamble involves offering the patient a hypothetical magic pill.[32] If the patient takes the pill, there is some chance that the patient will immediately receive perfect health, but there is 1 minus this chance that the patient will die immediately. Thus, with standard gamble, the assessment evaluates how much risk the patient is willing to take for a chance of perfect health relative to his current health. The standard gamble utility is then calculated as 1 minus the maximum chance of death that the patient was willing to risk with the magic pill. Because it involves uncertainty with associated probabilities, the standard gamble is the only true utility measure.[36] Uncertainty captures the subject's risk attitude, which could be risk-averse, risk-neutral, or risk-seeking. However, it has been found empirically that people are risk-averse for large gains, risk-seeking for small gains, and risk-seeking for losses.[37]

While utility is well suited to addressing quality of life issues when comparing outcomes across treatments, it does not address all important issues related to QoL. For questions targeted to specific quality of life issues, domain-specific questionnaire scales are remarkably valuable. Moreover, it may be difficult to envision how routinely measuring utilities in a series of patients would benefit future patients at the individual patient level. However, one particular application would seem beneficial, and that is predicted quality-adjusted survival. If baseline characteristics and utilities were measured in a cohort of patients, the resulting data set could then potentially be used to derive prediction models. For the future patient having difficulty with an important treatment decision, his or her baseline characteristics could be inserted into prediction models to obtain the predicted QALYs for each treatment option.

Characteristics of health-related quality of life measures

For scientifically rigorous investigations, HRQoL measures, whether health profile or utility assessment, must meet the same criteria of meaningfulness and dependability that are used to evaluate other assessment measures. These measurement criteria are typically referred to as reliability and validity.

Reliability

Hobart et al.[38] described reliability as the demonstration that results produced by a measure are accurate, consistent, stable and reproducible. They described four types of reliability including internal consistency, test–retest reliability, rater reliability (inter- and intra-rater), and parallel forms. Each of these assesses a different source of random error, and all are important in establishing the value of a measure. Guyatt et al.[6] suggested an additional form of reliability, "signal-to-noise ratio," which they defined as the ability to detect actual changes in a measure over time (the signal) in relation to error that occurs in any measurement process (the noise). For measures that evaluate change over time, they referred to the signal-to-noise ratio as "responsiveness." While it cannot be directly measured, responsiveness theoretically is the size of the difference in scores between subjects who have actually experienced change and those who have not. A significant threat to reliability occurs when measures demonstrate floor and ceiling effects. This could occur, for example, when a measure designed for a seriously ill population is implemented in less ill individuals. In that situation, respondents will cluster at the top of the scale and share the maximum score, but may in fact differ in their states of well-being. The difference is not demonstrated because the measure is not sensitive at that range of difference.

Validity

Validity is the second necessary attribute of a HRQoL measure, and refers to the relationship between the concept that is being measured and the instrument that assesses it. Typical categories of validity include content-related, construct-related, predictive ability, and criterion-related validity.[38] Methods used to establish the validity of an instrument are drawn from clinical and experimental psychology. Content validity addresses the extent to which the items in the instrument relate to the domain

being measured. Content validity typically is established by comprehensive literature reviews and surveying patients and heath-care professionals. As Guyatt et al.[6] discuss, Feinstein integrates face validity, that is the degree to which a measure appears to evaluate that which it is intended to measure. and content validity into the construct "sensibility," which relates to the applicability of a measure, its clarity and simplicity, likelihood of bias, comprehensiveness and the inclusion of redundant items.[39] Construct validity refers to the extent that the instrument under consideration performs as expected in relation to other measures. Closely related to construct validity is a measure's capacity to predict future health states, termed predictive validity. Because there is no gold standard for demonstrating the real level of HRQoL, it is not possible to establish criterion validation for HRQoL measures.[40] Although there is evidence that HRQoL measures correlate with white matter lesions and brain atrophy[41] and changes in Expanded Disability Status Scale (EDSS) and MS Functional Composite (MSFC),[42] these biological or clinician-assessed measures are not to be considered gold standards for criterion validation of HRQoL measures.

Item response theory and computer adaptive testing

Item response theory (IRT) and computer adaptive testing (CAT) are somewhat newer methods that can be used to construct and validate HRQoL scales.[43–46] IRT is based on the idea that a person's response on a test can be modeled to each item in the assessment because the response is function of that person's position on a latent trait, i.e. the probability of a specific response is a function of both the test item and the person taking the assessment. IRT models are sometimes referred to as latent trait models because they take into account a specific trait(s) or ability of the person (the person parameter); these may include a broad range of domains from positive psychological functioning to upper extremity functioning. Item parameters include discrimination and difficulty. Discrimination involves a determination of the item's mathematical slope and indicates how well an item can discriminate between different levels of an assessment domain (e.g. ambulates independently, requires unilateral support, and requires bilateral support). Difficulty refers to the threshold at which a person is more likely than not to answer an item in a specific way and is related to the individual's position on a particular trait. Computer adaptive testing (CAT) is a method of test administration in which a computer-based assessment adapts to the individual's performance level. For example, if an individual indicates seldom having trouble with independent dressing, the next question presented would be about a more challenging activity rather than a less changing activity Thus, CAT is a means of maximizing the assessment precision.

Neuro-QoL is a project funded by the National Institute of Neurological Disorders and Stroke, with the goal of creating measures specific to assessing HRQoL in adults and children with common neurological conditions,[47] including MS. Both IRT and CAT are used in Neuro-QoL to develop test item banks, calibrate them, and then develop the final Neuro-QoL assessment forms. For calibration, items are fit into an IRT model and the item parameters are estimated. Once they are calibrated, the item parameters can be used to develop CAT assessments and create the final assessment tool. At this time, 13 item banks and short forms have been developed, tested and released. When finished, Neuro-QoL will provide a platform for consistent assessment of important aspects of quality of life across neurological conditions and varied research approaches. As with other neurological HRQoL measures, this assessment platform captures patients' perceptions of their physical functional status which, as has been demonstrated, is distinct from clinicians' perspectives[7] but also assesses important patient domains, such as fatigue and emotional and social functioning, that can be affected by clinical interventions but are not captured by traditional clinical parameters.

Uses of health-related quality of life data

HRQoL data are used for three general purposes: to classify or group patients by levels of disease severity, to predict the health of subjects at a future point in time, and as outcome variables. A discriminative index is used to differentiate among groups or individuals along a given dimension, as may be done in an epidemiological study when no gold standard is available to use as a validation criterion. For example, assessing the HRQoL of persons with MS in comparison with persons with rheumatoid arthritis and inflammatory bowel disease requires a discriminative instrument. So does a study that compares MS patients who were divided among three levels of disability according to, for example, EDSS score. MS studies that include a HRQoL measure for discriminative purposes include those by Rudick et al., which used the generic Farmer HRQoL measure to compare the HRQoL of patients with MS, inflammatory bowel disease (IBD), and rheumatoid arthritis. They determined that patients with IBD had better HRQoL that the other two groups and that those with MS had the worst.[48] Another by Hermann et al.[49] reported MS patients scored significantly worse than those with diabetes and epilepsy on five of the eight SF-36 scales.

A predictive index is used to classify individuals into pre-established present or future categories. An appropriate use of a HRQoL measure for predictive purposes would be to determine whether changes in patients' self-reports indicate a current need for rehabilitative services or future job loss due to disability. Such a study was conducted by Nortvedt et al.,[50] who, in a prospective cohort study, found that independent of clinical status and MRI activity, MS patients with low scores on the SF-36 were correlated with worsened EDSS scores one year later. In another sense, a measure also can be considered predictive when it is highly correlated with a longer-term or more cumbersome measure that is believed to assess the same construct as does the new measure.[51]

Evaluative indexes are those that measure the amount of change in an individual or group over time as the result of disease progression or treatment intervention. MS treatment trials that included HRQoL end-points are discussed below. Sugano et al.[52] noted that these three types of instruments (discriminative, predictive, and evaluative) represent a continuum from epidemiological measures that are a static means of classification (discriminative) through risk factors (predictive) to outcome or response measurements (evaluative).

Epidemiological studies

Much has been learned about the natural history of MS through observational and epidemiological studies. Using the same principles, important information can be gained about the evolution of HRQoL in the MS population. Generic health profile measures are particularly useful in epidemiological studies that monitor the health of a diverse population, or of individuals with a medical condition that has a diverse set of signs and symptoms associated with it, such as MS. Epidemiological data using a disease-specific measure can determine how changes in HRQoL relate to change in employability. These data can be used for hypothesis generation, such as proposing interventions that improve quality of life. Cross-sectional data can be used to construct statistical norms for generic measures that allow the comparison of one disease group with other illness groups or the general population. Longitudinal assessments can help to delineate the temporal associations among biological, clinical and HRQoL measures in MS. For instance, a longitudinal epidemiological study might reveal a delay between biological indications of disease activity and their manifestation in clinical and HRQoL outcomes. This information would be important in designing clinical trials, providing indications for the timing of assessments in relation to interventions and the frequency at which assessments should be made, as well as how long studies must be continued in order to demonstrate a hypothesized change. The Sonja Slifka Longitudinal Multiple Sclerosis Study,[53] which began in 2000, recently demonstrated lower scores on the SF-12 in the 2109 persons with MS included in the database identified modifiable demographic, disease, and health services factors that influence HRQoL.[54]

Health services research

The Agency for Healthcare Quality and Research defines health services research as "the study of ways people get access to health care, how much care costs, and what happens to patients as a result of this care."[55] More recently, interest has been increasing in comparative effectiveness research. While much health service research is conducted using the same methods as those employed in randomized clinical trials, a subset of this research, outcomes studies, is intended to investigate or improve the usual processes of care. These outcomes studies take place in "usual practice" settings, and they place as much emphasis on patient perceptions as on clinical assessments.[56] For example, one of the authors recently completed a randomized trial of a telehealth intervention[57] to determine whether subjects who routinely monitor their HRQoL have better health outcomes as measured by the Multiple Sclerosis Quality of Life Inventory, an MS-specific HRQoL instrument.[58] Outcomes studies can indicate the potential for generic and disease-specific HRQoL measures to serve as screening instruments for patients who report changes in symptom severity or functional ability that signal the need for rehabilitative interventions.[59] Econometric HRQoL measures can be used in outcomes studies to examine how quality-of-life data can be used to involve patients and families in clinical decision-making.[12] On a larger scale, econometric HRQoL measures are often used by policy makers to allocate finite health care resources.[60]

Clinical trials

Clinical trials provide essential information about potential therapeutic interventions when the optimal treatment for a condition is unknown.[60] In chronic conditions with unknown cause and no cure, the goals of treatment are to prevent the disease worsening, reduce the severity and duration of relapses, and provide symptom management. When multiple interventions are equally effective in achieving these goals, it is important to compare their side-effect profiles on disease-specific HRQoL to determine optimal treatment. There are many reasons why HRQoL measures should be included in MS clinical trials.[61] The first of these is to determine whether the intervention has an impact on subjective well-being, such as Cohen *et al.* recently reported.[62] This information can be a particularly important end-point in conditions that do not affect mortality.

Given the progressive nature of MS, it is important that the direction and magnitude of the expected impact on HRQoL are clearly specified. In the case of interventions intended to provide symptom relief, the impact may be an immediate improvement in HRQoL. Alternatively, interventions intended to slow or halt disease progression may not improve the HRQoL for study subjects. Rather, they are intended to slow the decline or sustain the well-being of subjects over a number of years.

Another reason for including HRQoL assessment in clinical trials is to determine the potential negative effects of the treatment for subjects, and to compare them with the benefits of treatment. As in the case of the available MS disease-modifying treatments, until the relative and ultimate benefits of the interventions are determined, the side effects of the medicines (e.g. severity of flu-like symptoms) and method of administration (e.g. injection) are crucial aspects in comparing the treatments. When such questions are under investigation, it is important for the investigator to weigh the benefits of using health profile, as defined in the introduction, or utility measures. In some cases, in which there are adequate resources, the decision may be to utilize both.

Because the costs of both lifelong disability from MS and the disease-modifying treatments can be very high, a third reason to include HRQoL assessments in clinical trials is to assess the cost–benefit and cost–utility of the treatments under study.

Because patient well-being is as important as morbidity and mortality in chronic illnesses, a number of regulatory bodies responsible for the approval of new interventions rely on HRQoL data in their deliberations. These data are considered so significant that the FDA has issued guidance on the use of patient-reported outcomes in clinical trials that must be followed in to make an accepted HRQoL claim for a approved medical product.[63]

Randomized clinical trials in MS that included HRQoL measures

MS-specific HRQoL measures have been included as endpoints in many clinical studies, including some randomized controlled clinical trials. To identify randomized clinical trials in MS that used MS-specific HRQoL measures, we conducted a review of randomized clinical trials that included the 12 MS-specific multidimensional HRQoL measures cited in a recent comprehensive review of the MS HRQoL literature.[64] Both Ovid and the Web of Science were searched using strategies specific to each database. The Ovid search include the terms "clinical trial," "multiple sclerosis," and "quality of life" (all terms exploded), which were then combined with the complete name and abbreviation for each HRQoL measure. The Web of Science search was conducted by first searching for the reference manuscript for each HRQoL measure and selecting all citing references, which were then limited by the term "clinical trial." With both searches, all resulting studies were reviewed to identify those that included a randomized or non-randomized design with controls, and a minimum of 20 subjects. Relevant data from the included studies are shown in Table 8.1.[65–89]

This review of the literature identified 15 unique randomized controlled trials that included any of the 12 MS-specific HRQoL measures as an end-point; however, only five of these 12 were included as trial end-points.[58,65,70,79,82] The majority of these randomized trials tested interventions intended to improve physical functioning.[67,69,71,73,75,81,83–85] HRQoL results ranged from significant effects favoring treatment, trends toward benefit, to no significant findings. One of these investigations, assessing the benefit of exercise,[71] included two HRQoL measures, the Functional Assessment of Multiple Sclerosis[70] and the MSIS-29,[82] and found benefit on the former but not the latter. Three studies assessed the impact of mental health interventions[66,68,80] and found limited benefit for HRQoL. Of the three studies of disease-modifying therapies,[62,72,76] only Cohen *et al.* found a treatment (interferon) benefit on an HRQoL measure: HRQoL improved in eight of the 11 MSQLI scales. We found no randomized controlled trials for the remaining MS-specific HRQoL instruments identified in the recent comprehensive review of the MS HRQoL literature.[64] This review suggests that, even with the increased inclusion of disease-specific measures in randomized controlled trials, the multiplicity of measures and differences in trial design and target interventions make conclusions about HRQoL outcomes difficult.

Table 8.1. *Review of randomized trials using MS-specific HRQoL measures**

Measure	Author	Year	N	Randomization	Type of intervention	Level of outcome	Results
MSQOL-54[65]							
	Sharafaddinzadeh [66]	2010	96	Randomized to (1) Treatment with low-dose naltresone or (2) placebo	Promote psychological well-being	Primary	Overall HRQoL did not improve
	McClurg[67]	2006	30	Randomized to (1) pelvic floor muscle training (PFMT), (2) PFMT and EMG biofeedback, or (3) neuromuscular electrical stimulation	Management of bladder dysfunction	Secondary	HRQoL variable within and across groups
	Hart[68]	2005	60	Randomized to (1) individualized weekly cognitive behavioral therapy or (2) supportive- expressive group psychotherapy, or (3) sertraline	Manage depression	Secondary	HRQoL "Effects were nil"
	Romberg[69]	2005	114	Randomized to (1) treatment including 2-week in-patient followed by home exercise program, or (2) control (no intervention	Exercise	Secondary	HRQoL had "limited effects"
FAMS[70]							
	McCullagh[71]	2008	30	Randomized to (1) twice weekly in-center exercise with once weekly home exercise, or (2) usual activity with no intervention	Exercise	Primary	Significant HRQoL between-group difference favoring treatment
	Kappos[72]	2007	487	Randomized to (1) IFNβ-1b s.c. injection 250 μg every other day or (2) IFNβ-1b s.c. injection 160 μg every other day or (3) placebo s.c. injection 250 μg every other day or (4) placebo s.c. injection 160 μg every other day	Disease-modifying therapy after clinically isolated syndrome	Secondary	No between-group difference and no change over time
	Johnson[73]	2006	23	Randomized to (1) treatment ginkgo biloba (EGb 761), 240mg or (2) placebo	Improve functional performance	Primary	Significant HRQoL between-group difference
DIP[74]							
	No studies identified						
MSQLI[58]							
	Goodman[75]	2008	206	Randomized to (1) 10 mg fampridine twice daily or (2) 15 mg fampridine twice daily or (3) 20 mg fampridine twice daily or (4) placebo	Improve in walking speed	Secondary	Not reported
	North American Study Group[76]	2004	939	Randomized to (1) IFNβ-1b s.c. injection 250 μg every other day or (2) IFNβ-1b s.c. injection 160 μg every other day or (3) placebo s.c. injection 250 μg every other day or (4) placebo s.c. injection 160 μg every other day	Disease-modifying therapy in secondary progressive MS	Tertiary	No HRQoL between-group difference
	Cohen[62]	2002	436	Randomized to (1) IFNβ-1a IM injection 60μg every week or (2) placebo IM injection every week	Disease modifying therapy in secondary progressive MS	Secondary	Significant HRQoL benefit to treatment group on 8 of 11 scales
RAYS[77]							
	No studies identified						
LMSQOL[78]							
	No studies identified						

(cont.)

Table 8.1. (cont.)

Measure	Author	Year	N	Randomization	Type of intervention	Level of outcome	Results
HAQUAMS[79]							
	Naseri[80]	2009	38	Randomized to (1) controlled, cross-over trial of MS$_{14}$ 50 mg/kg/day) (an Iranian herbal marine compound and is equivalent to food), or (2) placebo	Improvement in quality of life	Primary	HRQoL results difficult to interpret
	Schulz[81]	2004	46	Randomized to (1) tailored 8-week bicycle ergometry program, or (2) control wait list	Exercise program	Tertiary	Small but statistical HRQoL improvement in treatment group in Total and 2 HAQUAMS sub-scales
MSIS-29[82]							
	Hughes[83]	2009	73	Randomized to (1) active treatment (precision reflexology), or (2) Control (sham reflexology	Pain relief	Secondary	No HRQoL between-group difference
	McClurg[84]	2008	74	Randomized to (1) pelvic floor muscle training, EMG biofeedback and placebo neuromuscular electrical stimulation or (2) pelvic floor muscle training, EMG biofeedback and active neuromuscular electrical stimulation	Reduction in urinary incontinence	Secondary	Both groups demonstrated a significant improvement in HRQoL. Between-group HRQoL differences were not described.
	McCullagh[71]	2008	30	Randomized to (1) treatment (twice weekly group exercise and once weekly home exercise), or (2) usual care	Exercise capacity	Primary	No HRQoL between-group difference
	Khan[85]	2007	101	Randomized to (1) individualized rehabilitation programe, or (2) control (wait list)	Functional performance	Secondary	No HRQoL between-group difference
MusiQoL[86]							
	No studies identified						
MSIP[87]							
	No studies identified						
PRIMUS[88]							
	No studies identified						
FILMS[89]							
	No studies identified						

* Measures included in Miller DM, Allen R. Quality of life in multiple sclerosis: determinants, measurement, and use in clinical practice. *Curr Neurol Neurosci* Rep 2010;10:397–406.

DIP = Disability and Impact Profile, FAMS = Functional Assessment of Multiple Sclerosis, FILMS = Functional Index for Living With Multiple Sclerosis, HAQUAMS = Hamburg Quality of Life Questionnaire in MS, LMSQOL = Leeds Multiple Sclerosis Quality of Life, MSIP = Multiple Sclerosis Impact Profile, MSIS-29 = Multiple Sclerosis Impact Scale, MSQLI = Multiple Sclerosis Quality of Life Inventory, MSQOL-54 = Multiple Sclerosis Quality of Life Health Survey-54, MusiQoL = Multiple Sclerosis International Quality of Life, PRIMUS = Patient-Reported Outcome Indices for Multiple Sclerosis, s.c. = subcutaneous, IM = intramuscular, EMG = electromyography.

While the use of disease-specific measures is increasing, an important place remains in MS clinical trials research for using generic HRQoL measures as outcomes as they allow broad assessment of treatment benefit. There have been three reported trials of approved MS disease modifying therapies that have used generic measures. In a trial of interferon β-1b with 781 patients with secondary progressive MS and using the Sickness Impact Profile as an end-point, Freeman *et al.*[90] reported that the treatment group demonstrated a slower rate of physical deterioration at each assessment point. Two trials of natalizumab, SENTINEL[91] and AFFIRM,[92] included the SF-36 and a assessment visual analog scale of general well-being as a tertiary end-point for 2113 subjects. As reported in the manuscript reporting the HRQoL end-points[93] in AFFRIM, natalizumab significantly improved the physical component summary (PCS) at week 24 and all time-points and the mental component summary (MCS) showed significant improvement at week 104. Patients treated with natalizumab in both the SENTINAL and AFFIRM trials showed clinically important improvement and were less likely to show clinically important deterioration with the SF-36 physical component summary. The visual analog scale was also significantly improved for those treated with natalizumab.

Conclusions

HRQoL is increasingly used as an end-point in MS research, including epidemiological investigations, health services research, and clinical trials. It is encouraging that we have entered an era when MS-specific measures are being used in clinical trials and other MS research. Neuro-QoL is another important development. The aspects of HRQoL assessment that focus more on function can support the relevance of clinician-assessed measures whereas the more emotional and social components enrich our understanding of the benefits and consequences of treatment. It is hoped that measures developed through Neuro-QoL will help investigators better assess the benefits and disadvantages of interventions under investigation. This is especially the case since there is concern that the most commonly used generic measure, the SF-36, may not be appropriate in many MS studies.[94–96]

HRQoL assessment in MS has focused on the use of health profiles. As more treatments become available that have positive benefit for disease course, but are associated with potentially severe adverse events, such as mitoxantrone[97] and natalizumab,[98] and there are more treatments among which physicians and patients must choose, the use of utility assessment becomes more relevant to the MS field.

Selection of the most appropriate disease-specific measures by investigators should be based on available validity and reliability data for those measures and the specific questions that the researcher hopes to answer. Investigators need to be mindful of the selected instrument's measurement characteristics. Is it to be used for discriminative, predictive, or evaluative purposes? Does it provide more or less information than is needed? Will study subjects accept the measure? While investigators are urged to use disease-specific measures, they are also encouraged to include an established generic measure in their investigations, both to help establish the properties of the disease-specific measures and to assure the interpretability of their data.

There are a number of other issues that must be considered if HRQoL data are to yield useful results and contribute the patient perspective to the practice of evidence-based medicine. A major advancement is the availability of the Neuro-QoL assessment platform, which will allow for consistent assessment of HRQoL across trials. Other issues include using methods for test administration that accommodate the physical disability of MS patients. Also, one must consider the effect that cognitive impairments may have on the assessment of HRQoL. Although we are able to determine the statistical significance of HRQoL scores, we need additional information concerning the clinical significance of the scores, or changes in scores. It is also essential that we become more precise in our hypotheses about HRQoL change. In some instances we will anticipate that HRQoL will improve in study patients compared with controls. In other studies, we may expect to see HRQoL initially stabilize and perhaps eventually improve, compared with control patients, depending on the amount of time it takes for the benefit of the intervention to be manifest. As we learn more about the HRQoL in MS patients, we will continue to learn the best ways to monitor it. Although this developmental approach will lead to some temporary imprecision, it is crucial that we systematically obtain patient reports of their well-being as it is affected by MS and its treatments.

References

1. Sackette DL. *Evidence-Based Medicine: How to Practice and Teach EBM*. New York: Churchill Livingstone, 1997.

2. Medicine Io. *Initial National Priorities for Comparative Effectiveness Research*. Washington, DC: The National Academies Press, 2009.

3. AHRQ. What is comparative effectiveness research? [online]. Available at: http://www.effectivehealthcare.ahrq.gov/index.cfm/what-is-comparative-effectiveness-research1/.

4. Slutsky JR, Clancy CM. Patient-centered comparative effectiveness research: essential for high-quality care. *Arch Intern Med* 2010;170:403–4.

5. Rose MR, Weinman J. Quality of life: listen to, change, or shoot the messenger? *Neurology* 2007;68:1095–6.

6. Guyatt GH, Jaeschke R, Feeny DH, Patrick DL, Spilker B. *Measurements in Clinial Trials: Choosing the Right Approach*. In Spilker B, ed. Philadelphia: Lippincott-Raven, 1996:41–8.

7. Rothwell PM, McDowell Z, Wong CK, Dorman PJ. Doctors and patients don't agree: cross sectional study of patients' and doctors' perceptions and assessments of disability in multiple sclerosis. *BMJ (Clin Res Ed)* 1997;314:1580–3.

8. Freeman JA, Langdon DW, Hobart JC, Thompson AJ. Inpatient rehabilitation in multiple sclerosis: do the benefits carry over into the community? *Neurology* 1999;52:50–6.

9. Kinkel RP, Conway K, Copperman L, *et al. Fatigue and Multiple Sclerosis: Evidence-Based Management Strategies for Fatigue in Multiple Sclerosis.*

Washington, DC: Paralyzed Veterans of America, 1998.

10. Guyatt GH, Feeny DH, Patrick DL. Measuring health-related quality of life. *Ann Intern Med* 1993;118:622–9.

11. Kaplan RM, Anderson JP, Spilker B. The general heath policy model: an integrated approach. In Spilker B, ed. *Quality of Life and Pharmacoeconomics in Clinical Trials*. Philadelphia: Lippincott Raven, 1996:309–22.

12. Kattan MW. Comparing treatment outcomes using utility assessment for health-related quality of life. *Oncology* 2003;17:1687–93.

13. Office of Communications DoDI, Center for Drug Evaluation and Research Food and Drug Administration. Guidance for Industry Patient-Reported Outcome Measures: Use in Medical Product Development

to Support Labeling Claims. Silver Spring, MD: Food and Drug Administration, December, 2009.

14. Norman GR, Wyrwich KW, Patrick DL. The mathematical relationship among different forms of responsiveness coefficients. *Qual Life Res* 2007;16:815–22.

15. Giordano A, Pucci E, Naldi P, *et al.* Responsiveness of patient reported outcome measures in multiple sclerosis relapses: the REMS study. *J Neurol Neurosurg Psychiatr* 2009;80:1023–8.

16. Traugott U. Evidence for immunopathogenesis. In: Cook S, ed. *Handbook of Multiple Sclerosis*. New York: Marcel Dekker, 1990;101–27.

17. World Health O. *International Classification of Impairments, Disabilities and Handicaps (ICIDH): A Manual for Classification*. Geneva: WHO, 1980.

18. Schipper H, Clinch JJ, Olweny CLM, Spilker. Quality of life studies: definitions and conceptual issues. In *Quality of Life and Pharmacoeconomics in Clinical Trials*. Philadelphia: Lippincott-Raven, 1996:11–24.

19. Glasziou PP, Simes RJ, Gelber RD. Quality adjusted survival analysis. *Stat Med* 1990;9:1259–76.

20. Weeks J. *Taking Quality of Life into Account in Health Economics Analysis*: National Cancer Institute, 1996.

21. Feeny DH, Torrance GW. Incorporating utility-based quality-of-life assessment measures in clinical trials. Two examples. *Med Care* 1989;27(3 Suppl):S190–204.

22. von Neumann J, Morgenstern O. *Theory of Games and Economic Behavior*. Princeton: Princeton University Press, 1944.

23. Weinstein MC, Fineberg HV. *Clinical Decision Analysis*. Philadelphia: W.B. Saunders, 1980.

24. Cole BF, Gelber RD, Goldhirsch A. Cox regression models for quality adjusted survival analysis. *Stat Med* 1993;12:975–87.

25. Glasziou PP, Cole BF, Gelber RD, Hilden J, Simes RJ. Quality adjusted survival analysis with repeated quality of life measures. *Stat Med* 1998;17:1215–29.

26. Hwang JS, Tsauo JY, Wang JD. Estimation of expected quality adjusted survival by cross-sectional survey. *Stat Med* 1996;15:93–102.

27. Shen LZ, Pulkstenis E, Hoseyni M. Estimation of mean quality adjusted survival time. *Stat Med* 1999;18:1541–54.

28. Fisk JD, Brown MG, Sketris IS, Metz LM, Murray TJ, Stadnyk KJ. A comparison of health utility measures for the evaluation of multiple sclerosis treatments. *J Neurol Neurosurg Psychiatr* 2005;76:58–63.

29. Kattan MW, Fearn NA, Miles BJ. Time trade-off utility modified to accommodate degenerative and life-threatening conditions. Presented at the 2001 American Medical Informatics Association Symposium, Washington, DC.

30. Bakker C, Rutten-van Molken M, Hidding A, van Doorslaer E, Bennett K, Van Der LS. Patient utilities in ankylosing spondylitis and the association with other outcome measures. *J Rheumatol* 1994;21:1298–304.

31. Bennett L, Hamilton R, Neutel CI, Pearson JC, Talbot B. Survey of persons with multiple sclerosis in Ottawa, 1974–75. *Can J Public Health* 1977;68:141–7.

32. Bosch JL, Hunink MG. The relationship between descriptive and valuational quality-of-life measures in patients with intermittent claudication. *Med Dec Making* 1996;16:217–25.

33. Froberg DG, Kane RL. Methodology for measuring health-state preferences–II: scaling methods. *J Clin Epidemiol* 1989;42:459–71.

34. Lenert LA, Cher DJ, Goldstein MK, Bergen MR, Garber A. The effect of search procedures on utility elicitations. *Med Dec Making* 1998;18:76–83.

35. Torrance GW. Utility approach to measuring health-related quality of life. *J Chronic Dis* 1987;40:593.

36. Revicki DA, Osoba D, Fairclough D, *et al.* Recommendations on health-related quality of life research to support labeling and promotional claims in the United States. *Qual Life Res* 2000;9:887–900.

37. Fischer G, Kamlet MS, Fienberg S, Schkade D. Risk preference for gains and losses in multiple objective decision making. *Manage Sci* 1986;31:1065–86.

38. Hobart JC, Thompson AJ, Polman C, Hohlfeld R. Measuring health outcomes in multiple sclerosis: why, which and how? In Thompson AJ, Polman C, Hohlfeld, eds. *Multiple Sclerosis: Clinical Challenges and Controversies*. St. Louis: Mosby, 1997:211–26.

39. Feinstein AR. *Clinimetrics*. New Haven: Yale University Press, 1987.

40. Spector WD, Spilker B. Functional disability scales. In *Quality of Life and Pharmacoeconomics in Clinical Trials*. Philadelphia: Lippincott Raven, 1996: 133–41.

41. Mowry EM, Beheshtian A, Waubant E, *et al.* Quality of life in multiple sclerosis is associated with lesion burden and brain volume measures. *Neurology* 2009;72:1760–5.

42. Miller DM, Cohen JA, Kooijmans M, Tsao E, Cutter G, Baier M. Change in clinician-assessed measures of multiple sclerosis and subject-reported quality of life: results from the IMPACT study. *Mult Scler* 2006;12:180–6.

43. Cella D, Riley W, Stone A, *et al.* The patient-reported outcomes measurement information System (PROMIS) developed and tested its first wave of adult self-reported health outcome item banks: 2005–2008. *J Clin Epidemiol* 2010;63:1179–94.

44. Walker J, Hnke, JR, Cerny T, Strasser F. Development of symptom assessments utilising item response theory and computer-adaptive testing–a practical method based on a systematic review. *Crit Rev Oncol-Hematol* 2010;73:47–67.

45. Bjorner JB, Chang C-H, Thissen D, Reeve BB. Developing tailored instruments: item banking and computerized adaptive assessment. *Qual Life Res* 2007;16 Suppl 1:95–108.

46. Chang C-H. Patient-reported outcomes measurement and management with innovative methodologies and technologies. *Qual Life Res* 2007;16 (Suppl 1):157–66.

47. Committee N-QE. Neuor-QoL: Progress report 2004–2007: NINDS, Evanston Northwestern Health Care, 2008.

48. Rudick RA, Miller D, Clough JD, Gragg LA, Farmer RG. Quality of life in multiple sclerosis. Comparison with inflammatory bowel disease and rheumatoid arthritis. *Arch Neurol* 1992;49:1237–42.

49. Hermann BP, Vickrey B, Hays RD, *et al.* A comparison of health-related quality of life in patients with epilepsy, diabetes and multiple sclerosis. *Epilepsy Res* 1996;25:113–18.

50. Nortvedt MW, Riise T, Myhr KM, Nyland HI. Quality of life as a predictor for change in disability in MS. *Neurology* 2000;55:51–4.

51. Shawaryn MA, Schiaffino KM, LaRocca NG, Johnston MV. Determinants of Health-Related Quality of Life in Multiple Sclerosis: The role of illness intrusiveness. *Mult Scler* 2002;8: 310–18.

52. Sugano DS, McElwee NE, Spilker B. An epidemiological perspective. In: Anonymous, ed. *Quality of Life and Pharmacoeconomics in Clinical Trials.* Philadelphia: Lippincott-Raven, 1996:555–62.

53. Minden SL, Frankel D, Hadden LS, Srinath KP, Perloff JN. Disability in elderly people with multiple sclerosis: an analysis of baseline data from the Sonya Slifka Longitudinal Multiple Sclerosis Study. *Neurorehabilitation* 2004;19:55–67.

54. Wu N, Minden SL, Hoaglin DC, Hadden L, Frankel D. Quality of life in people with multiple sclerosis: data from the Sonya Slifka Longitudinal Multiple Sclerosis Study. *J Health Hum Serv Admin* 2007;30:233–67.

55. Quality AfHRa. *Helping the Nation with Health Services Research.* Rockville: US Department of Health and Human Services, 2002.

56. Spilker B. Introduction. In: Anonymous, ed. *Quality of Life and Pharacoeconomics in Clinical Trials.* Philadelphia, New York: Lippincott-Raven, 1996:1–10.

57. Miller D, Moore S, Fox R, *et al.* Web-based self-management for patients with multiple sclerosis: a practical randomized trial. *Telemed e-Health* 2010; 17: 5–13.

58. National Multiple Sclerosis S, Consortium of Multiple Sclerosis C. *Multiple Sclerosis Quality of Life Inventory: A User's Manual.* New York: National Multiple Sclerosis Society, 1997.

59. Rubenstein LV, Spilker B. Using quality of life tests for patient diagnosis or screening, or to evaluate treatment. In Spilker B, ed. *Clinical Trials and Pharmacoeconomics in Clinical Trials.*

Philadelphia: Lippincott-Raven, 1996:363–74.

60. Hays RD, Sherbourne CD, Bozzette SA, Spilker B. Pharmacoeconomics and quality of life research beyond the randomized clinical trial. In Spilker B, ed. *Quality of Life Research and Pharamcoeconomics in Clinical Trials.* Philadelphia: Lippincott-Raven, 1996:155–60.

61. LaRocca NG, Ritvo PG, Miller DM, *et al.* Quality of life assessment in multiple sclerosis clinical trials: current status and strategies for improving multiple sclerosis clinical trial designs. In Goodkin DE, Rudick RA, eds. *Multiple Sclerosis: Advances in Clinical Trial Design, Treatment and Future Perspectives.* London: Springer, 1996:145–60.

62. Cohen JA, Cutter GR, Fischer JS, *et al.* Benefit of interferon beta-1a on MSFC progression in secondary progressive MS. *Neurology* 2002;59:679–87.

63. Office of Communications DoDI, Center for Drug Evaluation and Research Food and Drug Administration. Guidance for Industry Patient-Reported Outcome Measures: Use in Medical Product Development to Support Labeling Claims. In. Silver Spring, MD: Office of Communications, Division of Drug Information, Center for Drug Evaluation and Research, Food and Drug Administration, 2009.

64. Miller DM, Allen R. Quality of life in multiple sclerosis: determinants, measurement, and use in clinical practice. *Curr Neurol Neurosci Rep* 2010;10:397–406.

65. Vickrey BG, Hays RD, Harooni R, Myers LW, Ellison GW. A health-related quality of life measure for multiple sclerosis. *Qual Life Res* 1995;4:187–206.

66. Sharafaddinzadeh N, Moghtaderi A, Kashipazha D, Majdinasab N, Shalbafan B. The effect of low-dose naltrexone on quality of life of patients with multiple sclerosis: a randomized placebo-controlled trial. *Mult Scler*; 16:964–9.

67. McClurg D, Ashe RG, Marshall K, Lowe-Strong AS. Comparison of pelvic floor muscle training, electromyography biofeedback, and neuromuscular electrical stimulation for bladder dysfunction in people with multiple sclerosis: a randomized pilot

study. *Neurourol Urodyn* 2006;25:337–48.

68. Hart S, Fonareva I, Merluzzi N, Mohr DC. Treatment for depression and its relationship to improvement in quality of life and psychological well-being in multiple sclerosis patients. *Qual Life Res* 2005;14:695–703.

69. Romberg A, Virtanen A, Ruutiainen J. Long-term exercise improves functional impairment but not quality of life in multiple sclerosis. *J Neurol* 2005;252:839–45.

70. Cella DF, Dineen K, Arnason B, *et al.* Validation of the functional assessment of multiple sclerosis quality of life instrument. *Neurology* 1996;47: 129–39.

71. McCullagh R, Fitzgerald AP, Murphy RP, Cooke G. Long-term benefits of exercising on quality of life and fatigue in multiple sclerosis patients with mild disability: a pilot study. *Clin Rehabil* 2008;22:206–14.

72. Kappos L, Freedman MS, Polman CH, *et al.* Effect of early versus delayed interferon beta-1b treatment on disability after a first clinical event suggestive of multiple sclerosis: a 3-year follow-up analysis of the BENEFIT study. *Lancet* 2007;370:389–97.

73. Johnson SK, Diamond BJ, Rausch S, Kaufman M, Shiflett SC, Graves L. The effect of Ginkgo biloba on functional measures in multiple sclerosis: a pilot randomized controlled trial. *Explore: J Sci Healing* 2006;2:19–24.

74. Lankhorst GJ, Jelles F, Smits RC, *et al.* Quality of life in multiple sclerosis: the disability and impact profile (DIP). *Neurol* 1996;243:469–74.

75. Goodman AD, Brown TR, Cohen JA, *et al.* Dose comparison trial of sustained-release fampridine in multiple sclerosis. *Neurology* 2008;71:1134–41.

76. Panitch H, Miller A, Paty D, Weinshenker B, North American Study Group on Interferon beta-1b in Secondary Progressive MS. Interferon beta-1b in secondary progressive MS: results from a 3-year controlled study. *Neurology* 2004;63:1788–95.

77. Rotstein Z, Barak Y, Noy S, Achiron A. Quality of life in multiple sclerosis: development and validation of the "RAYS" scale and comparison with the SF-36. *Int J Qual Health Care* 2000;12:511–7.

78. Ford HL, Gerry E, Tennant A, Whalley D, Haigh R, Johnson MH. Developing a disease-specific quality of life measure for people with multiple sclerosis. *Clin Rehabil* 2001;15:247–58.

79. Gold SM, Heesen C, Schulz H, *et al.* Disease specific quality of life instruments in multiple sclerosis: validation of the Hamburg Quality of Life Questionnaire in Multiple Sclerosis (HAQUAMS). *Mult Scler* 2001;7:119–30.

80. Naseri M, Ahmadi A, Gharegozli K, *et al.* A double blind, placebo-controlled, crossover study on the effect of MS14, an herbal-marine drug, on quality of life in patients with multiple sclerosis. *J Med Plant Res* 2009;3:271–5.

81. Schulz K-H, Gold SM, Witte J, *et al.* Impact of aerobic training on immune-endocrine parameters, neurotrophic factors, quality of life and coordinative function in multiple sclerosis. *J Neurol Sci* 2004;225: 11–18.

82. Hobart J, Lamping D, Fitzpatrick R, Riazi A, Thompson A. The Multiple Sclerosis Impact Scale (MSIS-29): a new patient-based outcome measure. *Brain* 2001;124:962–73.

83. Hughes CM, Smyth S, Lowe-Strong AS. Reflexology for the treatment of pain in people with multiple sclerosis: a double-blind randomised sham-controlled clinical trial. *Mult Scler* 2009;15:1229–338.

84. McClurg D, Ashe RG, Lowe-Strong AS. Neuromuscular electrical stimulation and the treatment of lower urinary tract dysfunction in multiple sclerosis – a double blind, placebo controlled, randomised clinical trial. *Neurourol Urodyn* 2008;27:231–7.

85. Khan F, Pallant JF, Brand C, Kilpatrick TJ. Effectiveness of rehabilitation intervention in persons with multiple sclerosis: a randomised controlled trial. *J Neurol Neurosurg Psychiatry* 2008;79:1230–5.

86. Simeoni M, Auquier P, Fernandez O, *et al.* Validation of the Multiple Sclerosis International Quality of Life questionnaire. *Multiple Sclerosis* 2008;14:219–30.

87. Wynia K, Middel B, de Ruiter H, van Dijk JP, de Keyser JHA, Reijneveld SA. Stability and relative validity of the Multiple Sclerosis Impact Profile (MSIP). *Disabil Rehabil* 2008;30:1027–38.

88. Doward LC, McKenna SP, Meads DM, Twiss J, Eckert BJ. The development of patient-reported outcome indices for multiple sclerosis (PRIMUS). *Mult Scler* 2009;15:1092–102.

89. Wesson JM, Cooper JA, Jehle LS, Lockhart SN, Draney K, Barber J. The functional index for living with multiple sclerosis: development and validation of a new quality of life questionnaire. *Mult Scler* 2009;15:1239–49.

90. Freeman JA, Thompson AJ, Fitzpatrick R, *et al.* Interferon-Beta1b in the treatment of secondary progressive MS: impact on quality of life. *Neurology* 2001;57:1870–5.

91. Rudick RA, Stuart WH, Calabresi PA, *et al.* Natalizumab plus interferon beta-1a for relapsing multiple sclerosis. *New Engl J Med* 2006;354:911–23.

92. Polman CH, O'Connor PW, Havrdova E, *et al.* A randomized, placebo-controlled trial of natalizumab for relapsing multiple sclerosis. *New Engl J Med* 2006;354:899–910.

93. Rudick RA, Miller D, Hass S, *et al.* Health-related quality of life in multiple sclerosis: effects of natalizumab. *Ann Neurol* 2007;62:335–46.

94. Hobart J, Freeman J, Lamping D, Fitzpatrick R, Thompson A. The SF-36 in multiple sclerosis: why basic assumptions must be tested. *J Neurol Neurosurg Psychiatry* 2001;71:363–70.

95. Freeman JA, Hobart JC, Langdon DW, Thompson AJ. Clinical appropriateness: a key factor in outcome measure selection: the 36 item short form health survey in multiple sclerosis. *J Neurol Neurosurg Psychiatry* 2000;68:150–6.

96. Hickey AM, Bury G, O'Boyle CA, Bradley F, O'Kelly FD, Shannon W. A new short form individual quality of life measure (SEIQoL-DW): application in a cohort of individuals with HIV/AIDS. *BMJ* 1996;313:29–33.

97. Zingler VC, Nabauer M, Jahn K, *et al.* Assessment of potential cardiotoxic side effects of mitoxantrone in patients with multiple sclerosis. *Eur Neurol* 2005;54:28–33.

98. Singer E. Tysabri withdrawal calls entire class into question. *Nature Med* 2005;11:359.

Measures of acute and chronic lesions visualized by conventional magnetic resonance imaging

Jack H. Simon and Jerry S. Wolinsky

Introduction

Magnetic resonance imaging (MRI) plays an essential role in the diagnosis of multiple sclerosis (MS), is useful as a prognostic aid, has been accepted as a primary outcome measure in exploratory trials of the development of new drugs for disease modification, is an essential supportive secondary outcome variable for drug registration, and is invaluable in the management of individual patients. This chapter will review the use of conventional MRI (cMRI) as generally available to the practitioner, touch on newer MR-based tools as they illuminate our understanding of MS pathology as defined by cMRI, and explore the justification of the use of cMRI in these settings.

One of the most profound changes in our modern conceptualization of MS pathogenesis arises from MRI. Serial imaging enabled recognition of how dynamic the changes are that underlie the evolution of lesions in MS patients in the absence of those clinical events that characterize relapsing and, to a lesser extent, progressive forms of the disease. This has led to a model of how lesions evolve over time that as a first approximation characterizes most of the evolving pathology of MS for many but not all patients, and for most but not all developing MRI-defined lesions. MRI-defined lesion evolution largely stems from observation of changes in the white matter expanses of the cerebral hemispheres, brain stem, and spinal cord. However, there are some differences in the signatures of these lesions as they occur in different brain topographies. Somewhat more elusive is the evolution of intracortical lesions in MS (Chapter 13).

A brief primer in the basis of MR as applied to MS

MR is extremely sensitivity to changes in regional proton relaxation times occurring with processes that alter tissue water content and constraints on hydrogen molecule motion, particularly those associated with tissue-bound and free-water molecules. The intensity of tissue signals is influenced by proton density and the rate at which nuclear MR signals decay in the static magnetic field of the scanner following application of a radiofrequency excitation pulse as characterized by T1 (longitudinal relaxation time) and T2 (transverse relaxation time). These three parameters (proton density, T1, and T2 relaxation times) determine much of the appearance of conventional MR images. Their relative influences can be altered by changing the imaging parameters.

Proton density and T2 weighted images are generated with long repetition times (TR). Image appearance at relatively short echo times (TE), is mainly determined by proton density while at relatively long TE, the T2 effect is increased. T1-weighted images are normally generated at relatively short TR and TE. Fluid-attenuating inversion recovery (FLAIR) uses an inversion pulse followed by a variable signal recovery time to maximize the contrast between tissues with different T1 values. Most clinically used FLAIR inversion pulses are designed to null the signal from cerebrospinal fluid (CSF) at long TE to provide a high degree of T2 weighting in order to increase lesion conspicuity. While each pulse sequence produces some variation in individual lesions and total T2-lesion burden of disease, the lesions and their total volumes are strongly correlated across any of these popular T2-weighted methodologies. Moreover, as T1 values of gray and white matter and CSF all differ, single and double inversion pulses can be applied to selectively null one or two of these tissue types.

Intravenously administered gadolinium (Gd) chelate based paramagnetic contrast agents markedly shorten the T1 of neighboring water protons. The result is an increase in the signal from tissue where there normally is no blood–brain barrier, such as in the choroid plexus and the pituitary, or where the barrier is significantly compromised to allow Gd to enter the brain abnormally. This effect is best monitored on T1-weighted images. Several approaches to increase the conspicuity of enhancement have been developed, each with advantages and disadvantages, including inclusion of an off-resonance pulse (see below). The magnitude, extent, and sometimes the numbers of enhancements may also increase on the dose of contrast, delay in the time-to image acquisition, and even potentially by the type of contrast selected.[1] However, with the recognition of nephrogenic sclerosing fibrosis (NSF) related to higher doses of MR contrast in some patients, there is a risk–benefit that should

Multiple Sclerosis Therapeutics, Fourth Edition, ed. Jeffrey A. Cohen and Richard A. Rudick. Published by Cambridge University Press.
© Cambridge University Press 2011.

be considered especially when the dose of contrast or frequency of MRI studies is increased in patients with impaired renal function (see www.acr.org/secondarymainmenucategories/quality_safety/contrast_manual.aspx).

Protons from water molecules that are tightly bound to tissue contribute little signal to images acquired with cMRI. When a narrow bandwidth radiofrequency pulse with a 1 kHz to 2 kHz frequency offset from the excitation pulse is used to saturate protons associated with the bound water pool, magnetization is transferred from the bound to the free water pool (the pool that contributes to cMRI), through an incompletely understood interaction. The result is attenuation of the free water signal proportional to the concentration of the bound water molecules, providing a practical estimate of tissue integrity. The off-resonance or magnetization transfer (MT) pulse does not directly affect the free water signal. In the case where the MT pulse is applied to post-Gd-T1 imaging, the signal from brain tissue is reduced and the Gd effect by comparison appears enhanced. Images obtained without and with the application of an MT pulse can be mathematically manipulated to be displayed as a map of the relative integrity of the imaged tissue, an MTR image (Chapter 10).

Water molecules are in perpetual and random motion referred to as diffusion. Their diffusion is unrestricted in free water, but is less free (decreased) in tissue; the relative restriction is described by an apparent diffusion coefficient (ADC). In free water diffusion is invariant with respect to direction (isotropic diffusion). In highly organized structures, water diffusion is directionally preferential; for example water molecular motions are less impeded along the length of axons. This directional preference is referred to as diffusion anisotropy; fractional anisotropy (FA) is a commonly used measure of the extent of diffusion anisotropy. When diffusion is anisotropic, complete characterization of diffusion can be described by symmetric three-dimensional matrixes, referred to as the diffusion tensor (Chapter 15).

Any mobile proton can contribute signal to MR, but the abundance of water in tissue overwhelms signals from protons associated with biochemicals and macromolecules of biologic significance. MRS is able to sample some of these signals and suppress the signals from water. The metabolites most readily recognized in brain include myoinositol, choline, creatine, N-acetyl aspartate (NAA), lactate, and lipids. Methods are available to capture anatomically correlated data using single voxel and two- and three-dimensional multivoxel procedures, or as an unlocalized signal from whole brain (Chapter 12).

What is considered "conventional" MRI has, and will, continue to evolve. A practical definition might be those MR approaches that lend to image reconstruction for viewing in real time, and that can be subjectively interpreted by an experienced clinician without the need for extensive off line data transformation, processing and analysis. For imaging patients suspect for or having MS, this consists of several series of image acquisitions based on generally available pulse sequences developed to provide optimal tissue contrast for defining lesions in the white matter of the central nervous system (CNS). One standardized approach to imaging individual MS patients developed by the Consortium of MS Centers includes sagittal FLAIR, axial dual echo proton density and T2-weighted (TE1 usually <30 ms and TE2 >80 ms), axial FLAIR, and axial Gd-enhanced T1-weighted image series,[2] and is similar to the protocol currently recommended for MS trials.[3]

Enhancing, T2-hyperintense and T1-hypointense lesions (T1-holes; T1-black holes) are the three classic measures of MS pathology visible by cMRI that are the cornerstone of MRI-based outcomes in MS clinical trials and individual patient management. The three lesion "types" are inter-related, yet complementary, and integral to fully appreciate analyses of the diffuse pathology disclosed by MRI-based measures of normal appearing brain tissue, and brain and spinal cord atrophy.[4] Since the focal pathology of cMRI contributes to the diffuse pathology in normal appearing tissue through secondary neuronal degeneration and other mechanisms, cMRI and advanced quantitative MRI (qMRI) measures are not entirely independent.

Evolution of individual lesions as seen by MRI
"Typical" lesion formation

Effectively, all new lesions that arise from previously normal appearing white matter on cMRI are announced by an area of Gd enhancement on T1-weighted images and are invariably associated with a high signal intensity lesion at the same location on the T2-weighted or FLAIR image.[5] The acute enhancement is visualized as a result of abnormal leakage of Gd-containing contrast material (molecular weight approx 500–800 daltons) across disrupted tight junctions of the vascular endothelium with subsequent accumulation of the Gd-chelate in the perivenular interstitial spaces of the CNS (Fig. 9.1). The blood level determined concentration gradient and permeability factors drive contrast across the blood–brain barrier.[6] This passive process and issues related to imaging (pulse sequence and timing), pathologic characteristics of individual lesions, their location, age, and size explains some of the variability observed for enhancement within and between individuals.

An intact blood–brain barrier is a component of controlled cell trafficking and immune surveillance. When disturbed by the multiple pathologic processes accompanying inflammation in MS, this barrier becomes permeable to small molecules and hematogenous cells.[7] Factors associated with the initial disruption of the barrier are complex, but central to this process is passage of activated T-cells through previously intact tight junctions of the capillary endothelium. Activated lymphocytes recognize CNS antigen and trigger a cytokine/chemokine cascade that further mediates barrier disruption.[8] MRI-pathology correlative studies support the utilization of contrast enhancement in MS as a convenient if imperfect (see below) marker for the events associated with

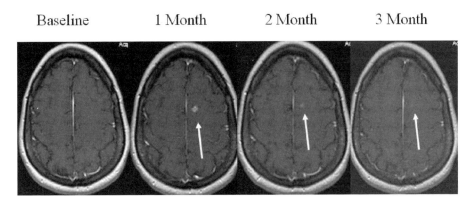

Baseline   1 Month   2 Month   3 Month

Fig. 9.1. Serial monthly MRI shows a new enhancing lesion on the one-month follow-up MRI (arrow, second panel). There is an expected decrease in enhancing area over the subsequent two months (arrows panel 3 and 4). MRI-histopathology correlation studies suggest that the decreased enhancement with time corresponds to reduction in inflammation and return of the integrity of the blood–brain barrier. While the enhancement in this case is nearly inconspicuous at three months, more optimal image display (below) showed that abnormal contrast leakage was still detected.

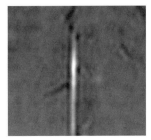

3 Month

macroscopic inflammation in MS.[9,10] Enhancement appears at the time inflammation can be observed under the microscope, and untreated last about 2–6 weeks in most cases with a range of less than 1 week to rarely 16 weeks or longer.[11,12] Further supporting the inflammation–enhancement association are studies from experimental demyelination based on experimental autoimmune encephalomyelitis (EAE) models, where a generally good temporal/spatial correlation has been established between enhancement and inflammation.[13]

Nearly three-quarters of the larger enhanced tissue regions appear hypointense on the T1-weighted image taken prior to the Gd injection. More than half of the T1-hypointensities associated with new enhancements spontaneously resolve within 4 weeks; about a third of those still evident at a month disappear over the next 2 to 5 months.[14] About a quarter of newly formed T1-hypointensities persist for at least 6 months.[15] Return to a T1-isointense state or mild T1-hypointensity may indicate extensive or partial remyelination.[16]

The size of the new T2-weighted or FLAIR visualized lesion usually contracts over weeks or months, and its intensity is reduced as edema resolves and some tissue repair occurs. Ultimately, the residual T2-hyperintensity remains as a convenient marker of past injury. These footprints of remote pathology rarely disappear completely in the hemispheric white matter; they more frequently become inconspicuous in the brain stem and spinal cord. Focal and confluent areas of residual T2-hyperintensity contribute to the total T2 disease burden, representing a useful qualitative and quantitative measure of the MS pathology, particularly in the earlier stages of disease. In later disease stages, the T2–hyperintensity burden becomes less sensitive to change as multifocal lesions become confluent due to proximity, and/or tissue shrinkage and the T2 burden may reach a volume plateau.[17,18]

Heterogeneity of enhancing lesions

Enhancement patterns vary more between rather than within patients,[19] which may support the concept of a heterogeneous pathology across MS patients.[20] Enhancement of individual lesions varies over time. Most enhancements are initially seen as small areas of nodular enhancement, with some progressing to rings, while others are ring enhancing when initially encountered on frequent serial imaging.[12] More aggressive lesions may show ring-like propagation of tissue enhancement over a few weeks or longer. These larger lesions associate with more complex architecture on T2-weighted images and a central spherical hypointensity on T1-weighted images, and have been reported to be more likely to persist,[21] but even rather large ring-enhanced lesions can show substantial resolution. The rings are associated with greater macrophage infiltration, larger size, longer duration, decreased magnetization transfer ratio,[22] and greater evolution to T1-holes.[23,24] However, recent long-term serial evaluations did not confirm a poor lesion outcome for ring enhancing lesions based on evolution to chronic T1-black holes or the persistence of chronic black holes.[25] The areas surrounding some of the larger T1-hypointense lesions may contract over time, indicating that this apparent repair is at the expense of surrounding tissue loss and regional atrophy with gliosis. This occurs in about 8%–9% of lesions followed for up to eight months.[14] Enhancing lesions seen only after triple dose tend to be smaller and less destructive than those detected following routine single dose (0.1 mmole/kg) contrast infusions.[26]

While the evolution of acute T1-hypointense lesions is intimately associated with enhancements, the relationship of enhancements to more chronic T1-hypointense lesion evolution is less compelling. Enhancement frequency is in part age dependent, being less frequent among older than younger patients with MS of all disease subtypes.[27] Yet, T1-hypointense lesions are more common with longer disease durations and among the progressive disease subtypes. The divergent behavior of these seemingly inter-related MRI metrics suggests that some T1-hypointense lesions result directly from new inflammatory events that are readily monitored by enhancements on MRI, while other T1-hypointense lesions evolve differently. Several groups have suggested that differences in the tendency between individual patients to form hypointense lesions might reflect different immunopathogenic or genetic traits.[28]

Lesion evolution appears even more complex with serial advanced MRI. Newly enhanced lesions that form within previously normal appearing white matter on cMRI have been used to identify informative regions of interest to explore tissue changes on serial MTR or MRS imaging that antedate the enhancement or occur with subsequent lesion evolution. Likely abnormalities in cMRI-defined normal appearing white matter precede many if not most enhancements and newly identified T2 lesions. These prelesional abnormalities include regional changes in MTR,[29] and focal increases in choline and the appearance of signals on MRS imaging consistent with alterations in lipids or other myelin-associated macromolecules that suggest that focal disruptions in tissue integrity anticipate lesion formation by several months.[30] These prelesional abnormalities could simply reflect another form of low grade inflammation,[31] although the basis for these abnormalities remains unclear. The most controversial postulate is that they more closely reflect the true primary abnormality in MS lesion pathogenesis and that this serves to target a subsequent secondary immune response that amplifies lesion formation, simplistically rendering the pathogenesis of MS to one that is "inside/out." More generally accepted is that these more subtle abnormalities reflect immune-mediated inflammatory lesional activity that will eventually rise to the threshold of detection by cMRI, the "outside/in" concept. While advanced MRI methods allow retrospective definition of regions at risk of cMRI-defined lesion formation, as yet only MRS imaging allows their prospective prediction.

Concomitant with tissue enhancement there is a dramatic fall in regional MTR, and drop in NAA. Other acute metabolic changes include increases in choline, signals from myelin breakdown products, and increases of myoinositol, glutamate plus glutamine, and lactate.[32] The biochemical changes are highly dynamic, and the concentrations of various metabolites and MTR tend to recover toward their normal values with time. Some of the observed early changes are in part explained by dilutional effects of acute vasogenic edema.[33] While MTR values are unlikely to fully normalize over time, a return toward normal is usually accompanied by resolution of accompanying T1-hypointense lesions.

Limitations of conventional contrast enhancement

While Gd enhancement is a convenient and effective imaging marker for blood–brain barrier leakage coincident with inflammation in MS, it has several well-recognized limitations. Transient leakage, present for a few weeks or less is not efficiently detected by monthly MRI.[11,12] Most methods used for tissue enhancement measures are based on intensity thresholding that define focal enhancement as either present or absent. Inherent sensitivity limitations assure that diffuse microscopic-level focal enhancement, and chronic low-grade enhancement from vascular leakage will go undetected.[34]

A controversial but important point relates to the interpretation of enhancement as indicative of damaging inflammation.[35] As discussed above, not all enhancement is equal in its deleterious "consequences;" some components of inflammation may be beneficial and even neuroprotective.[36] Unfortunately, no imaging techniques are available to confirm this hypothesis in vivo.

Experimental approaches to cellular imaging based on ultra-small particles of iron oxide (USPIO) incorporated in vivo into macrophages,[37] ex vivo in specific cell types,[38] or in vivo into specific cell types,[39] may provide a more cell type-specific and informative measure of inflammation in MS. Details of barrier injury can potentially be probed with multiple molecules of varying size and other useful characteristics, and based on standard and potentially more informative modeling approaches.[40]

Lesions that remain mildly T1-hypointense with intermediate MTR values show evidence of partial or more extensive remyelination on histological examination.[16] Diminished NAA within persistently T1-hypointense lesions indicates irreversible axonal loss and permanently T1-hypointense lesions have increased myoinositol content indicative of gliosis. Enhanced lesions generally have increased diffusion, decreased FA, and altered diffusion tensor values, and these alterations persist to a variable extent in those lesions that have the most severely altered tissue matrix.[41] The specialized anatomy of brain results in alterations at a distance related to disruption along connected pathways that traverse focal lesions, and Wallerian degeneration along highly organized pathways may be reflected in altered diffusion eigenvalues.[42] These distributed effects may explain some of the quantitative change that is rather consistently found in cMRI-defined normal appearing white matter.[43]

"Atypical" lesion formation (see also Chapter 13)

Intracortical lesions can be considered to be a special case of lesion formation that might, once better understood, also illuminate pre-enhancement events that underlie lesion formation in the white matter. MRS imaging defines dynamic metabolite change compatible with alterations in mobile lipids in cMRI normal appearing cortical gray matter,[44] which follows a pattern similar to that seen in normal appearing white matter with several exceptions. First, cMRI has thus far failed to identify subsequent cortical lesion evolution for all but those

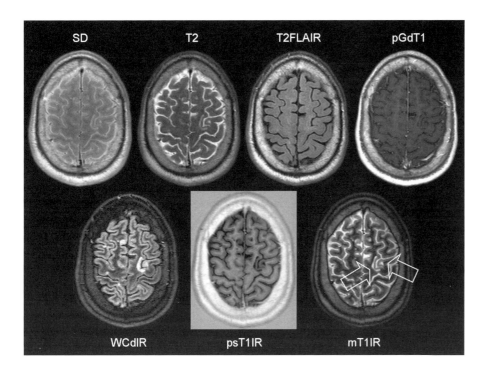

Fig. 9.2. This 50-year-old, Caucasian male has SPMS that began nine years prior to imaging with an episode of optic neuritis. He was reimaged after three years of steady gait deterioration despite disease-modifying drugs, when his most prominent finding on examination was a spastic paraparesis; he was still able to walk unassisted. Spin density (SD) and T2-weighted imaging without (T2) and with fluid attenuation by inversion recovery (T2 FLAIR), post-gadolinium T1-weighted (pGd T1), white matter and cerebrospinal fluid dual inversion recover (WCdIR), phase-sensitive T1 inversion recovery (ps T1IR), and magnitude mode T1 inversion recovery (m T1IR) are shown. All images were obtained at 3 tesla and slice thickness was 3 mm. The arrows on the m T1IR images point to two of the more prominent juxtacortical lesions; intracortical lesions are also present at other locations on this slice. The juxtacortical lesions, which are best identified on the WCdIR, ps T1IR and m T1IR images, can also be found on the SD and T2 images, but are not evident by T2 FLAIR.

intracortical lesions that have an adjacent juxtacortical white matter component. Second, even acute juxtacortical lesions that show enhancement with cMRI fail to show an extension of the enhancement into the cortical ribbon. These observations are consistent with the known occurrence and specialized histopathology of cortical plaques.[45] These lesions show little evidence of perivascular inflammation, and where present, perivascular inflammation in adjacent white matter does not extend into the cortex despite microglial cell-associated intracortical demyelination.

There are a number of possible reasons why intracortical and subpial lesions are poorly resolved by cMRI. These include similarity in the relaxation properties of intracortical lesions and normal gray matter, partial volume effects with adjacent CSF that obscure altered tissue relaxation times between subpial cortical lesions and subjacent normal cortex, and image resolution among others. Moreover, differences in the cortical and white matter microvascular architecture may influence the quantitative and qualitative (compartment differences) factors affecting contrast-enhancement conspicuity, as would the known limited inflammatory change in gray matter. Fortunately, visualization of intracortical lesions can be improved with techniques such as dual inversion recovery (suppression of signal from both white matter and CSF),[46] and T1-FLAIR,[47] compared to spin density, T2-weighted or conventional FLAIR imaging (Fig. 9.2). At ultrahigh fields (7–8T) in post-mortem material, T2* gradient echo MR sequences provides sensitivity in specimens, which approaches that of histopathology for macroscopic lesions.[48] We do not know as yet if these ultrahigh field T2* approaches can be translated to lower field strengths and in vivo imaging through adaptation of pulse sequences.

"Tumefactive" lesion formation

Another type of atypical lesion is the large "tumefactive" lesion seen in some patients with otherwise clinically typical MS. Often these individuals may have classic MS lesions at the time of presentation, or during their subsequent disease course.[49] When these patients with early clinical symptoms are imaged the lesions may not show enhancement, but often do so in a heterogeneous way over the next several weeks.[50] These are often large lesions at first imaging, and the subsequent enhancement is generally widespread across the cMRI-defined T2 lesion.

Evolution of cMRI-monitored disease

There are four cMRI components readily visible to the clinician considering the extent of MS pathology in individual patients that might be compared with the extent of MRI-defined pathology from group data derived from natural history or clinical trial cohorts. These include (1) the presence, number and quality of enhancements, (2) the aggregate number and volume of lesions defined on T2-weighted images, (3) the number and volume of T1-weighted hypointense lesions, and (4) net tissue loss or atrophy (Chapter 11). These provide useful indicators of how that individual fared to a particular point in time, and how they may be expected to behave in the future; information most useful at clinical presentation. Each of these measures has a time course of evolution that differs, and the complexity of their interplay over time is further compounded by as yet poorly explored individual-dependent variations. Nonetheless, all of these measures are quite useful across study populations to determine the effects of therapy on progression of the pathology of the disease.

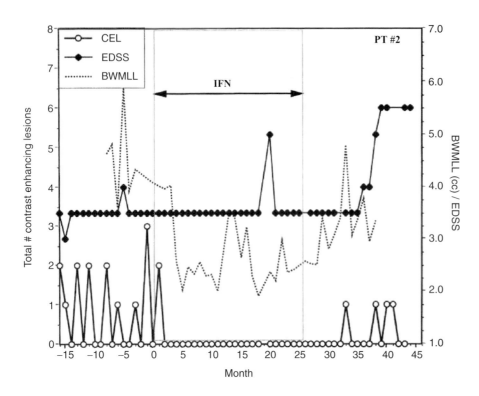

Fig. 9.3. This monthly MRI series from an individual followed over 60 months illustrates several important features. These include general activity trends prior to treatment, with fluctuations in Gd-enhancing lesions (open circles) between 0 and 3 with about half of the scans showing no enhancing lesions. With treatment, activity decreased over 1–2 months and stayed quite low over the next 2 years, but returned after some delay following cessation of therapy. T2-hyperintense lesion load (dashed line) fluctuated markedly from month to month, but also showed a trend generally consistent with enhancing lesion activity. The EDSS score (solid triangles) was relatively stable despite MRI activity, as the pathology depicted by MRI is mostly subclinical. BWMLL, brain white matter lesion load; IFN, interferon beta 1b. From Richert et al.,[53] with permission.

From the perspective of the clinician struggling with the meaning of MRI-defined change of disease activity, there is only one measure of interest: how many new lesions have occurred since the person was last imaged, both those caught at the time of imaging as enhanced and those that are unenhanced, but which clearly have appeared or greatly enlarged since the prior imaging session. This activity measure is readily accessible from well-acquired serial imaging and might be used to judge the likelihood that the new activity exceeds that expected of an adequate response to a disease modifying therapy, or to estimate future disease activity in the short and long term.

Enhanced lesion activity
Enhanced lesion behavior over time

Early natural history studies showed that the extent of subclinical activity as defined by Gd-enhancements greatly exceeded the number of clinical relapses by a factor of 5–10.[51] Far greater ratios of MRI to clinical events have been found in individuals. A meta-analysis of cross-sectional data from over 1300 relapsing subjects selected for recent clinical and sometimes also for subclinical enhancements showed that the presence of one or more enhancements on a single scan was predicted by the clinical phenotype (relapsing remitting MS (RRMS), or secondary progressive MS (SPMS) with or without ongoing clinical relapses), the subject's age at disease onset, the number of clinical attacks in the last one to two years, and the T2-defined disease burden on the images.[52] Factors of no significant predictive importance included gender, monosymptomatic, or polysymptomatic presentation, and Expanded

Disability Status Scale (EDSS) score. Clinical factors that retained predictive value after multivariate logistical regression modeling (age at first symptoms, disease course, and disease duration), are the more important predictors available to the clinician. Those patients with well-established RRMS are more likely to show activity on any given scan than those at first clinical presentation, or those in the secondary progressive phase of their disease. When the quantitative T2 cerebral disease burden was known, disease course was not retained as an important factor among the multivariate predictors. As a rough guide, when the T2 burden of disease is below 5 ml, the likelihood of an enhancement is 20%–40%, rising to 40%–60% for T2 lesion load between 5 and 15 ml, and over 60% for a lesion load above 15 ml. This prediction is then modified by the other remaining important predictors of age at disease onset and disease duration. These findings are generally consistent with previously developed caricatures of the disease course that showed enhancement frequency highest in relapsing patients, with higher activity among younger subjects, peak activity at mid disability levels, and waning activity among SPMS patients.[27]

In individuals. the expectation is to observe a variation in lesion number and volume from week-to-week and month-to-month, and in both individuals and populations a generalization can be made for a trend toward decreased activity with progression to SPMS. Even less activity is found in PPMS than the other MS phenotypes. Figure 9.3 illustrates the marked fluctuations in enhancing lesion number over short intervals that may be seen in some individuals with relatively active disease as described in a classic monthly MRI study conducted at the

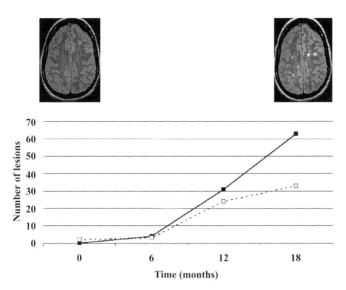

Fig. 9.4. MRI results from one untreated patient from the CHAMPS trial (Controlled High-Risk Subjects Avonex® Multiple Sclerosis Prevention Study). Enhancing lesions (open squares) and/or new or enlarging T2-hyperintense lesions (filled squares) disclosed marked activity; 63 new or enlarging T2 lesions developed, including 33 enhancing lesions over the 18-month MRI study. Nevertheless, there were no new clinical events over the same interval.

National Institutes of Health. This and numerous other studies showed that one could not accurately predict the number of enhancing lesions at a point in time based on an individual's prior activity profile.[31,54,55] However, general activity trends and patterns in lesion frequency can be discerned in individuals and populations, with high activity in some individuals over most intervals (Fig. 9.4), while others tend to have no or few lesions at most evaluations. Similar patterns have been observed for annual or 6-monthly MRI evaluations, where in untreated patients enhancement predicts subsequent enhancement.[56]

In clinical trials enhancing lesion counts provide sufficient stability over time to be an informative and important outcome measure. Typically, in Phase 2 trials multiple points in time are sampled, most commonly by monthly MRI, and the results summarized by monthly and cumulative enhancing lesion counts.[57] In Phase 3 trials, the large sample size limits sampling of enhancing lesion counts or enhancing lesion volume to relatively infrequent intervals (annual or semi-annually).

Following presentation with a CIS, patients with a positive MRI are at high risk for a subsequent clinical or MRI event, and those with a number of T2 lesions only some of which show Gd-enhancement can now be considered early MS.[58–60] In a trial of weekly intramuscular interferon beta-1a, 30% of patients with a monosymptomatic clinical presentation exhibited one or more enhancing lesions shortly after presentation; likely an underestimate of enhancing activity as all patients had received standardized high-dose corticosteroids prior to their baseline MRI study.[61] In a trial of weekly subcutaneous interferon beta-1a, which included patients with a wider interval between onset of their CIS and first on trial MRI and patients with a polysymptomatic presentation, 59% had enhancing lesions.[62]

In relapsing stages of MS, the frequency of contrast enhancement in untreated patients was reported to range from about 50% to 65% in larger studies,[27] with mean lesion counts varying from about one to five lesions, the variability related to entry criteria (see below). However, the frequency of enhancement at study entry has fallen for recent trials.[63,64]

Enhancing lesion frequency decreases in later disease stages, roughly in parallel with the decrease described in relapse rate with increasing disease duration and age.[65] Estimates for proportions of patients with enhancing lesions enrolled in SPMS from large multicenter trials range from about 35%–50%.[66–68] In contrast to relapsing MS, the acute lesions of PPMS appear to be less intensely inflammatory based on histopathology,[69] and reduced numbers of enhancing lesions are seen in population studies by MRI.[70] Frequencies of enhancing lesions at baseline range from only about 14% of patients in the trial of glatiramer acetate,[71] to 25% in the rituximab study.[72] Enhancement frequencies were somewhat higher for those PPMS subjects required to have CSF findings typical for MS.[72] The frequencies also may vary in part by the methodology used to detect the lesions, as some enhancements in PPMS may have relatively lower conspicuity compared to those seen in relapsing forms of MS. Our experience in PPMS trials supports that new T2 lesions are less likely to be accompanied by enhancement, and lesion expansion may occur more frequently with little or no new enhancement, or by subtle enhancement at the lesion's edge. Despite quantitative difference, most cases of PPMS show otherwise typical imaging features as compared to relapsing MS.[73]

Enhancing lesions in monitoring MS therapy

Enhancing lesions are used as an entry requirement to enrich for patients likely to show subsequent disease activity, as a randomization factor to achieve balance in trial arms, as a safety measure incorporated into stopping rules in Phase 1 and Phase 2 trials, as a primary outcome measure in Phase 2 and as a secondary outcome measure in Phase 3 trials.

Enrichment

Individual patients show MRI activity or inactivity trends. Since initially inactive subjects may not contribute much to measuring efficacy over time, many trials rely on a design including an enrichment strategy based on enhancement on one, or sometimes multiple screening MRI studies.[74] The yield for finding a positive MRI is limited after a first negative screening MRI, although not zero.[55] The requirement of clinical disease activity in the preceding one or two years prior to entry has a similar effect as MRI enrichment, but is not as effective when the goal is to enter patients with high enhancing lesion counts. Combined strategies are based on having either clinical or MRI activity in the preceding 1 to 2 years. The downside to strategies relying on enrichment is compromised extrapolation of results and their applicability to average patient populations that may not have similar activity levels. MRI-based enrichment has been a successful strategy in parallel group trials, but is problematic in crossover trials where decreased activity based on regression to the mean can confound "efficacy."

Randomization

For Phase 2 trials with enhancing lesions or other MRI measures as the primary outcome, balance at baseline for enhancing lesion activity can be critical for trial success and validity. In theory, an imbalance can be controlled for by statistical correction, but this involves assumptions that are not always straightforward (Chapter 16). As an example, in one large prospective trial, untreated patients presenting with enhancing lesions showed a median two-year increment in T2-hyperintense lesion volume of 2.98 ml compared to 0.67 ml for patients with no enhancements on their initial MRI study, and the enhanced lesion rate was about five-fold greater for untreated patients with enhancing lesions on their baseline MRI study.[56]

Safety measure

Monthly enhancing lesion counts and volumes have become increasingly utilized in Phase 1 dose escalation/safety trials as a biomarker for inflammation or subclinical disease activity. Stopping or red flag rules in Phase 1 and 2 trials that might precipitate an ad hoc external Data Safety Committee review may be recommended and often are based on a pre-determined level beyond expected change in MRI activity.[3,75] Here, an absolute or statistically determined threshold of increased enhancing lesions observed on one or two monthly MRI studies would be compared to one or multiple baseline or preceding study values.

Sample size based on enhancing lesions

Several studies have addressed the appropriate sample sizes for Phase 2 trials based on enhanced lesion activity. Sample size is dependent on design, enrichment for activity, disease duration, disability stage, MS phenotype, expectations of the activity levels in the comparison group, and treatment effect size.[76]

Clinical and pathologic significance of enhancing lesions

Enhancing lesions and relapses

Many consider enhancing activity to be an MRI equivalent of clinical relapse. In one meta-analysis of 204 subjects with adequate data to determine the concomitant correlation of total enhancements over six months and relapses over the same interval, and the predictive correlation of enhancements over six months with relapses over 12 months, correlation coefficients explained only about 5% of the variability in the associations between the MR and clinical metrics.[77] These observations suggest caution in using enhancement activity on a single scan as a predictive measure of near-term clinical outcome.

High enhancement numbers may be useful, but low enhancement numbers and enhanced tissue volumes are not strongly predictive.

Viewed from a different perspective, one might anticipate a higher than projected enhancement frequency among subjects imaged at the time of presentation with new clinical symptoms if enhancing activity and relapses were well correlated. This does not appear to be the case. In patients with CIS or CDMS who participated in controlled trials of methylprednisolone for acute optic neuritis,[78] or MS relapses who agreed to MRI evaluations before the onset of therapy,[79] only 62% had one or more enhancements found.[80] The proportion with enhancements was higher in those with CDMS (75%) than those with CIS (36%). All subjects were seen within four weeks of new symptoms onset, which could be interpreted to suggest that enhancements were already on the wane. Yet, in an unreported trial where patients were required to be randomized within seven days of an acute relapse, and where the results of the baseline cerebral imaging were not used as criteria for trial eligibility, only 53% of the 43 subjects entered had enhancing activity at baseline (JS Wolinsky, unpublished observations).

Moreover, population studies show only modest correlation between enhancing lesions and clinical relapse rates,[51,81] and in individual cases there may be no relationship even over many years when focal disease activity occurs in clinically silent regions of the CNS. However, when enhancing lesions occur in functionally sensitive regions, the imaging findings, symptoms and electrophysiological disturbances occur with a similar time course.[82] A correlation has been noted between periods of clinical worsening and periods of increasing enhancing lesion frequency.[83] In one CIS trial cohort, at the 18 months' follow-up of patients without on-study clinical relapses, 42% had one or more enhancing lesions on the "snapshot" MRI, and at least 82% had new T2-lesions over the ensuing asymptomatic 18-month interval.[84] Such discrepancies underscore the strength of enhanced lesion counts as a subclinical measure of disease activity in clinical trial patients and should serve to bedevil the clinician dealing with an individual patient's treatment decision.

In a comprehensive meta-analysis based on nearly 6600 subjects enrolled in 63 arms of 23 randomized, placebo-controlled trials, an impressive correlation was found between the magnitude of effect of the active treatment on relapses and the treatment effect on MRI lesional activity (adjusted $r^2 = 0.81$).[85] This type of correlation was independently confirmed using trial data from recently completed trials of oral disease modifying agents.[86] These studies support the use of new lesional activity measures as a biological marker of importance in MS therapeutics, even if the marker has limitations when applied to individual patients.

Enhancing lesions and disability

Most studies show little or no correlation between enhancing lesions and composite disability measures at one point in time, or over a few years. Yet, some studies that suggest that early enhancing lesion activity relates to delayed expression of disability.[87] An example of this is provided by an open-label trial of alemtuzumab, where disability, as well as brain atrophy progressed despite a marked reduction in the number of enhancing lesions. The factor that predicted disability (and atrophy) was the temporally remote inflammation in the brain before initiation of treatment, as judged by enhancing lesion activity,[87] with similar observations made in other studies.[88] Moreover, a quite recent meta-analysis based on slightly more than 10 000 RRMS subjects enrolled in 44 arms of 19 randomized, placebo-controlled trials, found a moderate but important correlation between the magnitude of effect of the active treatment on confirmed EDSS worsening and the treatment effect on MRI lesional activity (adjusted $r^2 = 0.57$).[89]

In PPMS, clinical deterioration occurs with little or no enhancement, underscoring the point that macroscopic inflammation alone, at least as measured by the enhancing lesions, is not a sufficient explanation for disability in MS. A more comprehensive model of injury, incorporating lesion characteristics, their anatomic location, host, and other factors may be both more appropriate and revealing.

Enhancing lesions and subsequent pathology

While the limited strength of the relationship between enhancing lesions and clinical expression of disease is disappointing, enhancing lesions nevertheless show important relationships with concurrent and subsequent injury.[90] As discussed above, the enhancing lesion can be characterized by a wide range in pathology, with blood–brain barrier leakage and inflammation of the central components. Variable degrees of edema, demyelination, and matrix disruption are expected. Axonal injury is now known to occur around the time of the early macroscopic inflammatory and presumably enhancing stages,[91–93] although little is known about the likely inter- and intra-individual variation in degree of axonal injury. Wallerian degeneration related to focal, enhancing MS lesions,[94] or acute MS lesions,[95] indicate that axonal injury from the focal pathology and its consequences are not infrequent even in early MS (Fig. 9.5). MR spectroscopy studies support concepts of early focal injury that may spread through the normal appearing white matter.[97] The immediate injury associated with enhancement over time is thought to contribute to temporally delayed injury, related to the initial disturbances of the oligodendrocyte–axon relationship, through demyelination and through loss of capacity for remyelination.

Despite month-to-month fluctuations, enhancing lesion activity predicts subsequent new and enlarging T2-lesions and T2-lesion volume increments in relapsing and progressive MS, and subsequent enhancing lesions over months to years.[56,98–100] The relationships between enhancing lesions and atrophy are weak, but contrast-enhancing lesion number predicts T1 black hole volume in subsequent years in both untreated,[101] and treated patients.[102]

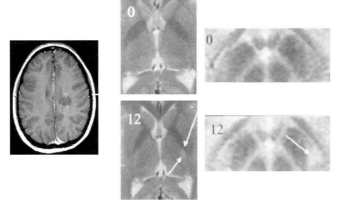

Fig. 9.5. A linkage of focal to diffuse and distant pathology in multiple sclerosis. The left panel shows a heterogeneously enhancing lesion in the white matter just above the mid portion of the left lateral ventricle in an image from a patient around the time of presentation as a clinically isolated syndrome; this was an asymptomatic lesion. The central panel, top, shows a normal posterior limb of the internal capsule, which on 3-month follow-up MRI was found to be abnormally T2-hyperintense (not shown), the T2-hyperintensity persisting on 12-month MRI (central panel, bottom, arrows). At the midbrain level, the initially normal corticospinal tract (right, top panel) was found to be abnormally T2-hyperintense at three months (not shown), the T2-hyperintensity persisting on 12-month MRI (right panel, bottom, arrow). These findings are presumed to reflect imaging correlates of Wallerian degeneration distal to the acute lesion in this case within motor pathways in the centrum semiovale. Multiple injuries similar to these are likely to occur throughout the brain, potentially contributing to abnormalities of the normal appearing brain tissue, and detected by "advanced" quantitative MRI techniques. From Simon et al.,[96] with permission.

Technical aspects of enhancing lesion measurement

Acquisition

Accurate measurement in clinical trials requires optimized acquisition techniques that provide high contrast-to-noise ratios (signal difference in tissues of interest to noise ratio). Practical considerations often dictate some compromise in technique to minimize scan time (long time is expensive and patient motion increases) and provide a common set of imaging parameters compatible with different MR instruments and software levels common in modern large multicenter trials. In the clinic, good imaging technique for individual patients should be very similar to that utilized in clinical trials.[2,3]

Contrast dose and scan timing

Contrast dose and timing are important variables for obtaining reproducible enhancement patterns and magnitude of enhancement for measurement by either qualitative or quantitative methods. Typically, for a standard contrast enhanced series, an explicit interval is set for injection (typically 30 seconds), and delay to start of scan (typically a set interval between five and ten minutes). Too short a delay interval will adversely affect lesion contrast; too long an interval may intensify a fraction of lesions, but some will develop blurry borders, and long scan times may be unacceptable, again for practical economic reasons. Most trials are based on conventional doses of the standard MR contrast agents at 0.1 mmole/kg. Triple doses and delayed imaging are well known to increase the number of enhancing lesions in relapsing and secondary progressive MS, on the order of 25 to 75% in most studies,[103] and increases the lesion yield in early PPMS where enhancement is less frequent.[104,105] Triple doses also increase lesion contrast, and to a lesser extent the fraction of patients with enhancing lesions, but potential safety issues, and increased variability in population studies that limit the statistical gain mitigate against the routine use of triple dose contrast.[3]

Pulse sequence

For clinical trials T1-weighted sequences are frequently based on classic two-dimensional (2D) spin-echo technique with short repetition time (TR) and short echo delay time (TE). Slices are typically 3 mm or 5 mm thick, without gaps with approximately 1 mm × 1 mm in plane resolution (pixel size). An alternative approach is to use three-dimensional (3D) T1-weighted acquisitions based on either a spoiled gradient echo methodology or magnetization prepared gradient echoes, both of which allow thin slices (known as partitions in 3D terminology).[106,107] With a 3D acquisition, partitions are typically 1 mm to 2 mm with no gaps, yet have good signal-to-noise. An advantage of the 3D acquisition is that it allows nearly seamless post-hoc image reconstruction in any scan plane, which may benefit image evaluation. A disadvantage is the potential for motion-related noise through the image. While the conspicuity of enhancing lesions can be increased by using a MT pulse sequence, most clinical trials have not used MT to increase enhancing lesion counts, as these images may be "noisy," more difficult to interpret, and MT pulse sequences vary within and between MR instruments even more so than do the conventional sequences. Combined approaches have been used for optimizing enhancing lesion counts, based on high doses of MR contrast and/or delayed imaging. These consistently improve lesion conspicuity, number of enhancing lesions, and percent of patients with enhancing lesions.[1] Despite the increased yield by the individual or combined methodologies, the effect on sample size in clinical trials may be inconsequential.

Accuracy of enhanced lesion counts

A major benefit of the use of enhancing lesion counts is the relative ease of identification by an experienced imager. Few studies have addressed the issue of the accuracy, inter- and intra-observer error, and measurement reproducibility over time. In one study, for scans with no activity, there was 100% agreement between observers. For scans with one or more lesions, there was agreement as to presence of lesions in 96% of the observations, with agreement on the exact number of lesions decreasing with increasing lesion numbers.[108] The agreement was 80% for scans with five or fewer lesions. In our expe-

rience, the agreement for no enhancing activity is less than 100%. Employing at least two experienced readers will decrease the missed lesion rate, and allows for consensus opinion in the three difficult scenarios of equivocal enhancement, vessel vs. enhancement, and motion (pulsation) artifact vs. enhancement. Enhanced lesion volume is also frequently measured in trials, as treatment may differentially impact enhanced lesion number and volume. However, lesion number and volume are highly correlated. Automated enhanced lesion detection has also been successfully applied in clinical trials, with outcomes based on total number of pixels with enhancement. The relative merit of the classical (lesion count) vs. computerized enhanced pixels has not been systematically evaluated, but both approaches have been used effectively in large trials.

T2-defined disease burden

T2-hyperintense lesions provide a complementary set of measures to enhancing lesions in both clinical trials (counts and volumetrics) and in the clinic (principally counts).[109] A variety of measures are utilized, including T2-hyperintense lesion volume (T2 burden of disease), new and/or enlarging T2 lesion numbers, and less frequently, interesting measures of new T2-abnormal pixels or new and/or enlarging T2 lesion volume. New T2 lesion counts in most circumstances are strongly correlated with enhancing lesion counts in high-frequency serial studies.[110] Their value increases in semi-annual to annual evaluations where enhancing lesions provide a measure of inflammation around the time of the MRI, and new T2 lesions provide a measure of disease activity over the interval. T2 lesion volume analyses provide a measure of accumulation of pathologic tissue, albeit non-specific regarding pathology.

T2 lesion behavior over time

After reaching a maximal lesion size over a period of about 2–8 weeks, individual T2-hyperintense lesions almost always shrink over a period of weeks to months,[111] leaving a smaller residual area, essentially a T2 footprint, related to the prior acute event. Occasionally, individual T2 lesions disappear, but this is uncommon. Lesion regression occurs due to loss of surrounding acute edema, and the core of the lesion contracts to a variable and unpredictable degree, which may reflect multiple factors such as type and severity of injury, location, and "healing." Once stabilized, after many months, the vast majority of chronic T2 lesions do not change in volume or other characteristics even when observed over many years. In those individual lesions that do change, several factors may contribute. Some expand through new activity along their periphery or less commonly through central activation. Reactivation of focal lesions is thought to be an important mechanism accounting for more severe cumulative pathology, including a lost capacity for remyelination.[112] An apparent increase in individual T2 lesion size often is the result of additional new, immediately adjacent or nearby lesions becoming confluent. Atrophy of tissue between lesions may also account for confluence.

Monthly MRI series show that the T2 burden of disease varies considerably between and within individuals. Monthly fluctuations on the order of 20% are not unusual, based on biological (true) variation, but with contributory measurement error.[113] However, in large populations and with sufficient intervals between scans, quantitation of T2 disease burden, despite its wide biological and technical variance, can be an effective measure of change disease. Over time, the total T2 lesion volume increases on average in the brain and/or spinal cord in the absence of treatment.

Some studies report change in T2 lesion burden expressed as a percentage increase in T2 lesion volume; change can also be reported as an absolute increase. The latter may be more meaningful in some circumstances, as in studies including individuals with small to modest lesion burdens, where small increments in lesion number may result in very large percentage increases in lesion burden, potentially biasing the analyses to these low lesion burden individuals. However, trial cohorts with large lesion burdens at entry may show very small percentage increase in T2 lesion volume over time, despite accumulating a number of new T2 lesions and new lesion volume over the same interval.

T2 lesion volume and number is often already substantial in the earliest stages of clinical disease, undoubtedly reflecting subclinical events that occurred prior to the single monosymptomatic or polysymptomatic clinical event that signaled the demyelinating disease. Across the CIS trials reported thus far, entry T2 volumes ranged from a median of 1.9–5.5 (range 0.2–54.1 ml), with an average of three to nine new T2 lesions developing in placebo cohorts over 24.[62,84,114,115] These studies all required some T2 lesions on cerebral MRI as trial entry criteria; as such they are not strictly applicable to all CIS patients at presentation.

Brain T2 lesion volume varies considerably in relapsing MS and is influenced by disease duration, disability range, prior activity criteria, and measurement technique. In the larger studies, volumes range from a low of about 2.6 ml to 48 ml.[27,56,63,116,117] With new diagnostic criteria for MS that allow new MRI activity to replace new clinical events for an earlier definitive MS diagnosis, smaller volume ranges may become more frequent in future studies.[118] Annual increases in T2 lesion volume in brain on the order of 5%–15% are typical in the relapsing stages of disease, with absolute increases on the order of 0.4 ml to 0.75 ml per year; these are highly dependent on baseline activity as judged by enhancing lesion status.[56] In secondary progressive MS, T2-lesion volumes also vary widely, ranging from about 3–28 ml,[66,119] but substantially higher volumes are common. Increases in T2 disease burdens range from about 0.1–2 ml per year or about 3.6%–9% per year. Large PPMS cohorts have had relatively low baseline mean T2 lesion burdens of about 8 ml, with untreated annual mean T2 volume increases of between 0.4–0.75 ml.[71,120]

T2-hyperintense lesions in monitoring therapy

Short-term clinical trials consistently document increases from trial entry in T2-weighted, MRI-defined disease burden over time among all patient cohorts and phenotypes. Increases are attenuated by current approved disease modifying therapies. Unfortunately, concomitant correlations between T2 lesion load and EDSS are generally poor. In part, this may be due to well-recognized problems with the EDSS (Chapter 6). Moreover, both T2 volumes and EDSS are subject to a complex mix of biologically based and measurement variability that may further erode the correlations. Meta-analysis using quantitative baseline T2 disease burden data pooled from a sub-sample of 1312 CIS, RR, and SPMS patients enrolled in 11 randomized controlled trials found weak to moderate correlations with age at disease onset, disease duration, disease course, EDSS (the most robust with $r = 0.35$, $P < 0.001$), relapse rate over the prior year, selected presenting symptoms, and the presence of Gd enhancement.[17] Perhaps most informative was an apparent plateau in an otherwise relatively linear relationship between increasing T2 disease burden and EDSS that occurred at EDSS values above 4.5. This suggests that the proportionate change in T2 disease burden should be most dynamic and best correlated with EDSS early in the course of relapsing disease, and become progressively less useful as the disease moves into a more progressive phase, particularly in those with clinically progressive disease who are increasingly gait impaired.[18]

In a meta-analysis of 650 SPMS patients, weak but significant predictive correlations between the number of new and enlarging "active" T2 lesions ($r = 0.16$, $P < 0.0001$), and percentage of T2 lesion volume change from baseline ($r = 0.13$, $P = 0.002$) over the first year with EDSS change over 3 years were found.[121] Limited attempts have been made to dissect information from clinical trial or natural history datasets to determine whether the extent of change can be used to predict subsequent clinical change or to define groups of patients at highest risk of clinical worsening, beyond the now well-established predictive value in the special case of CIS patients (see below).

Annual T2 lesion increases are suppressed by effective therapy, and the total T2 burden of disease may decrease below baseline values even with partially effective therapy. This may be related to elimination of reversible, edema-related components of T2-hyperintensity, but could also reflect improved reparative responses and gliosis both contributing to lesion contraction that occurs weeks to months after acute lesion development.

T2 lesion counts

While T2 lesion volume provides a measure of total non-specific lesion pathology over time, T2 lesion counts over 6- to 12-month intervals provide complementary, but distinct information. Each new or enlarged T2 lesion is an indication of interval activity that might otherwise be missed if one only depended on Gd enhancements at infrequent imaging intervals. In

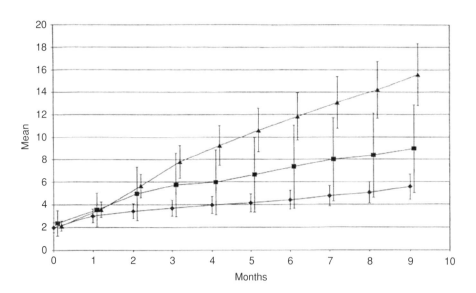

Fig. 9.6. Combined unique lesion accumulation on monthly scans. While most new lesions are detected by monthly enhancing lesion counts alone, this approach is more comprehensive in capturing additional T2-hyperintense lesions that do not enhance at the time of the MRI, from Li *et al.*,[119] with permission.

addition, although technically challenging, each new or enlarging T2 lesion followed over time to stable size could provide measures of the volume of new pathology independent of transient edema.

T2 lesions have been classified, similar to enhancing lesions as new lesions not seen on prior examinations (either baseline, or subsequent as explicitly defined in a study). Recurring lesions, defined as lesions reappearing in a location that had become normal are rare, and it may be very difficult to determine if these are truly new or reactivated. Enlarging lesions have been variably defined as those showing some increase in size from a prior examination. Typical guidelines require an increase in one diameter of at least 50% if the original lesion is <5 mm diameter, or at least 20% if the original lesion diameter is more than 5 mm. The best way to approach determination of new or enlarged T2 lesions in the absence of enhancing activity is through comparison of sets of well-registered scans. This can be done through similarly acquired images from well-positioned patients, but this can be exceedingly frustrating to misleading. Image processing approaches to register image sets prior to analysis, or registration of images and then digital subtraction of the paired image sets is clearly preferable.[122–124]

The sizes of individual T2 lesions are highly variable for unknown reasons. In theory, measures of individual lesion contraction could provide information related to resolution of the inflammatory process and its consequences. Prior studies of this nature, however, have been limited, and largely supplanted by analyses of conversion to T1 black holes (see below) or based on magnetization transfer values over time.

Are enhancing lesion and T2 lesion counts equivalent?

Given the linkage between new enhancing lesions and new T2 hyperintense lesions, there is some overlap in using these two outcomes to determine disease activity in MS clinical trials. The correlation between new T2 lesions and new enhancing lesions is strong in weekly, monthly, and alternate month MRI series.[103,125] In theory, for trials with monthly MRI, T2 lesion counts could be substituted for enhancing lesion counts after the baseline inflammatory activity is established with an enhancing lesion analyses, although with the penalty of decreased new lesion detection. In one series, 15% of new T2 lesions were missed due to small size and another 5% were missed because of their periventricular location.[126] The converse situation, in which a new lesion is detected on a T2 weighted image but not detected as an enhancing lesion is less frequent, but more likely in progressive MS.

A disadvantage of T2 lesion counts is the greater expertise required compared to enhancing lesions. Determining new T2 lesion counts is more easily applied in MS subjects with initial low T2 lesion burden where lesions less frequently overlap anatomically. New T2 lesion counts are increasingly more challenging and complicated in more advanced subjects where confluent and closely spaced lesions make T2 counts less reliable. For trials in which the scan interval is six-monthly or longer, new T2 counts provide a good index of interval activity, while enhancing lesion counts would only provide an index of inflammatory activity around the time of the MRI. Monthly serial studies that included both Gd-enhanced and T2-weighted image sets show that counts from either method alone will miss a fraction of new lesions. The enhanced lesion counts miss relatively short duration enhancements; the T2 lesion counts have reduced sensitivity to new lesions by virtue of tissue contrast, as some lesions are difficult to visualize with confidence, while others occur adjacent to prior lesions or within prior lesions and may readily be missed. A popular index of combined unique lesions was introduced by the University of British Columbia group to account for the fraction of missed new MS lesions;[119] this combines the number of Gd-enhancements with the number of unenhanced new T2 and enlarged T2 lesions (Fig. 9.6).

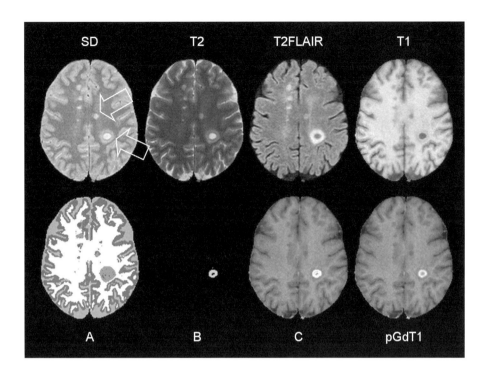

Fig. 9.7. Marked lesion heterogeneity is evident across these conventional 3 mm images obtained at 1.5 Tesla as part of a clinical trial. Illustrated are spin density (SD), T2-weighted without (T2) and with fluid attenuation by inversion recovery (T2FLAIR), and pre-(T1) and post-gadolinium T1-weighted (pGd T1) images, together with a segmented image (a) where gray matter is color coded as gray, white matter as white, T2-weighted lesion component as pink, and T1-hypointense non-enhanced tissue component as red; a threshold image (b) of the enhanced tissue volume, and (c) a localization of the enhanced tissue region on the pGd T1 image. The upper arrow points to a subcortical lesion that is not enhanced; the lower to a ring enhanced lesion. In this case, the total T2 lesion volume was 13.9 ml, the total T1-hypointense lesion volume 2.44 ml; while the enhanced lesion contributed 7.3 ml to the total lesion burden and 0.74 ml of the enhanced tissue. The amount of cerebrospinal fluid accounted for 324 with the non-CSF intracranial contents accounting for 1002 ml of total intracranial volume (see also color plate section).

Clinical and pathological significance of T2-weighted lesions

The clinical significance of the T2-hyperintense lesion

Multiple studies found no, or poor, correlation between T2-hyperintense lesion volume in the brain and composite disability measures, most notably the EDSS. Correlation coefficient are generally on the order of $r = 0.2$ in relapsing MS cohorts; in individuals, the relationship between lesion burden and disability can be strikingly poor. The MRI-disability discrepancy most likely is multifactorial, and as discussed below related to the lack of pathologic specificity of the T2 lesion. T2 lesion load does not take into consideration abnormality in normal appearing brain tissue, both gray and white matter,[4] although some but not all studies suggest a relationship between the focal and diffuse pathology. Another problem with correlations between T2 and disability is that the two may be dissociated in time. For example, reasonable correlation was seen between increasing T2 lesion load at five years from presentation as CIS and evolution to progressive disease and important disability at 20 years of follow-up.[127]

The pathologic substrate

The T2-hyperintense focal areas observed on MRI in both acute and chronic MS lesions in the brain and spinal cord are known from neuropathology studies to reflect a wide range of abnormalities, and are therefore pathologically non-specific. T2-hyperintensity can result from edema, demyelination, axonal loss, matrix disruption, and astrogliosis. The T2-weighted image and monoexponential T2-relaxation time measures are insensitive to the mix of these various pathologies. Neuropathology–MRI correlative studies have emphasized the limited histopathologic information contained within a T2-weighted image.[10,128] Yet the T2-weighted metrics do provide a simple and valuable measure of new disease over time.

In acute macroscopic MS lesions depicted by MRI, the T2-hyperintensity is often not homogeneous through the lesion, reflecting multiple components of pathology (Fig. 9.7). The outer portions of lesion are most likely predominantly simple interstitial fluid (edema); this T2-hyperintense area most often will completely regress after several weeks. Central hyperintensity is thought to be the result of water space changes that may reflect variable degrees of demyelination, astrogliosis, matrix disruption, and axonal injury or loss.[10] The T2 lesion areas may also include zones of active remyelination,[16] which is present more in early rather than in later stages. Zones of T2-hypointensity (dark on T2-weighted images) which may be related to T1-hyperintense areas are occasionally observed, potentially related to macrophage infiltration and/or free radical or other products.[129]

The pathology underlying T2 lesions is likely variable across patients, probably more so than within patients.[20] The heterogeneous pathology and variable severity characteristic of T2-hyperintense lesions accounts in part for the poor correlation between T2 lesion volume and disability that is so striking in individuals, but also in populations. Other factors also contribute to this poor correlation, including lesion location, redundancy in neural pathways, alternative functional pathways and functional reorganization responses to injury,[130,131] as well as limitations in the disability scoring systems.

Another source of T2-hyperintensity is that related to fiber tract degeneration.[132] Neuronal tract degeneration patterns are seen as relatively subtle T2-hyperintensity extending from focal MS lesions,[96] that can contribute to the overall burden of disease (Fig. 9.5). The mechanism presumed to underlie these injuries is Wallerian degeneration, predicated on early axonal injury and loss, and sometimes evident only after many months to years of myelin loss.[133]

Technical aspects of T2 lesion measurement

Acquisition

High-quality studies are a necessary step for optimal segmentation of T2 lesions. Current standards include 3 mm slice thickness, no interslice gaps, and good signal and contrast-to-noise. While most trials to date have been based on 2D acquisitions, 3D image acquisitions will likely become the standard in the future, as these can provide equal to greater image quality at higher resolution and fine multi-planar reformatting provided optimal quality control is implemented. As field strength improves the signal-to-noise, high field imaging at 1.5 T to 3 T has become standard. Irrespective of the range of instruments, field strength, and software level, key to clinical trial analyses by MRI is consistent use of the same, consistently well-maintained, instrument over multiple examinations, the assumption being that intra-individual changes will outweigh the inter-individual variation that can be expected related to these factors.

Pulse sequence

There is a wide range of pulse sequences that can be utilized as the basis for MRI acquisition for T2-lesion analyses. Typically, multiple pulse sequences provide multiple tissue contrasts, most commonly a multiecho series generating a proton density and more heavily T2-weighted dual echo series, and/or a FLAIR series is acquired. Historically, most MRI analyses were based on conventional spin-echo technique; however, RARE sequences (fast or turbo) have become routine. As mentioned above, moves to volumetric acquisitions are particularly attractive,[134] provided that optimal quality control of hardware systems and pulse sequence software is routinely upgraded in a multicenter environment.

Segmentation

Methodologies for segmentation are numerous and varied, making a comprehensive description of available algorithms outside the scope of this chapter and book. Algorithms vary on dimensionality (2D vs. 3D segmentation), user interaction (manual, supervised, or unsupervised), and fuzziness (assignment of a voxel to one category vs. allowing it to be considered a member of multiple categories or tissue classes). The most common approaches include manual tracing, voxel intensity thresholding, region growing (based on connectedness and edge detection), classifiers (Parzen window or nearest neighbor), clustering (k-means and fuzzy c-means), artificial neural networks, Markov Random Fields, deformable models (active contours or "snakes"), and atlas-based approaches. These techniques may also be combined with various pre-processing steps such as smoothing, bias field correction, and image registration or warping. It is not uncommon for an image processing pipeline to incorporate several of these algorithms in order to overcome the limitations of any one particular approach.[135] Furthermore, multispectral data are often used to take advantage of tissue contrast differences inherent in multi-echo echo sequences (such as spin-echo or FSE) and between scanning protocols.

The goal is to provide accurate classifications of tissue, not only in ideally acquired cases (one site, one time, optimized instrumentation), but in view of the realistic complexities of a multicenter clinical trial (many sites, many times, suboptimal instrumentation), and through software and hardware upgrades that are common in the timeframe of an MS clinical trial. A number of factors make this problematic, including suboptimal tissue contrast (resulting from inherent tissue properties, pulse sequence design or field strength), partial volume effects, image resolution, inhomogeneity artifacts (susceptibility effects, magnetic, and RF field inhomogeneities), noise, and image distortion. As all volumetric measures lack an absolute standard of truth, an expert reviewer is often utilized in the analysis pipeline to correct and/or validate a computerized segmentation. Efforts have focused on providing a statistical validation of quality based on the spatial overlap of multiple segmentations, providing a framework for estimating the "true" segmentation map.[136] Other assessments of segmentation methodology typically rely on some measure of precision, such as intra- and inter-observer variability, or scan–rescan reproducibility. These measures are most useful when discussed in the context of accuracy, as one can be completely precise and yet produce a completely incorrect result.

The analysis of different methodologies has been discussed, and multiple optimal measures proffered. The requirement of any segmentation technique is that its error is reasonable relative to true change. For annual changes of about 5%–10% per year, a measurement error (coefficient of variation) of about 1% to 7.5% in the clinical trials setting is adequate to detect substantial group differences,[108] but the upper range in error would be inadequate for detecting smaller effect sizes.

T1-hypointense disease burden

Qualitative or quantitative side-by-side comparison of T2- and T1-weighted images show that, for most MS patients and many MS lesions, about 80%–95% of T2 lesion area is isointense to normal white matter on T1-weighted images. A smaller fraction of the T2 lesions (~5%–20%) is hypointense compared to normal white matter on T1-weighted images. When persistent for 6–12 months or more, this T1-hypointense lesion fraction is the classic T1-"black hole" fraction. This lesion component is important as it represents white matter that has suffered relatively more severe and mostly irreversible tissue injury.[136]

T1-hypointense lesions are rarely seen in normal brain. Relatively simple water spaces from intraparenchymal CSF cysts, Virchow–Robbin spaces, mature cystic infarctions, or cavitary areas from matured areas of trauma may all be chronically T2-hyperintense and T1-hypointense, but these can usually be distinguished from MS T1-hypointense lesions, as they are often CSF-like on all pulse sequences, including proton density sequences. While T1-hypointense lesions do occur as a consequence of small vessel ischemia or infarction these are relatively uncommon, but can increase with age.

Similar to T2-lesions, T1-hypointense lesion volume increases with disease duration, is greater in established relapsing compared to the earliest stages of MS, and is greater in secondary compared to relapsing stages of disease. T1-hypointense lesion volume can be measured over yearly intervals, and is expected to increase at all stages and in all disease phenotypes, although increments may be small in advanced MS.

Even in early disease stages, some subjects already have T1-hypointense brain lesions. In the weekly intramuscular interferon beta-1a CIS study, 50% of patients with a positive entry MRI (at least two lesions) showed one or more T1-hypointense lesions, although their volume was small and possibly overestimated due to the use of standardized high dose corticosteroid treatment (which can suppress contrast enhancement) before the baseline MRI was obtained.[138] The ratio of T1-hypointense to total T2 lesion volume is potentially an informative measure of more severe pathology in individuals and populations.

In evaluating an MR image, it is important to distinguish acute T1-hypointense areas, which are T1-hypointense on the basis of edema, and may show considerable or complete recovery, from chronic T1-hypointense lesions (Fig. 9.7). Since serial studies are not always available, chronicity is often assumed based on T1-hypointensity in the absence of enhancement following contrast administration. High-dose corticosteroids can confound this interpretation by rapidly suppressing enhancement. In actuality, acute lesions with associated T1-hypointensity often evolve slowly over many months to their final T1-isointense or hypointense state, the latter occurring in individual lesions about 14%–41% of the time.[15,19] Transition of an acute T1-hypointense MS lesion to normal signal intensity in large part reflects recovery from the acute edematous stage. It is also likely that partial remyelination may also contribute to signal recovery.[16,112]

The evolution of individual T1-hypointense lesions and their aggregate behavior over time in a given individual and across cohorts is complex. Simplistically, the aggregate evolution could be viewed as a three component model, with one reflecting a dynamically evolving contribution from recently formed lesions, a second derived from a relatively stable pool of T1-hypointense lesions that have achieved maximal repair, and possibly a most important third contribution from those T2 lesions whose T1-hypointense regions are expanding in the absence of any captured re-enhancement. The last component is the least studied.

Genetic factors such as apolipoprotein E4-ε4 have been associated with greater T1-hypointense to T2 lesion ratios,[139] but relationships of this genotype to other severity measures in larger MS cohorts have not been evident.[140] Larger lesions, lesions with longer duration enhancement, and ring enhancing lesions have been considered risk factors for T1-hypointensities as discussed above.[141]

T1-hypointense lesions are infrequently observed in the spinal cord. Their infrequency in the spinal cord may be related to structure, possibly a local collapse of more severely injured tissue making them less apparent despite episodes of severe focal injury. But differing mechanisms of injury and repair in brain vs. spinal cord cannot be excluded. T1-hypointense lesions are also relatively infrequent in the cerebellum and brainstem.

T1-hypointense lesion behavior over time

The net increase in T1-hypointense disease burden has been reported as high as 23% over six months,[142] to 29% over 24 months in RRMS cohorts,[101] to as low as 4.2% over 12 months in progressive patients.[143] This variation may reflect shifts from disproportionate contributions from dynamically evolving newly enhanced tissue regions in the relapsing cohorts toward dominance of late lesion evolution in the more progressive cohorts. In support of this are data from primary progressive disease where enhanced lesion activity is low. In a large trial, the T1-hypointense lesion volume increased between 13%–14% over one and two years of follow-up among untreated subjects, and may have exceeded the proportionate growth of T2 lesion volume over the same interval (JS Wolinsky, unpublished observations). If something like a three-component model does fit T1-hypointense behavior and is related to disease stage, a better understanding of its genesis may be important in the staging and monitoring of the disease. Unfortunately, it is quite likely that a fourth component of T1 lesion exists that further complicates interpretation of these lesions; some T1-lesions appear to lose volume to regional tissue atrophy.[144]

T1-Hypointense lesions in monitoring therapy

A third measure is based on the fraction of new or enhancing lesions that evolve into T1-hypointense lesions.[14,145] Selection of the new lesions to evaluate (typically new lesions despite therapy), the follow-up interval (months to determine that a lesion is chronic rather than transient), and the potential selection bias for the limited number of lesions with more aggressive inflammatory characteristics make this a challenging measure.

Clinical and pathological significance of T1-hypointense lesions
Clinical significance of T1-hypointense lesions

Cross-sectional and longitudinal population correlations between T1-hypointense lesions and disability are weak to modest for most studies. While the correlations are generally stronger than those between T2-lesions and disability,[101,146,147] the differences are small, potentially related to disease stage, and may be highly dependent on the study population. Nevertheless, chronic T1-hypointense lesions serve as an indication of severe, irreversible injury, much of which is subclinical in individuals, and this measure is valued by clinicians as a disease assessment parameter.[148]

Pathology of T1-hypointense lesions

Post-mortem specimens show that areas identified as T1-hypointensities by ex vivo MRI are characterized microscopically by reduced axonal density, decreased myelin and greater tissue disruption,[149] compared to adjacent tissue. Several in vivo analyses suggest that T1-hypointensities have attributes expected for more severe tissue injury, including relatively reduced magnetization transfer ratios,[150] and reduced *N*-acetylaspartate, a neuronal marker.[151] Quantitative magnetization transfer experiments,[152] suggest that the changes in these lesions are related to a reduced semisolid macromolecular pool, presumably associated with demyelination and loss of tissue integrity, and to a lesser degree related to the density of the liquid pool (edema). However, T1-hypointense lesions are heterogeneous by multiple measures.[153]

Technical aspects of T1-hypointense lesion measurement

T1- hypointense lesion volumes

Global T1-hypointense volume is predominantly a measure of these lesions in supratentorial white matter. Acquisition parameters influence the relative T1-hypointensity and will affect the yield of T1-hypointense lesions. MR field strength (increased T1 relaxation time with increasing field), pulse parameters (TR/TE), pulse sequence (spin echo T1-holes vs. gradient echo T1-holes differ) are all important factors in standardizing measures in populations and individuals.

Measurement methods are generally similar to those used for T2-hyperintense lesion volume, and include manual trace, user-guided but semi-automated threshold-based techniques using seed points,[154] semi-automated contour methods based on a local threshold or intensity gradient,[155] and automated methods for lesion detection with fuzzy connectivity utilized for lesion segmentation.[156] Segmentation can also be based on T1-relaxation values; a methodology capable of detecting conventional focal T1-black holes, and abnormality in the normal appearing white matter based on tissue relaxation characteristics.[157]

Atrophy

By definition, atrophy is a loss of tissue that implies degeneration from the normal. Cross-sectional and longitudinal studies document that cerebral atrophy in MS is found in early patient cohorts and is progressive over time. Group data support global cerebral atrophy at rates of about 1% annually, at least among subjects recruited to clinical trials where selection criteria may enrich for higher short-term rates in all clinical and MRI metrics.[158] Tracking individual cases suggests that the rate of tissue loss is not likely to be uniform overtime, but rather show intervals when tissue loss is accelerated and other intervals when brain volumes are relatively stable. The structural basis for atrophy is likely to be complex, and only the regional components of global tissue loss seem to be reasonably well defined, based on the evolution of local lesions (See Chapter 11).

References

1. Wolansky LJ, Finden SG, Chang R, *et al*. Gadoteridol in multiple sclerosis patients. A comparison of single and triple dose with immediate vs. delayed imaging. *Clin Imaging* 1998;22: 385–92.

2. Traboulsee A, Simon J, Stone L, *et al*. Recommendations of the CMSC task force for a standardized MRI protocol and clinical guidelines for the diagnosis and follow up of multiple sclerosis: 2010 revision. *Int J MS Care* 2011;13: in press.

3. Barkhof FK, Simon J, Fazekas F, *et al*. Efficient monitoring of immuno-modulation in relapse–onset multiple sclerosis clinical trials using MRI. *Lancet Neurol*. 2011: submitted.

4. Miller DH, Thompson AJ, Filippi M. Magnetic resonance studies of abnormalities in the normal appearing white matter and grey matter in multiple sclerosis. *J Neurol* 2003;250:1407–19.

5. Cadavid D, Wolansky LJ, Skurnick J, *et al*. Efficacy of treatment of MS with IFNβ-1b or glatiramer acetate by monthly brain MRI in the BECOME study. *Neurology* 2009;72:1976–83.

6. Kermode AG, Tofts PS, Thompson AJ, *et al*. Heterogeneity of blood-brain barrier changes in multiple sclerosis: an MRI study with gadolinium-DTPA enhancement. *Neurology* 1990;40:229–35.

7. Kirk J, Plumb J, Mirakhur M, McQuaid S. Tight junctional abnormality in multiple sclerosis white matter affects all calibres of vessel and is associated with blood–brain barrier leakage and active demyelination. *J Pathol* 2003;201:319–27.

8. Prat A, Antel J. Pathogenesis of multiple sclerosis. *Curr Opin Neurol* 2005;18:225–30.

9. Nesbit GM, Forbes GS, Scheithauer BW, Okazaki H, Rodriguez M. Multiple sclerosis: histopathologic and MR and/or CT correlation in 37 cases at biopsy and three cases at autopsy. *Radiology* 1991;180:467–74.

10. Bruck W, Bitsch A, Kolenda H, Bruck Y, Stiefel M, Lassmann H. Inflammatory central nervous system demyelination: correlation of magnetic resonance imaging findings with lesion pathology. *Ann Neurol* 1997;42:783–93.

11. Lai M, Hodgson T, Gawne-Cain M, *et al*. A preliminary study into the sensitivity of disease activity detection by serial weekly magnetic resonance imaging in multiple sclerosis. *J Neurol Neurosurg Psychiatry* 1996;60:339–41.

12. Cotton F, Weiner HL, Jolesz FA, Guttmann CR. MRI contrast uptake in new lesions in relapsing–remitting MS followed at weekly intervals. *Neurology* 2003;60:640–6.

13. Hawkins CP, Munro PM, MacKenzie F, *et al.* Duration and selectivity of blood-brain barrier breakdown in chronic relapsing experimental allergic encephalomyelitis studied by gadolinium-DTPA and protein markers. *Brain* 1990;113(2):365–78.

14. Filippi M, Rovaris M, Rocca MA, Sormani MP, Wolinsky JS, Comi G. Glatiramer acetate reduces the proportion of new MS lesions evolving into "black holes." *Neurology* 2001;57:731–3.

15. Dalton CM, Miszkiel KA, Barker GJ, *et al.* Effect of natalizumab on conversion of gadolinium enhancing lesions to T1 hypointense lesions in relapsing multiple sclerosis. *J Neurol* 2004;251:407–13.

16. Barkhof F, Bruck W, De Groot CJ, *et al.* Remyelinated lesions in multiple sclerosis: magnetic resonance image appearance. *Arch Neurol* 2003;60:1073–81.

17. Li DK, Held U, Petkau J, *et al.* MRI T2 lesion burden in multiple sclerosis: a plateauing relationship with clinical disability. *Neurology* 2006;66: 1384–9.

18. Sormani MP, Rovaris M, Comi G, Filippi M. A reassessment of the plateauing relationship between T2 lesion load and disability in MS. *Neurology* 2009;73:1538–42.

19. Minneboo A, Uitdehaag BM, Ader HJ, Barkhof F, Polman CH, Castelijns JA. Patterns of enhancing lesion evolution in multiple sclerosis are uniform within patients. *Neurology* 2005;65:56–61.

20. Lucchinetti C, Bruck W, Parisi J, Scheithauer B, Rodriguez M, Lassmann H. Heterogeneity of multiple sclerosis lesions: implications for the pathogenesis of demyelination. *Ann Neurol* 2000;47:707–17.

21. Bagnato F, Jeffries N, Richert ND, *et al.* Evolution of T1 black holes in patients with multiple sclerosis imaged monthly for 4 years. *Brain* 2003;126:1782–9.

22. Filippi M, Rocca MA, Comi G. Magnetization transfer ratios of multiple sclerosis lesions with variable durations of enhancement. *J Neurol Sci* 1998;159:162–5.

23. van Waesberghe JH, van Buchem MA, Filippi M, *et al.* MR outcome parameters in multiple sclerosis: comparison of surface-based thresholding segmentation and magnetization transfer ratio histographic analysis in relation to disability (a preliminary note). *Am J Neuroradiol* 1998;19:1857–62.

24. Ciccarelli O, Giugni E, Paolillo A, *et al.* Magnetic resonance outcome of new enhancing lesions in patients with relapsing–remitting multiple sclerosis. *Eur J Neurol* 1999;6:455–9.

25. Davis M, Auh S, Riva M, *et al.* Ring and nodular multiple sclerosis lesions: A retrospective natural history study. *Neurology* 2010;74:851–6.

26. Filippi M, Rovaris M, Gasperini C, *et al.* A preliminary study comparing the sensitivity of serial monthly enhanced MRI after standard and triple dose gadolinium-DTPA for monitoring disease activity in primary progressive multiple sclerosis. *J Neuroimaging* 1998;8:88–93.

27. Wolinsky JS, Narayana PA, Noseworthy JH, *et al.* Linomide in relapsing and secondary progressive MS: part II: MRI results. MRI Analysis Center of the University of Texas-Houston, Health Science Center, and the North American Linomide Investigators. *Neurology* 2000;54:1734–41.

28. Bielekova B, Kadom N, Fisher E, *et al.* MRI as a marker for disease heterogeneity in multiple sclerosis. *Neurology* 2005;65:1071–6.

29. Richert ND, Ostuni JL, Bash CN, Leist TP, McFarland HF, Frank JA. Interferon beta-1b and intravenous methylprednisolone promote lesion recovery in multiple sclerosis. *Mult Scler* 2001;7:49–58.

30. Wolinsky JS, Narayana PA. Magnetic resonance spectroscopy in multiple sclerosis: window into the diseased brain. *Curr Opin Neurol* 2002;15:247–51.

31. Wuerfel J, Bellmann-Strobl J, Brunecker P, *et al.* Changes in cerebral perfusion precede plaque formation in multiple sclerosis: a longitudinal perfusion MRI study. *Brain* 2004;127:111–19.

32. Sajja BR, Wolinsky JS, Narayana PA. Proton magnetic resonance spectroscopy in multiple sclerosis. In Filippi M, ed. *Neuroimaging* Clinics

of North America: Elsevier, 2009: 45–58.

33. Helms G, Stawiarz L, Kivisakk P, Link H. Regression analysis of metabolite concentrations estimated from localized proton MR spectra of active and chronic multiple sclerosis lesions. *Magn Reson Med* 2000;43:102–10.

34. Vos CM, Geurts JJ, Montagne L, *et al.* Blood–brain barrier alterations in both focal and diffuse abnormalities on postmortem MRI in multiple sclerosis. *Neurobiol Dis* 2005;20:953–60.

35. Filippi M, Falini A, Arnold DL, *et al.* Magnetic resonance techniques for the in vivo assessment of multiple sclerosis pathology: consensus report of the white matter study group. *J Magn Reson Imaging* 2005;21:669–75.

36. Azoulay D, Urshansky N, Karni A. Low and dysregulated BDNF secretion from immune cells of MS patients is related to reduced neuroprotection. *J Neuroimmunol* 2008;195:186–93.

37. Dousset V, Brochet B, Deloire MS, *et al.* MR imaging of relapsing multiple sclerosis patients using ultra-small-particle iron oxide and compared with gadolinium. *Am J Neuroradiol* 2006;27:1000–5.

38. Anderson SA, Shukaliak-Quandt J, Jordan EK, *et al.* Magnetic resonance imaging of labeled T-cells in a mouse model of multiple sclerosis. *Ann Neurol* 2004;55:654–9.

39. Pirko I, Johnson A, Ciric B, *et al.* In vivo magnetic resonance imaging of immune cells in the central nervous system with superparamagnetic antibodies. *FASEB J* 2004;18:179–82.

40. Yankeelov TE, Rooney WD, Huang W, *et al.* Evidence for shutter-speed variation in CR bolus-tracking studies of human pathology. *NMR Biomed* 2005;18:173–85.

41. Castriota-Scanderbeg A, Fasano F, Hagberg G, Nocentini U, Filippi M, Caltagirone C. Coefficient D (av) is more sensitive than fractional anisotropy in monitoring progression of irreversible tissue damage in focal nonactive multiple sclerosis lesions. *Am J Neuroradiol* 2003;24:663–70.

42. Henry RG, Oh J, Nelson SJ, Pelletier D. Directional diffusion in relapsing–remitting multiple sclerosis: a possible in vivo signature of Wallerian degeneration. *J Magn Reson Imaging* 2003;18:420–6.

43. Ciccarelli O, Werring DJ, Barker GJ, *et al.* A study of the mechanisms of normal-appearing white matter damage in multiple sclerosis using diffusion tensor imaging–evidence of Wallerian degeneration. *J Neurol* 2003;250:287–92.

44. Sharma R, Narayana PA, Wolinsky JS. Grey matter abnormalities in multiple sclerosis: proton magnetic resonance spectroscopic imaging. *Mult Scler* 2001;7:221–6.

45. Bo L, Vedeler CA, Nyland H, Trapp BD, Mork SJ. Intracortical multiple sclerosis lesions are not associated with increased lymphocyte infiltration. *Mult Scler* 2003;9:323–31.

46. Geurts JJ, Pouwels PJ, Uitdehaag BM, Polman CH, Barkhof F, Castelijns JA. Intracortical lesions in multiple sclerosis: improved detection with 3D double inversion-recovery MR imaging. *Radiology* 2005;236: 254–60.

47. Nelson F, Poonawalla AH, Hou P, Huang F, Wolinsky JS, Narayana PA. Improved identification of intracortical lesions in multiple sclerosis with phase-sensitive inversion recovery in combination with fast double inversion recovery MR imaging. *Am J Neuroradiol* 2007;28:1645–9.

48. Pitt D, Boster A, Pei W, *et al.* Imaging Cortical Lesions in Multiple Sclerosis With Ultra-High-Field Magnetic Resonance Imaging. *Arch Neurol* 2010;67:812–8.

49. Lucchinetti CF, Gavrilova RH, Metz I, *et al.* Clinical and radiographic spectrum of pathologically confirmed tumefactive multiple sclerosis. *Brain* 2008;131:1759–75.

50. Enzinger C, Strasser-Fuchs S, Ropele S, Kapeller P, Kleinert R, Fazekas F. Tumefactive demyelinating lesions: conventional and advanced magnetic resonance imaging. *Mult Scler* 2005;11:135–9.

51. Barkhof F, Scheltens P, Frequin ST, *et al.* Relapsing–remitting multiple sclerosis: sequential enhanced MR imaging vs clinical findings in determining disease activity. *Am J Roentgenol* 1992;159:1041–7.

52. Barkhof F, Held U, Simon JH, *et al.* Predicting gadolinium enhancement status in MS patients eligible for randomized clinical trials. *Neurology* 2005;65:1447–54.

53. Richert ND, Zierak MC, Bash CN, Lewis BK, McFarland HF, Frank JA. MRI and clinical activity in MS patients after terminating treatment with interferon beta-1b. *Mult Scler* 2000;6:86–90.

54. Nauta JJ, Thompson AJ, Barkhof F, Miller DH. Magnetic resonance imaging in monitoring the treatment of multiple sclerosis patients: statistical power of parallel-groups and crossover designs. *J Neurol Sci* 1994;122:6–14.

55. Bagnato F, Tancredi A, Richert N, *et al.* Contrast-enhanced magnetic resonance activity in relapsing remitting multiple sclerosis patients: a short term natural history study. *Mult Scler* 2000;6:43–9.

56. Simon JH, Jacobs LD, Campion M, *et al.* Magnetic resonance studies of intramuscular interferon beta-1a for relapsing multiple sclerosis. The Multiple Sclerosis Collaborative Research Group. *Ann Neurol* 1998;43:79–87.

57. Healy BC, Ikle D, Macklin EA, Cutter G. Optimal design and analysis of phase I/II clinical trials in multiple sclerosis with gadolinium-enhanced lesions as the endpoint. *Mult Scler* 2010;16:840–7.

58. Miller D, Barkhof F, Montalban X, Thompson A, Filippi M. Clinically isolated syndromes suggestive of multiple sclerosis, part I: natural history, pathogenesis, diagnosis, and prognosis. *Lancet Neurol* 2005;4:281–8.

59. Montalban X, Tintore M, Swanton J, *et al.* MRI criteria for MS in patients with clinically isolated syndromes. *Neurology* 2010;74:427–34.

60. Polman CH, Reingold SC, Banwell B, *et al.* Diagnostic Criteria for Multiple Sclerosis: 2010 Revisions to the "McDonald Criteria." *Ann Neurol* 2011:in press.

61. Simon JH, the CHAMPS Study Group. MRI predictors of early conversion to clinically definite MS in the CHAMPS placebo group. *Neurology* 2002;59:998–1005.

62. Comi G, Filippi M, Barkhof F, *et al.* Effect of early interferon treatment on conversion to definite multiple sclerosis: a randomised study. *Lancet* 2001;357:1576–82.

63. Kappos L, Radue E-W, O'Connor P, *et al.* A placebo-controlled trial of oral fingolimod in relapsing multiple sclerosis. *N Engl J Med* 2010;362:387–401.

64. Giovannoni G, Comi G, Cook S, *et al.* A placebo-controlled trial of oral cladribine for relapsing multiple sclerosis. *N Engl J Med* 2010;362:416–26.

65. Filippi M, Wolinsky JS, Sormani MP, Comi G. Enhancement frequency decreases with increasing age in relapsing–remitting multiple sclerosis. *Neurology* 2001;56:422–3.

66. Miller DH, Molyneux PD, Barker GJ, MacManus DG, Moseley IF, Wagner K. Effect of interferon-beta1b on magnetic resonance imaging outcomes in secondary progressive multiple sclerosis: results of a European multicenter, randomized, double-blind, placebo-controlled trial. European Study Group on Interferon-beta1b in secondary progressive multiple sclerosis. *Ann Neurol* 1999;46:850–9.

67. Cohen JA, Cutter GR, Fischer JS, *et al.* Benefit of interferon beta-1a on MSFC progression in secondary progressive MS. *Neurology* 2002;59:679–87.

68. Fazekas F, Sorensen PS, Filippi M, *et al.* MRI results from the European Study on Intravenous Immunoglobulin in Secondary Progressive Multiple Sclerosis (ESIMS). *Mult Scler* 2005;11:433–40.

69. Revesz T, Kidd D, Thompson AJ, Barnard RO, McDonald WI. A comparison of the pathology of primary and secondary progressive multiple sclerosis. *Brain* 1994;117(Pt 4): 759–65.

70. Montalban X. Primary progressive multiple sclerosis. *Curr Opin Neurol* 2005;18:261–6.

71. Wolinsky JS, Narayana PA, O'Connor P, *et al.* Glatiramer acetate in primary progressive multiple sclerosis: results of a multinational, multicenter, double-blind, placebo-controlled trial. *Ann Neurol* 2007;61:14–24.

72. Hawker K, O'Connor P, Freedman MS, *et al.* Rituximab in patients with primary progressive multiple sclerosis: Results of a randomized double-blind placebo-controlled multicenter trial. *Ann Neurol* 2009;66:460–71.

73. Kremenchutzky M, Lee D, Rice GP, Ebers GC. Diagnostic brain MRI findings in primary progressive multiple sclerosis. *Mult Scler* 2000;6:81–5.

74. Comi G, Filippi M, Wolinsky JS, European/Canadian Glatiramer Acetate

Study Group. European/Canadian multicenter, double-blind, randomized, placebo-controlled study of the effects of glatiramer acetate on magnetic resonance imaging – measured disease activity and burden in patients with relapsing multiple sclerosis *Ann Neurol* 2001;49:290–7.

75. Frank JA, McFarland HF. How to participate in a multiple sclerosis clinical trial. *Neuroimaging Clin N Am* 2000;10:817–30.

76. Zhao Y, Traboulsee A, Petkau AJ, Li D. Regression of new gadolinium enhancing lesion activity in relapsing–remitting multiple sclerosis. *Neurology* 2008;70:1092–7.

77. Petkau J, Reingold SC, Held U, *et al.* Magnetic resonance imaging as a surrogate outcome for multiple sclerosis relapses. *Multiple Sclerosis* 2008;14:770–8.

78. Sellebjerg F, Nielsen HS, Frederiksen JL, Olesen J. A randomized, controlled trial of oral high-dose methylprednisolone in acute optic neuritis. *Neurology* 1999;52: 1479–84.

79. Sellebjerg F, Frederiksen JL, Nielsen PM, Olesen J. Double-blind, randomized, placebo-controlled study of oral, high-dose methylprednisolone in attacks of MS. *Neurology* 1998;51:529–34.

80. Sellebjerg F, Jensen CV, Larsson HB, Frederiksen JL. Gadolinium-enhanced magnetic resonance imaging predicts response to methylprednisolone in multiple sclerosis. *Mult Scler* 2003;9:102–7.

81. Weiner HL, Guttmann CR, Khoury SJ, *et al.* Serial magnetic resonance imaging in multiple sclerosis: correlation with attacks, disability, and disease stage. *J Neuroimmunol* 2000;104:164–73.

82. Youl BD, Turano G, Miller DH, *et al.* The pathophysiology of acute optic neuritis. An association of gadolinium leakage with clinical and electrophysiological deficits. *Brain* 1991;114(6):2437–50.

83. Smith ME, Stone LA, Albert PS, *et al.* Clinical worsening in multiple sclerosis is associated with increased frequency and area of gadopentetate dimeglumine-enhancing magnetic resonance imaging lesions. *Ann Neurol* 1993;33:480–9.

84. Jacobs LD, Beck RW, Simon JH, *et al.* Intramuscular interferon beta-1a therapy initiated during a first demyelinating event in multiple sclerosis. CHAMPS Study Group. *N Engl J Med* 2000;343:898–904.

85. Sormani MP, Bonzano L, Roccatagliata L, Cutter GR, Mancardi GL, Bruzzi P. Magnetic resonance imaging as a potential surrogate for relapses in multiple sclerosis: a meta-analytic approach. *Ann Neurol* 2009;65:268–75.

86. Sormani M, Bonzano L, Roccatagliata L, de Stefano N. Magnetic resonance imaging as surrogate for clinical endpoints in multiple sclerosis: data on novel oral drugs. *Multi Scler* 2011:in press.

87. Coles AJ, Cox A, Le Page E, *et al.* The window of therapeutic opportunity in multiple sclerosis: evidence from monoclonal antibody therapy. *J Neurol* 2006;253:98–108.

88. Fisher E, Rudick RA, Simon JH, *et al.* Eight-year follow-up study of brain atrophy in patients with MS. *Neurology* 2002;59:1412–20.

89. Sormani MP, Bonzano L, Roccatagliata L, Mancardi GL, Uccelli A, Bruzzi P. Surrogate endpoints for EDSS worsening in multiple sclerosis: A meta-analytic approach. *Neurology* 2010;75:302–9.

90. Simon JH. MRI in multiple sclerosis. *Phys Med Rehabil Clin N Am* 2005;16:383–409, viii.

91. Ferguson B, Matyszak MK, Esiri MM, Perry VH. Axonal damage in acute multiple sclerosis lesions. *Brain* 1997;120(Pt 3):393–9.

92. Trapp BD, Peterson J, Ransohoff RM, Rudick R, Mork S, Bo L. Axonal transection in the lesions of multiple sclerosis. *N Engl J Med* 1998;338:278–85.

93. Bitsch A, Schuchardt J, Bunkowski S, Kuhlmann T, Bruck W. Acute axonal injury in multiple sclerosis. Correlation with demyelination and inflammation. *Brain* 2000;123(6):1174–83.

94. Simon JH, Jacobs L, Kinkel RP. Transcallosal bands: a sign of neuronal tract degeneration in early MS? *Neurology* 2001;57:1888–90.

95. Bjartmar C, Kinkel RP, Kidd G, Rudick RA, Trapp BD. Axonal loss in normal-appearing white matter in a patient with acute MS. *Neurology* 2001;57:1248–52.

96. Simon JH, Kinkel RP, Jacobs L, Bub L, Simonian N. A Wallerian degeneration pattern in patients at risk for MS. *Neurology* 2000;54:1155–60.

97. Narayanan S, Francis SJ, Sled JG, *et al.* Axonal injury in the cerebral normal-appearing white matter of patients with multiple sclerosis is related to concurrent demyelination in lesions but not to concurrent demyelination in normal-appearing white matter. *Neuroimage* 2006;29:637–42.

98. Koudriavtseva T, Thompson AJ, Fiorelli M, *et al.* Gadolinium enhanced MRI predicts clinical and MRI disease activity in relapsing–remitting multiple sclerosis. *J Neurol Neurosurg Psychiatry* 1997;62:285–7.

99. Molyneux PD, Filippi M, Barkhof F, *et al.* Correlations between monthly enhanced MRI lesion rate and changes in T2 lesion volume in multiple sclerosis. *Ann Neurol* 1998;43:332–9.

100. Tubridy N, Coles AJ, Molyneux P, *et al.* Secondary progressive multiple sclerosis: the relationship between short-term MRI activity and clinical features. *Brain* 1998;121(Pt 2): 225–31.

101. Simon JH, Lull J, Jacobs LD, *et al.* A longitudinal study of T1 hypointense lesions in relapsing MS: MSCRG trial of interferon beta-1a. Multiple Sclerosis Collaborative Research Group. *Neurology* 2000;55:185–92.

102. Morgen K, Crawford AL, Stone RD, *et al.* Contrast-enhanced MRI lesions during treatment with interferonbeta-1b predict increase in T1 black hole volume in patients with relapsing–remitting multiple sclerosis. *Mult Scler* 2005;11:146–8.

103. Filippi M, Rovaris M, Capra R, *et al.* A multi-centre longitudinal study comparing the sensitivity of monthly MRI after standard and triple dose gadolinium-DTPA for monitoring disease activity in multiple sclerosis. Implications for phase II clinical trials. *Brain* 1998;121(Pt 10):2011–20.

104. Ingle GT, Sastre-Garriga J, Miller DH, Thompson AJ. Is inflammation important in early PPMS? a longitudinal MRI study. *J Neurol Neurosurg Psychiatry* 2005;76:1255–8.

105. Nilsson P, Sandberg-Wollheim M, Norrving B, Larsson EM. The role of MRI of the brain and spinal cord, and

CSF examination for the diagnosis of primary progressive multiple sclerosis. *Eur J Neurol* 2007;14:1292–5.

106. Filippi M, Yousry T, Horsfield MA, *et al.* A high-resolution three-dimensional T1-weighted gradient echo sequence improves the detection of disease activity in multiple sclerosis. *Ann Neurol* 1996;40:901–7.

107. Li D, Haacke EM, Tarr RW, Venkatesan R, Lin W, Wielopolski P. Magnetic resonance imaging of the brain with gadopentetate dimeglumine-DTPA: Comparison of T1-weighted spin-echo and 3D gradient-echo sequences. *J Magn Res Imaging* 1996;6:415–24.

108. Barkhof F, Filippi M, Miller DH, Tofts P, Kappos L, Thompson AJ. Strategies for optimizing MRI techniques aimed at monitoring disease activity in multiple sclerosis treatment trials. *J Neurol* 1997;244:76–84.

109. Simon JH, Li D, Traboulsee A, *et al.* Standardized MR imaging protocol for multiple sclerosis: Consortium of MS Centers consensus guidelines. *Am J Neuroradiol* 2006;27:455–61.

110. Bonzano L, Roccatagliata L, Mancardi G, Sormani M. Gadolinium-enhancing or active T2 magnetic resonance imaging lesions in multiple sclerosis clinical trials? *Multi Scler* 2009;15:1043–7.

111. Guttmann CR, Ahn SS, Hsu L, Kikinis R, Jolesz FA. The evolution of multiple sclerosis lesions on serial MR. *Am J Neuroradiol* 1995;16:1481–91.

112. Bruck W, Kuhlmann T, Stadelmann C. Remyelination in multiple sclerosis. *J Neurol Sci* 2003;206:181–5.

113. Stone LA, Albert PS, Smith ME, *et al.* Changes in the amount of diseased white matter over time in patients with relapsing–remitting multiple sclerosis. *Neurology* 1995;45:1808–14.

114. Comi G, Martinelli V, Rodegher M, *et al.* Effect of glatiramer acetate on conversion to clinically definite multiple sclerosis in patients with clinically isolated syndrome (PreCISe study): a randomised, double-blind, placebo-controlled trial. *Lancet* 2009;374:1503–11.

115. Kappos L, Polman CH, Freedman MS, *et al.* Treatment with interferon beta-1b delays conversion to clinically definite and McDonald MS in patients with clinically isolated syndromes. *Neurology* 2006;67:1242–9.

116. Li DK, Paty DW. Magnetic resonance imaging results of the PRISMS trial: a randomized, double-blind, placebo-controlled study of interferon-beta1a in relapsing–remitting multiple sclerosis. Prevention of Relapses and Disability by Interferon-beta1a Subcutaneously in Multiple Sclerosis. *Ann Neurol* 1999;46:197–206.

117. Freedman MS, Once Weekly Interferon for MS Study Group. Evidence of interferon beta-1a dose response in relapsing–remitting MS: the OWIMS Study. *Neurology* 1999;53:679–86.

118. Swanton JK, Rovira A, Tintore M, *et al.* MRI criteria for multiple sclerosis in patients presenting with clinically isolated syndromes: a multicentre retrospective study. *Lancet Neurol* 2007;6:677–86.

119. Li DK, Zhao GJ, Paty DW. Randomized controlled trial of interferon-beta-1a in secondary progressive MS: MRI results. *Neurology* 2001;56:1505–13.

120. Hawker KS, O'Connor P, Freedman MS, *et al.* Efficacy and safety of rituximab in patients with primary progressive multiple sclerosis: results of a randomized, double-blind, placebo-controlled, multicenter trial. *Multi Scler* 2008;14:S299.

121. Sormani MP, Bruzzi P, Beckmann K, *et al.* MRI metrics as surrogate endpoints for EDSS progression in SPMS patients treated with IFN beta-1b. *Neurology* 2003;60:1462–6.

122. Tao G, He R, Datta S, Narayana PA. Symmetric inverse consistent nonlinear registration driven by mutual information. *Comput Methods Programs Biomed* 2009;95:105–15.

123. Moraal B, van den Elskamp IJ, Knol DL, *et al.* Long-interval T2-weighted subtraction magnetic resonance imaging: a powerful new outcome measure in multiple sclerosis trials. *Ann Neurol* 2010;67:667–75.

124. Moraal B, Wattjes MP, Geurts JJ, *et al.* Improved detection of active multiple sclerosis lesions: 3D subtraction imaging. *Radiology* 2010;255:154–63.

125. Wolansky LJ, Haghighi MH, Sevdalis E, *et al.* Safety of serial monthly administration of triple-dose gadopentetate dimeglumine in multiple sclerosis patients: preliminary results of the BECOME trial. *J Neuroimaging* 2005;15:289–90.

126. Stone LA, Frank JA, Albert PS, *et al.* The effect of interferon-beta on blood-brain barrier disruptions demonstrated by contrast-enhanced magnetic resonance imaging in relapsing–remitting multiple sclerosis. *Ann Neurol* 1995;37:611–19.

127. Fisniku LK, Brex PA, Altmann DR, *et al.* Disability and T2 MRI lesions: a 20-year follow-up of patients with relapse onset of multiple sclerosis. *Brain* 2008;131:808–17.

128. Bot JC, Blezer EL, Kamphorst W, *et al.* The spinal cord in multiple sclerosis: relationship of high-spatial-resolution quantitative MR imaging findings to histopathologic results. *Radiology* 2004;233:531–40.

129. Powell T, Sussman JG, Davies-Jones GA. MR imaging in acute multiple sclerosis: ringlike appearance in plaques suggesting the presence of paramagnetic free radicals. *Am J Neuroradiol* 1992;13:1544–6.

130. Rocca MA, Colombo B, Falini A, *et al.* Cortical adaptation in patients with MS: a cross-sectional functional MRI study of disease phenotypes. *Lancet Neurol* 2005;4:618–26.

131. Goodin DS. Magnetic resonance imaging as a surrogate outcome measure of disability in multiple sclerosis: have we been overly harsh in our assessment? *Ann Neurol* 2006;59:597–605.

132. Simon JH, Zhang S, Laidlaw DH, *et al.* Identification of fibers at risk for degeneration by diffusion tractography in patients at high risk for MS after a clinically isolated syndrome. *J Magn Reson Imaging* 2006;24:983–8.

133. Bjartmar C, Trapp BD. Axonal and neuronal degeneration in multiple sclerosis: mechanisms and functional consequences. *Curr Opin Neurol* 2001;14:271–8.

134. Mills RJ, Young CA, Smith ET. 3D MRI in multiple sclerosis: a study of three sequences at 3 T. *Br J Radiol* 2007;80:307–20.

135. Sajja BR, Datta S, He R, *et al.* Unified approach for multiple sclerosis lesion segmentation on brain MRI. *Ann Biomed Eng* 2006;34:142–51.

136. Molyneux PD, Tofts PS, Fletcher A, *et al.* Precision and reliability for measurement of change in MRI lesion volume in multiple sclerosis: a comparison of two computer assisted

techniques. *J Neurol Neurosurg Psychiatry* 1998;65:42–7.

137. Barkhof F, McGowan JC, van Waesberghe JH, Grossman RI. Hypointense multiple sclerosis lesions on T1-weighted spin echo magnetic resonance images: their contribution in understanding multiple sclerosis evolution. *J Neurol Neurosurg Psychiatry* 1998;64Suppl 1:S77–9.

138. Simon JH, and the CHAMPS Study Group. Baseline MRI characteristics of patients at high risk for multiple sclerosis: results from the CHAMPS trial. Controlled High-Risk Subjects Avonex Multiple Sclerosis Prevention Study. *Mult Scler* 2002;8:330–8.

139. Enzinger C, Ropele S, Smith S, *et al.* Accelerated evolution of brain atrophy and "black holes" in MS patients with APOE-epsilon 4. *Ann Neurol* 2004;55:563–9.

140. van der Walt A, Stankovich J, Bahlo M, *et al.* Apolipoprotein genotype does not influence MS severity, cognition, or brain atrophy. *Neurology* 2009;73:1018–25.

141. van Waesberghe JH, van Walderveen MA, Castelijns JA, *et al.* Patterns of lesion development in multiple sclerosis: longitudinal observations with T1-weighted spin-echo and magnetization transfer MR. *Am J Neuroradiol* 1998;19:675–83.

142. Gasperini C, Pozzilli C, Bastianello S, *et al.* Interferon-beta-1a in relapsing–remitting multiple sclerosis: effect on hypointense lesion volume on T1 weighted images. *J Neurol Neurosurg Psychiatry* 1999;67:579–84.

143. Filippi M, Rovaris M, Rice GP, *et al.* The effect of cladribine on T(1) 'black hole' changes in progressive MS. *J Neurol Sci* 2000;176:42–4.

144. Arnold DL. Changes observed in multiple sclerosis using magnetic resonance imaging reflect a focal pathology distributed along axonal pathways. *J Neurol* 2005;252 (Suppl 5):v25–9.

145. Filippi M, Rocca MA, Camesasca F, *et al.* Interferon beta-b and glatiramer acetate effects on permanent black hole evolution. *Neurology* 2011;76: in press.

146. Truyen L, van Waesberghe JH, van Walderveen MA, *et al.* Accumulation of hypointense lesions ("black holes") on T1 spin-echo MRI correlates with disease progression in multiple sclerosis. *Neurology* 1996;47:1469–76.

147. van Walderveen MA, Barkhof F, Hommes OR, *et al.* Correlating MRI and clinical disease activity in multiple sclerosis: relevance of hypointense lesions on short-TR/short-TE (T1-weighted) spin-echo images. *Neurology* 1995;45:1684–90.

148. Barkhof F, Calabresi PA, Miller DH, Reingold SC. Imaging outcomes for neuroprotection and repair in multiple sclerosis trials. *Nat Rev Neurol* 2009;5:256–66.

149. van Walderveen MA, Kamphorst W, Scheltens P, *et al.* Histopathologic correlate of hypointense lesions on T1-weighted spin-echo MRI in multiple sclerosis. *Neurology* 1998;50:1282–8.

150. Loevner LA, Grossman RI, Cohen JA, Lexa FJ, Kessler D, Kolson DL. Microscopic disease in normal-appearing white matter on conventional MR images in patients with multiple sclerosis: assessment with magnetization-transfer measurements. *Radiology* 1995;196:511–15.

151. van Waesberghe JH, Kamphorst W, De Groot CJ, *et al.* Axonal loss in multiple sclerosis lesions: magnetic resonance imaging insights into substrates of disability. *Ann Neurol* 1999;46:747–54.

152. Levesque I, Sled JG, Narayanan S, *et al.* The role of edema and demyelination in chronic T1 black holes: a quantitative magnetization transfer study. *J Magn Reson Imaging* 2005;21:103–10.

153. Li BS, Regal J, Soher BJ, Mannon LJ, Grossman RI, Gonen O. Brain metabolite profiles of T1-hypointense lesions in relapsing–remitting multiple sclerosis. *Am J Neuroradiol* 2003;24:68–74.

154. Adams HP, Wagner S, Sobel DF, *et al.* Hypointense and hyperintense lesions on magnetic resonance imaging in secondary-progressive MS patients. *Eur Neurol* 1999;42:52–63.

155. Molyneux PD, Brex PA, Fogg C, *et al.* The precision of T1 hypointense lesion volume quantification in multiple sclerosis treatment trials: a multicenter study. *Mult Scler* 2000;6:237–40.

156. Datta S, Sajja BR, He R, Wolinsky JS, Gupta RK, Narayana PA. Segmentation and quantification of black holes in multiple sclerosis. *Neuroimage* 2006;29:467–74.

157. Parry A, Clare S, Jenkinson M, Smith S, Palace J, Matthews PM. White matter and lesion T1 relaxation times increase in parallel and correlate with disability in multiple sclerosis. *J Neurol* 2002;249:1279–86.

158. Bakshi R, Dandamudi VS, Neema M, De C, Bermel RA. Measurement of brain and spinal cord atrophy by magnetic resonance imaging as a tool to monitor multiple sclerosis. *J Neuroimaging* 2005;15:30S–45S.

Chapter

10

Measures of magnetization transfer

Massimo Filippi, Joseph C. McGowan, and Maria A. Rocca

Introduction

Although conventional magnetic resonance imaging (MRI) can detect multiple sclerosis (MS) lesions with high sensitivity, it is not without relevant limitations. First, MRI is not specific with regard to the heterogeneous pathological substrates of individual lesions, which include edema, inflammation, demyelination, remyelination, gliosis, and axonal loss. Second, MRI does not delineate tissue damage occurring in the gray matter (GM) and in the normal-appearing white matter (NAWM), which is known to be damaged in these patients.[1] These limitations are to some degree overcome by the use of gadolinium-enhancing (Gd-enhancing) T1-weighted images, which distinguish active from inactive lesions, since enhancement occurs as a result of increased blood–brain barrier (BBB) permeability and corresponds to areas with ongoing inflammation.[2] However, the activity of the lesions as demonstrated on post-contrast T1-weighted imaging still provides only limited information on tissue damage. Chronically hypointense areas on T1-weighted images correspond to areas where severe tissue disruption has occurred,[3] and their extent is correlated with the clinical severity of the disease and its evolution over time. Still, the extent of T1-hypointense lesions does not correspond to the severity of intrinsic lesion pathology and provides no information about NAWM and GM damage. Finally, the definition of hypointense is by nature highly subjective.

A number of non-conventional MRI techniques have been developed and applied in efforts to improve understanding of the evolution of MS.[1] These techniques, including magnetization transfer (MT) MRI, are designed to provide quantitative information with regard to MS microscopic and macroscopic lesion burdens with a higher pathological specificity to the most destructive aspects of MS than conventional MRI.

Physical basis of MT-MRI

All MRI techniques exploit the enhanced absorption of energy experienced by certain nuclei when exposed to radio-frequency energy at a particular (resonance) frequency. The historically rapid incorporation of MRI into routine clinical use was based upon the earlier observation that the recovery to equilibrium of such "excited" spins can be described by two relaxation times, T1 and T2.[4] Thus, a tissue being investigated with MRI of, for example, water protons can be characterized in terms of nuclear spin density, T1 and T2, and images can be produced that reflect primarily one or the other of these variables. So-called conventional MRI techniques incorporate the assumption that a region of tissue may be fully described using only those three variables, and thus, for example, a region of hyperintensity on T2-weighted imaging may be attributed to relatively longer T2. Since conventional MRI does not typically offer absolute quantitation of intensity, a region may be described as hyperintense without any conclusions being drawn about the magnitude of change in T2 that was responsible for the observation.

MT techniques in MRI are based upon an assumption that more than one relaxation time may influence the MR-observed characteristics of a region. As such, tissue is treated as a more complicated structure that includes non-water protons associated with proteins and other large molecules. These non-water protons cannot be detected directly, but MT theory holds that they may be probed via their effects on the water protons.

The premise of MT-MRI is that proton spins, having well-known relaxation properties, can exchange spin magnetization with protons of much larger molecules, such as myelin or other proteins. The consequence of these exchange processes in MRI is that observed proton relaxation times may reflect the characteristics of the macromolecular environment. Additionally, MRI acquisition techniques have been devised to provide contrast which reflects the magnitude of the transfer effect. In these studies the exchange process is relied upon to transfer magnetic saturation into the water proton spins, reducing or destroying the signal from affected spins. Quantitation in these MT-MRI studies arises from the ability to compare images reflecting the exchange of magnetization with those obtained as controls. Thus, MT techniques can provide quantitative information, a potential advantage over conventional methodology. More importantly, MT techniques represent a potential window into the structure of tissue.

Multiple Sclerosis Therapeutics, Fourth Edition, ed. Jeffrey A. Cohen and Richard A. Rudick. Published by Cambridge University Press.
© Cambridge University Press 2011.

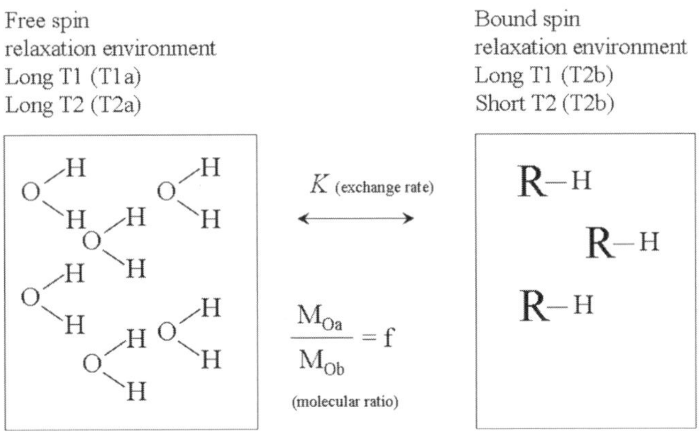

Free spin
relaxation environment
Long T1 (T1a)
Long T2 (T2a)

Bound spin
relaxation environment
Long T1 (T2b)
Short T2 (T2b)

K (exchange rate)

$$\frac{M_{Oa}}{M_{Ob}} = f$$

(molecular ratio)

Fig. 10.1. A two-site model for magnetization transfer (MT), demonstrating the six variables which are required for full characterization. The free spin environment corresponds to water, and the bound environment corresponds to large molecules, symbolized as a proton attached to the rest (R) of the molecule. See text for further details.

A two-site exchange model for MT

In biological tissue, water protons constitute the bulk of MR-visible nuclei. These are characterized by relatively long values of T1 and T2. The relaxation environment for protons attached to macromolecules is by comparison more solid-like, with correspondingly short transverse relaxation (T2) times. Direct observation of these spins is not currently feasible as the signal decay is very fast with respect to the time required to acquire the MR signal. A distinct and further complication is that the frequency of the signal from the water protons is very close to that of the signal from the protons associated with macromolecules. A two-site model demonstrating the exchange possibilities and characteristic variables is diagrammed in Fig. 10.1. It is assumed that each compartment has associated with it intrinsic relaxation times T1 and T2. These should be distinguished from observed relaxation times that are measured with standard techniques. With the addition of a rate constant k and a molecular ratio f, the exchange characteristics of the two-site system can be completely described using six variables. More complex models are possible but difficult to characterize with available techniques, and clinical applications to date have not mandated the incorporation of more than two sites.

Selective saturation

A fundamental requirement for detecting the effects of one type of spin (macromolecular) as opposed to those of another (water) is the ability to perform an MR study that is selective with respect to the spin of interest. Saturation of spin magnetization is perhaps the most straightforward method for this purpose, and was first employed in the "double resonance" experiments of Forsen and Hoffman[5] using a system of two chemically exchanging substances where the resonance frequencies differed in the two spin systems. Briefly, saturating radio-frequency excitation was applied at each spin resonance in turn, while the magnetization of the opposite spin resonance

was measured. The data obtained allowed the full characterization of the system. The first MT images employed continuous off-resonance saturation,[6] the efficacy of which can be demonstrated using Bloch's equations.[7] Modern techniques exploiting MT may use either inversion or, more frequently, saturation of the macromolecular spins with pulsed off-resonance or on-resonance saturation methods.[8] As in the pioneering methods cited above, two studies are performed and compared in order to associate quantitative information with each point or region of the image. This information is typically a number representing the amount of saturation effect measured in the water protons, often expressed as MT ratio (MTR).[9]

The pathological basis of MT-MRI changes in MS

Low MTR indicates a reduced capacity of the molecules in the brain tissue matrix to exchange magnetization with the surrounding (MRI-visible) water molecules. Post-mortem studies of lesions and NAWM have shown consistently that marked MTR reduction corresponds to severe tissue damage.[10,11] van Waesberghe et al.[10] demonstrated a strong correlation between MTR and both the percentage of residual axons and the degree of demyelination (Fig. 10.2). Schmierer et al.[11] found a strong correlation between MTR and myelin content, which in turn correlated strongly with axonal count. This study also showed that remyelinated lesions have higher MTR values than demyelinated lesions,[11] suggesting the potential of MT-MRI to monitor remyelination in MS.

Markedly reduced MTR values were also measured in the "pure" demyelinating lesions of patients with progressive multifocal leukoencephalopathy (PML)[12,13] or central pontine myelinolisis[14] and in the affected optic nerves of patients with optic neuritis where they were correlated with an increased latency of the visual evoked potentials (VEP),[15] which is in turn correlated to the extent and severity of demyelination.[16] A one-year follow up study of patients with an acute optic neuritis showed that MTR of the diseased optic nerves declined over time with a nadir at about 240 days after clinical onset, and then appeared to rise,[17] again suggesting a role for MT-MRI to monitor demyelination and remyelination in MS. The relationship between MTR decrease and myelin loss is consistent with the correlation found between MT-MRI derived metrics and the myelin water fraction from multicompartmental T2 analysis (which is believed to originate from water trapped between the myelin bilayers).[18,19] The relationship between reduced MTR values and axonal loss is consistent with the strong correlation found in MS lesions between MTR and N-acetyl-aspartate (NAA) levels,[20] signal intensity on T1-weighted images,[21] and mean diffusivity.[22]

Analysis of MT-MR images

The first step in the quantitative analysis of MT-MR images is the creation of calculated MT images or MTR maps, which are

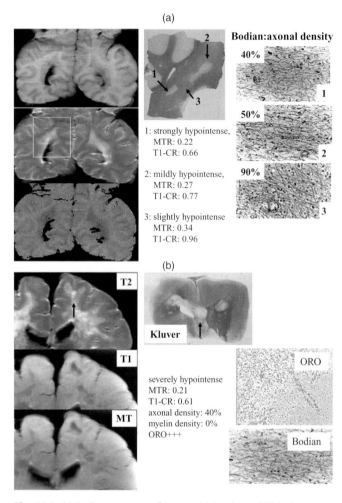

(a)

Bodian:axonal density

40%

1: strongly hypointense,
MTR: 0.22
T1-CR: 0.66

50%

2: mildly hypointense,
MTR: 0.27
T1-CR: 0.77

90%

3: slightly hypointense
MTR: 0.34
T1-CR: 0.96

(b)

T2

Kluver

T1

severely hypointense
MTR: 0.21
T1-CR: 0.61
axonal density: 40%
myelin density: 0%
ORO+++

MT

ORO

Bodian

Fig. 10.2. (a) An illustrative case of three multiple sclerosis (MS) lesions (arrows) showing that the magnetization transfer ratio (MTR) is lower when the density of residual axons is reduced. (b) An illustrative case of one MS lesion (arrow) showing that its MTR and myelin density are both very low. Courtesy of Drs. J.H. vanWaesberghe and F. Barkhof.

derived from two MR images, acquired without and with an off-resonance saturation pulse. MTR maps are derived, on a pixel-by-pixel basis, according to the following equation:

$$\text{MTR} = (1 - M_S/M_0) * 100\%,$$

in which M_0 is the intensity of a given pixel without the saturation pulse, and M_S is the intensity of the same pixel when the saturation pulse is applied (Fig. 10.3). Thus, MTR represents the fraction of signal loss due to the complete or partial saturation of the bound proton pool, and ranges from near zero in the cerebrospinal fluid (CSF) to about 50% in tissue that contains a high proportion of bound water molecules (Fig. 10.3). MS lesions, which usually have lower MTR than NAWM,[23] appear as areas of hypointensity on MTR maps. The degree of hypointensity is related to the amount of tissue destruction in the examined area.

Several approaches can be adopted to analyze MS-related abnormalities on MTR maps:

(1) Region of interest (ROI) analysis of specific tissues. This approach allows the study of individual MS lesions and discrete areas of the NAWM and GM.
(2) Analysis of the average MTR of T2 lesions. This approach allows the investigator to obtain information about the severity of tissue damage of the overall lesion population. The average lesion MTR can be formed, according to:

$$\text{Average lesion MTR} = \frac{\sum_i A_i \times \text{MTR}_i}{\sum_i A_i},$$

in which A_i is the area of lesion i, and MTR_i is the average MTR within that lesion. Thus the contribution that each lesion makes to the average is weighted by the size of the lesion. Clearly, such an approach can be applied to study lesions with more severe tissue damage.

(3) Contour plotting of MTR. This approach consists in displaying the MTR values as an overlay on MR images.[24] In this way, it is possible to detect gradients and boundaries of abnormal MTR that are too subtle to be detected by conventional reading of the MTR maps.

(4) Histogram analysis of large portions of brain tissue. This strategy encompasses both microscopic and macroscopic lesion burdens of the examined tissues.[25] However, it is possible to mask lesions before the production of histograms, thus assessing only normal-appearing tissues. For each histogram, several parameters can be calculated,[25] including the height and position of the histogram peak (i.e. the most common MTR value in the brain) and the average MTR. MTR histograms can be obtained for the whole brain, WM, GM, or for specific regions (e.g. frontal lobe, cerebellum, and brain stem), which can be segmented according to standard neuroanatomical references. MTR histogram analysis is a highly automated technique and, as a consequence, intra-rater, inter-rater, and scan–rescan variabilities of MTR histogram-derived metrics are low.[26,27]

(5) Voxel-wise statistical analysis of MTR images. This approach, which is based on the use of standardized anatomical spaces and a voxel-by-voxel analysis, allows the investigator to obtain an overall assessment of macroscopic and microscopic damages from the entire brain or specific brain tissues, such as the GM or the NAWM without *a-priori* knowledge about damage distribution.[28,29]

MT-MRI to assess tissue damage within macroscopic white matter lesions of MS

Although conventional T2-weighted scans play a major role in the assessment of MS lesion burden, cross-sectional[30] and longitudinal studies[31] have demonstrated that the magnitude of the correlation between clinical disability and brain T2-weighted lesion load is only modest. This observation is likely due, at least in part, to the extremely variable extent of the intrinsic tissue damage of MS lesions visible on conventional MRI scans. Using

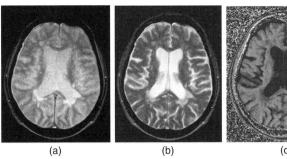
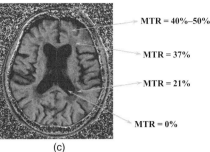

MTR = 40%–50%

MTR = 37%

MTR = 21%

MTR = 0%

(a)   (b)   (c)

Fig. 10.3. Axial gradient-echo images of the brain without (a) and with (b) the magnetization transfer (MT) pulse applied from a patient with multiple sclerosis (MS). The corresponding MT ratio (MTR) map obtained from the two previous images is shown in (c). MTR values of different brain regions are shown. MS lesions have highly variable MTR values.

MTR, it is possible to grade the extent of intrinsic tissue damage of individual MS lesions and, as a consequence, of aggregates of MS lesions. Monitoring individual lesion evolution may be relevant for the understanding of MS pathophysiology, and as a new strategy for assessing treatment efficacy. Different approaches have been used to estimate the severity of intrinsic tissue damage of aggregates of macroscopic WM lesions from individual MS patients or groups of MS patients, including the measurement of the load of the lesions visible as hypointense areas on the MTR maps (MT-MRI lesion load) and the analysis of the average MTR of T2 lesions (average lesion MTR).

MT-MRI changes in active MS lesions

In MS, lesions enhancing on MRI scans after Gd injection represent areas with a damaged BBB and ongoing inflammation.[2,32] However, "active" MS lesions may have different patterns (i.e. homogeneous or ring-like), different durations of enhancement, or may enhance only when using highly sensitive approaches, such as the administration of a triple dose of Gd[33] or the application of an MT pulse to a post-contrast T1-weighted image.[34,35] This enhancement variability suggests that the pathological nature of MS enhancing lesions and the severity of the associated changes in the inflamed tissue may widely vary. MT-MRI studies of individual enhancing lesions tend to be confirmatory of this hypothesis. Homogeneously enhancing lesions, which may represent new active lesions, have significantly higher MTR values than ring-enhancing lesions,[36,37] which may represent old, reactivated lesions. In the latter lesions, the central portions, which probably represent the most damaged tissue, have the lowest MTR values.[37] A longitudinal study[38] also confirmed that ring-like enhancing lesions had the lowest MTR, both at baseline and at follow-up, after enhancement ceased. The duration of enhancement is also associated with different degrees of MTR changes in new MS lesions: lesions enhancing on at least two consecutive monthly scans have lower MTR than those enhancing on a single scan,[39] indicating that a longer enhancement in MS lesions may be related to a more severe tissue damage. That a less damaged BBB is associated with a milder tissue damage is also indicated by the demonstration that new lesions enhancing after the injection of a standard dose of Gd have significantly lower MTR values than

those enhancing only after a triple dose[40] and that large enhancing lesions tend to have greater MTR reductions than smaller lesions.[36]

Using MT-MRI and variable frequencies of scanning, several authors have investigated the structural changes of new enhancing MS lesions for periods of time ranging from three to 36 months.[36,38,40–46] The results of all these studies consistently show that, on average, MTR drops dramatically when the lesions start to enhance and may show a partial or complete recovery in the subsequent 1 to 6 months. Studies which evaluated the evolution of individual lesions showed that a large proportion (33%–44%) of newly formed Gd-enhancing lesions had a marked MTR increase over months following their formation; a small fraction (2%–12%) showed a progressive MTR decrease, whereas the majority (50%–54%) of these lesions tended to maintain relatively stable MTR values.[38,44,46] In the study of Filippi et al.[46] the classification of the lesions after the first month of follow up strongly predicted the classification at the end of the follow up. New lesions enhancing only after the injection of a triple dose of Gd have a similar short-term recovery profile.[40] However, at each time point of the follow-up, MTR in triple dose enhancing lesions is significantly higher than in standard dose lesions,[40] confirming the relative mildness of tissue damage in those lesions with less severe BBB disruption. Chen et al.[47] developed a method to monitor the evolution of MTR in individual lesion voxels and found significant changes that followed different temporal patterns within the same lesion.

The most likely pathological mechanisms underlying the short-term changes in MTR of newly enhancing MS lesions might be demyelination and remyelination. The relative preservation of axons which is typical in acute MS lesions,[2,48] and the rapid and marked increase of the MTR are indeed consistent with demyelination and remyelination, but not with axonal loss. Nevertheless, edema and its subsequent resolution may also give rise to the observed pattern of MTR behaviour, due to the diluting effect of extra-tissue water. However, it seems unlikely that edema alone is sufficient to explain these findings, since edema in the absence of demyelination results in only modest MTR reductions.[23] The effect of gliosis on MTR is likely to be marginal, if any, since a post-mortem study was unable to detect any correlation between MTR and NAWM gliosis.[10] Regardless of the underlying pathological substrates, short-term MTR changes in newly formed MS lesions can be detected by image

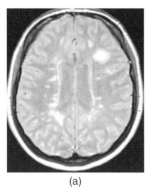
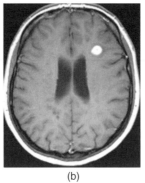
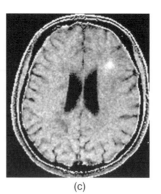

(a)   (b)   (c)

Fig. 10.4. (a) Proton-density weighted image showing several MS lesions. (b) Corresponding post-contrast T1-weighted image showing that one of these lesions is enhancing. (c) Magnetization transfer ratio (MTR) image obtained by an image combination method using follow-up MT-MRI scans (without gadolinium administration) showing that the enhancing lesion visible in (b) can be detected as an area of 'pseudo-enhancement'.

combination methods using serial MT-MRI scans as areas of "pseudo-enhancement," thus providing information about the acute events in MS that is usually derived from post-contrast T1-weighted images (Fig. 10.4).[49]

These results also suggest that the balance between damaging and reparative mechanisms may be highly variable during the early phases of MS lesion formation. Different proportions of lesions with different degrees of structural changes may, therefore, contribute to the evolution of the disease and may explain why previous studies found poor correlations between the number of enhancing lesions and the long-term disease evolution.[50] At present, however, there are few data supporting such a concept. A three year follow up study[45] showed that newly-enhancing lesions from patients with secondary progressive MS (SPMS) compared to those from patients with RRMS had lower MTR at the time of their appearance and presented a more severe and significant MTR reduction during the follow-up.

MT-MRI changes in established MS lesions

The vast majority of the enhancing lesions are associated with T2 abnormalities and a significant proportion of them may appear hypointense on T1-weighted scans. MTR values for MS lesions visible on T2-weighted scans are significantly lower than those for NAWM[11,51–54] and those of lesions from elderly patients,[55] or from patients with small-vessel disease,[53] systemic immune-mediated diseases,[56] human immunodeficiency virus (HIV)-encephalitis,[12] central nervous system (CNS) tuberculosis,[57] traumatic brain injury,[58] and migraine.[59] In contrast, reductions of MTR values with a magnitude comparable to that seen in MS lesions have been found in WM lesions of patients with vascular dementia,[60] amyotrophic lateral sclerosis,[61] PML,[12] central pontine myelinolisis,[14] cerebral autosomal dominant arteriopathy with subcortical infarcts and leukoencephalopathy (CADASIL),[62] LHON,[63] and acute disseminated encephalomyelitis (ADEM).[64] MT-MRI might also help to distinguish between tumefactive dyemilinating lesions and brain tumors.[65]

Lower MTR has been reported in hypointense lesions compared to lesions that are isointense to NAWM on T1-weighted scans,[11,37,38] and MTR has been found to be inversely correlated with the degree of hypointensity.[11,66] In a longitudinal monthly study,[38] MS lesions that changed from T1 hypointense to T1 isointense when Gd enhancement ceased also had a significant MTR increase, whereas a strongly decreased MTR at the time of initial enhancement was predictive of a persistent T1-weighted hypointensity and lower MTR after 6 months.

Decreased MTR has also been found in NAWM areas that are adjacent to focal T2-weighted MS lesions[51,52,54] and in WM areas characterized by subtle, and diffuse signal intensity changes on T2-weighted MR images, referred as "dirty-appearing" WM.[67] MTR progressively increased with distance from MS lesions to the cortical GM, and MTR was lower for patients with more disabling MS courses.[51]

MT-MRI to assess intrinsic tissue damage in aggregates of macroscopic MS lesions
MT-MRI lesion load

With this approach the total volume of tissue occupied by lesions which appear hypointense on MTR maps is measured. Several studies[68–70] have shown that MT-MRI, T2- and T1-weighted lesion loads differ considerably, and the measurement reproducibilities also differ. This is likely due to two main technical limitations of this approach. First, the identification of MS lesions on MT-MRI scans is subjective, albeit confirmed by the presence of corresponding abnormalities on T2-weighted images. Second, calculated MTR images have a poor contrast-to-noise ratio (CNR) and MS lesions with low MTR may show varying degrees of hypointensity, whereas areas of WM which are isointense on T2-weighted images may also have reduced MTR[51,52] and, therefore, appear relatively hypointense on MT-MRI scans. A "conservative" approach leads to an MT-MRI lesion load that is lower than the corresponding T2-weighted lesion load, with a similar measurement repeatability.[71] On the other hand, the inclusion of diffuse WM abnormalities extending beyond the borders of focal lesions weakens the pathological specificity of MT-MRI findings, leading to MT-MRI lesion load higher than T2-weighted lesion load,[69] and also to a poorer measurement reproducibility. On the basis of these

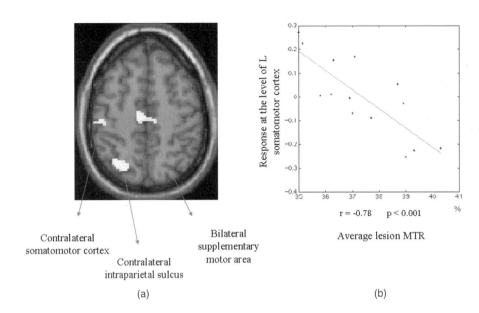

Fig. 10.5. (a) Relative cortical activation in right-handed relapsing–remitting multiple sclerosis patients during a simple motor task with their clinically unimpaired, right hand as compared to matched healthy volunteers. (b) Correlation between relative activation of the contralateral primary sensorimotor cortex and average lesion magnetization transfer ratio (MTR).

studies, the volume of hypointense lesions on MT-MRI scans would seem not to be a reliable measure of lesion burden in MS. The limited value of MT-MRI lesion load as an outcome measure in MS is confirmed by its modest correlations with clinical disability.[68,71]

Average lesion MTR

The analysis of average lesion MTR requires several post-processing steps, including the preliminary identification of MS lesions on T2-weighted scans, the coregistration of T2-weighted and MTR scans, and the superimposition of T2 lesion outlines onto the coregistered MTR scans. Compared to the measurement of the MT-MRI lesion load, this approach has two major advantages. First, it bases lesion identification on T2-weighted scans, which are characterized by a much better CNR than calculated MTR images. Second, it enables one to obtain a quantitative estimate of intrinsic tissue damage in the whole of the macroscopically diseased WM. That average lesion MTR may give additional information on MS tissue damage over that provided by other MRI measures of disease burden is suggested by the weak correlations reported between average lesion MTR and lesion load or brain volume.[72] The moderate correlations that have been found between average lesion MTR and other measures of intrinsic lesion damage derived from diffusion tensor (DT) MRI[22,54,72] and proton MR spectroscopy (^{1}H-MRS),[19] albeit stronger than those with MRI measures of macroscopic MS disease burden, also support this concept.

Even though the average lesion MTR was found to be the best discriminant between patients with MS and those with CNS symptoms or signs of systemic immune-mediated disorders, independent of the burden of MRI lesions,[56] the correlation between average lesion MTR and the clinical manifestations of MS are somewhat disappointing.[72] Patients with cognitive impairment have a significantly lower average lesion

MTR than those without, but average lesion MTR was found to explain only 35% of the total variance in neuropsychological test performance.[73] Similar average lesion MTR values have been found in patients with SPMS and primary progressive MS (PPMS), matched for the degree of disability.[74] Consistent with their clinical evolution, patients with SPMS have a faster decline of their average MTR values than all the other clinical phenotypes of the disease.[75] Average lesion MTR was found to be lower in patients with RRMS compared to those at presentation with clinically isolated syndromes (CIS) suggestive of MS,[76] but it was not significantly different between patients with RRMS and those with benign (B) MS or SPMS,[77] nor between patients with and without fatigue.[78] On the contrary, average lesion MTR percentage change over one year was found to be an independent predictor of accumulation of disability in the subsequent seven years in a cohort of patients with CIS, RRMS, and SPMS.[79] The only partial correlation found between the degree of intrinsic lesion damage, measured using average lesion MTR, and the clinical manifestations of MS might be due, on the one hand, to the variable extent of tissue damage outside T2 lesions and, on the other, by the fact that intrinsic lesion damage can induce adaptive cortical changes (Fig. 10.5),[80,81] which in turn have the potential to limit the clinical consequences of subcortical WM damage.[82]

MT-MRI to assess damage of MS tissues appearing normal on conventional MRI scans

MTR analysis has been extensively used to achieve reliable in-vivo estimates of the extent of tissue damage occurring outside T2 lesions, to increase our understanding of the mechanisms leading to the progressive accumulation of irreversible disability in MS and, as a consequence, to improve the magnitude of the clinical/MRI correlations.

Normal-appearing white matter and normal-appearing brain tissue

Post-mortem studies showed that abnormalities can be detected in the NAWM from patients with MS.[83,84] These abnormalities include diffuse astrocytic hyperplasia, patchy edema and perivascular cellular infiltration, abnormally thin myelin,[85] and axonal damage.[86] Such pathological abnormalities modify the relative proportions of mobile and immobile protons of the diseased tissue and, therefore, it is not surprising that MT-MRI is able to show microscopic damage in the NAWM which is not detected by conventional imaging.[51,52,54,87]

Variable degrees of NAWM changes may precede new lesion formation in MS.[41,42,88] There are several possible pathological substrates which may contribute to the changes seen to occur in NAWM before the appearance of new MS lesions, including edema, marked astrocytic proliferation, perivascular inflammation, and demyelination. All of these processes may account for an increased amount of unbound water and, as a consequence, determine MTR changes. A study based on multiparametric MT-MRI measurements, showed that about four months before the appearance of a new MS lesion a reduction of macromolecular material and a focal increase of free water are detected in the corresponding NAWM, which suggest that primary myelin damage might be the leading event.[88]

Using ROI analysis, several studies have shown that NAWM MTR values are altered in all the major phenotypes of MS and that these alterations span multiple cerebral regions.[51,52,54,87,89] Reduced MTR values have been found in several NAWM regions even in patients with clinically definite MS and no or only very few T2 lesions.[89,90] These observations have indicated the need to obtain more accurate estimates of the overall extent of NAWM damage in MS and, as a consequence, have led to the application of histogram analysis to all brain pixels classed as normal on conventional MRI.[91] Using such an approach, Tortorella et al. showed that MTR histogram abnormalities in the normal-appearing brain tissue (NABT) are present in all the main MS clinical phenotypes, and are more pronounced in patients with SPMS (Fig. 10.6).[91] These findings were confirmed by a subsequent study.[92] In RRMS patients, average MTR of the NABT was found to be highly correlated with cognitive impairment,[73] but not with fatigue.[78] NABT-MTR was found to be moderately correlated with disability in a mixed group of relapse-onset MS patients.[92] The NABT-MTR histogram characteristics of PPMS patients do not significantly differ from those of SPMS patients.[74] A significant decline of NABT-MTR over time has been shown to occur at a faster rate in patients with SPMS than in patients with other clinical phenotypes.[75] Reduced MTR values have also been detected in the NABT from patients with CIS[76] and the extent of these abnormalities has been found in one study to be an independent predictor of subsequent disease evolution.[76] NABT-MTR was found to be normal in patients with pediatric MS.[93]

In MS patients, NABT-MTR values are only partially correlated with the extent of macroscopic lesions and the severity

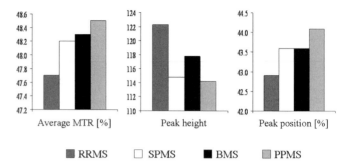

Fig. 10.6. Mean magnetization transfer ratio (MTR) histogram-derived metrics of the normal-appearing brain tissue (NABT) from patients with relapsing-remitting (RR) multiple sclerosis (MS), secondary progressive (SP) MS, benign (B) MS, and primary progressive (PP) MS. The MTR histogram from patients with RRMS has the lowest average MTR and peak position, and the highest peak height when compared with those from all the other MS phenotypes. This suggests small, discrete lesions beyond the resolution of conventional scanning as the most likely change occurring in a relatively large portion of the NABT. Compared with RRMS, SPMS patients had a dramatically reduced MTR histogram peak height, whereas no difference was found between RRMS and SPMS patients. This suggests that, among other factors, a progressive reduction of cerebral tissue with truly normal MTR may be responsible for the evolution from RRMS to SPMS. Patients with PPMS have the lowest peak height when compared with those from all the other MS phenotypes, whereas the average histogram MTR and peak position are similar to those from control subjects. This suggests that the amount of residual normal brain tissue is much lower in PPMS and suggests widespread but mild changes as the most likely underlying pathology.

of intrinsic lesion damage, thus suggesting that NABT changes do not only reflect Wallerian degeneration of axons traversing large focal abnormalities.[62,74,91] On the contrary, a strong correlation has been found between NABT-MTR and brain volume, suggesting that NABT damage is involved in determining irreversible tissue loss in MS.[91] More recently, in patients with RRMS[80] and PPMS,[94] moderate to strong correlations have also been found between the severity of MT-MRI changes of the NABT and the relative functional MRI activations of several cortical areas located in a widespread network for sensorimotor and multimodal integration.

Data coming from histogram analysis of NAWM taken in isolation confirm those obtained from the analysis of the NABT.[95–97] Using voxel-based analysis in CIS patients, Ranjeva et al.[29] found abnormally low MTR values in several NAWM regions, which correlated with measures of clinical impairment. A strong correlation has also been found between baseline NAWM-MTR and disability accumulation over five years in a preliminary study of a small group of MS patients.[98]

The role of NAWM-MTR changes in the diagnostic work-up of patients suspected of having MS remains to be elucidated, but it is likely to be modest, since MTR changes of NABT/NAWM are not disease-specific. Indeed, reduced NAWM-MTR values can also be found in patients with other neurological conditions associated with WM lesions on T2-weighted images, such as neuro-SLE,[56] CADASIL,[62] PML,[12] HIV-encephalitis,[12] LHON,[63] and cerebrotendinous xanthomatosis.[99] On the contrary, MTR changes of the NAWM have not been found in patients with other conditions, such as migraine,[59] neuromyelitis optica (NMO),[100] ADEM,[64] and neuroborreliosis.[101]

Gray matter

Post-mortem studies have shown that MS pathology does not spare cerebral GM.[102–104] Consistent with this, numerous studies have shown reduced MTR values in the GM from MS patients, using ROI[95], histogram,[95–97,105] or voxel-wise[28,29] analysis. Reduced MTR values have been demonstrated in the brain GM from patients with different MS phenotypes,[95–97,105] including those at the earliest clinical stages of the disease.[106,107] MTR abnormalities in the GM, NAWM, and lesions were less pronounced in patients with BMS vs. those with early RRMS.[108] MTR abnormalities in the GM were found to be correlated with disease duration, and, as a consequence, were more pronounced in patients with PPMS or SPMS than in those with other clinical phenotypes.[74] GM MTR changes correlate with clinical disability[97,105,107,109,110] and cognitive impairment,[29,111] whereas no correlation with fatigue has emerged.[112] Thalamic MTR abnormalities, occurring within the first five years of the disease in RRMS, also correlate with the Expanded Disability Status Scale (EDSS) score.[113] In addition, in patients with relapsing–onset MS, GM MTR was found to be an independent predictor of the accumulation of disability over the subsequent eight years.[79] In PPMS patients, GM MTR decline was shown to reflect the rate of clinical deterioration over three years.[114]

Voxel-based analysis of MTR images from CIS patients has revealed abnormalities in several GM areas.[28] In CIS patients with a previous optic neuritis, a selective reduction of MTR values in the occipital cortex has been found.[115] In PPMS, significant correlations between regional decrease of MTR values of cortical areas of the motor network and the EDSS scores as well as between MTR values in cortical areas of the cognitive network and the PASAT scores were found.[116] Significant correlations have also been reported between GM-MTR and T2 lesion volume.[95,105,113] This fits with the notion that at least part of GM pathology in MS is secondary to retrograde degeneration of fibers traversing WM lesions. Reduced GM-MTR values have also been demonstrated in patients with NMO,[117] and in those with cerebrotendinous xanthomatosis.[99]

MT-MRI to assess overall tissue damage of the brain in MS

As reviewed in the previous sections, there is evidence that the extent and nature of the damage of T2 abnormalities, NAWM, and GM all contribute to the accumulation of irreversible neurological disability in MS. Consistent with this view, there has been an increasing use of MR metrics with the potential to provide a complete assessment of MS pathology in the brain. Such MR metrics would be of particular interest in the context of clinical trials, where it would be unrealistic to monitor treatment efficacy by measuring the extent of tissue damage from several structures and tissues. One of the simplest and

most robust approach to generate MR metrics able to assess and grade overall tissue damage in MS is the production of MTR histograms of the whole of the brain tissue. However, this approach is not without limitations. First, by constructing an MTR histogram, one gives up spatial information present in an image and instead looks at the distribution of MTR values. Second, cerebral atrophy can lead to an increase in the contamination of the signal from parenchyma by signal from CSF. Due to the presence of diffuse demyelination and axonal loss, MS patients typically have lower whole-brain average MTR, as well as lower peak height and position of the whole-brain MTR histogram than normal subjects.[22,25,74,75,77,118,119] MTR histogram parameters also differ between the various clinical forms of MS.[74,77,118,119] Patients with SPMS have the lowest whole-brain MTR histogram-derived measures.[74,77,118,119] In patients with SPMS, whole-brain MTR histogram metrics also appear to be particularly sensitive to disease changes over relatively short periods of time.[75] This exquisite sensitivity could make these MTR-derived quantities appealing as outcome measures for assessing the efficacy of new experimental treatments in patients with SPMS. The potential of whole-brain MTR for contributing to treatment monitoring of MS is highlighted by recent findings showing that whole-brain MTR percentage change over 1 year predicts the accumulation of clinical disability in the subsequent 4 years in patients with definite MS.[120] Preliminary work has also suggested a potential role of whole-brain MTR histograms in the diagnostic work-up of individual cases suspected of having MS, especially in the absence of "typical" conventional MRI changes.[121]

Correlations between MTR histogram parameters and clinical outcome have been widely tested.[22,25,72,74,76,77,118,119,122,123] Whole-brain MTR/clinical correlations were found to be stronger in patients with RRMS and SPMS than in other clinical phenotypes of the disease,[118,119] whereas no significant correlations were found when patients with PPMS were considered in isolation.[74,118,119] Whole-brain MTR histogram metrics are also correlated with the presence of neuropsychological impairment in MS patients.[68,122,123]

Other studies have assessed the impact of overall tissue damage of specific brain structures on the corresponding clinical manifestations.[68,123,124] These studies have shown that MTR histogram parameters from the whole of the cerebellum and brain stem are strongly correlated with the impairment of the corresponding functional systems,[123] and that MTR histogram parameters of the whole of the frontal lobes are lower in patients with cognitive impairment compared to those without.[68,124]

MT-MRI studies of the cervical cord and optic nerve in MS

MT-MRI of the cervical cord and optic nerve presents technical difficulties, mainly because of the sizes of these two structures, and their tendency to move during imaging. Nevertheless, recent work has shown that it is possible to acquire

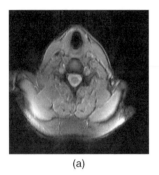 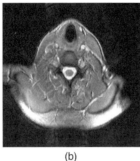 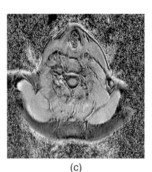

(a)   (b)   (c)

Fig. 10.7. Axial gradient-echo images of the cervical cord without (a) and with (b) the magnetization transfer (MT) pulse applied. The corresponding MT ratio (MTR) map obtained from the two previous images is shown in (c).

MT-MR images of the cervical cord[17,125,126] (Fig. 10.7) and optic nerve[15,17,127,128] of good quality.

Preliminary studies, using ROI,[129,130] or histogram[126] analysis and small cohorts of patients, found that the cervical cord of MS patients had lower MTR values than that of controls. Filippi *et al.* evaluated the contribution made by the cervical cord to the clinical manifestations of MS in a group of 96 patients with different MS phenotypes using MTR histogram analysis.[131] The entire cohort of patients with MS had significantly lower average MTR of the overall cervical cord tissue than control subjects. Compared with control subjects, patients with RRMS had similar cervical cord MTR histogram-derived measures, whereas those with PPMS had significantly lower average MTR and peak height. Patients with SPMS had lower MTR histogram peak height than those with RRMS. The peak height and position of the cervical cord MTR histogram were independent predictors of the probability of having locomotor disability. Another study compared cervical cord MTR histogram metrics of patients with PPMS and SPMS and found no significant difference between these two groups.[74] In PPMS, a model including cord area and cord MTR histogram peak height was significantly, albeit modestly, associated with the level of disability.[74] Rovaris *et al.*[132] evaluated 45 patients at the earliest clinical stage of MS and did not find any difference in cervical cord MTR between patients and healthy controls. Recently, using a 3.0 Tesla scanner, CSF normalized MT signal of the dorsal and lateral columns was correlated with sensorimotor impairment in MS patients with the major clinical phenotypes.[133]

Either no or at most moderate correlations have been found between brain T2 lesion load[131] or average brain MTR[134] and cervical cord MTR histogram metrics. This suggests that MS pathology in the cord is not solely a reflection of brain pathology (as it is the case for other conditions, such as CADASIL).[135] As a consequence, measuring cord pathology in MS offers the potential to strengthen the correlation between MRI findings and the clinical status. Another study[100] found no significant difference between any of the cervical cord MTR histogram metrics of patients with MS and NMO, despite the fact that macroscopic lesions in the cervical cord of patients with NMO were longer and had a conventional MRI appearance suggesting more severe intrinsic damage when compared with MS.

In MS patients with optic neuritis, Thorpe *et al.*[15] found significant differences in MTR between affected and unaffected nerves, as well as between affected nerves in patients and unaffected nerves in control subjects. Boorstein *et al.*[127] also reported a reduction of MTR values in the affected nerve of patients with acute unilateral optic neuritis independent of the presence of T2 lesions. Inglese *et al.*[136] have shown that MTR of the optic nerves from MS patients with incomplete or no recovery from a previous episode of acute optic neuritis is significantly lower than the corresponding quantities of the optic nerves from MS patients with complete functional recovery after an episode of acute optic neuritis, but not different from those of the optic nerves from patients with LHON. In contrast, MTR values of the affected optic nerves from patients with recovery did not differ from the corresponding quantities in clinically unaffected optic nerves, which had MTR values similar to those of the optic nerves from healthy volunteers.[136] In a 1-year follow-up study of patients with acute optic neuritis, Hickman *et al.*[17] showed a progressive decline of average MTR of the affected optic nerve which reached the nadir after about eight months despite rapid initial visual recovery; such an MTR reduction was then followed by partial recovery. More recently, patients with a first episode of acute optic neuritis were evaluated, using conventional and MT-MRI at baseline and after three and 12 months.[137] At the onset of acute optic neuritis, MTR values in the affected optic nerve were significantly higher than those of the healthy optic nerve, suggesting the presence of inflammatory cellular infiltrates due to the breakdown of the blood–optic nerve barrier. During follow up, MTR values of affected optic nerve progressively decreased over time, without a subsequent increase, suggesting a progression of optic nerve damage despite the early visual recovery.[137] Recent work at 3.0 T has shown that high-resolution MTR images of the intracranial portion of the optic nerve, optic chiasm and optic tract can reliably be obtained in healthy individuals.[128]

MT-MRI and clinical trials of MS

The limited ability of conventional MRI to characterize and quantify the features of pathology in MS has prompted the neuroimaging community to define more sensitive and more specific MRI measures for use in the monitoring of MS clinical trials. At present, none of the available MR techniques is able to provide metrics which fulfill all the requisites for being considered the dominant surrogate of MS pathology.[138] Nevertheless,

MT-MRI holds substantial promise for several reasons, including: (1) it can provide quantitative metrics with some specificity to MS-related irreversible tissue loss; (2) it enables to assess the entire brain, an important aspect when considering that MS is a widespread disease affecting all the CNS tissues; (3) quantities derived from MT-MRI are reproducible, correlated with the degree of disability and cognitive impairment, sensitive to disease changes and relatively cost-effective; and (4) MT-MRI is likely to be more easily implementable than other quantitative MR methods across the many centers that typically are involved in large-scale clinical trials of MS.[139] A consensus conference of the White Matter Study Group of the International Society for MR in Medicine has indeed recommended the use of MT-MRI in the context of large-scale MS trials as an adjunctive measure to monitor disease evolution;[140] as a consequence, ad-hoc guidelines for implementing MT-MRI as a part of multicenter clinical trials are strongly recommended.[141] Despite this, at present, only a few studies are based on an optimized acquisition of MT-MRI across different centers.[139,142]

Several MS clinical trials have incorporated MT-MRI, with a view to assessing the impact of treatment on demyelination and axonal loss. To our knowledge, MT-MRI has been used in Phase 2 and Phase 3 trials for RRMS (injectable and oral interferon beta-1a, interferon beta-1b, and oral glatiramer acetate and intravenous methylprednisolone), and SPMS (interferon beta-1b and intravenous immunoglobulins – IVIG). Some of these studies were conducted at single centers with small numbers of patients[143–146] and, as a consequence, they were not confronted with problems of standardization of MT-MRI acquisition and post-processing. In multicentre trials,[147,148] MT-MRI acquisition has been limited to highly-specialized MR centers and only subgroups of patients (about 50–100 per trial) have been studied. Two of these studies with a baseline-versus-treatment design have shown that treatment with interferon beta-1b[144] or interferon beta-1a[145] favorably modifies the recovery of MTR values which follows the cessation of Gd-enhancement in newly-formed lesions from RRMS patients. On the contrary, Richert *et al.*[144] did not find any significant difference in the MTR values of NAWM ROIs or in parameters derived from whole-brain MTR histograms[143] in a larger cohort of RRMS patients before or during interferon beta-1b therapy. In the latter study, month-to-month fluctuations of the histogram peak height persisted during the treatment period despite the almost complete suppression of contrast-enhanced MRI activity. A course of intravenous methylprednisolone was unable to modify favorably the changes of average lesion MTR and whole-brain MTR from 10 MS patients followed for eight weeks.[146] Two studies assessed MT-MRI changes in a relatively large cohort of interferon beta-1b[147] and IVIG treated[148] SPMS patients participating to multicenter placebo-controlled trials. Both interferon beta-1b and IVIG did not show an overall effect on worsening of MT-MRI measures. Taken all together, these findings confirm that MT-MRI has the potential to improve the ability to investigate the mechanisms of action of experimental treatments on the different aspects of MS pathology.

Two recent multicenter studies used MT-MRI to interrogate GM damage in patients with CIS[149] and PPMS.[150] In both studies, GM MTR derived measures showed a significant inter-centre heterogeneity. However, after correcting for the acquisition centre, pooled average MTR values of the GM were found to be different between both patient groups and controls, indicating the feasibility of such quantification in the context of treatment trials. Finally, using data from placebo-controlled multicenter trials, recent studies have estimated the sample sizes needed to demonstrate significant modifications of MT-MRI parameters with treatment. [151,152]

There are several possible explanations for the limited number of clinical trials where MT-MRI was applied to evaluate treatment efficacy. These include the careful standardization of the acquisition strategies, monitoring of scanner stability over time, and normative values as a reference. In addition, this technique is not routinely applied, and trained personnel are required.

Recently, it has been suggested that measures derived from MT-MRI might be useful to monitor demyelination and remyelination in patients with MS. As previously discussed, Chen et al. developed a method that allows a regional quantification of MTR changes within MS lesions in vivo.[47] Such a method demonstrated high scan/rescan reproducibility. Furthermore, its specificity and sensitivity towards myelin damage has been validated in a postmortem analysis of a single case.[153] By showing a correlation between data derived from MT-MRI and those from quantitative MT-MRI, a method that distinguishes changes in water content and macromolecular content, Giacomini *et al.* supported the use of MTR as a marker of demyelination and remyelination which can easily be applied in the clinical context.[154]

Conclusions

Conventional MRI has markedly increased the detection of macroscopic abnormalities of the brain and spinal cord associated with MS. New quantitative MR approaches with increased sensitivity to subtle NAWM and GM changes and increased specificity to the heterogeneous pathological substrates of MS lesions give complementary information to conventional MRI. MT-MRI offers the possibility of obtaining measures of MS tissue damage in a non-invasive manner. MTR histograms provide a means of estimating the relative volumes of tissues characterized by specific ranges of MTR, and allow conclusions to be drawn regarding both focal and diffuse aspects of the disease. This indicates the potential of MT-MRI for detecting relevant changes of pathology during experimental treatment of MS patients. Refinements in the techniques and equipment used for acquisition of MT-MR images should result in more precise measures of the MT effect, and eventually in more specific techniques for non-invasive MR-based evaluation of MS patients. Nevertheless, other quantitative techniques, such as ^{1}H-MRS and DT-MRI, are also contributing significantly to the understanding of MS pathophysiology. Since MT-MRI and

DT-MRI have the potential to provide relevant and complementary information on the structural changes occurring within and outside T2 lesions and ^{1}H-MRS could add information on the biochemical correlates of such changes, multiparametric MRI studies are now warranted to better define the nature of the pathological damage in MS,[155] and, hopefully, to evaluate the efficacy of experimental treatment in preventing the accumulation of "disabling" pathology.

References

1. Filippi M, Agosta F. Imaging biomarkers in multiple sclerosis. *J Magn Reson Imaging* 2010;31:770–88.

2. Katz D, Taubenberger JK, Cannella B, McFarlin DE, Raine CS, McFarland HF. Correlation between magnetic resonance imaging findings and lesion development in chronic, active multiple sclerosis. *Ann Neurol* 1993;34:661–9.

3. van Walderveen MA, Kamphorst W, Scheltens P, *et al*. Histopathologic correlate of hypointense lesions on T1-weighted spin-echo MRI in multiple sclerosis. *Neurology* 1998;50:1282–8.

4. Bloch F. Nuclear induction. *Phys Rev* 1946;70:460–74.

5. Forsen S, Hoffman R. Exchange rates by nuclear magnetic multiple resonance. III. Exchange reactions in systems with several nonequivalent sites. *J Chem Phys* 1964;40:1189–96.

6. Wolff SD, Balaban RS. Magnetization transfer contrast (MTC) and tissue water proton relaxation in vivo. *Magn Reson Med* 1989;10:135–44.

7. McGowan JC, Leigh JS, Jr. Selective saturation in magnetization transfer experiments *Magn Reson Med* 1994;32:517–22.

8. McGowan JC, 3rd, Schnall MD, Leigh JS. Magnetization transfer imaging with pulsed off-resonance saturation: variation in contrast with saturation duty cycle. *J Magn Reson Imaging* 1994;4:79–82.

9. Dousset V, Grossman RI, Ramer KN, *et al*. Experimental allergic encephalomyelitis and multiple sclerosis: lesion characterization with magnetization transfer imaging. *Radiology* 1992;182:483–91.

10. van Waesberghe JH, Kamphorst W, De Groot CJ, *et al*. Axonal loss in multiple sclerosis lesions: magnetic resonance imaging insights into substrates of disability. *Ann Neurol* 1999;46:747–54.

11. Schmierer K, Scaravilli F, Altmann DR, Barker GJ, Miller DH. Magnetization transfer ratio and myelin in postmortem multiple sclerosis brain. *Ann Neurol* 2004;56:407–15.

12. Dousset V, Armand JP, Lacoste D, *et al*. Magnetization transfer study of HIV encephalitis and progressive multifocal leukoencephalopathy. Groupe d'Epidemiologie Clinique du SIDA en Aquitaine. *Am J Neuroradiol* 1997;18:895–901.

13. Kasner SE, Galetta SL, McGowan JC, Grossman RI. Magnetization transfer imaging in progressive multifocal leukoencephalopathy. *Neurology* 1997;48:534–36.

14. Silver NC, Barker GJ, MacManus DG, Miller DH, Thorpe JW, Howard RS. Decreased magnetisation transfer ratio due to demyelination: a case of central pontine myelinolysis, *J Neurol Neurosurg Psychiatry* 1996;61:208–9.

15. Thorpe JW, Barker GJ, Jones SJ, *et al*. Magnetisation transfer ratios and transverse magnetisation decay curves in optic neuritis: correlation with clinical findings and electrophysiology. *J Neurol Neurosurg Psychiatry* 1995;59:487–92.

16. McDonald WI, Miller DH, Barnes D. The pathological evolution of multiple sclerosis, *Neuropathol Appl Neurobiol* 1992;18:319–34.

17. Hickman SJ, Toosy AT, Jones SJ, *et al*. Serial magnetization transfer imaging in acute optic neuritis. *Brain* 2004;127:692–700.

18. Moore GR, Leung E, MacKay AL, *et al*. A pathology-MRI study of the short-T2 component in formalin-fixed multiple sclerosis brain. *Neurology* 2000;55:1506–10.

19. Tozer DJ, Davies GR, Altmann DR, Miller DH, Tofts PS. Correlation of apparent myelin measures obtained in multiple sclerosis patients and controls from magnetization transfer and multicompartmental T2 analysis. *Magn Reson Med* 2005;53:1415–22.

20. Kimura H, Grossman RI, Lenkinski RE, Gonzalez-Scarano F. Proton MR spectroscopy and magnetization transfer ratio in multiple sclerosis: correlative findings of active versus irreversible plaque disease. *AJNR Am J Neuroradiol* 1996;17:1539–47.

21. Loevner LA, Grossman RI, McGowan JC, Ramer KN, Cohen JA. Characterization of multiple sclerosis plaques with T1-weighted MR and quantitative magnetization transfer. *Am J Neuroradiol* 1995;16:1473–9.

22. Cercignani M, Iannucci G, Rocca MA, Comi G, Horsfield MA, Filippi M. Pathologic damage in MS assessed by diffusion-weighted and magnetization transfer MRI. *Neurology* 2000;54:1139–44.

23. Filippi M, Tortorella C, Bozzali M. Normal-appearing white matter changes in multiple sclerosis: the contribution of magnetic resonance techniques. *Mult Scler* 1999;5:273–82.

24. McGowan JC, McCormack TM, Grossman RI, *et al*. Diffuse axonal pathology detected with magnetization transfer imaging following brain injury in the pig. *Magn Reson Med* 1999;41:727–33.

25. van Buchem MA, McGowan JC, Kolson DL, Polansky M, Grossman RI. Quantitative volumetric magnetization transfer analysis in multiple sclerosis: estimation of macroscopic and microscopic disease burden. *Magn Reson Med* 1996;36:632–6.

26. Sormani MP, Iannucci G, Rocca MA, *et al*. Reproducibility of magnetization transfer ratio histogram-derived measures of the brain in healthy volunteers. *Am J Neuroradiol* 2000;21:133–6.

27. Inglese M, Horsfield MA, Filippi M. Scan-rescan variation of measures derived from brain magnetization transfer ratio histograms obtained in healthy volunteers by use of a semi-interleaved magnetization transfer sequence *Am J Neuroradiol* 2001;22:681–4.

28. Audoin B, Ranjeva JP, Au Duong MV, *et al*. Voxel-based analysis of MTR images: a method to locate gray matter abnormalities in patients at the earliest stage of multiple sclerosis. *J Magn Reson Imaging* 2004;20:765–71.

29. Ranjeva JP, Audoin B, Au Duong MV, *et al*. Local tissue damage assessed with

statistical mapping analysis of brain magnetization transfer ratio: relationship with functional status of patients in the earliest stage of multiple sclerosis. *AJNR Am J Neuroradiol* 2005;26:119–27.

30. Gawne-Cain ML, O'Riordan JI, Coles A, Newell B, Thompson AJ, Miller DH. MRI lesion volume measurement in multiple sclerosis and its correlation with disability: a comparison of fast fluid attenuated inversion recovery (fFLAIR) and spin echo sequences. *J Neurol Neurosurg Psychiatry* 1998;64:197–203.

31. Brex PA, Ciccarelli O, O'Riordan JI, Sailer M, Thompson AJ, Miller DH. A longitudinal study of abnormalities on MRI and disability from multiple sclerosis. *N Engl J Med* 2002;346:158–64.

32. Kermode AG, Tofts PS, Thompson AJ, *et al.* Heterogeneity of blood-brain barrier changes in multiple sclerosis: an MRI study with gadolinium-DTPA enhancement. *Neurology* 1990;40:229–35.

33. Filippi M, Rovaris M, Capra R, *et al.* A multi-centre longitudinal study comparing the sensitivity of monthly MRI after standard and triple dose gadolinium-DTPA for monitoring disease activity in multiple sclerosis. Implications for phase II clinical trials. *Brain* 1998;121:2011–20.

34. Bastianello S, Gasperini C, Paolillo A, *et al.* Sensitivity of enhanced MR in multiple sclerosis: effects of contrast dose and magnetization transfer contrast. *Am J Neuroradiol* 1998;19:1863–7.

35. Silver NC, Good CD, Sormani MP, *et al.* A modified protocol to improve the detection of enhancing brain and spinal cord lesions in multiple sclerosis *J Neurol* 2001;248:215–24.

36. Silver NC, Lai M, Symms MR, Barker GJ, McDonald WI, Miller DH. Serial magnetization transfer imaging to characterize the early evolution of new MS lesions. *Neurology* 1998;51:758–64.

37. Petrella JR, Grossman RI, McGowan JC, Campbell G, Cohen JA. Multiple sclerosis lesions: relationship between MR enhancement pattern and magnetization transfer effect. *Am J Neuroradiol* 1996;17:1041–9.

38. van Waesberghe JH, van Walderveen MA, Castelijns JA, *et al.* Patterns of lesion development in multiple sclerosis: longitudinal observations with T1-weighted spin-echo and magnetization transfer MR. *Am J Neuroradiol* 1998;19:675–83.

39. Filippi M, Rocca MA, Comi G. Magnetization transfer ratios of multiple sclerosis lesions with variable durations of enhancement. *J Neurol Sci* 1998;159:162–5.

40. Filippi M, Rocca MA, Rizzo G, *et al.* Magnetization transfer ratios in multiple sclerosis lesions enhancing after different doses of gadolinium. *Neurology* 1998;50:1289–93.

41. Filippi M, Rocca MA, Martino G, Horsfield MA, Comi G. Magnetization transfer changes in the normal appearing white matter precede the appearance of enhancing lesions in patients with multiple sclerosis. *Ann Neurol* 1998;43:809–14.

42. Goodkin DE, Rooney WD, Sloan R, *et al.* A serial study of new MS lesions and the white matter from which they arise. *Neurology* 1998;51:1689–97.

43. Lai HM, Davie CA, Gass A, *et al.* Serial magnetisation transfer ratios in gadolinium-enhancing lesions in multiple sclerosis. *J Neurol* 1997;244:308–11.

44. Dousset V, Gayou A, Brochet B, Caille JM. Early structural changes in acute MS lesions assessed by serial magnetization transfer studies. *Neurology* 1998;51:1150–5.

45. Rocca MA, Mastronardo G, Rodegher M, Comi G, Filippi M. Long-term changes of magnetization transfer-derived measures from patients with relapsing–remitting and secondary progressive multiple sclerosis. *Am J Neuroradiol* 1999;20:821–7.

46. Filippi M, Rocca MA, Sormani MP, Pereira C, Comi G. Short-term evolution of individual enhancing MS lesions studied with magnetization transfer imaging. *Magn Reson Imaging* 1999;17:979–84.

47. Chen JT, Collins DL, Atkins HL, Freedman MS, Arnold DL. Magnetization transfer ratio evolution with demyelination and remyelination in multiple sclerosis lesions. *Ann Neurol* 2008;63:254–62.

48. Lassmann H, Suchanek G, Ozawa K. Histopathology and the blood-cerebrospinal fluid barrier in multiple sclerosis. *Ann Neurol* 1994;36 Suppl:S42–6.

49. Horsfield MA, Rocca MA, Cercignani M, Filippi M. Activity revealed in MRI of multiple sclerosis without contrast agent. A preliminary report. *Magn Reson Imaging* 2000;18:139–42.

50. Kappos L, Moeri D, Radue EW, *et al.* Predictive value of gadolinium-enhanced magnetic resonance imaging for relapse rate and changes in disability or impairment in multiple sclerosis: a meta-analysis. Gadolinium MRI Meta-analysis Group. *Lancet* 1999;353:964–9.

51. Filippi M, Campi A, Dousset V, *et al.* A magnetization transfer imaging study of normal-appearing white matter in multiple sclerosis, *Neurology* 1995;45:478–82.

52. Loevner LA, Grossman RI, Cohen JA, Lexa FJ, Kessler D, Kolson DL. Microscopic disease in normal-appearing white matter on conventional MR images in patients with multiple sclerosis: assessment with magnetization-transfer measurements. *Radiology* 1995;196:511–515.

53. Gass A, Barker GJ, Kidd D, *et al.* Correlation of magnetization transfer ratio with clinical disability in multiple sclerosis. *Ann Neurol* 1994;36:62–7.

54. Guo AC, Jewells VL, Provenzale JM. Analysis of normal-appearing white matter in multiple sclerosis: comparison of diffusion tensor MR imaging and magnetization transfer imaging. *Am J Neuroradiol* 2001;22:1893–900.

55. Wong KT, Grossman RI, Boorstein JM, Lexa FJ, McGowan JC. Magnetization transfer imaging of periventricular hyperintense white matter in the elderly. *Am J Neuroradiol* 1995;16:253–8.

56. Rovaris M, Viti B, Ciboddo G, *et al.* Brain involvement in systemic immune mediated diseases: magnetic resonance and magnetisation transfer imaging study. *J Neurol Neurosurg Psychiatry* 2000;68:170–7.

57. Gupta RK, Kathuria MK, Pradhan S. Magnetization transfer MR imaging in CNS tuberculosis. *Am J Neuroradiol* 1999;20:867–75.

58. Bagley LJ, Grossman RI, Galetta SL, Sinson GP, Kotapka M, McGowan JC. Characterization of white matter lesions in multiple sclerosis and

traumatic brain injury as revealed by magnetization transfer contour plots. *Am J Neuroradiol* 1999;20:977–81.

59. Rocca MA, Colombo B, Pratesi A, Comi G, Filippi M. A magnetization transfer imaging study of the brain in patients with migraine. *Neurology* 2000;54:507–9.

60. Tanabe JL, Ezekiel F, Jagust WJ, *et al*. Magnetization transfer ratio of white matter hyperintensities in subcortical ischemic vascular dementia. *Am J Neuroradiol* 1999;20:839–44.

61. Kato Y, Matsumura K, Kinosada Y, Narita Y, Kuzuhara S, Nakagawa T. Detection of pyramidal tract lesions in amyotrophic lateral sclerosis with magnetization-transfer measurements. *Am J Neuroradiol* 1997;18:1541–7.

62. Iannucci G, Dichgans M, Rovaris M, *et al*. Correlations between clinical findings and magnetization transfer imaging metrics of tissue damage in individuals with cerebral autosomal dominant arteriopathy with subcortical infarcts and leukoencephalopathy, *Stroke* 2001;32:643–8.

63. Inglese M, Rovaris M, Bianchi S, *et al*. Magnetic resonance imaging, magnetisation transfer imaging, and diffusion weighted imaging correlates of optic nerve, brain, and cervical cord damage in Leber's hereditary optic neuropathy. *J Neurol Neurosurg Psychiatry* 2001;70:444–9.

64. Inglese M, Salvi F, Iannucci G, Mancardi GL, Mascalchi M, Filippi M. Magnetization transfer and diffusion tensor MR imaging of acute disseminated encephalomyelitis. *AJNR Am J Neuroradiol* 2002;23:267–272.

65. Enzinger C, Strasser-Fuchs S, Ropele S, Kapeller P, Kleinert R, Fazekas F. Tumefactive demyelinating lesions: conventional and advanced magnetic resonance imaging. *Mult Scler* 2005;11:135–9.

66. van Waesberghe JH, Castelijns JA, Scheltens P, *et al*. Comparison of four potential MR parameters for severe tissue destruction in multiple sclerosis lesions. *Magn Reson Imaging* 1997;15:155–62.

67. Ge Y, Grossman RI, Babb JS, He J, Mannon LJ. Dirty-appearing white matter in multiple sclerosis: volumetric MR imaging and magnetization transfer ratio histogram analysis. *Am J Neuroradiol* 2003;24:1935–40.

68. Rovaris M, Filippi M, Falautano M, *et al*. Relation between MR abnormalities and patterns of cognitive impairment in multiple sclerosis. *Neurology* 1998;50:1601–08.

69. van Waesberghe JH, van Buchem MA, Filippi M, *et al*. MR outcome parameters in multiple sclerosis: comparison of surface-based thresholding segmentation and magnetization transfer ratio histographic analysis in relation to disability (a preliminary note). *Am J Neuroradiol* 1998;19:1857–62.

70. Filippi M, Rocca MA, Horsfield MA, Comi G. A one year study of new lesions in multiple sclerosis using monthly gadolinium enhanced MRI: correlations with changes of T2 and magnetization transfer lesion loads, *J Neurol Sci* 1998;158:203–8.

71. Rovaris M, Filippi M, Calori G, *et al*. Intra-observer reproducibility in measuring new putative MR markers of demyelination and axonal loss in multiple sclerosis: a comparison with conventional T2-weighted images. *J Neurol* 1997;244:266–70.

72. Iannucci G, Rovaris M, Giacomotti L, Comi G, Filippi M. Correlation of multiple sclerosis measures derived from T2-weighted, T1-weighted, magnetization transfer, and diffusion tensor MR imaging. *Am J Neuroradiol* 2001;22:1462–7.

73. Filippi M, Tortorella C, Rovaris M, *et al*. Changes in the normal appearing brain tissue and cognitive impairment in multiple sclerosis. *J Neurol Neurosurg Psychiatry* 2000;68:157–61.

74. Rovaris M, Bozzali M, Santuccio G, *et al*. In vivo assessment of the brain and cervical cord pathology of patients with primary progressive multiple sclerosis. *Brain* 2001;124:2540–9.

75. Filippi M, Inglese M, Rovaris M, *et al*. Magnetization transfer imaging to monitor the evolution of MS: a 1-year follow-up study. *Neurology* 2000;55:940–6.

76. Iannucci G, Tortorella C, Rovaris M, Sormani MP, Comi G, Filippi M. Prognostic value of MR and magnetization transfer imaging findings in patients with clinically isolated syndromes suggestive of multiple sclerosis at presentation. *Am J Neuroradiol* 2000;21: 1034–8.

77. Filippi M, Iannucci G, Tortorella C, *et al*. Comparison of MS clinical phenotypes using conventional and magnetization transfer MRI. *Neurology* 1999;52:588–94.

78. Codella M, Rocca MA, Colombo B, Rossi P, Comi G, Filippi M. A preliminary study of magnetization transfer and diffusion tensor MRI of multiple sclerosis patients with fatigue. *J Neurol* 2002;249:535–7.

79. Agosta F, Rovaris M, Pagani E, Sormani MP, Comi G, Filippi M. Magnetization transfer MRI metrics predict the accumulation of disability 8 years later in patients with multiple sclerosis. *Brain* 2006;129:2620–7.

80. Rocca MA, Falini A, Colombo B, Scotti G, Comi G, Filippi M. Adaptive functional changes in the cerebral cortex of patients with nondisabling multiple sclerosis correlate with the extent of brain structural damage. *Ann Neurol* 2002;51:330–9.

81. Filippi M, Rocca MA. Cortical reorganisation in patients with MS. *J Neurol Neurosurg Psychiatry* 2004;75:1087–9.

82. Filippi M, Rocca MA. Functional MR imaging in multiple sclerosis. *Neuroimaging Clin N Am* 2009;19:59–70.

83. Adams CW. Pathology of multiple sclerosis: progression of the lesion. *Br Med Bull* 1977;33:15–20.

84. Allen IV, McKeown SR. A histological, histochemical and biochemical study of the macroscopically normal white matter in multiple sclerosis. *J Neurol Sci* 1979;41:81–91.

85. Arstila AU, Riekkinen P, Rinne UK, Laitinen L. Studies on the pathogenesis of multiple sclerosis. Participation of lysosomes on demyelination in the central nervous system white matter outside plaques. *Eur Neurol* 1973;9:1–20.

86. Bjartmar C, Kinkel RP, Kidd G, Rudick RA, Trapp BD. Axonal loss in normal-appearing white matter in a patient with acute MS. *Neurology* 2001;57:1248–52.

87. Rovaris M, Filippi M. The value of new magnetic resonance techniques in multiple sclerosis. *Curr Opin Neurol* 2000;13:249–54.

88. Fazekas F, Ropele S, Enzinger C, Seifert T, Strasser-Fuchs S. Quantitative magnetization transfer imaging of

pre-lesional white-matter changes in multiple sclerosis. *Mult Scler* 2002;8:479–84.

89. De Stefano N, Narayanan S, Francis SJ, *et al.* Diffuse axonal and tissue injury in patients with multiple sclerosis with low cerebral lesion load and no disability, *Arch Neurol* 2002;59:1565–71.

90. Filippi M, Rocca MA, Minicucci L, *et al.* Magnetization transfer imaging of patients with definite MS and negative conventional MRI. *Neurology* 1999;52:845–8.

91. Tortorella C, Viti B, Bozzali M, *et al.* A magnetization transfer histogram study of normal-appearing brain tissue in MS. *Neurology* 2000;54:186–93.

92. Traboulsee A, Dehmeshki J, Peters KR, *et al.* Disability in multiple sclerosis is related to normal appearing brain tissue MTR histogram abnormalities. *Mult Scler* 2003;9:566–73.

93. Mezzapesa DM, Rocca MA, Falini A, *et al.* A preliminary diffusion tensor and magnetization transfer magnetic resonance imaging study of early-onset multiple sclerosis. *Arch Neurol* 2004;61:366–8.

94. Filippi M, Rocca MA, Falini A, *et al.* Correlations between structural CNS damage and functional MRI changes in primary progressive MS. *Neuroimage* 2002;15:537–46.

95. Cercignani M, Bozzali M, Iannucci G, Comi G, Filippi M. Magnetisation transfer ratio and mean diffusivity of normal appearing white and grey matter from patients with multiple sclerosis. *J Neurol Neurosurg Psychiatry* 2001;70:311–17.

96. Ge Y, Grossman RI, Udupa JK, Babb JS, Mannon LJ, McGowan JC. Magnetization transfer ratio histogram analysis of normal-appearing gray matter and normal-appearing white matter in multiple sclerosis. *J Comput Assist Tomogr* 2002;26:62–8.

97. Dehmeshki J, Chard DT, Leary SM, *et al.* The normal appearing grey matter in primary progressive multiple sclerosis: a magnetisation transfer imaging study. *J Neurol* 2003;250:67–74.

98. Santos AC, Narayanan S, de Stefano N, *et al.* Magnetization transfer can predict clinical evolution in patients with multiple sclerosis. *J Neurol* 2002;249:662–8.

99. Inglese M, DeStefano N, Pagani E, *et al.* Quantification of brain damage in cerebrotendinous xanthomatosis with magnetization transfer MR imaging *Am J Neuroradiol* 2003;24:495–500.

100. Filippi M, Rocca MA, Moiola L, *et al.* MRI and magnetization transfer imaging changes in the brain and cervical cord of patients with Devic's neuromyelitis optica. *Neurology* 1999;53:1705–10.

101. Agosta F, Rocca MA, Benedetti B, Capra R, Cordioli C, Filippi M. MR imaging assessment of brain and cervical cord damage in patients with neuroborreliosis. *Am J Neuroradiol* 2006;27:892–4.

102. Brownell B, Hughes JT. The distribution of plaques in the cerebrum in multiple sclerosis. *J Neurol Neurosurg Psychiatry* 1962;25:315–20.

103. Kidd D, Barkhof F, McConnell R, Algra PR, Allen IV, Revesz T. Cortical lesions in multiple sclerosis, *Brain* 1999;122 (1):17–26.

104. Peterson JW, Bo L, Mork S, Chang A, Trapp BD. Transected neurites, apoptotic neurons, and reduced inflammation in cortical multiple sclerosis lesions. *Ann Neurol* 2001;50:389–400.

105. Ge Y, Grossman RI, Udupa JK, Babb JS, Kolson DL, McGowan JC. Magnetization transfer ratio histogram analysis of gray matter in relapsing–remitting multiple sclerosis. *Am J Neuroradiol* 2001;22:470–5.

106. Fernando KT, Tozer DJ, Miszkiel KA, *et al.* Magnetization transfer histograms in clinically isolated syndromes suggestive of multiple sclerosis. *Brain* 2005;128:2911–25.

107. Ramio-Torrenta L, Sastre-Garriga J, Ingle GT, *et al.* Abnormalities in normal appearing tissues in early primary progressive multiple sclerosis and their relation to disability: a tissue specific magnetisation transfer study. *J Neurol Neurosurg Psychiatry* 2006;77:40–5.

108. De Stefano N, Battaglini M, Stromillo ML, *et al.* Brain damage as detected by magnetization transfer imaging is less pronounced in benign than in early relapsing multiple sclerosis. *Brain* 2006;129:2008–16.

109. Oreja-Guevara C, Charil A, Caputo D, Cavarretta R, Sormani MP, Filippi M. Magnetization transfer magnetic resonance imaging and clinical changes in patients with relapsing–remitting multiple sclerosis. *Arch Neurol* 2006;63:736–40.

110. Hayton T, Furby J, Smith KJ, *et al.* Grey matter magnetization transfer ratio independently correlates with neurological deficit in secondary progressive multiple sclerosis. *J Neurol* 2009;256:427–435.

111. Amato MP, Portaccio E, Stromillo ML, *et al.* Cognitive assessment and quantitative magnetic resonance metrics can help to identify benign multiple sclerosis, *Neurology* 2008;71:632–8.

112. Codella M, Rocca MA, Colombo B, Martinelli-Boneschi F, Comi G, Filippi M. Cerebral grey matter pathology and fatigue in patients with multiple sclerosis: a preliminary study. *J Neurol Sci* 2002;194:71–4.

113. Davies GR, Altmann DR, Rashid W, *et al.* Emergence of thalamic magnetization transfer ratio abnormality in early relapsing–remitting multiple sclerosis. *Mult Scler* 2005;11:276–81.

114. Khaleeli Z, Altmann DR, Cercignani M, Ciccarelli O, Miller DH, Thompson AJ. Magnetization transfer ratio in gray matter: a potential surrogate marker for progression in early primary progressive multiple sclerosis. *Arch Neurol* 2008;65:1454–9.

115. Audoin B, Fernando KT, Swanton JK, Thompson AJ, Plant GT, Miller DH. Selective magnetization transfer ratio decrease in the visual cortex following optic neuritis. *Brain* 2006;129:1031–9.

116. Khaleeli Z, Cercignani M, Audoin B, Ciccarelli O, Miller DH, Thompson AJ. Localized grey matter damage in early primary progressive multiple sclerosis contributes to disability. *Neuroimage* 2007;37:253–61.

117. Rocca MA, Agosta F, Mezzapesa DM, *et al.* Magnetization transfer and diffusion tensor MRI show gray matter damage in neuromyelitis optica. *Neurology* 2004;62:476–8.

118. Dehmeshki J, Ruto AC, Arridge S, Silver NC, Miller DH, Tofts PS. Analysis of MTR histograms in multiple sclerosis using principal components and multiple discriminant analysis. *Magn Reson Med* 2001;46:600–9.

119. Kalkers NF, Hintzen RQ, van Waesberghe JH, *et al.* Magnetization transfer histogram parameters reflect all dimensions of MS pathology,

including atrophy. *J Neurol Sci* 2001;184:155–62.

120. Rovaris M, Agosta F, Sormani MP, *et al.* Conventional and magnetization transfer MRI predictors of clinical multiple sclerosis evolution: a medium-term follow-up study. *Brain* 2003;126:2323–32.

121. Rovaris M, Holtmannspotter M, Rocca MA, *et al.* Contribution of cervical cord MRI and brain magnetization transfer imaging to the assessment of individual patients with multiple sclerosis: a preliminary study. *Mult Scler* 2002;8: 52–8.

122. van Buchem MA, Grossman RI, Armstrong C, *et al.* Correlation of volumetric magnetization transfer imaging with clinical data in MS. *Neurology* 1998;50:1609–17.

123. Iannucci G, Minicucci L, Rodegher M, Sormani MP, Comi G, Filippi M. Correlations between clinical and MRI involvement in multiple sclerosis: assessment using T(1), T(2) and MT histograms. *J Neurol Sci* 1999;171:121–9.

124. Comi G, Rovaris M, Falautano M, *et al.* A multiparametric MRI study of frontal lobe dementia in multiple sclerosis. *J Neurol Sci* 1999;171:135–44.

125. Bozzali M, Rocca MA, Iannucci G, Pereira C, Comi G, Filippi M. Magnetization-transfer histogram analysis of the cervical cord in patients with multiple sclerosis. *Am J Neuroradiol* 1999;20:1803–8.

126. Hickman SJ, Hadjiprocopis A, Coulon O, Miller DH, Barker GJ. Cervical spinal cord MTR histogram analysis in multiple sclerosis using a 3D acquisition and a B-spline active surface segmentation technique. *Magn Reson Imaging* 2004;22:891–5.

127. Boorstein JM, Moonis G, Boorstein SM, Patel YP, Culler AS. Optic neuritis: imaging with magnetization transfer. *AJR Am J Roentgenol* 1997;169:1709–12.

128. Vinogradov E, Degenhardt A, Smith D, *et al.* High-resolution anatomic, diffusion tensor, and magnetization transfer magnetic resonance imaging of the optic chiasm at 3T. *J Magn Reson Imaging* 2005;22:302–306.

129. Silver NC, Barker GJ, Losseff NA, *et al.* Magnetisation transfer ratio measurement in the cervical spinal cord: a preliminary study in multiple sclerosis. *Neuroradiology* 1997;39:441–445.

130. Lycklama a Nijeholt GJ, Castelijns JA, Lazeron RH, *et al.* Magnetization transfer ratio of the spinal cord in multiple sclerosis: relationship to atrophy and neurologic disability. *J Neuroimaging* 2000;10:67–72.

131. Filippi M, Bozzali M, Horsfield MA, *et al.* A conventional and magnetization transfer MRI study of the cervical cord in patients with MS. *Neurology* 2000;54:207–13.

132. Rovaris M, Gallo A, Riva R, *et al.* An MT MRI study of the cervical cord in clinically isolated syndromes suggestive of MS. *Neurology* 2004;63:584–5.

133. Zackowski KM, Smith SA, Reich DS, *et al.* Sensorimotor dysfunction in multiple sclerosis and column-specific magnetization transfer-imaging abnormalities in the spinal cord. *Brain* 2009;132:1200–9.

134. Rovaris M, Bozzali M, Santuccio G, *et al.* Relative contributions of brain and cervical cord pathology to multiple sclerosis disability: a study with magnetisation transfer ratio histogram analysis. *J Neurol Neurosurg Psychiatry* 2000;69:723–7.

135. Rocca MA, Filippi M, Herzog J, Sormani MP, Dichgans M, Yousry TA. A magnetic resonance imaging study of the cervical cord of patients with CADASIL. *Neurology* 2001;56:1392–4.

136. Inglese M, Ghezzi A, Bianchi S, *et al.* Irreversible disability and tissue loss in multiple sclerosis: a conventional and magnetization transfer magnetic resonance imaging study of the optic nerves. *Arch Neurol* 2002;59:250–5.

137. Melzi L, Rocca MA, Marzoli SB, *et al.* A longitudinal conventional and magnetization transfer magnetic resonance imaging study of optic neuritis. *Mult Scler* 2007;13:265–8.

138. Barkhof F, Calabresi PA, Miller DH, Reingold SC. Imaging outcomes for neuroprotection and repair in multiple sclerosis trials. *Nat Rev Neurol* 2009;5:256–66.

139. Ropele S, Filippi M, Valsasina P, *et al.* Assessment and correction of B1-induced errors in magnetization transfer ratio measurements. *Magn Reson Med* 2005;53:134–40.

140. Filippi M, Dousset V, McFarland HF, Miller DH, Grossman RI. Role of magnetic resonance imaging in the diagnosis and monitoring of multiple sclerosis: consensus report of the White Matter Study Group. *J Magn Reson Imaging* 2002;15:499–504.

141. Horsfield MA, Barker GJ, Barkhof F, Miller DH, Thompson AJ, Filippi M. Guidelines for using quantitative magnetization transfer magnetic resonance imaging for monitoring treatment of multiple sclerosis. *J Magn Reson Imaging* 2003;17:389–97.

142. Samson RS, Wheeler-Kingshott CA, Symms MR, Tozer DJ, Tofts PS. A simple correction for B1 field errors in magnetization transfer ratio measurements, *Magn Reson Imaging* 2006;24:255–263.

143. Richert ND, Ostuni JL, Bash CN, Duyn JH, McFarland HF, Frank JA. Serial whole-brain magnetization transfer imaging in patients with relapsing–remitting multiple sclerosis at baseline and during treatment with interferon beta-1b. *Am J Neuroradiol* 1998;19:1705–13.

144. Richert ND, Ostuni JL, Bash CN, Leist TP, McFarland HF, Frank JA. Interferon beta-1b and intravenous methylprednisolone promote lesion recovery in multiple sclerosis. *Mult Scler* 2001;7:49–58.

145. Kita M, Goodkin DE, Bacchetti P, Waubant E, Nelson SJ, Majumdar S. Magnetization transfer ratio in new MS lesions before and during therapy with IFNbeta-1a. *Neurology* 2000;54: 1741–5.

146. Fox RJ, Fisher E, Tkach J, Lee JC, Cohen JA, Rudick RA. Brain atrophy and magnetization transfer ratio following methylprednisolone in multiple sclerosis: short-term changes and long-term implications. *Mult Scler* 2005;11:140–5.

147. Inglese M, van Waesberghe JH, Rovaris M, *et al.* The effect of interferon beta-1b on quantities derived from MT MRI in secondary progressive MS. *Neurology* 2003;60:853–60.

148. Filippi M, Rocca MA, Pagani E, *et al.* European study on intravenous immunoglobulin in multiple sclerosis: results of magnetization transfer magnetic resonance imaging analysis. *Arch Neurol* 2004;61:1409–12.

149. Rocca MA, Agosta F, Sormani MP, *et al.* A three-year, multi-parametric MRI study in patients at presentation with CIS. *J Neurol* 2008;255:683–91.

150. Rovaris M, Judica E, Sastre-Garriga J, *et al*. Large-scale, multicentre, quantitative MRI study of brain and cord damage in primary progressive multiple sclerosis *Mult Scler* 2008;14:455–64.

151. Mesaros S, Rocca M, Sormani M, *et al*. Bimonthly assessment of magnetization transfer magnetic resonance imaging parameters in multiple sclerosis: a 14-month, multicentre, follow-up study, *Mult Scler* 2010;16:325–31.

152. Van Den Elskamp IJ, Knol DL, Vrenken H, *et al*. Lesional magnetization transfer ratio: a feasible outcome for remyelinating treatment trials in multiple sclerosis, *Mult Scler* 2010;16:660–9.

153. Chen JT, Kuhlmann T, Jansen GH, *et al*. Voxel-based analysis of the evolution of magnetization transfer ratio to quantify remyelination and demyelination with histopathological validation in a multiple sclerosis lesion. *Neuroimage* 2007;36:1152–8.

154. Giacomini PS, Levesque IR, Ribeiro L, *et al*. Measuring demyelination and remyelination in acute multiple sclerosis lesion voxels. *Arch Neurol* 2009;66:375–81.

155. Mainero C, De Stefano N, Iannucci G, *et al*. Correlates of MS disability assessed in vivo using aggregates of MR quantities. *Neurology* 2001;56:1331–4.

Chapter

11

Measurement of CNS atrophy

Elizabeth Fisher

Introduction

Brain atrophy has become part of the standard repertoire of magnetic resonance imaging (MRI) measurements commonly performed in MS studies. As a non-specific marker of tissue loss, atrophy provides additional information on disease severity not captured by lesion measures.[1] Its principal appeal stems from the idea that atrophy primarily reflects irreversible damage, including axonal loss and neurodegeneration, which result from pathological processes occurring in MS, and which underlie progressive MS disability. Studies over the past decade have shown that atrophy begins early in the course of MS, correlates with concurrent level of disability, and has predictive value for future disability. Brain atrophy is also attractive as an outcome measure from a technical standpoint because it can be measured from conventional MRIs.

This chapter describes methods and issues associated with measurement of atrophy in the central nervous system (CNS) in MS. Atrophy findings are summarized from cross-sectional and longitudinal studies in different MS subgroups. The relationship of tissue loss to other MRI-based measures of MS, as well as the relationship of tissue loss to disability is also reviewed. The last section discusses the use of atrophy measurements in clinical trials and the effects of various treatments on tissue loss. Regarding the terminology, atrophy is typically measured as volume loss; however, not all decreases in volume represent actual tissue loss or atrophy because water content can also affect volume measurements. In this chapter, the terms "atrophy," "tissue loss," and "volume loss," will be used interchangeably in most sections due to the fact that currently there is no way to distinguish different underlying sources of volume loss.

Methods for estimation of atrophy

CNS atrophy has been recognized as a common feature in patients with long-standing MS since the early days of CT and MR imaging.[2,3] However, the fact that atrophy begins early in the course of MS only became evident following the application of computerized image analysis techniques. In relapsing-remitting (RR) MS patients, the typical rate of brain tissue

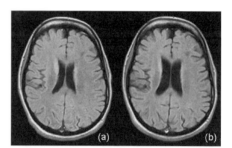
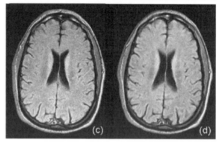

Fig. 11.1. Examples of MS atrophy over one year in two different patients: (a) Baseline image slice of Patient A; (b) Year 1 image of Patient A, after co-registration with baseline and resampling to obtain the same slice; enlargement of the lateral ventricles and sulci is clearly evident. Patient A is an extreme case, with 2.9% brain tissue loss. (c) Baseline image slice of Patient B; (d) Year 1 image of Patient B, after co-registration with baseline and resampling to obtain the same slice. Patient B is a typical case, with 0.87% brain tissue loss and atrophy is more difficult to detect visually.

loss is approximately 0.5%–1.0% per year, which is not readily visible on annual MRIs even if the slice positions and orientations are well matched (Fig. 11.1). Therefore, quantitative measurements are required to assess atrophy progression over time. Fortunately, these measurements do not require specialized MRI pulse sequences or equipment. The primary requirement is image analysis software, which is not typically included on standard MRI consoles. With acquisition of the standard MRI sequence recommended for use with the analysis software, careful attention to consistency in the image acquisition parameters, and image analysis performed by a trained operator, brain atrophy can be consistently detected in serial MRIs obtained 6 months to 1 year apart in MS patients at all stage of disease.

Several quantitative methods exist for estimating tissue loss in MRIs. The techniques vary considerably according to level of

Multiple Sclerosis Therapeutics, Fourth Edition, ed. Jeffrey A. Cohen and Richard A. Rudick. Published by Cambridge University Press.
© Cambridge University Press 2011.

automation, scale, and conceptual basis. The level of automation, or conversely, the degree of operator interaction required to perform the measurements, ranges from manual outlining of specific structures to fully automated volumetric calculations. The scale of atrophy measurements ranges from highly localized measurements of third ventricular width (on the order of 3 mm) to global measurements of whole brain volume (on the order of 1200 cm³). Methods also differ significantly according to conceptual approach. Segmentation-based methods estimate atrophy as a change in volume measurements over time. Registration-based methods calculate change directly from the shifts in the edges of the brain between two serially acquired images. Voxel-based morphology and deformation-based methods use spatial normalization to compare groups or to calculate volume differences from the deformation required to warp an image to a standard space.

Important considerations for any methodology are measurement reliability and sensitivity to change. Reliability is typically expressed in terms of accuracy, reproducibility, or inter-rater agreement, and is especially important for techniques to be used in longitudinal studies. The coefficient of variation (COV) between repeated measurements is often used to report reproducibility. To calculate COV, repeated measurements performed on scan–rescan data simulate conditions in serial studies and provide a better estimate of measurement variability than repeated measurements on the same image data. Ideally, the measurement variability should be small in relation to the size of the expected changes, which is less than 1.0% per year for whole brain volume in MS patients.

Manual methods

Subjective rating of atrophy on an ordinal scale based on visual inspection of MR images is a semi-quantitative approach that can be applied without specialized software or equipment. Comparison of patient images to those of age- and sex-matched controls from a large normative database demonstrated very good intra-observer agreement and moderate to very good inter-observer agreement.[4] The ordinal rating scale approach is limited in terms of sensitivity and, therefore, is not very useful in detecting changes over time.

Image analysis software allows for quantitative estimation of widths, areas, and/or volumes of CNS structures directly from digital images. The calculation of distances between manually selected anatomic landmarks is readily available on reading consoles and can be used to estimate the sizes of particular structures, such as the third ventricle width, lateral ventricle width, and brain width.[5–7] Many generic image analysis packages include tracing tools that can be used to manually delineate structures of interest so that volumes can be calculated by simply multiplying the sum of voxels included in the region by the voxel size.[8] Manual tracing by an expert observer yields accurate segmentation, but it is also the most time-consuming approach, and measurement variability is relatively high.

Semi-automated and automated methods for estimation of brain atrophy

Semi-automated and automated programs offer more rapid and reproducible assessments of atrophy. These methods are commonly used to calculate lateral ventricle volume,[9–12] CSF volume,[13,14] whole or partial brain volumes,[15–22] volume change,[23,24] and differences between groups of patients.[25] There are many different site-specific algorithms currently in use for MS applications. Atrophy measurement methods can be broadly classified into segmentation-based approaches, registration-based, and deformation-based approaches.

Segmentation-based approaches

Segmentation-based methods for quantification of brain parenchymal volumes typically consist of two basic steps: (1) separation of tissue from CSF and background, usually based on intensity, and (2) separation of the brain tissue from other cranial structures, usually by manual delineation, connectivity analysis, morphologic operations, edge detection, and/or knowledge-based anatomic operations (Fig. 11.2). One example of a semi-automated algorithm requires the user interactively to choose low and high thresholds that cover the intensity range of brain parenchyma, and then select a seed point within the parenchyma on a slice-by-slice basis.[20] A region is automatically grown around the seed point that includes all connected pixels within the given range of intensities. Boundaries are drawn manually when necessary to prevent the region from growing outside the brain and into other structures. The intra-observer COV for this technique calculated from re-segmentation of ten images is 1.9% for whole brain volume.

To reduce manual interaction and measurement variability, these steps have been automated to different extents using a variety of algorithms.[15–18] In one variation on this approach, the segmentation is restricted to a central 20 mm thick slab of tissue to calculate the central cerebral volume.[15] Limiting the segmentation to the central slices helps to avoid excessive manual editing, speeds up the processing, and increases sensitivity to change by focusing on the region in the brain around the ventricles. The COV is 0.56%, as determined by a scan–rescan test. A potential disadvantage of slice-based approaches is that the same central slab must be selected in each image through careful repositioning of the patient before each scan. In contrast, whole-brain segmentation methods[16–18,26,27] have less dependence on accurate repositioning and have been implemented as semi-automated programs (with only minor editing requirements) or fully automated programs. Measurement variability with these techniques is consistently below 1%. While fully automated software is desirable for studies involving large numbers of images, semi-automated techniques may offer higher accuracy because corrections can be made through user interaction. Several studies designed to directly compare semi-automated vs. fully automated segmentation methods have confirmed the benefits of automated atrophy measurement in

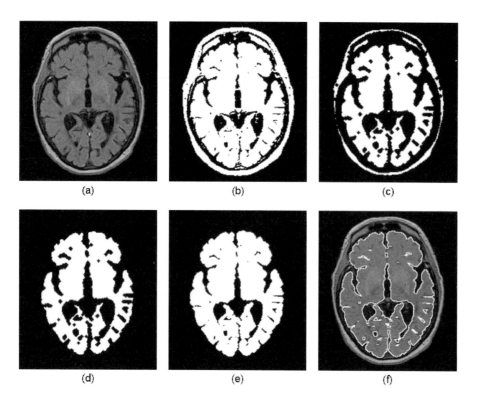

Fig. 11.2. Generic automated brain segmentation algorithm:[17] a) Slice from the original PD/T2 dual echo image (early echo minus late echo); (b) Optimal thresholding to separate tissue from background and CSF; (c) Morphological erosion with a 5 × 5 × 5 diamond-shaped kernel to disconnect connected structures; (d) Identification of the largest connected component, the brain parenchyma; (e) Morphological dilation with a 5 × 5 × 5 diamond-shaped kernel to recover the original shape; (f) Boundaries of final segmentation superimposed on the original image. The whole brain volume for this example is 946.4 ml.

MS, demonstrating that, although the values are indistinguishable from those calculated with semi-automated segmentation, the reproducibility is higher.[28-30]

Another important distinction between different types of atrophy measurements is whether the structure size is reported as an absolute volume or as a head-size normalized volume. A common approach for normalizing whole-brain volume is to calculate as the ratio of brain parenchymal volume to the intra-cranial volume. Normalized brain volume calculated in this way is referred to as the brain to intracranial cavity volume ratio (BICVR), percent brain parenchyma volume (PBV), brain parenchymal fraction (BPF),[31] brain-to-intracranial-cavity ratio (BICCR), or parenchymal fraction (PF).[12] COVs for normalized brain volume range from 0.2% to 2%, depending on the level of automation in the segmentation. Calculation of these quantities usually involves independent segmentation operations to determine the volumes used in the numerator and the denominator, which can compound measurement errors. In order to reduce this type of variability, one approach for BPF calculation[31] normalizes the volume of brain parenchyma by the total volume within a smoothed outer surface of the brain, which is generated during an intermediate step of the brain segmentation algorithm (Fig. 11.3). The scan–rescan COV for this BPF method is 0.2%.

Head-size normalization is particularly important in cross-sectional studies in which normal biological variation in head size can easily obscure subtle disease-related volume differences. In normal healthy controls, normalized brain volume is fairly consistent between the ages of 20 and 55.[32] Therefore, normalized brain volumes also provide a means to estimate the

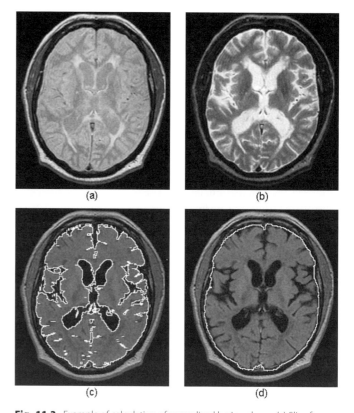

Fig. 11.3. Example of calculation of normalized brain volume: (a) Slice from original proton density-weighted image; (b) Slice from original T2-weighted image; (c) Segmented brain parenchymal volume. Volume calculated by multiplying number of segmented voxels by the voxel size is 1262.9 ml; (d) Segmented intracranial contents (brain parenchyma + CSF). Volume is 1633.9 ml. The normalized brain volume for this example is 0.773.

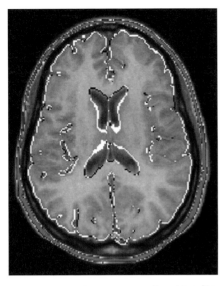

Fig. 11.4. Example output image from SIENA.[24] Input images were from an MS patient at baseline and year 4 follow-up. White points along the brain boundary indicate regions of tissue loss; black points indicate tissue expansion. This patient had a 1.72% decrease in normalized brain volume overall.

total amount of atrophy that has occurred up to the time of the scan, by comparison with an age-matched healthy control group. Normalization is also important in placebo-controlled longitudinal trials where it is necessary to establish that two groups of patients are comparable at baseline. Using absolute brain volumes, it is not possible to ensure that the placebo group and the treated groups do not have different amounts of atrophy at the start of a trial.

Registration-based approaches

Another class of atrophy estimation methods calculates brain volume changes directly from images acquired serially over time.[23,24] This approach involves registration of the images followed by change detection. SIENA (structural image evaluation using normalization of atrophy) is a commonly used registration-based software package for automatic calculation of percentage brain volume change (PBVC).[24] The software uses registration to align the skull in the two images, and then calculates the minute shifts in the brain edge at each point using the derivative of intensity profiles oriented perpendicular to the brain boundary (Fig. 11.4). PBVC is then derived from the sum of all edge point shifts normalized for the number of points and multiplied by the ratio of brain surface area to brain volume. The median atrophy error for SIENA is 0.15%, as calculated by a scan–rescan test of 16 normal volunteers.[33]

SIENAX is an adaptation of SIENA for cross-sectional measurements of normalized brain volume (NBV). SIENAX realigns the input image to a standard anatomic space and classifies extracted brain voxels as gray matter, white matter, or CSF to determine tissue volumes. Normalization for head size is achieved through the registration to standard space, which

provides a scaling factor for each subject. Results are reported in milliliters rather than as a ratio. The test–retest error for NBV calculated with SIENAX is 1%.[33]

Deformation-based methods

Voxel-based morphometry (VBM) and tensor-based morphometry (TBM) belong to a third class of image analysis techniques used to detect brain. In VBM, the images from individual subjects are spatially normalized to a common reference space prior to segmentation so that differences between groups of subjects can be assessed on a voxel by voxel basis.[25] This approach has been applied in MS patient subgroups to identify differences in regional volumes without the need to define structures of interest a priori.[34-36] TBM is similar, but once the non-linear deformation is determined, rates of tissue loss are derived through analysis of the deformation required to bring the images into alignment, without the need for tissue segmentation.[37] TBM has not been widely applied in multiple sclerosis, possibly because it requires adaptation to handle white matter lesions.[38]

Methods for measurement of gray matter and white matter atrophy

Differentiation of brain tissue into white matter and gray matter allows for additional specificity in atrophy measurements. Although it has been considered primarily a white matter disease, MS affects the gray matter extensively.[39,40] Post-mortem studies have shown that cortical lesions are plentiful, although for the most part, these lesions are not detectable with conventional MRI sequences. Retrograde axonal degeneration and neuronal loss secondary to distant white matter lesions contribute to gray matter pathology in MS. Both gray matter lesions and neurodegeneration secondary to white matter lesions are likely to result in gray matter atrophy.

Methods to quantify gray matter atrophy include volumetric analyses based on tissue classification to calculate fractional gray matter,[41-45] and techniques to estimate cortical thickness.[46-48] A commonly used software package to estimate gray matter fraction is SPM,[25] which calculates probabilities for each brain voxel of belonging to gray matter, white matter, or CSF (Fig. 11.5). Fractional gray matter can be calculated as the number of voxels labeled as gray matter divided by the sum of white matter, gray matter, CSF, and lesion voxels. The scan–rescan COV for calculating fractional gray matter using SPM is 0.4%.[22] SIENAX, the cross-sectional version of SIENA, is another commonly used software package for calculating gray matter volume.[24] All of these methods utilize anatomic information in addition to intensity information to accurately classify voxels into their appropriate tissue types. However, MS lesions can still be problematic and may lead to segmentation errors if not taken into account by the software. A segmentation program designed specifically for measurement of gray matter fraction in MS patients has been developed to circumvent the issues

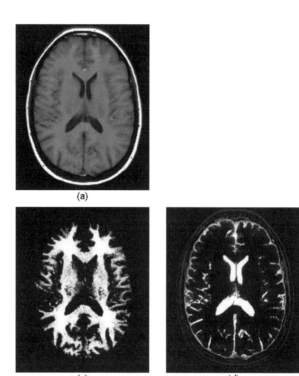

(a)

(b) (c) (d)

Fig. 11.5. Example of atrophy analysis using SPM99.[25] (a) Original T1-weighted input image; (b) Output gray matter probabilities; (c) Output white matter probabilities; and (d) Output cerebrospinal fluid probabilities.

encountered with lesions.[44] A direct comparison of several different methods for automated gray matter segmentation was performed to evaluate the strengths and weaknesses of each approach.[49]

Regional and global cortical thickness measurements are commonly performed using a program called FreeSurfer.[50] This software measures cortical thickness at every point by creating a surface at the leuko-cortical junction and deforming it outward to find the surface at the cortical–pial junction. The cortical thickness at each point is calculated as the shortest distance between the two continuous surfaces. Inflation of the cortical surface map effectively unfolds the cortex to allow visualization of thickness measurements over the entire surface and mapping of structures across individuals. A similar approach uses linked vertices between the inner and outer cortical surfaces to estimate cortical thickness.[51,52] To detect the very small changes in cortical thickness over time, a longitudinal deformation algorithm (CLADA) has been developed and tested in MS patients.[48] A modification of SIENA has also been used to estimate changes in cortical thickness in MS patients.[46] Studies utilizing the various tools available for quantification of cortical thickness and fractional tissue volumes are currently under way to clarify the significance of gray and white matter atrophy in MS.

Methods for measurement of atrophy in brain structures and lobes

Many of the earliest studies of MRI-based quantification of CNS atrophy in MS patients focused on measurements of particular

regions of the brain, such as corpus callosum area,[53] third ventricle width,[5] lateral ventricular volume,[54] 4- or 7-slice central cerebral volume,[15,20] bicaudate ratio,[55] or other brain regional volumes[8,20] primarily because these measurements were more practical to perform than whole-brain measurements with the tools available at that time. As automated segmentation- and registration-based methods became more widely available, the focus shifted to measurements of whole-brain atrophy. However, global techniques do not account for the spatial location of brain volume changes. Localized measurements of morphometric changes would be expected to show greater correlations to specific functional deficits and may indicate patterns across patients of particular regions being more susceptible to tissue destruction than others over the course of disease.

The investigation of regional atrophy across many different anatomic structures requires delineation of regions preferably through spatial normalization or anatomic labeling techniques, although it can also be accomplished with manual tracing in small cross-sectional studies. In general, manual tracing is considered to be prohibitively time-consuming for studies involving large numbers of patients and not reproducible enough for longitudinal analyses. Spatial normalization is the process of deforming a patient's MRI to match a standard image,[24,25] whereas anatomic labeling works in the opposite direction by deforming the standard image to the patient's MRI.[56] For regional atrophy applications, one could use an average brain,[57] or a brain atlas[58] as the standard image. As long as the deformation or non-linear registration results in accurate alignment between homologous structures across the brain, then the anatomic labels can be directly applied to the patient's MRI. Spatial normalization and anatomic labeling are challenging in MS because of the significant structural differences caused by atrophy.

Normalization of the brain to standard space is inherent to several algorithms, including FreeSurfer and VBM, and therefore gray matter atrophy results derived from these approaches are automatically reported as regional measurements. Analyses of the anatomic differences in patterns of atrophy between different subgroups of patients are typically done via this class of techniques.[34–36,52,59] To segment single regions of interest, more structure-specific approaches are required. Recent examples that have been applied to MS are a rule-based manual method to segment the hippocampus and its subregions[60] and manual methods for medulla oblongata volume and corpus callosum parcellation.[61,62]

Methods for measurement of spinal cord atrophy

Tissue loss due to MS pathologic processes is also detectable in the spinal cord with MRI.[10,63–66] In one of the first studies of spinal cord atrophy, a comparison of MS patients and normal controls found that atrophy affected 40% of the patients.[63] Histopathologic analyses of MS spinal cords post-mortem have demonstrated that axonal degeneration, as opposed to tissue loss within focal cord lesions, is the main pathologic substrate of cord atrophy,[67] and that cord tissue loss occurs primarily within the white matter.[68]

Reliable measurement of spinal cord atrophy is challenging. The cord is small in relation to the image resolutions typically used, so partial volume effects are significant. For some methods, care must be taken to align the imaging planes exactly perpendicular to the cord and to select consistent landmarks (vertebral discs, usually) to frame measurements. An example of a semi-automated method to estimate cord cross-sectional area at the level of C2/C3 requires the operator to trace regions of CSF and cord in the top slice and to select a seed point on each subsequent slice.[64] Then the boundary between cord and CSF is determined for each slice automatically and cord cross-sectional area is calculated as the mean over five consecutive slices. Volumetric segmentation of the spinal cord using edge detection[69] and active surfaces[70,71] requires less time and operator interaction, plus it enables cross-sectional measurements oriented perpendicular at any point along the cord. The importance of normalization for cord measurements is still an open question.[69,72] A direct comparison of normalized vs. absolute cord volumes suggested that the absolute volumes were more reproducible and more strongly correlated to disability.[69] The increasing availability of better coils and faster imaging times may make it possible to incorporate cord atrophy measures into more MS MRI protocols.

Comparisons of atrophy measurement methods

The lack of an accepted standardized method for measurement of brain atrophy complicates the interpretation of results because the numerical values cannot be compared directly across studies. However, in studies where more than one whole brain atrophy measure was applied to the same dataset, the main findings are generally consistent, even though between-group differences may not always reach statistical significance.[29] A few studies have been conducted to directly compare techniques in terms of the sample sizes required for clinical trials with atrophy as the outcome measure. In a direct comparison of atrophy results obtained with SIENA and a semi-automated thresholding technique, the between-patient variability was significantly lower with SIENA, indicating that the statistical power for detecting differences between groups is higher.[73] To investigate this further, a series of studies were conducted using MRIs from small groups of patients where each was analyzed with multiple atrophy measurement techniques. Sample sizes were again lower for SIENA as compared to semi-automated brain segmentation, brain boundary shift integral, and ventricular enlargement in RRMS[74] and for SIENA as compared to central cerebral volume and SIENAX normalized brain volume in SPMS.[75] According to these calculations, approximately 40–50 patients per arm would be required to detect a 50% reduction in atrophy rate at the 5% significance level with 90% power in a 2-year study using SIENA. A separate power analysis using SIENA measurements from multicenter MRI data estimated the sample size to be approximately 100 patients per arm.[76] In a larger clinical trial dataset, blinded analysis by separate MRI reading centers using either SIENA or automated BPF measurements demonstrated similar trends in the overall trial results, but between-patient variability was lower for BPF change than for SIENA, indicating higher power for detecting differences using BPF.[77] Comparisons between normalized measures of whole-brain volume vs. gray matter volume and white matter volume (all obtained with SIENAX) showed that sample sizes were lowest for gray matter volume, mainly because this compartment had the greatest amount of change.[78,79] All of these studies suggest that brain atrophy (either whole brain, or gray matter) is a suitable outcome measure for proof-of-concept trials of neuroprotective agents, with relatively low sample size requirements for a 2-year study duration.

Confounding issues in atrophy measurements

Regardless of the method used, atrophy measurements from MRIs can be affected by technical and biological factors that may further complicate interpretation of the results. Technical factors include patient positioning, scanner hardware and software upgrades, partial volume effects, lesion changes, motion artifacts, dental artifacts, voxel size calibration, intensity inhomogeneities, and protocol or sequence variations. Three-dimensional, or volumetric measures can reduce the effects of patient re-positioning on atrophy measurements. Scanner upgrades and voxel size drift can be partially corrected using phantoms and consistent calibration procedures throughout the course of longitudinal studies, or by use of normalized volumes (i.e. BPF and NBV). Partial volume effects can be minimized by decreasing slice thickness and/or accounting for partial volume effects in volume calculations.

MS white matter lesions can affect brain volume measurements for both technical and biological reasons. Technically, a common issue encountered when using T1-weighted images for brain volume measurements is the misclassification of T1 black holes as CSF. In particular, if a T1 hypointense lesion is present at baseline but disappears at follow-up, e.g. as gadolinium-enhancing lesions typically do, then the space originally occupied by the disappearing lesion may be counted as brain "growth" by the software. Lesion changes can present a problem for all three classes of atrophy measurement techniques[80–82] and can affect gray matter and white matter segmentation in subtle ways beyond misclassification.[44] Therefore, it is important to account for lesions or, at least to verify that their effects on the algorithm are negligible, when measuring brain atrophy.

Biologically, new white matter lesions indicate MS disease activity and inflammation, which can have complex effects on atrophy measurements. Changes in brain volume can occur due to inflammatory edema and fluctuations in tissue water content. Although related to MS disease pathology, the volume decreases resulting from resolution of edema do not represent true tissue loss, and therefore, this phenomenon is referred to as "pseudoatrophy." A study performed to model the sources of variability in brain atrophy measurements suggested that changes related to lesion activity had a much greater effect on BPF than either technical factors (i.e. patient repositioning) or physiological factors (i.e. hydration status).[83] In a 2-year study in RRMS patients, there was a decrease in white matter fraction in the half of patients who had the largest decrease in enhancing lesion volume, whereas white matter fraction actually increased in the other subgroup of patients who had a net increase in enhancing lesion volume.[84] These findings have important implications for the design and interpretation of clinical trials. Whether or not pseudoatrophy truly is benign and reversible, and how it should be accounted for, are still under investigation.

Other (patho-) biological factors that affect atrophy measurements include normal aging, alcoholism, anorexia, dehydration, diabetes, cerebral vascular disease, and steroid treatment. An experiment designed to quantify the influence of hydration state on brain volume measurements demonstrated that lack of fluid intake for 16 hours had a significant effect (−0.55%) on brain volume change measurements, as did rehydration (+0.72%).[85] Normal aging has a well-studied affect on brain atrophy, which tends to accelerate with age.[86] In an older population 65–75 years of age, the rate of BPF change is −0.55%/year, which is similar to mean rates of change in MS patients. Typically, the effects of MS pathology outweigh the normal aging process, but age matching and proper exclusion criteria are important considerations for atrophy studies. It is also important to postpone atrophy measurements until at least 4 weeks following steroid administration due to the reversible

effects that steroids have been shown to have on brain volumes.[87]

Natural history of atrophy in MS

Tissue destruction begins early in the course of MS. Immuno-histochemical analysis of MS brain tissue has shown that axonal transection and severe damage occur in new inflammatory lesions.[88] MR spectroscopy of patients with less than 5 years' disease duration demonstrated reduced N-acetylaspartate indicative of axonal damage or loss.[89] MRI atrophy findings in very early MS are consistent with these studies. In several different longitudinal studies of patients with clinically isolated syndromes (CIS),[11] brain atrophy was significantly higher in the patients who progressed to clinically definite MS over the course of the 1–6 year studies, than in the patients who did not develop MS.[11,90–93] These findings were consistent despite different measurement techniques, patient groups, and follow-up durations. In a cross-sectional study, CIS patients with MRI lesions had significantly thinner cortex than CIS patients without MRI lesions.[94] In these patients, the mean cortical thickness was closer to RRMS patients than healthy controls, suggesting that gray matter damage may begin very early in the course of MS. Studies that applied VBM analyses in CIS patients reported contradictory results. While two VBM studies demonstrated evidence of early gray matter damage, primarily in the thalamus, deep gray matter structures, and cerebellum[36] and in the limbic system,[35] a smaller study found no evidence of gray matter tissue loss in CIS.[59] There is some evidence that spinal cord atrophy might also begin at the earliest stage of MS,[66] but findings vary across studies.

In RRMS patients, brain volumes have been shown to be consistently lower than in age-matched healthy controls. Atrophy does not appear to be confined to particular structures, even at this stage of disease. Cross-sectionally, significant volume differences between RRMS patients and controls have been found for whole brain,[12,43,84,95] central cerebral volume,[96] gray matter fraction,[91] lateral ventricles,[12] corpus callosum,[96] brain stem,[8] thalamus, widespread cortical regions,[97] and cerebellum.[98] Interestingly, white matter atrophy is not a consistent finding in RRMS. Longitudinal studies have shown that brain atrophy rates are higher in RRMS patients than age-matched normal healthy controls.[20,23,84,91,97,99] The mean rate of whole brain atrophy in RRMS is approximately 0.5%–1.5% per year, but atrophy rates vary considerably between patients and across different measurement techniques (Table 11.1). Even using the same measurement technique (SIENA), the atrophy rate in untreated RRMS patients varies from −0.49% to −1.2% per year across MRI analysis centers.[76,77] Most studies have not found significant differences in spinal cord cross-sectional area between RRMS patients and healthy controls.[64,65,69]

Patients with secondary-progressive (SP) MS have significantly more brain and cord atrophy than RRMS patients when

Table 11.1. *Annualized mean (and standard deviation, if published) percent decrease in brain volume in untreated MS patients*

Study	Atrophy measure	CIS	RRMS	SPMS	PPMS
Losseff 1996	CCV		−1.12	(13 RR, 16 SP)	
Rudick 1999	BPF		−0.61 (0.65) (n = 72)		
Ge 2000	WBV		−1.5 (n = 27)	−2.0 (n = 9)	
Fox 2000*	BBSI		−0.8 (n = 6)	−0.6 (n = 6)	−0.9 (n = 9)
Rovaris 2000†	WBV		−1.3 (n = 50)		
Molyneux 2000	CCV			−1.3 (1.2) (n = 46)	
Rovaris 2001	CCV		−0.9 (n = 114)		
Kalkers 2002	PF		−0.7	−0.8	
	VF		3.9 (n = 42)	3.9 (n = 21)	
Filippi 2004	PBVC	−0.83 (1.1) (n = 98)			
Sormani 2004	PBVC		−0.9 (1.2)		
	WBV		−0.8 (2.2) (n = 105)		
Tiberio 2005‡	BPF		−0.75		
	GMF		−1.1		
	WMF		−0.09 (n = 21)		
Anderson 2007§	WBV	−0.25 (1.04)	−0.76 (1.38)		
	BBSI	−0.22 (0.48)	−0.72 (0.60)		
	PBVC	−0.32 (0.47) (n = 37)	−0.78 (0.59) (n = 30)		
Jasperse 2007	PBVC		−0.8 (0.8) (n = 56)		
Miller 2007	BPF		−0.43 (n = 315)		
Mesaros 2008	CCV		−2.0 (2.8) (n = 466)		
Healy 2009	NBV (SIENAX)		−0.94		
	NGMV		−3.57		
	NWMV		−0.093 (n = 116)		
Kapoor 2010	CCV			−2.48 (−0.97)	
	PBVC			−0.59	
	GMF			−9.24 (−1.47)	
	WMF			0.41 (0.10) (n = 57)	
DiFilippo 2010	PBVC	−0.38 (0.55) (n = 92)			
Barkhof 2010	PBVC		−1.20 (1.15) (n = 90)		
Kappos 2010	PBVC		−0.65 (1.05) (n = 383)		
De Stefano 2010	PBVC	−0.40 (0.47) (n = 157)	−0.49 (0.65) (n = 579)	−0.64 (0.68) (n = 139)	−0.56 (0.55) (n = 88)

Abbreviations: BBSI = brain boundary shift integral, BPF = brain parenchymal fraction, CCV = central cerebral volume (4-slice or 7-slice), CIS = clinically isolated syndrome, GMF = grey matter fraction, NBV = normalized brain volume, NGMF = normalized gray matter volume, NWMV = normalized white matter volume, PBVC = percent brain volume change (SIENA), PF = parenchymal fraction, PPMS = primary progressive multiple sclerosis, RRMS = relapsing-remitting multiple sclerosis, SPMS = secondary progressive multiple sclerosis, VF = ventricular fraction, WBV = whole brain volume, WMF = white matter fraction.
* Annual atrophy rate in 26 normal controls was −0.3%.
† Annual atrophy rate in 5 normal controls was −0.07%.
‡ Annual rates calculated from 2-year rates of change. Changes in 10 healthy controls were: BPF −0.3%, gray matter fraction −0.5%, white matter fraction −0.09%.
§ Atrophy rates in 16 healthy controls were: WBV 0.51(1.32), BBSI −0.04 (0.52), PBVC −0.07 (0.34).

groups are compared cross-sectionally, as expected.[10,100,101] Most longitudinal studies of SPMS patients indicate that brain atrophy continues to progress in SPMS at about the same rate or faster compared with RRMS, when subgroups of patients are compared directly.[23,76,91,95,102–104] The long-term kinetics of CNS tissue loss are not known, however. A 4-year study comparing brain atrophy rates in healthy controls, CIS, RRMS, and SPMS subgroups from a single site suggested that atrophy

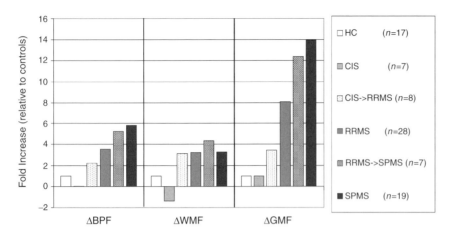

Fig. 11.6. Atrophy rates in MS patient subgroups expressed as a fold increase relative to healthy controls. Percent change in brain parenchymal fraction was calculated from annual scans acquired for a four-year longitudinal study of MS patients and healthy subjects.(adapted from Fisher et al.[91]) Whole brain and gray matter atrophy rates increased with disease progression/severity whereas white matter atrophy rates remained relatively constant across groups.

might accelerate with disease progression.[91] Furthermore, atrophy acceleration was due entirely to increased rates of gray matter atrophy whereas white matter atrophy rates were found to be relatively consistent across the groups. The gray matter atrophy rate was approximately eight-fold higher in RRMS than in normal healthy controls and 14-fold higher in SPMS (Fig. 11.6). In contrast, a large study 963 patients with MRI data pooled across multiple centers (and multiple MRI acquisition protocols) showed that differences in atrophy rates between patient subgroups disappeared after correcting for baseline brain volume.[76] Both studies had limitations; therefore, whether atrophy rates remain stable or accelerate over the disease course is still unclear. Further investigation with longer term follow-up in individual subjects is needed to determine the kinetics of atrophy over the lifespan of MS.

Brain and cord atrophy have also been measured in patients with primary progressive MS.[12,23,103,105–107] In cross-sectional studies that compare atrophy across MS subtypes, PPMS patients appear to have approximately the same amount of brain atrophy as SPMS patients of the same disease duration or similar disability levels, despite the significantly lower lesion load in PPMS patients. Longitudinally, brain atrophy appears to progress at a rate similar to SPMS and RRMS. In a longitudinal study of 42 RRMS, 21 SPMS, and 20 PPMS patients followed over 2–4 years, there were significant decreases in parenchymal fractions and corresponding increases in ventricular fractions in all three subgroups, but there were no differences between the groups.[102] More recently, VBM demonstrated regional thalamic atrophy in patients in the early stage of PPMS compared to healthy controls.[34] Gray matter atrophy in the deep gray matter, cortical, and infratentorial areas was detected over 1-year follow-up.

Patterns of regional atrophy differ across the clinical phenotypes of MS. VBM has been used to map differences in gray matter atrophy across subgroups of patients.[59] Compared with CIS, RRMS patients had significant gray matter atrophy in the pre- and postcentral gyri. SPMS patients demonstrated more widespread atrophy in all of the major lobes, cerebellum, and deep gray matter structures compared to RRMS, and compared to PPMS, SPMS patients had more gray matter atrophy in a few

specific gyri, thalamus, and cerebellum. Interestingly, PPMS patients did not have more gray matter atrophy than SPMS patients in any region. A 15-month longitudinal study also showed different patterns of regional atrophy among patients with RR, SP, and PP MS.[108] Although all groups in this study exhibited atrophy around the lateral fissure, the insula, and in regions of the temporal, frontal, parietal and occipital lobes, the predominant region for atrophy in the RRMS patients was the ventricular system. In contrast, the SPMS and PPMS patients tended to have more atrophy in specific cortical and subcortical gray matter regions. Similarly, a comparison of regional cortical thickness in MS patients grouped by disease duration showed cortical atrophy was already apparent focally in the temporal lobes in patients within three years of diagnosis, spreading to multiple areas including the motor cortex in patients with greater than 5 years' disease duration.[47] Using a different approach that restricted analysis to a few specific structures, a classification tree based only on atrophy of medulla oblongata and corpus callosum atrophy measures correctly classified patients into RRMS, SPMS, or PPMS with 80% accuracy.[61] Together, these studies suggest that, although tissue loss becomes increasingly more global as the disease progresses, structures with a high degree of interconnectivity tend to be more severely affected, even early in the disease.

Correlations between atrophy and other MRI measurements

The major pathologic substrates of atrophy in MS are believed to be demyelination and axonal loss; therefore, it is reasonable to hypothesize that the amount of tissue loss is related to other MRI markers of pathology, including lesions, magnetization transfer ratio (MTR), and diffusion tensor imaging (DTI) measures. However, results from correlational analyses have been inconclusive, particularly the relationship between enhancing lesions and atrophy.

Gadolinium-enhancing lesions have been implicated as the initiating events that lead to severe tissue damage and atrophy in MS.[109] This hypothesis is supported by evidence in some studies where enhancing lesions at baseline were predictive of subsequent atrophy.[5,91,104,110–114] However, other studies have found no association between enhancing lesions and atrophy.[15,43,103,115–119] Multiple regression analyses to identify independent MRI predictors of atrophy also report inconsistent findings. The presence of enhancing lesions at baseline was an independent predictor of subsequent atrophy over 4 years in RRMS,[91] but not over 14 months in a very large population ($n =$ 466)[119] and not over two years in newly diagnosed patients.[118] The discrepancy in findings may be related to pseudoatrophy and the complex effects inflammation and edema have on brain tissue volume. In addition, enhancing lesions are pathologically heterogenous, they only enhance for 2–4 weeks, and they occur less frequently over the course of disease. Most clinical trials have shown that brain atrophy slows but continues to progress despite effective suppression of inflammation,[117] possibly implicating other disease processes not linked to inflammation.

If atrophy is the final step in a pathologic cascade initiated by inflammation, then the unknown and variable time lag between inflammatory damage and subsequent atrophy also contribute to inconsistent findings. A three-year trial with monthly MRIs noted that changes in brain volume appeared to lag behind changes in the enhancing lesions by 3–6 months.[120] Frequent scans with triple-dose gadolinium revealed that the cumulative volume of new enhancing lesions in the first six months was not predictive of concurrent changes in brain volume, but strongly correlated with brain atrophy over a period of 18 months.[121] In an eight-year follow-up study of RRMS patients, the number of enhancing lesions at year 2 was a significant predictor of the subsequent atrophy from year 2 to year 8.[122] However, together with T2 lesion volume at year 2, lesion measurements only accounted for 27% of the variance in subsequent brain atrophy.

Hyperintense lesions on T2-weighted scans are non-specific markers of MS pathology including edema, inflammation, demyelination, axonal loss, and/or gliosis. Despite lack of pathologic specificity, correlations between T2 lesions and atrophy have been demonstrated consistently. To some extent, both measures reflect the net result of previous damage, which may explain the association. In longitudinal studies of RRMS patients, T2 lesions at baseline and changes in T2 lesions predict subsequent brain atrophy.[5,91,112,118,119,123] Notably, a 14-year follow-up study of patients with CIS demonstrated that early changes in T2 lesion load from baseline to year five were predictive of subsequent brain atrophy measurements 14 years later.[124] T2 lesion volumes were also correlated to subsequent atrophy in patients followed over shorter time periods ranging from 14 months to eight years. However, white matter lesions typically account for less than 30% of the variance in subsequent whole brain atrophy.

Surprisingly, white matter lesion load seems to be more strongly correlated to gray matter atrophy than to white matter atrophy.[42,43,81,84,99,101,125,126] Correlations between T2 lesion volume and gray matter fraction support the hypothesis that gray matter atrophy is partly due to retrograde neurodegeneration secondary to focal tissue damage in the white matter.[38,97] Interestingly, there are no correlations between T2 lesion volume and gray matter atrophy in PPMS patients,[127,128] perhaps implicating different underlying mechanisms for atrophy in the different disease phenotypes. The MRI predictors of gray matter atrophy may also differ for RRMS and SPMS.[91] A 4-year longitudinal study reported that change in T2 lesion volume along with normal-appearing brain tissue MTR and lesion MTR could account for 62% of the variance in gray matter atrophy in RRMS patients, whereas there were no significant MRI predictors of gray matter atrophy found in SPMS patients. It is possible that cortical lesions, which are not visible on conventional MRIs, become the main determinant of gray matter atrophy in the later stage of disease.

The nature of the association between focal white matter damage and gray matter atrophy is a topic of great interest. The proportion of cortical tissue loss that stems from neurodegeneration secondary to pathology in white matter vs. that which arises from focal pathology in the gray matter is unknown. Regional analysis methods have been applied to investigate this question. Cross-sectional VBM and regional cortical thickness studies have both demonstrated significant associations between cortical atrophy and T2 lesions in the nearby white matter,[52,59] suggesting a connection between the pathologic processes in white matter and the cortex, but the direction and extent of this interaction has not been studied.

T1 hypointense lesions, or T1 black holes, represent regions of severe tissue damage and axonal loss,[129] and therefore, would be expected to correlate more strongly with atrophy than non-specific T2 lesions. However, in most studies, the strength of the correlations between atrophy and T1 lesions has turned out to be surprisingly similar to that between atrophy and T2 lesions.[43,84,96,112,116,123,130] In a mixed group of RR, SP, and PPMS patients, both T1 lesion volume and diffuse tissue damage, as measured by MTR peak height, were correlated to atrophy to varying degrees in the different subgroups.[131] A cross-sectional study in SPMS patients found that T1 lesion volume was the only independent correlate of gray matter fraction, accounting for 52% of the variance.[132] Studies of regional gray matter atrophy have also demonstrated correlations with T1 hypointensities. Atrophy in the thalamus and hippocampus was correlated with overall T1 lesion load[36] and atrophy in the lateral geniculate nuclei was correlated with T1 lesions along the optic radiations.[34] Both studies provide further evidence that Wallerian degeneration secondary to damage in focal white matter lesions is a significant factor in gray matter atrophy.

The association between MTR and atrophy has not been as extensively studied as that between atrophy and lesions. Decreased MTR is mainly due to demyelination and axonal loss within focal lesions, and diffuse abnormalities and axonal degeneration in normal-appearing white matter.[133,134] Since these are the same factors believed to be responsible for tissue loss, MTR would be expected to correlate robustly with atrophy measures. Cross-sectionally, various MTR parameters, including mean MTR and MTR histogram peak height, were correlated with central cerebral volume.[135] Correlations between mean whole brain MTR and normalized brain volume measures are also relatively strong ($r = 0.6 - 0.7$).[136] In a four-year longitudinal study, both lesion MTR and mean MTR in normal-appearing brain tissue at baseline were significant independent predictors of subsequent atrophy in RRMS patients.[91] The MTR variables remained in the multiple regression models whether the dependent variable was whole brain, gray matter, or white matter atrophy. Brain atrophy appears to be more strongly correlated with whole-brain MTR than with lesions,[131] which is consistent with the hypothesis that both measures are sensitive to diffuse damage in normal-appearing tissue and possibly have common pathological substrates in RRMS.

Atrophy correlations have also been investigated using other types of MRI data. N-acetylaspartate (NAA), a marker of neuronal/axonal injury, was found to be correlated with brain atrophy in relapse–onset patient subgroups[137,138] but not in primary progressive MS patients,[139] suggesting different underlying pathologic mechanisms of tissue loss. T2 hypointensities possibly due to iron deposition in subcortical gray matter have been shown to be correlated to brain atrophy both cross-sectionally and longitudinally,[140] indicating that iron accumulation may be related to tissue loss in MS. DTI, which measures white matter fiber tract integrity through characterization of directional water diffusion, has also been used to understand mechanisms of atrophy. In particular, DTI has been used to further probe the link between white matter tissue damage and gray matter atrophy. A one-year longitudinal DTI study in CIS patients found that baseline fractional anisotropy along white matter fiber tracts was the only significant predictor of subsequent change in gray matter volume.[141] Taken together, the observed correlations between MRI abnormalities and atrophy suggest that both focal white matter lesions and diffuse damage in the normal-appearing brain tissue contribute to tissue loss in MS, but current MRI measures cannot account for all of the variance in atrophy. In the future, longer-term longitudinal studies and inclusion of cortical lesion measurements should help to clarify the relative contributions of white matter and gray matter lesions and diffuse tissue damage to CNS tissue loss.

Correlations between atrophy and disability

Measures of atrophy are more closely related to neurologic disability in MS patients than are conventional lesion measurements (Table 11.2). The strength of the correlations depend on the type of atrophy measure, type of disability measure, and type of MS. Cross-sectionally, correlations between EDSS and brain volume are typically modest ($r = 0.2 - 0.5$). This may be related to limitations of the EDSS, which is heavily weighted toward ambulation and does not account for cognitive impairment. Correlations between brain atrophy and the

MS Functional Composite (MSFC)[142] are consistently stronger than the atrophy / EDSS correlations.[130,143,144]

Comparison of results across studies indicates that normalized atrophy measures, which correct for head size, appear to be more strongly correlated to disability than absolute volume measurements. Several longitudinal studies indicate that patients with greater rates of atrophy are more likely to worsen clinically[15,104,143,145,146] and vice versa.[147] In an eight-year follow-up study of patients with established RRMS (entry EDSS ≤ 3.5,) 56% of patients in the quartile with the highest rate of atrophy in the first 2 years had reached EDSS 6 or greater at the eight-year follow-up, whereas only 14% of patients in the lowest quartile had reached this milestone.[122] Even at the earliest stage of disease, brain atrophy has been shown to predict subsequent disability.[90,145,146] A six-year follow-up study of CIS patients found that whole-brain atrophy over the first year predicted conversion to clinically definite MS by year 6. As with the relationships between atrophy and lesions, the relationship between atrophy and disability may be complicated by a possible time lag between tissue injury and when this injury is detectable as atrophy on MRI. Furthermore, the brain may be able to compensate for tissue injury early in the disease when there is still sufficient functional reserve and capacity for tissue repair, leading to a long dissociation in time between atrophy and disability. Data demonstrating higher atrophy-disability correlations later on in the disease or in SPMS as compared to RRMS support this hypothesis.[95,143]

Multiple studies suggest that gray matter atrophy is more closely related to neurological or neuropsychological disability than white matter atrophy or T2 lesions. In a large cross-sectional study involving 597 MS patients, multivariate analysis showed that gray matter fraction was the only MRI variable that predicted EDSS.[101] In patients imaged 20 years after their first attack, there were highly significant differences between CIS, RRMS, and SPMS subgroups in normalized gray matter volume but not in normalized white matter volume.[126] Furthermore, gray matter, but not white matter, atrophy was correlated to EDSS and MSFC. The relevance of gray matter atrophy is more clearly evident in longitudinal studies. In a group of CIS patients followed for three years, gray matter atrophy was significantly higher in the patients who converted to clinically definite MS than in those that did not, whereas there were no detectable changes in WM volumes, highlighting the significance of gray matter atrophy in the earliest stage of MS.[90] Longitudinal measurement of CTh over just one year in RR and SPMS patients found higher rate of cortical atrophy in patients with disability progression as compared to patients who remained stable over that year.[46] Similarly, in a longer-term follow-up study of 70 RR- and SPMS patients, patients who progressed on MSFC over 6.5 years had more gray matter (but not white matter) atrophy than those who remained stable.[144] The stronger correlation between gray matter atrophy and disability may be related to the possibility that neuronal damage has a greater impact on disability than does demyelination and axonal loss, or it may be primarily technical. That is, it might be much more difficult to reliably

Table 11.2. *Cross—sectional correlations between atrophy and disability, grouped by atrophy measure*

Study	Atrophy measure	n MS type	Disability measure	r	P
Losseff 1996	Cord area	30 RR, 15 SP, 15 PP	EDSS	−0.7	<0.001
Lycklama à Nijeholt 1998	Cord area	28 RR, 32 SP, 31 PP	EDSS	−0.34	0.001
Stevenson 1999	Cord area	158 PP, 33 TP	EDSS	−0.30	<0.001
Liu 1999	Cord area	20 RR, 20 SP	EDSS	−0.37	0.023
Zivadinov 2008	Cervical cord volume	11 CIS, 34 RR, 14 SP, 7 PP	EDSS	−0.51	<0.0001
Horsfield 2010	Normalized cord area	20 RR, 20 SP	EDSS	−0.59	<0.001
Lycklama à Nijeholt 1998	Ventricle volume	28 RR, 32 SP, 31 PP	EDSS	No correlation	
Losseff 1996	CCV	13 RR, 16 SP	EDSS	No correlation	
Stevenson 1999	CCV	158 PP, 33 TP	EDSS	−0.20	0.006
			Timed walk	−0.39	<0.001
Molyneux 2000	CCV	95 SP	EDSS	0.18	0.018
Liu 1999	Cerebral WM	20 RR, 20 SP	EDSS	−0.37	0.018
Filippi 2000	WBV	11 RR, 4 SP	EDSS	No correlation	
Fisher 2000	BPF	134 RR	EDSS	−0.42	<0.001
			MSFC	0.50	<0.0001
Kalkers 2001	PF and VF	80 RR, 36 SP, 21 PP	EDSS	−0.25	<0.01
			MSFC	−0.40	<0.01
Bermel 2003	BPF	60 RR, 18 SP	EDSS	−0.39	0.0006
Rovaris 2007	NBV	142 RR	EDSS	−0.29	0.0007
	PBVC/y			−0.18	0.04
Jasperse 2007	PBVC/y	79 RR	EDSS	−0.32	0.004
			MSFC	0.45	<0.001
Chard 2002	BPF, GMF, WMF	26 RR	EDSS	No correlation	
Quarantelli 2003	GMF, WMF	50 RR	EDSS	No correlation	
Sanfilipo 2005	GMF	35 RR, 6 SP	EDSS	−0.46	0.004
Fisher 2008	GMF	36 RR, 26 SP	EDSS	−0.48	
			MSFC	0.52	
			T25FW	−0.43	
			9HPT	0.46	
			PASAT	0.43	
Fisniku 2008	GMF	33 RR, 11 SP	EDSS	−0.41	0.005
			MSFC	0.55	<0.001
			T25FW	−0.40	0.001
			9HPT	0.44	0.003
			PASAT	0.32	0.038
Sailer 2003	Cortical thickness	11 RR, 9 SP	EDSS	−0.56	0.01
Charil 2007	Cortical thickness	425 RR	EDSS	−0.28	<0.0001
De Stefano 2003	Normalized cortical volume	65 RR, 25 PP	EDSS	−0.27	0.04
				−0.64	<0.0001
Tao 2009	Regional GM atrophy	88 RR	EDSS		
	Thalamus			−0.51	<0.0001
	Caudate			−0.43	<0.0001
	Putamen			−0.36	<0.001
	Pons			−0.29	<0.01

Abbreviations: 9HPT = Nine-Hole Peg Test, BBSI = brain boundary shift integral, BPF = brain parenchymal fraction, CCV = central cerebral volume (4-slice or 7-slice), CIS = clinically isolated syndrome, EDSS = Expanded Disability Status Scale, GMF = gray matter fraction, MS = multiple sclerosis, MSFC = Multiple Sclerosis Functional Composite, NBV = normalized brain volume, NGMF = normalized gray matter volume, NWMV = normalized white matter volume, PASAT = Paced Auditory Serial Addition Test, PBVC = percent brain volume change (SIENA), PF = parenchymal fraction, PP = primary progressive, RR = relapsing-remitting, SP = secondary progressive, T25FW = Timed 25-foot Walk, TP = transitional progressive, VF = ventricular fraction, WBV = whole brain volume, WM = white matter, WMF = white matter fraction.

measure tissue loss in the white matter due to ongoing inflammatory activity and edema that confound the measurements. Preliminary evidence from clinical trials supports the latter explanation.

Regional brain atrophy is related to specific aspects of clinical dysfunction.[148] A two-year SIENA VBM analysis demonstrated that even in patients with minimal disability, worse ambulatory function was associated with atrophy in the central brain regions, while poor hand function (nine-hole peg test) was associated with atrophy in both central and peripheral regions. Cortical thickness patterns were found to differ according to disability level.[47] In patients with mild disability (EDSS <3), there was significant focal cortical thinning in the superior temporal gyrus, whereas patients with moderate disability (EDSS 3.5–6.0) had additional focal areas of cortical atrophy in the parietal, and frontal medial gyri. Patients with severe disability (EDSS >6) demonstrated similar cortical thinning in the temporal, parietal and frontal regions, plus areas of significant atrophy along the motor cortex. EDSS correlated significantly with the mean cortical thickness of the motor cortex.

Brain atrophy has also been shown to be related to cognitive impairment,[54,149–152] depression,[153] fatigue,[154,155] and quality of life[4,147] in MS patients. An early study of chronic progressive MS patients[149] demonstrated that performance on memory and intelligence tests was correlated to degree of ventricle enlargement. In patients followed over one year, cognitive change was related to baseline normalized brain atrophy measures.[150] Multiple regression analysis showed that brain atrophy accounts for more variance in cognitive impairment than do lesions.[156] Relative to whole-brain atrophy, gray matter atrophy is an even more sensitive marker of cognitive impairment. A cross-sectional study comparing cognitively impaired vs. cognitively preserved RRMS patients found that normalized cortical volume was significantly lower in the cognitively impaired group, and that cortical atrophy was moderately correlated to measures of verbal memory, verbal fluency, and attention/concentration.[157] Cortical atrophy was more closely correlated to cognitive performance scores than whole brain atrophy or T2 lesions. In a follow-up study of these patients after 2.5 years, patients with cognitive deterioration had significantly higher changes in cortical volume than those who remained cognitively stable or improved.[158] A separate study that also measured cortical lesions reported that normalized cortical volume and cortical lesions were independent predictors of cognitive impairment.[159] Regional atrophy analysis has also been used to gain a better understanding of cognitive impairment in MS. One study found that memory dysfunction was best predicted by temporal lobe atrophy, which was the only MRI variable retained in a linear regression model.[160] Processing speed was related to both global and regional atrophy measures and learning consistency was related to frontal atrophy. A subsequent study found that deep gray matter atrophy was related to impairment in new learning and free recall, whereas mesial temporal lobe atrophy had a distinctly different association with performance on delayed recognition tests.[161]

Spinal cord atrophy has been shown to be correlated with disability in all studies, despite differences in atrophy measurement techniques, patient characteristics, and clinical disability measures. Correlations between EDSS and spinal cord tissue loss are not only more consistent but also stronger than correlations between EDSS and brain atrophy.[12,65,107] This finding is likely to be attributable to characteristics of the EDSS, which is heavily weighted toward ambulation, and thus it would be expected to correlate more strongly with tissue damage in the spinal cord than in the brain. In studies that included measures of both brain and cord atrophy, both measures independently predicted disability.[162]

Atrophy in MS clinical trials

The proven clinical and biological relevance of tissue loss, along with the feasibility of measuring volume loss from conventional MRIs, have led to recommendations to use atrophy measurement as a marker of neuroprotection in clinical trials.[163] The treatment effect on atrophy, whether through primary or secondary neuroprotective mechanisms, is now recognized as a key assessment for all potential therapies. Atrophy measures provide information on disease severity that is complementary to lesion-based disease activity measures. Therefore, both atrophy and lesion measures are now typically included as outcome measures in MS clinical trials. (Table 11.3). The results are not easy to compare across trials, mainly because different types of atrophy measures have been used. Some early studies found no treatment effects on atrophy,[103,112,164–166] while others detected possible effects that were difficult to interpret. For example, a two-year Phase 3 trial of IFNβ-1a in RRMS demonstrated a significant treatment effect on whole brain atrophy in the second year of the trial; however, there was no difference in atrophy rates in the first year.[167] Brain atrophy results from placebo-controlled trials of natalizumab[168] and glatiramer acetate (GA)[29] in RRMS demonstrated similar patterns to those observed in the IFN trials (Fig. 11.7): minimal difference between treatment arms over the initial study period, followed by reduced atrophy rate in the active treatment arm compared to placebo in subsequent time periods. Taken together, these studies suggest that anti-inflammatory drugs may have a *delayed* treatment effect on atrophy.

The apparent delay in treatment effects on atrophy may be related to the more immediate effects on inflammation. The resolution of edema that accompanies anti-inflammatory effects may manifest as *accelerated* volume loss, or pseudoatrophy, that stabilizes after the first few months. The accelerated volume loss might mask any early effects on true tissue loss. The delay may also be due to a time lag between inflammatory activity that occurred prior to treatment, and the subsequent destructive processes already in progress after initiation of treatment. Results from several other studies support these hypotheses. A small open-label cross-over trial of IFNβ-1b in RRMS demonstrated that the rate of brain atrophy lessened after the first year of treatment.[120] In a 3-year European trial of IFNβ-1b in

Table 11.3. *Atrophy outcomes in clinical trials, grouped by MS subtype*

Study	Atrophy measure	Subjects	Duration (months)	Study design	Atrophy results
Filippi 2004 IFNβ-1a (s.c.) ETOMS	PBVC	263 CIS	24	Double-blind, plc controlled	Treatment effect on atrophy ($P = 0.003$)
Rudick 1999 IM IFNβ-1a	BPF	140 RR	24	Double-blind, plc controlled	Treatment effect on atrophy only in second year ($P = 0.03$)
Jones 2001 IFNβ-1a (s.c.) PRISMS	WBR	519 RR	24	Double-blind, plc controlled	No treatment effect on atrophy
Hardmeier 2005 IFNβ-1a (IM) dose comparison	BPF	386 RR	36	Randomized to high or low dose	No difference between doses. Reduced atrophy in second and third years compared to year 1.
Frank 2004 IFNβ-1b	WBV	30 RR	36	Open-label, baseline vs. treatment	Reduced atrophy rate in second and third years compared to baseline
O'Connor 2009 IFNβ-1b vs. GA BEYOND	PBVC	2096 early RR	36	Single-blind, randomized to low or high-dose IFN or GA	No differences between treatments. Reduced atrophy in second and third years compared to year 1.
Ge 2000 GA	WBV	27 RR	24	Double-blind, plc controlled	Treatment effect on atrophy
Wolinsky 2001 GA (open-label extension)	Normalized CSF volume	135 RR	82	Open-label long-term follow-up	Reduced atrophy in original GA-treated group compared to original plc group ($P = 0.04$)
Rovaris 2001 GA	CCV	227 RR	18	9m blind, plc controlled, + 9m open label	No treatment effect on atrophy
Sormani 2004 GA	PBVC	207 RR	18	9m blind, plc controlled, + 9m open label	Treatment effect on atrophy in second 9 months ($P = 0.015$)
Zivadinov 2001 IVMP	WBV	88 RR	60	Single-blind controlled	Treatment effect on atrophy ($P = 0.003$)
Miller 2007 natalizumab AFFIRM	BPF	942 RR	24	Double-blind, plc controlled	Treatment effect on atrophy only in second year ($P = 0.004$)
The CAMMS223 Trial Investigators 2009 alemtuzumab vs. IFNβ-1a (s.c.)	CCV	333 RR	36	Single-blind, active arm comparison, high- and low-dose alemtuzumab	Greater treatment effect on atrophy ($P = 0.05$) in alemtuzumab group
Kappos 2010 fingolimod vs. plc, FREEDOMS	PBVC	1033 RR	24	Double-blind, plc controlled, high- and low-dose fingolimod	Treatment effect on atrophy ($P < 0.001$)
Cohen 2010 fingolimod vs. IFNβ-1a (IM) TRANSFORMS	PBVC	1153 RR	24	Double-blind, active arm comparison, high and low dose fingolimod	Greater treatment effect on atrophy ($P < 0.001$) in fingolimod group
Barkhof 2010 Ibudilast (Phase 2)	PBVC	248 RR	12	Double-blind, plc controlled, high and low dose	Dose-dependent treatment effect on atrophy ($P = 0.04$)
Lin 2003 s.c. IFNβ-1a	Spinal cord area	20 RR, 18 SP	48	Double-blind, plc controlled for 2–3 years, + open label	No treatment effect on atrophy
Molyneux 2000 IFNβ-1b	CCV	95 SP	36	Double-blind, plc controlled	No treatment effect on atrophy In subgroup without gad lesions at baseline, more atrophy in plc
Paolillo 1999 Campath1H	CCV	29 SP	18	Crossover	No treatment effect on atrophy Atrophy strongly correlated to gad lesions pre-treatment
Kapoor 2010 lamotrigine	CCV	108 SP	24	Double-blind, plc controlled	No treatment effect on atrophy Greater atrophy in lamotrigine group in year 1
Filippi 2000 cladribine	WBV	159 SP & PP	12	Double-blind, plc controlled	No treatment effect on atrophy
Killestein 2005 riluzole	Spinal cord area + PF	16 PP	24	Run-in vs. treatment pilot	Reduced rate of cord atrophy; minimal change in PF

Abbreviations: BPF = brain parenchymal fraction, CCV = central cerebral volume (4-slice or 7-slice), CIS = clinically isolated syndrome, GA = glatiramer acetate, IFNβ = interferon beta, IM = intramuscular, IVMP = intravenous methylprednisolone, PBVC = percent brain volume change (SIENA), PF = parenchymal fraction, plc = placebo, PP = primary progressive, RR = relapsing-remitting, s.c. = subcutaneous, SP = secondary progressive, WBR = whole brain ratio, WBV = whole brain volume.

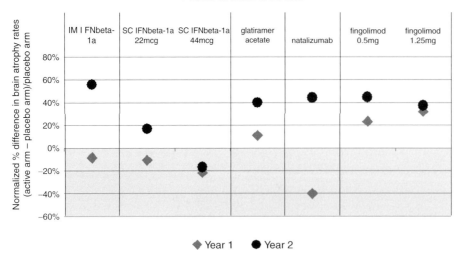

Reductions in atrophy rates relative to placebo in Phase III trials in RRMS

Fig. 11.7. Effects of approved therapies on whole brain atrophy based on published data from Phase 3 placebo-controlled trials in RRMS[29, 31, 166, 168, 178]. Each marker represents the percent difference in mean atrophy rates between the active arm and the placebo arm. A positive value indicates less atrophy in the active arm relative to placebo. In most instances, the treatment effects tended to be higher in the second year compared to the first year, which is consistent with pseudoatrophy effects and/or a delayed observable effect on atrophy because of the kinetics of the pathological process. (Note: The differences in rates are not directly comparable across studies because different techniques were used to calculate atrophy.)

SPMS,[169] there was no treatment effect for the group overall, but stratification by the presence of gadolinium-enhancing lesions at baseline revealed that in the subgroup without enhancing lesions, the treated group had significantly less atrophy than the placebo group.

Studies completed more recently also show evidence of pseudoatrophy. The large head-to-head comparison study of low- and high-dose IFNβ-1b versus GA (BEYOND) found that volume loss as measured with SIENA PBVC was greater in the IFNβ-1b arms compared with GA in the first year, but there were no differences in atrophy between treatment arms over 3 years.[170] Comparison of the reported atrophy rates year-to-year suggested higher rates of volume loss in year 1 compared with years 2 and 3. In years 2 and 3, the mean brain volume changes reported for all three arms were actually positive rather than negative, possibly indicating a partial reversal of the early volume loss, although this was not observed in previous trials of IFNs or GA. Similarly, in the Phase 2 trial of low- and high-dose alemtuzumab vs. IFNβ-1a (CAMMS232), the median changes in central cerebral volume were negative in year 1, but positive in years 2 and 3 in the alemtuzumab groups.[171] Overall, there was a significant reduction in brain atrophy in the combined alemtuzumab arms compared with the IFNβ-1a arm. The positive changes in brain tissue volume reported in years 2 and 3 in both of these studies are not yet understood, and may be related to technical issues. However, the overall pseudoatrophy pattern is consistent with other trials of anti-inflammatory drugs.

The pattern of accelerated volume loss in the first year was not observed in all clinical trials. The ETOMS study of weekly subcutaneous IFNβ-1a in patients with CIS demonstrated a treatment effect on brain atrophy over two years, but PBVC was consistent in year 1 and year 2 in the IFN arm.[172] It is possible that pseudoatrophy is less prominent in the CIS stage of disease or with the dose of subcutaneous IFNβ-1a or dosage interval

used in the ETOMS study, or that steroids administered prior to the baseline scan pre-empted an IFN-induced volume loss. In the large Phase 3 trials of fingolimod (FREEDOMS and TRANSFORMS), there were significant treatment effects on both brain atrophy and gadolinium-enhancing lesions, but no evidence of pseudoatrophy.[173,174] The reduction in the rate of volume loss was already apparent in the first six months of treatment. The lack of even a trend toward pseudoatrophy in a drug with prominent anti-inflammatory effects has not been previously observed, and possibly indicates additional effects separate from reduced inflammation. Explanation for the fingolimod atrophy effects requires further investigation.

The Phase 2 trial of ibudilast offers another example of a compound that demonstrated a treatment effect of atrophy in the first year and no evidence of pseudoatrophy.[175] In this case, the lack of pseudoatrophy is not surprising because there was no effect on inflammatory activity as measured by either relapses or gadolinium-enhancing lesions, the primary outcome measure. Possible neuroprotective effects of ibudilast were further supported by a reduction in the number of enhancing lesions that evolved into persistent black holes. Although the trial was negative based on primary outcome, important data were reported regarding the detection of neuroprotective effects using atrophy and other supporting measures of severe tissue destruction. To date, there has only been one randomized placebo-controlled study prospectively designed to detect neuroprotection through effects on brain atrophy: the lamotrigine study in SPMS.[176] This trial was also negative in that there were no differences in brain atrophy observed between groups. Interestingly, the lamotrigine group had a higher rate of volume loss than the placebo group in year 1, but the kinetics were not entirely consistent with pseudoatrophy as the greatest difference occurred between six and 12 months and there were no concurrent differences in lesion activity observed. Post-study central cerebral volume measurements revealed that the accelerated volume loss in the lamotrigine group was partially reversible upon cessation of treatment. This study highlights the complexity of brain volume measurements and their interpretation in the presence of treatment- and/or MS-induced fluid shifts. More research is needed to derive methods to factor out water changes from true tissue loss.

The lamotrigine study was also one of the few clinical trials that measured gray matter and white matter volumes separately. In that study, the accelerated volume loss was prominently confined to the white matter and there were no differences in gray matter atrophy between groups. This finding is consistent with other recent gray matter atrophy studies, which suggest that therapies may have differential effects on gray matter vs. white matter, that the mechanisms of tissue destruction may differ, and that white matter may be more susceptible to volumetric changes due to fluid shifts, such as pseudoatrophy. A three-year open-label study of IM IFNβ-1a vs. no treatment suggested that IFN had a treatment effect on gray matter but not white matter atrophy.[177] This finding held up in a re-analysis of the MRIs from the Phase 3 placebo-controlled trial of IM IFNβ-1a in which there was less gray matter atrophy in the IFN group compared with placebo, but no differences in white matter atrophy between the groups.[178] There was a more prominent pseudoatrophy effect in white matter compared to gray matter, as evidenced by a higher rate of white matter tissue loss in year 1 in the IFN-treated group. Therefore, gray matter atrophy may provide a better marker of neuroprotection than whole-brain atrophy because the changes are more closely related to true tissue loss as opposed to changes in edema.

Atrophy is attractive as an outcome measure for MS clinical trials because it provides a highly feasible means to test the ability of treatments to halt tissue destruction. The optimal use of atrophy measurements to measure neuroprotection is an important area of ongoing research.

Conclusions

Various reliable techniques have been developed to estimate CNS atrophy. Although atrophy is not pathologically specific, it primarily reflects irreversible tissue loss due to MS, and therefore, it is a valuable marker of disease severity. Brain atrophy can be detected very early in the course of MS, and appears to progress almost from disease onset. Current evidence suggests that atrophy correlates better with neurologic measures of disability than do conventional lesion measurements. Both cross-sectional and longitudinal measurements of atrophy provide important information on disease severity and progression. Atrophy measurement over time in RRMS detects underlying tissue destruction "between relapses", which is not expressed clinically due to functional reserve capacity. Finally, atrophy measurement in SPMS may provide an indication of ongoing tissue destruction not necessarily related inflammatory events in this later stage of the disease.

Atrophy is an attractive component of an MRI-based outcome assessment in MS clinical trials because it reflects diffuse pathologic processes that are not accounted for by lesion measurements, and yet it can still be measured from images acquired with conventional MRI pulse sequences. Gray matter atrophy has emerged as a topic of particular interest because it shows greater clinical and biological relevance than white matter atrophy. Cortical pathology is extensive in MS, and since gray matter lesions cannot be detected with conventional MRI, gray matter atrophy may provide a feasible measure of the extent of cortical pathology. Several areas related to CNS atrophy are still not well-understood: the time course of atrophy following tissue damage, the relationship between focal inflammation and tissue loss in the white matter and in the gray matter, the optimal method for factoring out the confounding effects of water content on atrophy measurements, and the precise pathologic mechanisms of atrophy at different stages of MS. These are all important areas for future research.

References

1. Miller DH, Barkhof F, Frank JA, Parker GJ, Thompson AJ. Measurement of atrophy in multiple sclerosis: pathological basis, methodological aspects and clinical relevance. *Brain* 2002;125(8):1676–95.

2. Gyldensted C. Computer tomography of the cerebrum in multiple sclerosis. *Neuroradiology* 1976;12(1):33–42.

3. Sheldon JJ, Siddharthan R, Tobias J, Sheremata WA, Soila K, Viamonte M, Jr. MR imaging of multiple sclerosis: comparison with clinical and CT examinations in 74 patients. *Am J Roentgenol* 1985;145(5):957–64.

4. Janardhan V, Bakshi R. Quality of life and its relationship to brain lesions and atrophy on magnetic resonance images in 60 patients with multiple sclerosis. *Arch Neurol* 2000;57(10):1485–91.

5. Simon JH, Jacobs LD, Campion MK, *et al.* A longitudinal study of brain atrophy in relapsing multiple sclerosis. The Multiple Sclerosis Collaborative Research Group (MSCRG). *Neurology* 1999;53(1):139–48.

6. Turner B, Ramli N, Blumhardt LD, Jaspan T. Ventricular enlargement in multiple sclerosis: a comparison of three-dimensional and linear MRI estimates. *Neuroradiology* 2001;43(8):608–14.

7. Martola J, Bergstrom J, Fredrikson S, *et al.* A longitudinal observational study of brain atrophy rate reflecting four decades of multiple sclerosis: a comparison of serial 1D, 2D, and volumetric measurements from MRI images. *Neuroradiology* 2010;52(2):109–17.

8. Filippi M, Mastronardo G, Rocca MA, Pereira C, Comi G. Quantitative volumetric analysis of brain magnetic resonance imaging from patients with multiple sclerosis. *J Neurol Sci* 1998;158(2):148–53.

9. Matthews PM, Pioro E, Narayanan S, *et al.* Assessment of lesion pathology in multiple sclerosis using quantitative MRI morphometry and magnetic resonance spectroscopy. *Brain* 1996;119 (3):715–22.

10. Nijeholt GJ, van Walderveen MA, Castelijns JA, *et al.* Brain and spinal cord abnormalities in multiple sclerosis. Correlation between MRI parameters, clinical subtypes and symptoms. *Brain* 1998;121 (4):687–97.

11. Brex PA, Jenkins R, Fox NC, *et al.* Detection of ventricular enlargement in patients at the earliest clinical stage of MS. *Neurology* 2000;54(8):1689–91.

12. Kalkers NF, Bergers E, Castelijns JA, *et al.* Optimizing the association between disability and biological markers in MS. *Neurology* 2001;57(7):1253–8.

13. Wolinsky JS, Narayana PA, Noseworthy JH, *et al.* Linomide in relapsing and secondary progressive MS: part II: MRI results. MRI Analysis Center of the University of Texas-Houston, Health Science Center, and the North American Linomide Investigators. *Neurology* 2000;54(9):1734–41.

14. Dastidar P, Heinonen T, Lehtimaki T, *et al.* Volumes of brain atrophy and plaques correlated with neurological disability in secondary progressive multiple sclerosis. *J Neurol Sci* 1999;165(1):36–42.

15. Losseff NA, Wang L, Lai HM, *et al.* Progressive cerebral atrophy in multiple sclerosis. A serial MRI study. *Brain* 1996;119 (6):2009–19.

16. Bedell BJ, Narayana PA. Automatic removal of extrameningeal tissues from MR images of human brain. *J Magn Reson Imaging* 1996;6(6):939–43.

17. Fisher E. Cothren RM. Tkach JA. Masaryk TJ. Cornhill JF. Knowledge-based 3D segmentation of MR images for quantitative MS lesion tracking. *SPIE Med Imaging* 1997;3034:19–25.

18. Goldszal AF, Davatzikos C, Pham DL, Yan MX, Bryan RN, Resnick SM. An image-processing system for qualitative and quantitative volumetric analysis of brain images. *J Comput Assist Tomogr* 1998;22(5):827–37.

19. Alfano B, Quarantelli M, Brunetti A, *et al.* Reproducibility of intracranial volume measurement by unsupervised multispectral brain segmentation. *Magn Reson Med* 1998;39(3):497–9.

20. Rovaris M, Inglese M, van Schijndel RA, *et al.* Sensitivity and reproducibility of volume change measurements of different brain portions on magnetic resonance imaging in patients with multiple sclerosis. *J Neurol* 2000;247(12):960–5.

21. Bermel RA, Sharma J, Tjoa CW, Puli SR, Bakshi R. A semiautomated measure of whole-brain atrophy in multiple sclerosis. *J Neurol Sci* 208;(1–2):57–65.

22. Chard DT, Parker GJ, Griffin CM, Thompson AJ, Miller DH. The reproducibility and sensitivity of brain tissue volume measurements derived from an SPM-based segmentation methodology. *J Magn Res Imaging* 2002;15(3):259–67.

23. Fox NC, Jenkins R, Leary SM, *et al.* Progressive cerebral atrophy in MS: a serial study using registered, volumetric MRI.[see comment]. *Neurology* 2000;54(4):807–12.

24. Smith SM, De SN, Jenkinson M, Matthews PM. Normalized accurate measurement of longitudinal brain change. *J Comput Assist Tomogr* 2001;25(3):466–75.

25. Ashburner J, Friston KJ. Voxel-based morphometry–the methods. *Neuroimage* 2000;11(6 pt 1):805–21.

26. Udupa JK, Wei L, Samarasekera S, Miki Y, van Buchem MA, Grossman RI. Multiple sclerosis lesion quantification using fuzzy-connectedness principles. *IEEE Trans Med Imaging* 1997;16(5):598–609.

27. Kikinis R, Guttmann CR, Metcalf D, *et al.* Quantitative follow-up of patients with multiple sclerosis using MRI: technical aspects. *J Magn Reson Imaging* 1999;9(4):519–30.

28. Horsfield MA, Rovaris M, Rocca MA, *et al.* Whole-brain atrophy in multiple sclerosis measured by two segmentation processes from various MRI sequences. *J Neurol Sci* 2003;216(1):169–77.

29. Sormani MP, Rovaris M, Valsasina P, Wolinsky JS, Comi G, Filippi M. Measurement error of two different techniques for brain atrophy assessment in multiple sclerosis. *Neurology* 2004;62(8):1432–4.

30. Sharma J, Sanfilipo MP, Benedict RH, Weinstock-Guttman B, Munschauer FE, III, Bakshi R. Whole-brain atrophy in multiple sclerosis measured by automated versus semiautomated MR imaging segmentation. *Am J Neuroradiol.* 2004;25(6):985–96.

31. Rudick RA, Fisher E, Lee JC, Simon J, Jacobs L. Use of the brain parenchymal fraction to measure whole brain atrophy in relapsing–remitting MS. Multiple Sclerosis Collaborative Research Group. *Neurology* 1999;53(8):1698–704.

32. Pfefferbaum A, Mathalon DH, Sullivan EV, Rawles JM, Zipursky RB, Lim KO. A quantitative magnetic resonance imaging study of changes in brain morphology from infancy to late adulthood. *Arch Neurol* 1994;51(9):874–87.

33. Smith SM, Zhang Y, Jenkinson M, *et al.* Accurate, robust, and automated longitudinal and cross-sectional brain change analysis. *Neuroimage* 2002;17(1):479–89.

34. Sepulcre J, Sastre-Garriga J, Cercignani M, Ingle GT, Miller DH, Thompson AJ. Regional gray matter atrophy in early primary progressive multiple sclerosis: a voxel-based morphometry study. *Arch Neurol* 2006;63(8):1175–80.

35. Audoin B, Zaaraoui W, Reuter F, *et al.* Atrophy mainly affects the limbic system and the deep grey matter at the first stage of multiple sclerosis. *J Neurol Neurosurg Psychiatry* 2010;81(6):690–5.

36. Henry RG, Shieh M, Okuda DT, Evangelista A, Gorno-Tempini ML, Pelletier D. Regional grey matter atrophy in clinically isolated syndromes at presentation. *J Neurol Neurosurg Psychiatry* 2008;79(11):1236–44.

37. Studholme C, Cardenas V, Schuff N, Rosen H, Miller B, Weiner M. Detecting spatially consistent structural differences in Alzheimer's and frontotemporal dementia using deformation morphometry. *MICCAI Proceedings* 2001: 41–8.

38. Tao G, Datta S, He R, Nelson F, Wolinsky JS, Narayana PA. Deep gray matter atrophy in multiple sclerosis: a tensor based morphometry. *J Neurol Sci* 2009;282(1–2):39–46.

39. Kidd D, Barkhof F, McConnell R, Algra PR, Allen IV, Revesz T. Cortical lesions in multiple sclerosis. *Brain* 1999;122 (1):17–26.

40. Peterson JW, Bo L, Mork S, Chang A, Trapp BD. Transected neurites, apoptotic neurons, and reduced inflammation in cortical multiple sclerosis lesions. *Ann Neurol* 2001; 50(3):389–400.

41. Alfano B, Quarantelli M, Brunetti A, *et al.* Reproducibility of intracranial volume measurement by unsupervised

multispectral brain segmentation.[see comment]. *Magn Reson Med* 1998;39(3):497–9.

42. Ge Y, Grossman RI, Udupa JK, Babb JS, Nyul LG, Kolson DL. Brain atrophy in relapsing–remitting multiple sclerosis: fractional volumetric analysis of gray matter and white matter. *Radiology* 2001; 220(3):606–10.

43. Chard DT, Griffin CM, Parker GJ, Kapoor R, Thompson AJ, Miller DH. Brain atrophy in clinically early relapsing–remitting multiple sclerosis. *Brain* 2002;125(2):327–37.

44. Nakamura K, Fisher E. Segmentation of brain magnetic resonance images for measurement of gray matter atrophy in multiple sclerosis patients. *Neuroimage* 2009;44(3):769–76.

45. Smith SM, Jenkinson M, Woolrich MW, *et al.* Advances in functional and structural MR image analysis and implementation as FSL. *Neuroimage* 2004;23 (Suppl 1):S208–19.

46. Chen JT, Narayanan S, Collins DL, Smith SM, Matthews PM, Arnold DL. Relating neocortical pathology to disability progression in multiple sclerosis using MRI. *Neuroimage* 2004; 23(3):1168–75.

47. Sailer M, Fischl B, Salat D, *et al.* Focal thinning of the cerebral cortex in multiple sclerosis. *Brain* 2003;126(8):1734–44.

48. Nakamura K, Fox R, Fisher E. CLADA: cortical longitudinal atrophy detection algorithm. *Neuroimage* 2011;54(1): 278–89.

49. Derakhshan M, Caramanos Z, Giacomini PS, *et al.* Evaluation of automated techniques for the quantification of grey matter atrophy in patients with multiple sclerosis. *Neuroimage* 2010;52(4):1261–7.

50. Fischl B, Dale AM. Measuring the thickness of the human cerebral cortex from magnetic resonance images. *Proc Natal Acad Sci USA* 2000; 97(20):11050–5.

51. Kim JS, Singh V, Lee JK, *et al.* Automated 3-D extraction and evaluation of the inner and outer cortical surfaces using a Laplacian map and partial volume effect classification. *Neuroimage* 2005;27(1):210–21.

52. Charil A, Dagher A, Lerch JP, Zijdenbos AP, Worsley KJ, Evans AC. Focal cortical atrophy in multiple sclerosis: relation to lesion load and disability. *Neuroimage* 2007;34(2):509–17.

53. Simon JH, Schiffer RB, Rudick RA, Herndon RM. Quantitative determination of MS-induced corpus callosum atrophy in vivo using MR imaging. *Am J Neuroradiol* 1987; 8(4):599–604.

54. Edwards SG, Liu C, Blumhardt LD. Cognitive correlates of supratentorial atrophy on MRI in multiple sclerosis. *Acta Neurol Scand* 2001;104(4):214–23.

55. Bermel RA, Bakshi R, Tjoa C, Puli SR, Jacobs L. Bicaudate ratio as a magnetic resonance imaging marker of brain atrophy in multiple sclerosis. *Arch Neurol* 2002;59(2):275–80.

56. Meier DS, Fisher E. Atlas-based anatomic labeling in neurodegenerative disease via structure-driven atlas warping. *J Neuroimaging* 2005;15(1):16–26.

57. Evans A, Collins L, Holmes C, *et al.* A 3D probabilistic atlas of normal human neuroanatomy. *Third International Conference on Functional Mapping of the Human Brain*; 1997: 349.

58. Kikinis R, Shenton ME, Iosifescu DV, *et al.* Digital brain atlas for surgical planning, model-driven segmentation and teaching. *IEEE Transa Visualization Comp Graphics* 1996;2:232–41.

59. Ceccarelli A, Rocca MA, Pagani E, *et al.* A voxel-based morphometry study of grey matter loss in MS patients with different clinical phenotypes. *Neuroimage* 2008;42(1):315–22.

60. Sicotte NL, Kern KC, Giesser BS, *et al.* Regional hippocampal atrophy in multiple sclerosis. *Brain* 2008;131(4):1134–41.

61. Sampat MP, Berger AM, Healy BC, *et al.* Regional white matter atrophy–based classification of multiple sclerosis in cross-sectional and longitudinal data. *Am J Neuroradiol* 2009;30(9):1731–9.

62. Audoin B, Davies G, Rashid W, Fisniku L, Thompson AJ, Miller DH. Voxel-based analysis of grey matter magnetization transfer ratio maps in early relapsing remitting multiple sclerosis. *Mult Scler* 2007;13(4): 483–9.

63. Kidd D, Thorpe JW, Thompson AJ, *et al.* Spinal cord MRI using multi-array coils and fast spin echo. II. Findings in multiple sclerosis. *Neurology* 1993;43(12):2632–7.

64. Losseff NA, Webb SL, O'Riordan JI, *et al.* Spinal cord atrophy and disability in multiple sclerosis. A new reproducible and sensitive MRI method with potential to monitor disease progression. *Brain* 1996;119 (3):701–8.

65. Stevenson VL, Leary SM, Losseff NA, *et al.* Spinal cord atrophy and disability in MS: a longitudinal study. *Neurology* 1998;51(1):234–8.

66. Brex PA, Leary SM, O'Riordan JI, *et al.* Measurement of spinal cord area in clinically isolated syndromes suggestive of multiple sclerosis. *J Neurol, Neurosurg Psychiatry* 2001;70(4):544–7.

67. Evangelou N, DeLuca GC, Owens T, Esiri MM. Pathological study of spinal cord atrophy in multiple sclerosis suggests limited role of local lesions. *Brain* 2005;128(1):29–34.

68. Gilmore CP, DeLuca GC, Bo L, *et al.* Spinal cord atrophy in multiple sclerosis caused by white matter volume loss. *Arch of Neurol* 2005;62(12):1859–62.

69. Zivadinov R, Banas AC, Yella V, Abdelrahman N, Weinstock-Guttman B, Dwyer MG. Comparison of three different methods for measurement of cervical cord atrophy in multiple sclerosis. *Am J Neuroradiol* 2008;29(2):319–25.

70. Coulon O, Hickman SJ, Parker GJ, Barker GJ, Miller DH, Arridge SR. Quantification of spinal cord atrophy from magnetic resonance images via a B-spline active surface model. *Magn Res Med* 2002;47(6):1176–85.

71. Horsfield MA, Sala S, Neema M, *et al.* Rapid semi-automatic segmentation of the spinal cord from magnetic resonance images: application in multiple sclerosis. *Neuroimage* 2010;50(2):446–55.

72. Song F, Huan Y, Yin H, *et al.* Normalized upper cervical spinal cord atrophy in multiple sclerosis. *J Neuroimaging* 2008;18(3):320–7.

73. Sormani MP, Rovaris M, Valsasina P, Wolinsky JS, Comi G, Filippi M. Measurement error of two different techniques for brain atrophy assessment in multiple sclerosis. *Neurology* 2004;62(8):1432–4.

74. Anderson VM, Bartlett JW, Fox NC, Fisniku L, Miller DH. Detecting treatment effects on brain atrophy in relapsing remitting multiple sclerosis: sample size estimates. *J Neurol* 2007; 254(11):1588–94.

75. Altmann DR, Jasperse B, Barkhof F, *et al.* Sample sizes for brain atrophy outcomes in trials for secondary progressive multiple sclerosis. *Neurology* 2009;72(7):595–601.

76. De Stebano N, Giorgio A, Battaglini M, *et al.* Assessing brain atrophy rates in a large population of untreated multiple sclerosis subtypes. *Neurology* 2010;74(23):1868–76.

77. Barkhof F, Fisher E, Van Den Elskamp I, *et al.* The effect of temsirolimus on brain atrophy. *Multi Scler* 2009;15, S140. (Abstract)

78. Mehta LR, Schwid SR, Arnold DL, *et al.* Proof of concept studies for tissue-protective agents in multiple sclerosis. *Mult Scler* 2009;15(5): 542–6.

79. Healy B, Valsasina P, Filippi M, Bakshi R. Sample size requirements for treatment effects using gray matter, white matter and whole brain volume in relapsing-remitting multiple sclerosis. *J Neurol Neurosurg Psychiatry* 2009;80(11):1218–23.

80. Chard DT, Parker GJ, Griffin CM, Thompson AJ, Miller DH. The reproducibility and sensitivity of brain tissue volume measurements derived from an SPM-based segmentation methodology. *J. Magn Reson Imaging* 2002;15(3):259–67.

81. Sanfilipo MP, Benedict RH, Sharma J, Weinstock-Guttman B, Bakshi R. The relationship between whole brain volume and disability in multiple sclerosis: a comparison of normalized gray vs. white matter with misclassification correction. *Neuroimage* 2005;26(4):1068–77.

82. Chard DT, Jackson JS, Miller DH, Wheeler-Kingshott CA. Reducing the impact of white matter lesions on automated measures of brain gray and white matter volumes. *J Magn Reson Imaging* 2010;32(1):223–8.

83. Sampat MP, Healy BC, Meier DS, Dell'Oglio E, Liguori M, Guttmann CR. Disease modeling in multiple sclerosis: assessment and quantification of sources of variability in brain parenchymal fraction measurements. *Neuroimage* 2010;52(4):1367–73.

84. Tiberio M, Chard DT, Altmann DR, *et al.* Gray and white matter volume changes in early RRMS: a 2-year longitudinal study. *Neurology* 2005;64(6):1001–7.

85. Duning T, Kloska S, Steinstrater O, Kugel H, Heindel W, Knecht S. Dehydration confounds the assessment of brain atrophy. *Neurology* 2005;64(3):548–50.

86. Enzinger C, Ropele S, Smith S, *et al.* Accelerated evolution of brain atrophy and "black holes" in MS patients with APOE-epsilon 4. *Ann Neurol* 2004; 55(4):563–9.

87. Fox RJ, Fisher E, Tkach J, Lee JC, Cohen JA, Rudick RA. Brain atrophy and magnetization transfer ratio following methylprednisolone in multiple sclerosis: short-term changes and long-term implications. *Mult Scler* 2005;11(2):140–5.

88. Trapp BD, Peterson J, Ransohoff RM, Rudick R, Mork S, Bo L. Axonal transection in the lesions of multiple sclerosis. *N Engl J Med* 1998;338(5):278–85.

89. De Stefano N, Narayanan S, Francis GS, *et al.* Evidence of axonal damage in the early stages of multiple sclerosis and its relevance to disability.[see comment]. *Arch Neurol* 2001;58(1):65–70.

90. Dalton CM, Chard DT, Davies GR, *et al.* Early development of multiple sclerosis is associated with progressive grey matter atrophy in patients presenting with clinically isolated syndromes. *Brain* 2004;127(5):1101–7.

91. Fisher E, Lee JC, Nakamura K, Rudick RA. Gray matter atrophy in multiple sclerosis: a longitudinal study. *Ann Neurol* 2008;64(3):255–65.

92. Anderson VM, Fernando KT, Davies GR, *et al.* Cerebral atrophy measurement in clinically isolated syndromes and relapsing remitting multiple sclerosis: a comparison of registration-based methods. *J Neuroimaging* 2007;17(1):61–8.

93. Di Filippo M, Anderson VM, Altmann DR, *et al.* Brain atrophy and lesion load measures over 1 year relate to clinical status after 6 years in patients with clinically isolated syndromes. *J Neurol Neurosurg Psychiatry* 2010;81(2): 204–8.

94. Calabrese M, Atzori M, Bernardi V, *et al.* Cortical atrophy is relevant in multiple sclerosis at clinical onset. *J Neurol* 2007;254(9):1212–20.

95. Ge Y, Grossman RI, Udupa JK, *et al.* Brain atrophy in relapsing-remitting multiple sclerosis and secondary progressive multiple sclerosis: longitudinal quantitative analysis. *Radiology* 2000;214(3):665–70.

96. Paolillo A, Pozzilli C, Gasperini C, *et al.* Brain atrophy in relapsing–remitting multiple sclerosis: relationship with 'black holes', disease duration and clinical disability. *J Neurol Sci* 2000;174(2):85–91.

97. Battaglini M, Giorgio A, Stromillo ML, *et al.* Voxel-wise assessment of progression of regional brain atrophy in relapsing–remitting multiple sclerosis. *J Neurol Sci* 2009;282(1–2):55–60.

98. Edwards SG, Gong QY, Liu C, *et al.* Infratentorial atrophy on magnetic resonance imaging and disability in multiple sclerosis. *Brain* 1999;122 (2):291–301.

99. Chard DT, Griffin CM, Rashid W, *et al.* Progressive grey matter atrophy in clinically early relapsing–remitting multiple sclerosis. *Multi Scler* 2004;10(4):387–91.

100. Lin X, Blumhardt LD, Constantinescu CS. The relationship of brain and cervical cord volume to disability in clinical subtypes of multiple sclerosis: a three-dimensional MRI study. *Acta Neurol Scand* 2003;108(6):401–6.

101. Tedeschi G, Lavorgna L, Russo P, *et al.* Brain atrophy and lesion load in a large population of patients with multiple sclerosis. *Neurology* 2005;65(2):280–5.

102. Kalkers NF, Ameziane N, Bot JC, Minneboo A, Polman CH, Barkhof F. Longitudinal brain volume measurement in multiple sclerosis: rate of brain atrophy is independent of the disease subtype. *Arch Neurol* 2002;59(10):1572–6.

103. Filippi M, Rovaris M, Iannucci G, Mennea S, Sormani MP, Comi G. Whole brain volume changes in patients with progressive MS treated with cladribine. *Neurology* 2000;55(11):1714–8.

104. Molyneux PD, Kappos L, Polman C, *et al.* The effect of interferon beta-1b treatment on MRI measures of cerebral atrophy in secondary progressive multiple sclerosis. European Study Group on Interferon beta-1b in secondary progressive multiple sclerosis. *Brain* 2000;123 (11):2256–63.

105. Stevenson VL, Miller DH, Rovaris M, *et al.* Primary and transitional progressive MS: a clinical and MRI cross-sectional study. *Neurology* 1999;52(4):839–45.

106. Rovaris M, Bozzali M, Santuccio G, *et al.* In vivo assessment of the brain and cervical cord pathology of patients with primary progressive multiple sclerosis. *Brain* 2001;124(12):2540–9.

107. Rovaris M, Judica E, Sastre-Garriga J, *et al.* Large-scale, multicentre, quantitative MRI study of brain and cord damage in primary progressive multiple sclerosis. *Mult Scler* 2008;14(4):455–64.

108. Pagani E, Rocca MA, Gallo A, *et al.* Regional brain atrophy evolves differently in patients with multiple sclerosis according to clinical phenotype. *Am J Neuroradiol* 2005;26(2):341–6.

109. Simon JH. From enhancing lesions to brain atrophy in relapsing MS. [Review]. *J Neuroimmunol* 1999;98(1):7–15.

110. Leist TP, Gobbini MI, Frank JA, McFarland HF. Enhancing magnetic resonance imaging lesions and cerebral atrophy in patients with relapsing multiple sclerosis. *Arch Neurol* 2001;58(1):57–60.

111. Luks TL, Goodkin DE, Nelson SJ, Majumdar S, Bacchetti P, Portnoy D, et al. A longitudinal study of ventricular volume in early relapsing–remitting multiple sclerosis. *Mult Scler* 2000;6(5):332–7.

112. Rovaris M, Comi G, Rocca MA, Wolinsky JS, Filippi M. Short-term brain volume change in relapsing–remitting multiple sclerosis: effect of glatiramer acetate and implications. *Brain* 2001;124(9): 1803–12.

113. Lin X, Blumhardt LD. Inflammation and atrophy in multiple sclerosis: MRI associations with disease course. *J Neurol Sci* 2001;189(1–2):99–104.

114. Paolillo A, Coles AJ, Molyneux PD, *et al.* Quantitative MRI in patients with secondary progressive MS treated with monoclonal antibody Campath 1H. *Neurology* 1999;53(4):751–7.

115. Saindane AM, Ge Y, Udupa JK, Babb JS, Mannon LJ, Grossman RI. The effect of gadolinium-enhancing lesions on whole brain atrophy in relapsing–remitting MS. *Neurology* 2000;55(1):61–5.

116. Rudick RA, Fisher E, Lee JC, Duda JT, Simon J. Brain atrophy in relapsing multiple sclerosis: relationship to relapses, EDSS, and treatment with

interferon beta-1a. *Mult Scler* 2000;6(6):365–72.

117. Inglese M, Mancardi GL, Pagani E, *et al.* Brain tissue loss occurs after suppression of enhancement in patients with multiple sclerosis treated with autologous haematopoietic stem cell transplantation. *J Neurol, Neurosurg Psychiatry* 2004;75(4):643–4.

118. Jasperse B, Minneboo A, de G, *et al.* Determinants of cerebral atrophy rate at the time of diagnosis of multiple sclerosis. *Arch Neurol* 2007;64(2): 190–4.

119. Mesaros S, Rocca MA, Sormani MP, Charil A, Comi G, Filippi M. Clinical and conventional MRI predictors of disability and brain atrophy accumulation in RRMS. A large scale, short-term follow-up study. *J Neurol* 2008;255(9):1378–83.

120. Frank JA, Richert N, Bash C, *et al.* Interferon-beta-1b slows progression of atrophy in RRMS: Three-year follow-up in NAb- and NAb+ patients. *Neurology* 2004;62(5):719–25.

121. Paolillo A, Piattella MC, Pantano P, *et al.* The relationship between inflammation and atrophy in clinically isolated syndromes suggestive of multiple sclerosis: a monthly MRI study after triple-dose gadolinium-DTPA. *J Neurol* 2004;251(4):432–9.

122. Fisher E, Rudick RA, Simon JH, *et al.* Eight-year follow-up study of brain atrophy in patients with MS. *Neurology* 2002;59(9):1412–20.

123. Zivadinov R, Rudick RA, De MR, *et al.* Effects of IV methylprednisolone on brain atrophy in relapsing–remitting MS. *Neurology* 2001;57(7):1239–47.

124. Chard DT, Brex PA, Ciccarelli O, *et al.* The longitudinal relation between brain lesion load and atrophy in multiple sclerosis: a 14 year follow up study. *J Neurol, Neurosurg Psychiatry* 2003;74(11):1551–4.

125. Quarantelli M, Ciarmiello A, Morra VB, *et al.* Brain tissue volume changes in relapsing-remitting multiple sclerosis: correlation with lesion load. *Neuroimage* 2003;18(2):360–6.

126. Fisniku LK, Chard DT, Jackson JS, *et al.* Gray matter atrophy is related to long-term disability in multiple sclerosis. *Ann Neurol* 2008;64(3):247–54.

127. De Stefano N, Matthews PM, Filippi M, *et al.* Evidence of early cortical atrophy

in MS: relevance to white matter changes and disability. *Neurology* 2003;60(7):1157–62.

128. Sastre-Garriga J, Ingle GT, Chard DT, *et al.* Grey and white matter volume changes in early primary progressive multiple sclerosis: a longitudinal study. *Brain* 2005;128(6):1454–60.

129. van Walderveen MA, Kamphorst W, Scheltens P, *et al.* Histopathologic correlate of hypointense lesions on T1-weighted spin-echo MRI in multiple sclerosis. *Neurology* 1998;50(5):1282–8.

130. Kalkers NF, Bergers E, Castelijns JA, *et al.* Optimizing the association between disability and biological markers in MS. *Neurology* 2001;57(7):1253–8.

131. Kalkers NF, Vrenken H, Uitdehaag BM, Polman CH, Barkhof F. Brain atrophy in multiple sclerosis: impact of lesions and of damage of whole brain tissue. *Multi Scler* 2002;8(5):410–4.

132. Furby J, Hayton T, Altmann D, *et al.* Different white matter lesion characteristics correlate with distinct grey matter abnormalities on magnetic resonance imaging in secondary progressive multiple sclerosis. *Mult Scler* 2009;15(6):687–94.

133. Brochet B, Dousset V. Pathological correlates of magnetization transfer imaging abnormalities in animal models and humans with multiple sclerosis. *Neurology* 1999;53(Suppl 3):S12–17.

134. Schmierer K, Scaravilli F, Altmann DR, Barker GJ, Miller DH. Magnetization transfer ratio and myelin in postmortem multiple sclerosis brain. *Ann Neurol* 2004;56(3):407–15.

135. Rovaris M, Bozzali M, Rodegher M, Tortorella C, Comi G, Filippi M. Brain MRI correlates of magnetization transfer imaging metrics in patients with multiple sclerosis. *J Neurol Sci* 1999;166(1):58–63.

136. Traboulsee A, Dehmeshki J, Peters KR, *et al.* Disability in multiple sclerosis is related to normal appearing brain tissue MTR histogram abnormalities. *Mult Scler* 2003;9(6):566–73.

137. De Stefano N, Iannucci G, Sormani MP, *et al.* MR correlates of cerebral atrophy in patients with multiple sclerosis. *J Neurol* 2002;249(8):1072–7.

138. Ge Y, Gonen O, Inglese M, Babb JS, Markowitz CE, Grossman RI. Neuronal

cell injury precedes brain atrophy in multiple sclerosis. *Neurology* 2004;62(4):624–7.

139. Rovaris M, Gallo A, Falini A, *et al.* Axonal injury and overall tissue loss are not related in primary progressive multiple sclerosis. *Arch Neurol* 2005; 62(6):898–902.

140. Bermel RA, Puli SR, Rudick RA, *et al.* Prediction of longitudinal brain atrophy in multiple sclerosis by gray matter magnetic resonance imaging T2 hypointensity. *Arch Neurol* 2005;62(9):1371–6.

141. Raz E, Cercignani M, Sbardella E, *et al.* Gray- and white-matter changes 1 year after first clinical episode of multiple sclerosis: MR imaging. *Radiology* 2010;257(2):448–54.

142. Rudick R, Antel J, Confavreux C, *et al.* Recommendations from the National Multiple Sclerosis Society Clinical Outcomes Assessment Task Force. *Ann Neurol* 1997;42(3):379–82.

143. Fisher E, Rudick RA, Cutter G, *et al.* Relationship between brain atrophy and disability: an 8-year follow-up study of multiple sclerosis patients. *Mult Scler* 2000;6(6):373–7.

144. Rudick RA, Lee JC, Nakamura K, Fisher E. Gray matter atrophy correlates with MS disability progression measured with MSFC but not EDSS. *J Neurol Sci* 2009;282(1–2):106–11.

145. Minneboo A, Jasperse B, Barkhof F, *et al.* Predicting short-term disability progression in early multiple sclerosis: added value of MRI parameters. *J Neurol Neurosurg Psychiatry* 2008;79(8):917–23.

146. Di FM, Anderson VM, Altmann DR, *et al.* Brain atrophy and lesion load measures over 1 year relate to clinical status after 6 years in patients with clinically isolated syndromes. *J Neurol Neurosurg Psychiatry* 2010;81(2):204–8.

147. Rudick RA, Cutter G, Baier M, *et al.* Use of the Multiple Sclerosis Functional Composite to predict disability in relapsing MS. *Neurology* 2001;56(10):1324–30.

148. Jasperse B, Vrenken H, Sanz-Arigita E, *et al.* Regional brain atrophy development is related to specific aspects of clinical dysfunction in multiple sclerosis. *Neuroimage* 2007;38(3):529–37.

149. Rao SM, Glatt S, Hammeke TA, *et al.* Chronic progressive multiple sclerosis.

Relationship between cerebral ventricular size and neuropsychological impairment. *Arch Neurol* 1985;42(7): 678–82.

150. Hohol MJ, Guttmann CR, Orav J, *et al.* Serial neuropsychological assessment and magnetic resonance imaging analysis in multiple sclerosis. *Arch Neurol* 1997;54(8):1018–25.

151. Benedict RH, Carone DA, Bakshi R. Correlating brain atrophy with cognitive dysfunction, mood disturbances, and personality disorder in multiple sclerosis. [Review]. *J Neuroimaging* 2004; 14(3 Suppl): 36S–45S.

152. Lazeron RH, Boringa JB, Schouten M, *et al.* Brain atrophy and lesion load as explaining parameters for cognitive impairment in multiple sclerosis. *Mult Scler* 2005;11(5):524–31.

153. Feinstein A, Roy P, Lobaugh N, Feinstein K, O'Connor P, Black S. Structural brain abnormalities in multiple sclerosis patients with major depression. *Neurology* 2004;62(4): 586–90.

154. Marrie RA, Fisher E, Miller DM, Lee JC, Rudick RA. Association of fatigue and brain atrophy in multiple sclerosis. *J Neurol Sci* 2005;228(2): 161–6.

155. Tedeschi G, Dinacci D, Lavorgna L, *et al.* Correlation between fatigue and brain atrophy and lesion load in multiple sclerosis patients independent of disability. *J Neurol Sci* 2007;263(1–2):15–19.

156. Benedict RH, Weinstock-Guttman B, Fishman I, Sharma J, Tjoa CW, Bakshi R. Prediction of neuropsychological impairment in multiple sclerosis: comparison of conventional magnetic resonance imaging measures of atrophy and lesion burden. *Arch Neurol* 2004;61(2):226–30.

157. Amato MP, Bartolozzi ML, Zipoli V, *et al.* Neocortical volume decrease in relapsing–remitting MS patients with mild cognitive impairment. *Neurology* 2004;63(1):89–93.

158. Amato MP, Portaccio E, Goretti B, *et al.* Association of neocortical volume changes with cognitive deterioration in relapsing–remitting multiple sclerosis. *Arch Neurol* 2007;64(8):1157–61.

159. Calabrese M, Agosta F, Rinaldi F, *et al.* Cortical lesions and atrophy associated with cognitive impairment in

relapsing-remitting multiple sclerosis. *Arch Neurol* 2009;66(9):1144–50.

160. Benedict RH, Zivadinov R, Carone DA, *et al.* Regional lobar atrophy predicts memory impairment in multiple sclerosis. *Am J Neuroradiol* 2005;26(7):1824–31.

161. Benedict RH, Ramasamy D, Munschauer F, Weinstock-Guttman B, Zivadinov R. Memory impairment in multiple sclerosis: correlation with deep grey matter and mesial temporal atrophy. *J Neurol Neurosurg Psychiatry* 2009;80(2):201–6.

162. Bonati U, Fisniku LK, Altmann DR, *et al.* Cervical cord and brain grey matter atrophy independently associate with long-term MS disability. *J Neurol Neurosurg Psychiatry* 2010;**82** (4): 471–2.

163. Barkhof F, Calabresi PA, Miller DH, Reingold SC. Imaging outcomes for neuroprotection and repair in multiple sclerosis trials. *Nat Rev Neurol* 2009;5(5):256–66.

164. Lin X, Tench CR, Turner B, Blumhardt LD, Constantinescu CS. Spinal cord atrophy and disability in multiple sclerosis over four years: application of a reproducible automated technique in monitoring disease progression in a cohort of the interferon beta-1a (Rebif) treatment trial.[see comment]. *J Neurol, Neurosurg Psychiatry* 2003;74(8):1090–4.

165. Wolinsky JS, Narayana PA, Johnson KP, Multiple Sclerosis Study Group and the MRI Analysis Center. United States open-label glatiramer acetate extension trial for relapsing multiple sclerosis: MRI and clinical correlates. Multiple Sclerosis Study Group and the MRI Analysis Center. *Multi Scler* 2001;7(1):33–41.

166. Jones CK, Riddehough A, Li DKB, *et al.* MRI cerebral atrophy in relapsing-remitting MS: results from the PRISMS trial. *Neurology* 2001;**56**[Suppl 3]: A379.

167. Rudick RA, Fisher E, Lee JC, Simon J, Jacobs L. Use of the brain parenchymal fraction to measure whole brain atrophy in relapsing-remitting MS. Multiple Sclerosis Collaborative Research Group. *Neurology* 1999;53(8):1698–704.

168. Miller DH, Soon D, Fernando KT, *et al.* MRI outcomes in a placebo-controlled trial of natalizumab in

relapsing MS. *Neurology* 2007;68(17): 1390–401.

169. Molyneux PD, Kappos L, Polman C, *et al.* The effect of interferon beta-1b treatment on MRI measures of cerebral atrophy in secondary progressive multiple sclerosis. European Study Group on Interferon beta-1b in secondary progressive multiple sclerosis. *Brain* 2000;123 (11): 2256–63.

170. O'Connor P, Filippi M, Arnason B, *et al.* 250 microg or 500 microg interferon beta-1b versus 20 mg glatiramer acetate in relapsing-remitting multiple sclerosis: a prospective, randomised, multicentre study. *Lancet Neurol* 2009;8(10): 889–97.

171. Coles AJ, Compston DA, Selmaj KW, *et al.* Alemtuzumab vs. interferon beta-1a in early multiple sclerosis. *N Engl J Med* 2008;359(17):1786–801.

172. Filippi M, Rovaris M, Inglese M, *et al.* Interferon beta-1a for brain tissue loss in patients at presentation with syndromes suggestive of multiple sclerosis: a randomised, double-blind, placebo-controlled trial. *Lancet* 2004; 364(9444):1489–96.

173. Kappos L, Radue EW, O'Connor P, *et al.* A placebo-controlled trial of oral fingolimod in relapsing multiple sclerosis. *N Engl J Med* 2010;362(5):387–401.

174. Cohen JA, Barkhof F, Comi G, *et al.* Oral fingolimod or intramuscular interferon for relapsing multiple sclerosis. *N Engl J Med* 2010;362(5):402–15.

175. Barkhof F, Hulst HE, Drulovic J, Uitdehaag BM, Matsuda K, Landin R. Ibudilast in relapsing-remitting multiple sclerosis: a neuroprotectant? *Neurology* 2010;74(13):1033–40.

176. Kapoor R, Furby J, Hayton T, *et al.* Lamotrigine for neuroprotection in secondary progressive multiple sclerosis: a randomised, double-blind, placebo-controlled, parallel-group trial. *Lancet Neurol* 2010;9(7):681–8.

177. Zivadinov R, Locatelli L, Cookfair D, *et al.* Interferon beta-1a slows progression of brain atrophy in relapsing-remitting multiple sclerosis predominantly by reducing gray matter atrophy. *Mult Scler* 2007;13(4):490–501.

178. Nakamura K, Rudick RA, Lee J-C, Foulds P, Fisher E. Effect of Intramuscular Interferon beta-1a on gray matter atrophy in relapsing-remitting multiple sclerosis. *Neurology* 2010; 74(Suppl 2); A 407.

12

Axonal pathology in patients with multiple sclerosis
Evidence from in vivo proton magnetic resonance spectroscopy

Sridar Narayanan, Zografos Caramanos, Paul M. Matthews, and Douglas L. Arnold

Introduction

The clinical course of multiple sclerosis (MS) is highly variable, and pathological changes that are seen with the disease are heterogeneous amongst individuals. In recent years, there has been increasing interest in the development of magnetic resonance imaging (MRI) approaches to characterizing the pathological substrates of disability in MS[1] with the objective of developing quantitative in vivo indices of pathology that could provide new insights into the pathogenesis of the disease, as well as provide more specific or sensitive end-points for treatment trials.

This chapter reviews results from studies that have used either proton magnetic resonance spectroscopy (^{1}H-MRS, a technique that allows for the acquisition of [1]H-MR spectra from single voxels) or [1]H-MR spectroscopic imaging (^{1}H-MRSI, a technique that allows for the simultaneous acquisition of [1]H-MR spectra from multiple voxels) to measure in vivo chemical pathology associated with impairment of axonal metabolic or structural integrity, and places these results in the context of relevant histopathological investigations. We will focus on an important hypothesis that has developed from these studies: that axonal pathology is central to the final common pathway leading to the progressive disability that is seen in individuals with this disease.

The case for the contribution of axonal pathology in patients with MS (see Chapter 2)
Demyelination alone cannot account for the chronic functional impairments in patients with MS

Compared with the inflammatory lesions of infectious encephalitides or ischemic infarction, microscopic examination of MS plaques shows demyelination with a relative preservation of axons. This observation, in conjunction with findings of conduction block following acute demyelination, led to an early focus on demyelination of the white matter (WM) of the central nervous system (CNS) as a unifying explanation for the range of functional impairments found in patients with MS.[2] However, demyelination alone does not seem to adequately explain the functional impairments and

their evolution in patients with MS (for a review, see Smith and McDonald[3]). For example, conduction can recover even in still segmentally demyelinated axons.[4] In patients with optic neuritis, even though there may be early conduction block after acute inflammation, conduction can recover across even chronically demyelinated regions of the optic nerve.[5] Furthermore, even though the propagation of action potentials in the optic nerve of the myelin-deficient rat is approximately five times slower than normal, this propagation is stable and has refractory and frequency-following properties that are similar to those of myelinated axons in the wild-type.[6]

This can be explained by the adaptive molecular changes found in the chronic condition. For example, mice deficient in class I MHC (i.e. β2-microglobulin deficient mice) that are infected with Theiler's murine encephalomyelitis virus develop extensive demyelination, but without neurological deficits.[7] Recovery in this model is associated with increased axonal sodium-channel density. By contrast, class II MHC-deficient mice develop paresis leading to death after infection and do not show axonal sodium channel up-regulation.

Mechanisms of acute conduction block are distinct from those responsible for chronic functional impairment

More generally, axonal adaptations (including the increased expression of new sodium channels) can contribute to the maintenance of axonal function with chronic demyelination.[8] It is important to distinguish pathophysiologically between the phenomena of acute and chronic impairment of axonal function with demyelination; mechanisms responsible for acute conduction block are different from those that cause chronic functional impairment.

Mechanisms of acute conduction block

Conduction block occurs acutely after demyelination in part because of the relatively sparse distribution of sodium channels in the newly exposed, but otherwise-intact, internodal axon membrane;[9] with adaptive up-regulation in the demyelinated axon, they become distributed spatially along the membrane to

Multiple Sclerosis Therapeutics, Fourth Edition, ed. Jeffrey A. Cohen and Richard A. Rudick. Published by Cambridge University Press.
© Cambridge University Press 2011.

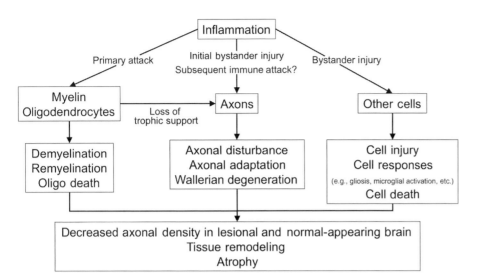

Fig. 12.1. Flow chart summarizing the bases and outcomes of axonal pathology in the lesional and normal-appearing brain tissue of patients with multiple sclerosis.

allow restoration of conduction.[10] There is evidence that insertion of new sodium channels in demyelinated axons also occurs in patients with MS: patients show up to a four-fold increase in saxitoxin binding (i.e. a measure of the density of sodium channels) in demyelinated regions of WM.[11]

The inflammatory response itself is probably partially responsible for some of the acute conduction block that is seen in MS. Local inflammation can lead to injury or dysfunction of axons even if the axons are not the direct auto-immune target by means of locally released inflammatory mediators (e.g. nitric oxide and other reactive oxygen species) that cause metabolic dysfunction and conduction block.[12,13] With exposures for only short periods of time or at low enough concentrations, these effects are reversible. This likely accounts in part for functional recovery with resolution of inflammation in patients within the initial relapsing–remitting (RR) stage of the disease.

Anti-neuronal antibodies may contribute to this potentially reversible dysfunction. For example, antibodies directed against GM1 gangliosides cause conduction block by suppressing the axonal sodium current necessary for depolarization.[14] Relative selectivity of antibodies for different subtypes of sodium channels may account for the apparent variability of conduction block between different classes of axons.[15]

Mechanisms of *chronic* functional impairment: the "axonal hypothesis"

Defining the pathological changes that are ultimately responsible for the chronic functional impairments that are seen in patients with MS is critical for the optimal targeting of new therapies. Indeed, trials of apparently effective anti-inflammatory therapies have highlighted an apparent dissociation between efficacy in the modulation of new inflammation and an impact on the short-term progression of disability.[16,17] In conjunction with evidence of the type cited above, such observations emphasize that acute demyelination cannot be the primary or proximate pathological substrate for chronic disability. As a result,

we have proposed an "axonal hypothesis" for the chronic disability: axonal injury or loss is required for – and the extent of axonal loss directly determines the degree of – chronic functional impairment and disability in MS.[18,19]

Figure 12.1 is an overview of the proposed pathogenesis of axonal injury in MS and the presumed associated changes in other tissue components of the brain. The primary attack in MS is presumed to be directed against myelin or oligodendrocytes, at least initially. Axons are thought to be injured as "innocent bystanders" as a result of the local effects of soluble inflammatory mediators. In the longer term, however, axons may also be targeted by a direct immune response that may develop as a secondary consequence of the chronic tissue injury. If the acute injury to myelin or axons is sublethal, there may be partial recovery of conduction associated with remyelination and/or axonal adaptations such as the insertion of new sodium channels. On the other hand, lethally injured and transected axons undergo Wallerian degeneration during which the distal, disconnected segments of axons and their myelin degenerate and are eventually removed.[20] This process results in decreased axonal density in both the lesional and the normal-appearing brain tissues of patients with MS, and would contribute to explaining the generalized brain and spinal cord atrophy observed in these patients.[21]

A prediction of the axonal hypothesis is that chronic, irreversible disability is associated with irreversible axonal loss. A second prediction is that reversible axonal injury should be associated with the functional recovery that is seen after a relapse. As we will see, evidence supporting both contentions has come from studies that have used ^{1}H-MRS or ^{1}H-MRSI (hereafter referred to as ^{1}H-MRS(I)) to investigate the brains of patients with MS.[22] Indeed, such studies have allowed for the quantitative and non-invasive in vivo assessment of axonal disturbance in such patients and, thereby, have furthered our understanding of the dynamic relationship between axonal pathology and clinical disability in patients with MS.

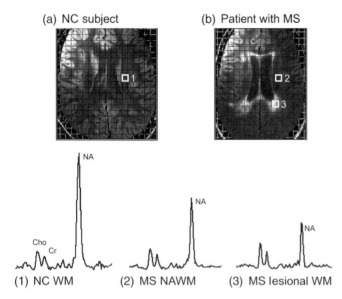

Fig. 12.2. Conventional MRI showing the phase-encoding grid for ¹H-MRSI studies in: (a) a normal control (NC) subject and (b) a patient with multiple sclerosis (MS). Below these are shown sample spectra acquired with an echo time of 272 ms from, as indicated in the images above: (1) a voxel of normal white matter (WM) in the NC subject; as well as (2) a voxel of homologous normal-appearing white matter (NAWM), and (3) a voxel of lesional WM in the patient with MS. Note the decreased NA peak in the voxel of MS NAWM as compared to that in the voxel of NC WM, and the even-further decreased NA peak in the voxel of MS lesional-WM.

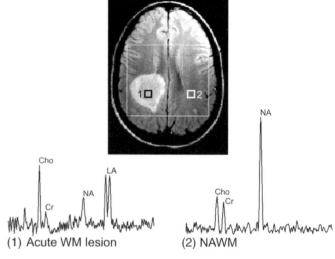

Fig. 12.3. Conventional MRI and the volume of excitation chosen for ¹H-MRSI in a patient with multiple sclerosis. Below are shown sample ¹H-MRSI spectra acquired with an echo time of 272 ms from, as indicated in the image above: (1) a voxel within a large, isolated, acute white matter (WM) lesion and (2) a voxel within the homologous, contralateral normal-appearing WM (NAWM). Note the increased Cho peak, the decreased NA peak, and the increased LA peak in the voxel of acute, lesional WM as compared to that in the voxel of NAWM.

¹H-MRS(I) evidence for axonal pathology in patients with MS

Introduction to ¹H-MRS(I)

A limitation of conventional MRI techniques (i.e. techniques such as T1- and T2-weighted imaging) is that the associated image contrast is affected by too many factors to allow for changes in such contrast to be interpreted in terms of specific pathological processes. ¹H-MRS(I) studies allow the acquisition of information about hydrogen nuclei (i.e. protons) from molecules other than water[23] and provide specific information regarding pathological changes in both the lesional and the normal-appearing brain tissue in patients with MS.[24] Importantly, as we will see below, these spectroscopic techniques seem to provide specific information regarding impairment of function or integrity of the neuro-axonal unit. Even though the low concentrations of intracellular metabolites that are being measured with ¹H-MRS(I) allow a spatial resolution for these spectroscopic methods that is much lower (i.e. on the order of 1 cm³) than for conventional MRI (which can readily be acquired at a spatial resolution on the order of 1 mm³), inferences based on the combination of these two types of imaging techniques can be both pathologically specific and usefully spatially well-resolved.

There are two major factors that determine whether metabolite resonances can be usefully studied by ¹H-MRS(I) of the brain in vivo: the correlation time (a measure of molecule mobility) and the concentration of the nuclei observed. In consequence: (i) only those molecules that are freely mobile give rise to well-defined, discrete resonances and (ii) only molecules that are relatively abundant (i.e. those with concentrations on the order of millimoles per liter) afford sufficient signal-to-noise for practical study in vivo. As shown in Figs. 12.2 and 12.3, the water-suppressed, localized ¹H-MRSI spectra of the human brain acquired at relatively-long echo times reveal major resonances of choline-containing phospholipids (Cho), the methyl-resonance of creatine and phosphocreatine (Cr), the methyl-resonance of N-acetyl-containing compounds (NA), and (under appropriate observational conditions) resonances from lactate and mobile lipids or macromolecules (LA). At shorter echo times, resonances from amino acids such as glutamate and γ-aminobutyric acid (GABA) and from sugars such as myo-inositol can also be identified (Fig. 12.4).

The NA resonance

In the adult mammalian CNS, the NA resonance primarily reflects the presence of N-acetylaspartate (NAA) and, to a lesser extent, N-acetylaspartylglutamate (NAAG). NAA is synthesized by neuronal mitochondria and is found at very high concentrations in the mammalian brain, second only to glutamate in terms of free amino acid concentrations.[25] NAA has been posited to have multiple roles, serving as (i) a source of acetyl groups necessary for the synthesis of myelin lipids,[26] (ii) a molecular water pump in myelinated neurons,[27] and (iii) a neuronal precursor for NAAG, which is the most prevalent and widely distributed neuropeptide in the mammalian nervous system.[28] NAAG is also thought to play multiple roles as

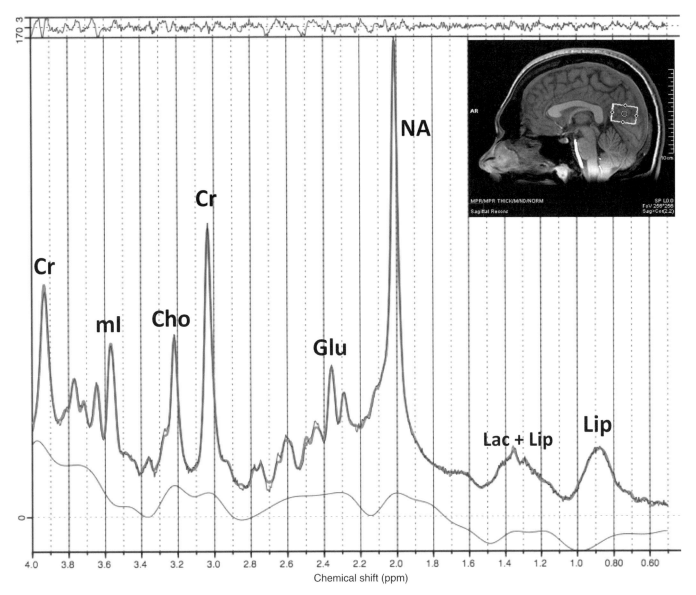

Fig. 12.4. Short-echo ¹H-MRS PRESS spectrum (TE = 30 ms) acquired at 3T from a 30 x 30 x 20 mm³ voxel over the posterior cingulate cortex, positioned as indicated by the inset. Compared to the long-echo spectra of Figs. 12.2 and 12.3, this spectrum shows many more metabolites, but also illustrates the complex baseline and overlapping resonances typical of short-echo spectra. Higher field (3T or greater) helps resolve overlapping resonances to some degree, but relatively sophisticated fitting techniques are needed for robust quantitation.

(i) a neurotransmitter,[29] (ii) a modulator of the effects of other neurotransmitters,[28] (iii) a source of extracellular glutamate[28] and (iv) – in conjunction with NAA – a cell-specific signaling molecule mediating communication among neurons, astrocytes, and oligodendrocytes.[30] In the adult CNS, these two molecules seem to both be localized almost exclusively to neurons and neuronal processes,[31,32] with only traces of NAA being seen in the glial cells, where it is metabolized. Because of the presence of its constituent metabolites in neurons and its prominence in the ¹H-MR spectrum, decreases in the integrated magnitude of the NA resonance have been widely used as an indicator of brain pathology and disease progression in a variety of CNS diseases, including MS.[19,33,34]

It should be noted that, although NAA has been found in cell cultures of oligodendroglial cell lineage,[35–37] this seems to be a phenomenon that is largely limited to in vitro cell cultures. NAA is not present in significant concentrations in astrocytes or mature oligodendrocytes that are harvested in vivo.[35,37] Evidence for the specificity of NAA as an axon-specific marker of mature WM in vivo – even in the presence of injury and a high density of oligodendroglial cell precursors – has been provided by a study directly relating biochemical and immunohistochemical changes after rat optic nerve transection.[38] The validity of NAA as a surrogate measure of axonal density in patients with MS has also been established by studies reporting strong correlations (i) between findings from in vivo

^{1}H-MRS and from histopathological analysis of cerebral biopsy specimens[39] and (ii) between findings from high-performance liquid chromatography and those from histopathological analysis of spinal cord biopsy specimens.[40]

Interpreting changes in NA

Because ^{1}H-MRS(I) spectra reflect the amount of NA within a voxel(s) of interest, decreases in the NA signal can occur as a result of any of the following within-voxel changes: (i) decreases in relative axonal density due to axonal loss or atrophy, (ii) decreases in neuro-axonal NA concentration due to mitochondrial metabolic dysfunction within the neurons and axons that are still present, (iii) dilution of NA secondary to edema or to infiltration with non-NA-containing cells, or (iv) some combination of these factors. As a result, depending on the nature of the pathology that is responsible, observed decreases in NA may be either irreversible or reversible.[41–44] Permanent axonal loss may result from axonal transection and Wallerian degeneration,[45] while reversible metabolic dysfunction may be associated with either sublethal injury associated with a reversible decrease in mitochondrial NA synthesis[46] or local tissue concentration changes with the resolution of acute edema.[47]

The Cr resonance

In the adult mammalian CNS, the Cr resonance reflects the presence of creatine and phosphocreatine – two molecules that are known to play an important role in energy metabolism, with phosphocreatine representing reserves of high-energy phosphates that provide for homeostasis and energy needs.[23,48,49] The Cr peak is present in both neurons and glial cells, but its concentration has been shown to be the highest in astrocytes and oligodendrocytes (at least when expressed in terms of nM/mg protein).[35]

NA/Cr ratios

Because Cr concentration is relatively constant throughout the brain and is also relatively resistant to change, one common approach to quantifying ^{1}H-MRS(I) data is to use the within-voxel resonance intensity of Cr as an internal standard for that of other metabolites.[50] For example, the use of within-voxel NA/Cr ratios as an index of neuro-axonal integrity now is increasingly common in the study of patients with MS.[24,33,51] However, while this intra-voxel normalization corrects for a multitude of technical difficulties that can affect absolute quantitation, as well as for dilution effects due to edema, this comes at the expense of introducing a dependency on changes in the concentration of Cr (which may be affected in patients with MS).[52] Nevertheless, tissue-specific changes in the mean NA/Cr values of patients with MS have been shown to be highly concordant with the changes in their mean NA concentrations within the same tissues.[52] Furthermore, NA/Cr values in patients with MS have been shown to have a high degree of convergent validity

as they are correlated strongly with measures of clinical disability,[53–55] as well as to changes in other imaging measures of MS neuropathology (e.g. cerebral atrophy[56] or functional measures of adaptive reorganization[57]).

The Glu and Gln resonances

Glutamate is the primary excitatory neurotransmitter in the brain. Neurons produce glutamate from glutamine via the enzyme glutaminase.[58] Glutamate released by neurons into the synaptic cleft during neurotransmission is transported into astrocytes, where it is aminated to glutamine that then is released for uptake into neurons as part of a neural–glial glutamate–glutamine cycle.[58,59] In the extrasynaptic WM of the CNS, oligodendrocytes are the cells largely responsible for glutamate clearance.[60,61] Measurement of glutamate in the brains of patients with MS is of interest given the observations that: (i) glutamate excitotoxicity is associated with neurodegeneration in other disorders such as Alzheimer's disease and amyotrophic lateral sclerosis,[62] (ii) glutamate also is produced by infiltrating lymphocytes and activated microglia,[63–65] and (iii) excess glutamate has been associated with axonal and oligodendrocyte damage.[63]

In patients with MS, glutamate re-uptake by oligodendrocytes appears to be impaired.[60] Furthermore, as measured in vivo with a novel J-resolved MRS technique,[66] total glutamate (both intracellular and extracellular) has been shown to be elevated in the acute lesions and in the normal-appearing WM of patients with MS, although not in their chronic lesions.[67] Recent work has also suggested that genetic factors associated with in vivo levels of glutamate in patients with MS may in turn be associated with lower brain NA values and brain volume,[68] supporting the hypothesis that glutamate toxicity may play a role in neurodegeneration in MS.

Measurement issues

While resonances from glutamate (Glu) and glutamine (Gln) are observable on short-echo ^{1}H-MRS, their quantification can be challenging. Because of its molecular structure and consequent interaction with the nuclei of other metabolites (J-coupling), the proton spectrum of glutamate is complex. At the conventional field strength of 1.5 T, the glutamate signal overlaps considerably with the signal from glutamine, GABA and NA, making reliable quantification of Glu difficult. As a result, studies at 1.5 T have generally reported the magnitude of the integrated C4 Glu + Gln (referred to as Glx) resonances, but this approach does not capture relative concentration changes associated with altered Glu–Gln cycling. Overlap of the two resonances is greatly reduced at higher field strengths such as 3 T, but appreciable overlap remains. Several fairly complex approaches have been developed to improve the selective quantification of Glu using 2D J-resolved spectral editing techniques.[66,69,70] However, it has been shown recently that by careful selection of the echo time (TE), measurement of Glu at

3 T using a standard PRESS (point resolved spectroscopy) technique is as reliable as the more complex techniques.[70,71] An echo time of 40 ms has been demonstrated to substantially reduce signal contributions from overlapping resonances to the 2.35 ppm (parts-per-million) C4 Glu resonance via J-modulation effects, while minimizing loss of signal and T2-weighting as compared to higher echo times (such as 80 ms) that may be more selective for Glu.[71] Another benefit of using a relatively short TE is that quantification of Gln and GABA is still possible, though with lower precision than for Glu or NA.[71]

^{1}H-MRS(I) evidence for substantial axonal disturbance in patients with MS

The most striking observation made by the initial ^{1}H-MRS studies of patients with MS was that the mean NA/Cr ratio in central slabs of their brains was lower than that in the homologous tissue of normal control (NC) subjects.[72] As the mean Cr/Cho ratio was normal in these patients, it was concluded that NA concentration in their brains must have been reduced, implying that there was a substantial loss of axonal integrity throughout the WM. This was confirmed subsequently by direct, quantitative neuropathological study.[73] The observation of low cerebral NA/Cr was then confirmed in numerous subsequent studies[51,74–81] and has now been shown to be present at even the earliest stages of the disease.[55,82,83]

Importantly, these earliest ^{1}H-MRS(I) studies of patients with MS showed substantial decreases in brain NA, even though lesions occupied only a small fraction of the ^{1}H-MRS(I) volume of interest. This suggested that axonal pathology was widespread in patients with MS and not restricted just to the T2-hyperintense lesions. Indeed, as can be seen in Fig. 12.2, decreases in NA resonance intensity of up to 50%[84] can be observed even in these patients' so-called "normal-appearing" WM (NAWM); that is, the WM that appears normal on both gross pathological examination and conventional MRI. Detailed examination of such NAWM has demonstrated not just histopathological evidence for axonal loss,[73,85–89] but also evidence consistent with potentially reversible functional impairments of mitochondria,[90] (iii) microglial activation,[91,92] and astrocytic proliferation.[91,92]

As can be seen in Figs. 12.2 and 12.3, the resonance intensity of NA in WM within regions of hyperintense T2 signal is lower than in the NAWM, with reductions of 80% or more being seen in extreme cases.[42] The spatial distribution of axonal pathology around large, acute lesions shows a gradient with greater injury (as suggested by decreasing NA/Cr values on ^{1}H-MRSI) closer to the center of a lesion relative to adjacent or more distant NAWM.[74] However, direct measurements of the absolute concentrations of these metabolites has confirmed that NA concentrations within both the lesional WM and NAWM of patients with MS are consistently reduced relative to those in the WM of NC subjects.[39,52,93] Furthermore, the relationship between decreases in NAA resonance intensities to decreases in axonal density in the subacute lesions of patients with MS has

been confirmed in brain-biopsy specimens that were obtained stereotactically[39] and in spinal-cord tissue samples obtained post-mortem.[40]

^{1}H-MRS(I)-measured values of NA within the gray matter (GM) of patients with MS have also been shown to be decreased relative to those in NC subjects – both in cortical[94–100] and subcortical[101–103] GM tissue. Importantly, a study that combined spectroscopic and histopathological analysis of the thalamus has provided evidence that neuronal loss could be responsible for a large proportion of the chronic reduction of NA that is seen in the thalamic GM of patients with MS.[101]

The overall consistency and magnitude of the findings from these and many other recent ^{1}H-MRS(I) studies is supported by the results of a meta-analysis that we recently performed to integrate information from all of the peer-reviewed studies to date.[52] We assessed the consensus of the mean absolute (or semi-absolute) concentrations of Cr and NA in the lesional WM, the non-lesional WM, and/or the GM of patients with MS and contrasted these values with those in the homologous tissues of normal control (NC) subjects. We found a large effect-size[104] for the decrease in mean concentrations of NA in patients' lesional WM relative to NC WM, a medium effect-size decrease in patients' non-lesional WM relative to NC WM and a medium effect-size decrease in patients' GM relative to NC GM. Across all studies, although some reported no difference in the mean NA concentration for patients relative to NC, none reported increases. We also evaluated the consensus evidence for changes in mean concentrations of brain Cr with MS. We found no statistically significant overall change in the patients' mean lesional WM Cr relative to NC mean WM Cr, although statistically significant increases and decreases were found in some studies. A medium effect-size for an increase of Cr in patients' non-lesional WM relative to NC WM was observed, but no statistically significant change of Cr was seen in patients' GM relative to NC GM. Importantly, the direction of change in the mean concentration of NA and the mean NA/Cr ratios was concordant in almost all of the contrasts for which both of these sets of data were available. Together, these results confirmed the presence of a widespread decrease in neuro-axonal integrity throughout the brains of patients with MS (as indicated by decreased concentrations of NA within the WM lesions, the NAWM, and the GM of such patients). These results also suggested that, even though within-voxel NA/Cr ratios are not simply indices of NA content, they do represent a practical compromise between technical complexity and general feasibility as an index of neuro-axonal integrity.[52]

^{1}H-MRS(I) findings agree with histopathological evidence of axonal damage in patients with MS

Despite the emphasis over the last several decades on the damage to myelin and oligodendrocytes in the brains of patients with MS, even the earliest neuropathological studies of such material demonstrated axonal injury and loss in and around the lesions of patients with this disease: what was "forgotten" in the emphasis on MS as a demyelinating disease in the latter half of the twentieth century is that Charcot[105] and other pathologists emphasized that there was a *relative* preservation of axons in patients with MS (thereby contrasting MS with other highly destructive inflammatory diseases such as encephalitis). Indeed, as we will now see, the aforementioned ^{1}H-MRS(I) evidence is consistent with recent histopathological findings in the lesional and normal-appearing brain tissues of patients with MS.

WM histopathology

The ^{1}H-MRS(I) findings of decreased NA in the lesional WM of patients with MS[52] are in agreement with findings from numerous histopathological studies that have shown axonal damage and loss in both the acute and chronic lesions of such individuals.[106–108] Interestingly, axonal loss varies considerably between lesions,[109] and axonal injury (at least as assessed via the expression of amyloid precursor protein) is far more extensive than is axonal transection.[110] Furthermore, the ^{1}H-MRS(I) findings of decreased NA in the NAWM of patients with MS[52] are also in agreement with recent histopathological findings – with numerous studies now showing that the axonal loss that is seen in the lesional WM also extends substantially into the NAWM.[73,85–89] For example, in one recent histopathological study of the corpora callosa of patients with MS,[73] axonal density was found to be decreased by a mean of 35% in the NAWM outside of lesions; moreover, these patients also demonstrated an overall loss of WM volume, implying an even greater total axonal loss.

GM histopathology

Despite the fact that cortical GM lesions have long been recognized in patients with MS on detailed histopathological examination,[111,112] until recently such GM pathology has routinely been underestimated because it has been difficult to detect using standard techniques.[113] For example, GM lesions are not evident on conventional post-mortem examinations[114,115] because cortical myelin is not readily apparent on routine histological staining with Luxol fast blue, and cortical lesions are not hypercellular and, therefore, are not readily identified on hematoxylin-eosin-stained sections. Furthermore, GM lesions are also not evident on conventional MRI examinations[116–118] because GM lesions are small or thin (when they are band-like, making them subject to partial volume effects on MRI) and they are associated with much less inflammation[114,119] and demyelination[119] than is typical of WM lesions, which means that they are associated with very little contrast on conventional T2-weighted or T1-weighted MRI. Nevertheless, a number of different types of GM lesions have now been described by histopathological analysis and these lesions have been shown to be much more widespread than was previously appreciated.[118–121] Indeed, a number of

post-mortem studies have now quantified the surprisingly high number of cortical lesions in MS.[111,112,116,118,119] For example, the prevalence of GM lesions can be inferred from the results of the study by Peterson *et al.*,[119] in which immunocytochemical analysis identified as many as 112 cortical lesions within 110 blocks of tissue from 50 patients with MS. Importantly, these GM lesions not only showed evidence of demyelination, but they also demonstrated axonal and dendritic transection, as well as neuronal apoptosis (particularly in neurons whose axons showed demyelination). It is also important to keep in mind that, in addition to this widespread lesional-GM pathology, GM that is not directly affected by macroscopic lesions in patients with MS may also be affected indirectly by neuronal and dendritic changes that may occur secondary to axonal injury within their lesional and normal-appearing WM.[108,110] Thus, the ^{1}H-MRS(I) findings of decreased NA in the GM of patients with MS[52,122] are also in agreement with findings from histopathological studies of the GM in such individuals.

The relationship between ^{1}H-MRS(I) findings and clinical disability

^{1}H-MRS(I) measurements of NA correlate with measures of clinical disability in patients with MS

The axonal hypothesis that we have proposed posits that chronic neuro-axonal pathology (however it may occur) is the major proximate cause of chronic functional impairment in patients with MS. If this is true, then one might expect a negative correlation between patients' ^{1}H-MRS(I)-measured levels of brain NA (indicative of neuro-axonal integrity) and levels of clinical disability – both cross-sectionally and longitudinally.

One of the first ^{1}H-MRSI studies of such patients suggested that this was indeed the case,[72] a demonstration that was followed by that of Davie *et al.*[123] who then showed that MS patients with high cerebellar dysfunction scores had lower cerebellar concentrations of NA than those with low cerebellar dysfunction scores, and that healthy controls had higher cerebellar concentrations of NA than either patient group. More recently, cross-sectional studies also have shown strong negative correlations between cerebral WM NA/Cr and disability in patients with relapsing–remitting MS (RR-MS).[34,84] Importantly, in a recent study that examined the results of a number of conventional and non-conventional MRI techniques, cerebral NA/Cr values were found to have the strongest relationship with measures of clinical disability.[53]

In addition to these cross-sectional findings, at least two studies have suggested that ^{1}H-MRS(I)-measured WM NA/Cr values are sensitive to the increasing axonal damage that is to be expected from increasing disease burden across time. In an early, serial study of patients with MS, single-voxel [1]H-MR spectra that were acquired from a volume centered on the corpus callosum demonstrated a decrease in NA/Cr that was found to progress over eighteen months.[75] This was confirmed in a follow-up study with a larger group of patients, although the mean rate of decrease of NA/Cr in the larger study was slower.[124] These and other studies have suggested that serial measurements of NA/Cr in the voxels that are typically included in ^{1}H-MRSI studies are reproducible to within 5–10%, and that changes of this magnitude can be readily detected even with relatively short-term follow-up. However, the mean changes in NA/Cr across time that are measured in groups of patients with MS can vary from 0%[125] to about 5%[84] per year, making the statistical power of such longitudinal ^{1}H-MRS(I) studies variable.

The importance of ^{1}H-MRS(I)-measured axonal disturbance in NAWM

Even though axonal loss and damage seem to be less severe in the NAWM of patients with MS than in individual WM lesions, the contribution of the axonal disturbance within the NAWM may be even more significant than that from within the lesional WM in terms of determining the chronic, non-relapse-related disability that is seen in such patients. This is because NAWM constitutes, by far, the greatest bulk of their WM.

One of the earliest studies to suggest the potential importance of such NAWM abnormalities compared changes on conventional MRI and ^{1}H-MRS(I) in both a group of patients with RR-MS and a group of patients with secondary progressive MS (SP-MS).[126] The degree of axonal disturbance (as assessed by decreases in their mean central-brain NA/Cr ratios) was significantly greater in the group of patients with SP-MS, who also had longer disease duration as well as more-severe clinical disability. In order to better understand these findings and the relationship between progression of chronic disability in patients with MS and the relative concentration of NA in their brains, statistical models were used to determine the correlations over time between the spatial distribution of chemical changes on ^{1}H-MRSI and the presence of lesions on conventional MRI.[84,127] In this way, the time course of NA/Cr changes could be followed with respect to the spatial distribution of NA/Cr across the brain and to the presence or absence of T2-weighted lesions in the same areas. This approach demonstrated that brain NA/Cr values were lower in SP-MS than in RR-MS patients because of a lower NA/Cr ratio in the NAWM for SP-MS patients rather than because of differences within T2-hyperintense lesions.[84] Furthermore, this approach confirmed earlier reports[75] that showed progressive decreases in NA/Cr with time and correlations between such decreases in NAWM NA/Cr values and progression of disability in patients with MS. The strong correlation of decreased NAWM NA/Cr with increasing disability has since been confirmed and extended with measurements of absolute concentrations of NA.[52,93]

The relationship between clinical remission and the recovery of ^{1}H-MRS(I)-measured NA

The remission of symptoms following exacerbations of MS is likely to be associated with multiple factors, including, e.g. the restoration of conduction in persisting axons[11] and the contribution of functional adaptations.[57,128] An initially unexpected observation was that acute MS lesions (Figs. 12.2 and 12.3) can also be associated with reversible decreases in NA/Cr.[41,74] Consistent with the neuro-axonal hypothesis, these reversible decreases are associated with a concomitant reversal of functional impairments.[41] For example, serial studies of individual ^{1}H-MRS(I) voxels have shown that initial NA/Cr decreases of 30%–80% within the centers of lesions can demonstrate variable recovery (sometimes even complete) after the acute phase of the patient's clinical exacerbation has passed – with such NA/Cr recovery being most rapid over the first few months after the relapse.[41] Furthermore, such reversible decreases in NA/Cr values can also be detected in the projection pathways of such acutely inflammatory demyelinating lesions.[44]

Given that the relative volumetric changes (even in large lesions) are smaller than the initial relative decrease in NA,[47] only a proportion of the apparent decrease and subsequent recovery of NA in these large lesions can be related to the formation and subsequent resolution of local edema. Other factors that could contribute to NA recovery after acute demyelination include reversible changes in axonal diameter associated with demyelination and remyelination,[129–131] and reversible suppression of axonal mitochondrial function by soluble factors associated with acute inflammation.[12] Furthermore, mitochondrial toxins have also been shown to be associated with reversible decreases in NAA,[132] and in vitro studies of a neuronal cell line have also demonstrated that decreases in NAA following serum deprivation can be fully reversed by further incubation in serum-containing medium.[133] Thus, the recovery of NA in such lesions can result, for example, from an increase in the relative within-voxel axonal volume, an increase in the concentration of NA within the remaining axons, or a combination of these these mechanisms. At this point, it is worth re-emphasizing that ^{1}H-MRS(I)-measured NA values do not only provide information regarding the loss or damage of neurons and their processes (including axons) as is traditionally assessed by histopathological investigation; rather, because the concentration of NA is very sensitive to mitochondrial dysfunction, ^{1}H-MRS(I)-measured NA values also provide information regarding the metabolic integrity of neurons and their processes.

Implications for understanding the natural history and treatment of patients with MS

As we have seen, evidence from histopathological and ^{1}H-MRS(I) studies of patients with MS suggest that chronic, progressive changes in the disability of such patients may reflect the chronic, progressive axonal pathology that is now appreciated to be a key feature of this disease.[9,113,134] Indeed, a principal conclusion of recent ^{1}H-MRS(I) studies is that neuro-axonal disturbance is manifest throughout the normal-appearing WM and the GM of the brains of patients with MS, not just in their focal WM lesions where the most prominent inflammatory changes occur.[52,84,93] Furthermore, axonal pathology in patients with MS is not restricted to only axonal transection and loss;

rather, axonal-metabolic dysfunction seems to also play a role in the acute, reversible functional impairments that are associated with relapses in patients with MS,[3] and such dysfunction may also play a role in the functional impairments that seem to be related to the diffuse, non-lesional pathology that is seen in these patients. These observations have a number of important implications for the understanding of MS and for the treatment of patients with this disease.

First, these observations suggest that a given treatment strategy may not be equally efficacious for all aspects of MS pathogenesis or for all patients. Indeed, if there is significant heterogeneity of pathological mechanisms between different stages of MS and between individuals, it may be rational to tailor treatments for particular pathological subgroups. Thus, it is hoped that a combination of conventional and non-conventional imaging methods could provide a clinically practical way of stratifying patients for different treatments based on degrees of, for example, inflammation, neuronal disturbance, myelin disturbance (e.g. as measured via short-T2 imaging[135] or magnetization transfer imaging[136,137]), and tissue loss (e.g. as quantified via measures of brain and spinal cord atrophy[138–144]).[145] Furthermore, there is a need to coordinate findings from histopathological studies with those from conventional and non-conventional MRI studies in order to better interpret the "in vivo pathology" that is suggested by the latter.

Second, there is a need for the development of new drugs or combinations of drugs that are targeted against the multiple mechanisms that seem to be responsible for the progression of CNS pathology in patients with MS. For example, although most currently used approaches are directed primarily towards limiting the acute inflammatory responses, new therapeutics development for MS is being targeted toward neuroprotection and mechanisms that could enhance functional re-organization of the brain.[146–150] While treatments such as axonal potassium-channel blockade by aminopyridines[151,152] may be expected to have their greatest impact over only a limited period in lesion evolution (i.e. during the period of acute conduction block), activity-dependent neurotrophic modulation[153] could translate into longer-lasting impact on the magnitude or quality of recovery after acute demyelination. Moreover, further development of strategies based on the use of neurotrophins and other neuronal survival factors may be important for enhancing axonal survival and the potential for recovery in the longer term. Finally, efforts to control specific mechanisms of axonal injury, such as those that might be mediated by sodium overload[154] or by antibodies directed against[155] sodium channels, also need to be explored.

A third major conclusion from the work reviewed above arises from the observation that axonal injury occurs even in acute lesions. With this in mind, the rationale for reducing relapse rate and treating acute relapses changes from that of short-term enhancement of the quality of life to that of preventing the accumulation of later, more-severe axonal loss and associated disability. The sensitivity of clinical measures in short trials for detecting such changes is understandably limited,

suggesting that the use of potentially more-sensitive surrogate markers (e.g. composite measures of inflammation, neuronal integrity, myelin integrity, and brain-tissue loss) may provide a practical approach to rapidly identifying new drugs that could limit the progression of axonal damage. Furthermore, an appreciation for the role of axonal injury in the progression of chronic disability and the mechanisms by which inflammation leads to axonal injury should enhance enthusiasm for early treatment of patients that is aimed at reducing inflammation.

The specificity of the NA signal to neuroaxonal integrity suggests the utility of ^{1}H-MRS(I) in assessing the effectiveness of new treatments targeting neuroaxonal protection. However, to date, ^{1}H-MRS(I) has not been used extensively in clinical trials, perhaps due to the complexities of performing standardized acquisition and analysis of ^{1}H-MRS(I) data in the context of a multicenter study. A number of single-center studies have been reported using ^{1}H-MRS(I) to evaluate MS therapies.[43,156–161] These open-label studies have generally included relatively small numbers of patients, but significant, beneficial effects on limiting or even reversing axonal injury have been shown for interferon beta-1b,[43,157] glatiramer acetate,[159,160] and fluoxetine,[161] suggesting that ^{1}H-MRS(I) measures of NA have sufficient power to be used in randomized, controlled trials.

Early cross-sectional, multicenter studies employing ^{1}H-MRS(I) constrained acquisition to a single scanner make to reduce cross-scanner variability, with the data analysis performed centrally.[56,163] These studies showed that NA/Cr ratios were comparable across centers when using the same scanner, sequences, and post-processing. The first use of ^{1}H-MRS(I) in a longitudinal, randomized, double-blind, multicenter, and *multi-scanner* study of a new MS therapeutic was performed as a sub-study of a phase 3 trial of oral glatiramer acetate.[164] A large, central-brain volume of interest containing mostly normal-appearing brain tissue was used to provide information on the effect of treatment on diffuse neuroaxonal pathology, complementing lesion-based data from MRI. Participation was not constrained to sites with a specific make of scanner in order to enable the enrollment of more patients. To minimize the impact of differences in metabolite ratios due to sequence implementation differences on different scanners, paired changes over time were compared across the treatment arms. The main MRS outcome was change of NA/Cr from baseline to termination (13 months). The data showed no change in metabolite ratios in either the treated or placebo group, and hence no treatment effect, in agreement with the other study outcomes,[165] a finding that was at least partially due to the generally inactive patient population recruited into this study. However, this sub-study did establish the feasibility of including ^{1}H-MRS(I) measures in a multicenter clinical trial, and suggested practical considerations that helped enable this. Building on this experience, ^{1}H-MRS then was used in the subsequent Phase 3, double-blind, randomized, placebo-controlled trial of glatiramer acetate for patients with clinically isolated syndromes (CIS). Data from a large, central-brain, single-voxel were acquired from 34 patients enrolled at ten clinical sites in seven countries with a standardized protocol. Paired changes of NA/Cr were significantly different between patients treated with glatiramer acetate compared to placebo after 12 months, providing class-A evidence of neuroaxonal protection by a disease-modifying therapy for MS. The MRS protocol used for this study was incorporated into published guidelines for the use of ^{1}H-MRS(I) in multicenter MS studies.[166]

Ultimately, the development of multiple, complementary methods for the definition and classification of the pathological changes that are seen within the CNS of patients with MS[1,113] may contribute towards rational approaches to the preparation of in vivo strategies for the simultaneous targeting of multiple pathological stages with combined therapy. Such approaches should also allow for improved trial designs, not only by increasing the precision with which trial end-points based on such biomarkers can be reached, but also by providing pathological specificity that should allow for trials of new agents even in populations that are already being treated with agents targeting other stages in the pathological progression of the disease.

Conclusions

The results of recent ^{1}H-MRS(I) and neuropathological studies of the brains of patients with MS have focused the attention of the MS research community on the importance of widespread axonal pathology in what has, until recently, been thought of primarily as a demyelinating disease of the WM. Early axonal injury is most likely the result of "innocent bystander"

damage that is associated with the inflammatory response directed against myelin and oligodendrocytes. However, given that axons depend on glia for trophic and other support, accumulating glial damage may ultimately lead to axonal atrophy, dysfunction, and subsequent transection. ^{1}H-MRS(I) studies of neuroaxonal NA levels have emphasized that axonal disturbance in the brains of patients with MS can be substantial and widespread – encompassing both the lesional and normal-appearing WM and GM – and that it can begin even early in the course of the disease. Furthermore, the ability to observe axonal disturbance in vivo that is made possible by ^{1}H-MRS(I) allows for correlations across time to be made between measures of axonal pathology and measures of clinical disability. The role of glutamate in mediating neuronal, axonal and oligodendrocyte damage in MS is a promising area of investigation enabled by ^{1}H-MRS(I), with potentially important implications for future therapies. Taken together, these observations suggest that ^{1}H-MRS(I) has an important role to play in the assessment of new treatments for MS that are directed towards either limiting the damage to the neuro-axonal CNS or to enhancing its recovery after inflammatory damage.

Acknowledgments

SN, ZC, and DLA are grateful for support from the Canadian Institutes for Health Research and the Multiple Sclerosis Society of Canada. PMM acknowledges support from the Medical Research Council of Great Britain and the Multiple Sclerosis Society of Great Britain and Northern Ireland and is a full-time employee of GlaxoSmithKline, Ltd.

References

1. Caramanos Z, Santos AC, Arnold DL. Magnetic resonance imaging and spectroscopy: Insights into the pathology and pathophysiology of multiple sclerosis. In McDonald WI, Noseworthy JH, eds. *Multiple Sclerosis 2, Blue Books of Practical Neurology Series (Vol. 27)*. USA: Butterworth-Heinemann, 2003:139–67.

2. Waxman SG. Membranes, myelin, and the pathophysiology of multiple sclerosis. *N Engl J Med* 1982;306(25):1529–33.

3. Smith KJ, McDonald WI. The pathophysiology of multiple sclerosis: the mechanisms underlying the production of symptoms and the natural history of the disease. *Philos Trans R Soc Lond B Biol Sci* 1999;354(1390):1649–73.

4. Felts PA, Baker TA, Smith KJ. Conduction in segmentally demyelinated mammalian central axons. *J Neurosci* 1997;17(19):7267–77.

5. Youl BD, Turano G, Miller DH, et al. The pathophysiology of acute optic neuritis. An association of gadolinium leakage with clinical and electrophysiological deficits. *Brain* 1991;114 (6):2437–50.

6. Utzschneider DA, Thio C, Sontheimer H, Ritchie JM, Waxman SG, Kocsis JD. Action potential conduction and sodium channel content in the optic nerve of the myelin-deficient rat. *Proc Biol Sci* 1993;254(1341):245–50.

7. Rivera-Quinones C, McGavern D, Schmelzer JD, Hunter SF, Low PA, Rodriguez M. Absence of neurological deficits following extensive demyelination in a class I-deficient murine model of multiple sclerosis. *Nat Med* 1998;4(2):187–93.

8. Waxman SG, Craner MJ, Black JA. Na$^+$ channel expression along axons in multiple sclerosis and its models. *Trends Pharmacol Sci* 2004;25(11):584–91.

9. Waxman SG. Demyelinating diseases – new pathological insights, new therapeutic targets. *N Engl J Med* 1998;338(5):323–5.

10. England JD, Gamboni F, Levinson SR, Finger TE. Changed distribution of sodium channels along demyelinated axons. *Proc Natl Acad Sci USA* 1990;87(17):6777–80.

11. Moll C, Mourre C, Lazdunski M, Ulrich J. Increase of sodium channels in demyelinated lesions of multiple sclerosis. *Brain Res* 1991;556(2):311–16.

12. Redford EJ, Kapoor R, Smith KJ. Nitric oxide donors reversibly block axonal conduction: demyelinated axons are especially susceptible. *Brain* 1997;120 (12):2149–57.

13. Brosnan CF, Litwak MS, Schroeder CE, Selmaj K, Raine CS, Arezzo JC. Preliminary studies of cytokine-induced functional effects on the visual pathways in the rabbit. *J Neuroimmunol* 1989;25(2–3):227–39.

14. Takigawa T, Yasuda H, Kikkawa R, Shigeta Y, Saida T, Kitasato H. Antibodies against GM1 ganglioside affect K⁺ and Na⁺ currents in isolated rat myelinated nerve fibers. *Ann Neurol* 1995;37(4):436–42.

15. Waxman SG. Sodium channel blockade by antibodies: a new mechanism of neurological disease? *Ann Neurol* 1995;37(4):421–3.

16. Panitch H, Miller A, Paty D, Weinshenker B. Interferon beta-1b in secondary progressive MS: results from a 3-year controlled study. *Neurology* 2004;63(10):1788–95.

17. Kappos L, Weinshenker B, Pozzilli C, *et al.* Interferon beta-1b in secondary progressive MS: a combined analysis of the two trials. *Neurology* 2004;63(10):1779–87.

18. Fu L, Matthews PM, De Stefano N, *et al.* Imaging axonal damage of normal-appearing white matter in multiple sclerosis. *Brain* 1998;121(1):103–13.

19. Matthews PM, De Stefano N, Narayanan S, *et al.* Putting magnetic resonance spectroscopy studies in context: axonal damage and disability in multiple sclerosis. *Semin Neurol* 1998;18(3):327–36.

20. Meyer R, Weissert R, Diem R, *et al.* Acute neuronal apoptosis in a rat model of multiple sclerosis. *J Neurosci* 2001;21(16):6214–220.

21. Simon JH. Brain and spinal cord atrophy in multiple sclerosis. *Neuroimaging Clin N Am* 2000;10(4):753–70,ix.

22. Arnold DL, Matthews PM, De Stefano N. MRI and proton MRS in the evaluation of multiple sclerosis. In Bachelard HS, ed. *Magnetic Resonance Spectroscopy and Imaging in Neurochemistry.* Vol 8. New York: Plenum Publishing Corp 1997:267–88.

23. Ross B, Bluml S. Magnetic resonance spectroscopy of the human brain. *Anat Rec* 2001;265(2):54–84.

24. Arnold DL, De Stefano N, Narayanan S, Matthews PM. Proton MR spectroscopy in multiple sclerosis. *Neuroimaging Clin N Am* 2000;10(4):789–89.

25. Birken DL, Oldendorf WH. N-acetyl-L-aspartic acid: a literature review of a compound prominent in 1H-NMR spectroscopic studies of brain. *Neurosci Biobehav Rev* 1989;13(1):23–31.

26. Chakraborty G, Mekala P, Yahya D, Wu G, Ledeen RW. Intraneuronal N-acetylaspartate supplies acetyl groups for myelin lipid synthesis: evidence for myelin-associated aspartoacylase. *J Neurochem* 2001;78(4):736–45.

27. Baslow MH. Evidence supporting a role for N-acetyl-L-aspartate as a molecular water pump in myelinated neurons in the central nervous system. An analytical review. *Neurochem Int* 2002;40(4):295–300.

28. Neale JH, Bzdega T, Wroblewska B. N-Acetylaspartylglutamate: the most abundant peptide neurotransmitter in the mammalian central nervous system. *J Neurochem* 2000;75(2):443–52.

29. Blakely RD, Coyle JT. The neurobiology of N-acetylaspartylglutamate. *Int Rev Neurobiol* 1988;30:39–100.

30. Baslow MH. Functions of N-acetyl-L-aspartate and N-acetyl-L-aspartylglutamate in the vertebrate brain: role in glial cell-specific signaling. *J Neurochem.* Aug 2000;75(2):453–459.

31. Simmons ML, Frondoza CG, Coyle JT. Immunocytochemical localization of N-acetyl-aspartate with monoclonal antibodies. *Neuroscience* 1991;45(1):37–45.

32. Moffett JR, Namboodiri MA, Cangro CB, Neale JH. Immunohistochemical localization of N-acetylaspartate in rat brain. *Neuroreport* 1991;2(3):131–34.

33. Arnold DL, Wolinsky JS, Matthews PM, Falini A. The use of magnetic resonance spectroscopy in the evaluation of the natural history of multiple sclerosis. *J Neurol Neurosurg Psychiatry* 1998; 64 Suppl 1: S94–101.

34. De Stefano N, Bartolozzi ML, Guidi L, Stromillo ML, Federico A. Magnetic resonance spectroscopy as a measure of brain damage in multiple sclerosis. *J Neurol Sci* 2005;233(1–2):203–8.

35. Urenjak J, Williams SR, Gadian DG, Noble M. Proton nuclear magnetic resonance spectroscopy unambiguously identifies different neural cell types. *J Neurosci* 1993;13(3):981–9.

36. Bhakoo KK, Pearce D. In vitro expression of N-acetyl aspartate by oligodendrocytes: implications for proton magnetic resonance spectroscopy signal in vivo. *J Neurochem* 2000;74(1):254–62.

37. Urenjak J, Williams SR, Gadian DG, Noble M. Specific expression of N-acetylaspartate in neurons, oligodendrocyte-type-2 astrocyte progenitors, and immature oligodendrocytes in vitro. *J Neurochem* 1992;59(1):55–61.

38. Bjartmar C, Battistuta J, Terada N, Dupree E, Trapp BD. N-acetylaspartate is an axon-specific marker of mature white matter in vivo: a biochemical and immunohistochemical study on the rat optic nerve. *Ann Neurol* 2002;51(1):51–8.

39. Bitsch A, Bruhn H, Vougioukas V, *et al.* Inflammatory CNS demyelination: histopathologic correlation with in vivo quantitative proton MR spectroscopy. *Am J Neuroradiol* 1999;20(9):1619–27.

40. Bjartmar C, Kidd G, Mork S, Rudick R, Trapp BD. Neurological disability correlates with spinal cord axonal loss and reduced N-acetyl aspartate in chronic multiple sclerosis patients. *Ann Neurol* 2000;48(6):893–901.

41. De Stefano N, Matthews PM, Antel JP, Preul M, Francis G, Arnold DL. Chemical pathology of acute demyelinating lesions and its correlation with disability. *Ann Neurol* 1995;38(6):901–9.

42. De Stefano N, Matthews PM, Arnold DL. Reversible decreases in N-acetylaspartate after acute brain injury. *Magn Reson Med* 1995;34(5):721–7.

43. Narayanan S, De Stefano N, Francis GS, *et al.* Axonal metabolic recovery in multiple sclerosis patients treated with interferon beta-1b. *J Neurol* 2001;248(11):979–86.

44. De Stefano N, Narayanan S, Matthews PM, Francis GS, Antel JP, Arnold DL. In vivo evidence for axonal dysfunction remote from focal cerebral demyelination of the type seen in multiple sclerosis. *Brain* 1999;122 (10):1933–9.

45. Bjartmar C, Battistuta J, Terada N, Dupree E, Trapp BD. N-acetylaspartate is an axon-specific marker of mature white matter in vivo: a biochemical and immunohistochemical study on the rat optic nerve. *Ann Neurol* 2002;51(1):51–8.

46. Dautry C, Vaufrey F, Brouillet E, *et al.* Early N-acetylaspartate depletion is a marker of neuronal dysfunction in rats

and primates chronically treated with the mitochondrial toxin 3-nitropropionic acid. *J Cereb Blood Flow Metab* 2000;20(5):789–99.

47. Helms G. Volume correction for edema in single-volume proton MR spectroscopy of contrast-enhancing multiple sclerosis lesions. *Magn Reson Med* 2001;46(2):256–63.

48. Wyss M, Kaddurah-Daouk R. Creatine and creatinine metabolism. *Physiol Rev* 2000;80(3):1107–213.

49. Miller BL. A review of chemical issues in 1H NMR spectroscopy: *N*-acetyl-L-aspartate, creatine and choline. *NMR Biomed* 1991;4(2):47–52.

50. De Stefano N, Narayanan S, Mortilla M, *et al.* Imaging axonal damage in multiple sclerosis by means of MR spectroscopy. *Neurol Sci* 2000;21(4 Suppl 2):S883–7.

51. Matthews PM, Francis G, Antel J, Arnold DL. Proton magnetic resonance spectroscopy for metabolic characterization of plaques in multiple sclerosis. *Neurology* 1991;41(8):1251–6.

52. Caramanos Z, Narayanan S, Arnold DL. 1H-MRS quantification of tNA and tCr in patients with multiple sclerosis: a meta-analytic review. *Brain* 2005; 128(11):2483–506.

53. Mainero C, De Stefano N, Iannucci G, *et al.* Correlates of MS disability assessed in vivo using aggregates of MR quantities. *Neurology* 2001;56(10): 1331–4.

54. Tartaglia MC, Narayanan S, Francis SJ, *et al.* The relationship between diffuse axonal damage and fatigue in multiple sclerosis. *Arch Neurol* 2004;61(2):201–7.

55. De Stefano N, Narayanan S, Francis GS, *et al.* Evidence of axonal damage in the early stages of multiple sclerosis and its relevance to disability. *Arch Neurol* 2001;58(1):65–70.

56. De Stefano N, Iannucci G, Sormani MP, *et al.* MR correlates of cerebral atrophy in patients with multiple sclerosis. *J Neurol* 2002;249(8):1072–7.

57. Reddy H, Narayanan S, Arnoutelis R, *et al.* Evidence for adaptive functional changes in the cerebral cortex with axonal injury from multiple sclerosis. *Brain* 2000;123 (11):2314–20.

58. Newsholme P, Lima MM, Procopio J, *et al.* Glutamine and glutamate as vital metabolites. *Braz J Med Biol Res* 2003; 36(2):153–63.

59. Sibson NR, Mason GF, Shen J, *et al.* In vivo (13)C NMR measurement of neurotransmitter glutamate cycling, anaplerosis and TCA cycle flux in rat brain during. *J Neurochem* 2001;76(4): 975–89.

60. Pitt D, Nagelmeier IE, Wilson HC, Raine CS. Glutamate uptake by oligodendrocytes: implications for excitotoxicity in multiple sclerosis. *Neurology* 2003;61(8):1113–20.

61. Ouardouz M, Coderre E, Zamponi GW, *et al.* Glutamate receptors on myelinated spinal cord axons: II. AMPA and GluR5 receptors. *Ann Neurol* 2009;65(2):160–6.

62. Doble A. The role of excitotoxicity in neurodegenerative disease: implications for therapy. *Pharmacol Ther* 1999; 81(3):163–221.

63. Werner P, Pitt D, Raine CS. Multiple sclerosis: altered glutamate homeostasis in lesions correlates with oligodendrocyte and axonal damage. *Ann Neurol* 2001;50(2):169–80.

64. Centonze D, Muzio L, Rossi S, Furlan R, Bernardi G, Martino G. The link between inflammation, synaptic transmission and neurodegeneration in multiple sclerosis. *Cell Death Differ* 2010;17(7):1083–91.

65. Piani D, Frei K, Do KQ, Cuenod M, Fontana A. Murine brain macrophages induced NMDA receptor mediated neurotoxicity in vitro by secreting glutamate. *Neurosci Lett* 1991; 133(2):159–62.

66. Hurd R, Sailasuta N, Srinivasan R, Vigneron DB, Pelletier D, Nelson SJ. Measurement of brain glutamate using TE-averaged PRESS at 3T. *Magn Reson Med* 2004;51(3):435–40.

67. Srinivasan R, Sailasuta N, Hurd R, Nelson S, Pelletier D. Evidence of elevated glutamate in multiple sclerosis using magnetic resonance spectroscopy at 3 T. *Brain* 2005; 128(5):1016–25.

68. Baranzini SE, Srinivasan R, Khankhanian P, *et al.* Genetic variation influences glutamate concentrations in brains of patients with multiple sclerosis. *Brain* 2010;133(9):2603–11.

69. Thompson RB, Allen PS. A new multiple quantum filter design procedure for use on strongly coupled spin systems found in vivo: its application to glutamate. *Magn Reson Med* 1998;39(5):762–71.

70. Schubert F, Gallinat J, Seifert F, Rinneberg H. Glutamate concentrations in human brain using single voxel proton magnetic resonance spectroscopy at 3 Tesla. *Neuroimage* 2004;21(4):1762–71.

71. Mullins PG, Chen H, Xu J, Caprihan A, Gasparovic C. Comparative reliability of proton spectroscopy techniques designed to improve detection of J-coupled metabolites. *Magn Reson Med* 2008;60(4):964–9.

72. Arnold DL, Matthews PM, Francis G, Antel J. Proton magnetic resonance spectroscopy of human brain in vivo in the evaluation of multiple sclerosis: assessment of the load of disease. *Magn Reson Med* 1990;14(1):154–9.

73. Evangelou N, Esiri MM, Smith S, Palace J, Matthews PM. Quantitative pathological evidence for axonal loss in normal appearing white matter in multiple sclerosis. *Ann Neurol* 2000;47(3):391–5.

74. Arnold DL, Matthews PM, Francis GS, O'Connor J, Antel JP. Proton magnetic resonance spectroscopic imaging for metabolic characterization of demyelinating plaques. *Ann Neurol* 1992;31(3):235–41.

75. Arnold DL, Riess GT, Matthews PM, *et al.* Use of proton magnetic resonance spectroscopy for monitoring disease progression in multiple sclerosis. *Ann Neurol* 1994;36(1):76–82.

76. Miller DH, Austin SJ, Connelly A, Youl BD, Gadian DG, McDonald WI. Proton magnetic resonance spectroscopy of an acute and chronic lesion in multiple sclerosis. *Lancet* 1991;337(8732): 58–9.

77. Van Hecke P, Marchal G, Johannik K, *et al.* Human brain proton localized NMR spectroscopy in multiple sclerosis. *Magn Reson Med* 1991;18(1): 199–206.

78. Bruhn H, Frahm J, Merboldt KD, *et al.* Multiple sclerosis in children: cerebral metabolic alterations monitored by localized proton magnetic resonance spectroscopy in vivo. *Ann Neurol* 1992;32(2):140–50.

79. Grossman RI, Lenkinski RE, Ramer KN, Gonzalez-Scarano F, Cohen JA. MR proton spectroscopy in multiple sclerosis. *Am J Neuroradiol* 1992;13(6):1535–43.

80. Davie CA, Hawkins CP, Barker GJ, *et al.* Serial proton magnetic resonance

spectroscopy in acute multiple sclerosis lesions. *Brain* 1994;117 (1): 49–58.

81. Husted CA, Goodin DS, Hugg JW, *et al.* Biochemical alterations in multiple sclerosis lesions and normal-appearing white matter detected by in vivo 31P and 1H spectroscopic imaging. *Ann Neurol* 1994;36(2):157–65.

82. Inglese M, Ge Y, Filippi M, Falini A, Grossman RI, Gonen O. Indirect evidence for early widespread gray matter involvement in relapsing-remitting multiple sclerosis. *Neuroimage* 2004;21(4):1825–9.

83. Rocca MA, Mezzapesa DM, Falini A, *et al.* Evidence for axonal pathology and adaptive cortical reorganization in patients at presentation with clinically isolated syndromes suggestive of multiple sclerosis. *Neuroimage* 2003; 18(4):847–55.

84. Fu L, Matthews PM, De Stefano N, *et al.* Imaging axonal damage of normal-appearing white matter in multiple sclerosis. *Brain* 1998;121 (1): 103–13.

85. Evangelou N, Konz D, Esiri MM, Smith S, Palace J, Matthews PM. Size-selective neuronal changes in the anterior optic pathways suggest a differential susceptibility to injury in multiple sclerosis. *Brain* 2001;124(9):1813–20.

86. Evangelou N, Konz D, Esiri MM, Smith S, Palace J, Matthews PM. Regional axonal loss in the corpus callosum correlates with cerebral white matter lesion volume and distribution in multiple sclerosis. *Brain* 2000;123 (9): 1845–9.

87. Ganter P, Prince C, Esiri MM. Spinal cord axonal loss in multiple sclerosis: a post-mortem study. *Neuropathol Appl Neurobiol* 1999;25(6):459–67.

88. Bjartmar C, Kinkel RP, Kidd G, Rudick RA, Trapp BD. Axonal loss in normal-appearing white matter in a patient with acute MS. *Neurology* 2001;57(7):1248–52.

89. Lovas G, Szilagyi N, Majtenyi K, Palkovits M, Komoly S. Axonal changes in chronic demyelinated cervical spinal cord plaques. *Brain* 2000;123 (2): 308–17.

90. Dutta R, McDonough J, Yin X, *et al.* Mitochondrial dysfunction as a cause of axonal degeneration in multiple sclerosis patients. *Ann Neurol* 2006;59:478–89.

91. Allen IV, McKeown SR. A histological, histochemical and biochemical study of the macroscopically normal white matter in multiple sclerosis. *J Neurol Sci* 1979;41(1):81–91.

92. Allen IV, Glover G, Anderson R. Abnormalities in the macroscopically normal white matter in cases of mild or spinal multiple sclerosis (MS). *Acta Neuropathol Suppl (Berl)* 1981;7:176–8.

93. Sarchielli P, Presciutti O, Pelliccioli GP, *et al.* Absolute quantification of brain metabolites by proton magnetic resonance spectroscopy in normal-appearing white matter of multiple sclerosis patients. *Brain* 1999;122 (3):513–21.

94. Adalsteinsson E, Langer-Gould A, Homer RJ, *et al.* Gray matter N-acetyl aspartate deficits in secondary progressive but not relapsing-remitting multiple sclerosis. *Am J Neuroradiol* 2003;24(10):1941–5.

95. Chard DT, Griffin CM, McLean MA, *et al.* Brain metabolite changes in cortical grey and normal-appearing white matter in clinically early relapsing-remitting multiple sclerosis. *Brain* 2002;125(10):2342–52.

96. Sarchielli P, Presciutti O, Tarducci R, *et al.* Localized (1)H magnetic resonance spectroscopy in mainly cortical gray matter of patients with multiple sclerosis. *J Neurol* 2002;249(7): 902–10.

97. Sastre-Garriga J, Ingle GT, Chard DT, *et al.* Metabolite changes in normal-appearing gray and white matter are linked with disability in early primary progressive multiple sclerosis. *Arch Neurol* 2005;62(4):569–73.

98. Sijens PE, Mostert JP, Oudkerk M, De Keyser J. (1)H MR spectroscopy of the brain in multiple sclerosis subtypes with analysis of the metabolite concentrations in gray and white matter: initial findings. *Eur Radiol* 2006; 16:489–95.

99. Staffen W, Zauner H, Mair A, *et al.* Magnetic resonance spectroscopy of memory and frontal brain region in early multiple sclerosis. *J Neuropsychiatry Clin Neurosci* 2005;17(3):357–63.

100. DiMaio S, Narayanan S, De Stefano N, Chen JT, Lapierre Y, Arnold DL. *In vivo* evidence of cortical neuronal injury in secondary progressive multiple sclerosis. *Proceedings of the 11th Scientific Meeting of the International Society for Magnetic Resonance in Medicine.* 2003;11:1998 (abstract).

101. Cifelli A, Arridge M, Jezzard P, Esiri MM, Palace J, Matthews PM. Thalamic neurodegeneration in multiple sclerosis. *Ann Neurol* 2002;52(5): 650–3.

102. Inglese M, Liu S, Babb JS, Mannon LJ, Grossman RI, Gonen O. Three-dimensional proton spectroscopy of deep gray matter nuclei in relapsing-remitting MS. *Neurology* 2004;63(1): 170–2.

103. Wylezinska M, Cifelli A, Jezzard P, Palace J, Alecci M, Matthews PM. Thalamic neurodegeneration in relapsing–remitting multiple sclerosis. *Neurology* 2003;60(12):1949–54.

104. Cohen J. A power primer. *Psychol Bull* 1992;112(1):155–9.

105. Charcot JM. Histologie de le sclerose en plaques. *Gazette des Hopitaux* 1868:554–558.

106. Bitsch A, Schuchardt J, Bunkowski S, Kuhlmann T, Bruck W. Acute axonal injury in multiple sclerosis. Correlation with demyelination and inflammation. *Brain* 2000;123 (6):1174–83.

107. Kuhlmann T, Lingfeld G, Bitsch A, Schuchardt J, Bruck W. Acute axonal damage in multiple sclerosis is most extensive in early disease stages and decreases over time. *Brain* 2002; 125(10):2202–12.

108. Trapp BD, Peterson J, Ransohoff RM, Rudick R, Mork S, Bo L. Axonal transection in the lesions of multiple sclerosis. *N Engl J Med* 1998;338(5): 278–85.

109. Barnes D, Munro PM, Youl BD, Prineas JW, McDonald WI. The longstanding MS lesion. A quantitative MRI and electron microscopic study. *Brain* 1991;114 (3):1271–80.

110. Ferguson B, Matyszak MK, Esiri MM, Perry VH. Axonal damage in acute multiple sclerosis lesions. *Brain* 1997; 120 (3):393–9.

111. Brownell B, Hughes JT. The distribution of plaques in the cerebrum in multiple sclerosis. *J Neurol Neurosurg Psychiatry* 1962;25:315–20.

112. Lumsden CE. The neuropathology of multiple sclerosis. In: Vinken PJ, Bryun QW, eds. *Handbook of Clinical Neurology.* Amsterdam: North Holland, 2001:217–309.

113. Peterson JW, Trapp BD. Neuropathobiology of multiple sclerosis. *Neurol Clin* 2005;23(1): 107–29.

114. Bo L, Vedeler CA, Nyland H, Trapp BD, Mork SJ. Intracortical multiple sclerosis lesions are not associated with increased lymphocyte infiltration. *Mult Scler* 2003;9(4):323–31.

115. Peterson JW, Trapp BD. Neuropathobiology of multiple sclerosis. *Neurol Clin* 2005;23(1): 107–29.

116. Geurts JJ, Bo L, Pouwels PJ, Castelijns JA, Polman CH, Barkhof F. Cortical lesions in multiple sclerosis: combined postmortem MR imaging and histopathology. *Am J Neuroradiol* 2005;26(3):572–7.

117. Geurts JJ, Pouwels PJ, Uitdehaag BM, Polman CH, Barkhof F, Castelijns JA. Intracortical lesions in multiple sclerosis: improved detection with 3D double inversion-recovery MR imaging. *Radiology* 2005;236(1): 254–60.

118. Kidd D, Barkhof F, McConnell R, Algra PR, Allen IV, Revesz T. Cortical lesions in multiple sclerosis. *Brain* 1999;122 (1):17–26.

119. Peterson JW, Bo L, Mork S, Chang A, Trapp BD. Transected neurites, apoptotic neurons, and reduced inflammation in cortical multiple sclerosis lesions. *Ann Neurol* 2001; 50(3):389–400.

120. Bo L, Vedeler CA, Nyland HI, Trapp BD, Mork SJ. Subpial demyelination in the cerebral cortex of multiple sclerosis patients. *J Neuropathol Exp Neurol* 2003;62(7):723–32.

121. Kutzelnigg A, Lucchinetti CF, Stadelmann C, *et al.* Cortical demyelination and diffuse white matter injury in multiple sclerosis. *Brain* 2005;128(11):2705–12.

122. Caramanos Z, DiMaio S, Narayanan S, Lapierre Y, Arnold DL. ¹H-MRSI evidence for cortical gray matter pathology that is independent of cerebral white matter lesion load in patients with secondary progressive multiple sclerosis. *J Neurol Sci* 2009; 282(1–2):72–9.

123. Davie CA, Barker GJ, Webb S, *et al.* Persistent functional deficit in multiple sclerosis and autosomal dominant cerebellar ataxia is associated with axon loss. *Brain* 1995;118 (6):1583–92.

124. De Stefano N, Matthews PM, Fu L, *et al.* Axonal damage correlates with disability in patients with relapsing-remitting multiple sclerosis. Results of a longitudinal magnetic resonance spectroscopy study. *Brain* 1998;121 (8):1469–77.

125. Narayanan S, De Stefano N, Pouwels PJ, Barkhof F, Filippi M, Arnold DL. The effect of oral glatiramer acetate treatment on axonal integrity in multiple sclerosis: results from the multicentre CORAL MRS sub-study. *Mult Scler* 2005;11(Suppl 1):S60.

126. Matthews PM, Pioro E, Narayanan S, *et al.* Assessment of lesion pathology in multiple sclerosis using quantitative MRI morphometry and magnetic resonance spectroscopy. *Brain* 1996;119 (3):715–22.

127. Fu L, Wolfson C, Worsley KJ, *et al.* Statistics for investigation of multimodal MR imaging data and an application to multiple sclerosis patients. *NMR Biomed* 1996;9(8): 339–46.

128. Reddy H, Narayanan S, Matthews PM, *et al.* Relating axonal injury to functional recovery in MS. *Neurology* 2000;54(1):236–9.

129. Prineas JW, Connell F. The fine structure of chronically active multiple sclerosis plaques. *Neurology* 1978; 28:68–75.

130. Prineas JW, Connell F. Remyelination in multiple sclerosis. *Ann Neurol* 1979;5(1):22–31.

131. Chang A, Tourtellotte WW, Rudick R, Trapp BD. Premyelinating oligodendrocytes in chronic lesions of multiple sclerosis. *N Engl J Med* 2002;346(3):165–73.

132. Bates TE, Strangward M, Keelan J, Davey GP, Munro PM, Clark JB. Inhibition of N-acetylaspartate production: implications for 1H MRS studies in vivo. *Neuroreport* 1996; 7(8):1397–400.

133. Matthews PM, Cianfaglia L, McLaurin J, *et al.* Demonstration of reversible decreases in N-acetylaspartate (NAA) in a neuronal cell line: NAA decreases as a marker of sublethal neuronal dysfunction [abstract]. *Proc Soc Magn Reson Med J1 – SMRM* 1995;1: 147.

134. Bjartmar C, Trapp BD. Axonal and neuronal degeneration in multiple sclerosis: mechanisms and functional consequences. *Curr Opin Neurol* 2001;14(3):271–8.

135. Laule C, Vavasour IM, Moore GR, *et al.* Water content and myelin water fraction in multiple sclerosis. A T2 relaxation study. *J Neurol* 2004;251(3): 284–93.

136. Sled JG, Pike GB. Quantitative imaging of magnetization transfer exchange and relaxation properties in vivo using MRI. *Magn Reson Med* 2001;46(5):923–31.

137. Narayanan S, Francis SJ, Sled JG, *et al.* Axonal injury in the cerebral normal-appearing white matter of patients with multiple sclerosis is related to concurrent demyelination in lesions but not to concurrent demyelination in normal-appearing white matter. *Neuroimage* 2006;29: 637–42.

138. Chard DT, Griffin CM, Parker GJ, Kapoor R, Thompson AJ, Miller DH. Brain atrophy in clinically early relapsing-remitting multiple sclerosis. *Brain* 2002;125(2):327–37.

139. Chen JT, Narayanan S, Collins DL, Smith SM, Matthews PM, Arnold DL. Relating neocortical pathology to disability progression in multiple sclerosis using MRI. *Neuroimage* 2004;23(3):1168–75.

140. Collins LD, Narayanan S, Caramanos Z, De Stefano N, Tartaglia MC, Arnold DL. Relation of cerebral atrophy in multiple sclerosis to severity of disease and axonal injury [abstract]. *Neurology* 2000;54(Suppl. 3):A17.

141. Fisher E, Rudick RA, Cutter G, *et al.* Relationship between brain atrophy and disability: an 8-year follow-up study of multiple sclerosis patients. *Mult Scler* 2000;6(6):373–7.

142. Fox NC, Jenkins R, Leary SM, *et al.* Progressive cerebral atrophy in MS: a serial study using registered, volumetric MRI. *Neurology* 2000;54(4):807–12.

143. Liu C, Edwards S, Gong Q, Roberts N, Blumhardt LD. Three dimensional MRI estimates of brain and spinal cord atrophy in multiple sclerosis. *J Neurol Neurosurg Psychiatry* 1999;66(3): 323–30.

144. Rudick RA, Fisher E, Lee JC, Simon J, Jacobs L. Use of the brain parenchymal fraction to measure whole brain atrophy in relapsing–remitting MS. Multiple Sclerosis Collaborative Research Group. *Neurology* 1999; 53(8):1698–704.

145. Bielekova B, Kadom N, Fisher E, *et al.* MRI as a marker for disease heterogeneity in multiple sclerosis. *Neurology* 2005;65(7):1071–6.

146. Payne N, Siatskas C, Barnard A, Bernard CC. The prospect of stem cells as multi-faceted purveyors of immune modulation, repair and regeneration in multiple sclerosis. *Curr Stem Cell Res Ther* 2011;6:50–62.

147. Tselis A, Khan OA, Lisak RP. Approaches to neuroprotective strategies in multiple sclerosis. *Expert Opin Pharmacother* 2010;11(17):2869–78.

148. Aktas O, Kieseier B, Hartung HP. Neuroprotection, regeneration and immunomodulation: broadening the therapeutic repertoire in multiple sclerosis. *Trends Neurosci* 2010;33(3):140–52.

149. Penner IK, Kappos L, Rausch M, Opwis K, Radu EW. Therapy-induced plasticity of cognitive functions in MS patients: insights from fMRI. *J Physiol Paris* 2006;99(4–6):455–62.

150. Yang Y, Liu Y, Wei P, *et al.* Silencing Nogo-A promotes functional recovery in demyelinating disease. *Ann Neurol* 2010;67(4):498–507.

151. Goodman AD, Brown TR, Krupp LB, *et al.* Sustained-release oral fampridine in multiple sclerosis: a randomised, double-blind, controlled trial. *Lancet* 2009;373(9665):732–8.

152. Thompson A, Polman C. Improving function: a new treatment era for multiple sclerosis? *Lancet* 2009;373(9665):697–8.

153. Kuczewski N, Porcher C, Lessmann V, Medina I, Gaiarsa JL. Activity-dependent dendritic release of BDNF and biological consequences. *Mol Neurobiol* 2009;39(1):37–49.

154. Stys PK. General mechanisms of axonal damage and its prevention. *J Neurol Sci* 2005;233(1–2):3–13.

155. Kapoor R. Sodium channel blockers and neuroprotection in multiple sclerosis using lamotrigine. *J Neurol Sci* 2008;274(1–2):54–6.

156. Sarchielli P, Presciutti O, Tarducci R, *et al.* 1H-MRS in patients with multiple sclerosis undergoing treatment with interferon beta-1a: results of a preliminary study. *J Neurol Neurosurg Psychiatry* 1998;64(2):204–12.

157. Schubert F, Seifert F, Elster C, *et al.* Serial 1H-MRS in relapsing-remitting multiple sclerosis: effects of interferon-beta therapy on absolute metabolite concentrations. *Magma* 2002;14(3):213–22.

158. Parry A, Corkill R, Blamire AM, *et al.* Beta-Interferon treatment does not always slow the progression of axonal injury in multiple sclerosis. *J Neurol* 2003;250(2):171–8.

159. Khan O, Shen Y, Caon C, *et al.* Axonal metabolic recovery and potential neuroprotective effect of glatiramer acetate in relapsing-remitting multiple sclerosis. *Mult Scler* 2005;11(6):646–51.

160. Khan O, Shen Y, Bao F, *et al.* Long-term study of brain 1H-MRS study in multiple sclerosis: effect of glatiramer acetate therapy on axonal metabolic function and feasibility of long-Term H-MRS monitoring in multiple sclerosis. *J Neuroimaging* 2008;18(3):314–19.

161. Mostert JP, Sijens PE, Oudkerk M, De Keyser J. Fluoxetine increases cerebral white matter NAA/Cr ratio in patients with multiple sclerosis. *Neurosci Lett* 2006;402(1–2):22–4.

162. De Stefano N, Narayanan S, Francis SJ, *et al.* Diffuse axonal and tissue injury in patients with multiple sclerosis with low cerebral lesion load and no disability. *Arch Neurol* 2002;59(10):1565–71.

163. Narayana PA, Wolinsky JS, Rao SB, He R, Mehta M. Multicentre proton magnetic resonance spectroscopy imaging of primary progressive multiple sclerosis. *Mult Scler* 2004;10 (Suppl 1):S73–8.

164. Narayanan S, De Stefano N, Pouwels PJW, Barkhof F, Filippi M, Arnold DL. The effect of oral glatiramer acetate treatment on axonal integrity in multiple sclerosis: results from the multicentre CORAL MRS sub-study. *Mult Scler* 2005;11(Suppl 1):S60.

165. Filippi M, Wolinsky JS, Comi G. Effects of oral glatiramer acetate on clinical and MRI-monitored disease activity in patients with relapsing multiple sclerosis: a multicentre, double-blind, randomised, placebo-controlled study. *Lancet Neurol* 2006;5(3):213–20.

166. De Stefano N, Filippi M, Miller D, *et al.* Guidelines for using proton MR spectroscopy in multicenter clinical MS studies. *Neurology* 2007;69(20):1942–52.

Chapter 13

Imaging of gray matter lesions in multiple sclerosis

Mike P. Wattjes, Jeroen J.G. Geurts, and Frederik Barkhof

Introduction

Multiple sclerosis (MS) is the most common immune-mediated chronic inflammatory disease of the central nervous system affecting young adults. MS is characterized by inflammation, demyelination, and neuroaxonal degeneration. In early histopathological studies, it was demonstrated that MS pathology occurs both in the white and in the gray matter. However, since demyelination in gray matter structures is difficult to visualize with conventional histochemistry, or with conventional magnetic resonance imaging (MRI) techniques, gray matter pathology in MS has until recently been disregarded. As a consequence, MS has been traditionally considered a "white matter disease". The introduction of newer histopathological staining methods such as myelin protein immunohistochemistry, as well as the implementation of more advanced and quantitative MRI techniques, has shed light on the importance of gray matter pathology in MS in many respects (Fig. 13.1).[1,2] In particular, the clinical relevance of gray matter lesions has become more obvious. For example, while global white matter damage have been attributed to more general clinical outcome measures, gray matter changes could also be related to more specific clinical manifestations including cognitive impairment within several different domains and to epilepsy. Gray matter pathology can be observed in early stages of MS, but generally grows more prominent with increasing disease duration.

Features of gray matter pathology in MS

In general, gray matter abnormalities can become manifest in two different ways, i.e. changes occurring primarily in the gray matter (e.g. focal and diffuse cortical demyelination) and gray matter changes secondary to white matter damage (e.g. Wallerian degeneration). In most patients, particularly in later disease stages, a combination of both can be observed. Different classification systems have been proposed for primary gray matter lesions.[3–6] The most accepted classification proposed by Bø et al. (2003)[5,6] distinguishes four different types: type I cortical lesions affect the cortical gray matter as well as the adjacent white matter (so-called "mixed white matter–gray matter lesions" or "leukocortical lesions"). Type II lesions are purely intracortical, neither affecting the subpial cortical layers nor the subcortical white matter; type III lesions start at the pial surface and work their way downwards, never reaching the white matter–gray matter boundary. Type IV lesions span the entire cortical gray matter including the subpial regions, but do not involve the adjacent subcortical white matter (for an overview of the Bø classification of cortical lesions, see Table 13.1 and Figs. 13.2 and 13.3). Cortical gray matter lesions can be observed throughout the brain, but they were reported to be more frequent in the cingulate gyrus, temporal, and frontal cortex and are less often observed in occipital and primary motor cortex.[6–9] In addition to the neocortex, archi- and paleocortical areas such as the hippocampus and insula may be involved, as well as the basal ganglia, thalamus, hypothalamus, dentate nucleus and spinal cord (Fig. 13.3).[10–12]

Histopathologically, cortical lesions differ from white matter lesions. Cortical lesions show only minor inflammation, with no complement deposition or blood–brain barrier disruption. A different pattern of inflammatory cells was observed, with substantially lower numbers of $CD3^+$ lymphocytes and $CD68^+$ macrophage-microglial cells. In cortical lesions, activated microglia, rather than (foamy) macrophages, may be present, especially at the lesion border.[4,6,13,14] Furthermore, regional differences in terms of inflammatory changes in the gray matter can be observed: hypothalamic lesions show a more inflammatory activity including the presence of foamy macrophages, whereas inflammation in hippocampal lesions, like in cortical lesions, is rare. The underlying reason for these regional differences of inflammation pattern is currently not understood. Different densities of myelin and regional differences in the duration of inflammation might be possible explanations for these differences in the inflammatory reaction.[7,10,12,15]

Several studies have shown that meningeal inflammation with presence of B-cell follicles may be observed in MS patients. However, whether meningeal inflammation is associated with cortical demyelinaton is still a matter of debate.[16,17] The presence of B-cell follicles, their relationship to Epstein–Barr virus, and their relationship to cortical demyelination are unresolved issues currently.

Multiple Sclerosis Therapeutics, Fourth Edition, ed. Jeffrey A. Cohen and Richard A. Rudick. Published by Cambridge University Press.

(a)

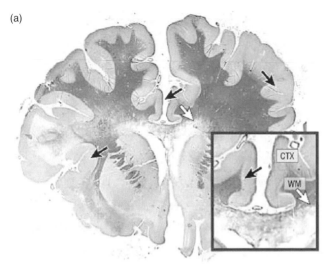

(b)

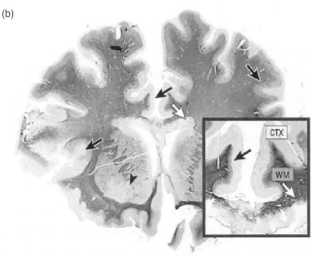

Fig. 13.1. Adjacent paraffin sections obtained from a MS patient with diffuse cortical subpial demyelination. The section is stained for myelin using Luxol fast-blue technique (a) and immunohistochemically for proteolipid protein (PLP) (b). Demyelination of the white matter such as the periventricular white matter and the corpus callosum is easily detectable (white arrows); cortical myelin is largely unstained. White matter lesions are also sharply delineated on the PLP stained specimen (green arrow). In the cortical gray matter, all areas show a superficial subpial myelin loss (black arrows). Please note also loss of myelin in deep gray matter structures such as the putamen (arrowhead). On higher magnification, a well delineated cortical lesion border (cingulate gyrus) is visible by PLP immunohistochemistry (b; inset, black arrow); the border not well detectable on the adjacent Luxol fast-blue stained section (a; inset, black arrow). Reproduced from Bö et al.,[2] with permission from the American Medical Association (see also color plate section).

Imaging of gray matter pathology
Conventional MRI

The high sensitivity of proton density (PD)/T2-weighted and fluid-attenuated inversion-recovery (FLAIR) pulse sequences in the detection of demyelinating lesions in the white matter has led to the incorporation of MRI into the diagnostic criteria of

Table 13.1. Classification of cortical lesions according to Bø et al., 2003[5,6]

Type I	Lesion involves both gray matter and the adjacent white matter (mixed white matter–gray matter lesion)
Type II	Lesion located in the cortex not involving the subpial cortex or the subcortical white matter
Type III	Lesion that is located in the subpial cortex
Type IV	Lesion affects the entire width of the cerebral cortex but not the adjacent white matter

MS. Hence, MRI is currently considered to be the most powerful paraclinical diagnostic tool for patients with suspected MS. However, sensitivity of conventional MRI (PD/ T2-weighted, FLAIR) for gray matter lesions is poor.

It has been shown that certain pulse sequences such as double inversion recovery (DIR), T1-weighted 3D spoiled gradient-recalled echo (SPGR), and phase-sensitive inversion recovery (PSIR) can substantially improve the detection of cortical lesions. DIR is an inversion recovery sequence which applies two consecutive inversion pulses leading to a simultaneous attenuation of the cerebrospinal fluid (CSF) and white matter which improves the contrast between gray and white matter. The advantage of DIR over conventional MRI techniques can be summarized as follows: first of all, DIR was shown to detect a significantly higher number of cortical lesions than FLAIR and/or PD/ T2-weighted imaging. Secondly, the increased GM/WM contrast leads to a better differentiation of juxtacortical (U fiber) lesions, mixed white matter–gray matter lesions and "purely" intracortical lesions (Figs. 13.4 and 13.5). In other words, DIR not only leads to a higher sensitivity concerning the detection of cortical lesions, but also to a higher specificity. However, despite these obvious advantages, DIR also shows a high propensity to artifacts, owing to flow and pulsation and a low signal-to-noise ratio. The implementation of multi-slab and later single-slab 3D DIR sequences have reduced artifacts, and have further increased image quality and hence detection rate of cortical gray matter lesions in MS. In addition, the combined use of DIR and T1-weighted SPGR or PSIR may allow for a reduction of false-positive and false-negative scorings and may further improve the reliability of cortical lesion detection in MS.[18–20] Guidelines for cortical lesion scoring were recently formulated in a multicenter consensus meeting, and post mortem verification of DIR lesions is under way.

Besides adaptation of image contrast, such as DIR, higher magnetic field strengths (>1.5 T) have been increasingly used to improve detection of both white matter and gray matter lesions. Due to the almost linear relationship of the magnetic field strength used and the signal-to-noise ratio (SNR), high field MRI benefits from the increased SNR in many aspects (e.g. higher spatial and temporal resolution, faster image acquisition, etc.). It has already been conclusively shown that high field MRI, operating at 3 T detects significantly more white

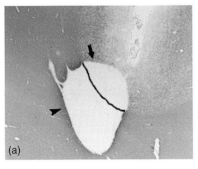

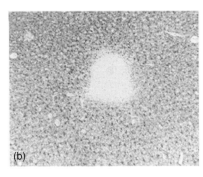

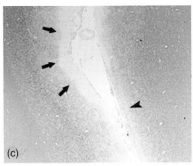

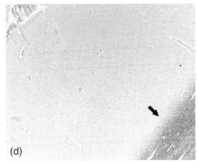

Fig. 13.2. Different types of cortical gray matter lesions on myelin immunohistochemistry, (proteolipid protein). Figures (a)–(d) show the different types of cortical according to the Bö classification. Type I lesion (a) represents mixed white matter-gray matter lesions. The black line represents the border between the cortex and the subcortical white matter. The gray matter part of the lesion is indicated by the arrow, the white matter part of the lesion is indicated by the arrow head. Type II (b) pure intracortical lesion surrounds a blood vessel. Type III (c) cortical lesion represents a subpial lesion (arrows), the adjacent cortex is not affected (arrowhead). Type IV (d) cortical lesion involves the entire width of the cortex. Arrow indicates the gray matter–white matter interface. Hippocampal lesions (e) can be frequently observed and involve most often the gray and white matter. The black arrow indicated the demyelinated areas and the white arrows indicate areas with preserved myelin. Spinal cord section (F) with a large demyelinated area and small areas with intact myelin (arrows). Reproduced from Geurts et al.,[10] and Geurts and Barkhof[1] with permission from Lippencott Williams and Wilkins and Elsevier (see also color plate section).

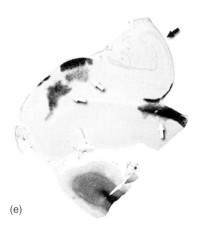

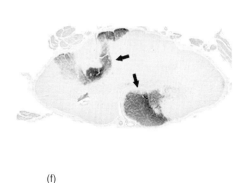

(e)

(f)

matter lesions in the perventricular, juxtacortical, and infratentorial white matter when compared to 1.5 T MRI.[21–23] Post-mortem studies show conflicting results, however. Using high field MRI operating 4.7 T, no significant increase of sensitivity in the detection of gray matter lesions could be observed. However, using ultra-high field MRI operating 8 T or even 9.4 T, cortical lesion load measurements increase substantially. In vivo studies have shown that the application of higher magnetic field strengths using conventional T2-weighted sequences does not necessarily lead to a significantly improved detection of cortical lesions.[24–26] However, the combination of higher magnetic field strengths (3 T) and DIR significantly improves the detection of purely intracortical and mixed white matter–gray matter lesions when compared to 1.5 (Fig. 13.6)[27] Recent in vivo MRI studies applying magnetic field strengths of 7 T with a submillimeter spatial high resolution have shown a further increased detection rate, possibly even allowing classification of cortical lesions according to neuropathology criteria.[28]

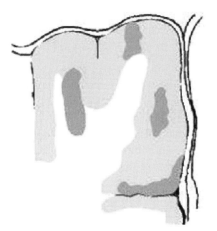

Fig. 13.3. Overview of the different types of cortical lesions according to the classification provided by Bø et al.,[56] 2003 (see also Table 13.1). Reproduced from Bö L. et al. Acta Neurol Scand 2006; 113 (Suppl. 183): 48–50 with permission from John Wiley & Sons Ltd.

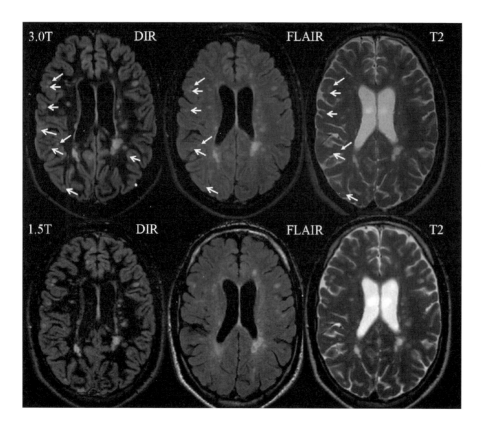

Fig. 13.4. Axial double inversion recovery (DIR), fluid attenuated-inversion recovery (FLAIR) and T2-weighted images through the supratentorial brain of a patient with relapsing remitting MS. Images were obtained at 1.5 T (bottom row) and 3.0 T (top row). DIR provide a better contrast between the gray and white matter as well as between the lesion and the gray/white matter. DIR images are more sensitive for the detection of gray matter lesions. In addition, it allows a better classification between lesion located in the juxtacortical white matter (arrows) and those lesions which are already involving the cortical gray matter (open head arrows). Please note also the higher signal and better lesion detectablity at higher magnetic field (3.0 T) when compared to 1.5 T.

Cortical lesions seen on MRI using DIR are mainly located in the frontal and temporal cortex, which corresponds well with histopathological findings (see above). From a clinical point of view, the detection of cortical lesions is important. It has been conclusively demonstrated that cortical lesions are associated with clinical disability measured by EDSS. In relapsing–remitting MS, cortical lesions accumulate over time and are associated with clinical disease progression. Cortical lesion volume predicts disability (EDSS) accumulation. In particular, cortical lesions are associated with cognitive impairment involving several domains. MS patients with cognitive decline have a higher cortical lesion load compared to patients who are cognitively normal.[29–32]

Quantitative MRI techniques

Despite advances in the detection of focal gray matter lesions, the detection and quantification of diffuse gray matter damage is currently beyond the range of detection of available qualitative MRI techniques. Diffuse gray matter damage in MS can occur primarily due to gray matter demyelination but also secondarily due to retrograde white matter damage. Quantitative MRI techniques are able to detect and to quantify primary and secondary gray matter abnormalities and provide further insights into disease progression and contribution of these changes to clinical outcome measures.

MR spectroscopy (Chapter 12)

Proton MR spectroscopy (^{1}H-MRS) is frequently used for the evaluation of normal appearing brain tissue in MS. Compared with conventional imaging techniques, data concerning the metabolic evaluation of gray matter pathology in MS are rather scarce. This is mainly due to the fact that ^{1}H-MRS of the gray matter (particularly cortical gray matter) is technically challenging because of the rather small voxel size and proximity to the cerebrospinal fluid.[33] Similar to findings in normal appearing white matter, substantial alterations in metabolic concentrations can be observed including *N*-acetyl-aspartate (NAA) indicating loss of axonal integrity, myo-inositol (Ins) indicating higher degree of glial cell activity, and choline (Cho) indicating increased membrane turnover. These changes in metabolite concentration have not only been observed in the cortical gray matter but also in deep gray matter structures such as thalamus and hippocampus.[34,35]

Compared to healthy controls, decrease in NAA concentration up 19%, and increase of Ins up to 31% have been observed in the thalamus (Fig. 13.7). In addition, higher Ins but normal NAA concentrations were found in the hippocampus of MS patients. The increase of Ins concentration in the thalamus as well as in the hippocampus correlated significantly with the T2 lesion load. The degree of Ins increase was more pronounced in advanced disease stages such as secondary progressive MS, and the largest NAA decrease was observed in primary-progressive MS. The decrease in NAA correlates with the thalamic volume.[36]

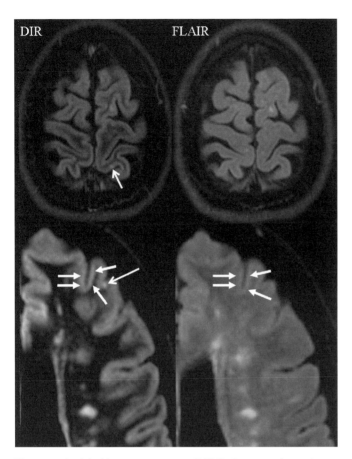

Fig. 13.5. Axial double inversion recovery (DIR), fluid attenuated-inversion recovery (FLAIR) images obtained from a 44-year old female with relapsing remitting MS. Note the higher sensitivity of pure intracortical gray matter lesions (open head arrows) on DIR when compared to FLAIR. Please note also areas of diffuse cortical gray matter demyelination (arrows).

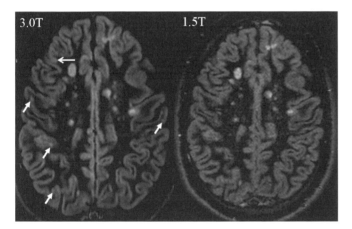

Fig. 13.6. Axial double inversion recovery (DIR) section obtained from a patient with relapsing remitting MS at 1.5 T (right) and 3.0 T (left). In vivo MRI at 3.0 T (arrows) shows significantly more focal cortical gray matter lesions compared to 1.5T but also areas with more diffuse demyelination (open head arrow).

The results concerning metabolic alterations in the cortical gray matter are not completely conclusive. Some groups have reported metabolic changes whereas others did not. Lower concentrations of NAA suggestive of axonal damage in the cortical gray matter of MS have been reported by several groups. These changes can be observed early in the disease, e.g. patients with disease duration of 2 years. Similar to observations in the normal appearing white matter and deep gray matter structures, the degree of metabolic changes, particularly NAA decline, becomes more pronounced in later and progressive disease stages. Interestingly, compared to NAA decline in the normal white matter, which is highly correlated with EDSS, NAA reduction in the gray matter does not correlate with EDSS or with MS functional composite scores. Although it is believed that gray matter pathology occurs at least to a certain extent independently of white matter damage, a relationship between enhancing white matter lesions and cortical metabolic changes (NAA and Cho) can be observed in clinically isolated syndromes suggestive of MS. This suggests that cortical neuronal/axonal damage as measured by ^{1}H-MRS is at least partially influenced by white matter pathology and is not exclusively based on primary neuronal damage.[33]

Diffusion tensor imaging (Chapter 15)

Diffusion tensor imaging (DTI) assesses the random movement of water molecules within the brain tissue. DTI is a measure of the size and geometry of water-filled spaces in the brain. Due to the architecture of white matter, restricted (anisotropic) water motion along the axis of axons can be observed. Anisotropic diffusion is also present in gray matter, but to lesser extent when compared to white matter. Important measures describing the degree of diffusion are mean diffusivity (MD) and fractional anisotropy (FA). DTI sensitively detects white matter demyelination in focal lesions but also in the NAWM leading to an increase in random water diffusion expressed by higher MD and lower FA values. Although challenging from the technical point of view, DTI enables also the detection cortical as well as deep gray matter damage in MS. Similar to metabolic changes measured by ^{1}H-MRS, DTI shows different dimensions of gray matter damage among different disease course and disease durations, and SPMS patients were shown to exhibit higher degrees of gray matter involvement than RRMS or CIS patients.[37–39] Clinically, a correlation can be observed between cognitive decline and MD values in RRMS as well as a correlation between GM diffusion measures and development of disability during the subsequent 5-years in PPMS patients.[40]

Magnetization transfer imaging (Chapter 10)

Magnetization transfer (MT) imaging is based on a magnetization interaction between free water protons and protons bound to macromolecular structures. Applying an off resonance radio frequency impulse to protons bound to macromolecular molecules induces saturation of these protons that

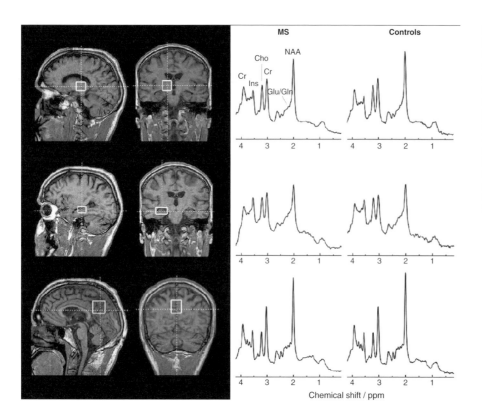

Fig. 13.7. Coronal and sagittal T1-weighted images obtained from an MS patient and healthy control indicating the voxel placement in the thalamus (upper row), hippocampus (middle row) and cortical gray matter (bottom row). The corresponding spectra show a substantial decrease of N-acetylaspartate (NAA) in the thalamus and to a lesser extent in the hippocampus of MS patients when compared to healthy controls indicating substantial axonal damage. In addition increased levels of (myo)inositol indicating increased glial cell activity could be observed in the thalamus of MS patients compared to healthy controls. Reproduced from Geurts et al.[35] with permission from John Wiley & Sons Ltd.

is then transferred to free water protons. This results in a signal decrease depending on the degree of MT between macromolecules and free water protons. The magnetization transfer ratio (MTR) is defined as the difference in signal intensity with or without MT. A lower MTR means reduced concentration protons in the macromolecular pool, relative to free water protons, and this reflects the degree of tissue damage.

Reduced MTR values in gray matter can be observed early in the disease, and increase with advancing disease. Voxel-based analysis of MTR values allows assessment of regional differences in MTR values. Patients presenting with CIS suggestive of MS had decreased MTR in the occipital cortices.[41] Regional differences were also observed in RRMS patients when compared to healthy controls. Lower MTR values were found in several GM regions such as the bilateral lentiform nuclei, bilateral insula, the cortex of the left posterior cingulate, and the right orbitofrontal cortex but not in the thalamus.[42,43]

MTR changes accumulate with time and are related to disease duration. Consequently, MTR changes in the GM are more pronounced in SPMS and PPMS patients. Similar to DTI measurements, the extent of MTR change correlates with clinical outcome measures such as disability and cognitive impairment, but not with fatigue. In addition, MTR change predicts accumulation of disability. In patients with RRMS, gray matter MTR was shown to be an independent predictor disability progression over the subsequent 8 years. In PPMS, gray matter MTR

reduction was associated with the rate of clinical deterioration over 3 years.[44,45]

Tissue relaxation time measurements

T1- and T2-relaxation time (RT) measurements allow the assessment and quantification of white matter and gray matter damage in various neurodegenerative and neuroinflammatory diseases. Increased T1-RT has been observed in the thalamus, and correlated with the degree of fatigue in RRMS patients. T2-based measurements of the basal ganglia structures are increasingly being performed in MS patients in order to detect iron deposition as a possible surrogate marker for neurodegeneration. Increased T2-hypointensity of deep gray matter structures such as the basal ganglia, thalamus red nucleus, and dentate nucleus suggestive of increased iron deposition can be observed in various disease courses and even in very early stages of MS including CIS and benign MS. T2-hypointensity is associated with enlargement of the third ventricle and higher T1- and T2-lesion load. The degree of T2-hypointensity is correlated with the extent of clinical disability and cognitive decline as well as a strong predictor of disability and clinical course.[46–49]

Functional MRI (Chapter 14)

Functional MRI (fMRI) allows assessment of physiological changes in cortex in MS patients. Several fMRI studies using different paradigms have shown that functional reorganization of cortical areas can be observed in different MS "phenotypes." Motor network studies in early disease have demonstrated increased recruitment of cortical areas involved in the performance of a specific task. These areas include primary sensorimotor cortex (SMC), and supplementary motor area. In more advanced disease stages, bilateral involvement of these cortical areas and activation of additional cortical areas has been observed. Activation of cortical areas in the unaffected hemisphere observed in MS patients presenting with acute motor syndromes can also disappear, and recovery of the primary SMC in the affected cortex may occur. This is associated with a good clinical outcome.[50,51]

In general, the ability to recruit "alternative" cortical networks plays a key role in limiting the functional consequences of tissues damage related to MS pathology. However, increased compensatory recruitment of other complex neuronal networks can also represent impairment or inefficiency of neuronal adaptive processes, and may be associated with fatigue or poor clinical recovery.[52]

Functional and conventional (structural) MRI findings are intercorrelated to a certain extent. It has been shown that the amount of T2-lesion load as well as the degree of pathologic changes in the NAWM, gray matter, and spinal cord seem to be correlated with the fMRI activity in (sub)cortical areas of several cerebral networks in movement and memory tasks.[53]

Imaging of gray matter atrophy (Chapter 11)

Reduced brain and spinal cord volume (atrophy) is a well-known pathologic feature in MS and is a reliable outcome measure for monitoring treatment effects in multicenter treatment trials.[54] Gray matter atrophy can be related to primary gray matter pathology (e.g. gray matter demyelination) but can also reflect neuronal degeneration secondary to white matter pathology with axonal transection. The annual rate of brain volume loss is in the range of 0.5% to 1% in MS patients, compared with 0.1% to 0.3% in age-matched healthy control subjects. Increased availability of high-resolution MR images and improved segmentation techniques has permitted more accurate and reproducible evaluation of gray matter volume changes in the brain. This has shed some light onto the important role of gray matter atrophy in MS, and its impact on clinical outcome measures.[55,56]

Reductions in gray matter volume occur in early disease stages. CIS patients developing MS during a follow-up period of 3 years showed a 3.3% decrease in gray matter fraction, whereas no white matter atrophy could be observed at that stage.[57] Longitudinal MRI studies have shown a similar significant reduction of gray matter loss in early RRMS, PPMS and SPMS patients, while white matter volumes remain rather stable. This indicates that gray matter atrophy is at least partially independent from white matter atrophy, at least in early disease stages. The rate of gray matter loss increases with disease

duration and differs between different disease categories. The degree of GM atrophy increases from CIS to RRMS patients and is most severe in SPMS patients.[58] Voxel-based techniques demonstrated a topographic distribution of gray matter damage, i.e. gray matter tissue damage follows certain patterns in terms of regional distribution according to clinical phenotype.[59] Patients presenting with CIS suggestive of MS show atrophy of deep gray matter structures such as the thalamus, hypothalamus, putamen, and caudate nucleus, whereas involvement of the frontotemporal lobes can be observed in RRMS. In PPMS patients, atrophy involving the thalami is present in the initial stage and subsequently extends to other structures including other deep gray matter structures and infratentorial gray matter. Pediatric MS patients primarily show atrophy of the thalami.[56]

Gray matter atrophy correlates significantly with clinical outcome. In particular, the degree of gray matter loss correlates with the severity of disability measured with EDSS and MSFC. Cognitive impairment involving several domains is strongly associated with gray matter atrophy. Cognitively impaired MS patients show significantly lower cortical gray matter volumes compared to cognitively normal MS patients. In addition, gray matter loss predicts verbal memory impairment and neurobehavioral symptoms. Certain atrophy patterns are linked to specific clinical manifestations. For example, hippocampal atrophy is strongly related to memory decline; fatigue is associated with frontal cortical atrophy; and cerebellar cortical volume loss was associated with decline in cerebellar function.[56]

Spinal cord imaging

Gray matter pathology also occurs in the spinal cord. From a clinical point of view, spinal cord pathology is highly relevant, as it is related both to clinical outcome and to diagnosis and differential diagnosis of MS. Spinal cord lesions can be observed in early stages of MS, although spinal cord involvement is more pronounced in later, progressive disease stages. On conventional MRI, focal and diffuse abnormalities can be observed, both of which affect white matter as well as gray matter. Compared to high sensitivity in the detection of demyelinating lesions in the brain, spinal cord imaging remains challenging due to technical difficulties mainly related CSF and vessel pulsation. Up to now, spinal cord MRI is performed with cardiac gated conventional T1- and T2-weighted (fast) spin echo sequences. Special pulse sequences, which provide a higher sensitivity in the detection of gray matter lesions in the brain, such as inversion recovery sequences, are not easy applicable to spinal cord imaging and provide rather poor lesion detection rates. Post-mortem high-resolution imaging at higher magnetic field strengths can provide a sensitivity of more than 70% for gray matter lesions and almost 90% for white matter lesions. (Fig. 13.8)[60] However, the applicability to in vivo imaging remains challenging and demands further investigation.

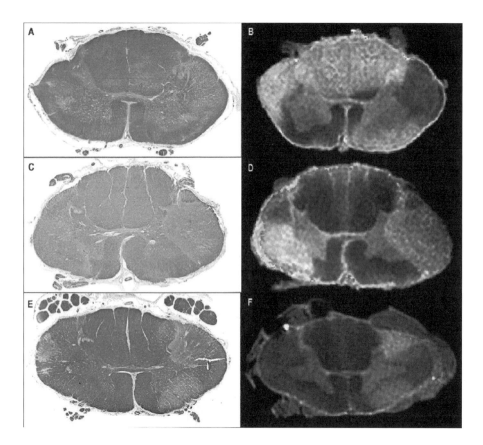

Fig. 13.8. Axial paraffin spinal cord sections of MS patients stained with immunohistochemically anti-myelin basic protein antibodies (a), (c), (e) and the corresponding proton-density-weighted MRI sections (b), (d), (f) at 4.7 T. Demyelinated lesions affect the white matter as well as the spinal cord gray matter. Reproduced from Gilmore *et al.*, 2009[60] with permission from SAGE publications (see also color plate section).

The technical challenges of advanced MRI techniques in the spinal cord are even more pronounced. However, recent studies involving ^{1}H-MRS, DTI and fMRI were able to detect and quantify disease activity in the spinal cord involving the gray matter including reduction of NAA concentration, decreased FA and increased MD, spinal cord atrophy, as well as functional changes.[61-64] A recent study by Ciccarelli *et al.* showed that NAA concentrations drop and recover over time following the development of a focal spinal cord lesion. However, the extent to which NAA recovers seemed to be dependent on disease duration, suggesting once more that the reparative capacity of the central nervous system is limited.[65-67]

Future perspectives

Gray matter involvement is an important pathological feature of MS pathology. It can occur as a primary event (e.g. focal and diffuse cortical demyelination) but also may be secondary to white matter pathology with axonal transaction and Wallerian degeneration. Although gray matter pathology is present in early disease stages, it accumulates and may accelerate with time, and is most severe in advanced and progressive disease. The in vivo assessment of gray matter changes is crucial since it has been conclusively shown that the presence and the extent of cortical pathology is strongly associated with clinical outcome, including neurological and neuropsychological impairment. The

in vivo detection of cortical lesions remains challenging, however. Clinical high field MRI operating at 3 T and the application of special pulse sequences (DIR, PSIR) has improved the sensitivity of cortical lesion detection. Compared with white matter lesions, however, the detection rate of cortical lesions remains rather poor. Future technical developments such has ultra-high field MRI application in combination with certain pulse sequence may further increase the ability to detect focal and diffuse gray matter demyelination. This is particularly important for prognostic (prediction of the conversion to definite MS) and for diagnostic purposes, and may lead to the incorporation of gray matter lesions into MRI and diagnostic criteria for MS.

Several advanced and quantitative MRI techniques are available for the evaluation of normal-appearing gray matter. All of these quantitative MRI techniques have conclusively shown that gray matter pathology is frequent and extensive, and almost certainly reflects pathology that is not seen on conventional MRI. Advances in MRI techniques such as higher magnetic field strengths might lead to benefits in terms of imaging protocols, which may increase the sensitivity of diffuse normal-appearing gray matter involvement in MS. In particular, MR spectroscopy will benefit from higher magnetic field strengths that allow detection and quantification of metabolites that more specifically reflect aspects of inflammation and neurodegeneration.

References

1. Geurts JJG, Barkhof F. Gray matter pathology in multiple sclerosis. *Lancet Neurol* 2008; 7: 841–51.

2. Bö L, Geurts JJG, Van Der Valk P, Polman C, Barkhof F. Lack of correlation between cortical demyelination and white matter pathologic changes in multiple sclerosis. *Arch Neurol* 2007; 64: 76–80.

3. Kidd D, Barkhof F, Mc Connell R *et al.* Cortical lesions in multiple sclerosis. *Brain* 1999; 122: 17–26.

4. Peterson JW, Bö L, Mörk SJ, *et al.* Transected neurites, apoptotic neurons, and reduced inflammation in cortical multiple sclerosis lesions. *Ann Neurol* 2001; 50: 389–400.

5. Bø L, Vedeler CA, Nyland HI *et al.* Subpial demyelination in the cerebral cortex of multiple sclerosis patients. *J Neuropathol Exp Neurol* 2003; 62: 723–32.

6. Bø L, Vedeler CA, Nyland H, Trapp BD, Mörk SJ. Intracortical multiple sclerosis lesions are not associated with increased lymphocyte infiltration. *Mult Scler* 2003; 9:323–31.

7. Kutzelnigg A, Lucchinetti CF, Stadelmann C, *et al.* Cortical demyelination and diffuse white matter injury in multiple sclerosis. *Brain* 2005; 128: 2705–12.

8. Gilmore CP, Donaldson I, Bö L, *et al.* Regional variations in the extent and pattern of grey matter demyelination in multiple sclerosis: a comparison between the cerebral cortex, cerebellar cortex, deep grey matter nuclei and the spinal cord. *J Neurol Neurosurg Psychiatry* 2009; 80: 182–7.

9. Albert M, Antel J, Brück W, *et al.* Extensive cortical remyelination in patients with chronic multiple sclerosis. *Brain Pathol* 2007; 17: 129–38.

10. Geurts JJG, Bö L, Roosendaal SD, *et al.* Extensive hippocampal demyelination in multiple sclerosis. *J Neuropathol Exp Neurol* 2007; 66: 819–27.

11. Gilmore Cp, Bö L, Owens T, *et al.* Spinal cord gray matter demyelination in multiple sclerosis – a novel pattern of residual plaque morphology. *Brain Pathol* 2006; 16:202–8.

12. Vercellino M, Plano F, Votta B, *et al.* Grey matter pathology in multiple sclerosis. *J Neuropathol Ex Neurol* 2005; 64: 1101–7.

13. Brink BP, Veerhuis R, Breij EC, *et al.* The pathology of multiple sclerosis is location-dependent: no significant complement activation is detected in purely cortical lesions. *J Neuropathol Exp Neurol* 2005; 64: 147–55.

14. van Horssen J, Brink BP, de Vries HE, *et al.* The blood-brain barrier in cortical multiple sclerosis lesions. *J Neuropathol Exp Neurol* 2007; 66: 321–8.

15. Kutzelnigg A, Faber-Rod JC, Bauer J, *et al.* Widespread demyelination in the cerebellar cortex in multiple sclerosis. *Brain Pathol* 2007; 17: 38–44.

16. Serafini B, Rosicarelli B, Magliozzi R *et al.* Detection of ectopic B-cell follicles with germinal centers in the meninges of patients with secondary progressive multiple sclerosis. *Brain Pathol* 2004; 14: 164–74.

17. Kooi EJ, Geurts JJ, van Horssen J, *et al.* Meningeal inflammation is not associated with cortical in chronic multiple sclerosis. *J Neuropathol Ex Neurol* 2009; 68: 1021–8.

18. Wattjes MP, Lutterbey GG, Gieseke J, *et al.* Double-inversion recovery brain imaging at 3 tesla: diagnostic value in the detection of multiple sclerosis lesions. *Am J Neuroradiol* 2007; 28: 54–9.

19. Geurts JJG, Pouwels PJW, Uitdehaag BMJ, *et al.* Intracortical lesions in multiple sclerosis: improved detection with double inversion recovery MR imaging. *Radiology* 2005; 236: 254–60.

20. Nelson F, Poonawalla AH, Huang F, Wolinsky JS, Narayana PA. Improved identification of intracortical lesions in multiple sclerosis with phase-sensitive inversion recovery in combination with fast double inversion recovery MR imaging. *Am J Neuroradiol* 2007; 28: 1645–9.

21. Wattjes MP, Lutterbey GG, Harzheim M, *et al.* Higher sensitivity in the detection of inflamatory brain lesions in patients with clinical isolated syndromes suggestive of multiple sclerosis using high field MRI: an intraindividual comparison of 1.5T with 3.0T. *Eur Radiol* 2006; 16: 2067–73.

22. Wattjes MP, Kuhl CK, Harzheim M, *et al.* Does high-field MRI have an influence on the classification of patients with clinically isolated syndromes according to current diagnostic magnetic resonance imaging criteria for multiple sclerosis. *Am J Neuroradiol* 2006; 27: 1794–98.

23. Wattjes MP, Barkhof F. High field MRI in the diagnosis of multiple sclerosis: high field–high yield? *Neuroradiology* 2009; 51: 279–92.

24. Geurts JJG, Blezer EL, Vrenken H, *et al.* Does high-field MR imaging improve cortical lesion detection in multiple sclerosis? *J Neurol* 2008; 255: 183–91.

25. Schmierer K, Parkes HG, So PW, *et al.* High field (9.4 Tesla) magnetic resonance imaging of cortical grey matter lesions in multiple sclerosis. *Brain* 2010; 133: 858–67.

26. Pitt D, Boster A, Pei W, *et al.* Imaging cortical lesions in multiple sclerosis with ultra-high-field magnetic resonance imaging. *Arch Neurol* 2010; 67: 812–18.

27. Simon B, Schmidt S, Lukas C, *et al.* Improved in vivo detection of cortical lesions in multiple sclerosis using double inversion recovery MR imaging at 3 Tesla. *Eur Radiol* 2010; 20: 1675–83.

28. Mainero C, Benner T, Radding A *et al.* In vivo imaging of cortical pathology in multiple sclerosis using ultra-high field MRI. *Neurology* 2009; 73:941–8

29. Calabrese M, De Stefano N, Atzori M *et al.* Extensive cortical inflammation is associated with epilepsy in multiple sclerosis. *J Neurol* 2008; 255:581–6

30. Calabrese M, Rocca MA, Atzori M, *et al.* A 3-year magnetic resonance imaging study of cortical lesions in relapse-onset multiple sclerosis. *Ann Neurol* 2010; 67: 376–83.

31. Calabrese M, Battaglini M, Giorgio A, *et al.* Imaging distribution and frequency of cortical lesions in patients with multiple sclerosis. *Neurology* 2010; 75: 1234–40.

32. Calabrese M, Filippi M, Gallo P. Cortical lesions in multiple sclerosis. *Nat Rev Neurol* 2010; 6: 438–44.

33. Sajja BR, Wollinsky JS, Narayana PA. Proton magnetic resonance spectroscopy in multiple sclerosis. *Neuroimaging Clin N Am* 2009; 19: 45–58.

34. Cifelli A, Arridge M, Jezzard P, *et al.* Thalamic neurodegeneration in multiple sclerosis. *Ann Neurol* 2002; 52: 650–3.

35. Geurts JJG, Reuling IE, Vrenken H, *et al.* MR spectroscopic evidence for thalamic and hippocampal, but not cortical damage in multiple sclerosis. *Magn Reson Med* 2006; 55: 478–83.

36. Wylezinska M, Cifelli A, Jezzard P, *et al.* Thalamic neurodegeneration in relapsing–remitting multiple sclerosis. *Neurology* 2003; 60: 1949–54.

37. Filippi M, Rocca MA. MR imaging of gray matter involvement in multiple sclerosis: implications for understanding disease pathophysiology and monitoring treatment efficacy. *Am J Neuroradiol* 2010; 31: 1171–7.

38. Vrenken H, Pouwels PJ, Geurts JJ, *et al.* Altered diffusion tensor in multiple sclerosis normal-appearing brain tissue: cortical diffusion changes seem related to clinical deterioration. *J Magn Reson Imaging* 2006; 23: 628–6.

39. Tortorella P, Rocca MA, Mezzapesa DM, *et al.* MRI quantification of gray and white matter damage in patients with early-onset multiple sclerosis. *J Neurol* 2006; 253: 903–7.

40. Rovaris M, Judica E, Gallo A, *et al.* Grey matter damage predicts the evolution of primary progressive multiple sclerosis at 5 years. *Brain* 2006; 129: 2628–34.

41. Audoin B Fernando KT, Swanton JK, *et al.* selective magnetization transfer ratio decrease in the visual cortex following optic neuritis. *Brain* 2006; 129: 1031–9.

42. Audion B Davies G, Rashid W, *et al.* Voxel-based analysis of grey matter magnetization transfer ratio maps in early relapsing remitting multiple sclerosis. *Mult Scler* 2007; 13: 483–9.

43. Davies GR, Altman DR, Rashid W *et al.* Emerge of thalamic magnetization transfer ratio abnormality in early relapsing–remitting multiple sclerosis. *Mult Scler* 2005; 11: 276–81

44. Agosta F, Rovaris M, Pagani E, *et al.* Magnetization transfer MRI metrics predict the accumulation of disability 8 years later in patients with multiple sclerosis. *Brain* 2006; 128: 2620–7.

45. Khaleeli Z, Altmann DR, Cercignami M, *et al.* Magnetization transfer ratio in gray matter: a potential surrogate marker for progression in early primary progressive multiple sclerosis. *Arch Neurol* 2008; 65: 1454–9.

46. Neema M, Stankiewicz J, Arora A *et al.* T1- and T2-based MRI measures of diffuse gray matter and white matter damage in patients with multiple sclerosis. *J Neuroimaging* 2007; 17 (Suppl 1): 16S–21S.

47. Niepel G, Tench ChR, Morgan PS *et al.* Deep gray matter and fatigue in MS: a T1 relaxation time study. *J Neurol* 2006; 253: 896–902.

48. Bakshi R, Benedict RH, Bermel RA, *et al.* T2 hypointensity in the deep gray matter of patients with multiple sclerosis. A quantitative magnetic resonance imaging study. *Arch Neurol* 2002; 59: 62–8.

49. Ceccarelli A, Rocca MA, Neema M, *et al.* Deep gray matter T2 hypointensity is present in patients with clinically isolated syndromes suggestive of multiple sclerosis. *Mult Scler* 2010; 16: 39–44.

50. Filippi M, Rocca MA. Functional MR imaging in multiple sclerosis. *Neuroimaging Clin N Am* 2009; 19: 59–70.

51. Rocca MA, Colombo B, Falini A, *et al.* Cortical adaptation in patients with MS: a cross-sectional functional MRI study of disease phenotypes. *Lancet Neurol* 2005; 4: 618–26.

52. Rocca MA, Agosta F, Colombo B, *et al.* fMRI changes in relapsing-remitting multiple sclerosis patients complaining of fatigue after IFNbeta-1a injection. *Hum Brain Map* 2007; 28: 373–82.

53. Filippi M, Rocca MA, Falini A, *et al.* Correlations between structural CNS damage and functional MRI changes in primary progressive MS. *Neuroimage* 2002; 15: 537–46.

54. Barkhof F, Calabresi PA, Miller DH, Reingold SC. Imaging outcomes for neuroprotection and repair inmultiple sclerosis trials. *Nat Rev Neurol* 2009; 5: 256–66.

55. Giorgio A, Battaglini M, Smith SM, De Stefano N. Brain atrophy assessment in multiple sclerosis: importance and limitations. *Neuroimaging Clin N Am* 2008; 18: 675–86.

56. Filippi M, Agosta F. Imaging biomarkers in multiple sclerosis. *J Magn Reson Imaging* 2010; 31:770–88.

57. Dalton CM, Chard DT, Davies GR, *et al.* Early development of multiple sclerosis is associated with progressive grey matter atrophy in patients presenting with clinically isolated syndromes. *Brain* 2004; 127: 1101–7.

58. Fisher E, Lee JC, Nakamura K, *et al.* Gray matter atrophy in multiple sclerosis: a longitudinal study. *Ann Neurol* 2008; 64: 255–65.

59. Ceccarelli A, Rocca MA, Pagani E, *et al.* A voxel-based morphometry study of grey matter loss in MS patients with different clinical phenotypes. *Neuroimage* 2008; 42: 315–22.

60. Gilmore CP, Geurts JJ, Evangelou N, *et al.* Spinal cord grey matter lesions in multiple sclerosis detected by post-mortem high field imaging. *Mult Scler* 2009; 15: 180–8.

61. Agosta F, Absinta M, Sormani MP, *et al.* In vivo assessment of cervical cord damage in MS patients: a longitudinal diffusion tensor MRI study. *Brain* 2007; 130: 2211–19.

62. Ciccarelli O, Wheeler-Kingshott CA, McLean MA, *et al.* Spinal cord spectroscopy and diffusion based tractography to assess acute disability in multiple sclerosis. *Brain* 2007; 130: 2220–31.

63. Agosta F, Valsasina P, Caputo D, Stroman PW, Filippi M. Tactile-associated recruitment of the cervical cord is altered in patients with multiple sclerosis. *Neuroimage* 2008; 15: 1542–8.

64. Agosta F, Pagani E, Caputo D, Filippi M. Association between cervical cord gray matter damage and disability in patients with multiple sclerosis. *Arch Neurol* 2007; 64: 1302–5.

65. Ciccarelli O, Altmann DR, McLean MA, *et al.* Spinal cord repair in MS: does mitochondrial metabolism play a role. *Neurology* 2010; 74:721–7.

66. Geurts JJ, van Horssen J. The brake on neurodegeneration: increased mitochondrial metabolism in the injured MS spinal cord. *Neurology* 2010; 74: 710–11.

67. Schoonheim MM, Geurts JJ, Barkhof F. The limits of functional reorganization in multiple sclerosis. *Neurology* 2010; 74: 1246–7.

Functional imaging in multiple sclerosis

Kyle C. Kern and Nancy L. Sicotte

Introduction

The development of magnetic resonance imaging (MRI) has greatly facilitated the diagnosis of multiple sclerosis (MS). However, the weak association between structural white matter findings and clinical disability has prompted the use of functional imaging techniques to further understand the physiological response to MS damage and to better predict clinical outcomes. This chapter will provide background on the use of functional imaging in MS research and the feasibility of applying these approaches to clinical therapeutic trials. A brief methodological description of the most revealing functional imaging modalities will highlight the potential benefits and limitations of applying these techniques to patient studies. In addition, recent functional neuroimaging literature will be reviewed that has led to significant advances in our understanding of several different domains of MS clinical disability. Finally, we will consider the integration of imaging modalities in investigating functional compensation and network dysfunction, with an emphasis on blood oxygen-level dependent (BOLD) functional magnetic resonance imaging (fMRI) which holds promise as a meaningful outcome measure for future trials of neuroprotective and regenerative therapies.

In recent years, the use of multiple imaging modalities in MS research has painted a much more complex picture of MS pathology that better explains the wide spectrum of clinical deficits. While MRI has long been used to monitor both acutely enhancing and chronic lesions, the lack of histopathological specificity of MRI hyperintensities allows only a weak correlation with progression of neurological disability.[1] However, additional imaging techniques such as magnetization transfer,[2] magnetic resonance spectroscopy,[3] and double inversion recovery[4] have revealed gray matter structural changes in MS as well (Chapters 11 and 13). Both cortical[5] and subcortical[6,7] gray matter changes provide more specific biomarkers linking potentially irreversible structural damage with early clinical disability. However, while MS-related pathology is heterogeneous, the brain's ability to adapt also varies between patients. The promise of dynamic, in vivo measurements of brain function provides the best hope for understanding the mechanisms of brain plasticity. Functional imaging in multiple sclerosis may better explain the discrepancy between structural damage and clinical function.

Adaptive cortical reorganization implies the redistribution of neural processing that maintains clinical function or minimizes loss in spite of pathological damage. This compensation can occur through altered morphology and function of neuronal interactions in response to experience or injury. Detecting and understanding these changes in vivo is the ultimate goal of functional imaging, so that we may monitor and promote these processes during treatment and recovery. While MS-related structural changes may coincide with altered functional imaging results, we must be careful in labeling these changes as adaptive compensation. Interpretation of functional imaging is complicated by the fact that the data are merely indirect measures of neuronal function, and that neural activity may be either excitatory or inhibitory. However, functional changes observed thus far in studies of MS patients has generally involved increased normal brain activity and/or additional areas of increased activity relative to healthy controls that is required to maintain normal performance on a task.[8]

Functional imaging methods

Several techniques have been used to assess brain function by measuring glucose metabolism,[9] receptor binding,[10] or cerebral blood flow.[11] Single photon emission computed tomography (SPECT) and positron emission tomography (PET) are among the earliest functional imaging techniques developed and are dependent on the injection of a radioactive tracer. Since the mid 1990s, fMRI has become the most commonly used method since it is completely non-invasive. The ability of any functional imaging study to reveal brain activity accurately is limited by the spatial and temporal resolution of the particular technique, the type of scanner used, and the parameters chosen for an individual scan. The choice of acquisition parameters must be considered when comparing functional activity across studies. Furthermore, "activity" must be carefully interpreted, since increased metabolism or blood flow is not exclusive to neuronal excitation.

Multiple Sclerosis Therapeutics, Fourth Edition, ed. Jeffrey A. Cohen and Richard A. Rudick. Published by Cambridge University Press.
© Cambridge University Press 2011.

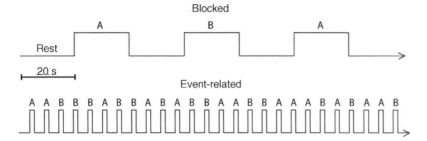

Fig. 14.1. Schematic examples of blocked and event-related fMRI experimental designs. In the blocked design (top), experimental conditions A and B occur for 20 seconds, alternating with rest periods. Localizing changes in the hemodynamic response is feasible as differing cerebral states are maintained for relatively long periods. In contrast, the event-related design (bottom) shows a pseudorandom ordering of individual trials for each condition. In this case, cortical responses can be sorted according to trial type or subject's behavioral response, and the time course of the hemodynamic response is determined by deconvolving the signal changes over time according to an algorithm.

Single photon emission computed tomography (SPECT)

SPECT images are acquired after administration of a radioactive compound that emits single photons that can be detected by gamma-cameras. Technetium-99m complexes are commonly injected intravenously and used to measure brain perfusion.[12] Other radioisotopes such as xenon-133 or iodine-123, or engineered radioligands can also be injected or inhaled to measure blood volume, metabolic function, or receptor binding.[13] SPECT acquires only relative image intensities, has a spatial resolution on the order of centimeters, and generally takes longer to acquire than PET since it uses longer tracer half-lives.

Positron emission tomography (PET)

Similar to SPECT, PET imaging also uses radioactive biotracers to monitor physiological processes. However, better localization is achieved in PET imaging, since the administered radioactive tracer emits positrons that collide with electrons to produce two gamma rays at 180 degrees, both of which are detected coincidently on the external detector ring. Coincident localization and the use of tomographic reconstruction allow for a better spatial resolution of about 5 mm. However, with PET the timing of the tracer administration is crucial since the tracers' half-lives are generally shorter. But an added benefit is that the amount of tracer in the blood can be sampled to determine its kinetics. As detector hits accumulate over time, absolute functional activity can be quantified. PET ligands have been engineered to investigate many physiological functions, including glucose metabolism,[9] receptor binding,[10] cerebral blood flow,[11] and even gene expression.[14]

Functional magnetic resonance imaging (fMRI)

Magnetic resonance imaging (MRI) uses a strong, standing magnetic field and measures the MR signal attenuation as polar molecules realign after the application of radiofrequency energy pulses. Because deoxygenated hemoglobin is paramagnetic and alters the $T2^*$ MR signal, MR pulse sequences can be optimized to detect the hemodynamic changes that result from increased neuronal function. In areas of increased brain activity, the ratio of oxyhemoglobin to deoxyhemoglobin increases as the hemodynamic response overcompensates for neuronal function. This response is detected as the blood oxygen level dependent (BOLD) signal.

The use of fMRI has exploded in the last two decades due to the fact that it is non-invasive, is widely available, involves no exposure to radioactivity and therefore lends itself to multiple acquisitions and longitudinal assessments. Compared to PET or SPECT, fMRI has a superior spatial resolution of 1–3 mm. The BOLD response has been shown to correlate closely to neuronal firing rate and synaptic activity.[15] Furthermore, functional localization determined by fMRI has been in agreement with electrophysiological and lesion studies.[16]

One of the major disadvantages to fMRI is that acquisition time is relatively long, so data quality is highly susceptible to motion in the scanner. This can be particularly problematic if the functional task requires movement, since task synchronous movement is difficult to distinguish from task-dependent activation. Aside from motion artifacts, tissue magnetic susceptibility distortion also affects the echo planar imaging pulse sequences used for fMRI. In regions where air interfaces with tissue, perturbations in the magnetic field can cause geometric distortions or signal dropout. All of these complications are concerning in fMRI since the BOLD signal intensity change due to neural activity typically only ranges from 0.5% to 5%.

fMRI can be used with several different experimental designs to answer distinct questions about brain function as shown in Fig. 14.1. The most straightforward is the task-dependent boxcar design, which is used to localize brain activity during a task with an on/off paradigm. Task stimuli are presented for 20 to 30 second intervals with rest or control periods interspersed between. The use of several blocks allows for signal averaging of the on/off contrast. Although seemingly straightforward, the analysis can be confounded by attenuation of the physiological response due to habituation or fatigue.

Another task-dependent use of fMRI is an event-related design. Stimuli are presented as brief, isolated events and the contrast paradigm is fit to these stimuli. Event-related designs are better for quantifying and characterizing graded responses since the temporal dynamics of the hemodynamic response are preserved. However, the lower statistical power of the design requires more repetitions, and the order of stimuli presentation must be carefully considered to avoid priming or bias effects.

Unlike the task-dependent designs, resting-state fMRI (rsfMRI) requires no stimulus presentation. Subjects are asked

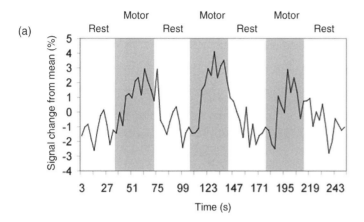

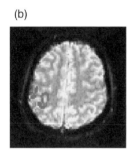

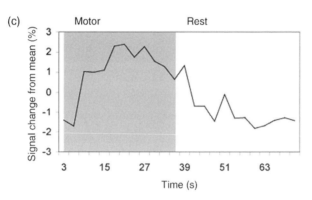

Fig. 14.2. Example of a blocked fMRI experimental design and data from a normal control subject. (a) BOLD signal changes in the most active voxel during a finger tapping motor paradigm. Gray background regions indicate motor task performance (36 s); white regions are rest (36 s). (b) The left hemisphere cortical region activated by performing the task in the right hand. (c) Average signal change in the same voxel as (a), over 3 cycles of the task. Data analysis was done using FEAT (FMRI Expert Analysis Tool) Version 5.1, part of FSL (FMRIB's Software Library, www.fmrib.ox.ac.uk/fsl).[19] Time series statistical analysis was carried out using FILM (FMRIB's Improved Linear Model).[20] Z statistic images were thresholded using voxel clusters determined by Z > 3.0 and a cluster significance threshold of P = 0.01.[21] Registration to standard images was carried out using FLIRT[22] (see also color plate section).

to try not to think about anything nor fall asleep for 5 to 10 minutes. The goal is to detect constitutive brain activity fluctuations of up to 3% that occur every 10 to 100 seconds.[17] Patterns in low-frequency BOLD fluctuations are analyzed using independent component analysis to determine networks of connectivity between different brain regions. Several different resting-state networks have been identified using this technique that are closely linked with underlying structural connectivity.[18]

Statistical techniques and image processing

Functional imaging data analysis is not for the computationally timid, but it does hold promise as a secondary outcome measure for clinical trials. Before any statistical analyses, the data must undergo an array of preprocessing steps to reduce mechanical and physiological noise. Usually motion correction is performed by aligning each volume of data to a single volume to account for minor changes in head position. Spatial and temporal filtering is applied to eliminate drifts. The use of independent component analysis is not always necessary but can help remove physiological patterns such as breathing and pulse. Alternatively, using cardiac gating to time the pulse sequence during acquisition can also help minimize such physiological interferences.

Statistical analyses can be performed on specific regions of interest (ROI) or across all voxels globally using voxel-wise techniques. At the individual level, task-dependent activity is measured relative to another experimental condition, a control task, or a resting period (see Fig. 14.2). However, when comparing across many voxels or multiple ROIs, stringent multiple comparison corrections must be applied.

To perform group analyses, individual functional data are first aligned to a structural image that also facilitates alignment to a common brain template. Standardized atlases are widely available and are useful for stereotaxic reporting of activation coordinates. These atlases include the Tailarach atlas[23] from a single hemisphere of one individual, and the MNI template,[24] which is an average of 452 normal brains. However, when studying diseased populations, a disease-specific or study-specific atlas is preferable to mitigate misalignment due to pathological structural changes.

Once the group data have been aligned to a common space, different analytical methods can be applied including fixed-effect models or random-effects models, depending on the clinical question. Independent component analysis (ICA), is applied to resting-state fMRI (rsfMRI) to identify regions of synchronous brain activity. Several anatomically distinct resting-state networks have been identified that can be engaged during specific types of brain activity.[25]

MS-specific challenges

MS disease-related brain changes including the presence of focal lesions and atrophy can complicate functional neuroimaging studies. Accounting for brain atrophy can be challenging, particularly in the alignment of the MS brain to the common

177

atlas. Varying amounts of atrophy and ventricular enlargement cause misalignment, reducing statistical power. For this reason, the use of a study-specific brain template may be preferable to a standard atlas of healthy brains. Also, longitudinal studies may detect functional changes that, in reality, are driven mostly by shifts in peak activation due to brain atrophy and imperfect alignment. Separately investigating the effects of total lesion load or global brain atrophy on functional activity may provide meaningful insight on how structural damage affects function.

Another potentially confounding factor with MS populations is the use of medications or disease-modifying therapies that may alter neural activity, perfusion, or the hemodynamic response. For example, IFNß-1a is known to increase relative blood flow to the basal ganglia in MS patients 6 hours after administration.[26] Patients also take muscle relaxants such as baclofen or benzodiazepines, which are known to reduce cerebral metabolism.[27] MS patients may also be on antiepileptic medication such as gabapentin or carbamezepine, or antidepressants such as SSRIs or tricyclics. The effects of these medications on functional activity have not been studied in isolation, and they could be misinterpreted as disease-related differences when a non-medicated control group is used for comparison. Several other variables that affect the BOLD response include caffeine intake,[28] lack of sleep,[29] circadian rhythm,[30] and menstrual cycle.[31] It is important to control for each of these factors when designing a functional imaging study.

While long-term brain structural damage can affect functional activity, episodic physiological changes such as inflammation may also affect blood flow and metabolism. Local changes in perfusion have been detected in lesion-forming locations including altered cerebral blood flow, volume, mean transit time, and the apparent diffusion coefficient.[32] Local perfusion and blood–brain barrier permeability are also affected.[33] In spite of these challenges, a wide variety of studies have successfully applied functional imaging in MS populations, revealing considerable differences from healthy controls. Several examples are discussed next.

Functional imaging in MS

In one of the earliest studies, Brooks et al. used PET to measure regional cerebral blood flow (rCBF) and oxygen extraction rate at rest, demonstrating decreased cerebral O_2 metabolism in the patient group.[34] Other studies have reported relative rCBF decreases in both gray and white matter, and that reduced O_2 metabolism is correlated with higher EDSS scores.[35] Lycke et al. used SPECT to show that frontal lobe gray matter rCBF is related to disability in both relapsing–remitting (RR) and secondary progressive (SP) MS.[36]

Studies investigating glucose metabolism using fluorodeoxyglucose (FDG) PET rather than O_2 metabolism report similar findings, demonstrating decreased metabolism in several brain regions in MS patients (see Fig. 14.3), but these reductions showed little to no correlations with disability.[37] In a cross-sectional study, Blinkenberg et al. found that decreases

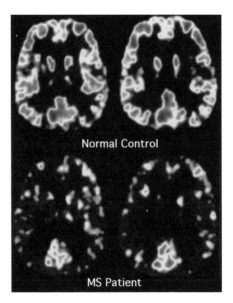

Fig. 14.3. Global decreases in brain activity in MS detected with FDG PET. Images from two slice locations in a normal control (top row) and a patient with MS (bottom row) displayed using the same scale. The MS patient scan demonstrates widespread reductions in cerebral glucose metabolism compared with the control scan. (From Bakshi et al.,[33] used with permission) (see also color plate section).

in cortical and subcortical glucose metabolism (CMRglu) were associated with increased total lesion area and cognitive dysfunction, but not EDSS.[38] In a longitudinal study, CMRglu in frontal and parietal cortices decreased over 2 years, and although this decrease was not correlated with other clinical changes, these results suggest that metabolic markers might be more sensitive to disease progression than other exam-based measures.[39]

Fatigue

Fatigue and depression occur frequently in MS and have a detrimental impact on patient quality of life. Functional imaging holds promise in the study of these poorly understood MS symptoms. Glucose metabolism as measured by CMRglu is decreased in the prefrontal, premotor, supplementary motor, and basal ganglia regions with increased fatigue severity score (FSS) in MS patients. Concurrently, increased CMRglu in the cerebellar vermis and anterior cingulate gyri was also associated with fatigue in MS.[40] The described changes were not associated with EDSS, lesion load, or brain atrophy, suggesting that functional alterations occur in the absence of detectable structural changes.

Filippi and colleagues used fMRI to assess a right-hand motor task in minimally disabled MS patients (EDSS < 2, no hand motor impairment) with and without fatigue. MS patients overall had increased activation in multiple contralateral motor areas and bilateral cingulate motor areas (CMA) compared to controls. But the fatigued patients had greater activation in the contralateral CMA and less activation in the contralateral thalamus and middle frontal gyrus, ipsilateral cerebellum,

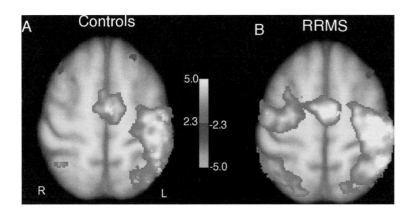

Fig. 14.4. Activated regions revealed by fMRI of healthy controls and MS patients performing a right-hand finger tapping motor task. Average fMRI activation (t-values) from one slice location in a group of 16 healthy controls (a) and a group of 24 early RRMS patients (EDSS < 3) (b), displayed using the same scale. A relative increase in cortical recruitment is evident in the MS group, demonstrated by extended activations in the left ipsilateral premotor, motor, and parietal cortices, as well as greater intensity activations in the right contralateral sensorimotor cortex and supplementary motor area (see also color plate section).

rolandic operculum, and precuneus. Increased FSS was associated with reduced activation in several areas, including the contralateral intraparietal sulcus, the ipsilateral rolandic operculum, and the thalamus. The authors suggested that fatigue might be related to impaired cortical-subcortical interactions of functionally related areas.[41]

DeLuca and colleagues monitored brain activity using fMRI to investigate cognitive fatigue in MS during four trials of a modified symbol digit modalities task. Several regions demonstrated a pattern of increasing activity over the length of the task in MS compared with controls despite maintained performance, including the basal ganglia, frontal lobes, parietal cuneus and precuneus regions, thalami, and occipital lobes. The study suggests that central fatigue is associated with the recruitment of greater functional resources over time, a theory that fits well with clinical descriptions of MS-related fatigue.[42]

Rocca and colleagues investigated the effects of interferon beta-1a injection on reversible fatigue and functional activity during a motor task. Patients who reported reversible fatigue after drug injection showed abnormally increased thalamic and frontal lobe activity during the task when compared to non-fatigued states or patients without fatigue. The authors conclude that abnormal recruitment of fronto-thalamic circuitry underlies interferon beta-1a induced fatigue.[43]

Depression

The effects of depression in MS can be difficult to isolate since they are often associated with fatigue and impaired cognition. In fact, very few studies have attempted to address the issue of depression in MS using functional imaging. Sabatini and colleagues used SPECT to show a unique association between asymmetrical limbic rCBF and depression. While there were no differences between global cognitive scores, EDSS, or regional lesion load between depressed and non-depressed patients, depressed patients had relative hyperperfusion in the left limbic lobe and hypoperfusion in the right limbic lobe.[40] Another fMRI study, not specific to depressed patients, found that altered emotional processing in MS was associated with impaired amygdala–frontal lobe connectivity.[41] Similar results implicating limbic dysfunction involvement in

unipolar depressed patients have been reported, but data suggest that antidepressive treatment can restore normal activity.[46] But to date these studies have not been done in MS patients with depression.

Motor system

The motor system has been extensively studied in MS patients and widespread structural and functional changes have been reported.[47] Simple foot, hand, or finger tasks all show increased cortical activity in MS patients with a decreased lateralization compared to healthy controls. The decreased lateralization of the response in MS is due to both decreased contralateral motor cortex activity and increased ipsilateral motor cortex activity relative to controls (see Fig. 14.4).[48] These patterns are seen in clinically isolated syndrome (CIS), RR, primary progressive (PP), and SP forms of the disease.[49,50] Activation has been shown to increase with task complexity,[51] though similar patterns are seen for both passive and active movements.[52] The brain regions involved include several normal areas of motor planning and execution, including the sensorimotor cortex (SMC), supplementary motor area (SMA), CMA, and cerebellum. Also, the somatotopic organization seen in healthy controls in the cerebrum and cerebellum is preserved in MS. However, motor activity in patients may also include more widespread networks generally reserved for more complex function such as the frontal lobe, the insula, and the thalamus. Slight shifts in peak activation have also been reported in MS patients.[51]

Often, the MS cohorts chosen for functional imaging studies have motor function within the normal range, and yet patterns of activity are already significantly altered. The increased activity is believed to be compensatory in that it is necessary to maintain normal function despite pathological damage. Rocca and colleagues demonstrated that increased fMRI motor network activity during hand motor tasks is associated with greater tissue damage. They showed that increased whole brain gray matter diffusivity in RRMS patients correlated with more ipsilateral SMA activity.[53] In another study, white matter damage, measured by T2 lesion volume, magnetization transfer ratio, and water diffusivity, was also linked to greater motor network activity. Associations were found in the contralateral SMC, ipsilateral SMA, bilateral CMA, and the contralateral intraparietal sulcus.[50] Similar but less extensive effects were seen in a study of CIS patients: greater axonal pathology, as measured by whole-brain NAA levels, correlated with increased contralateral SMC activity during the hand motor task.[55] The authors conclude that increased cortical recruitment over a distributed motor network can limit the functional impact of MS pathology.

These studies and others reveal a pattern of cortical reorganization that varies with disease stage. Early on when tissue damage is minimal, patients may have increased activity in areas typically activated in healthy controls. As disease progresses, patients may engage bilateral motor areas, and then in late-stage disease, they may recruit higher order regions that are normally reserved for complex or novel tasks.[56]

The long-term temporal patterns of functional motor changes in MS patients have only been studied cross-sectionally, but a few longitudinal studies have shown dynamic functional changes even acutely. In a study following a single patient after a relapse leading to hemiparesis, abnormally increased bilateral fMRI motor activity progressively decreased and lateralized (normalized) in the remitting phase in conjunction with increasing corticospinal tract NAA levels.[53] A similar pattern of change after a motor relapse was detected in a series of 12 patients with pseudotumoral lesions: initial increased recruitment of the unaffected hemisphere that normalized over time, but only in patients that recovered clinically.[57,58] Finally, another longitudinal study following a group of nine patients over 15 to 26 months showed that abnormally increased ipsilateral SMA and contralateral cerebellar activity, on average, normalized over time, but that such normalization was hindered in older or more progressed patients.[59]

Only two studies thus far have used fMRI to monitor motor dysfunction using treatment or an intervention in MS. In one, patients were subjected to motor training between multiple fMRI acquisitions during a thumb flexion task. Patients exhibited increased contralateral dorsal premotor activity before and after training, and did not show the practice-dependent signal reduction seen in healthy controls, consistant with a reduced capacity to optimize motor network recruitment through practice in MS.[60] In the second study, a group of 12 MS patients were scanned before and after taking 3,4-diaminopyridine, a potassium channel blocker known to improve motor function and reduce fatigue. Compared to functional activity under placebo, activations increased in the ipsilateral SMC and SMA following drug administration. Transcranial magnetic stimulation also showed that the drug reduced inhibition and increased excitation intracortically, suggesting that 3,4-diaminopyridine may work by increasing brain excitability.[61] This study shows how functional imaging in conjunction with other electrophysiological modalities can be used to measure improvements in neuronal transmission in relevant pathways.

Vision

During active optic neuritis (ON), reductions in BOLD response may be seen in the visual cortex, concurrent with reduced amplitude and latency of visual evoked potentials (VEPs). Toosy and colleagues reported reduced BOLD responses in the visual cortices of patients one month after ON, the degree of which was correlated with optic nerve gadolinium-enhanced lesion length.[62] By 3 months, however, this relationship reversed, and an increased response was observed in the number and size of extrastriate cortical areas responding to visual stimulation. An increased response was still present 1 year later, and patients with the largest cortical activations tended to improve the most in visual acuity. Such recruitment involved a large network of extraoccipital areas, including the insula-claustrum, the lateral temporal and posterior parietal cortices, and the thalamus.[63] These areas are known to have extensive visual connections and are believed to be involved in multimodal sensory integration. This recruitment may underlie improvement in acuity that occurs after ON in spite of continued VEP abnormalities and optic nerve damage.[63]

Cognition

Forty to sixty percent of MS patients suffer cognitive deficits,[64] which may be due to damage to any of a variety of overlapping functional networks. Affected cognitive domains include attention, memory, executive function, visuospatial abilities, problem solving, abstract reasoning, and language. However, conventional MRI data such as T2 lesion volumes[65] are only weakly linked to cognition in MS. Although measures of cortical lesions and atrophy may be more sensitive measures, the application of functional imaging to the study of cognitive dysfunction in MS has obvious appeal.

SPECT and PET studies have shown that cognitive dysfunction is linked to reduced cerebral blood flow and hypometabolism. Pozzilli and colleagues demonstrated frontal and left temporal hypometabolism in cognitively impaired MS patients using SPECT associated with greater third ventricular width and periventricular lesion volume.[66] Frontal lobe hypometabolism as measured by CMRglu has also been seen in cognitively impaired MS patients, along with decreases in the basal ganglia, thalami, and hippocampi related to memory impairment.[67]

Functional MRI studies of MS patients have utilized a variety of cognitive tasks, making it difficult to generalize across results. However, despite the unique cortical regions engaged by tasks such as the PVSAT, PASAT, 2-Back, N-Back or word recall tasks, some general patterns are seen. Patients with preserved or only mildly impaired cognition have increased cortical activity relative to controls including areas normally activated, and in many cases additional brain regions as well.[68] When cognitive function becomes significantly impaired, relative brain activity is diminished, suggesting a loss of compensatory processes associated with more severe structural damage (see Fig. 14.5).[69,70]

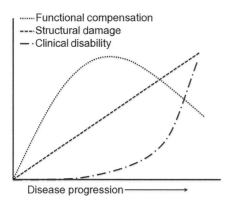

Fig. 14.5. Schematic of the hypothesized relationship between structural damage, functional compensation, and clinical disability with MS disease progression. In early stages of disease, such as CIS, BMS, and very early RRMS, subtle structural damage elicits an increasing response in functional activity without much obvious clinical disability. However, as structural damage accumulates further, functional activity plateaus and clinical disability becomes more apparent. As disease progresses even further and irreversible structural damage persists, such as in SPMS or PPMS, functional activity declines and clinical disability is widespread. Adapted from Schoonheim et al., 2010.[70]

Functional imaging has also been used to study the effects of drug treatment on cognition and brain activity. Two studies used Rivastigmine, a cholinesterase inhibitor, in conjunction with fMRI during an attention and executive function paradigm, the counting Stroop task. In the first study, MS patients off treatment showed greater left medial prefrontal activity and less right frontal activity relative to controls that was associated with disease burden. Low-dose acute administration of Rivastigmine in MS patients normalized these differences, leading to less left prefrontal activity and more right frontal activity. However treatment did not result in improved performance.[71] The second study used high-dose chronic administration of Rivastigmine and confirmed that treatment increased right frontal lobe activity with a trend for improved performance. Furthermore, the second study demonstrated that Rivastigmine also increased functional connectivity between several brain regions involved during an N-back test.[72] The authors suggest that cholinergic agonism may restore functional efficiency by increasing neuronal responsiveness to excitatory input.

Interpretation of cortical reorganization

As functional imaging becomes more popular in MS clinical research, there is still uncertainty in the interpretation of the physiological significance of brain activity changes. Recent studies have combined functional imaging with multimodal structural imaging techniques to more fully understand how cortical activation patterns reflect the brain's response to injury and recovery and how these approaches may lend themselves as readouts for therapeutic interventions. Novel functional imaging paradigms such as rsfMRI have prompted new theories

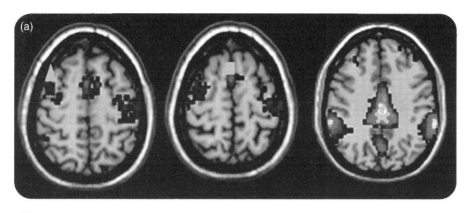

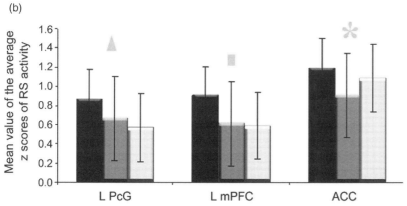

Fig. 14.6. Differences in default mode network (DMN) activity in progressive multiple sclerosis patients relative to healthy controls. Panel (a) shows three axial images demonstrating DMN activity measured by resting state fMRI activity in multiple sclerosis patients relative to healthy controls. Patterns of resting state activity differed significantly in the left precentral gyrus (triangle), medial prefrontal cortex (square), and anterior cingulate cortex (asterisk). Panel (b) shows averaged resting state activity in graphical form across the three groups studied. (Black bars = controls, dark gray bars = primary progressive MS, light gray = secondary progressive MS). (From Rocca et al., 2010,[78] used with permission) (see also color plate section).

on the mechanisms of functional compensation and cortical reorganization.

The most established interpretation of fMRI changes in MS propose that increased activity in areas normally engaged by the task as well as bilateral increases and recruitment of additional areas are adaptive and contribute to maintaining adequate performance. However, other data suggest that increases in detectable activity are not always compensatory. For example, greater ipsilateral motor cortical activity is associated with damage to transcallosal fibers, as measured by diffusion tensor imaging (DTI) and transcranial magnetic stimulation (TMS), suggesting that the loss of inhibitory input rather than compensation may underlie this change.[73] On the other hand, corticospinal damage is linked to increased contralateral SMC activity, which may be more likely to reflect adaptive compensation.[74]

rsfMRI has been used in only a few MS studies to date but holds great promise as a useful measure of axonal and myelin integrity and could serve as a biomarker in clinical trials of remyelination approaches. Lowe *et al.* used rsfMRI in MS in the motor system to demonstrate changes in functional connectivity between the primary SMCs that correlated with tract specific DTI alterations.[75] Roosendaal and colleagues recently demonstrated reduced hippocampal functional connectivity in MS, associated with hippocampal atrophy.[76]

Whole-brain resting-state connectivity analyses have revealed alterations in the default mode network (DMN) in MS that are detectable in CIS patients without measurable impairment or structural damage.[77] Decreased functional connectivity was also seen in the anterior cingulate cortex associated with both cognitive impairment and white matter damage (see Fig. 14.6).[78] Theories on the DMN propose that it is more active than other brain regions during rest or passive thought, but that it is increasingly suppressed during effortful tasks in proportion to task difficulty.[79] In some sense, resting state DMN activity may reflect available resources for task activation, especially since it is known to decrease with increasing prefrontal recruitment.[25] Since connectivity within the DMN network is critical for proper function, white matter damage in MS may reduce the capacity for functional compensation.

fMRI studies using working memory tasks have shown that DMN suppression in MS patients is associated with increased T2 lesion load and poor cognitive performance.[80]

Future directions

Despite many advances, the use of functional imaging in understanding MS disease pathophysiology and progression has been limited to date, and reserved primarily for the research realm. The use of functional imaging to evaluate therapeutic responses will be challenging, but increasingly relevant as neuroprotective and regenerative approaches are developed. Longitudinal studies are needed to establish the reliability of the technique as well as determine the extent of normal variation in brain responses.[81] Incorporating functional imaging paradigms with informative multimodal structural biomarkers such as DTI or cortical thickness will be critical. Improvements in resolution and novel functional imaging techniques such as resting state fMRI will allow us to circumvent many of the limitations of working with functionally impaired patient populations. Furthermore, using other predictive biomarkers such as genotype, endocrine function, or electrophysiological data may improve our understanding of how functional activity is modulated.

Conclusions

Functional imaging studies in MS patients may help resolve the discrepancy between traditional MR measures and clinical outcome. The brain's innate capacity to adapt can limit the expression of the disease process in MS. However, this capacity is not infinite. The prognosis of neurological insult varies with location in the nervous system and the severity of tissue loss. Early functional changes are seen before measurable disability occurs, indicating that gray matter damage, either direct or indirect, may be involved from disease onset. Finally, fMRI in MS patients offers a unique opportunity to study both human brain plasticity and neurodegenerative disease. As our understanding of altered brain activity develops, functional imaging will play a much larger role in clinical trials for MS involving remyelination, cell grafts, neuroprotective treatments, and in illuminating the mechanisms of progressive disease.

References

1. Nijeholt GJ, van Walderveen MA, Castelijns JA, *et al.* Brain and spinal cord abnormalities in multiple sclerosis. Correlation between MRI parameters, clinical subtypes and symptoms. *Brain* 1998;121:687–97.

2. Wolff S, Balaban R. Magnetization transfer contrast (MTC) and tissue water proton relaxation in vivo. *Magn Reson Med* 1989;10:135–44.

3. Frahm J, Bruhn H, Gyngell M, Merboldt K, H‰nicke W, Sauter R. Localized high-resolution proton NMR spectroscopy using stimulated echoes:

initial applications to human brain in vivo. *Magn Reson Med* 1989;9:79–93.

4. Redpath TW, Smith FW. Technical note: use of a double inversion recovery pulse sequence to image selectively grey or white brain matter. *Br J Radiol* 1994;67:1258–63.

5. Sailer M, Fischl B, Salat D, *et al.* Focal thinning of the cerebral cortex in multiple sclerosis. *Brain*. 2003;126:1734–44.

6. Cifelli A, Arridge M, Jezzard P, Esiri MM, Palace J, Matthews PM. Thalamic

neurodegeneration in multiple sclerosis. *Ann Neurol* 2002;52:650–3.

7. Sicotte NL, Kern KC, Giesser BS, *et al.* Regional hippocampal atrophy in multiple sclerosis. *Brain*. 2008;131:1134–41.

8. Audoin B, Ibarrola D, Ranjeva JP, *et al.* Compensatory cortical activation observed by fMRI during a cognitive task at the earliest stage of MS. *Hum Brain Mapp* 2003;20:51–8.

9. Mazziotta JC, Phelps ME, Halgren E. Local cerebral glucose metabolic

response to audiovisual stimulation and deprivation: studies in human subjects with positron CT. *Hum Neurobiol* 1983;2:11–23.

10. Bahn MM, Huang SC, Hawkins RA, *et al.* Models for in vivo kinetic interactions of dopamine D2-neuroreceptors and 3-[18F]fluoroethyl)spiperone examined with positron emission tomography. *J Cereb Blood Flow Metab* 1989;9:840–9.

11. Mazziotta JC, Huang SC, Phelps ME, Carson RE, MacDonald NS, Mahoney K. A noninvasive positron computed tomography technique using oxygen-15–labeled water for the evaluation of neurobehavioral task batteries. *J Cereb Blood Flow Metab* 1985;5:70–8.

12. Leonard JP, Nowotnik DP, Neirinckx RD. Technetium-99m-d, 1-HM-PAO: a new radiopharmaceutical for imaging regional brain perfusion using SPECT–a comparison with iodine-123 HIPDM. *J Nucl Med* 1986;27:1819–23.

13. Kauppinen T, Yang J, Kilpelainen H, Kuikka JT. Quantitation of neuroreceptors: a need for better SPECT imaging. *Nuklearmedizin* 2001;40:102–6.

14. Sun X, Annala AJ, Yaghoubi SS, *et al.* Quantitative imaging of gene induction in living animals. *Gene Ther* 2001;8:1572–9.

15. Logothetis NK, Pauls J, Augath M, Trinath T, Oeltermann A. Neurophysiological investigation of the basis of the fMRI signal. *Nature* 2001;412:150–7.

16. Mukamel R, Gelbard H, Arieli A, Hasson U, Fried I, Malach R. Coupling between neuronal firing, field potentials, and FMRI in human auditory cortex. *Science* 2005;309:951–4.

17. Damoiseaux JS, Rombouts SA, Barkhof F, *et al.* Consistent resting-state networks across healthy subjects. *Proc Natl Acad Sci USA* 2006;103:13848–53.

18. Greicius MD, Supekar K, Menon V, Dougherty RF. Resting-state functional connectivity reflects structural connectivity in the default mode network. *Cereb Cortex* 2009;19:72–8.

19. Smith SM, Jenkinson M, Woolrich MW, *et al.* Advances in functional and structural MR image analysis and implementation as FSL. *Neuroimage* 2004;23Suppl 1:5208–19.

20. Woolrich MW, Ripley BD, Brady M *et al.* Temporal autocorrelation in univariate linear modeling of fMRI data *Neuroimage* 2001;14(6):1370–86.

21. Friston KJ. Analysis of fMRI time-series revisited [see comment]. *Neuroimage* 1995;2(1):45–53.

22. Jenkinson M, Bannister P, Brady M, Smith S. Improved optimization for the robust and accurate linear registration and motion correction of brain images *Neuroimage* 2002;17(2):825–41.

23. Talairach J, Tournoux P. *Co-planar Stereotaxic Atlas of the Human Brain: 3-Dimensional Proportional System: An Approach to Cerebral Imaging*: Thieme; 1988.

24. Mazziotta JC. A probabilistic atlas and reference system for the human brain: International Consortium for Brain Mapping (ICBM). *Phil Trans R Soc Lond B Biol Sci* 2001;356:1293–322.

25. Greicius MD, Krasnow B, Reiss AL, Menon V. Functional connectivity in the resting brain: a network analysis of the default mode hypothesis. *Proc Natl Acad Sci USA* 2003;100:253–8.

26. Mackowiak PA, Siegel E, Wasserman SS, Cameron E, Nessaiver MS, Bever CT. Effects of IFN-beta on human cerebral blood flow distribution. *J Interferon Cytokine Res* 1998;18: 393–7.

27. de Wit H, Metz J, Wagner N, Cooper M. Effects of diazepam on cerebral metabolism and mood in normal volunteers. *Neuropsychopharmacology* 1991;5:33–41.

28. Liu TT, Behzadi Y, Restom K, *et al.* Caffeine alters the temporal dynamics of the visual BOLD response. *Neuroimage* 2004;23:1402–13.

29. Mu Q, Nahas Z, Johnson KA, *et al.* Decreased cortical response to verbal working memory following sleep deprivation. *Sleep* 2005;28:55–67.

30. Buysse DJ, Nofzinger EA, Germain A, *et al.* Regional brain glucose metabolism during morning and evening wakefulness in humans: preliminary findings. *Sleep* 2004;27:1245–54.

31. Dietrich T, Krings T, Neulen J, Willmes K, Erberich S, Thron A, *et al.* Effects of blood estrogen level on cortical activation patterns during cognitive activation as measured by functional MRI. *Neuroimage* 2001;13:425–32.

32. Werring DJ, Brassat D, Droogan AG, *et al.* The pathogenesis of lesions and normal-appearing white matter changes in multiple sclerosis: a serial diffusion MRI study. *Brain* 2000;123:1667–76.

33. Chavarria A, Alcocer-Varela J. Is damage in central nervous system due to inflammation? *Autoimmun Rev* 2004;3:251–60.

34. Brooks DJ, Leenders KL, Head G, Marshall J, Legg NJ, Jones T. Studies on regional cerebral oxygen utilisation and cognitive function in multiple sclerosis. *J Neurol Neurosurg Psychiatry* 1984;47:1182–91.

35. Sun X, Tanaka M, Kondo S, Okamoto K, Hirai S. Clinical significance of reduced cerebral metabolism in multiple sclerosis: a combined PET and MRI study. *Ann Nucl Med* 1998;12:89–94.

36. Lycke J, Wikkelso C, Bergh AC, Jacobsson L, Andersen O. Regional cerebral blood flow in multiple sclerosis measured by single photon emission tomography with technetium-99m hexamethylpropyleneamine oxime. *Eur Neurol* 1993;33:163–7.

37. Bakshi R, Miletich RS, Kinkel PR, Emmet ML, Kinkel WR. High-resolution fluorodeoxyglucose positron emission tomography shows both global and regional cerebral hypometabolism in multiple sclerosis. *J Neuroimaging* 1998;8:228–34.

38. Blinkenberg M, Rune K, Jensen CV, *et al.* Cortical cerebral metabolism correlates with MRI lesion load and cognitive dysfunction in MS. *Neurology* 2000;54:558–64.

39. Blinkenberg M, Jensen CV, Holm S, Paulson OB, Sorensen PS. A longitudinal study of cerebral glucose metabolism, MRI, and disability in patients with MS. *Neurology* 1999;53:149–53.

40. Roelcke U, Kappos L, Lechner-Scott J, *et al.* Reduced glucose metabolism in the frontal cortex and basal ganglia of multiple sclerosis patients with fatigue: a 18F-fluorodeoxyglucose positron emission tomography study. *Neurology* 1997;48:1566–71.

41. Filippi M, Rocca MA, Colombo B, *et al.* Functional magnetic resonance imaging correlates of fatigue in multiple sclerosis. *Neuroimage* 2002;15:559–67.

42. DeLuca J, Genova HM, Hillary FG, Wylie G. Neural correlates of cognitive

fatigue in multiple sclerosis using functional MRI. *J Neurol Sci* 2008;270:28–39.

43. Rocca MA, Agosta F, Colombo B, *et al.* fMRI changes in relapsing-remitting multiple sclerosis patients complaining of fatigue after IFNbeta-1a injection. *Hum Brain Mapp* 2007;28:373–82.

44. Sabatini U, Pozzilli C, Pantano P, *et al.* Involvement of the limbic system in multiple sclerosis patients with depressive disorders. *Biol Psychiatry* 1996;39:970–5.

45. Passamonti L, Cerasa A, Liguori M, *et al.* Neurobiological mechanisms underlying emotional processing in relapsing-remitting multiple sclerosis. *Brain* 2009;132:3380–91.

46. Kennedy SH, Evans KR, Kruger S, *et al.* Changes in regional brain glucose metabolism measured with positron emission tomography after paroxetine treatment of major depression. *Am J Psychiatry* 2001;158:899–905.

47. Lee M, Reddy H, Johansen-Berg H, *et al.* The motor cortex shows adaptive functional changes to brain injury from multiple sclerosis. *Ann Neurol* 2000;47:606–13.

48. Pantano P, Iannetti GD, Caramia F, *et al.* Cortical motor reorganization after a single clinical attack of multiple sclerosis. *Brain* 2002;125: 1607–15.

49. Filippi M. Linking structural, metabolic and functional changes in multiple sclerosis. *Eur J Neurol* 2001;8:291–7.

50. Rocca MA, Gavazzi C, Mezzapesa DM, *et al.* A functional magnetic resonance imaging study of patients with secondary progressive multiple sclerosis. *Neuroimage* 2003;19:1770–7.

51. Filippi M, Rocca MA, Mezzapesa DM, *et al.* Simple and complex movement-associated functional MRI changes in patients at presentation with clinically isolated syndromes suggestive of multiple sclerosis. *Hum Brain Mapp* 2004;21:108–17.

52. Reddy H, Narayanan S, Woolrich M, *et al.* Functional brain reorganization for hand movement in patients with multiple sclerosis: defining distinct effects of injury and disability. *Brain* 2002;125:2646–57.

53. Rocca MA, Pagani E, Ghezzi A, *et al.* Functional cortical changes in patients with multiple sclerosis and nonspecific findings on conventional magnetic resonance imaging scans of the brain. *Neuroimage* 2003;19:826–36.

54. Rocca MA, Falini A, Colombo B, Scotti G, Comi G, Filippi M. Adaptive functional changes in the cerebral cortex of patients with nondisabling multiple sclerosis correlate with the extent of brain structural damage. *Ann Neurol* 2002;51:330–9.

55. Rocca MA, Mezzapesa DM, Falini A, *et al.* Evidence for axonal pathology and adaptive cortical reorganization in patients at presentation with clinically isolated syndromes suggestive of multiple sclerosis. *Neuroimage* 2003;18:847–55.

56. Rocca MA, Colombo B, Falini A, *et al.* Cortical adaptation in patients with MS: a cross-sectional functional MRI study of disease phenotypes. *Lancet Neurol* 2005;4:618–26.

57. Reddy H, Narayanan S, Matthews PM, *et al.* Relating axonal injury to functional recovery in MS. *Neurology* 2000;54:236–9.

58. Mezzapesa DM, Rocca MA, Rodegher M, Comi G, Filippi M. Functional cortical changes of the sensorimotor network are associated with clinical recovery in multiple sclerosis. *Hum Brain Mapp* 2008;29:562–73.

59. Pantano P, Mainero C, Lenzi D, *et al.* A longitudinal fMRI study on motor activity in patients with multiple sclerosis. *Brain* 2005;128:2146–53.

60. Morgen K, Kadom N, Sawaki L, *et al.* Training-dependent plasticity in patients with multiple sclerosis. *Brain* 2004;127:2506–17.

61. Mainero C, Inghilleri M, Pantano P, *et al.* Enhanced brain motor activity in patients with MS after a single dose of 3,4-diaminopyridine. *Neurology* 2004;62:2044–50.

62. Toosy AT, Hickman SJ, Miszkiel KA, *et al.* Adaptive cortical plasticity in higher visual areas after acute optic neuritis. *Ann Neurol* 2005;57:622–33.

63. Werring DJ, Bullmore ET, Toosy AT, *et al.* Recovery from optic neuritis is associated with a change in the distribution of cerebral response to visual stimulation: a functional magnetic resonance imaging study. *J Neurol Neurosurg Psychiatry* 2000;68:441–9.

64. Rao SM, Leo GJ, Bernardin L, Unverzagt F. Cognitive dysfunction in multiple sclerosis. I. Frequency, patterns, and prediction. *Neurology* 1991;41:685–91.

65. Rao SM, Leo GJ, Haughton VM, St Aubin-Faubert P, Bernardin L. Correlation of magnetic resonance imaging with neuropsychological testing in multiple sclerosis. *Neurology* 1989;39:161–6.

66. Pozzilli C, Passafiume D, Bernardi S, *et al.* SPECT, MRI and cognitive functions in multiple sclerosis. *J Neurol Neurosurg Psychiatry* 1991;54:110–15.

67. Paulesu E, Perani D, Fazio F, *et al.* Functional basis of memory impairment in multiple sclerosis: a[18F]FDG PET study. *Neuroimage* 1996;4:87–96.

68. Staffen W, Mair A, Zauner H, *et al.* Cognitive function and fMRI in patients with multiple sclerosis: evidence for compensatory cortical activation during an attention task. *Brain* 2002;125:1275–82.

69. Mainero C, Caramia F, Pozzilli C, *et al.* fMRI evidence of brain reorganization during attention and memory tasks in multiple sclerosis. *Neuroimage* 2004;21:858–67.

70. Schoonheim MM, Geurts JJ, Barkhof F. The limits of functional reorganization in multiple sclerosis. *Neurology* 2010;74:1246–7.

71. Parry AM, Scott RB, Palace J, Smith S, Matthews PM. Potentially adaptive functional changes in cognitive processing for patients with multiple sclerosis and their acute modulation by rivastigmine. *Brain* 2003;126:2750–60.

72. Cader S, Palace J, Matthews PM. Cholinergic agonism alters cognitive processing and enhances brain functional connectivity in patients with multiple sclerosis. *J Psychopharmacol* 2009;23:686–96.

73. Lenzi D, Conte A, Mainero C, *et al.* Effect of corpus callosum damage on ipsilateral motor activation in patients with multiple sclerosis: a functional and anatomical study. *Hum Brain Mapp* 2007;28:636–44.

74. Pantano P, Mainero C, Iannetti GD, *et al.* Contribution of corticospinal tract damage to cortical motor reorganization after a single clinical attack of multiple sclerosis. *Neuroimage* 2002;17:1837–43.

75. Lowe MJ, Beall EB, Sakaie KE, *et al.* Resting state sensorimotor functional

connectivity in multiple sclerosis inversely correlates with transcallosal motor pathway transverse diffusivity. *Hum Brain Mapp* 2008;29:818–27.

76. Roosendaal SD, Hulst HE, Vrenken H, *et al.* Structural and functional hippocampal changes in multiple sclerosis patients with intact memory function. *Radiology* 2010;255:595–604.

77. Roosendaal SD, Schoonheim MM, Hulst HE, *et al.* Resting state networks

change in clinically isolated syndrome. *Brain* 2010;133:1612–21.

78. Rocca MA, Valsasina P, Absinta M, *et al.* Default-mode network dysfunction and cognitive impairment in progressive MS. *Neurology* 2010;74:1252–9.

79. Singh KD, Fawcett IP. Transient and linearly graded deactivation of the human default-mode network by a visual detection task. *Neuroimage* 2008;41:100–12.

80. Genova HM, Hillary FG, Wylie G, Rypma B, Deluca J. Examination of processing speed deficits in multiple sclerosis using functional magnetic resonance imaging. *J Int Neuropsychol Soc* 2009;15:383–93.

81. Cardinal KS, Wilson SM, Giesser BS, Drain AE, Sicotte NL. A longitudinal fMRI study of the paced auditory serial addition task. *Mult Scler* 2008;14:465–71.

Chapter

15

Diffusion imaging in multiple sclerosis

Stephen E. Jones and Michael D. Phillips

Introduction

Diffusion imaging is a special MRI technique that has been used extensively since the early 1990s to evaluate a wide variety of neurological processes. Although best known for its essential role in imaging acute infarction, diffusion imaging is also applied to many other conditions, including multiple sclerosis (MS). Its widespread use is a reflection of the power and sensitivity of this technique to provide new information regarding the underlying structure of the brain, which can often reflect pathologic processes at their earliest stages. One method of diffusion imaging called diffusion tensor imaging (DTI) is unique in its ability to delineate and investigate specific white matter pathways within the brain. Its relevance to our understanding of MS has been demonstrated clearly through a broad array of research applications. Diffusion imaging is sensitive to all stages of the disease process in MS and may provide a new approach to differentiate ongoing inflammation from neurodegeneration. For example, applied to specific pathways, DTI measures can be compared directly to pathway-specific function as well as other pathway-specific functional imaging metrics such as functional MRI (fMRI) and functional connectivity, often demonstrating strong correlations that outperform conventional MR techniques.

Despite the clear research applications for diffusion imaging, it has not been consistently applied in the clinical arena or within therapeutic trials. Reasons for this include perceived and real uncertainties regarding performance and reproducibility, particularly across platforms and institutions. Recent studies have demonstrated, however, that DTI can be performed consistently across centers with good sensitivity for longitudinal changes in MS. This suggests that DTI will in the future play a larger role in both clinical decision-making and therapeutic trials.

Diffusion imaging: the basics

For an excellent review of the basics of diffusion imaging the reader is referred to LeBihan et al.[1] Diffusion imaging is exquisitely sensitive to the net movement or displacement of a population of water molecules within a given imaging voxel.

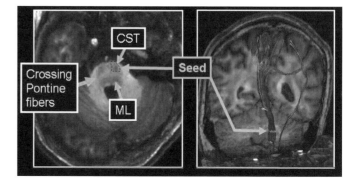

Fig. 15.1. Example of deterministic fiber tracking derived from DTI imaging data. The left panel shows an axial section of a colorized FA map through the level of the brainstem. The bilateral corticospinal tracks (CST) are visualized as purple regions in the anterior pons (the left CST is outlined by dashed lines, and forms an ROI for the "seeding" of fibertracks). Also seen are the crossing pontine fibers (orange) and the medial longitudinal fasciculus (purple). The right panel shows fiber tracks generated using the left CST ROI, using an anterior coronal 3D view. Several features are noteworthy: deterministic tracking of the CST always fails to find tracks extending to the lateral margins of the brain, secondary to strong effects of crossing fibers in the corona radiata; aberrant tracks are included that are not anatomic (for example crossing to contralateral side); while coarse features of tracks are anatomically reasonable, numerous details of the tracks are highly variable (not shown) and very sensitive to specified user input values (see also color plate section).

Although this information can be used to make very compelling images of white matter "tracks" (Fig. 15.1) and subsequently derive insights to the underlying structure of the brain, it is essential to remember that the only thing actually being measured is the movement of water. The most commonly applied diffusion imaging method works by simply adding an additional pulse of strong magnetic gradient within a T2 weighted echo planar imaging (EPI) sequence. Note that gradients are completely described by a magnitude and a single direction in space. All modern MRI machines are engineered so that the direction of the gradient can be applied in any specified direction within 4π steradians, in addition to varying strengths. During the echo sequence, water molecules moving along the direction of the gradient experience maximal dephasing, in comparison to water molecules that are not moving in the direction of the gradient. This dephasing of water molecules results in a net loss of signal during formation of the echo, which is

Multiple Sclerosis Therapeutics, Fourth Edition, ed. Jeffrey A. Cohen and Richard A. Rudick. Published by Cambridge University Press.
© Cambridge University Press 2011.

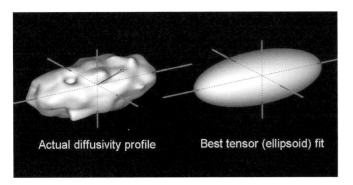

Actual diffusivity profile   Best tensor (ellipsoid) fit

Fig. 15.2. The left panel shows a schematic of a possible diffusivity profile, which forms a three-dimensional surface in diffusion space. The surface is formed such that the distance from the origin to any point on the surface (for example, along the arrow connecting the origin to the small circle on the surface) is the measured diffusivity obtained from a DTI acquisition using a diffusion gradient along that same direction. For an isotropic media such as CSF this surface would be a sphere, whereas for a complex media the surface can be elongated and highly irregular. Note that to generate such a smooth surface requires an infinite number of diffusion gradients, which is not practical. At the other extreme, the best minimum description of the diffusivity profile is achieved with a best-fit ellipsoid, mathematically described as a second-rank tensor, and only requires 6 different diffusion gradient acquisitions. Modern techniques using more directions, for example 71 directions and higher, do not use the tensor fit and can probe more details of the diffusivity profile, which are termed High Angular Resolution Diffusion Imaging (HARDI).

roughly proportional to the distance traveled while the gradient is applied. This signal loss can be directly related to the mean diffusivity of water *along that direction*. To more fully interrogate the three-dimensional nature of diffusion, multiple directions are required. In fact, if infinite directions could be acquired over all 4π steradians, a smooth diffusivity profile could be computed in the form of a closed surface around the origin (Fig 15.2), such that the distance from the origin along a line to any point on the surface would represent the diffusivity along that direction. For large CSF spaces, water freely diffuses equally in all directions, and this surface becomes a sphere representing isotropic diffusivity. In distinction, within tissue, water diffusion is decreased or restricted by barriers such as cell membranes, and the shape of the diffusivity surface can significantly change in both size and sphericity. For example, in white matter, myelin is hydrophobic and forms a strong barrier to water diffusion, resulting in highly anisotropic diffusion that occurs primarily parallel to axons. Correspondingly, relatively little diffusion occurs perpendicular to axons as the movement of water in this direction is restricted by myelin. During the typical EPI sequence, water molecules have the opportunity to move approximately 10 to 15 μm during the time of acquisition. In theory, this makes diffusion imaging sensitive to ultrastructural changes within the brain on the order of 10 to 15 μm, which explains the highly sensitive nature of diffusion imaging. It also offers some explanation for the very non-specific nature of diffusion results. Any pathology that alters the ultra-structure of the brain also produces changes in diffusion as is evidenced by the thousands of papers published over the broad spectrum of neurologic diseases using diffusion imaging. Although diffusion gradients can be applied in any direction to form a

diffusivity profile, it is not practical to probe every direction. The trade-off for fewer directions is decreased resolution of the diffusivity profile. The lowest limit is six different directions, such that the resulting diffusivity profile is in effect a best-fit ellipsoid (Fig. 15.2) to the real underlying profile, and mathematically this forms a second-rank tensor.[1] Imaging based on this methodology is known as diffusion tensor imaging (DTI), in distinction to the simplest form of diffusion imaging, diffusion-weighted imaging or DWI, which forgoes any directional information about diffusion and only provides mean diffusion values such as the apparent diffusion constant (ADC). In DTI, it is simplest to think of the diffusion tensor as an ellipsoid, with the three principal axes determined by the three eigenvectors (Fig. 15.3). The principal eigenvector forms the long axis of the ellipsoid and can be considered the diffusion direction with the greatest magnitude inside the voxel. The secondary and tertiary eigenvectors are perpendicular to the principal eigenvector and represent short axes of diffusion. A reasonable hypothesis in strongly organized white matter is that the principal eigenvector aligns parallel with major white matter tracts (see Fig. 15.3) and the secondary and tertiary eigenvectors are perpendicular to the white matter tracts. This allows DTI measurements to provide a good description of diffusion direction or anisotropy. The DTI diffusion properties most commonly reported are the mean diffusivity (MD), which is the average diffusion along the directions of the eigenvectors; the fractional anisotropy (FA), which is a rough measurement of the degree of diffusion directionality; parallel or axial diffusivity ($\lambda_{\parallel}$), which is simply the principal eigenvector measurement; and transverse or radial diffusivity ($\lambda_{\perp}$), which is the average of the secondary and tertiary eigenvectors. In highly organized white matter tracts, $\lambda_{\parallel}$ is parallel to the course of axons and $\lambda_{\perp}$ is oriented perpendicular to the course of the pathway. FA, $\lambda_{\perp}$, and $\lambda_{\parallel}$ are relatively well described in highly organized pathways; however, within regions of crossing fibers, or in areas of low anisotropy such as gray matter or within lesions, caution is required to interpret these measurements. Although DTI measurements have become the primary method used for MS research, the initial diffusion imaging observations in MS were performed with DWI, which remains the most commonly applied clinical diffusion sequence.

DWI in MS

Early evaluations of MS with diffusion imaging focused on the most basic form of diffusion imaging, DWI, which is relatively easy to perform using only acquisitions in the three cardinal imaging planes.[2–10] This simple method only allows for computation of the scalar apparent diffusion coefficient (ADC), and cannot evaluate reliable directional variation. Despite this, DWI consistently demonstrates *increased* ADC values within MS lesions.[2–10] Furthermore, there are significant differences in ADC values among acute, subacute, and chronic MS lesions.[4,6,9] ADC values discriminate between different types of MS (relapsing–remitting vs. secondary progressive),[2,7] correlate

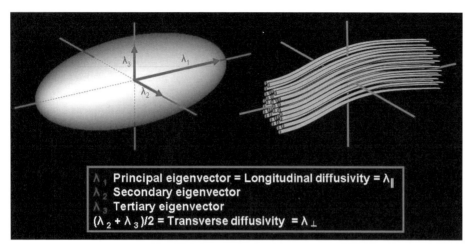

λ_1 **Principal eigenvector = Longitudinal diffusivity = $\lambda_\parallel$**
λ_2 **Secondary eigenvector**
λ_3 **Tertiary eigenvector**
$(\lambda_2 + \lambda_3)/2$ = Transverse diffusivity = $\lambda_\perp$

Fig. 15.3. Graphical example of a diffusion tensor ellipsoid, showing the three principal axes as formed by the three eigenvectors. The lengths of these vectors reflect the diffusivity along those directions, with that of the longest vector termed the longitudinal diffusivity. The transverse diffusivity is formed from the average of the secondary and tertiary diffusivity. The mean diffusivity (MD) is formed from the average of all three eigenvalues. The fractional anisotropy (FA) is a measure of the deviation of the ellipsoid from sphericity. The right panel depicts the underlying hypothesis that the principal eigenvector is parallel to the major direction of an axonal bundle. Although appealing, this relationship becomes very weak in multiple areas of the brain, for example in regions of crossing fibers. Thus, it is always essential to remember that visualized tracts resulting from DTI analysis actually reflect the movement of water, and do not necessarily represent underlying tracts.

with clinical measurements of disease severity,[2] and demonstrate a strong inverse correlation with magnetization transfer (MT) measurements of disease burden.[3] Additionally, there are ADC changes in normal appearing white matter (NAWM) of MS patients similar to those seen on MT, suggesting that DWI may be sensitive to disease burden not seen on conventional MRI imaging.[3–5,10–12] Focal *decreases* in ADC measurements can be seen in regions of NAWM several weeks before the MS lesions become visible on subsequent conventional MR images, again suggesting the increased sensitivity of diffusion imaging for disease detection.[8,12] In addition to focal ADC abnormalities associated with MS lesions, more global abnormalities can be computed using whole-brain histograms of ADC values, in effect measuring global MS disease burden.[2,7] Interestingly, diffusion pathway-specific changes in MS were initially demonstrated using DWI. Werring *et al.* showed increased ADC values of NAWM within homologous white matter contralateral to a focal acute MS lesion, which may share a common pathway.[12] ADC changes demonstrated a similar progression to those seen within the new white matter lesion. These findings suggest that diffusion imaging may be sensitive to acute pathway changes related to the appearance of new MS lesions within the pathway.[12] In contrast to DWI, DTI imaging is more technically difficult to perform, but has improved ability to delineate anisotropy within white matter tracts and allows for white matter fiber tracking.

DTI in MS: MD and FA lesion and whole-brain approaches

DTI has been employed extensively to evaluate MS. The simplest non-spherical model of a full three-dimensional diffusion profile is described by a second-rank tensor, and geometrically takes the form of a best-fit ellipse. DTI employs diffusion gradients applied in at least six unique directions to fully describe the diffusion tensor.[1] The advantage of DTI over DWI is that it provides a simple measure of diffusional anisotropy, and the resulting directional preference can be used for fiber tracking.[1,13–17] Useful mathematical parameters that emerge from the tensor include the geometric axes of the tensor ellipsoid, the mean diffusivity (MD), fractional anisotropy (FA), and the parallel and perpendicular diffusivity, $\lambda_\parallel$ and $\lambda_\perp$, respectively. Multiple authors have shown that DTI can accurately detect MS lesions. Typical MS lesions demonstrate a reduction in FA and an increase in MD.[18–22] Additionally, DTI measures may predict the progression of early gadolinium enhancing MS lesions. Specifically, FA and $\lambda_\perp$ measurements may predict the likelihood that a lesion will progress to a black hole.[23,24] These metrics may also provide some evidence of remyelination and/or repair both within lesions and NAWM during the course of therapy.[23] Several studies have also demonstrated that DTI can detect lesion burden within NAWM.[10,18–22,25–30] NAWM demonstrates a reduction in FA and an increase in MD in comparison to the white matter of age match controls.[18–22,25–27,29,31,32] In addition to tracking disease in relapsing remitting and progressive MS, DTI changes are found in patients with clinically isolated syndrome suggestive of MS and so-called benign MS.[33–41,42–45]. Given the sensitivity of DTI to both focal MS lesions and lesion burden within NAWM, DTI has been proposed as a sensitive measure of global disease burden. Whole-brain evaluations of DTI, often expressed as histograms, demonstrate global changes in FA and MD in MS.[46–48] Of particular clinical value, these global changes demonstrate a moderate correlation with MS disability.[19,22,46] After segmenting histogram analyses in terms of normal appearing brain tissue (NABT),

NAWM and NAGM, a wide variety of studies have explored the relationship between white and gray matter lesion burden, as well as the relationship to disability and disease progression for lesions within the gray and white matter compartments.[29,30,39,40,47,49–56]

In addition to white matter pathology, DTI measurements are also sensitive to MS changes within both deep and cortical gray matter structures. Both MD and ADC are commonly used in gray matter and typically demonstrate increased values in both deep and cortical gray matter.[29,30,32,39,40,47,49–58] Regarding FA, although changes within the white matter consistently suggest decreased FA with disease progression, measurements in gray matter are less consistent with both increased and decreased FA reported.[29,30,32,39,40,47,49–58] This likely reflects the variability in FA measurements in areas of low anisotropy such as gray matter. Small changes in noise can alter both the direction and magnitude of the principal eigenvector as well as the secondary and tertiary eigenvectors from which FA is calculated. Hence, FA is a less reliable measurement within gray matter. Gray matter DTI measurements correlate with other measures of function and the degree of disease burden within white matter.[29,30,32,39,40,47,49–58] Gray matter changes appear to be present even at the earliest stages of MS; however, during the early stages of disease gray matter DTI metrics do not demonstrate a strong correlation with disease progression or function.[39,40] Gray matter changes appear to predict clinical worsening in primary progressive MS and appear to be a hallmark of the later stages of disease demonstrating a strong correlation with disability.[50–52]

Voxel-wise comparisons (VWC) and track-based spatial statistics (TBSS)

Several investigators have proposed evaluating diffusion imaging data using voxel-wise comparisons (VWC), demonstrating significant differences in the distribution pattern of white matter abnormalities within subtypes of MS.[43,59–61] However, applying DTI to VWC is difficult with several potential technical pitfalls including the need for rigorous spatial registration and appropriate spatial smoothing. For example, different smoothing algorithms can significantly affect the consistency of results.[62,63] Given these caveats, Smith et al. proposed a new VWC method to address these issues called tract-based spatial statistics (TBSS).[64] The method produces a "skeleton" of major white matter tracts that permits a relatively robust method of coregistration between subjects and groups, which allows reliable comparisons. This method has been used in multiple studies of MS showing regional differences in white matter FA values that correspond to specific functional disabilities, differ between specific disease types of multiple sclerosis, and correspond to regional gray matter volume loss.[34,35,60,65–67] Although TBSS addresses many of the problems with VWC, potential pitfalls remain. For example, focal lesions within a white matter track can alter the selection of the FA "skeleton," and the skeleton itself may be misregistered.[63]

Histopathology, electrophysiology, and DTI measurements: $\lambda_\perp$ and $\lambda_\parallel$

There are several lines of evidence suggesting that DTI measurements correlate well with the burden of histopathology and physiologic measures in MS, for both animal models of demyelination and in human MS. Human histopathology in MS usually implies a post-mortem analysis, and correlational studies comparing imaging and histopathology are difficult to perform due to several technical factors. DTI metrics are affected by temperature and pulsatile motion, which differ in the post-mortem condition. In addition, peri-mortem ischemia or other insults can alter DTI measurements. Despite these drawbacks, Schmierer et al. were able compare post-mortem MR with histopathology in MS brain slices,[68] demonstrating a strong correlation between MD/FA values and direct measurements of myelin content and axonal counts. In addition to human studies, there are data from animal studies supporting pathological specificity of diffusion measurements. Song et al. used a variety of animal models of axonal injury and demyelination to demonstrate correlations between DTI values and underlying histopathology,[28,69–75] specifically showing a strong correlation between increased $\lambda_\perp$ and demyelination as measured by luxol fast blue staining. In addition, they consistently demonstrated that $\lambda_\parallel$ is strongly correlated with axonal damage as determined by APP measurements.[28,69–75] Concha et al. demonstrated DTI changes after surgical callosotomy,[76] showing that FA and $\lambda_\parallel$ were abnormal early after surgery in fiber tracts affected by the callosotomy, whereas follow-up imaging demonstrated normalization in FA and $\lambda_\parallel$ with relatively increased $\lambda_\perp$. These findings suggest that DTI, particularly $\lambda_\perp$, is a sensitive marker of white matter disconnection, likely reflecting the loss of both axons and myelin. Animal studies have also demonstrated similar changes in $\lambda_\perp$ that are associated with Wallerian degeneration comprising loss of both axons and myelin.[77] Additionally, there is a report of similar $\lambda_\perp$ changes in Wallerian degeneration associated with stroke in humans.[78] It remains unclear as to whether changes in $\lambda_\perp$ are specific to axonal disconnection and Wallerian degeneration, or are reflective of a more generalized process.[79,80] Using MR spectroscopy, DTI metrics also correlate spatially with measurements of NAA, a known marker of axonal loss.[81,82] Additionally, studies of visual evoked potentials in MS patients with optic neuritis have demonstrated a strong correlation between $\lambda_\perp$ and electrophysiologic measures of pathway conduction, suggesting changes related to demyelination and axonal loss.[83,84]

While it is tempting to simplistically associate $\lambda_\perp$ and $\lambda_\parallel$ abnormalities directly with specific neuropathology, it should be remembered that these measurements simply reflect the movement of water within a specific voxel, which can be altered by many factors. A recent study by Wheeler-Kingshott and Cercignani points out many caveats and pitfalls for the acquisition and interpretation of $\lambda_\perp$ and $\lambda_\parallel$ measurements.[85] Measurements can be particularly affected in regions of crossing fibers, in addition to regions of severe MS pathology where the

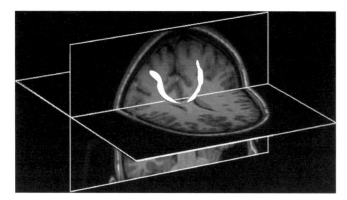

Fig. 15.4. Example of probabilistic fiber tracking, in distinction to the deterministic fiber tracking example shown in Figs. 15.1. In this case, a seed region was placed in the right-hand region of the motor strip, with a target region in the contralateral side. The resulting track-density map, shown in white, correctly shows the known anatomic connection, which is difficult to derive using deterministic tracking.

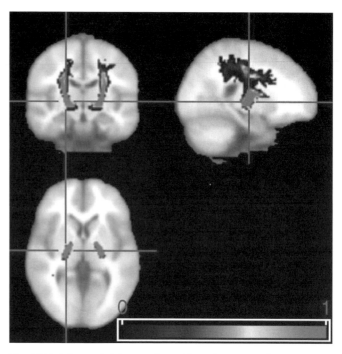

Fig. 15.5. A fiber probability map formed from deterministic fiber tracking on a group of normal humans. These tracts can then be co-registered in MS patients to allow identification of the track in the presence of disease (Reproduced with permission from Pagani, et al., 2005) (see also color plate section).

orientation of the principal eigenvectors, and subsequent measurements of $\lambda_\perp$ and $\lambda_\parallel$, can vary significantly.[85] These measurements may be more reliable, however, in well-organized fiber pathways with a relatively well-understood orientation for the primary eigenvector. This can be potentially accomplished by making measurements within well-identified organized pathways using DTI fiber tracking. Investigators have utilized these methods to show correlations between pathway specific $\lambda_\perp$ values and measures of pathway-specific function as well as functional connectivity.[86,87]

DTI fiber tracking and identification of pathways in MS

DTI is unique in its ability to identify white matter pathways in the brain. The ability of DTI to identify the principal direction of highly organized white matter led naturally to the development of methods to identify connected axonal pathways in the white matter of the brain.[14,88] Research in this area of neuroimaging is particularly vigorous, with many avenues of investigation currently being explored by many groups.[89] Approaches can be broken up into two main categories: *deterministic*, and *probabilistic*. The deterministic approach uses various methods to establish a continuous fiber track from one point in the brain to another, as shown in the example of Fig. 15.1. Probabilistic approaches view the voxel-level directional water diffusion characteristics as a probability density function that is integrated to determine probabilistic pathways between anatomic regions in the brain, as shown in the example of Fig. 15.4. The majority of MS studies have used a deterministic approach for fiber tracking to directly identify pathways.[87,90,91] The major drawback of this approach is that MS lesions result in decreased FA, resulting in uncertainty of the orientation for the primary eigenvector.[92] In addition, deterministic tracks will frequently stop within lesions. Often times this approach leads to tracking of normal appearing white matter excluding portions of the fiber pathway that may contain

lesions.[87,90,91] An alternative approach used by many investigators is to perform deterministic tracking on normal individuals, and thereby build a probability map for the position of specific fiber tracts (Fig. 15.5).[93] These tracts are then co-registered to MS patients to allow identification of the track in the presence of disease.[93,94–97] While this methodology does allow for identification of tracks in MS patients, it may also include brain regions outside the tracks due to misregistration, in addition to uncertainty created by the relatively broad definition of tracks resulting from combining multiple normal individuals. In contrast to deterministic tracking, probabilistic fiber tracking approaches have also been applied to MS, which allows for direct identification of the complete track despite the presence of lesions (Fig. 15.6).[86,98] Probabilistic methods effectively track through MS lesions and thereby permit accurate determination of complete fiber pathway characteristics.[86,98] These methods have been increasingly applied over the last several years with good results. On the whole, pathway-specific track-based DTI measurements demonstrate excellent correlation with pathway function, pathway specific electrophysiological measurements, functional MRI, and functional connectivity.

DTI enabled pathway-specific measurements in MS

One of the principal drawbacks to conventional MR measures of disease burden in MS is the lack of pathway specificity.

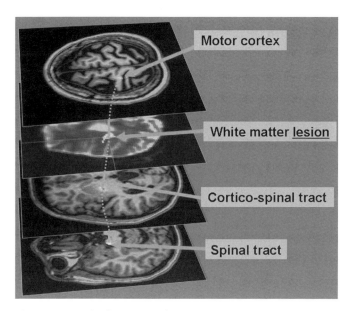

Motor cortex

White matter lesion

Cortico-spinal tract

Spinal tract

Fig. 15.6. Example of probabilistic fiber tracking through a lesion in an MS patient. A seed region was placed in the corticospinal tract, with a target region in the contralateral motor strip. The resulting tract density map correctly followed the expected anatomic course of the CST, and intersected a known white matter lesion in the corona radiata. Tract-based values using this path showed significant DTI differences compared to a symmetrical control path on the contralateral side, reflecting the long-range influence of the white matter lesion to diffusion properties along the entire associated tract (see also color plate section).

Most current measurements of disease burden such as T2 lesion volume, new gadolinium enhancing lesions, and brain atrophy are performed as global assessments of disease burden. These measurements treat all lesions equally regardless of their geographic position within the brain. Such global assessments are then compared with functional assessments of disability such as multiple sclerosis functional composite and the Kurtzke EDSS, which test relatively few pathways. Hence, significant lesion burden outside of the tested pathways may remain undetected, possibly accounting in part for the relatively modest correlation of conventional imaging measures with disability in MS. In contrast, DTI enabled pathway specific measurements can be compared directly to pathway function. Early studies demonstrated a clear improvement in the correlation between disability and disease burden when a pathway specific approach was employed.[91,99] Lesion burden was assessed using T1 measures[91] and a novel fiber-track-based diffusion tensor measurement.[99] These measures of lesion burden were compared with both the general Kurtzke EDSS score and the pyramidal Kurtzke functional systems score – a more motor-pathway specific score. Measurements within the descending motor pathway produced a strong positive correlation for T1 lesion burden ($r = 0.64$, $P = 0.0007$)[91] and an inverse correlation for DTI-based methods ($r = -0.75$, $P < 0.0001$)[99] compared with the pyramidal Kurtzke functional systems score.[91,99] Pathway lesion burden demonstrated a more modest correlation with non-pathway-specific overall Kurtzke EDSS score ($r = 0.55$, $P = 0.005$) in the case of T1 measurements[91] and ($r = -0.48$, $P < 0.05$)

in the case of DTI-based methods.[99] Note that global conventional MR measures of T1 and T2 lesion burden gathered on the same group of patients demonstrated no correlation with disability.[91,99] Similarly, one early study demonstrated strong correlations between pathway-specific measurements of $\lambda_\perp$ and functional impairment in the transcallosal motor pathway.[87] Multiple additional studies have demonstrated correlations between DTI pathway measures of disease burden and pathway function.[59,100–111] These studies have probed multiple functional systems including motor, language, vision, memory, executive function, and other cognitive domains. Typically, these studies have demonstrated significantly better correlation between function and pathway-specific imaging measures than have been typically achieved using global imaging measures – suggesting increased sensitivity to disease progression for pathway-specific methods.[59,100–111]

DTI measures also correlate with electrophysiologic measures of pathway function including visual evoked potentials and transcranial magnetic stimulation with electromyography.[83,84,105] DTI measurements have also been made in conjunction with fMRI and functional connectivity measurements. Note that fMRI requires a task performance and is therefore a functional pathway-specific test. Multiple studies have demonstrated changes in fMRI cortical activity that is correlated to the degree of injury within the associated white matter pathways as measured by DTI. Typically, these studies have demonstrated relatively increased activation within cortical structures which correlates with the degree of white matter injury as manifest by increased MD and decreased FA.[95,106,112,113] Measures of functional network connectivity have also demonstrated strong correlations with the degree of white matter injury as determined by DTI, using both functional connectivity derived from fMRI activation studies[95–97] and resting state functional connectivity.[86,114] eMRI activation methods tend to show increased connectivity, reflecting the increased activation seen on fMRI studies in MS. This increase inactivation is usually correlated with increased pathway specific injury as measured by increased MD and decreased FA.[95–97] In contrast, functional connectivity in the resting state is typically decreased in MS, demonstrating reduced connectivity with increased white matter injury (Fig. 15.7).[86,114]

DTI is unique in its ability to provide pathway-based measures of white matter integrity, demonstrating strong correlations between lesion burden and specific functions. Combined with other functional imaging techniques, a new picture is emerging in which pathways and networks within the brain can be assessed both in terms of structure and function. The most intriguing feature of combining DTI and resting state functional connectivity is that they provide information about network function without requiring patients to perform a task. Hence they can be applied to a broad range of MS subjects regardless of the level of disability. Importantly, although DTI and resting state connectivity provide pathway-specific information, they are whole brain imaging techniques capable of

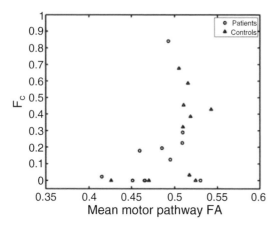

Fig. 15.7. Comparison of resting-state connectivity in MS patients compared with controls, as measured in major motor pathways. A total of 10 MS patients and 10 controls underwent resting-state fMRI. The *y*-axis shows the temporal correlation coefficient, which significantly separates the two populations and shows the MS population having reduced connectivity. A similar, but less significant separation is seen with tract-based values of the mean FA. (Reproduced with permission from Lowe *et al.*, 2008[86]).

producing a global assessment of network and pathway function. In short, pathway-specific methods have strong potential for adding new information to our understanding of MS and possibly providing new metrics for assessment of therapeutic efficacy in clinical trials.

Diffusion imaging in routine clinical care and clinical trials

Despite the clear sensitivity of DTI and its potential for pathway-specific measurements of disease burden, it is rarely if ever used in the clinical assessment of MS. While initially this may have been due to lack of availability of DTI sequences and analysis, all major MR manufacturers today provide standard sequences with multiple diffusion direction capability. Further, standardized output with ADC maps, FA maps, and colorized FA maps are readily available, all of which are automatically generated by the scanner. Additionally, fiber tracking software is widely available both from the major MR manufacturers and from third parties. Yet, even with present improvements in availability and implementation, DTI remains essentially unused in the clinical decision-making process. The simplest explanation is that DTI images provide relatively little information regarding disease progression and severity on simple visual inspection, especially when compared to the striking changes readily seen on standard T2, FLAIR, and post-contrast T1 sequences, which are relatively easy to understand and interpret. Visualization of changes in DTI typically requires an additional level of analysis, for example, ROI analysis, whole-brain histogram analysis, or sophisticated analysis of fiber tracts. Further, the long-standing experience with conventional MR imaging gives the provider the sense that they know what a particular lesion means in the context of the disease in underlying pathology. Similarly, *quantitative* measures of atrophy, T2 lesion burden, and T1 enhancing lesion volume are also not used routinely in daily clinical decision making; however, they have long-standing use in clinical trials. Arguably, if conventional quantitative MR measures can be used on a routine clinical basis, so could advanced DTI measures.

The more difficult question to answer is why diffusion imaging has not been used routinely in clinical trials, especially given its demonstrated sensitivity to all aspects of disease progression and arguably superior correlation with function. This absence may stem from earlier concerns regarding the ability of individual sites to reproducibly perform the examination over time, the variability of DTI results across imaging platforms, and potential issues regarding a uniform method for analysis. Today, many of these issues have been addressed and recent data suggest that DTI may perform at a level close to that of other quantitative MR measures. Data acquisition for diffusion imaging has also become rapidly more uniform with relatively standard imaging packages available from all MR manufacturers.

It should also be recognized that, despite extensive use in clinical trials, there are relatively little published data regarding multisite and multiplatform accuracy and reproducibility of T2 lesion burden, atrophy, and new enhancing lesion burden measurements. Additionally, there is no community agreement regarding a standard for image analysis software, and today there exist a multitude of different methods being applied in clinical trials. Nevertheless, of all these measurements the best studied is atrophy, particularly using the SEINA and SIENAX methodologies.[115–121] These studies suggest good reproducibility *within* individual centers on single machines for measurements of atrophy with good sensitivity over relatively short time frames for disease progression.[115–121] These studies do not provide data regarding reproducibility across multiple platforms in centers with subjects scanned across multiple machines. Realistically, this may not be that important in typical therapeutic trials as the purpose is to determine the change over time at individual sites for specific patients. There are multiple studies in the literature regarding accuracy of DTI acquisitions both within a given site and platform and across sites and platforms.[56,122–129] The majority of the studies have used the same subjects as "human phantoms" to assess the reproducibility of studies. These studies, on the whole, suggest relatively robust reproducibility for DTI measurements within single sites and imaging platforms, as well as across sites with multiple imaging platforms. Coefficients of variance for FA measurements in these studies have varied between 0.8% and 6.2% using a wide variety of imaging platforms and analysis techniques.[56,122–124,126–130] On the whole, these studies suggest that careful attention to image acquisition parameters, evaluation of data quality, and analysis techniques dramatically reduces variability of results. As expected, all studies have demonstrated the best results in terms of reproducibility when images are performed on the same imaging platform with coefficients of variance ranging from 0.8% to 3.0%.[56,122–124,126–129]

A recent study using human phantoms across five different imaging platforms performed over a 3-year time span suggested a high level of concordance despite platform upgrades during the course of the study. The concordance correlation coefficient (CCC) for FA values ranged between 0.94 and 0.96, which is comparable with inter-site atrophy studies using SIENAX (0.94) and SIENA (0.95).

A recent study has demonstrated a high level of sensitivity for detection of disease progression in MS using DTI.[131] Harrison et al. studied 78 patients with relapsing–remitting MS with three MRIs over a 2-year period, showing in the corpus callosum a decreasing FA of 1.7% per year and decreasing $\lambda_\perp$ of 1.2% per year. These results supported a power analysis indicating a sample size of about 40 participants per arm over a 1–2-year clinical trial is required to detect a 50% reduction in disease progression with 80% power.[131] This compares favorably with previous estimates of the sample size required for therapeutic trials in relapsing remitting MS using SIENA. Anderson et al.[116] demonstrated that 69 subjects per arm would be required to detect a 50% reduction in progression as measured by atrophy with 90% power.

Conclusions

Diffusion imaging has rapidly developed since its first applications for MS in the early 1990s. Techniques have progressed from simple global assessments using DWI to sophisticated fiber tracking based pathway-specific measurements, which can be combined with functional imaging technologies to provide a relatively complete picture of structural and functional changes in MS. Despite the progress made in diffusion imaging, it remains rarely used for clinical decision-making or therapeutic trials. However, recent data suggest that diffusion imaging is a robust and reliable technique capable of rapidly detecting changes in MS, and requiring relatively small sample sizes. Given the sensitivity and robust nature of diffusion imaging, a strong argument can be made for its increased use in both the clinical and research setting.

References

1. Le Bihan D, Mangin JF, Poupon C, et al. Diffusion tensor imaging: concepts and applications. *J Magn Reson Imaging* 2001; 13:534–46.

2. Castriota Scanderbeg A, Tomaiuolo F, Sabatini U, Nocentini U, Grasso MG, Caltagirone C. Demyelinating plaques in relapsing–remitting and secondary-progressive multiple sclerosis: assessment with diffusion MR imaging. *Am J Neuroradiol* 2000; 21:862–68.

3. Cercignani M, Iannucci G, Rocca MA, Comi G, Horsfield MA, Filippi M. Pathologic damage in MS assessed by diffusion-weighted and magnetization transfer MRI. *Neurology* 2000; 54:1139–44.

4. Christiansen P, Gideon P, Thomsen C, Stubgaard M, Henriksen O, Larsson HB. Increased water self-diffusion in chronic plaques and in apparently normal white matter in patients with multiple sclerosis. *Acta Neurol Scand* 1993; 87:195–9.

5. Filippi M, Iannucci G, Cercignani M, Assunta Rocca M, Pratesi A, Comi G. A quantitative study of water diffusion in multiple sclerosis lesions and normal-appearing white matter using echo-planar imaging. *Arch Neurol* 2000; 57:1017–21.

6. Nusbaum AO, Lu D, Tang CY, Atlas SW. Quantitative diffusion measurements in focal multiple sclerosis lesions: correlations with appearance on TI-weighted MR images. *Am J Roentgenol* 2000; 175:821–5.

7. Nusbaum AO, Tang CY, Wei T, Buchsbaum MS, Atlas SW. Whole-brain diffusion MR histograms differ between MS subtypes. *Neurology* 2000; 54:1421–7.

8. Rocca MA, Cercignani M, Iannucci G, Comi G, Filippi M. Weekly diffusion-weighted imaging of normal-appearing white matter in MS. *Neurology* 2000; 55:882–4.

9. Roychowdhury S, Maldjian JA, Grossman RI. Multiple sclerosis: comparison of trace apparent diffusion coefficients with MR enhancement pattern of lesions. *Am J Neuroradiol* 2000; 21:869–74.

10. Tievsky AL, Ptak T, Farkas J. Investigation of apparent diffusion coefficient and diffusion tensor anisotrophy in acute and chronic multiple sclerosis lesions. *Am J Neuroradiol* 1999; 20:1491–9.

11. Rocca MA, Mastronardo G, Rodegher M, Comi G, Filippi M. Long-term changes of magnetization transfer-derived measures from patients with relapsing-remitting and secondary progressive multiple sclerosis. *Am J Neuroradiol* 1999; 20:821–7.

12. Werring DJ, Brassat D, Droogan AG, et al. The pathogenesis of lesions and normal-appearing white matter changes in multiple sclerosis: a serial diffusion MRI study. *Brain* 2000; 123 (8):1667–76.

13. Basser PJ, Pajevic S, Pierpaoli C, Duda J, Aldroubi A. In vivo fiber tractography using DT-MRI data. *Magn Reson Med* 2000; 44:625–32.

14. Conturo TE, Lori NF, Cull TS, et al. Tracking neuronal fiber pathways in the living human brain. *Proc Natl Acad Sci USA* 1999; 96:10422–7.

15. Jones DK, Simmons A, Williams SC, Horsfield MA. Non-invasive assessment of axonal fiber connectivity in the human brain via diffusion tensor MRI. *Magn Reson Med* 1999; 42:37–41.

16. Poupon C, Clark CA, Frouin V, et al. Regularization of diffusion-based direction maps for the tracking of brain white matter fascicles. *Neuroimage* 2000; 12:184–95.

17. Xue R, van Zijl PC, Crain BJ, Solaiyappan M, Mori S. In vivo three-dimensional reconstruction of rat brain axonal projections by diffusion tensor imaging. *Magn Reson Med* 1999; 42:1123–7.

18. Bammer R, Augustin M, Strasser-Fuchs S, et al. Magnetic resonance diffusion tensor imaging for characterizing diffuse and focal white matter abnormalities in multiple sclerosis. *Magn Reson Med* 2000; 44:583–91.

19. Ciccarelli O, Werring DJ, Wheeler-Kingshott CA, et al. Investigation of MS normal-appearing brain using diffusion tensor MRI with

clinical correlations. *Neurology* 2001; 56:926–33.

20. Filippi M, Cercignani M, Inglese M, Horsfield MA, Comi G. Diffusion tensor magnetic resonance imaging in multiple sclerosis. *Neurology* 2001; 56:304–11.

21. Guo AC, MacFall JR, Provenzale JM. Multiple sclerosis: diffusion tensor MR imaging for evaluation of normal-appearing white matter. *Radiology* 2002; 222:729–36.

22. Werring DJ, Clark CA, Barker GJ, Thompson AJ, Miller DH. Diffusion tensor imaging of lesions and normal-appearing white matter in multiple sclerosis. *Neurology* 1999; 52:1626–32.

23. Fox RJ, Cronin T, Lin J, *et al.* Measuring myelin repair and axonal loss with diffusion tensor imaging. *Am J Neuroradiol*; 2011; 32:85–91.

24. Naismith RT, Xu J, Tutlam NT, *et al.* Increased diffusivity in acute multiple sclerosis lesions predicts risk of black hole. *Neurology* 2010; 74:1694–701.

25. Coombs BD, Best A, Brown MS, *et al.* Multiple sclerosis pathology in the normal and abnormal appearing white matter of the corpus callosum by diffusion tensor imaging. *Mult Scler* 2004; 10:392–7.

26. Ge Y, Law M, Johnson G, *et al.* Preferential occult injury of corpus callosum in multiple sclerosis measured by diffusion tensor imaging. *J Magn Reson Imaging* 2004; 20:1–7.

27. Guo AC, Jewells VL, Provenzale JM. Analysis of normal-appearing white matter in multiple sclerosis: comparison of diffusion tensor MR imaging and magnetization transfer imaging. *Am J Neuroradiol* 2001; 22:1893–900.

28. Kim JH, Budde MD, Liang HF, *et al.* Detecting axon damage in spinal cord from a mouse model of multiple sclerosis. *Neurobiol Dis* 2006; 21:626–32.

29. Rocca MA, Iannucci G, Rovaris M, Comi G, Filippi M. Occult tissue damage in patients with primary progressive multiple sclerosis is independent of T2-visible lesions–a diffusion tensor MR study. *J Neurol* 2003; 250:456–60.

30. Rovaris M, Bozzali M, Iannucci G, *et al.* Assessment of normal-appearing white and gray matter in patients with primary progressive multiple sclerosis: a diffusion-tensor magnetic resonance imaging study. *Arch Neurol* 2002; 59:1406–412.

31. Caramia MD, Palmieri MG, Desiato MT, *et al.* Brain excitability changes in the relapsing and remitting phases of multiple sclerosis: a study with transcranial magnetic stimulation. *Clin Neurophysiol* 2004; 115:956–65.

32. Rovaris M, Iannucci G, Falautano M, *et al.* Cognitive dysfunction in patients with mildly disabling relapsing-remitting multiple sclerosis: an exploratory study with diffusion tensor MR imaging. *J Neurol Sci* 2002; 195:103–9.

33. Absinta M, Rocca MA, Moiola L, *et al.* Brain macro- and microscopic damage in patients with paediatric MS. *J Neurol Neurosurg Psychiatry* 2010; 81:1357–62.

34. Raz E, Cercignani M, Sbardella E, *et al.* Gray- and white-matter changes 1 year after first clinical episode of multiple sclerosis: MR imaging. *Radiology* 2010; 257:448–54.

35. Raz E, Cercignani M, Sbardella E, *et al.* Clinically isolated syndrome suggestive of multiple sclerosis: voxelwise regional investigation of white and gray matter. *Radiology* 2010; 254:227–34.

36. Caramia F, Pantano P, Di Legge S, *et al.* A longitudinal study of MR diffusion changes in normal appearing white matter of patients with early multiple sclerosis. *Magn Reson Imaging* 2002; 20:383–8.

37. Ranjeva JP, Pelletier J, Confort-Gouny S, *et al.* MRI/MRS of corpus callosum in patients with clinically isolated syndrome suggestive of multiple sclerosis. *Mult Scler* 2003; 9:554–65.

38. Bester M, Heesen C, Schippling S, *et al.* Early anisotropy changes in the corpus callosum of patients with optic neuritis. *Neuroradiology* 2008; 50:549–57.

39. Rovaris M, Judica E, Ceccarelli A, *et al.* A 3-year diffusion tensor MRI study of grey matter damage progression during the earliest clinical stage of MS. *J Neurol* 2008; 255:1209–14.

40. Yu CS, Lin FC, Liu Y, Duan Y, Lei H, Li KC. Histogram analysis of diffusion measures in clinically isolated syndromes and relapsing-remitting multiple sclerosis. *Eur J Radiol* 2008; 68:328–34.

41. Henry RG, Shieh M, Amirbekian B, Chung S, Okuda DT, Pelletier D. Connecting white matter injury and thalamic atrophy in clinically isolated syndromes. *J Neurol Sci* 2009; 282: 61–6.

42. Rocca MA, Ceccarelli A, Rodegher M, *et al.* Preserved brain adaptive properties in patients with benign multiple sclerosis. *Neurology* 2010; 74:142–9.

43. Ceccarelli A, Rocca MA, Pagani E, *et al.* The topographical distribution of tissue injury in benign MS: a 3T multiparametric MRI study. *Neuroimage* 2008; 39:1499–509.

44. Rovaris M, Riccitelli G, Judica E, *et al.* Cognitive impairment and structural brain damage in benign multiple sclerosis. *Neurology* 2008; 71:1521–6.

45. Ceccarelli A, Filippi M, Neema M, *et al.* T2 hypointensity in the deep gray matter of patients with benign multiple sclerosis. *Mult Scler* 2009; 15:678–86.

46. Cercignani M, Inglese M, Pagani E, Comi G, Filippi M. Mean diffusivity and fractional anisotropy histograms of patients with multiple sclerosis. *Am J Neuroradiol* 2001; 22:952–8.

47. Rashid W, Hadjiprocopis A, Griffin CM, *et al.* Diffusion tensor imaging of early relapsing–remitting multiple sclerosis with histogram analysis using automated segmentation and brain volume correction. *Mult Scler* 2004; 10:9–15.

48. Rocca MA, Falini A, Colombo B, Scotti G, Comi G, Filippi M. Adaptive functional changes in the cerebral cortex of patients with nondisabling multiple sclerosis correlate with the extent of brain structural damage. *Ann Neurol* 2002; 51:330–9.

49. Poonawalla AH, Hasan KM, Gupta RK, *et al.* Diffusion-tensor MR imaging of cortical lesions in multiple sclerosis: initial findings. *Radiology* 2008; 246:880–6.

50. Pulizzi A, Rovaris M, Judica E, *et al.* Determinants of disability in multiple sclerosis at various disease stages: a multiparametric magnetic resonance study. *Arch Neurol* 2007; 64:1163–8.

51. Vrenken H, Pouwels PJ, Geurts JJ, *et al.* Altered diffusion tensor in multiple sclerosis normal-appearing brain tissue: cortical diffusion changes seem related to clinical deterioration. *J Magn Reson Imaging* 2006; 23:628–36.

52. Rovaris M, Judica E, Gallo A, *et al.* Grey matter damage predicts the evolution of

primary progressive multiple sclerosis at 5 years. *Brain* 2006; 129:2628–34.

53. Rovaris M, Gallo A, Valsasina P, *et al.* Short-term accrual of gray matter pathology in patients with progressive multiple sclerosis: an in vivo study using diffusion tensor MRI. *Neuroimage* 2005; 24:1139–46.

54. Oreja-Guevara C, Rovaris M, Iannucci G, *et al.* Progressive gray matter damage in patients with relapsing-remitting multiple sclerosis: a longitudinal diffusion tensor magnetic resonance imaging study. *Arch Neurol* 2005; 62:578–84.

55. Rocca MA, Pagani E, Ghezzi A, *et al.* Functional cortical changes in patients with multiple sclerosis and nonspecific findings on conventional magnetic resonance imaging scans of the brain. *Neuroimage* 2003; 19:826–36.

56. Cercignani M, Bammer R, Sormani MP, Fazekas F, Filippi M. Inter-sequence and inter-imaging unit variability of diffusion tensor MR imaging histogram-derived metrics of the brain in healthy volunteers. *Am J Neuroradiol* 2003; 24:638–43.

57. Bozzali M, Cercignani M, Sormani MP, Comi G, Filippi M. Quantification of brain gray matter damage in different MS phenotypes by use of diffusion tensor MR imaging. *Am J Neuroradiol* 2002; 23:985–8.

58. Zhou F, Zee CS, Gong H, Shiroishi M, Li J. Differential changes in deep and cortical gray matters of patients with multiple sclerosis: a quantitative magnetic resonance imaging study. *J Comput Assist Tomogr* 2010; 34: 431–6.

59. Hecke WV, Nagels G, Leemans A, Vandervliet E, Sijbers J, Parizel PM. Correlation of cognitive dysfunction and diffusion tensor MRI measures in patients with mild and moderate multiple sclerosis. *J Magn Reson Imaging*; 31:1492–98.

60. Bodini B, Khaleeli Z, Cercignani M, Miller DH, Thompson AJ, Ciccarelli O. Exploring the relationship between white matter and gray matter damage in early primary progressive multiple sclerosis: an in vivo study with TBSS and VBM. *Hum Brain Mapp* 2009; 30:2852–61.

61. Ceccarelli A, Rocca MA, Valsasina P, *et al.* A multiparametric evaluation of regional brain damage in patients with

primary progressive multiple sclerosis. *Hum Brain Mapp* 2009; 30:3009–19.

62. Jones DK, Symms MR, Cercignani M, Howard RJ. The effect of filter size on VBM analyses of DT-MRI data. *Neuroimage* 2005; 26:546–54.

63. Jones DK, Cercignani M. Twenty-five pitfalls in the analysis of diffusion MRI data. *NMR Biomed* 2010; 23:803–20.

64. Smith SM, Jenkinson M, Johansen-Berg H, *et al.* Tract-based spatial statistics: voxelwise analysis of multi-subject diffusion data. *Neuroimage* 2006; 31:1487–505.

65. Roosendaal SD, Schoonheim MM, Hulst HE, *et al.* Resting state networks change in clinically isolated syndrome. *Brain* 2010; 133:1612–21.

66. Cader S, Johansen-Berg H, Wylezinska M, *et al.* Discordant white matter N-acetylasparate and diffusion MRI measures suggest that chronic metabolic dysfunction contributes to axonal pathology in multiple sclerosis. *Neuroimage* 2007; 36:19–27.

67. Dineen RA, Vilisaar J, Hlinka J, *et al.* Disconnection as a mechanism for cognitive dysfunction in multiple sclerosis. *Brain* 2009; 132:239–49.

68. Schmierer K, Wheeler-Kingshott CA, Boulby PA, *et al.* Diffusion tensor imaging of post mortem multiple sclerosis brain. *Neuroimage* 2007; 35:467–77.

69. Drobyshevsky A, Song SK, Gamkrelidze G, *et al.* Developmental changes in diffusion anisotropy coincide with immature oligodendrocyte progression and maturation of compound action potential. *J Neurosci* 2005; 25:5988–97.

70. Song SK, Kim JH, Lin SJ, Brendza RP, Holtzman DM. Diffusion tensor imaging detects age-dependent white matter changes in a transgenic mouse model with amyloid deposition. *Neurobiol Dis* 2004; 15:640–7.

71. Song SK, Sun SW, Ju WK, Lin SJ, Cross AH, Neufeld AH. Diffusion tensor imaging detects and differentiates axon and myelin degeneration in mouse optic nerve after retinal ischemia. *Neuroimage* 2003; 20:1714–22.

72. Song SK, Sun SW, Ramsbottom MJ, Chang C, Russell J, Cross AH. Dysmyelination revealed through MRI as increased radial (but unchanged axial) diffusion of water. *Neuroimage* 2002; 17:1429–36.

73. Song SK, Yoshino J, Le TQ, *et al.* Demyelination increases radial diffusivity in corpus callosum of mouse brain. *Neuroimage* 2005; 26: 132–40.

74. Sun SW, Liang HF, Trinkaus K, Cross AH, Armstrong RC, Song SK. Noninvasive detection of cuprizone induced axonal damage and demyelination in the mouse corpus callosum. *Magn Reson Med* 2006; 55:302–8.

75. Sun SW, Neil JJ, Song SK. Relative indices of water diffusion anisotropy are equivalent in live and formalin-fixed mouse brains. *Magn Reson Med* 2003; 50:743–8.

76. Concha L, Gross DW, Wheatley BM, Beaulieu C. Diffusion tensor imaging of time-dependent axonal and myelin degradation after corpus callosotomy in epilepsy patients. *Neuroimage* 2006; 32:1090–9.

77. Beaulieu C, Does MD, Snyder RE, Allen PS. Changes in water diffusion due to Wallerian degeneration in peripheral nerve. *Magn Reson Med* 1996; 36:627–31.

78. Pierpaoli C, Barnett A, Pajevic S, *et al.* Water diffusion changes in Wallerian degeneration and their dependence on white matter architecture. *Neuroimage* 2001; 13:1174–85.

79. Henry RG, Oh J, Nelson SJ, Pelletier D. Directional diffusion in relapsing-remitting multiple sclerosis: a possible in vivo signature of Wallerian degeneration. *J Magn Reson Imaging* 2003; 18:420–6.

80. Oh J, Henry RG, Genain C, Nelson SJ, Pelletier D. Mechanisms of normal appearing corpus callosum injury related to pericallosal T1 lesions in multiple sclerosis using directional diffusion tensor and 1H MRS imaging. *J Neurol Neurosurg Psychiatry* 2004; 75:1281–6.

81. Assaf Y, Chapman J, Ben-Bashat D, *et al.* White matter changes in multiple sclerosis: correlation of q-space diffusion MRI and (1)H MRS. *Magn Reson Imaging* 2005; 23:703–10.

82. Sijens PE, Irwan R, Potze JH, Mostert JP, De Keyser J, Oudkerk M. Analysis of the human brain in primary progressive multiple sclerosis with mapping of the spatial distributions using 1H MR spectroscopy and diffusion tensor imaging. *Eur Radiol* 2005; 15:1686–93.

83. Hickman SJ, Wheeler-Kingshott CA, Jones SJ, et al. Optic nerve diffusion measurement from diffusion-weighted imaging in optic neuritis. Am J Neuroradiol 2005; 26:951–6.

84. Trip SA, Wheeler-Kingshott C, Jones SJ, et al. Optic nerve diffusion tensor imaging in optic neuritis. Neuroimage 2006; 30:498–505.

85. Wheeler-Kingshott CA, Cercignani M. About "axial" and "radial" diffusivities. Magn Reson Med 2009; 61:1255–60.

86. Lowe MJ, Beall EB, Sakaie KE, et al. Resting state sensorimotor functional connectivity in multiple sclerosis inversely correlates with transcallosal motor pathway transverse diffusivity. Hum Brain Mapp 2008; 29:818–27.

87. Lowe MJ, Horenstein C, Hirsch JG, et al. Functional pathway-defined MRI diffusion measures reveal increased transverse diffusivity of water in multiple sclerosis. Neuroimage 2006; 32:1127–33.

88. Mori S, Crain BJ, Chacko VP, van Zijl PC. Three-dimensional tracking of axonal projections in the brain by magnetic resonance imaging. Ann Neurol 1999; 45:265–9.

89. Mori S, van Zijl PC. Fiber tracking: principles and strategies – a technical review. NMR Biomed 2002; 15:468–80.

90. Tench CR, Morgan PS, Wilson M, Blumhardt LD. White matter mapping using diffusion tensor MRI. Magn Reson Med 2002; 47:967–72.

91. Vaithianathar L, Tench CR, Morgan PS, Wilson M, Blumhardt LD. T1 relaxation time mapping of white matter tracts in multiple sclerosis defined by diffusion tensor imaging. J Neurol 2002; 249:1272–8.

92. Pagani E, Bammer R, Horsfield MA, et al. Diffusion MR imaging in multiple sclerosis: technical aspects and challenges. Am J Neuroradiol 2007; 28:411–20.

93. Pagani E, Filippi M, Rocca MA, Horsfield MA. A method for obtaining tract-specific diffusion tensor MRI measurements in the presence of disease: application to patients with clinically isolated syndromes suggestive of multiple sclerosis. Neuroimage 2005; 26:258–65.

94. Lin F, Yu C, Jiang T, Li K, Chan P. Diffusion tensor tractography-based group mapping of the pyramidal tract in relapsing-remitting multiple sclerosis

patients. Am J Neuroradiol 2007; 28:278–82.

95. Rocca MA, Absinta M, Valsasina P, et al. Abnormal connectivity of the sensorimotor network in patients with MS: a multicenter fMRI study. Hum Brain Mapp 2009; 30:2412–25.

96. Rocca MA, Pagani E, Absinta M, et al. Altered functional and structural connectivities in patients with MS: a 3-T study. Neurology 2007; 69:2136–45.

97. Rocca MA, Valsasina P, Ceccarelli A, et al. Structural and functional MRI correlates of Stroop control in benign MS. Hum Brain Mapp 2009; 30:276–90.

98. Pine AB, Jones S, Lowe MJ, Sakaie K, Phillips MD. Fiber-tracking through multiple sclerosis lesions using probabilistic tracking. In 17th Annual Meeting of the International Society for Magnetic Resonance in Medicine. Honolulu, 2009.

99. Wilson M, Tench CR, Morgan PS, Blumhardt LD. Pyramidal tract mapping by diffusion tensor magnetic resonance imaging in multiple sclerosis: improving correlations with disability. J Neurol Neurosurg Psychiatry 2003; 74:203–7.

100. Audoin B, Guye M, Reuter F, et al. Structure of WM bundles constituting the working memory system in early multiple sclerosis: a quantitative DTI tractography study. Neuroimage 2007; 36:1324–30.

101. Bonzano L, Tacchino A, Roccatagliata L, Abbruzzese G, Mancardi GL, Bove M. Callosal contributions to simultaneous bimanual finger movements. J Neurosci 2008; 28:3227–33.

102. Bonzano L, Tacchino A, Roccatagliata L, Mancardi GL, Abbruzzese G, Bove M. Structural integrity of callosal midbody influences intermanual transfer in a motor reaction-time task. Hum Brain Mapp 2011; 32:218–28.

103. Fox RJ, McColl RW, Lee JC, Frohman T, Sakaie K, Frohman E. A preliminary validation study of diffusion tensor imaging as a measure of functional brain injury. Arch Neurol 2008; 65:1179–84.

104. Freund P, Wheeler-Kingshott C, Jackson J, Miller D, Thompson A, Ciccarelli O. Recovery after spinal cord relapse in multiple sclerosis is predicted by radial diffusivity. Mult Scler 2010; 16:1193–202.

105. Kolbe S, Chapman C, Nguyen T, et al. Optic nerve diffusion changes and atrophy jointly predict visual dysfunction after optic neuritis. Neuroimage 2009; 45:679–86.

106. Lenzi D, Conte A, Mainero C, et al. Effect of corpus callosum damage on ipsilateral motor activation in patients with multiple sclerosis: a functional and anatomical study. Hum Brain Mapp 2007; 28:636–44.

107. Roca M, Torralva T, Meli F, et al. Cognitive deficits in multiple sclerosis correlate with changes in fronto-subcortical tracts. Mult Scler 2008; 14:364–9.

108. Warlop NP, Achten E, Debruyne J, Vingerhoets G. Diffusion weighted callosal integrity reflects interhemispheric communication efficiency in multiple sclerosis. Neuropsychologia 2008; 46:2258–64.

109. Fink F, Eling P, Rischkau E, et al. The association between California Verbal Learning Test performance and fibre impairment in multiple sclerosis: evidence from diffusion tensor imaging. Mult Scler 2010; 16: 332–41.

110. Ozturk A, Smith SA, Gordon-Lipkin EM, et al. MRI of the corpus callosum in multiple sclerosis: association with disability. Mult Scler 2010; 16: 166–77.

111. Lin X, Tench CR, Morgan PS, Constantinescu CS. Use of combined conventional and quantitative MRI to quantify pathology related to cognitive impairment in multiple sclerosis. J Neurol Neurosurg Psychiatry 2008; 79:437–41.

112. Bonzano L, Pardini M, Mancardi GL, Pizzorno M, Roccatagliata L. Structural connectivity influences brain activation during PVSAT in Multiple Sclerosis. Neuroimage 2009; 44:9–15.

113. Ceccarelli A, Rocca MA, Valsasina P, et al. Structural and functional magnetic resonance imaging correlates of motor network dysfunction in primary progressive multiple sclerosis. Eur J Neurosci 2010; 31:1273–80.

114. Rocca MA, Valsasina P, Absinta M, et al. Default-mode network dysfunction and cognitive impairment in progressive MS. Neurology 2010; 74:1252–9.

115. Altmann DR, Jasperse B, Barkhof F, et al. Sample sizes for brain atrophy

outcomes in trials for secondary progressive multiple sclerosis. *Neurology* 2009; 72:595–601.

116. Anderson VM, Bartlett JW, Fox NC, Fisniku L, Miller DH. Detecting treatment effects on brain atrophy in relapsing remitting multiple sclerosis: sample size estimates. *J Neurol* 2007; 254:1588–94.

117. Smith SM, Zhang Y, Jenkinson M, *et al.* Accurate, robust, and automated longitudinal and cross-sectional brain change analysis. *Neuroimage* 2002; 17:479–89.

118. Pelletier D, Garrison K, Henry R. Measurement of whole-brain atrophy in multiple sclerosis. *J Neuroimaging* 2004; 14:11S–9S.

119. Jasperse B, Valsasina P, Neacsu V, *et al.* Intercenter agreement of brain atrophy measurement in multiple sclerosis patients using manually-edited SIENA and SIENAX. *J Magn Reson Imaging* 2007; 26:881–5.

120. Sharma S, Noblet V, Rousseau F, Heitz F, Rumbach L, Armspach JP. Evaluation of brain atrophy estimation algorithms using simulated ground-truth data. *Med Image Anal* 2010; 14:373–89.

121. Neacsu V, Jasperse B, Korteweg T, *et al.* Agreement between different input image types in brain atrophy measurement in multiple sclerosis using SIENAX and SIENA. *J Magn Reson Imaging* 2008; 28:559–65.

122. Bisdas S, Bohning DE, Besenski N, Nicholas JS, Rumboldt Z. Reproducibility, interrater agreement, and age-related changes of fractional anisotropy measures at 3T in healthy subjects: effect of the applied b-value. *Am J Neuroradiol* 2008; 29:1128–33.

123. Bonekamp D, Nagae LM, Degaonkar M, *et al.* Diffusion tensor imaging in children and adolescents: reproducibility, hemispheric, and age-related differences. *Neuroimage* 2007; 34:733–42.

124. Ciccarelli O, Parker GJ, Toosy AT, *et al.* From diffusion tractography to quantitative white matter tract measures: a reproducibility study. *Neuroimage* 2003; 18:348–59.

125. Fox RJ, Sakaie K, Lee JC, *et al.* A validation study of multi-centre diffusion tensor imaging. *Mult Scler* 2007; 13:S76.

126. Heiervang E, Behrens TE, Mackay CE, Robson MD, Johansen-Berg H.

Between session reproducibility and between subject variability of diffusion MR and tractography measures. *Neuroimage* 2006; 33:867–77.

127. Jansen JF, Kooi ME, Kessels AG, Nicolay K, Backes WH. Reproducibility of quantitative cerebral T2 relaxometry, diffusion tensor imaging, and 1H magnetic resonance spectroscopy at 3.0 Tesla. *Invest Radiol* 2007; 42:327–37.

128. Pfefferbaum A, Adalsteinsson E, Sullivan EV. Replicability of diffusion tensor imaging measurements of fractional anisotropy and trace in brain. *J Magn Reson Imaging* 2003; 18:427–33.

129. Vollmar C, O'Muircheartaigh J, Barker GJ, *et al.* Identical, but not the same: intra-site and inter-site reproducibility of fractional anisotropy measures on two 3.0T scanners. *Neuroimage* 2010; 51:1384–94.

130. Pagani E, Hirsch JG, Pouwels PJ, *et al.* Intercenter differences in diffusion tensor MRI acquisition. *J Magn Reson Imaging* 2010; 31:1458–68.

131. Harrison DM, Caffo BS, Shiee N, *et al.* Longitudinal changes in diffusion tensor-based quantitative MRI in multiple sclerosis. *Neurology* 2011; 76:179–86.

Chapter

16

The use of MRI in multiple sclerosis clinical trials

Robert A. Bermel, Elizabeth Fisher, Peter B. Imrey, and Jeffrey A. Cohen

Introduction

Clinical trials of any new therapeutic agent depend on sensitive indices of disease activity to detect benefit. Surrogate measures, which ideally are directly linked to the mechanism of disease, are not available for many neurological diseases. In multiple sclerosis (MS) clinical trials, MRI markers of inflammatory disease activity have been crucial to rapid acceleration in development of MS therapeutics. MRI measures will likely be central to development of drugs for primary neuroprotection and repair as well. In this chapter, we briefly review standard and newer MRI measures (more detailed coverage can be found in other chapters in this book), address the role of MRI in monitoring safety in clinical trials, discuss statistical considerations when baseline characteristics are imbalanced or when the distribution of MRI data is skewed, and discuss practical operational aspects when using MRI in multicenter clinical trials.

Rationale for MRI as an outcome measure in MS clinical trials

The principal impetus for utilization of MRI as an outcome measure in MS clinical trials is the potential for increased sensitivity to change and treatment effects compared to clinical measures. The ultimate goal of MS disease therapy is to prevent relapses and accumulation of neurologic disability, and demonstration of benefit on clinical outcomes is required for regulatory approval of new treatments. The direct relevance to patient outcome is at the expense of efficiency, however. Even if trials are enriched for participants at high risk of relapse or disability progression, Phase 3 trials require relatively prolonged follow-up and large sample sizes on the order of a thousand patients. This renders Phase 3 trials resource intensive. In addition, in a number of neurological diseases including MS, clinical manifestations are delayed from disease onset, sometimes until after substantial irreversible tissue damage has already accumulated. In Phase 2 trials both treatment-related adverse events and placebo-related disease activity remain risks. Outcome measures with greater sensitivity can help to reduce the required sample size and therefore the number of participants exposed to those risks. The inefficiency of clinical outcomes is of

Table 16.1. *Advantages of MRI-derived outcome measures in MS trials*

Feature	Advantage
Increased sensitivity to disease activity	Smaller sample sizes; improved safety monitoring
Relatively easy blinding of MRI raters to treatment and clinical status	Reduced expectation bias
Greater reproducibility over clinical measures	Smaller sample sizes
Can provide continuous variables on linear scales	Smaller sample sizes
Potential retrieval of raw data for post-hoc analyses	Potential development of new data in the future
More closely represents underlying pathology	Possible mechanistic understanding of drug effects

even greater concern in an era of active treatment comparator studies, which require larger sample sizes, or more sensitive outcome measures, or both.[1] Thus, there is great impetus to develop more sensitive outcome measures.[2]

MRI lesion activity in MS exceeds the rate of relapses 5–10-fold, providing a much more sensitive measure of the disease process.[3] Statistical power is further enhanced by the continuous nature of some MRI variables. When analyzed by a blinded "central reading center" within a clinical trial, MRI data provide an independent, quantitative means to supplement potentially subjective clinical ratings.[4] MRI raw data can be archived and reanalyzed to assess for reproducibility or even extract new variables, which were unrecognized at the initial time of the study.

For these reasons, MRI has received substantial consideration as a potential surrogate measure for MS clinical trials (Table 16.1). Although current MRI-based MS outcome measures do not satisfy stringent, formal criteria for a surrogate measure,[5] there are many advantages to using an MRI measure of MS activity (1) as primary end-point in early trials assessing preliminary evidence of efficacy, and (2) using both MRI activity and burden of disease as secondary end-points to corroborate clinical measures in pivotal efficacy trials (Table 16.1). At all stages of drug development, MRI provides data on safety and mechanism of action.

Multiple Sclerosis Therapeutics, Fourth Edition, ed. Jeffrey A. Cohen and Richard A. Rudick. Published by Cambridge University Press.
© Cambridge University Press 2011.

Table 16.2. *Relative strengths of different MRI-based outcome measures*

Modality	Pathology assessed	Specificity	Multicenter feasibility
Measures of Inflammatory Activity			
T2 lesions	combined	+	++++
Gd-enhancing lesions	acute inflammation	++	++++
Measures of Axonal/Neuronal Integrity			
T1 "black holes"	axons/myelin	++	++++
Whole brain atrophy	combined	+	++++
GM atrophy	combined	++	+++
MTR	myelin	+++	++
MRS	axons	++++	++
DTI	axons/myelin	+++	++
fMRI	function	++	+

GM = gray matter; MTR = magnetization transfer ratio; MRS = magnetic resonance spectroscopy; DTI = diffusion tensor imaging; fMRI = functional magnetic resonance imaging

Standard MRI assessment in MS clinical trials includes measures of lesion activity (gadolinium-enhancing (Gd-enhancing) lesions, new or enlarged T2-hyperintense lesions) and measures of disease severity or burden (total T2-hyperintense lesion volume, total T1-hypointense lesion volume, and whole-brain atrophy). Substantial experience has accumulated in implementing these measures in multicenter clinical trials, estimating sample sizes, conducting statistical analysis of the data generated, and interpreting results of these analyses. Newer MRI parameters potentially provide additional sensitivity or pathologic specificity (magnetization transfer imaging [MTI], diffusion tensor imaging [DTI], gray matter atrophy measures, proton magnetic resonance spectroscopy [^{1}HMRS], and functional MRI [fMRI], among others) (Table 16.2).

Standard MRI measures of disease activity
Gadolinium-enhancing lesions
Lesions that are hyperintense on T1 images after intravenous administration of gadolinium chelate represent focal areas of blood–brain barrier (BBB) disruption, which in MS are presumed to represent areas of active inflammation. MS lesions typically have an acute inflammatory stage lasting 2–4 weeks, after which they cease to enhance.[6] Therefore, Gd-enhancing activity on a single scan provides information on disease activity over a relatively narrow time window. When scans are performed at frequent intervals (e.g. monthly), the total number or volume of Gd-enhancing lesions provides a cumulative measure of disease activity over the entire interval. Periods of clinical worsening correlate with increased Gd-enhancing lesion burden.[7] The relationship between Gd-enhancing lesion activity and neurologic disability is weak over short intervals, but stronger over longer intervals. Three factors likely account for the poor correlation: (1) lesions frequently occur in

non-eloquent regions of brain, (2) concurrent remyelination, repair, and functional adaptation may reduce the clinical manifestations of new lesions, and (3) inflammatory lesion accrual tends to occur early in the disease when functional reserve is high, and progressive disability may not occur until later in the disease, after the accumulation of new inflammatory lesions has slowed.

Several technical factors must be addressed to ensure valid analysis of Gd-enhancing lesions in clinical trials. The dose of gadolinium, time from injection to scanning, and acquisition parameters must be standardized. Higher contrast doses (e.g. triple dose) and a planned delay to imaging increase the sensitivity of enhancing lesion detection.[8,9] However, it remains uncertain whether the Gd-enhancing lesions detected with different doses of contrast represent comparable pathological processes. Scan acquisition and pulse sequence should be designed to minimize the intrusion of T2 effects into the post-contrast scans, which could lead to false-positives. Image processing software must allow review by the operator to "veto" pixels incorrectly identified as Gd-enhancing lesions, e.g. blood vessels. In general, total Gd-enhancing lesion number and volume are highly correlated. However, a therapeutic agent conceivably could alter lesion evolution but not lesion initiation, and as a result decrease Gd-enhancing volume but not number, dissociating the two measures. Though to our knowledge this is yet to occur, both parameters should be measured in a clinical trial.

New or enlarged T2-hyperintense lesion number
Because of their transient nature, Gd-enhancing lesions on a single scan indicate disease activity at that timepoint only. Because Gd-enhancing lesions are virtually always associated with longer-lasting T2-hyperintensity,[10] enumerating the number of T2 lesions that are new or enlarged on a follow-up scan compared to baseline provides a measure of lesion activity over that time period. T2 lesions comprise a variety of tissue changes including edema, inflammation, demyelination, remyelination, axon loss, and gliosis. The variability of these processes leads to significant month-to-month fluctuation in T2 lesion volume, on the order of 20% within subjects.[11] The criteria for lesion enlargement must take this into account and be defined in advance of data analysis. A typical definition is to classify a lesion as enlarged if it has a 50% increase in diameter (if smaller than 5 mm) or a 20% increase in diameter for a lesion larger than 5 mm.[12] To avoid double-counting T2 lesions which are also Gd-enhancing, the parameter "combined, unique, active lesions" is useful.[13] Registration and subtraction methods have been developed for improved detection of new T2 lesions.[14]

A comprehensive meta-analysis of 23 randomized, double-blind, placebo-controlled MS clinical trials, confirms that MRI lesion activity is an accurate surrogate for relapses. More than 80% of the variance in the effect on relapses between trials was explained by the variance in MRI effects. The authors concluded that short trials with MRI lesion activity as the primary outcome measure are effective at efficiently screening treatments eventually targeted at decreasing the relapse rate.[15]

Standard MRI measures of disease severity

T2-hyperintense lesion volume

The most useful method of quantifying the overall "burden of disease" is total volume of abnormal T2-hyperintensity. Despite its lack of pathologic specificity, T2 lesion burden early in the disease is the best known MRI predictor of long-term disability and brain atrophy.[16,17] When implementing T2 lesion burden in a clinical trial, acquisition parameters must be standardized and optimized to maximize sensitivity and reproducibility. Reliable, longitudinal detection of small T2 lesions requires protocols with thin tissue slices (generally 3 mm) without interslice gaps. Cerebrospinal fluid (CSF)-suppressed sequences such as fluid-attenuated inversion recovery (FLAIR) increase sensitivity for periventricular and juxtacortical lesions compared to traditional T2-weighted or proton density-weighted sequences.[18] The T2-weighted acquisition sequence (conventional spin-echo vs. rapid acquisition with relaxation enhancement (RARE) vs. a fluid-suppressed sequence) must be standardized at all sites and held constant through the trial.[19] Because lesion boundaries are indistinct, semi-automated segmentation approaches are preferable to manual methods to minimize operator variability. Conversely, with automated techniques, approaches to limit misclassification of lesions are necessary, because certain lesions can have signal intensity similar to brain tissue or CSF depending on lesion stage and MRI pulse sequence.[20]

T1-hypointense lesions (black holes)

A proportion of T2-hyperintense lesions (5%–20%) are hypointense on T1-weighted images – so-called "T1 black holes" representing areas with more severe tissue loss and axonal destruction.[21] Total T1 black hole volume correlates more strongly than T2 lesion volume with physical disability and brain atrophy in most cross-sectional analyses, though the absolute magnitude of these correlations remains modest.[22,23]

Approximately half of Gd-enhancing lesions evolve into chronic T1 black holes, making baseline Gd-enhancing lesion number a strong predictor of subsequent T1 black holes.[24] The proportion of Gd-enhancing lesions that convert to black holes has been utilized as a surrogate measure of neuroprotection.[25,26]

Brain atrophy

MRI lesion measures are useful as a surrogate for relapses and for measuring the inflammatory and focal components of MS. However, inflammation alone, as currently defined by lesions visible with conventional MRI, accounts incompletely for disability progression.[27,28] In studies of agents in secondary progressive MS, neurologic disability and brain atrophy

progress despite effective inhibition of MRI lesion activity.[29,30] Therefore, the MRI outcomes presented up to this point are not sufficient for testing treatments targeting the progressive or degenerative component of MS, including potential neuroprotective or reparative strategies.

Tissue loss can be viewed as the final common pathway for the wide variety of pathologic processes that occur in MS, and can be captured by measurement of whole-brain atrophy. The lack of specificity is both an advantage and a shortcoming of brain atrophy as an outcome measure. Whole-brain atrophy becomes very apparent in the mid to late stages of the disease,[31,32] but is detectable even in the earliest stages of the disease, suggesting substantial subclinical pathology.[33,34] Short-term whole-brain atrophy progression predicts longer-term disability.[35]

Multiple techniques have been developed to measure brain atrophy,[36] including manual, linear measurement of central or regional atrophy,[37] semi-automated or automated methods of measuring whole-brain atrophy using segmentation-based techniques,[22,38,39] and registration-based techniques to identify changes in brain volume over time.[40–42] Brain atrophy progression and treatment effects can be detected in two-year clinical trials when precise automated techniques that normalize brain volume are utilized.[22,43] Sample size estimates to demonstrate treatment benefit on whole-brain atrophy progression are similar to those required for lesion analyses, and roughly an order of magnitude below those required for clinical outcomes.[44]

An important issue with the use of brain atrophy in clinical trials is that the magnitude of change is small in short-term trials and different measures can produce conflicting results due to differences in reproducibility, susceptibility to artifacts, geometry as a function of anatomic site, and biologic factors determining the rate of atrophy in different structures.[45–47] In addition, brain volume fluctuates as a result of tissue water content related to hydration status and inflammatory activity. This issue is especially relevant to high-dose corticosteroids, which can induce "pseudoatrophy" depending on the timing of their use relative to scan acquisition.[48] Anti-inflammatory effects of MS disease-modifying agents cause initial acceleration in the rate of brain volume loss at the initiation of therapy.[22] Therefore, when using normalized brain atrophy as a key outcome measure in a clinical trial of an agent expected to have anti-inflammatory activity, it may be useful to establish a stable baseline some months after the intervention is started. Even treatments which may not have known primary anti-inflammatory effects may be found to reduce brain volume initially, as was the case during a recent trial of lamotrigine in secondary progressive MS.[49]

Exploratory MRI measures for clinical trials

Several imaging approaches have been proposed to provide additional pathologic specificity with greater ability to monitor tissue integrity both within lesions visible on standard imaging, normal appearing brain tissue (NABT), and gray matter (GM).

Magnetization transfer imaging

MTI quantifies the interaction between MRI-visible free water protons and MR-invisible protons associated with macromolecules (proteins and lipids), providing a measure of tissue integrity, particularly myelin. Magnetization transfer ratio (MTR) is defined as the relative difference in signal intensities in images acquired with and without an off-resonance magnetization pulse. Demyelination and reduced axonal density are associated with decreased MTR.[50] Whole-brain MTR correlates with T2 lesion volume and with whole-brain atrophy,[51] raising some question of its added value in clinical trials. However, MTI provides information on preservation of tissue structure, distinguishing it from these other measures.

Disease-related alterations of whole-brain MTR are frequently assessed using histogram analysis. Whereas normal controls have a narrow range of MTR values, MS patients have a higher proportion of voxels with low values, resulting in a lower mean MTR and higher variance.[52–54] Whole-brain histogram analysis on a relatively large scale (82 patients from 5 centers) failed to show an effect on MTR for interferon beta-1b in secondary progressive MS.[55] An alternative approach is to measure MTR in defined regions, such as lesions, NABT, white matter, gray matter, etc. Measuring MTR in the cortex may be one method for detecting subpial, or intra-cortical demyelinating lesions.[56] Stablization of MTR in individual lesions over time may suggest preservation of myelin and axons; improvement may suggest remyelination or repair. Longitudinal MTR measures are thus a potential method to test neuroprotective or repair strategies.[57] Benefit was demonstrated in small studies for intravenous methylprednisolone and interferon-beta using this approach.[58,59]

Inclusion of MTI in large-scale multicenter trials has been limited by technical issues and difficulty with standardization across sites. Guidelines for incorporation of MTI into trials recently were published,[60] which will hopefully lead to more data from multicenter studies.

Diffusion tensor imaging

With DTI, the diffusivity of water molecules is quantified in multiple spatial directions to determine the orientation and integrity of fiber tracts. As fiber tracts degenerate, decreased restriction allows water molecules to diffuse more equally in all directions. This is manifest as increased mean diffusivity and decreased fractional anisotropy. DTI quantification can be performed on white matter, within pathway specific tracts, or on lesions. All approaches can be applied longitudinally over time. A preliminary study suggested that DTI can be performed reproducibly at high field strength across multiple study sites.[61] DTI appears sensitive to disease-related changes in NABT, even over short time periods.[62–64] A recent longitudinal study of 78 patients with MS identified tract-specific DTI measures as potentially more sensitive to short-term changes than whole-brain or ROI-based DTI measures.[65] Measurement of fractional anisotropy in the corpus callosum was more sensitive to change over the two year study than other DTI measures and more sensitive than brain volume change in this cohort. The study authors estimate 26 subjects per arm would be required to show a 25% treatment effect on FA in the corpus callosum when three scans are acquired over a two-year study.[65]

Proton magnetic resonance spectroscopy

^{1}HMRS is a technique that derives a nuclear MR spectrum from a volume of tissue, yielding relative concentrations of the major proton-yielding metabolites. The most prominent peak in the spectrum from the CNS is N-acetyl aspartate (NAA), almost exclusively contained within neurons and their processes. The concentration of NAA, measured most commonly as a ratio of NAA to Creatine (Cr), decreases when there is neuronal dysfunction, damage, or axonal or neuronal loss.[66] Decreased NAA/Cr was demonstrated within MS lesions[67] as well as NABT.[68] Use of ^{1}HMRS in clinical trials has been limited, but studies of both interferon-beta[69,70] and glatiramer acetate[71] demonstrated treatment benefit.

Issues complicating the use of ^{1}HMRS in multicenter trials include the need for standardization of techniques across centers, and the limitations of single-voxel techniques (which are difficult to precisely reproduce over time within patients). With the growing capability of whole-brain MRS techniques,[72,73] some of these issues may be overcome. Recommendations were published to facilitate the use of ^{1}HMRS in multicenter clinical trials.[74]

Gray matter atrophy

It is possible to separate brain volumes into different compartments, using automated or manual parcellation software. One distinction of particular interest is gray vs. white matter. GM pathology is widespread in MS, but GM lesions are largely MR-invisible using current imaging techniques (Chapters 2,11,13). Selective GM atrophy has been noted early in relapsing-remitting (RR) and progressive MS, is among the best correlates of physical disability, and accelerates later in the disease.[75,76] Tissue water shifts underlying the confounding phenomenon of pseudoatrophy appear confined primarily to the white matter compartment,[77,78] making GM atrophy potentially useful as an outcome measure in shorter duration trials. Gray matter atrophy is an attractive outcome measure for testing neuroprotective therapies in progressive MS (Table 16.3).

Lobar atrophy

Measurement of lobar brain atrophy also is feasible, and may correlate best with specific cognitive measures.[79,80]

Spinal cord atrophy

A significant portion of the physical disability in MS results from spinal cord involvement and associated upper extremity and gait impairment. Patients with MS were shown to have up to 40% spinal cord volume loss compared to normal controls,

Table 16.3. *Advantages of gray matter (GM) atrophy as an outcome measure*

Appeal of gray matter (GM) atrophy as an outcome measure in clinical trials of anti-inflammatory or neuroprotective therapies
• At all stages of MS, GM atrophy correlates better with disability than any other MRI metric, including whole-brain and white matter atrophy.   • The rate of GM atrophy equals white matter atrophy in early stages of MS, and exceeds it in more progressive stages.   • GM pathology is widespread in MS, but focal GM lesions are invisible on current multicenter clinical trial MRI protocols.   • GM atrophy is a currently available, reliable measure of GM pathology which is able to be utilized in multicenter trials.   • Pseudoatrophy appears to occur primarily in the white matter compartment, making GM atrophy potentially useful as an outcome measure in shorter duration trials.

particularly in PPMS, where spinal cord atrophy was found to progress over periods as short as 1 year.[81] Spinal cord atrophy has not yet been used as a supportive outcome in a major clinical trial, primarily because of poor reproducibility of current techniques. Spinal cord atrophy is of great interest in trials of progressive MS, particularly as newer, more reproducible techniques are developed.[82]

Functional MRI

Focal damage in MS elicits not only attempted tissue repair but also neural plasticity with reassignment of function to other anatomic sites. fMRI can be used to study the effects MS on specific pathways and provides a way to interrogate these compensatory mechanisms. Most methods utilize the different magnetic properties of oxygenated and deoxygenated hemoglobin to identify regions of increased or decreased cerebral blood flow (termed the blood oxygen level-dependent or BOLD technique). There may be particular utility in using fMRI to study effects on fatigue, a consequence of the disease which thus far has been difficult to objectively quantify.[83] fMRI protocols are highly dependent on a standardized methodology as implemented by technicians and other study staff, rendering it challenging to implement longitudinally in multicenter trials.

Purposes served by MRI in clinical trials

Some of the measures discussed above are now routinely incorporated into clinical trials at all stages of drug development, where they serve multiple purposes. However, the emphasis is different in Phase 1, Phase 2, and Phase 3 studies.

Subject selection

MRI is commonly used to support the diagnosis of MS in clinical practice and, likewise, for enrollment in clinical trials. Increasingly, trials allow diagnosis of MS by criteria in which dissemination of pathology anatomically or over time is confirmed by MRI.[84] This effectively expands the pool of subjects eligible for clinical trials. MRI is also helpful in excluding subjects with other neurologic diagnoses mimicking MS.

Studies have been enriched with subjects more likely to experience ongoing disease activity during the trial by requiring Gd-enhancing lesions as an inclusion criterion. This predicts MRI activity and relapses during the trial, results in higher on-study event rates, and reduces required sample sizes. However, because of regression to the mean, high activity periods may be followed by low activity periods even without therapy.[85] Therefore, determining the magnitude of benefit still requires a parallel comparison group.

If randomization is successful in large-scale trials, treatment groups should be matched for MRI parameters at baseline. Randomization may be less successful for smaller trials, which are most likely to rely on MRI as an outcome measure. A screening MRI allows stratification for variables of interest, limiting potential confounders in small studies. It is also possible to compensate for potential imbalances statistically, but results of this approach may be difficult to interpret (see Statistical considerations with use of MRI in trials).

Assessment of efficacy

Given their increased sensitivity over clinical outcomes, MRI measures of MS disease activity are ideally suited to preliminary trials aimed at exploring efficacy of agents expected to have a rapid and prominent effect on lesion activity. Use of MRI outcomes allows smaller sample size and shorter study duration, with less exposure of study populations to an agent with which there may be limited experience.

The effect of a novel treatment on cumulative disease severity can also be assessed by MRI. Quantifying the overall volume of T2 lesions is the most routinely performed measure of overall burden of disease, though whole-brain atrophy is becoming increasingly common. Measures of cumulative disease severity can also include T1 black hole volume as well as advanced MRI techniques.

Even in initial small-scale trials, a treatment's relative effect on different MRI measures can yield information about the kinetics and mechanism of action of the tested therapy. For instance, potent suppression of Gd-enhancing lesions implies an anti-inflammatory mechanism of action. Improvement on MTI or ^{1}HMRS-derived metrics would suggest myelin or axonal preservation. The timing of an agent's biologic effect, impacted by both its pharmacokinetics and pharmacodynamics, is often first identified in a Phase 1 or Phase 2 study utilizing frequent MRI to closely monitor for the outcome of interest.

Monitoring safety

In initial studies of novel therapies, scans obtained shortly after treatment onset can be used to monitor for unexpected increase in disease activity suggesting "reverse efficacy," as was seen in trials of interferon-gamma, altered peptide ligand, and tumor necrosis factor alpha antagonists.[86–88] Increased tissue damage can occur despite a therapeutic decrease in inflammation, for example, the increased rate of brain atrophy as seen following immunoablation with bone marrow transplantation

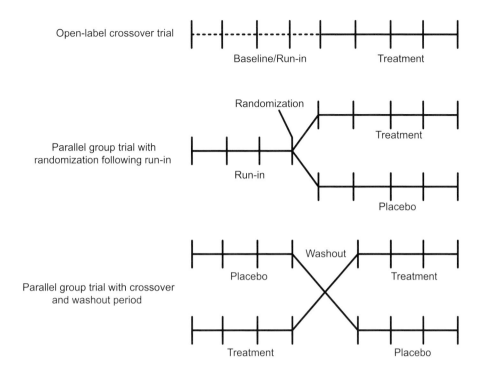

Fig. 16.1. Example designs of possible Phase 2 studies using gadolinium-enhancing lesions on magnetic resonance imaging (MRI) as the primary outcome measure. Vertical lines signify MRI scans.

rescue.[78] With emerging potent immunomodulatory therapies, neoplasia and opportunistic infection, e.g. progressive multifocal leukoencephalopathy,[89] are concerns. Thus, MRI also functions as an important safety outcome measure. During development of the protocol, it must be decided where MRI scans will be monitored for safety issues: at the central reading center or at the individual sites. Likewise, a plan for dealing with incidental findings on brain MRI should be included in the study protocol and discussed as part of the informed consent process.[90] Incidental findings are reported in between 2% and 8% of individuals from the general population volunteering for research studies, with older patients and those with more medical comorbidities carrying a greater risk of discovering unexpected non-MS pathology in the course of a clinical trial.[91]

MRI in Phase 1 trials

Phase 1 trials aim to expose a relatively small number of subjects (sometimes healthy individuals) to a new medication for a short period of time, monitoring primarily for safety concerns. In Phase 1 trials, MRI is used primarily to determine eligibility and monitor adverse effects of therapy. MRI also can be incorporated to provide preliminary information on efficacy, but due to the typically short duration and small sample size of such trials, clear-cut evidence of efficacy is not expected.

MRI in Phase 2 trials

At early stages of drug development, information about the magnitude and kinetics of benefit, side effects, and optimal dose need to be generated to guide future definitive studies.

In addition, exposure of subjects to a novel agent of unproven safety and efficacy needs to be minimized, as does exposure to placebo. Clinical outcomes (relapses and disability progression) are insufficiently sensitive to accomplish these goals in preliminary studies.

As a result, MRI-based studies have become standard for Phase 2 (proof-of-concept) trials of disease modification in MS. The most common approaches (Fig. 16.1) include frequent (most often monthly) scanning of subjects with active RRMS and enumeration of Gd-enhancing lesions over periods ranging from three to 12 months. There now is substantial experience in the field with such designs, including trial conduct, subject selection, sample size estimation, and data analysis.[92,93] Natalizumab is one of several agents shown to be effective on MRI-based outcomes in a Phase 2 proof-of-concept trial,[94] followed by successful Phase 3 pivotal clinical trials.[95,96]

The timing of MRI scans in the trial must be laid out to capture the expected effect on Gd-enhancing lesions, based on knowledge of the pharmacokinetics and pharmacodynamics of the tested agent. Assuming rapid onset of therapeutic effect, follow-up for three months may be adequate to show efficacy, though a six month endpoint is the most common. Less frequent (bimonthly) MRI follow-up may be possible and cost effective without sacrificing analysis power.[97] For an agent expected to have a delayed effect on Gd-enhancing, early scans can be included to look for evidence of a deleterious increase in disease activity, but principal scans for analysis should be later, after a delay. Also, longer and more frequent follow-up often is desirable to avoid missing less-prominent or more gradual benefit, confirm persistent efficacy, and provide additional safety data.

Data on which to base sample size estimates are available from a natural history cohort plus subjects involved in the placebo arms of clinical trials.[98] A number of methods are often employed to increase the number of on-study events and hopefully improve power. One recruitment tactic selects for active subjects by requiring one or more Gd-enhancing lesions on screening MRI. This approach usually is effective, but can impede enrollment. In addition, some subjects may have decreased on-study activity following an active scan due to 'regression to the mean.' Other useful selection criteria (which probably are inter-related) are young age, short disease duration, and recent relapses. Another way potentially to augment on-study events is to increase gadolinium dose (e.g. triple-dose) and delay scanning after gadolinium administration.[99] However, the additional lesions detected by this approach have unclear pathogenic significance, and it is uncertain that this method actually improves the ability to detect differences between treatment groups.

The intermittent use of intravenous methylprednisolone (IVMP) to treat relapses can confound use of Gd-enhancing as an outcome. IVMP suppresses Gd-enhancing lesions for 4–8 weeks.[100] Delaying a protocol-dictated MRI scan to avoid this effect complicates visit scheduling and data analysis. If possible, the preferred approach is to obtain the scheduled scan prior to administration of IVMP.

A final decision involves whether to include a placebo-treated comparison group. A single arm cross-over design has the advantage that all subjects receive active therapy (after a pre-baseline run-in period). However, interpretation of the results assumes that Gd-enhancing lesion activity would have remained constant in the absence of treatment, which is a questionable assumption. Interpretation of a parallel-group placebo-controlled design is usually more straightforward, but there are practical and ethical issues with including a placebo arm. Namely, effective treatments are available for patients with active RRMS.

Phase 2 designs based on enumeration of Gd-enhancing lesions work well for agents with a rapid and prominent effect on inflammatory activity. If this is not the case, one runs the risk of erroneously discarding a potentially useful agent. There are a number of immunomodulatory agents expected to have modest or gradual effect on BBB integrity. From a practical perspective, this shortcoming also applies to testing agents with putative neuroprotective or reparative mechanisms of action. It remains uncertain how to conduct preliminary studies of such agents to obtain data supporting proof-of-concept prior to undertaking large-scale pivotal trials. Potential approaches include MTI, DTI, or ^{1}HMRS applied to lesions, specific pathways, or the whole brain.

MRI in Phase 3 trials

Primary outcomes for Phase 3 (pivotal) trials, which may lead to regulatory submission for new agents, remain relapses and disability progression. MRI metrics serve as important supportive measures, corroborating efficacy.[101] In all of the most recent pivotal trials of new therapies, the effect size on imaging metrics has paralleled or exceeded clinical outcomes.[95,96,102] MRI also provides important information for interpreting the results of the study, including characteristics of the population, assessing whether the treatment groups were well matched at baseline, identifying factors predicting responders and non-responders, and analyzing the effects of factors that can interfere with efficacy, e.g. neutralizing antibodies.

Phase 3 trials in MS typically are large, based on the expected statistical power of clinical end-points. In most trials, all subjects undergo standard MRI at entry and exit (or annually). Cost and logistics preclude frequent MRI of all subjects. Therefore, when included in Phase 3 trials, more frequent or advanced MRI usually is performed in a cohort of subjects at selected sites as a substudy. If this approach is taken, separate power analyses are conducted to determine the size of the subset needed to show efficacy on MRI end-points.[103] Similarly, substudies of advanced MRI techniques, which are important to advance the field, can be performed at selected sites with the necessary technical resources and expertise.

Statistical considerations with use of MRI in trials (see also Chapter 21)

Clinical trial results are most readily accepted when baseline variables, particularly characteristics that affect outcome, are comparable or when analyses adjust for baseline inequities by a well-accepted method. Otherwise, results may defy clear interpretation due to statistical confounding of apparent treatment effects with baseline differences. In principle, randomization of very large trials is very likely to balance the net effect of all identified, unmeasured, and even unknown baseline prognostic factors. However, few MS trials are large enough to justify reliance on this principle, and treatment groups of smaller MS studies, such as Phase 2 MRI-based trials, commonly differ noticeably on one or more prognostic factors, including MRI parameters. Constrained randomization using key MRI prognostic parameters, such as by stratified permuted block randomization[104] or minimization[105] can help avoid this. Local or central evaluation of baseline scans for this purpose pose practical but manageable hurdles.

There are three distinct considerations in the use of MRI for MS trials: (1) considerations related to the specific scan technique or protocol(s), e.g. FLAIR scan; (2) extraction of MRI summary parameters, e.g. total T2-hyperintense lesion volume, from the scan at the reading center; and (3) computation and statistical analysis of outcome measures, e.g. change in total T2-hyperintense lesion volume from baseline to study end in oder to make statistical inferences about treatment effects. Each step of this sequence should be precisely defined and tailored to the population being studied and biologic question asked, and implemented with careful quality control. The primary outcome in Phase 2 studies has been a cumulative number of Gd-enhancing lesions, sometimes accumulated only after a lag period. A similar approach has been used in frequent MRI sub-studies of Phase 3 trials. The most common analytic target for lesion volumes and atrophy measurements in Phase 3 studies has been absolute change or percent change from baseline to study end.

The specific choice of outcome measure affects the options for probability modeling and statistical analysis. Gd-enhancing lesion counts take discrete values, only a predictable few of which occur frequently in trials. T2 lesion volume and brain atrophy data are continuous, potentially taking any value in a wide range. Many MRI measures such as lesion counts and volumes exhibit highly positively-skewed distributions, which are also often overdispersed or heavy-tailed. "Overdispersed" and "heavy-tailed" describe ways in which outer percentiles of data may be more extreme relative to center values than commonly used biostatistical methods assume. Lesion volume subtraction methods (e.g. end-point-baseline) or change ratios are also susceptible to these complications when negligible baseline values occur. For instance, the very high coefficients of variation ($CV = SD/mean$) for inherently positive MRI measures, as seen in the Avonex Combination Trial (ACT)[106] and many other MS trials, commonly reflect extreme skewing.

With such data, a few patients with very high lesion counts and/or volumes can easily dominate standard parametric statistical analyses, including t-tests, ordinary least-squares analysis of variance and covariance, and linear and Poisson regression. This increases the risk of missing a true benefit or inferring benefit when none exists. Moreover, clinical impact measures (e.g. low N-to-treat per clinical relapse or new/enlarged T2-hyperintense lesion) require different interpretation if they may reflect dramatic reductions in only a few highly active patients rather than more widespread benefit.

Numerous analytic alternatives are available for alleviating the statistical effects of relatively few highly active patients. Negative binomial regression is an overdispersion-adjusted generalization of Poisson regression analysis that has been used to analyze MRI lesion counts in many recent trials including ACT,[106] a recent Phase 3 trial of oral fingolimod,[102] and a dose comparison trial of glatiramer acetate.[107] Several methodologically oriented studies using actual or simulated MS MRI lesion counts have generally supported the appropriateness of negative binomial regression,[97,109–110] except possibly when studies select samples enriched for disease activity.[108] Quasi-likelihood adjustment and other generalizations of Poisson regression accommodating overdispersion may also be used for analyzing MRI counts. Other gamma generalized linear models (a class of statistical models including negative binomial regression) may be useful for analysis of MRI volumes and volume change ratios. Ordinal categorical data analyses were used to analyze lesion counts in a Phase 3 trial of natalizumab,[111] and are often used with pooling of extreme observations into an upper category. Non-parametric methods and statistically "robustified" modifications of standard analyses can be used with or without categorization, as used in ACT for lesion volumes and volume changes.[106] Non-parametric covariance analyses,[112] were also used in ACT for lesion volumes and volume changes.[106] Preliminary logarithmic, cube root, or other Box–Cox data transformation, or replacing high with lower observed values ("Winsorization"), are simple tactics that can sometimes allow use of more standard continuous data methods.[113] Very high values may also be truncated and treated as right-censored, allowing use of survival analytic tools to study lesion volumes. Focusing on absolute rather than relative changes in lesion volumes can ease both analyses and interpretation of accumulating lesion burdens. Since choice of analytic method influences statistical power and sample size, and how the strength of treatment effect is expressed when interpreting results, it must not be considered in isolation.

For studies with periodic MRI examinations, where the time course of an MRI parameter may provide mechanistic insight, serial observations are best analyzed jointly rather than singly at each time, using a comprehensive approach that accounts for correlations among repeated studies of the same patient, and controls for multiple comparisons. Such approaches include mixed statistical models, possibly robustified;[114–116] multivariate generalized linear models analyzed using generalized estimating equations;[117] and hidden Markov models.[118]

Regardless of confounding, statistical adjustment for baseline predictors can increase statistical power. While such a gain is assured and readily estimated for ordinary least-squares modeling, the situation is more complex for other analytic approaches, and simulation may be required. Statistical adjustment of randomized trial data is scientifically appropriate strategy but, since opportunistic post-hoc variable selection can introduce bias, it is desirable to select predictors in advance, or by an explicit, blinded method that precludes this concern.

Adaptive clinical trial designs, incorporating structured interim fine-tuning of trial design parameters based on accumulating data, constitute an active area of biostatistical investigation, with ramifications for many clinical areas including multiple sclerosis. MRI parameters are expected to play prominent roles in such designs.[119,120]

Practical aspects of image analysis in trials

Ensuring the technical rigor of the MRI aspect of a clinical trial can be difficult. The expertise of a multidisciplinary team with members from neurology, radiology, MRI physics, biomedical engineering, computer science, and biostatistics is necessary to guarantee accurate acquisition and analysis of the data (Table 16.4). Fig. 16.2 depicts the typical workflow of MRI data in a multicenter clinical trial.

First, the acquisition protocol must generate images that can be quantified reliably and accurately, yet be technically feasible at the participating study sites and tolerable to subjects. The MRI reading center must be able to reliably receive, read, and analyze data from the scanners utilized at the sites, which may come from a variety of manufacturers, use different software packages or versions, and have different field strengths. A test scan usually is required from each study site prior to

Table 16.4. *Steps to ensure high-quality MRI data in a clinical trial*

Pre-study	MRI analysis center personnel	Participating site personnel
Design MRI protocol with appropriate pulse sequences and consideration of: Ease of standardization across sites Reasonable acquisition time High tissue contrast / lesion conspicuity Resolution / slice thickness / coverage	PI, RE	
Select and evaluate MRI analysis software to ensure: High accuracy and reproducibility Functionality in multicenter studies Feasibility for a large number of scans (automation, user time required per scan)	RE	
Setup image analysis database, data handling, documentation, and standard operating procedures	RE, SC	
Train MRI analysis center personnel	RE, Tech	
Provide MRI manual to participating sites	SC	
Train participating sites (investigators meeting)	RE, Tech	PI, SC, Tech
Evaluate site performance (MRI dummy scans)	RE, SC	SC, Tech
During study		
Communicate frequently with sites to ensure: Scans are sent to reading center in a timely manner Same scanner and protocol are used throughout the study Scans approved or rejected	SC	SC
Evaluate study scans for: Complete and error-free electronic transfer Adherence to protocol Consistency with previous scans Image quality	SC, RE, Tech	SC, Tech
Repeat acquisition of rejected images	SC	PI, SC, Tech
Monitor and account for scanner hardware and software upgrades (prospectively or retrospectively)	SC, Tech	Tech
Analyze scans according to pre-specified procedures with consideration of: Consistent operator for a given patient (semi-automated software) Consistent parameters used for a given patient (automated software)	SC, Tech	
Review and visually verify analysis results	SC, RE	
Post-study		
Perform final quality assurance on analysis results	PI, RE	
Archive raw MRI data	SC, Tech	SC, Tech
Archive MRI analysis results	SC, Tech	

Abbreviations: PI = Study or Site Principal Investigator, RE = Radiologist / Imaging Engineer / Physicist in charge of the central MRI analysis center, Tech = MRI Technologist or other technical personnel, SC = Study Coordinator.

enrolling study subjects to ensure appropriate scan acquisition and data transfer procedures. Use of the same scanner or at least same model and software at a particular site is very important; scanner changes during a trial can have significant effects on the data acquired, for which even complex corrective postprocessing approaches may inadequately compensate.[19,121,122] However, scanner upgrades and replacement usually are not under control of the study investigators. Table 16.3 lists additional quality control measures and the responsible parties at either the study site or the central MRI analysis center.

Data flow between the individual sites and the analysis center should be as rapid and seamless as possible. Accurate tracking of data and prompt assessment of transmitted studies allow

efficient feedback to study sites. Analysis of imaging data on an ongoing basis is preferable to batch analysis at the end of a trial, so that technical errors can be corrected before they are repeated. This approach also facilitates the provision of preliminary MRI data to the study team and data safety monitoring board.

Volumetric measurements can be performed by a number of techniques,[36] including manual tracing methods, semi-automated methods where a user places a seed point at the edge of the structure of interest,[38,123,124] or automated methods based on signal intensities and spatial information.[125–127] Automated methods (as depicted in Fig. 16.3) are generally preferable in that (once established) they are less time and

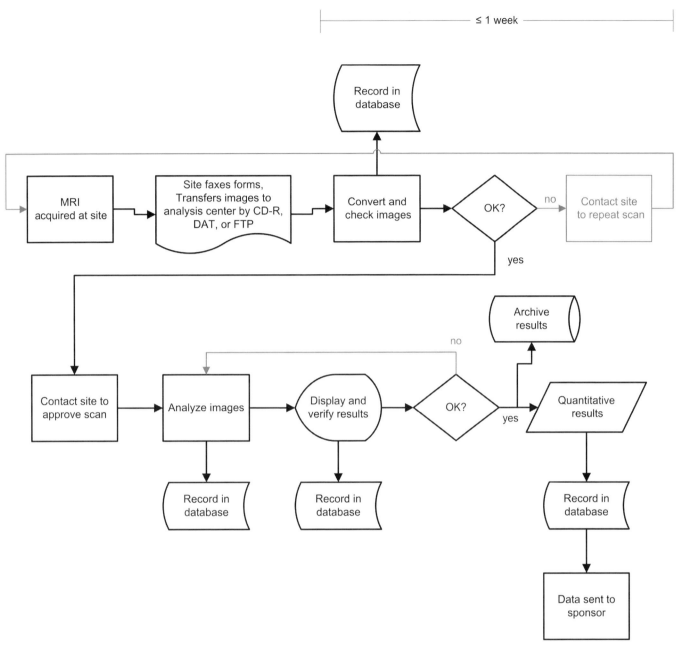

Fig. 16.2. Example MRI workflow for clinical trials.

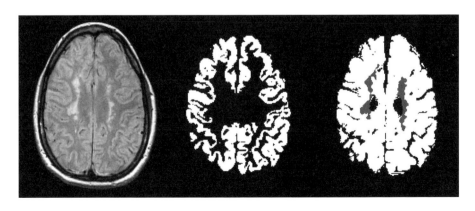

Fig. 16.3. Example of image analysis results using automated segmentation for a single slice. Left to right are the proton density-weighted image, gray matter, and brain lesion mask.

labor-intensive, unbiased, and have higher reproducibility.[128] However, any method which does not utilize human oversight for error checking runs the risk of misclassifying tissue types.[20,129]

When individual lesions or regional atrophy are tracked over time, image registration is necessary. Consistent slice angle and level can be reproduced by repositioning of the subject in the scanner at each imaging session. However, this method is imprecise and labor intensive. Image registration through post-processing is more accurate, places less demand on MRI personnel and subjects, and also can compensate for changes in magnetic field homogeneity. The latter issue is particularly relevant to newer, echo-planar sequences, such as those used in DTI.

Conclusions

MRI is an integral part of MS clinical trials. It provides the primary efficacy outcome of preliminary proof-of-concept studies and important corroborating data as secondary and exploratory outcomes in pivotal trials. At all stages of drug development, MRI provides important information on the kinetics and magnitude of treatment effect and insight into potential mechanisms of action. Attention to issues in scan acquisition, quantitative image processing, and statistical analysis are critical to generate high-quality data. Though it is unlikely that one single outcome measure will capture all aspects of the MS disease process, there is potential for MRI outcomes to evaluate both inflammatory and degenerative components within clinical trials.

References

1. Polman CH, Reingold SC, Barkhof F, *et al*. Ethics of placebo-controlled clinical trials in multiple sclerosis: a reassessment. *Neurology* 2008;70(13, 2): 1134–40.

2. Sormani MP, Rovaris M, Bagnato F, *et al*. Sample size estimations for MRI-monitored trials of MS comparing new vs standard treatments. *Neurology* 2001;57(10):1883–5.

3. Paty DW, McFarland H. Magnetic resonance techniques to monitor the long term evolution of multiple sclerosis pathology and to monitor definitive clinical trials. *J Neurol, Neurosurg Psychiatry* 1998;64(Suppl 1): S47–51.

4. Martinelli Boneschi F, Rovaris M, Comi G, *et al*. The use of magnetic resonance imaging in multiple sclerosis: lessons learned from clinical trials. *Mult Scler* 2004;10(4):341–7.

5. Prentice RL. Surrogate endpoints in clinical trials: definition and operational criteria. *Stat Med* 1989;8(4):431–40.

6. Stone LA, Frank JA, Albert PS, *et al*. Characterization of MRI response to treatment with interferon beta-1b: contrast-enhancing MRI lesion frequency as a primary outcome measure. *Neurology* 1997;49(3):862–9.

7. Smith ME, Stone LA, Albert PS, *et al*. Clinical worsening in multiple sclerosis is associated with increased frequency and area of gadopentetate dimeglumine-enhancing magnetic resonance imaging lesions. *Ann Neurol* 1993;33(5):480–9.

8. Filippi M, Rovaris M, Capra R, *et al*. A multi-centre longitudinal study comparing the sensitivity of monthly MRI after standard and triple dose gadolinium-DTPA for monitoring disease activity in multiple sclerosis. Implications for phase II clinical trials. *Brain* 1998;121 (Pt 10): 2011–20.

9. Silver NC, Good CD, Sormani MP, *et al*. A modified protocol to improve the detection of enhancing brain and spinal cord lesions in multiple sclerosis. *J Neurol* 2001;248(3):215–24.

10. Molyneux PD, Filippi M, Barkhof F, *et al*. Correlations between monthly enhanced MRI lesion rate and changes in T2 lesion volume in multiple sclerosis. *Ann Neurol* 1998; 43(3):332–9.

11. Stone LA, Albert PS, Smith ME, *et al*. Changes in the amount of diseased white matter over time in patients with relapsing-remitting multiple sclerosis. *Neurology* 1995;45(10):1808–14.

12. Simon JH, Miller DE. Measures of gadolinium enhancement, T1 black holes and T2-hyperintense lesions on magnetic resonance imaging. In Cohen JA, Rudick RA, eds. London, UK: Informa Healthcare, 2007;113, 114–142.

13. Li DK, Paty DW. Magnetic resonance imaging results of the PRISMS trial: a randomized, double-blind, placebo-controlled study of interferon-beta1a in relapsing–remitting multiple sclerosis. Prevention of relapses and disability by interferon-beta1a subcutaneously in multiple Sclerosis. *Ann Neurol* 1999;46(2):197–206.

14. Moraal B, Van Den Elskamp IJ, Knol DL, *et al*. Long-interval T2-weighted subtraction magnetic resonance imaging: a powerful new outcome measure in multiple sclerosis trials. *Ann Neurol* 2010;67(5):667–75.

15. Sormani MP, Bonzano L, Roccatagliata L, *et al*. Magnetic resonance imaging as a potential surrogate for relapses in multiple sclerosis: a meta-analytic approach. *Ann Neurol* 2009;65(3): 268–75.

16. Sormani MP, Rovaris M, Comi G, *et al*. A reassessment of the plateauing relationship between T2 lesion load and disability in MS. *Neurology* 2009; 73(19):1538–42.

17. Rudick RA, Lee JC, Simon J, *et al*. Significance of T2 lesions in multiple sclerosis: A 13-year longitudinal study. *Ann Neurol* 2006;60(2):236–42.

18. Bakshi R, Ariyaratana S, Benedict RH, *et al*. Fluid-attenuated inversion recovery magnetic resonance imaging detects cortical and juxtacortical multiple sclerosis lesions. *Arch Neurol* 2001 May; 58(5):742–8.

19. Filippi M, Rocca MA, Gasperini C, *et al*. Interscanner variation in brain MR lesion load measurements in multiple sclerosis using conventional spin-echo, rapid relaxation-enhanced, and fast-FLAIR sequences. *Am J Neuroradiol* 1999;20(1):133–7.

20. Sanfilipo MP, Benedict RH, Sharma J, *et al*. The relationship between whole brain volume and disability in multiple sclerosis: a comparison of normalized gray vs. white matter with misclassification correction. *Neuroimage* 2005;26(4):1068–77.

21. van Walderveen MA, Kamphorst W, Scheltens P, *et al*. Histopathologic

correlate of hypointense lesions on
T1-weighted spin-echo MRI in multiple
sclerosis. *Neurology* 1998;50(5):1282–8.

22. Rudick RA, Fisher E, Lee JC, *et al.* Use
of the brain parenchymal fraction to
measure whole brain atrophy in
relapsing-remitting MS. Multiple
Sclerosis Collaborative Research
Group. *Neurology* 1999;53(8):1698–704.

23. Paolillo A, Pozzilli C, Gasperini C, *et al.*
Brain atrophy in relapsing-remitting
multiple sclerosis: relationship with
'black holes', disease duration and
clinical disability. *J Neurol Sci* 2000;
174(2):85–91.

24. Simon JH, Lull J, Jacobs LD, *et al.* A
longitudinal study of T1 hypointense
lesions in relapsing MS: MSCRG trial of
interferon beta-1a. Multiple Sclerosis
Collaborative Research Group.
Neurology 2000; 55(2):185–92.

25. Filippi M, Rovaris M, Rocca MA, *et al.*
Glatiramer acetate reduces the
proportion of new MS lesions evolving
into "black holes". *Neurology* 2001;
57(4):731–3.

26. Barkhof F, Hulst HE, Drulovic J, *et al.*
Ibudilast in relapsing-remitting
multiple sclerosis: a neuroprotectant?
Neurology 2010;74(13):1033–40.

27. Kappos L, Moeri D, Radue EW, *et al.*
Predictive value of gadolinium-
enhanced magnetic resonance imaging
for relapse rate and changes in disability
or impairment in multiple sclerosis: a
meta-analysis. Gadolinium MRI
Meta-analysis Group. *Lancet* 1999;
353(9157):964–9.

28. Sormani MP, Bruzzi P, Comi G, *et al.*
MRI metrics as surrogate markers for
clinical relapse rate in relapsing-
remitting MS patients. *Neurology*
2002;58(3):417–21.

29. Paolillo A, Coles AJ, Molyneux PD,
et al. Quantitative MRI in patients with
secondary progressive MS treated with
monoclonal antibody Campath 1H.
Neurology 1999;53(4):751–7.

30. Rice GP, Filippi M, Comi G. Cladribine
and progressive MS: clinical and MRI
outcomes of a multicenter controlled
trial. Cladribine MRI Study Group.
Neurology 2000;54(5):1145–55.

31. Miller DH, Barkhof F, Frank JA, *et al.*
Measurement of atrophy in multiple
sclerosis: pathological basis,
methodological aspects and clinical
relevance. *Brain* 2002;125(8):
1676–95.

32. Bermel RA, Bakshi R. The
measurement and clinical relevance of
brain atrophy in multiple sclerosis.
Lancet Neurol 2006;5(2):158–70.

33. Paolillo A, Piattella MC, Pantano P,
et al. The relationship between
inflammation and atrophy in clinically
isolated syndromes suggestive of
multiple sclerosis: a monthly MRI study
after triple-dose gadolinium-DTPA. *J
Neurol* 2004;251(4):432–9.

34. Brex PA, Jenkins R, Fox NC, *et al.*
Detection of ventricular enlargement in
patients at the earliest clinical stage of
MS. *Neurology* 2000;54(8):1689–91.

35. Fisher E, Rudick RA, Cutter G, *et al.*
Relationship between brain atrophy
and disability: an 8-year follow-up
study of multiple sclerosis patients.
Mult Scler 2000;6(6):373–7.

36. Pelletier D, Garrison K, Henry R.
Measurement of whole-brain atrophy
in multiple sclerosis. [Review] [53 refs].
J Neuroimaging 2004;14(3 Suppl):
11S–9S.

37. Simon JH. Linear and regional
measures of brain atrophy in multiple
sclerosis. In Zivadinov R, Bakshi R,
eds. Hauppauge: Nova Science; 2004:
15–27.

38. Bermel RA, Sharma J, Tjoa CW, *et al.* A
semiautomated measure of whole-brain
atrophy in multiple sclerosis. *J Neurol
Sci* 2003;208(1–2):57–65.

39. Smith SM, Zhang Y, Jenkinson M, *et al.*
Accurate, robust, and automated
longitudinal and cross-sectional brain
change analysis. *Neuroimage* 2002;
17(1):479–89.

40. Ge Y, Grossman RI, Udupa JK, *et al.*
Brain atrophy in relapsing-remitting
multiple sclerosis and secondary
progressive multiple sclerosis:
longitudinal quantitative analysis.
Radiology 2000;214(3):665–70.

41. Smith SM, De Stefano N, Jenkinson M,
et al. Normalized accurate
measurement of longitudinal brain
change. *J Comput Assist Tomogr*
2001;25(3):466–75.

42. Fox NC, Jenkins R, Leary SM, *et al.*
Progressive cerebral atrophy in MS: a
serial study using registered, volumetric
MRI. *Neurology* 2000;54(4):807–12.

43. Kappos L, Radue EW, O'Connor P,
et al. A placebo-controlled trial of oral
fingolimod in relapsing multiple
sclerosis. *N Engl J Med* 2010;362(5):
387–401.

44. Anderson VM, Bartlett JW, Fox NC,
et al. Detecting treatment effects on
brain atrophy in relapsing remitting
multiple sclerosis: sample size
estimates. *J Neurol* 2007;254(11):
1588–94.

45. Filippi M, Rovaris M, Inglese M, *et al.*
Interferon beta-1a for brain tissue loss
in patients at presentation with
syndromes suggestive of multiple
sclerosis: a randomised, double-blind,
placebo-controlled trial. *Lancet* 2004;
364(9444):1489–96.

46. Jones CK, Riddehough A, Li DKB, *et al.*
MRI cerebral atrophy in relapsing-
remitting MS: results from the PRISMS
trial [abstract]. *Neurology* 2001;56
(Suppl 3):A379.

47. Zivadinov R, Grop A, Sharma J, *et al.*
Reproducibility and accuracy of
quantitative magnetic resonance
imaging techniques of whole-brain
atrophy measurement in multiple
sclerosis. *J Neuroimaging* 2005;
15(1):27–36.

48. Fox RJ, Fisher E, Tkach J, *et al.* Brain
atrophy and magnetization transfer
ratio following methylprednisolone in
multiple sclerosis: short-term changes
and long-term implications. *Mult Scler*
2005;11(2):140–5.

49. Kapoor R, Furby J, Hayton T, *et al.*
Lamotrigine for neuroprotection in
secondary progressive multiple
sclerosis: a randomised, double-blind,
placebo-controlled, parallel-group
trial. *Lancet Neurol* 2010;9(7):
681–8.

50. van Waesberghe JH, Kamphorst W, De
Groot CJ, *et al.* Axonal loss in multiple
sclerosis lesions: magnetic resonance
imaging insights into substrates of
disability. *Ann Neurol* 1999;46(5):
747–54.

51. Phillips MD, Grossman RI, Miki Y,
et al. Comparison of T2 lesion volume
and magnetization transfer ratio
histogram analysis and of atrophy and
measures of lesion burden in patients
with multiple sclerosis. *Am J
Neuroradiol* 1998;19(6):1055–60.

52. Cercignani M, Iannucci G, Rocca MA,
et al. Pathologic damage in MS assessed
by diffusion-weighted and
magnetization transfer MRI. *Neurology*
2000;54(5):1139–44.

53. Filippi M, Iannucci G, Tortorella C,
et al. Comparison of MS clinical
phenotypes using conventional and

magnetization transfer MRI. *Neurology* 1999;52(3):588–94.

54. Kalkers NF, Hintzen RQ, van Waesberghe JH, *et al.* Magnetization transfer histogram parameters reflect all dimensions of MS pathology, including atrophy. *J Neurol Sci* 2001; 184(2):155–62.

55. Inglese M, van Waesberghe JH, Rovaris M, *et al.* The effect of interferon beta-1b on quantities derived from MT MRI in secondary progressive MS. *Neurology* 2003;60(5):853–60.

56. Chen JT, Schneider C, Nakamura K, *et al.* Validation of MRI-based measurements of subpial cortical demyelination in an MS brain. *Mult Scler* 2010;16(S10):S107.

57. van Waesberghe JH, van Walderveen MA, Castelijns JA, *et al.* Patterns of lesion development in multiple sclerosis: longitudinal observations with T1-weighted spin-echo and magnetization transfer MR. *AJNR Am J Neuroradiol* 1998;19(4): 675–83.

58. Richert ND, Ostuni JL, Bash CN, *et al.* Interferon beta-1b and intravenous methylprednisolone promote lesion recovery in multiple sclerosis. *Mult Scler* 2001;7(1):49–58.

59. Kita M, Goodkin DE, Bacchetti P, *et al.* Magnetization transfer ratio in new MS lesions before and during therapy with IFNbeta-1a. *Neurology* 2000;54(9): 1741–5.

60. Horsfield MA, Barker GJ, Barkhof F, *et al.* Guidelines for using quantitative magnetization transfer magnetic resonance imaging for monitoring treatment of multiple sclerosis. *J Magn Reson Imaging* 2003;17(4):389–97.

61. Fox RJ, Sakaie K, Lee JC, *et al.* A validation study of multi-centre diffusion tensor imaging. *Mult Scler* 2007;13(S7):S76.

62. Rocca MA, Cercignani M, Iannucci G, *et al.* Weekly diffusion-weighted imaging of normal-appearing white matter in MS. *Neurology* 2000;55(6): 882–4.

63. Werring DJ, Brassat D, Droogan AG, *et al.* The pathogenesis of lesions and normal-appearing white matter changes in multiple sclerosis: a serial diffusion MRI study. *Brain* 2000;123: 1667–76.

64. Fox RJ. Picturing multiple sclerosis: conventional and diffusion tensor

imaging. *Semin Neurol* 2008;28(4): 453–66.

65. Harrison DM, Caffo BS, Shiee N, *et al.* Longitudinal changes in diffusion tensor–based quantitative MRI in multiple sclerosis. *Neurology* 2011; 76(2):179–86.

66. Bjartmar C, Battistuta J, Terada N, *et al.* N-acetylaspartate is an axon-specific marker of mature white matter in vivo: a biochemical and immunohistochemical study on the rat optic nerve. *Ann Neurol* 2002;51(1): 51–8.

67. Matthews PM, Pioro E, Narayanan S, *et al.* Assessment of lesion pathology in multiple sclerosis using quantitative MRI morphometry and magnetic resonance spectroscopy. *Brain* 1996;119 (3):715–22.

68. Fu L, Matthews PM, De Stefano N, *et al.* Imaging axonal damage of normal-appearing white matter in multiple sclerosis. *Brain* 1998;121 (1): 103–13.

69. Sarchielli P, Presciutti O, Tarducci R, *et al.* ¹H-MRS in patients with multiple sclerosis undergoing treatment with interferon beta-1a: results of a preliminary study. *J Neurol Neurosurg Psychiatry* 1998;64(2):204–12.

70. Parry A, Corkill R, Blamire AM, *et al.* Beta-Interferon treatment does not always slow the progression of axonal injury in multiple sclerosis. *J Neurol* 2003;250(2):171–8.

71. Khan O, Shen Y, Caon C, *et al.* Axonal metabolic recovery and potential neuroprotective effect of glatiramer acetate in relapsing-remitting multiple sclerosis. *Mult Scler* 2005;11(6): 646–51.

72. Inglese M, Ge Y, Filippi M, *et al.* Indirect evidence for early widespread gray matter involvement in relapsing-remitting multiple sclerosis. *Neuroimage* 2004;21(4):1825–9.

73. Rovaris M, Gambini A, Gallo A, *et al.* Axonal injury in early multiple sclerosis is irreversible and independent of the short-term disease evolution. *Neurology* 2005;65(10):1626–30.

74. De Stefano N, Filippi M, Miller D, *et al.* Guidelines for using proton MR spectroscopy in multicenter clinical MS studies. *Neurology* 2007;69(20): 1942–52.

75. Sailer M, Fischl B, Salat D, *et al.* Focal thinning of the cerebral cortex in

multiple sclerosis. *Brain* 2003;126(8):1734–44.

76. Fisher E, Lee JC, Nakamura K, *et al.* Gray matter atrophy in multiple sclerosis: a longitudinal study. *Ann Neurol* 2008;64(3):255–65.

77. Dalton CM, Chard DT, Davies GR, *et al.* Early development of multiple sclerosis is associated with progressive grey matter atrophy in patients presenting with clinically isolated syndromes. *Brain* 2004;127(5):1101–7.

78. Chen JT, Collins DL, Atkins HL, *et al.* Brain atrophy after immunoablation and stem cell transplantation in multiple sclerosis. *Neurology* 2006; 66(12):1935–7.

79. Benedict RH, Ramasamy D, Munschauer F, *et al.* Memory impairment in multiple sclerosis: correlation with deep grey matter and mesial temporal atrophy. *J Neurol Neurosurg Psychiatry* 2009;80(2):201–6.

80. Sanfilipo MP, Benedict RH, Weinstock-Guttman B, *et al.* Gray and white matter brain atrophy and neuropsychological impairment in multiple sclerosis. *Neurology* 2006; 66(5):685–92.

81. Stevenson VL, Leary SM, Losseff NA, *et al.* Spinal cord atrophy and disability in MS: a longitudinal study. *Neurology* 1998;51(1):234–8.

82. Horsfield MA, Sala S, Neema M, *et al.* Rapid semi-automatic segmentation of the spinal cord from magnetic resonance images: application in multiple sclerosis. *Neuroimage* 2010; 50(2):446–55.

83. Filippi M, Rocca MA, Colombo B, *et al.* Functional magnetic resonance imaging correlates of fatigue in multiple sclerosis. *Neuroimage* 2002;15(3): 559–67.

84. Polman CH, Reingold SC, Banwell B, *et al.* Diagnostic criteria for multiple sclerosis: 2010 revisions to the McDonald Criteria. *Ann Neurol* 2011;69(2):292–302.

85. Martinez-Yelamos S, Martinez-Yelamos A, Martin Ozaeta G, *et al.* Regression to the mean in multiple sclerosis. *Mult Scler* 2006;12(6):826–9.

86. Panitch HS, Hirsch RL, Schindler J, *et al.* Treatment of multiple sclerosis with gamma interferon: exacerbations associated with activation of the immune system. *Neurology* 1987; 37(7):1097–102.

87. TNF neutralization in MS: results of a randomized, placebo-controlled multicenter study. The Lenercept Multiple Sclerosis Study Group and The University of British Columbia MS/MRI Analysis Group. *Neurology* 1999;53(3):457–65.

88. Bielekova B, Goodwin B, Richert N, *et al.* Encephalitogenic potential of the myelin basic protein peptide (amino acids 83–99) in multiple sclerosis: results of a phase II clinical trial with an altered peptide ligand. *Nat Med* 2000;6(10):1167–75.

89. Ransohoff RM. Natalizumab and PML. *Nat Neurosci* 2005;8(10):1275.

90. Illes J, Kirschen MP, Edwards E, *et al.* Practical approaches to incidental findings in brain imaging research. *Neurology* 2008;70(5):384–90.

91. Morris Z, Whiteley WN, Longstreth WT, *et al.* Incidental findings on brain magnetic resonance imaging: systematic review and meta-analysis. *BMJ*; 339.

92. Kappos L, Antel J, Comi G, *et al.* Oral fingolimod (FTY720) for relapsing multiple sclerosis. *N Engl J Med* 2006;355(11):1124–40.

93. Hauser SL, Waubant E, Arnold DL, *et al.* B-cell depletion with rituximab in relapsing-remitting multiple sclerosis. *N Engl J Med* 2008;358(7):676–88.

94. O'Connor P, Miller D, Riester K, *et al.* Relapse rates and enhancing lesions in a phase II trial of natalizumab in multiple sclerosis. *Mult Scler* 2005;11(5): 568–72.

95. Polman CH, O'Connor PW, Havrdova E, *et al.* A randomized, placebo-controlled trial of natalizumab for relapsing multiple sclerosis. *N Engl J Med* 2006;354(9):899–910.

96. Rudick RA, Stuart WH, Calabresi PA, *et al.* Natalizumab plus interferon beta-1a for relapsing multiple sclerosis. *N Engl J Med* 2006;354(9):911–23.

97. Healy BC, Ikle D, Macklin EA, *et al.* Optimal design and analysis of phase I/II clinical trials in multiple sclerosis with gadolinium-enhanced lesions as the endpoint. *Mult Scler* 2010;16(7): 840–7.

98. Sormani MP, Miller DH, Comi G, *et al.* Clinical trials of multiple sclerosis monitored with enhanced MRI: new sample size calculations based on large data sets. *J Neurol Neurosurg Psychiatry* 2001;70(4):494–9.

99. Filippi M, Yousry T, Campi A, *et al.* Comparison of triple dose versus standard dose gadolinium-DTPA for detection of MRI enhancing lesions in patients with MS. *Neurology* 1996; 46(2):379–84.

100. Gasperini C, Pozzilli C, Bastianello S, *et al.* The influence of clinical relapses and steroid therapy on the development of Gd-enhancing lesions: a longitudinal MRI study in relapsing-remitting multiple sclerosis patients. *Acta Neurol Scand* 1997;95(4):201–7.

101. Goodin DS. Magnetic resonance imaging as a surrogate outcome measure of disability in multiple sclerosis: have we been overly harsh in our assessment? *Ann Neurol* 2006; 59(4):597–605.

102. Cohen JA, Barkhof F, Comi G, *et al.* Oral fingolimod or intramuscular interferon for relapsing multiple sclerosis. *N Engl J Med* 2010;362(5): 402–15.

103. Molyneux PD, Miller DH, Filippi M, *et al.* The use of magnetic resonance imaging in multiple sclerosis treatment trials: power calculations for annual lesion load measurement. *J Neurol* 2000;247(1):34–40.

104. Matts JP, Lachin JM. Properties of permuted-block randomization in clinical trials. *Control Clin Trials* 1988;9(4):327–44.

105. Begg CB, Iglewicz B. A treatment allocation procedure for sequential clinical trials. *Biometrics* 1980;36(1):81–90.

106. Cohen JA, Imrey PB, Calabresi PA, *et al.* Results of the Avonex Combination Trial (ACT) in relapsing–remitting MS. *Neurology* 2009;72(6):535–41.

107. Comi G, Cohen JA, Arnold DL, *et al.* Phase III dose-comparison study of glatiramer acetate for multiple sclerosis. *Ann Neurol* 2011;69(1):75–82.

108. Morgan CJ, Aban IB, Katholi CR, *et al.* Modeling lesion counts in multiple sclerosis when patients have been selected for baseline activity. *Mult Scler* 2010;16(8):926–34.

109. Van Den Elskamp I, Knol D, Uitdehaag B, *et al.* The distribution of new enhancing lesion counts in multiple sclerosis: further explorations. *Mult Scler* 2009;15(1):42–9.

110. Aban IB, Cutter GR, Mavinga N. Inferences and power analysis concerning two negative binomial

distributions with an application to MRI lesion counts data. *Comput Stat Data Anal* 2009;53(3):820–33.

111. Radue EW, Stuart WH, Calabresi PA, *et al.* Natalizumab plus interferon beta-1a reduces lesion formation in relapsing multiple sclerosis. *J Neurol Sci* 2010;292(1–2):28–35.

112. Koch GG, Tangen CM, Jung JW, *et al.* Issues for covariance analysis of dichotomous and ordered categorical data from randomized clinical trials and non-parametric strategies for addressing them. *Stat Med* 1998; 17(15–16):1863–92.

113. Li DK, Held U, Petkau J, *et al.* MRI T2 lesion burden in multiple sclerosis: a plateauing relationship with clinical disability. *Neurology* 2006;66(9):1384–9.

114. Lange KL, Little RJA, Taylor JMG. Robust Statistical Modeling Using the Distribution. *J Am Stat Assoc* 1989; 84(408):pp. 881–96.

115. Lin TI, Lee JC. A robust approach to linear mixed models applied to multiple sclerosis data. *Stat Med* 2006;25(8): 1397–412.

116. Gill PS. A robust mixed linear model analysis for longitudinal data. *Stat Med* 2000;19(7):975–87.

117. D'yachkova Y, Petkau J, White R. Longitudinal analyses for magnetic resonance imaging outcomes in multiple sclerosis clinical trials. *J Biopharm Stat* 1997;7(4):501–31.

118. Altman RM, Petkau AJ. Application of hidden Markov models to multiple sclerosis lesion count data. *Stat Med* 2005;24(15):2335–44.

119. Chataway J, Nicholas R, Todd S, *et al.* A novel adaptive design strategy increases the efficiency of clinical trials in secondary progressive multiple sclerosis. *Mult Scler* 2011; 17(1): 81–8.

120. Friede T, Schmidli H. Blinded sample size reestimation with negative binomial counts in superiority and non-inferiority trials. *Methods Inf Med* 2010;49(6):618–24.

121. Gasperini C, Rovaris M, Sormani MP, *et al.* Intra-observer, inter-observer and inter-scanner variations in brain MRI volume measurements in multiple sclerosis. *Mult Scler* 2001;7(1): 27–31.

122. Han X, Jovicich J, Salat D, *et al.* Reliability of MRI-derived

measurements of human cerebral cortical thickness: the effects of field strength, scanner upgrade and manufacturer. *Neuroimage* 2006; 32(1):180–94.

123. Molyneux PD, Wang L, Lai M, *et al.* Quantitative techniques for lesion load measurement in multiple sclerosis: an assessment of the global threshold technique after non uniformity and histogram matching corrections. *Eur J Neurol* 1998;5(1):55–60.

124. Raff U, Rojas GM, Hutchinson M, *et al.* Quantitation of T2 lesion load in patients with multiple sclerosis: a novel semiautomated segmentation

technique. *Acad Radiol* 2000;7(4): 237–47.

125. Alfano B, Brunetti A, Larobina M, *et al.* Automated segmentation and measurement of global white matter lesion volume in patients with multiple sclerosis. *J Magn Reson Imaging* 2000;12(6):799–807.

126. Anbeek P, Vincken KL, van Osch MJ, *et al.* Automatic segmentation of different-sized white matter lesions by voxel probability estimation. *Med Image Anal* 2004;8(3):205–15.

127. Wu Y, Warfield SK, Tan IL, *et al.* Automated segmentation of multiple

sclerosis lesion subtypes with multichannel MRI. *Neuroimage* 2006;32(3):1205–15.

128. Achiron A, Gicquel S, Miron S, *et al.* Brain MRI lesion load quantification in multiple sclerosis: a comparison between automated multispectral and semi-automated thresholding computer-assisted techniques. *Magn Reson Imaging* 2002;20(10):713–20.

129. Nakamura K, Fisher E. Segmentation of brain magnetic resonance images for measurement of gray matter atrophy in multiple sclerosis patients. *Neuroimage* 2009;44(3):769–76.

Chapter

17

Optical coherence tomography to monitor axonal and neuronal integrity in multiple sclerosis

Kristin M. Galetta and Laura J. Balcer

Introduction

Axonal and neuronal degeneration are important features of multiple sclerosis (MS) that may lead to permanent neurological and visual impairment.[1-5] Optical coherence tomography (OCT) (Figs. 17.1 and 17.2) is a non-invasive imaging technique that allows for precise anatomic measurement of the retinal nerve fiber layer (RNFL), a structure that contains ganglion cell axons that form the optic nerves, chiasm, and optic tracts.[5-32] Within the retina, these axons are non-myelinated, so the RNFL is an ideal structure to monitor neurodegeneration and the effects of neuroprotective agents. In contrast to the peripapillary RNFL, which contains axons, the macula contains a large proportion of retinal ganglion cell neurons (about 34% of total macular volume) (Fig. 17.3).[21] About 1200 μm in diameter, the macula is easily identified within the retina. The application of newer MRI techniques such as magnetization transfer imaging, magnetic resonance spectroscopy, and diffusion tensor imaging (Chapters 10, 12, and 15) has led to only modest achievements in linking imaging data with clinical measures of disease severity. Therefore, recent MS clinical trials and observational studies have incorporated OCT as an exploratory outcome measure in order to achieve a greater understanding of the relationship between changes in retinal structure and patient reported outcomes of visual function.[33-36]

This chapter describes the applications and advances in development of OCT as a novel technology that enables the use of the retina as an eloquent model of neurodegeneration in MS and optic neuritis (ON). OCT allows rapid, reproducible, non-invasive assessment of the structural composition of the retina. Ultimately, OCT could substantially increase our understanding of the mechanisms of tissue injury in MS, and could be used to identify new therapeutic strategies focused on neuroprotection of central axonal and neuronal structures. RNFL and macular thickness measurements could also be useful for detecting and monitoring neurorestoration, a treatment goal not yet within the capability of the neurologist.[23-28]

Features and advantages of OCT imaging

Huang et al.[37] first reported use of OCT in 1991. In vivo retinal imaging was first demonstrated in 1993,[38,39] and early studies in 1995 provided the first demonstration of OCT imaging of the normal retina[40] and of macular pathology.[41] OCT is analogous to ultrasound imaging but uses light instead of sound waves. Unlike ultrasound, ocular interferometry does not require contact with the tissue examined.[5,24-28] The OCT interferometer resolves retinal structures by measuring the echo delay times of light reflected and backscattered from different microstructural features in the retina (Fig. 17.1A). From multiple axial scans (A-scans) at different retinal locations, two-dimensional, cross-sectional images are obtained (Fig. 17.1B). OCT provides real-time cross-sectional images and quantitative analyses of RNFL thickness, macular thickness/volume and optic disc topography. With OCT, high-resolution cross-sectional or three-dimensional images of the internal retinal structure are generated by an optical beam being scanned across the retina and the magnitude and echo time delay of backscattered light being measured.[5,24-28]

Early OCT systems were based on low coherence interferometry. In this technique, measurements are performed using a Michelson type interferometer with a low-coherence-length, superluminescent diode light source. One arm of the interferometer directs light on to the sample and collects the backscattered signal. A second reference arm has a reflecting mirror, which is mechanically scanned to vary the time delay and measure interference. The use of a low-coherence-length light source means that interference occurs only when the distance traveled by the light in the sample and reference arms of the interferometer matches to within the coherence length. This enables measurement of the echo delays of the light from the tissue with extremely high temporal accuracy. The resulting data set is a two-dimensional or three-dimensional array, which represents the optical backscattering in a cross-section or volume of the tissue. These data can be processed and displayed as a two-dimensional or volumetric gray-scale or false-color image.[5]

Multiple Sclerosis Therapeutics, Fourth Edition, ed. Jeffrey A. Cohen and Richard A. Rudick. Published by Cambridge University Press.
© Cambridge University Press 2011.

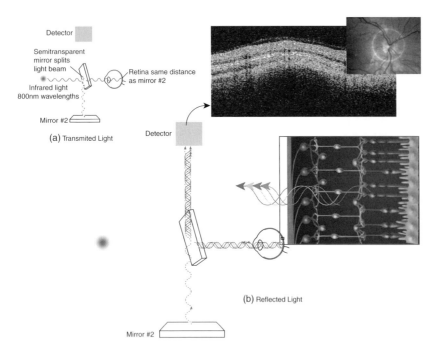

Fig. 17.1. Images of the internal retinal structure taken with optical coherence tomography (OCT), demonstrating the processes involved in using this technology. (a) Low-coherence infrared light is transmitted into the eye through use of an interoferometer. (b) The infrared light is transmitted through the pupil and then penetrates through the transparent nine layers of the retina. Subsequently, the light backscatters and returns through the pupil, where detectors can analyze the interference of light returning from the layers of the retina compared with light traveling a reference path (mirror #2). An algorithm mathematically uses this information to construct a gray-scale or false-color image representing the anatomy of the retina (shown in the upper right portion of the figure). (From Frohman EM *et al. Nat Clin Pract Neurol* 2008,[5] with permission.) (see also color plate section).

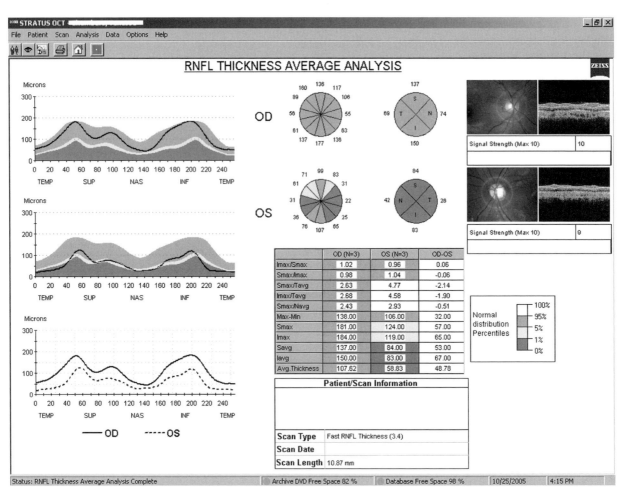

Fig. 17.2. A typical optical coherence tomography (OCT) report from a patient with MS, generated by Zeiss Stratus OCT3TM with software 4.0 (Carl Zeiss Meditec, Inc). On the upper left, retinal nerve fiber layer (RNFL) thickness is plotted (Y axis) with respect to a circumferential retinal map on the X axis (temporal-superior-nasal-inferior-temporal (TSNIT) quadrants of the RNFL). Note the normal 'double-hump' appearance of the topographic map of the right eye (OD), signifying the thicker RNFL measures derived from the superior and inferior retina compared with the nasal and temporal regions. Also note the quadrant and clockface sector measures of RNFL thickness (upper middle illustration). The table (lower middle) compiles the quantitative data, including the average RNFL thickness (bottom row). This patient experienced an episode of left optic neuritis 6 months before this study. Note the marked reduction in RNFL thickness across all quadrants (red region denoting values below 1% of what would be expected when compared with a reference population), multiple sectors, and with respect to the average RNFL thickness (bottom row of table). Abbreviations: OD, right eye; OS, left eye. (From Frohman EM *et al. Nat Clin Pract Neurol* 2008,[5] with permission.) (see also color plate section).

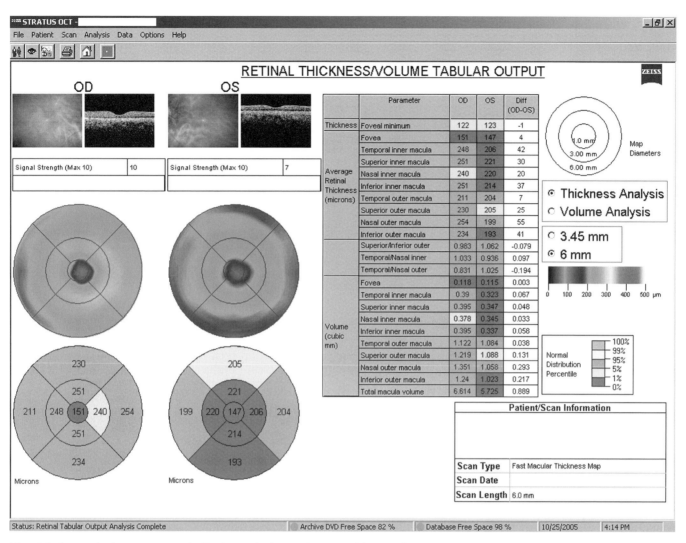

Fig. 17.3. An optical coherence tomography (OCT) report for the macular region of the retina from the same MS patient shown in Fig. 17.2. Note the volume reductions in the foveola (central macula) and the parafoveal quadrants on the left of the report. Whereas the reductions in retinal nerve fiber layer thickness implicate loss of ganglion cell axons, macular changes implicate losses of the ganglion cell neurons themselves. While the patient has had no history of optic neuritis in the right eye, there are some subtle macular changes on that side, suggesting occult involvement of this eye as well. Abbreviations: OD, right eye; OS, left eye. (From Frohman EM *et al. Nat Clin Pract Neurol* 2008,[5] with permission.) (see also color plate section).

More recently, the development of "Fourier domain" (or spectral domain) detection has revolutionized OCT technology (Figs. 17.4 and 17.5).[42] Spectral domain OCT detects light echoes by measuring the interference spectrum from an interferometer with a stationary reference arm. A spectrometer and high-speed line-scan camera record the interference spectrum, which is Fourier transformed to obtain the magnitude and echo time delay of the light (the axial scan). By comparison to time domain OCT, which measures light echoes sequentially, spectral domain OCT detects all light echoes simultaneously, leading to increased speed and sensitivity while imaging.[43,44] Retinal imaging with spectral domain OCT became possible only with recent advances in camera technology. The first retinal images with this technique were reported in 2002,[45] and high-speed, high-resolution retinal imaging was demonstrated in 2003.[46,47] The technology became commercially available in 2006; most commercial instruments achieve axial image resolution of 5–7 μm with imaging speeds of 25 000 axial scans per second, approximately 50 times faster than the previous generation of time domain OCT technologies.[5,24–28,39–48]

Various features and advantages of OCT are listed in Table 17.1. Retinal imaging technologies such as OCT can rapidly evaluate the integrity of the RNFL and the macula for the purpose of tracking disease progression, and may be advantagous for monitoring the effects of neuroprotection therapy. Decreasing RNFL thickness (assessed by average, quadrant, and clock-face sector analyses) has been associated with declines in visual function, as measured by low-contrast letter acuity and visual field testing.[5–9,11,14,24–28,31]

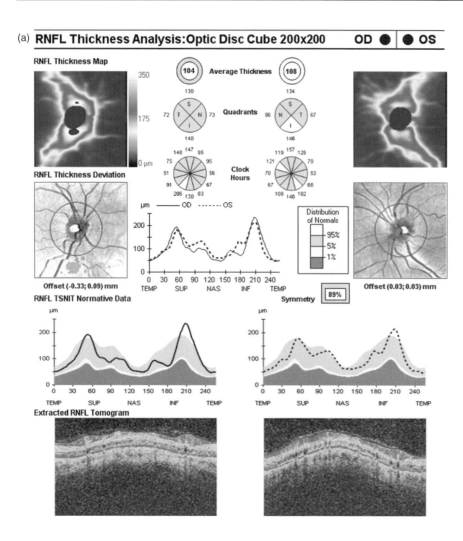

Fig. 17.4. (a) Example of a high-resolution, Fourier domain optical coherence tomography (OCT) report from a patient with neuromyelitis (NMO), generated by Zeiss Stratus Cirrus high-resolution Fourier domain OCT (Carl Zeiss Meditec, Inc.). The patient had bilateral mild disc hyperemia and edema in the setting of subacute visual loss. (See also color plate section). (b) MRI of the orbits with fat-saturation and gadolinium showed bilateral optic nerve enhancement and an enhancing lesion in the midbrain. (see also color plate section).

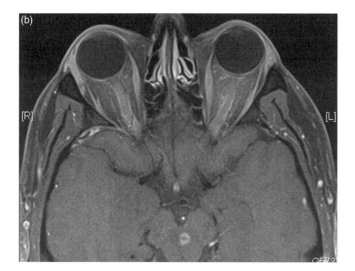

Multiple sclerosis and optic neuritis as specific models for visual pathway axonal loss

Bedside visualization of optic atrophy became possible following the introduction of the hand-held ophthalmoscope by Helmholtz in 1851.[49] Using a hand-held ophthalmoscope more than a century later in 1974, Frisén and Hoyt reported their subjective analysis of thinning of the RNFL, in patients with MS.[50] A post-mortem study demonstrated atrophy of the RNFL (typically containing about 80% axons and 20% glia) in 35 out of 49 eyes of patients with MS. While this study supported Frisén and Hoyt's findings,[51] it was not sufficiently quantitative to enable a full appreciation of the relationship between vision, RNFL thickness, and integrity of the approximately 1.2 million axons that make up the optic nerve.

In recent years, we have observed the emergence of "quantitative ophthalmoscopes" such as Heidelberg Retinal Tomography (HRT), laser polarimetry with variable corneal compensation (GDx-VCC), and OCT, all of which can be used to efficiently and objectively measure changes in structural architecture within the retina.[5,29,52] Measures derived from these modalities have been shown to directly and reliably relate

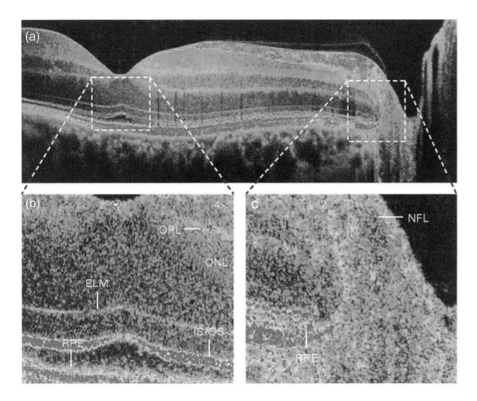

Fig. 17.5. High-definition, ultra-high-resolution optical coherence tomography (OCT) scans. The high data acquisition speeds available with spectral domain detection enable the acquisition of high-definition images with large numbers of transverse pixels. (a) A 10 000 axial scans per second image of the papillomacular axis acquired in 0.6 s. The axial image resolution is approximately 3 μm. The image may be zoomed in the (b) foveal or (c) optic disc regions to visualize details of internal retinal morphology. OCT has been termed "optical biopsy," and ultra-high-resolution OCT imaging can provide excellent visualization of retinal architecture. Abbreviations: ELM, external limiting membrane; IS/OS, junction between inner and outer photoreceptor segments; NFL, nerve fiber layer; ONL, outer nuclear layer; OPL, outer plexiform layer; RPE, retinal pigment epithelium. (Figure adapted from Drexler W and Fujimoto JG. *Prog Retin Eye Res* 2008;27:45–88,[42] published by Elsevier Ltd.) (see also color plate section).

to visual function and seem to parallel the pathological changes that occur in the brains of patients with MS.

Recent studies have demonstrated that MS and ON provide useful clinical models with which to couple clinical measures of visual function with validated and objective structural and physiological correlates of MS.[5,24–28,36] The anterior visual pathway is a frequent target of the MS disease process. During the course of disease, between 30% and 70% of patients with MS will experience ON.[53,54] However, almost all patients with MS will be found to have characteristic changes in the retina and optic nerve on post-mortem analysis, even if they never experienced acute ON.[2,24–28,55,56] These data suggest that the visual system has a very high predilection for developing disease-related disability and could be used effectively to measure and monitor the pathology of the disease process.

In contrast with occult optic neuropathy in MS, which is a largely subclinical manifestation of disease in the anterior visual system, most cases of acute ON are associated with pain and visual disturbances, including diminished vision, color desaturation, poor low-contrast acuity, and field abnormalities.[53] ON can, therefore, be evaluated with clinical and neurophysiological techniques, such as patient-reported acuity (high and low contrast) and sensitivity, visual field analysis, and visual evoked responses.[53,54] Furthermore, coronal, fat-suppressed, T1-weighted gadolinium-enhanced MRI will reveal enhancement in the optic nerve in over 90% of ON cases, confirming a breach in the integrity of endothelial tight junctions at the blood–brain barrier.[57] Studies with conventional MRI have shown that the optic nerve area declines subsequent to

an event of ON, when compared with the companion eye.[58] Retinal imaging techniques have added greatly to our knowledge of this area, revealing changes in retinal architecture that reflect alterations in visual system physiology and function.[5,24–28]

Visual function has been shown to be directly related to the integrity of retinal anatomy. In particular, abnormalities in the retina following ON produce corresponding clinical deficits in patient performance on vision tests.[29] However, since visual function is a measure of both anterior and posterior visual pathways, novel imaging approaches that are specific to the retina and optic nerve may enable more specific quantification of axon injury related to ON.[59]

Role for OCT in modeling axonal and neuronal loss in MS

The earliest application of OCT technology to the study of MS was reported by Parisi *et al.* in 1999.[6] In this study, which utilized first-generation OCT technology, 14 patients with MS who had completely recovered from a previous event of acute ON were analyzed. The thickness of the RNFL was shown to be reduced by 46% in the ON eyes vs. healthy control eyes ($P < 0.01$), and by 28% when ON eyes were compared with the "unaffected" eyes of the same patient ($P < 0.01$). Even in the supposedly unaffected eyes of the patients, however, there was a 26% reduction in RNFL thickness when compared with healthy control eyes ($P < 0.01$).

Table 17.1. *Features and advantages of optical coherence tomography (OCT) imaging*

Physical properties
1. Optical analog of ultrasound
2. Generates cross-sectional images measuring back-reflected echoes of light
3. Interferometric methods used to detect echoes since times are too fast for direct detection
4. Current technology has 8–10 μm resolution; new technology has 5–7 μm resolution

Imaging metrics (current technology)
1. Average retinal nerve fiber layer (RNFL) thickness
2. Quadrant and clockface sector analyses
3. Total macular volumes
4. Quadrant assessment of parafoveal areas
5. Inferior and superior RNFL are thickest (double hump waveform on temporal-superior-nasal-inferior-temporal [TSNIT] analyses)

Imaging metrics (new technology)
1. RNFL mapping
2. Mapping intraretinal layers in the macula
3. 3D-OCT of optic nerve head topography and internal structure
4. Technology is new and metrics remain to be defined

Biomarker features and validation
1. Correlates with high-contrast and low-contrast visual acuity
2. Pathological distribution predicts visual field changes
3. OCT metrics predict brain atrophy
4. Subtypes of multiple sclerosis predict severity of RNFL thinning
5. Measures of laser polarimetry with variable corneal compensation (GDx-VCC) corroborate OCT evidence of axonal degeneration

Application features
1. Testing performance is quick and easy
2. Pupil dilation is typically not required
3. Low coefficient of variation for repeated measures
4. Low interindividual and intra-individual variation
5. Low variability across different centers using the same device
6. Scan quality can be assured with disc centering and adequate signal strength

Adapted from Frohman EM, *et al. Nat Clin Pract Neurol* 2008,[5] with permission.

In 2005, Trip and colleagues[7] reported their observations with OCT in 11 patients with MS and 14 patients with clinically isolated syndrome (CIS), all of which individuals had a history of a single episode of ON. The study was a cross-sectional analysis with duration after the ON event ranging from 1 to 9 years. Corroborating the previous findings by Parisi *et al.*, the investigators found a 33% reduction in RNFL thickness in the eyes of the patients when compared with the eyes of matched controls, and a 27% reduction when the affected and unaffected eyes of the same MS patient were compared ($P < 0.001$). Trip *et al.*[7] extended the utility of OCT by also showing that the macular volume was reduced by 11% in the eyes of patients with a history of ON when compared with control eyes ($P < 0.001$), and by 9% in the affected vs. the unaffected eye of the same MS patient ($P < 0.001$).

An important finding of these studies was that the apparently unaffected eyes of patients with MS were in fact significantly abnormal when compared with the eyes of matched healthy control individuals, but were less abnormal than the eye with a history of ON. In a recent meta-analysis of published data for OCT in MS and ON, 27 studies compared eyes with a history of ON with unaffected fellow eyes in patients with MS. Differences in RNFL thickness from control eyes were substantial, showing that ON eyes were 14.57 μm thinner (95% CI-16.5–12.63), on average, compared with controls. MS eyes without a history of acute ON were also reduced with regard to RNFL thickness compared with controls.[60] These findings illustrate that ON, by comparison with less perceptible changes like that of glaucoma, results in rapid and more acute changes histopathologically.

As a validation of the axonal basis of OCT metrics in the RNFL, Trip and colleagues[7] showed that such measures correlated better with visual evoked potential P100 amplitudes (a measure of axonal integrity or function) than with P100 latency (typically a reflection of myelin integrity). It is now generally accepted that disruption of myelin has a direct impact on the function and preservation of axons[61] (Chapter 2). During the pathological process, however, these two structural elements can become temporarily uncoupled. The axon might be intact – albeit vulnerable – for a short period during inflammation and myelin disruption. A demyelinated but intact axon has a number of potential destinies. The axon may remyelinate if viable adult oligodendrocytes in the vicinity can provide new concentric lamellar internodes, or recovery can also be provided by oligodendrocyte progenitors terminally differentiating into adult process-bearing myelinating cells. Even partial remyelination might be protective.

The impact of acute ON on RNFL thickness was investigated by Costello and colleagues in 2006.[8] They reported that the majority of patients with MS who had ON (about 75%) sustained 10–40 μm of RNFL loss within a period of only about 3–6 months following ON. This finding is striking given that the RNFL is only about 110–120 μm thick by the age of 15 years, and that most individuals without a history of glaucoma or macular degeneration lose only about 0.017% per year in retinal thickness, which equates to approximately 10–20 μm over 60 years.[62] Costello *et al.*[8] also provided compelling evidence identifying an injury threshold; thinning of the RNFL below about 75 μm led to a corresponding decay in visual function, as measured by automated perimetry.

The development of validated measures of visual functioning has greatly facilitated the exploration for a structural marker for neurodegeneration in MS. Balcer, Baier and colleagues[63,64] utilized performance on low-contrast letter acuity charts to compare retinal structure with visual function in patients with MS, who have MS pathology in the anterior visual system. As mentioned, MS patients with a history of ON have lower RNFL thickness measures than MS patients with no prior history of ON, or individuals without a history of ON or MS. The fact that severity of visual loss (as confirmed by performance on automated perimetry or low-contrast letter acuity) is a predictor of abnormal retinal architecture is further evidence that OCT can be used as a non-invasive approach to monitor the course of disease in patients with MS and to detect and monitor the efficacy of new therapies targeting mechanisms that might promote neuroprotective effects on retinal axons and ganglion cell neurons.[5]

While axonal and neuronal loss may be anticipated in patients presenting with ON, more recent studies have looked at the relationship between low-contrast acuity and RNFL thickness in heterogeneous MS cohorts without a history of ON.[9] Among 90 patients (180 eyes) and 36 MS-free control individuals (72 eyes), the average RNFL thickness was significantly reduced in the eyes of patients with MS. As expected, eyes from patients with a known history of one or more attacks of ON had significantly lower RNFL thickness (85 SD 17 μm) than did the eyes of patients with MS who did not have a prior ON history (96 SD 14 μm; $P < 0.001$). RNFL thickness was also reduced in the eyes of patients with MS without an ON history compared with normal control eyes (105 μm; $P = 0.03$). With use of normative data included in the OCT 4.0 software for the OCT-3, only 40 (22%) of 180 eyes from patients with MS had "abnormal" average RNFL thickness. In view of the fact that the OCT 4.0 normative database considers the fifth percentile for age to be the cut-off for abnormal values, however, abnormalities in RNFL thickness are likely to be of substantially greater prevalence in the eyes of patients with MS and ON.

Results from this study also suggested that the "unaffected" eyes of patients with a history of ON are at a similar risk for axonal loss as MS eyes in general; both MS groups have more axonal loss than age-matched control individuals.[9] It was also found that low-contrast letter acuity scores were significantly correlated with overall average RNFL thickness in the eyes of patients with MS ($P < 0.001$ by use of generalized estimating equation models accounting for age and adjusting for within-patient, inter-eye correlations); for every one-line change in low-contrast letter acuity score, an average RNFL thickness difference of 4 μm was noted. Average overall RNFL thickness also declined with increasing degrees of overall neurological impairment and disability in the MS cohort, and it was significantly associated with EDSS score and disease duration ($P = 0.03$).

The recent meta-analysis by Petzold et al.[60] reviewed the relation between loss of RNFL and change in the Expanded Disability Status Scale (EDSS). Higher (worse) EDSS scores were associated with thinner RNFL in six studies, with linear correlations ranging from $r = -0.30$ to $r = -0.7$. Two further studies showed similar results with increasing EDSS percentiles relating to RNFL thickness changes. The remaining four studies did not observe a correlation.[60]

It has now been shown that an RNFL thickness stratification can be achieved when MS is segregated into its various subtypes.[5,11,13] In particular, patients with greater brain atrophy, as measured by metrics such as brain parenchymal fraction, have more RNFL loss.[14,65] Thus, the eye would seem to be an appropriate model for mechanisms of neurodegeneration, and could even be used to detect and monitor neuroprotection in MS. Specifically, with OCT we can measure the integrity of both neurons and their axonal projections within the retina. Further, the severity of retinal damage directly correlates with

visual dysfunction clinically, and with both the severity of MS-related brain pathology (i.e. atrophy), and MS clinical subtype designations (as stratified by disease progression status).[5]

While prior studies have emphasized the association between worse visual function and reductions in OCT-measured RNFL thickness[9] and macular volume[21] at a single time point, longitudinal studies have also demonstrated progressive thinning of the RNFL over time, even among eyes with no history of acute ON.[31] Patients at three academic centers underwent OCT-3 (Stratus) measurement of RNFL thickness at 6-month intervals during a mean follow-up of 18 months. Vision was assessed using low-contrast letter acuity (2.5%, 1.25% contrast) and high-contrast visual acuity (VA). Among 593 eyes of 299 MS patients with ≥6 months follow-up, eyes with visual loss showed greater RNFL thinning compared to eyes with stable vision (low-contrast acuity, 2.5%: $P < 0.001$; VA: $P = 0.005$). RNFL thinning increased over time, with average loss of 2.9 μm at 2–3 years and 6.1 μm at 3–4.5 years ($P < 0.001$ vs. 0.5–1-year follow-up interval). These patterns were observed for eyes with or without prior history of ON. Proportions of eyes with RNFL loss greater than test-retest variability (≥6.6 μm) increased from 11% at 0–1 year to 44% at 3–4.5 years ($P < 0.001$). This study thereby provides compelling evidence that progressive RNFL thinning occurs as a function of time in MS, even in the absence of a history of ON, and is associated with clinically significant visual loss. These findings are consistent with sub-clinical axonal loss in the anterior visual pathway in MS, and support the use of OCT and low-contrast acuity as methods to evaluate the effectiveness of putative neuroprotection protocols.[31] Further, the recent meta-analysis performed by Petzold et al., indicates two other studies had similar findings with RNFL thinning correlating with reduced high-contrast visual acuity.[60]

Reproducibility is an important aspect of longitudinal investigations involving OCT technologies, including clinical trials and observational studies. Previous work by Cettomai et al.[16] showed good levels of inter-rater and test–retest reliability for OCT-3 (Stratus) measurements of RNFL thickness in patients with MS and disease-free controls. A more recent study, however, demonstrated that high-resolution Fourier domain OCT techniques afford an even greater degree of reproducibility of RNFL thickness and macular volume assessments.[32] This prospective study of inter-visit, inter-rater, and intra-rater reproducibility was performed using Cirrus high-resolution OCT. Among 58 patients with MS and 32 healthy controls, there was excellent reproducibility of average and quadrantic RNFL thickness values, average macular thickness, and total macular volume; intraclass correlation coefficients (ICCs) ranged from 0.92–0.97 for inter-visit, 0.94–0.99 for inter-rater, and 0.83–0.99 for intra-rater reproducibility.

The authors suggested that, in addition to implementing high-resolution Fourier domain technology, the utilization of specific procedures such as reading algorithms and quality control, can serve to optimize the quality of OCT data.[32] OCT reading centers have been a key ingredient to the recent introduction of these technologies into MS clinical trials. Several phase 2 and 3 MS treatment trials have incorporated OCT-3 measures of RNFL and macular thickness as exploratory outcomes. In a sub-study of a trial of the compound dirucotide for secondary progressive MS, the feasibility of using OCT as well as low-contrast letter acuity and visual acuity was first demonstrated, and emphasized the importance of quality control and data collection methods provided by an established OCT and vision reading center. In the phase 3 trial of fingolimod, all patients underwent OCT-3 imaging of the peripapillary RNFL and macula. Results of this large-scale trial will provide a critical complement to observational longitudinal study data on OCT and visual function in MS. Emerging data from the fingolimod trials will not only further establish the feasibility of OCT and vision testing in MS trials, but will show whether or not OCT measures can detect treatment effects within the time span of a two-year randomized study of patients with active relapsing MS.

While MS is classically considered to be a disorder involving central nervous system white matter, recent pathologic and MRI studies of brain tissue have confirmed that neuronal apoptosis and gray matter degeneration occur in MS. The retina has proven to be no exception to these findings, and results of a recent post-mortem analysis of 82 patients reported retinal atrophy with shrunken neurons.[66] There was dropout of retinal ganglion cells in 79% of eyes, and inner nuclear layer atrophy (amacrine and bipolar cells) in 40% of eyes of patients with MS. The severity of retinal atrophy was significantly associated with post-mortem brain weight, with a trend towards association with disease duration. This report by Green and colleagues[66] provided the first description of inner nuclear layer cell loss in MS, and supports a role for forthcoming OCT studies that incorporate segmentation technologies to determine thicknesses of specific retinal layers and structures. Future investigations of segmentation capability in high-resolution OCT may make it possible to visualize changes on the cellular level. Understanding these changes may also give insight into the pathophysiology of MS.

Electrophysiologic measures of the visual pathway, including visual evoked potentials (VEPs), are generally regarded as complementary to clinical measures of function and structural measures of axonal and neuronal integrity. Naismith et al.[67] systematically evaluated the utility of OCT and VEPs to detect the presence of clinical and subclinical ON, and examined the relation of these measures to visual function. This retrospective, cross-sectional study evaluated 65 subjects ($n = 96$ eyes) with MS ($n = 40$), clinically isolated syndrome (CIS, $n = 1$), neuromyelitis optica (NMO, $n = 20$) and idiopathic demyelination ($n = 4$). Patients had at least one episode of ON ≥ 6 months prior to enrollment. VEPs detected ON in 81% of patients (32% of subclinical ON in unaffected eyes and 75% of all subclinical ON). In contrast, using their criteria, they found that OCT identified 60% of eyes with ON, and less than 20% of subclinically affected eyes. The authors concluded that OCT is "less sensitive than VEPs in ON." On the other hand, to the extent that this study focused on patients and eyes with relatively poor vision, there were likely floor effects with regard to OCT RNFL thickness.

The future of retinal imaging in MS

The hypothesis that measures of the RNFL are causally related to visual performance has been corroborated by recent experiments by our group utilizing another type of quantitative ophthalmoscope, GDx-VCC (Table 17.1).[5] GDx, which is based on the projection of polarized light and its retardation when propagating through a birefringent medium (such as the RNFL), can be used to measure both the thickness and the integrity of the nerve fiber layer.[17] The physical properties of this technology also permit us to examine the retinal substructure in order to assess the integrity of axonal microtubules. While it is common to refer to the intensity of the retardation pictured in the GDx-VCC printout as correlating with nerve fiber layer thickness, it is implicit that this is only in normal retinal tissue, and one of the strengths of GDx is that it would seem to denote the quantitative distribution of the nerve fiber regardless of thickness due to edema.[68]

Notwithstanding these differences, we have confirmed that OCT and GDx metrics yield very similar findings with respect to visual loss in patients with MS who have ON.[17] Like OCT, GDx produces measures that correlate with performance on low-contrast letter acuity and with changes in visual field; however, GDx can additionally detect abnormalities even when they are highly restricted to a particular distribution.

OCT is also, however, undergoing improvements. The new high-resolution OCT devices, such as Cirrus OCT, offer automated disc centering and have longitudinal co-registration to minimize scan-to-scan variability. This device also has correction for eye movement, which will reduce retinal slip and image quality degradation. The high image acquisition speeds afforded by the Fourier domain instruments enable the generation of high-definition OCT images with increased numbers of transverse pixels and improved coverage of the retina, as well as the acquisition of three-dimensional OCT (3D-OCT) data sets. 3D-OCT imaging is especially promising, because projection image data can be summed to provide a virtual fundus image, which enables precise and reproducible registration of individual OCT images to fundus features.[69,70] Together, these features promise to improve the reproducibility of RNFL thickness measurements and other morphometric measurements. Furthermore, 3D-OCT data can be processed to generate virtual circumpapillary scans, which can be registered to retinal features in post processing (Fig. 17.5). Volumetric 3D-OCT data also provide comprehensive information about the optic disc. RNFL-thickness maps (analogous to retardance maps from the GDx), or topographic maps (similar to those from Heidelberg Retinal Tomography), can be generated.[70]

Some important issues remain to be addressed. Different OCT instruments have different measurement protocols as well as different data analysis methods, so careful quantitative

Table 17.2. *Clinical features that distinguish acute demyelinating optic neuritis (ON) from non-arteritic anterior ischemic optic neuropathy (NAION)*

	Acute demyelinating optic neuritis (ON)[a]	Non-arteritic anterior ischemic optic neuropathy (NAION)
Age, Sex	20–50 years; typically women (3:1)	>50 years; men or women
Pain	Present in more than 90%; exacerbated by eye movement; resolves within 1 week	Uncommon (less than 10%); headache occurs in temporal arteritis
Pattern of visual loss	Progression over hours to days, 7 to 10 days maximum; unilateral in adult patients; signs of optic neuropathy (visual acuity, color vision, and visual field defects)	Sudden onset, often noted upon awakening; unilateral in adult patients; signs of optic neuropathy (visual acuity, color vision, and visual field defects)
Optic disk appearance	Optic disk swelling in 1/3 of patients, retrobulbar in remainder; absence of hemorrhages/exudates	Optic disk swelling, sectoral involvement, hemorrhages; fellow eye disk crowded with small or no cup
Visual field defects	Typically central, but may be arcuate (radiate from physiologic blind spot); cecocentral (involve central vision and physiologic blind spot); hemianopic (involve area to right or left of vertical)	Typically altitudinal (involve area above or below horizontal)
Pattern of visual recovery	Begins within 2 to 4 weeks, generally favorable overall (20/20 or better in 75 % with baseline normal vision)	Modest improvement over months in approximately 40 % (by 3 lines or more on Snellen chart)
OCT findings	Acute retrobulbar: Normal RNFL Acute papillitis: Elevated RNFL Chronic (>3 months): reduced RNFL thickness by 20 to 40% in majority of patients	Acute phase: Elevated RNFL, decreased cup to disc ratio in fellow eye Chronic phase: Reduced RNFL in the majority of patients

[a] Absence of these typical features should suggest other causes of inflammatory optic neuropathy or alternative diagnoses such as sarcoidosis, systemic lupus and other vasculitides, paraneoplastic disease, syphilis, Lyme disease, and *Bartonella henselae* infection (associated with cat scratch neuroretinitis), ischemic optic neuropathy, or Leber's hereditary optic neuropathy.

studies must be performed to compare morphometry results and to establish consistent normative baselines. In addition, questions remain about which protocols or visualization methods are best suited for a given application. The improved visualization and performance of new OCT technology suggests that it will have an increasingly important role in assessing the processes of axonal and neuronal degeneration in neurological disease in general and for MS in particular.

Role for OCT in distinguishing other optic neuropathies

For the neurologist, separation of acute demyelinating ON from other causes of optic nerve dysfunction or visual loss is essential. The emergence of OCT technologies have allowed measurements of RNFL and macular thickness that complement the history and clinical examination in distinguishing forms of acute optic neuropathy and retinal disease.[24–28] The age of onset of ON is typically between 20 to 50 years, and ON occurs three times more frequently in women (Table 17.2).[55] Visual loss in ON is most often unilateral in adults, although a bilateral presentation may occur more frequently in children. The temporal profile of the visual loss and subsequent visual recovery are important features of ON. Patients with typical ON usually lose vision over 7–10 days. In fact, progression of visual loss beyond two weeks is unusual.[71] Pain is an important feature of ON and its absence should raise a question of whether the patient has an alternative etiology for their optic neuropathy. In the Optic Neuritis Treatment Trial (ONTT), greater than 90% of patients had pain, particularly with eye movements.[72]

The pain usually persists for 1 to 2 weeks. Finally, some recovery of vision should occur within 30 days of onset of ON. On examination in ON, there is reduced acuity in one eye and an afferent pupillary defect is almost always present (unless a matched conduction defect is present in the fellow eye). There is impaired color vision, particularly to red–green objects, but occasionally to blue ones. Visual field defects are common and almost any type of field defect may occur in ON. Diffuse visual field loss and central scotomas are common in typical ON, particularly early in the course. Altitudinal defects are less commonly observed in ON and should raise the possibility of anterior ischemic optic neuropathy (AION) when optic disc swelling is present. In acute ON, optic disc swelling occurs in one-third of patients. The remainder of patients with ON will have retrobulbar inflammation, in which the optic nerve head will initially appear normal. Features of atypical ON include the presence of neuroretinitis (swollen optic nerve head with retinal inflammation or exudates), a markedly swollen nerve, retinal hemorrhages, retinal exudates, and the presence of no-light-perception (NLP) vision at onset.[55] Patients with these features have a lower risk of developing MS, particularly when a baseline brain MRI is normal.[55,73] The distinction of ON from other causes of optic neuropathy is primarily based on the clinical features outlined above. The following are entities that commonly appear in the differential diagnosis of ON, with emphasis on OCT findings.

Neuromyelitis optica (NMO)

Patients with severe visual acuity loss (worse than 20/200) have an increased probability of having a positive NMO antibody test. In fact, the visual prognosis for patients with severe acuity loss is far worse for those who are NMO positive (over 60% are 20/200 or less in one eye within 5 years).[74] Patients with NMO usually a greater degree of RNFL loss when compared to ON and control patients. In one study, the average RNFL thickness for eyes of NMO patients was 63 μm compared to 88 μm for ON eyes and 102 for controls.[75] Using linear regression analysis, a diagnosis of NMO was associated with 24 μm greater RNFL loss than for those patients with ON associated with relapsing remitting MS (RRMS). These findings also correlated well with more severe visual loss in the NMO group. Finally, NMO eyes may have more diffuse loss of RNFL compared to the temporal (papillomacular bundle) nerve fiber loss that predominates with ON in the setting of RRMS.

Conclusions

Rapid advancements in OCT technologies have allowed for improved visualization of the retina. High-resolution Fourier domain OCT has allowed for rapid imaging of the retina as well as three-dimensional imaging and improved volumetric measurements.[70] Ongoing studies of OCT in clinical trials and research will further examine patterns of axonal degeneration and visual loss over time, and will establish the role for OCT and other ocular imaging modalities as structural markers. With the emergence of a variety of OCT techniques, including Fourier Domain OCT, future studies will also help establish the protocols for data analysis to provide meaningful information about changes in structure from baseline. OCT is likely to play an increasing role in MS trials for measuring both axonal integrity and neuronal preservation.

Acknowledgments

This work was supported by the National Multiple Sclerosis Society (RG 4212-A-4; TR 3760-A-3); NIH/ National Eye Institute (R01 EY 019473; K24 EY 018136); the DAD's Foundation, and the McNeill Foundation. We are grateful to Dr. Steven Galetta for helpful input and expertise regarding this manuscript.

References

1. Trapp BD, Peterson J, Ransohoff RM, et al. Axonal transection in the lesions of multiple sclerosis. N Engl J Med 1998; 338: 278–85.

2. Evangelou N, Konz D, Esiri MM, et al. Size-selective neuronal changes in the anterior optic pathways suggest a differential susceptibility to injury in multiple sclerosis. Brain 2001; 124:1813–20.

3. DeLuca GC, Williams K, Evangelou N, et al. The contribution of demyelination to axonal loss in multiple sclerosis. Brain 2006; 129: 1507–16.

4. Sepulcre J, Goñi J, Masdeu JC, et al. Contribution of white matter lesions to gray matter atrophy in multiple sclerosis: evidence from voxel-based analysis of T1 lesions in the visual pathway. Arch Neurol. 2009; 66: 173–9.

5. Frohman EM, Fujimoto JG, Frohman TC, et al. Optical coherence tomography: a window into the mechanisms of multiple sclerosis. Nat Clin Pract Neurol 2008; 4: 664–75.

6. Parisi V, Manni G, Spadaro M, et al. Correlation between morphological and functional retinal impairment in multiple sclerosis patients. Invest Ophthalmol Vis Sci 1999; 40: 2520–7.

7. Trip SA, Schlottmann PG, Jones SJ, et al. Retinal nerve fiber layer axonal loss and visual dysfunction in optic neuritis. Ann Neurol 2005; 58: 383–91.

8. Costello F, Coupland S, Hodge W, et al. Quantifying axonal loss after optic neuritis with optical coherence tomography. Ann Neurol 2006; 59: 963–9.

9. Fisher JB, Jacobs DA, Markowitz CE, et al. Relation of visual function to retinal nerve fiber layer thickness in multiple sclerosis. Ophthalmology 2006; 113: 324–32.

10. Cheng H, Laron M, Schiffman JS, Tang RA, Frishman LJ. The relationship between visual field and retinal nerve fiber layer measurements in patients with multiple sclerosis. Invest Ophthalmol Vis Sci 2007; 48; 5798–805.

11. Pulicken M, Gordon-Lipkin E, Balcer LJ, et al. Optical coherence tomography and disease subtype in multiple sclerosis. Neurology 2007; 69: 2085–92.

12. Costello F, Hodge W, Pan YI, et al. Differences in retinal nerve fiber layer atrophy between multiple sclerosis subtypes. J Neurol Sci 2009; 281: 74–9.

13. Henderson AP, Trip SA, Schlottmann PG, et al. An investigation of the retinal nerve fibre layer in progressive multiple sclerosis using optical coherence tomography. Brain 2008; 131: 277–87.

14. Gordon-Lipkin E, Chodkowski B, Reich DS, et al. Retinal nerve fiber layer is associated with brain atrophy in multiple sclerosis. Neurology 2007; 69: 1603–9.

15. Sepulcre J, Murie-Fernandez M, Salinas-Alaman A, et al. Diagnostic accuracy of retinal abnormalities in predicting disease activity in MS. Neurology 2007; 68: 1488–94.

16. Cettomai D, Pulicken M, Gordon-Lipkin E, et al. Reproducibility of optical coherence tomography in multiple sclerosis. Arch Neurol 2008; 65: 1218–22.

17. Zaveri M, Conger A, Salter A, et al. Retinal imaging by laser polarimetry corroborates optical coherence tomography evidence of axonal degeneration in multiple sclerosis. Arch Neurol 2008; 65: 924–8.

18. Salter AR, Conger A, Frohman TC, et al. Retinal architecture predicts pupillary reflex metrics in MS. Mult Scler 2008; 15: 479–86.

19. Pueyo V, Ara JR, Almarcegui C, et al. Sub-clinical atrophy of the retinal nerve fibre layer in multiple sclerosis. Acta Ophthalmol 2010; 88: 748–52.

20. Costello F, Hodge W, Pan YI, Metz L, Kardon RH. Retinal nerve fiber layer and future risk of multiple sclerosis. Can J Neurol Sci 2008; 35: 482–7.

21. Burkholder BM, Osborne B, Loguidice MJ, et al. Macular volume by optical coherence tomography as a measure of neuronal loss in multiple sclerosis. Arch Neurol 2009; 66: 1366–72.

22. Kolappan M, Henderson APD, Jenkins TM, *et al.* Assessing structure and function of the afferent visual pathway in multiple sclerosis and associated optic neuritis. *J Neurol* 2009; 256: 305–19.

23. Barkhof F, Calabresi P, Miller DH, Reingold SC. Imaging outcomes for neuroprotection and repair in multiple sclerosis trials. *Nat Rev Neurol* 2009; 5: 256–66.

24. Jindahra P, Hedges TR, Mendoza-Santiesteban CE, Plant GT. Optical coherence tomography of the retina: applications in neurology. *Curr Opin Neurol* 2010; 23: 16–23.

25. Lameril C, Newman N, Biousse V. The use of optical coherence tomography in neurology. *Rev Neurol Dis* 2009; 6: E105–20.

26. Sakata LM, DeLeon-Ortega J, Sakata V, Girkin CA. Optical coherence tomography of the retina and optic nerve – a review. *Clin Exp Ophthalmol* 2009; 37: 90–9.

27. Glisson CC, Galetta SL. Nonconventional optic nerve imaging in multiple sclerosis. *Neuroimag Clin N Am* 2009; 19: 71–9.

28. Kallenbach K, Frederiksen J. Optical coherence tomography in optic neuritis and multiple sclerosis: a review. *Eur J Neurol* 2007; 14: 841–9.

29. Frohman E, Costello F, Zivadinov R, *et al.* Optical coherence tomography in multiple sclerosis. *Lancet Neurol* 2006; 5: 853–63.

30. Burkholder BM, Osborne B, Loguidice MJ, *et al.* Macular volume determined by optical coherence tomography as a measure of neuronal loss in multiple sclerosis. *Arch Neurol* 2008; 66:1366–72.

31. Talman LS, Bisker ER, Sackel DJ, *et al.* Longitudinal study of vision and retinal nerve fiber layer thickness in multiple sclerosis. *Ann Neurol* 2010; 67: 749–60.

32. Syc SB, Warner CV, Hiremath GS, *et al.* Reproducibility of high-resolution optical coherence tomography in multiple sclerosis. *Mult Scler* 2010; 16: 829–39.

33. Traboulsee A, Dehmeshki J, Peters KR, *et al.* Disability in multiple sclerosis is related to normal appearing brain tissue MTR histogram abnormalities. *Mult Scler* 2003; 9: 566–73.

34. Frohman EM, Zhang H, Kramer PD, *et al.* MRI characteristics of the MLF in MS patients with chronic internuclear ophthalmoparesis. *Neurology* 2001; 57: 762–8.

35. Frohman EM, Frohman TC, O'Suilleabhain P *et al.* Quantitative oculographic characterization of internuclear ophthalmoparesis in multiple sclerosis: the versional dysconjugacy index Z score. *J Neurol Neurosurg Psychiatry* 2002; 73: 51–5.

36. Fox RJ, McColl RW, Lee JC, *et al.* A preliminary validation study of diffusion tensor imaging as a measure of functional brain injury. *Arch Neurol* 2008; 65: 1179–84.

37. Huang D, Swanson EZ, Lin CP, *et al.* Optical coherence tomography. *Science* 1991; 254: 1178–81.

38. Swanson EA, Izatt JA, Hee MR, *et al.* In vivo retinal imaging by optical coherence tomography. *Opt Lett* 1993; 18: 1864–6.

39. Fercher AF, Hitzenberger CK, Drexler W, *et al.* In vivo optical coherence tomography. *Am J Ophthalmol* 1993; 116: 113–14.

40. Hee MR, Puliafito CA, Wong C, *et al.* Optical coherence tomography of the human retina. *Arch Ophthalmol* 1995; 113: 325–32.

41. Puliafito CA, Hee MR, Lin CP, *et al.* Imaging of macular diseases with optical coherence tomography. *Ophthalmology* 1995; 102: 217–29.

42. Drexler W and Fujimoto JG. State-of-the-art retinal optical coherence tomography. *Prog Retin Eye Res* 2008; 27: 45–88.

43. de Boer JF, Cense B, Park BH, *et al.* Improved signal-to-noise ratio in spectral-domain compared with time-domain optical coherence tomography. *Opt Lett* 2003; 28: 2067–9.

44. Leitgeb R, Hitzenberger A, Fercher C. Performance of Fourier domain vs. time domain optical coherence tomography. *Opt Express* 2003; 11: 889–94.

45. Wojtkowski M, Leitgeb R, Kowalczyk A, Bajraszewski T, Fercher AF. In vivo human retinal imaging by Fourier domain optical coherence tomography. *J Biomed Opt* 2002; 7:457–63.

46. Nassif N, Cense B, Park BH, *et al.* In vivo human retinal imaging by ultrahigh-speed spectral domain optical coherence tomography. *Opt Lett* 2004; 29: 480–2.

47. Wojtkowski M, Srinivasan V, Ko T, Fujimoto J, Kowalczyk A, Duker J. Ultrahigh-resolution, high-speed, Fourier domain optical coherence tomography and methods for dispersion compensation. *Opt Express* 2004; 12: 2404–22.

48. Choma MA, Sarunic M, Yang C, Izatt J. Sensitivity advantage of swept source and Fourier domain optical coherence tomography. *Opt Express* 2003; 11: 2183–9.

49. Keeler CR. The ophthalmoscope in the lifetime of Hermann von Helmholtz. *Arch Ophthalmol* 2002; 120: 194–201.

50. Frisén L, Hoyt WF. Insidious atrophy of retinal nerve fibers in multiple sclerosis. Funduscopic identification in patients with and without visual complaints. *Arch Ophthalmol* 1974; 92: 91–7.

51. Kerrison JB, Flynn T, Green WR. Retinal pathologic changes in multiple sclerosis. *Retina* 1994; 14: 445–51.

52. Frohman EM, Costello F, Stüve O, *et al.* Modeling axonal degeneration within the anterior visual system: implications for demonstrating neuroprotection in multiple sclerosis. *Arch Neurol* 2008; 65: 26–35.

53. Balcer LJ. Clinical practice. Optic neuritis. *N Engl J Med* 2006; 354: 1273–80.

54. Frohman EM, Frohman TC, Zee DS, McColl R, Galetta S. The neuro-ophthalmology of multiple sclerosis. *Lancet Neurol* 2005; 4: 111–21.

55. Ikuta F, Zimmerman HM. Distribution of plaques in seventy autopsy cases of multiple sclerosis in the United States. *Neurology* 1976; 26: 26–8.

56. Toussaint D, Périer O, Verstappen A, Bervoets S. Clinicopathological study of the visual pathways, eyes, and cerebral hemispheres in 32 cases of disseminated sclerosis. *J Clin Neuro-Ophthalmol* 1983; 3: 211–20.

57. Kupersmith MJ, Alban T, Zeiffer B, Lefton D. Contrast-enhanced MRI in acute optic neuritis: relationship to visual performance. *Brain* 2002; 125: 812–22.

58. Hickman SJ, Toosy AT, Jones SJ, *et al.* A serial MRI study following optic nerve mean area in acute optic neuritis. *Brain* 2004; 127: 2498–505.

59. Wu GF Schwartz ED, Lei T, *et al.* Relation of vision to global and regional

brain MRI in multiple sclerosis. *Neurology* 2007; 69: 2128–35.

60. Petzold A, de Boer JF, Schippling S, *et al.* Optical coherence tomography in multiple sclerosis: a systematic review and meta-analysis. *Lancet Neurol* 2010; 9: 921–32.

61. Frohman EM, Racke MK, Raine CS, *et al.* Multiple sclerosis—the plaque and its pathogenesis. *N Engl J Med* 2006; 354: 942–55.

62. Kanamori A, Escano MF, Eno A, *et al.* Evaluation of the effect of aging on retinal nerve fiber layer thickness measured by optical coherence tomography. *Opthalmologica* 2003; 217: 273–8.

63. Balcer LJ, Baier ML, Cohen JA, *et al.* Contrast letter acuity as a visual component for the Multiple Sclerosis Functional Composite. *Neurology* 2003; 61: 1367–73.

64. Baier ML, Cutter GR, Rudick RA, *et al.* Low-contrast letter acuity testing captures visual dysfunction in patients with multiple sclerosis. *Neurology* 2005; 64: 992–5.

65. Grazioli E, Zivadinov R, Weinstock-Guttman B, *et al.* Retinal nerve fiber layer thickness is associated with brain MRI outcomes in multiple sclerosis. *J Neurol Sci* 2008; 268: 12–17.

66. Green A, McQuaid S, Hauser SL, Allen IV, Lyness R. Ocular pathology in multiple sclerosis: retinal atrophy and inflammation irrespective of disease duration. *Brain* 2010; 133: 1591–601.

67. Naismith RT, Tutlam NT, Xu J, *et al.* Optical coherence tomography is less sensitive than visual evoked potentials in optic neuritis. *Neurology* 2009; 73: 46–52.

68. Banks MC, Robe-Collignon NJ, Rizzo JF 3rd, *et al.* Scanning laser polarimetry of edematous and atrophic optic nerve heads. *Arch Ophthalmol* 2003; 121: 484–90.

69. Jiao S, Knighton R, Huang X, *et al.* Simultaneous acquisition of sectional and fundus ophthalmic images with spectral-domain optical coherence tomography. *Opt Express* 2005; 13: 444–52.

70. Wojtkowski M, Srinivasan V, Fugimoto J, *et al.* Three-dimensional retinal imaging with high-speed ultrahigh-resolution optical coherence tomography. *Ophthalmology* 2005; 112: 1734–46.

71. Beck RW, Cleary PA, Anderson MM, *et al.* A randomized, controlled trial of corticosteroids in the treatment of acute optic neuritis. *N Engl J Med* 1992; 326: 581–8.

72. Optic Neuritis Study Group: The clinical profile of optic neuritis. Experience of the Optic Neuritis Treatment Trial. *Arch Ophthalmol* 1991; 109: 1673–8.

73. Optic Neuritis Study Group. High risk and low risk profiles for the development of multiple sclerosis within 10 years after optic neuritis: Experience of the Optic Neuritis Treatment Trial. *Arch Ophthalmol* 2003; 121: 944–9.

74. Wingerchuk DM, Hogancamp WF, O'Brien PC, Weinshenker BG. The clinical course of neuromyelitis optica (Devic's syndrome). *Neurology* 1999; 53: 1107–14.

75. Ratchford JN, Quigg ME, Conger A, *et al.* Optical coherence tomography helps differentiate neuromyelitis optica from MS optic neuropathies. *Neurology* 2009; 73: 302–8.

Chapter 18

The process of drug development and approval in the United States, the European Union, and Asia

Nadine Cohen, Ann Dodds-Frerichs, Tammy Phinney, and Paula Sandler

Introduction

The process for drug development and approval is complex, lengthy, and costly. The average time frame from discovery to registration has been estimated to be 12–15 years with costs ranging from 800 million to 2 billion dollars.[1] Throughout this process, regulatory agencies play a critical role. Charged with the responsibility of ensuring the safety of subjects during clinical trial testing, these regulators define the requirements for preclinical testing, drug manufacture and quality testing, subject inclusion and exclusion in studies, subject monitoring, and study conduct. Once pivotal trials are completed, and a sponsor seeks regulatory approval for the investigational product, the responsible authorities will review the submitted data to ascertain whether sufficient evidence has been generated to prove the safety and efficacy of the drug, and to establish that the benefit risk profile for the studied entity is positive. Reviews are usually lengthy, in depth, and can entail considerable communication between the sponsor and the regulatory agency prior to garnering an approval.

Importantly, the perspectives of regulatory agencies regarding drug development and approval can vary dramatically between countries and regions, adding further complexity to the process. Recent data, for example, indicate that the US and European authorities disagree regarding product approvals as often as 20% of the time.[2] The following discussion outlines the role of the regulators in drug development and approval in the United States, Europe, and in some emerging international markets.

Drug review and approval process in the United States

Structure of the Food and Drug Administration

The process of drug approval in the United States is regulated by the Food and Drug Administration (FDA). Applications for new drugs and therapeutic proteins are reviewed and approved by the Center for Drug Evaluation and Research (CDER) and applications for new vaccine, gene therapy, and blood products are reviewed and approved by the Center for Biologics Evaluation and Research (CBER).

Regulation of clinical trials

The Investigational New Drug application

The sponsoring company must first obtain FDA's permission to begin clinical testing. A company must compile and submit preclinical information, manufacturing information, and clinical plans to the FDA in the form of an Investigational New Drug application (IND). The FDA assesses the information to determine if the product is reasonably safe for testing in humans. Clinical investigations cannot begin until 30 days after the FDA's receipt of the IND unless the sponsor is notified otherwise.

In addition, sponsors are required to ensure details of each controlled clinical trial, are posted on Clinicaltrials.gov. except for Phase 1 investigations. This database is intended to be a central resource providing current information on clinical trials to patients and others.

As clinical drug development proceeds, FDA requires sponsors to submit new clinical protocols, changes to protocols, new toxicology information, as well as changes to chemistry and manufacturing processes. FDA allows for, and encourages, sponsors to meet with FDA at appropriate times during the development process to seek feedback.

As part of drug development, FDA requires sponsors to assess products in the pediatric population in order to inform drug labeling. Based on the drug profile or disease, FDA may defer the requirement to study products in children until data are available in adults. In certain cases the requirement may be waived, for example, if the disease state being targeted is not prevalent in children. To date, FDA has waived the pediatric requirement for multiple sclerosis (MS); however, FDA has indicated that they are rethinking this position and may require studies in children in the future.

Institutional Review Boards and informed consent

The FDA regulates clinical testing by setting minimum standards for clinical trials known as good clinical practices (GCP). GCPs also include the requirement for obtaining the informed consent of clinical subjects. Informed consent ensures that patients voluntarily participate in a clinical trial and understand the benefits and risks of participation. Institutional Review

Multiple Sclerosis Therapeutics, Fourth Edition, ed. Jeffrey A. Cohen and Richard A. Rudick. Published by Cambridge University Press.
© Cambridge University Press 2011.

Boards (IRBs) are used to ensure the rights and welfare of people participating in clinical trials.[3] IRBs ensure that participants are fully informed of risks of study participation and have given their written consent before studies ever begin.

Fast Track

A sponsor can apply to the FDA to obtain Fast Track designation for a product. Fast track designation can aid the development, as well as accelerate the review and approval process for a product. This designation can only be accorded to new drugs that are intended to treat serious or life-threatening conditions and, in addition, address an unmet medical need.

Fast track designation can be requested at any time from the original IND submission until marketing approval is granted. There are several advantages of fast track designation, including more frequent meetings with FDA to discuss the drug development program, and "rolling review," meaning that companies can submit portions of a marketing application for FDA review before the entire application is completed. Additionally, products with fast track designation would normally receive a "priority" review by FDA, meaning that the target approval time is 6 months instead of the usual 10 months.

Marketing authorization application

In order for a company to market a new drug or biologic, the FDA must approve an application to market the product, known, respectively, as a new drug application (NDA) or biologics license application (BLA).[4,5] The sponsor must file an NDA or BLA, which consists of non-clinical and clinical data, chemical and biological information, and product manufacturing and control information as well as pay a filing fee unless the product has received orphan designation. The standard review time for a new application is 10 months, which includes a 60-day screening period. The FDA determines if the product is safe and effective for its indicated use, if the benefits of using the product outweigh the risks, and whether the methods used in manufacturing and quality control are adequate to preserve the product's identity, strength, quality, potency, and purity. The FDA also determines if the proposed labeling is appropriate.[6] The labeling should constitute a summary of the essential scientific information needed for the safe and effective use of the product. The labeling also sets out boundaries or limits as to what the sponsoring company may say in advertising its product.

Accelerated approval

One means by which FDA can expedite product approval is through accelerated approval which allows for approval based on a surrogate end-point, e.g. a laboratory measurement, or physical sign. This status is granted to certain new drug products that have been studied for their safety and effectiveness in treating serious or life-threatening conditions and are believed to provide a meaningful benefit to patients over existing therapies. Under the provisions of accelerated approval, marketing approval is granted by FDA on the basis of clinical

trials that establish that the product has an effect on a surrogate end-point that is reasonably likely to predict clinical benefit. The approval requires that the applicant conduct a study post-approval to demonstrate a real clinical benefit of the product. FDA can withdraw approval if the post-marketing clinical study fails to show clinical benefit or if the applicant fails to adhere to any of the post-marketing agreements.

Priority review

FDA can expedite the review process for a marketing application or supplement by granting priority review. This status is granted for an application if the product is thought to be a major advancement in treatment, or a treatment where no adequate therapy is available. *Priority review* status is accorded to drugs that are used to treat serious diseases as well as to drugs for less serious illnesses. Priority applications and efficacy supplements have a target review time of 6 months in contrast to a standard review time of 10 months.

Inspections

The FDA conducts on-site inspections of facilities and clinical sites prior to approval of a new drug. These inspections focus on good laboratory practices (GLPs), good clinical practices (GCPs), and good manufacturing practices (GMPs), and are designed to ensure that clinical and preclinical studies were conducted in accordance with regulations and that the product is manufactured in accordance with GMPs.

Maintaining the marketing authorization license

After approval, there are a number of requirements to which the sponsor must adhere. These requirements include safety reporting, periodic summaries of safety reports, post-marketing commitments, and reporting changes to the product manufacturing process or labeling. Additionally, FDA conducts inspections of manufacturing facilities on a regular basis. These inspections can be either prearranged or unannounced and focus on quality systems, adverse event reporting, and GMPs.

The FDA requires two types of post-marketing safety reporting, 15-day alert reports and periodic adverse experience reports. A 15-day alert report is submitted to FDA within 15 days of initial receipt of information for an adverse experience that is both serious and unexpected. Periodic adverse experience reports include a summary of the 15-day alert reports submitted during the reporting period as well as a listing of the other adverse drug experiences that were reported to the sponsor during that period. Periodic adverse experience reports are required to be submitted quarterly for the first three years after approval and then annually. Based on these safety reports, labeling may need to be revised to reflect the current benefit risk profile of the product.

Prior to gaining product approval a Sponsor must agree to the post-marketing commitments delineated by FDA. These commitments could include additional clinical or analytical studies. The FDA requires that reports on the status of clinical post-marketing commitments and information on the distribution of product be submitted on an annual or semi-annual basis after product approval.

Additionally, subsequent to product approval, the company is required to report any changes regarding manufacturing or testing of a product as well as any changes to the product label. Depending on the magnitude of these changes, the sponsor may or may not be required to submit a supplement to FDA for approval before implementation of the change. Promotional material is also required to be submitted at time of dissemination or prior to distribution for a product granted accelerated approval.

Drug review and approval process in the European Union

Structure of the European Union and its regulatory bodies

The European Union (EU) includes 27 Member States: Austria, Belgium, Bulgaria, Cyprus, Czech Republic, Denmark, Estonia, Finland, France, Germany, Greece, Hungary, Ireland, Italy, Latvia, Lithuania, Luxembourg, Malta, The Netherlands, Poland, Portugal, Romania, Slovakia, Slovenia, Spain, Sweden, United Kingdom.

Each Member State has its own national regulatory agency responsible for the approval of clinical trial and marketing applications and also for pharmacovigilance in its territory. Their activities are coordinated by three central bodies:

- The European Medicines Agency (EMA) – coordinates scientific resources across the EU to assess new drugs, develop efficient regulatory approval procedures, and create an effective pharmacovigilance network
- The Committee for Medicinal Products for Human Use (CHMP) – is a scientific advisory committee that provides opinions to the European Commission (EC) on the safety, quality, and efficacy of medicines, and guidance on the development of new medicines.
- The European Commission – is responsible for implementing common policies across Europe and granting marketing authorizations based on the recommendations of the CHMP.

Regulation of clinical trials

Investigational medicinal product dossier and ethics committees

To start a clinical trial in the EU, it is necessary to obtain, in each country where the study will be undertaken, both an Ethics Committee and a regulatory agency approval. A regulatory agency approval is obtained by submitting an investigational medicinal product dossier (IMPD) to each Member State where the clinical trial will be conducted.[7] The IMPD

consists of a summary of preclinical information, manufacturing information, and any previous clinical experience. Additional requirements are necessary for biotechnological and biological products in certain countries (e.g. viral safety committee submissions in France).

Guidance documents issued by the regulators outline the various documents and data necessary for Ethics Committee[8] or regulatory agency[9] approval. The specific requirements do vary to some extent amongst Member States. The sponsor is also required to ensure that specific details of each interventional clinical trial are registered in a database (EudraCT). This database, maintained by the EMA, provides the EMA and the national regulatory agencies information on all clinical trials in the EU and facilitates the exchange of information if there are any significant safety or quality issues affecting a study.

In contrast to the US, FDA, the EMA, and the CHMP are not charged with the responsibility of oversight of products in clinical trials. However, the CHMP offers a scientific advice procedure whereby a company can request advice on specific development issues. In addition, sponsors can seek advice from individual national regulatory agencies.

The CHMP also issues guidance documents to assist sponsors in the development of medicines for certain diseases, such as multiple sclerosis.[10] The guidance documents include information on the design of studies, the methods to assess efficacy and the selection of patients.

In January 2007, the EU introduced sweeping new legislation on the development and approval of pediatric medicines, with the goal of providing better protection of the health of children in the EU.[11] Marketing applications for new drugs must now include results of studies conducted in the pediatric population (up to age 17), unless the EMA grants a deferral. If granted, pediatric development is deferred until the efficacy and safety of the product is shown in adults (waivers may also be granted for products targeting diseases that do not impact children, such as Parkinson's disease). A pediatric investigation plan (PIP) must be submitted to, and agreed upon with, the EMA Pediatric Committee prior to filing a marketing authorization. This plan should describe the studies to be conducted in children. Once approved, products with pediatric data are eligible for a 6-month patent extension.

Marketing authorization application

There are four procedures that can be used for obtaining marketing authorizations in the EU:

- the National Procedure whereby a marketing authorization is only granted in a single Member State;
- the Mutual Recognition Procedure, in which a marketing authorization is granted by the regulatory agency of a Member State for its own territory that is subsequently recognized by other Member States;
- the Decentralized Procedure whereby Member States grant national marketing authorizations in a coordinated manner; and

- the Centralized Procedure, in which a marketing authorization is granted by the European Commission for enforcement in the entire EU and is under the control of the EMA.

Companies are required to utilize the Centralized Procedure for all products developed for multiple sclerosis.

Centralized Procedure

The Centralized Procedure is used to obtain a single marketing authorization for a medicine that is valid in all Member States. A single application is submitted to the EMA, who coordinates the review and approval process. The scientific assessment is completed by two Member States who are referred to as rapporteurs. The rapporteurs provide their assessment and recommendation to the CHMP. The CHMP then renders an opinion. If the CHMP provides a positive opinion, it is made legally binding across all Member States by a decision from the European Commission. Subsequently, the Commission issues the marketing authorization.

The Centralized Procedure is compulsory for biotechnology products derived from recombinant DNA technology or from manipulation of genetic material. In addition, orphan medicinal products and products that are intended to treat autoimmune diseases and viral diseases must follow the Centralized Procedure.[12] For new active substances and other innovative medicinal products, the choice of the Centralized Procedure is optional.

Accelerated approval

In the EU it is possible to have an accelerated evaluation of some marketing authorization applications through the Centralized Procedure.[13] There have to be compelling public health reasons to do this, according to the following criteria:

(1) the seriousness of the disease,
(2) the absence of appropriate alternative therapeutic approaches, and
(3) the anticipation of exceptional high therapeutic benefit.

An accelerated evaluation can result in a CHMP opinion within 120 days vs. 210 days for a standard approval. It is important to note that there is no provision to reduce the regulatory requirements and it is likely that the approval will also require the company to commit to follow up studies to gain further data post-marketing.

Inspections

The EMA's Inspections Sector coordinates inspections of facilities and documentation for good clinical practices (GCPs), good laboratory practices (GLPs), and good manufacturing practices (GMPs). Member States in the European Union provide the expertise to undertake the inspections. These inspections are conducted prior to marketing approval and on a regular basis, thereafter.

Maintaining the marketing authorization license

Once a medicinal product has been approved, the sponsor is responsible for a variety of post-approval activities, such as periodic safety update reports (PSUR), risk management plans (RMP), follow-up measures, post-marketing commitments, and reporting changes.

Products that receive conditional approval through the Centralized Procedure are subject to annual reassessment of the benefit–risk ratio. The annual reassessment involves summarizing the status of the post-marketing commitments and follow-up measures and continues until the sponsor has fulfilled the obligations. Products that receive a standard approval must have their marketing authorization renewed after 5 years; after this point the marketing authorization will be valid for an unlimited period, unless a further 5-year renewal is required on grounds of pharmacovigilance.

The sponsor may wish to alter or improve the product or to add additional safeguard measures for a variety of reasons. In order to do this, a formal variation that contains information describing the change must be filed. The sponsor must also ensure that promotional materials are approved in accordance with regulations in the individual countries.

Drug review and approval process in Asia

Clinical studies to support drug development are increasingly becoming more global in nature as trial subjects are recruited from countries throughout the world. Recent data suggest that for many products greater than 30% of patients in trials come from regions outside of the US and Europe.[14] Expanding clinical trials to include sites in countries such as India and China is attractive because of their highly trained investigators, fast patient accrual, and low per patient trial costs. In addition, inclusion of subjects in these regions may expedite the subsequent approval for the product in these countries.

The increased clinical trial and marketing applications in these "new regions" have resulted in quickly evolving regulatory environments there, as regulatory agencies build infrastructure and expertise. In the last 5 to 10 years the roles, responsibilities, and authorities of the Chinese SFDA, and Indian Central Drug Authority have dramatically changed. New processes are being established with the intention to harmonize the approaches and standards with those of the West. Despite this, additional requirements may still be imposed by these regulators as part of the clinical trial application process. For example, in China the sponsor may need to provide clinical study data demonstrating the pharmacokinetic profile of the product in patients who are of Chinese or Asian descent in order to gain approval of the clinical trial application.

This approach of expanding the global reach of clinical trial studies is not without its challenges. During the approval process regulatory authorities in various countries may question the impact of including patients from disparate geographies. New analyses may be required to clarify that the patients in the studies show similar demographics across regions regarding disease characteristics and background treatments. And, fundamentally, questions may be raised seeking evidence that enrollment of patients in these regions does not impact the overall efficacy and safety findings.

Emerging topics in the regulatory environment

The regulatory environment is very dynamic as global health authorities grapple with innovations in science and technology in addition to changes in health policy in their respective countries. This results in the generation of new regulations, guidances, and practices as well as new initiatives. The following topics highlight some of the more recent initiatives.

Focus on post-marketing safety

High-profile, safety issues of prescription drugs in recent years has led to an increased focus on post-marketing safety monitoring. Increased patient exposure can reveal safety signals that are not observed in carefully controlled clinical programs with limited patient exposure data and controlled patient populations.

Amid such issues, FDA implemented the drug safety initiative in 2004, which outlined transformations to patient and prescriber information resources, reorganized CDER, established the Drug Safety Oversight Board, and made improvements to risk communication.

Further enhancing FDA's ability, the Food and Drug Administration Amendments Act of 2007 (FDAAA) was enacted which increased FDA's enforcement capabilities by authorizing FDA to require post-approval clinical trials and demand safety labeling changes to product labels. FDA also posts online quarterly safety reports, which notify the public of any new drug safety information.

Biosimilars

One issue that may impact MS treatments over the next period of time is the development of biosimilars, i.e. generic versions of currently available biologic treatments. In order to obtain regulatory approval of a biosimilar product, manufacturers would need to prove comparability to the original product. Achieving this regulatory hurdle may be difficult. Comparability would require that the biosimilar product be similar to the reference product and demonstrate no clinically meaningful differences that could impact the safety, purity, and or potency of the product. Since biologics have complex structures, small differences could result in changes in these characteristics that may only be evident in substantive clinical studies. In 2010 the US Health Care Reform Act was passed which included provisions for FDA to approve biosimilar therapeutics in the USA. The FDA has been mandated by Congress to create guidance for the pharmaceutical industry outlining the requirements that would be necessary in order to obtain approval of a biosimilar product. The FDA is currently in the process of developing such guidance.

The European Medicines Agency (EMA) issued a guidance document on biosimilars in 2005, stating that biosimilars are not interchangeable with current available products, as well as delineating requirements for comparability studies. The EMA considers every biosimilar a new product. However, for some products waivers may be granted for aspects of the development process.

Given the complexity of developing biosimilars, it may be difficult to hasten or simplify the development process without impacting safety and efficacy. The emerging regulations in addition to the experiences of the pharmaceutical industry will likely determine the success of biosimilars.

FDA transparency

FDA's transparency initiative is designed to explain agency operations, how it makes decisions, and the drug approval process. The goal of this initiative is to better explain the FDA's actions by providing information to the public that supports clinical medicine, biomedical innovation, and public health. The first phase was established to provide basic information about FDA and how the agency works. To support this phase, the agency launched a web-based resource known as "FDA Basics," which includes online sessions hosted by FDA officials addressing specific topics and answering questions from the public.

The second phase is in regard to the scope, nature, and boundaries of FDA's proactive disclosure of information it has in its possession. The goal is to make information about agency activities and decision-making more transparent, useful, and understandable to the public, while appropriately protecting confidential information. In May 2010 the FDA's transparency task force announced a series of sweeping draft proposals that would significantly increase the information available to the public about pending investigational and marketing applications. This would include, for example, disclosure of correspondence with sponsors when FDA rejects a new product application, or release of summary data on the safety and effectiveness of pending product applications. With these disclosures, however, FDA's intent is to maintain the confidentiality of a company's trade secrets and of individually identifiable patient information. These proposals are likely to be further pared down and prioritized with time. Implementation of many of the proposals could not occur without major revisions to FDA regulations and relevant statutes.

The third and final phase of the initiative is slated to address ways that FDA can become more transparent to regulated industry, in order to foster a more efficient and cost-effective regulatory process.

Food and Drug Administration Amendments Act of 2007

The Food and Drug Administration Amendments Act (FDAAA) were signed into law in September 2007. Under this law, the Prescription Drug User Fee Act (PDUFA) and the Medical Device User Fee and Modernization Act (MDUFMA) have been reauthorized and expanded. These programs ensure that FDA has additional resources needed to conduct the comprehensive reviews necessary to approve new drugs and medical devices.

Also included was authority for FDA to require a risk evaluation and mitigation strategy (REMS) for certain drugs and biological products, to ensure the benefits of such products outweighed the risks. A REMS is a risk-management plan that applies only to prescription drugs and biologics that have a significant risk associated with their use and requires the use of certain risk minimization tools beyond routine labeling. The elements of a REMS are designed based on the safety profile of the drug. Required elements can include a medication guide, educational tools for health care providers and patients, as well as elements to ensure safe use, such as restricted distribution. If a manufacturer does not comply, FDA can prohibit the drug from being commercially available. FDA has the authority to require a REMS during the pre-approval phase or post-approval phase if FDA becomes aware of new safety information once the product is on the market.

Conclusions

With the increasing focus on globalization, there has been further emphasis on cooperation among world-wide regulatory agencies. As an indication of this approach, at this time FDA has over 100 formal agreements with its counterparts in 29 countries. These agreements allow for more open dialog on emerging issues, exchange of information on processes, policy development, and enforcement in many areas.

Cooperation amongst regulators in regional health authorities has also been advanced through engagement in the International Conference on Harmonization (ICH). This body brings together regulators from the European Union, Japan, and the United States, as well as technical experts from the pharmaceutical industry in these three regions. Their goal is to produce a single set of technical requirements for the registration of new drugs and biologics, in order to allow for more economical use of human, animal and material resources, and eliminate unnecessary delay in the global development and availability of new medicines.

In spite of efforts to harmonize the guidance, regulations, and requirements for drug development and approval across geographies, clear differences remain. The variability can be attributed to reasons based on the populations studied, the disease, and the therapy itself. However, other overarching factors may also come into play such as, fundamental dissimilarities in the systems of health care delivery throughout the world, distinctions in the roles and responsibilities accorded to the regulatory agencies themselves, as well as changes in the political environment and priorities which may influence and/or affect regulators. The regulations and requirements also continue to evolve as further strides are made in the understanding of diseases and the relevant tools, approaches, and therapies for the management of those diseases. Given these drivers, the development and approval process for pharmaceuticals will likely continue to be a complex and costly process for the foreseeable future.

Acknowledgments

We would like to acknowledge Simon Bennett, Cyndie Gangi, Cristina Diramio, Anisha Grover, and Rita Shah for their contributions to the researching and writing of this chapter.

References

1. Masia N. The cost of developing a new drug. In Clack G, Neely M, eds. *Focus on Intellectual Property Rights*. US Department of State Publication, 2006; 84–5.

2. Jenkins J. New Drug Review 2009 Update. *December 3, 2009* http://www.fda.gov/downloads/ AboutFDA/CentersOffices/CDER/ UCM192786.pdf (Accessed October 7, 2010).

3. United States Federal Government. Code of Federal Regulations, Title 21, Part 50. Office of the Federal Register, *National Archives and Records Administration*: Washington, DC, April 1, 2010.

4. United States Federal Government. Code of Federal Regulations, Title 21, Part 314. *Office of the Federal Register, National Archives and Records Administration*: Washington, DC, April 1, 2010.

5. United States Federal Government. Code of Federal Regulations, Title 21, Part 600. *Office of the Federal Register, National Archives and Records Administration*: Washington, DC, April 1, 2010.

6. United States Federal Government. Code of Federal Regulations, Title 21, Part 201.57. *Office of the Federal Register, National Archives and Records Administration*: Washington, DC, April 1, 2010.

7. Council of European Communities. Council Directive 2001/20/EC of 4 April 2001 on the approximation of laws, regulations, and administrative provisions of member states relating to the implementation of good clinical practice in the conduct of clinical trials on medicinal products for human use. Brussels, 4 April 2001.

8. European Commission. Detailed guidance on the application format and documentation to be submitted in an application for an ethics committee opinion on the clinical trial on medicinal products for human use. *Brussels*, rev.1, April 2004.

9. European Commission. Detailed guidance for the request for authorization of a clinical trial on a medicinal product for human use to the competent authorities, notification of substantial amendments and declaration of the end of the trial. *Brussels*, April 2003.

10. European Medicines Agency for the Evaluation of Medicinal Products. Note for guidance on clinical investigation of medicinal products for the treatment of

multiple sclerosis. *CPMP/EWP/561/98 Rev* 1, 16 November 2006.

11. Regulation (EC) of the European Parliament and of the Council of 12 December 2006 on Medicinal Products for Paediatric Use. *EC 1901/2006*, 12 December 2006.

12. Regulation (EC) No 726/2004 of the European Parliament and of the Council of 31 March 2004 laying down Community procedures for the authorisation and supervision of medicinal products for human and veterinary use and establishing a European Medicines Agency.

13. European Medicines Agency for the Evaluation of Medicinal Products. Accelerated evaluation of products indicated for serious diseases (life threatening or heavily disabling diseases). *CPMP/495/96 rev*. 1, September 2001.

14. Levinson D. Challenges to FDA's ability to monitor and inspect foreign clinical trials. June 2010. http://oig.hhs.gov/oei/reports/oei-01-08-00510.pdf (Accessed October 7, 2010).

Chapter

19

Selection, interpretation, and development of end-points for multiple sclerosis clinical trials

Marc K. Walton

Introduction

Multiple sclerosis (MS) research in recent years has identified an increasing number of potential therapeutic products that can be evaluated. Particularly when there are multiple compounds that might be evaluated, efficient clinical evaluation programs are important. Selection of appropriate study end-points can significantly contribute to successfully advancing clinical development programs to ultimately result in widespread availability of effective therapies.

This chapter will consider the types of patient assessments used in studies within a clinical development program, emphasizing how study goals and assessment characteristics influence the selection of the endpoints. Also highlighted are the potential for inadequately understood end-points to lead a clinical development program astray, and the potential to develop improved end-points when currently available end-points are suboptimal.

Types of end-points

Two major types of study end-points can be distinguished: clinical efficacy end-points and biomarkers. Clinical end-points are those that directly measure a meaningful aspect of the clinical status of the patient (i.e. how the patient feels, functions, or survives). Clinical end-points are essential in the later stages of drug development which provide the definitive evidence of effectiveness to support marketing approval. Effectiveness of a drug is established by demonstrating a meaningful treatment-related effect either directly on a clinical end-point or on an end-point that is an indirect measure that has previously been shown to predict clinically meaningful effects (e.g. blood pressure, serum cholesterol).

In contrast to efficacy end-points, biomarker end-points measure drug activity by assessing a biochemical or biological process. They include biochemical measurements that report on the first step in a drug's action (e.g. ligand-receptor binding), biochemical measures that are thought to measure the level of ongoing disease pathophysiologic activity (e.g. certain serum cytokine levels, or some CNS imaging techniques), and assessments that may reflect the patient's clinical status (either current or in the future) but are not a direct measure of the patient's function (e.g. certain other CNS imaging techniques).

Terminology and concepts for biomarker assessments now widely used have been described by a Biomarkers Definitions Working Group.[1] A biomarker is an objective laboratory-measured patient parameter that is believed to be informative in some specific way, but is not an intrinsically interpretable measure of the patient's clinical status. Some biomarkers may be prognostic of the patient's future clinical course or a post-measurement therapeutic intervention or predictive of the potential for a patient to respond to an intervention. Biomarkers of these types are measured only once at the start of a clinical trial, and are not within the scope of this chapter. Relevant biomarkers for this chapter reveal the patient's response to a treatment, i.e. pharmacodynamic biomarkers. The biomarker may assess a proximal biological response to the investigational product or may measure something thought to be associated with the disease process. Biological responses not known to be related to the disease process may also be used for some purposes. Neuroimaging studies such as MRI, CT, and others are laboratory measures for the purposes of this discussion, and are the most widely known biomarkers in MS. In general, a patient does not perceive a change in the quantity or level of the assessed biomarker in itself, but may perceive clinical changes if clinical function changes occur simultaneously.

A surrogate end-point is a biomarker used as an explicit substitute for a clinical efficacy end-point, and is expected to predict the clinical effect of the treatment. As noted by the Biomarkers Working Group, this use requires specification of the clinical end-point for which the substitution is being effected. While all surrogate end-points are biomarkers, only a small fraction of biomarkers will be suitable for use as surrogate end-points. To accept a biomarker as a surrogate end-point, data must be developed that rigorously establish the relationship between the biomarker and the specified clinical end-point, and the data must be relevant to the manner in which the biomarker is used in the study being designed or analyzed.

For purposes of this chapter the general term end-point means a specific outcome assessment (clinical or laboratory) measured at a specific time in the clinical trial, and the data analyzed using a specified statistical method. Some methods will use multiple sequential time-points of evaluation (e.g. repeated measures designs) or the study-time when a specified event

Multiple Sclerosis Therapeutics, Fourth Edition, ed. Jeffrey A. Cohen and Richard A. Rudick. Published by Cambridge University Press.
© Cambridge University Press 2011.

occurs (e.g. as in time to event analyses). The usefulness within drug development studies of a specific type of outcome measurement is not solely an intrinsic characteristic of the measurement, but can depend also upon the measurement frequency, timing, and statistical analysis components that define the end-point. How a particular measurement is used in a study can be as important as what the measurement is.

Structure of clinical development programs: study goals and end-points

The ultimate goal of a drug development program is to establish that, when used in a specified manner in a described patient population, the drug has a favorable effect upon the patient and has risks that are acceptable in light of the benefit (i.e. a favorable risk–benefit comparison). The studies that provide this evidence are chiefly those in later stages of the development program. Nonetheless, the early (Phase 1) and intermediate (Phase 2) studies are essential parts of a development program. They are used to reach decisions whether the subsequent longer and larger studies are reasonable to pursue and to optimize the design of late-stage (confirmatory, Phase 3) studies.

The questions posed in clinical studies during clinical development about a potential therapy change as the development program progresses. The nature of clinical trial end-points consequently also shifts across the successive trials. While accurately and adequately understanding the safety profile of a new therapy is important, this chapter is focused on end-points used to assess the therapeutic activity of new products rather than safety.

The small Phase 1 studies provide a coarse, initial, safety assessment. Phase 1 studies often evaluate pharmacokinetics and may, in some cases, offer preliminary insight into the biological activity of the product. If the drug's mechanism of action is adequately understood and assays sensitive to this mechanism are available, assessment of laboratory parameters (i.e. biomarkers) of, or proximate to, the drug's molecular action may be useful to identify doses and regimens that achieve the intended cellular-action goal. Because of patient variability in responses, end-points evaluating processes distant from the drug's molecular activity may be unable to provide the "proof of concept" that might be sought; this is even more the case for clinical end-points. Generally, these studies can confirm the in vivo occurrence of the expected cellular interaction, and identify a broad dose-regimen range suitable for further evaluation, but not the precise optimal dose.

Phase 2 studies typically seek a deeper assessment of the product's activity profile. Response to a range of doses and/or regimens can provide evidence that a clinical efficacy effect is reasonably plausible for this product. Phase 2 study end-points are often biologic effects occurring subsequent to the immediate cellular action that are plausible indicators for a clinical benefit. In some cases patient functional assessments may also be useful tools. Sensitive functional assessments may show that there is an effect upon the integrated function of the neurologic

system. Assessment tools which have this sensitivity, however, may not have well-established clinical interpretability (see following section) and thus cannot serve as a clinical efficacy end-point. Nonetheless, they can provide the evidence that further development of the drug is warranted and guide Phase 3 study design. Disadvantages of the available true clinical benefit end-points, discussed below, often render them inefficient for moderate size Phase 2 studies. Phase 2 studies, however, can serve as excellent testing grounds for clinical efficacy end-point assessments for which there is limited prior experience in clinical trials. Assessing the practicality and performance characteristics of unfamiliar assessment tools will guide selection of the efficacy end-point of the Phase 3 study.

Phase 3 studies are designed to be adequate and well-controlled studies that provide the convincing evidence of clinical efficacy on specific identified features of MS. The conclusion is chiefly based on the study's primary end-point(s), but secondary end-points also contribute to forming conclusions regarding clinical effectiveness. Thus Phase 3 study designers select end-points capable of providing definitive evidence of a clinically meaningful benefit. Marketing approval of a drug is based on benefit–risk comparisons, and the clinical import of the demonstrated benefit must be understood. Without such, it may be difficult or infeasible to determine if the observed benefits outweigh the observed or expected risks of the therapy.

Biomarkers are also often included as secondary end-points of Phase 3 studies. Confidence in the objective nature of the biomarker, or biomarker confirmation of the expected therapeutic mechanism, may strengthen the conclusion of clinical effectiveness that the primary end-point is intended to establish.

Clinical end-points

MS therapies may be intended to affect the underlying pathologic processes of the disease or to affect the existing physiologic function of the nervous system in a temporary way. The latter are regarded as symptomatic treatments and typically achieve their effect in a relatively prompt manner. Symptomatic therapeutic effects can usually be assessed by observable alterations of functional abilities in studies of modest duration. Although many assessment types may be appropriate to establish either symptomatic benefits or effects on long-term outcome, it is likely that the study time-point used to formulate the end-point, and perhaps the analysis method, will be different. Concerns regarding reliability, sensitivity, and interpretability are relevant to any use of the assessment tools as efficacy end-points.

MS is a central nervous system-wide disease; many different neurologic systems are affected. Therapies that are expected to alter the underlying disease process would be expected to provide benefits in a broad range of neurologic functions. Such therapies can potentially be evaluated by assessment of any, or a combination of several, neurologic systems that are damaged and cause disability.

As noted previously, a clinical end-point is one that describes how a patient feels, functions, or survives. Patients with MS can have sensations such as pain or localized dysesthesia or feelings of systemic fatigue; thus a valid assessment of how the patient feels can be used as a clinical efficacy end-point. While some patients are severely affected, this is not a dominant feature of MS for most patients most of the time. Symptomatic therapies may, however, be more practically targeted to these types of MS features than therapies intended to alter the disease pathophysiologic process. In general, assessments of how patients feel are not typically used as the primary effectiveness end-point for drugs that will alter the course of the disease. Similarly, since very early mortality is not typical for MS patients, this has also not been an end-point suitable for studies of reasonable length. An exception might be for studies of very late-stage patients, but most therapy development does not primarily target this patient population. Therefore, most MS drug development programs use an assessment of patients' functional abilities as the clinical end-point.

Clinical effectiveness of a drug is demonstrated by showing an effect on a clinical end-point evaluating some functional ability of patients that is impaired by the disease. Explicitly characterizing the full range of disabilities caused by MS that may be important to patients can aid consideration of the range of possible assessments. Characteristics of the disability such as the frequency of occurrence in MS patients, the range of severity, the rate of worsening, day-to-day or week-to-week variability of the disability should be considered as these will affect the utility of an assessment focused on a specific type of disability. Identifying the assessment tools that have been developed that measure each type of disability, and understanding the measurement characteristics of each tool is also important. The sensitivity of the tool is one important characteristic, i.e. whether small changes can be detected or only large changes in the patient's functional ability. Characteristics such as the intrapatient reliability, the inter-rater reliability, the burden on the patient to undergo the assessment (which alone can influence patient dropout and missing data) are among those important to understand. The disease characteristics for the particular disability and the tool's characteristics will combine to influence whether a particular tool is well suited for a particular study. For example, a tool sensitive only to large changes in neurologic function (e.g. an interval scale with coarse steps between grades) may be very reliable, but unsuitable for a short study where there is not expected to be substantial change in the patient's functional ability in that domain.

A characteristic requiring careful consideration is the clinical interpretability of the measurement. Evaluation of changes in how a patient functions is meaningful when the change in the measure can describe or imply changes that have meaning to the patient in typical day-to-day life. For purposes of this chapter, clinical end-points intended to assess functional abilities can be broken into two broad categories. In one category are assessments that directly address the patient's

functioning in actual daily life. These are reports of the patient's activities, either recorded by the patient during the course of daily life, or a questionnaire administered in the clinic relying on recall of ability in daily life activities. Patient questionnaires of actual typical activities are termed patient reported outcomes (PROs). Because these are intended to directly evaluate meaningful patient function, PROs can conceptually have great sensitivity and maintain interpretability. PROs have not been widely used in MS drug-development effectiveness studies as primary end-points because there are not yet well-established PROs that are qualified for that purpose and widely accepted.

A second broad category of function evaluations are rating scales for which the patient performs a precisely defined task (or tasks) in the clinic and some aspect of the performance is measured. These are indirect measures of the conceptually targeted functional ability. Tests such as the timed 25-foot walk or visual acuity are common examples, and many other defined-task assessments for performance in the clinic have been developed. While walking and accurately identifying objects at a moderate distance are part of every patient's daily life, the underlying ability is not employed in daily life as performed in these tests. A valuable aspect of these performance tests is that the test can depend on integrating the same neurologic systems, but the artificial nature of the task makes it important to understand what change in the measured test result translates into a change in a day-to-day activity that is perceptible and meaningful to a patient.

When carefully performed and properly analyzed, some tests may be capable of reliably demonstrating small changes in the patient's neurologic impairments. For some tools, small changes are detected, but only larger changes can be confidently interpreted as being clinically meaningful. This does not mean that the tool should not be used, rather that this should be considered when selecting the tool for a particular study. Small, reliably detected changes in neurologic function can be a valuable indicator for use in Phase 2 dose-ranging studies, for example, where demonstration of efficacy is not a goal but showing a drug effect within a limited duration study can be important. The same tool might be a less useful choice for Phase 3 studies if the study population's rate of change in function for that specific domain, coupled with the study duration, leads to expecting that only few patients will have changes sufficiently large to be confidently interpreted as a meaningful change. In this circumstance only a few patients will have opportunity to contribute to showing an effectiveness difference between the drug and the control treatment.

Persistent (sustained) increases in physical impairments are typically the more concerning aspect of MS for patients. They may occur with a rapid onset or increase in impairment (a relapse which incompletely resolves), or a slowly accruing decline in function. The intermittent relapses with good recovery may be a more prominent feature in the early stages of MS. Relapses (brisk but mostly transient increases in physical disability) and persistent physical disability have been the clinical features most commonly examined in clinical trials.

Selection of an end-point may also require particular additional study design features to ensure validity for the purpose to which the end-point is to be applied. For example, because these clinical assessments are not entirely objective, blinding of patients and physicians to assigned treatment has been important. Since some treatments may have recognized side effects, many studies are designed with separate patient management physicians (who may become treatment-unblinded by patient symptoms, physical examination, or laboratory values) and outcome evaluation physicians to better assure unbiased evaluations.

Relapse outcome

Many Phase 3 studies have evaluated the effect of a treatment on frequency of relapses, including the studies for all the currently approved chronic MS immune system modulator treatments. Relapse data from a clinical study may be analyzed in a variety of ways and provide a good illustration of the importance of selecting the analysis method to best suit the study goals. For example, the number of relapses per patient over a defined period (e.g. 2 years) can be analyzed, or the proportion of patients who have had no relapses. Alternatively, the time to first on-study relapse can analyzed. Some newer statistical techniques may permit using the time-to-next-relapse for each of a patient's relapses during a defined period in an analysis. The analytic method used to define the end-point should be chosen with consideration of the specifics of the study design, including the goal for study result interpretation and application. Some of these analytic methods may give greater statistical power for shorter duration studies, but be more difficult to interpret with regard to the clinical meaning of the resulting statistic. Such methods may be well suited to exploratory studies (e.g. early dose ranging studies) but less so for the adequate and well-controlled studies. Carefully selecting the analysis method is equally important when assessments of unremitting disability are used in an end-point.

The analysis method can influence what aspects of the therapeutic effects are most important to the analysis result. For example, there is a growing interest in comparative effectiveness studies evaluating two or more different treatments. Different therapies may have different time-courses of onset of effect so that the effect of one appears greater in short timeframes, but might have little difference in the effect size over an extended time-period; alternatively, the reverse might be true. An end-point of time to first relapse may be particularly sensitive to differences in time course of onset, but less sensitive to the later occurring overall degree of effect. The number of relapses experienced by a patient over an extended period is more important than the timing (early vs. later within the period) of the first relapse experienced. Thus, if it is the effect over extended periods of treatment that is of greatest interest, a time to first relapse end-point may be less useful than a frequency of relapses end-point. The manner in which the relapse events are analyzed can

be attuned towards the therapeutic aspects of greatest interest and the study objective.

The expected mechanism of drug action will also affect whether relapses are an appropriate end-point in a particular study. Flares of the inflammatory disease process occurring in a CNS location to which patient function is sensitive are thought to cause relapses. Therapeutics that decrease disease-related inflammatory activity may have an impact upon relapse occurrence. Research is also being directed to identifying potential therapeutics that may be neuroprotective or promote neural repair.[2] Such therapies are not intended to alter the inflammatory process and thus may not alter the occurrence of relapses. In these cases, assessment of relapses as the chief efficacy end-point may not be fruitful.

Physical disability outcome

The Kurtzke Expanded Disability Status Scale[3] (EDSS) has been employed as the chief physical disability measure in development programs for many of the currently available therapies. The manner in which EDSS has been used in these studies illustrates additional considerations that should be applied in using a patient assessment in an efficacy end-point. Related in part to the definition of the scale, and in part to the observed reproducibility of the assessment process, changes of 1 point or greater in the EDSS have been accepted as reliable and clinically meaningful (although the latter may be questionable at the very low end of the scale). An analysis that examines the fraction of patients who show increased disability of least 1 point, or compares the time to progression of at least 1 point is a common formulation of an efficacy endpoint based on EDSS. MS patients, however, may exhibit month-to-month variation in function that can confound interpretation of these EDSS data as well as increase the statistical variance of the data. Because the interest has been in (presumed) irreversible disability, to decrease uncertainty in data interpretation, it has been typical to require that the EDSS increases be confirmed as sustained in a second EDSS evaluation several months later. The two-evaluation method to decrease variation and ensure that the assessment can be interpreted as irreversible disability can also be employed whether the end-point is a comparison of EDSS at a fixed time after randomization or time to EDSS increase.

The EDSS has a number of recognized weaknesses, such as suboptimal sensitivity to small but meaningful loss of a patient's abilities, particularly in the upper region of the scale (e.g. scores above 6), and a shift from evaluation of multiple neurologic systems in the low score portions of the scale to a focus on ambulation in the upper region of the scale. Despite these weaknesses, EDSS remains the most successfully employed assessment for a physical disability end-point in past clinical trials. An important strength is the widespread acceptance that changes in EDSS can be interpreted as validly describing clinically meaningful changes in a patient's condition.

Other evaluations of functional ability have also been used as outcome measures in clinical studies to evaluate efficacy, such as walking times for a defined distance. The dalfampridine development program used the 25-foot walk time as the primary efficacy end-point for this symptomatic treatment drug. The analysis for the two Phase 3 studies involved categorizing each patient individually as a responder or a non-responder, based on an algorithm that included examination of five evaluations prior to treatment and four on-treatment evaluations. Subsequent exploration of the data analyzing the fraction of patients with specified (e.g. 10%, 20%, 30%) increases in walking speed were also important to understanding the clinical meaning of the drug effect.

Selection of which evaluation to use depends on the study patient population and expectations for the treatment effect during the study period. For example, reliance upon just a walking measure requires an expectation that, despite the within-patient variation in severity of impairment across the different anatomic regions of the body, the treatment effect will be well represented in most or all patients by examining only ambulation. If that cannot be relied upon, then tests of walking ability will not be an optimal evaluation tool. In some cases, the patient population eligible for the study can be narrowed to only those patients for whom this expectation appears appropriate.

Other functional ability assessments may also be subject to the month-to-month variation in patient function. These measures can also be applied in a double measurement manner of some form (e.g. average or best score of two assessments) as is typically done with EDSS to damp-out some of the within-patient variation. This component of the end-point specification may take the expected therapeutic objective into account to ensure interpretation of the result is not confounded. For example, a study of a therapy intended to promote CNS repair leading to disability improvement during the study is different from the prevention of decline in function objective for studies of anti-inflammatory therapies. The two-evaluation method for confirmation of change in function will still be valuable, but consideration of using a worst score of two successive function evaluations may be necessary.

Clinical end-points and labeling claims

An important aspect of drug development is determining what drug benefits should be claimed in the approved drug labeling. The clinical efficacy study results are the evidence that justify the labeling claims. The labeling claims state what benefits have been well demonstrated and identify to patients and physicians the benefits that may be expected when the drug is used. More comprehensive knowledge (e.g. addressing multiple domains of clinical function) aids patients and physicians to more confidently make decisions regarding whether to use the drug, or which among several drugs to use. Consequently, drug developers often will consider the desired labeling claims for the particular drug being developed, and select efficacy end-points for the Phase 3 studies that will support the desired claims in addition to the drug approval decision. For this purpose also,

clinical end-points that enable one to clearly convey the meaning and value of the observed benefit are important.

As stated earlier, the term *end-point* in this chapter includes a specification of the statistical analytic method applied to the data values collected during the study. Interpretability of the end-point can be affected by the selected analytic method, and should be considered when making that selection. Some analytic methods may combine patient measurements in ways that obscure the clinical meaning of the final statistical parameter, to which the *P*-value applies. While such methods may be statistically valid, and appropriate as evidence that a treatment effect has occurred, they may be very difficult to explain in labeling without implying benefits that have not actually been demonstrated. For example, some statistical methods will take clinical measurements of several different types, and combine them into an overall statistical parameter (e.g. a global odds ratio or other score) with a *P*-value for that parameter testing the null hypothesis. Success on the global statistic does not mean that benefit has been demonstrated on each of the component measurements. Each of the components must be individually examined to understand the treatment effect on that domain.

Other clinical evaluations and development of new end-points

Previous chapters in this volume have discussed a variety of other clinical assessment measures and many more are described in the medical literature. Many of these have not been widely used in clinical drug intervention trials as the chief outcome evaluation or adequately evaluated. They may nonetheless deserve further consideration as they may have superior characteristics for some clinical trial settings and objectives. It is important to recognize that new clinical outcome assessment tools can be developed into accepted efficacy end-points and may justify the effort if they offer advantages over existing tools. Careful formulation of the tool, coupled with testing, can bring new tools to clinical trials as outcome assessments. Adequate testing to ensure they are reliable and have clinical meaning is important prior to adoption as the primary efficacy end-point of a Phase 3 trial.

For example, there has been interest in improving upon the EDSS to gain greater sensitivity to change and to be more comprehensive of a patient's functional abilities. One of these proposed new tools is the multiple sclerosis functional composite (MSFC),[4,5] which incorporates a specified performance test in each of several domains and is discussed more fully in an earlier chapter of this volume. The initial formulation included tests of ambulation, upper limb function, and cognitive function that are combined in a specified manner into a single score for each patient at each evaluation. This tool remains under evaluation and is not at the present time sufficiently validated to recommend for use as the primary end-point of clinical efficacy trials.

The developing experience with MSFC illustrates the magnitude of effort necessary to develop a new assessment tool, particularly the process of testing the new measurement tool for reliability and clinical meaning. Creation of new clinical outcome tools is best considered as a separate tool development program, apart from the development program for any specific potential new therapeutic product. End-point tool development may be best undertaken by a collaborative group rather than by a single investigator. When regulatory decisions are intended to rely on data from a new tool, consultation with regulatory agencies along the course of development is advisable. This program will need to plan to define the new tool and test the reliability of the assessment and the meaningfulness (clinical interpretability) when used as an outcome end-point. Reformulating the tool, followed by retesting, may be needed to address weaknesses discerned in the testing process. While an end-point development program is conceptually separate from any specific drug product's development program, clinical trials of new drugs can incorporate the procedures and evaluations necessary to obtain data that advance the end-point development, in effect piggy-backing the end-point development upon a number of different drug development programs.

The experience with the MSFC also illustrates a number of aspects in defining and testing a tool that will be generally applicable to any other new clinical evaluation being considered. An important aspect as already discussed is the clinical interpretability of the end-point. The first proposed formulation of the MSFC included three assessments recorded as a continuous measure, each component for each patient is then translated into a z-score (number of standard deviations from a population mean, typically the study population at baseline) and the three component z-scores averaged for an overall patient z-score at that time-point. This is a complex transformation and combination of the primary observed data, and a number of difficulties with this formulation have contributed to it not becoming accepted as an efficacy end-point.[6] The chief difficulty is an inability to interpret the clinical meaning of any particular size change in the overall z-score due to the mathematical formulation, with further contribution from the inherent change in general weighting among the components across different studies when each study uses its own study population as the reference, and complex differential weighting of the components across patients within the same study depending on the location of their baseline assessment within the population distribution for each component (but not directly the absolute severity of the baseline impairment). This illustrates that complex transformations and combinations of the primary assessments can render interpretation difficult.

This formulation of MSFC, however, does retain the continuous nature of the evaluations in the final end-point and consequently may have the ability to indicate small changes in patient function, even if of unknown clinical meaning. If that possibility is realized, this form of MSFC may have value in Phase 2 studies as a measure that shows drug effect on the integrated neurologic function involved in these assessments, and provides a proof of concept demonstration, or guides selection doses for testing in Phase 3 studies. Use in this manner is predicated upon an assumption that continued drug treatment will

lead to continually accumulating drug effect, and that at some time in the future the accumulated drug affect will be sufficient to be a clinically meaningful amount. Demonstrating that greater amount of accumulated drug effect will be the objective of the Phase 3 studies establishing effectiveness.

The initial concept for the MSFC was more flexible than this single form and the concept offers potential for other formulations that may have different performance characteristics. The MSFC illustrates an assessment intended to measure several domains of patient disability by incorporating several different component tests, and this choice can be revised to suit the objectives. Patients suffer impairment in additional neurologic systems beyond the three domains that have been included, such as visual difficulties. A visual ability measure might also be included into a revised MSFC to broaden it.[6-8] The performance characteristics of the individual tests may affect which specific tests will yield an optimal MSFC. For example, the test typically used as the cognitive test, paced auditory serial addition test (PASAT), is known to have practice-improvement effects that might cloud demonstration of the drug effects. Substitution with a different cognitive test with lessened learning effect may yield an improved MSFC, and some efforts to identify better cognitive tests have been published.[9-13] Candidate tests should be well evaluated for their properties (e.g. reliability, sensitivity, interpretability) prior to adoption.

How the components are combined in the data analysis may also be changed to adjust the characteristics of the overall measure. For example, composite-event end-points have been used successfully in many disorders, and could be considered here as explored by Rudick et al.[6] Transforming each of the components into an "event" indicating a change of at least a specified size (as is done with EDSS when using a time to event analysis) allows creation of a composite event form of MSFC. All domains remain included, but each is more readily interpreted in how it influences the composite. If each of the individual domain "events" has been defined as a change of at least a specified amount (or percentage) externally demonstrated to be clinically meaningful, then the composite event also is a clinically meaningful event irrespective of which component within the composite gave rise to the event for a particular patient. This formulation can be used in a comparison of incidence of events or time to event analyses for an efficacy analysis, and remain a clinically interpretable finding.

In this event-oriented approach the criterion for a change-event should be carefully selected to ensure acceptance that it is clinically meaningful. That criterion is determined from tool-development studies focused on that question. It is important to distinguish between a change-size that is reliably determined and a change-size that is confidently interpreted as clinically meaningful. The question of a reliably determined change is often easier to study than the meaningful change, and is the more commonly studied aspect in published studies.[14-16] There have, however, been studies that work towards understanding meaningful change.[15,17,18] The minimum reliably determined change may be greater or less than the demonstrated minimum clinically meaningful change for some tools. A good assessment suitable for an efficacy end-point in clinical studies will need to have both aspects understood. Precisely how the test is administered may affect these aspects.[15]

When a tool or component of a tool is evaluated for clinical meaningfulness, it is important to understand that a clinical efficacy end-point is used to demonstrate that a meaningful effect has occurred at the time-point of the assessment. An end-point that predicts a meaningful effect for some time in the future, but not at that time, is a surrogate end-point and not a true direct efficacy end-point. The approach to demonstrating acceptability of a surrogate end-point is different than for a direct efficacy end-point.

It is also important to ensure that the data supporting the interpretability of the tool apply to how it will be used in the study. An incomplete list of important questions includes:

(1) The similarity, in any characteristics potentially related to performance, of the patients supplying the validation data to the patients to be enrolled in the clinical trial. This can, for example, create a change in the portion of the measure's range that will be used in the study or the impact of floor or ceiling limits of the measure
(2) Whether the setting of the validation data collection is similar to the setting of the clinical study
(3) The reliability of the tool, both inter-rater and intra-patient
(4) Whether the test was conducted in the validation study in the same way as planned in the clinical study.

Differences in any aspect between the source of the validation data and the clinical trial use of the test should be considered carefully, and may need re-evaluation if there is concern of a significant difference. For example, in considering the addition of visual acuity testing to MSFC in an event composite formulation, reduced contrast eye chart vision testing may be promising.[7,8] For high contrast vision testing, the number-of-letters change necessary to be both reliably determined and clinically meaningful has been established. That determination will come from studies specifically of low contrast testing, as the high contrast results will not automatically transfer to testing with reduced contrast eye charts.[19]

There is considerable interest in PROs as outcome assessments because they have the potential to provide a more comprehensive evaluation of a patient, greater ease to communicate interpretation, address aspects of patient function difficult to measure in observed performance rating tests[20,21] or be more sensitive to meaningful change. Regulatory agencies, including FDA, have seen PROs increasingly proposed for multiple disorders and have offered guidance to persons or collaborative groups seeking to develop PROs for clinical study efficacy end-points.[22] PROs will require well-planned development programs to define, refine, and then demonstrate suitability of new PRO. A variety of PROs have been proposed for MS, but none has yet been adequately evaluated to justify adoption as a primary efficacy end-point. Further development of these tools may ultimately enable relying on this type of end-point.

Biomarkers as outcome measures

Ultimately, only clinically meaningful drug effects are important to patients. Well-recognized difficulties with relying only on clinical end-points in all studies throughout the drug development program, however, make this approach infeasible. Biomarkers have the potential to be informative on a number of different aspects of biological responses in much shorter time and fewer patients, and therefore importantly contribute to feasible and successful drug development.

Useful biomarkers measure an aspect of the biological mechanism of the treatment's activity or of the pathogenesis of MS that predict a clinical response. For most biomarkers the quantitative relationship of biomarker level to clinical outcome may be only imprecisely known, or perhaps only assumed in some uses. If the biomarker is completely unpredictive of the patient's clinical outcome, there is no utility for the biomarker to be a response indicator in the therapy development. Any plans to rely on a biomarker effect at any stage of drug development should be predicated upon an assessment of the knowledge relating the biomarker to an expected clinical outcome and whether it is sufficient to justify the drug development decisions that will be made based on the biomarker results. In some cases, concurrently examining several biomarkers that assess successive steps in the presumed mechanism leading to clinical effects may be useful if they show concurring effects.

Uses of biomarkers in different stages of clinical development are briefly discussed earlier in this chapter. A complete discussion of how best to use biomarkers to construct effective clinical development programs is beyond the scope of this chapter. The earlier discussion highlights the fact that several biomarkers that assess different portions of the therapeutic response process can serve different purposes along the course of clinical development. The biomarkers best suited to any particular stage of development may also differ between drugs that rely on different mechanisms of action. For example, in evaluating effects of anti-inflammatory therapies, a biomarker of gadolinium-enhanced MRI lesion count (an effect many steps distant from the drug-receptor binding) has demonstrated great value. Therapies hypothesized to provide neuroprotection or promote repair, however, will likely need a different biomarker, although the optimal selection remains unclear.[23,24]

Biomarkers can continue to play an important role in Phase 3 studies as secondary endpoints where the biomarker effects may add to the totality of the data supporting a drug's effectiveness. An objectively measured biomarker end-point may alleviate some concerns relating to a subjectively influenced primary efficacy end-point. A robust result on a biomarker secondary end-point may help to strengthen the conclusion from a primary efficacy end-point result that is positive but not highly robust, particularly if the biomarker is thought to be informative of late steps in the treatment mechanism. A biomarker measurement that has greater precision than the clinical assessment may aid concluding that the treatment-associated benefit applies broadly to the study population. Alternatively, a biomarker may suggest a population subset, which may have notably greater or lesser response than the overall study result. While a post-hoc subset analysis will usually require confirmation, this observation may lead to improvement in the risk–benefit relationship for the drug.

Surrogate end-points

There is great interest in the possibility that a biomarker end-point might serve as the basis for establishing drug effectiveness, i.e. be a surrogate end-point because it predicts future clinical effects well. At best, only a few biomarkers will perform this well, and fewer still can be shown to do so. Effects on biomarkers that have been adequately validated as predicting clinical status may be used for this purpose. The relationship of the biomarker to the specifically identified clinical outcome must be sufficiently well understood to permit the biomarker to stand in the place of the clinical outcome of interest. Careful consideration of the actual strength and extent of knowledge of the biomarker–clinical outcome relationship is critical prior to adopting this approach. At present, there are no biomarkers generally accepted for use as surrogate primary efficacy end-points in clinical trials in MS.

FDA regulations describe certain circumstances in which a product may be marketed, based on an effect on a less then fully validated surrogate end-point, called accelerated approval. Typically for accelerated approval, the unvalidated surrogate end-point is the primary endpoint in a Phase 3 study or studies intentionally designed to support this objective. These regulations apply to treatments for serious or life-threatening diseases that provide an important advance over existing therapies, if any. The regulation is stated in 21CFR601.41 for biological products where a Biologics License Application (BLA) approval is sought; similar language at 21CFR314.510 applies to drug products where a new drug application (NDA) approval is sought:

Sec. 601.41 Approval based on a surrogate end-point or on an effect on a clinical endpoint other than survival or irreversible morbidity.

FDA may grant marketing approval for a biological product on the basis of adequate and well-controlled clinical trials establishing that the biological product has an effect on a surrogate end-point that is reasonably likely, based on epidemiologic, therapeutic, pathophysiologic, or other evidence, to predict clinical benefit or on the basis of an effect on a clinical end-point other than survival or irreversible morbidity. Approval under this section will be subject to the requirement that the applicant study the biological product further, to verify and describe its clinical benefit, where there is uncertainty as to the relation of the surrogate endpoint to clinical benefit, or of the observed clinical benefit to ultimate outcome. Post-marketing studies would usually be studies already under way. When required to be conducted, such studies must also be adequate and well controlled. The applicant shall carry out any such studies with due diligence.

In this setting, an effect on an incompletely validated surrogate end-point that is deemed "reasonable likely…to predict clinical benefit" is the substantial evidence of effectiveness needed to support marketing approval. A discussion by Katz[25] provides a more in-depth discussion of the regulatory context for this approach to marketing approval. A full discussion of the circumstances where this approach can be successful is beyond the scope of this chapter. This approach provides the potential for bringing a therapy to wide availability earlier than if the true clinical benefit were relied upon, but some disadvantages of this approach have been discussed by Fleming.[26] Use of a biomarker in this role requires that there be a strong, but not yet definitive understanding of the relationship to the expected clinical outcome. Early engagement with regulatory authorities to plan for applying this circumstance is important.

Understanding biomarkers and hazards of incorrect assumptions

MS is a complex disease with inadequately understood pathogenesis, and variable disease course between different patients and over time within an individual patient. These disease aspects will also make interpreting biomarker results complex. Use of biomarkers, however, brings the need to carefully assess the quantitative knowledge regarding the relationship between effects on the biomarker and clinical status. As noted above, assessing the strength of knowledge describing this relationship prior to use of a biomarker at any stage of development is warranted.

Disparity between drug effects on the biomarker and the clinical outcome can cause either under- or over-estimation of the true clinical effect. If unrecognized, this can lead to poor choices of which drug development programs to continue or terminate, or of what dose, regimen, population, or sample size to use in the design of the definitive efficacy study (and lead to the study failing to provide robust evidence of efficacy even for an effective drug).

Prentice[27] described the ideal relationship between a clinical outcome and a biomarker for a surrogate end-point. An ideal biomarker shows effect whenever the intervention has an effect upon the true clinical end-point; that is the biomarker is sensitive to the intervention's clinical effects. An ideal biomarker also does not show an effect unless the intervention has a corresponding effect upon the clinical outcome, i.e. the biomarker is specific for clinical effects. For biomarkers intended to be used as surrogate end-points, a well-defined relationship is important, while diffuse evidence suggesting a qualitative adherence may be insufficient support. Validation of biomarkers as surrogate end-points is a topic that cannot be covered in this discussion, but numerous authors have discussed various aspects of this, often from the statistical standpoint.[27–30] As noted in one discussion,[30] the statistical issues alone are not sufficient to enable conclusions on validation. Understanding the medical and biological background and context will have critical roles in reaching an assessment. As noted by Fleming and DeMets,[31] validating the biomarker can be very difficult.

Epidemiologic observations alone may not be sufficient to determine a biomarker's validity as a surrogate end-point,

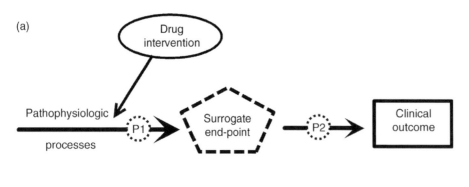

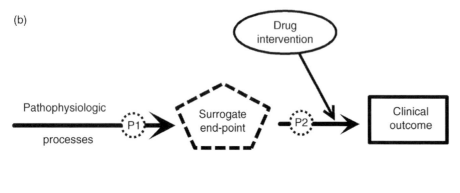

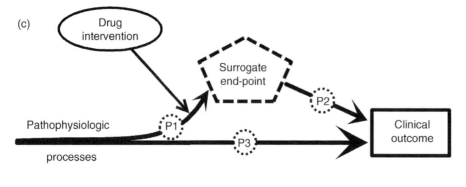

Sequential order of processes

Fig. 19.1. Disease process paths with sites of surrogate endpoint and drug intervention. (a) Single pathway of sequential processes. The surrogate is located within this chain of processes prior to the clinical outcome, and the site of drug intervention is prior to the surrogate. (b) Single pathway as in (a) with drug intervention after the surrogate. (c) Multiple simultaneous pathways of disease activity, with opportunity for multiple sites of drug intervention. Figure modified from ref. 31, with permission.

as seen in some cases where the biological background was thought to be well understood. While cardiac ventricular premature beat (VPB) rate post-infarction appeared to be associated with mortality risk, in the CAST study[32] suppression of VPBs failed to decrease mortality. Another cautionary example is that fluoride treatment improved bone density in osteoporosis patients, but did not lead to reduction in bone fracture rates.[33] Biomarkers may also fail in the inverse manner. Patients with chronic granulomatous disease treated with interferon gamma experienced a reduction in clinical infections despite absence of the expected increase in the biomarker of superoxide production.[34] Temple has addressed additional uses in cardiovascular disorders.[35]

Fleming and DeMets[26] have discussed the conceptual basis for biomarkers failing as surrogate end-points. Divergence between the biomarker and the clinical outcome can arise because the biomarker is not as integral to the disorder's pathophysiologic pathway as assumed or because the intervention's mechanism of action is not as expected. The idealized mechanistic relationship between a proposed surrogate and the clinical outcome is often thought of as a single set of sequential processes in a causal chain with the surrogate integrally located prior to the clinical outcome (Fig. 19.1(a)). This permits an intervention which acts on a process prior to the surrogate (P1) to have effects upon both the surrogate and the clinical outcome.

If the assumptions regarding the site of drug action or of the simplicity of a single causal chain of processes are not correct, however, the association between the proposed surrogate and the clinical outcome can fail in a variety of different ways. If, instead, the biomarker is located prior to the site of drug action (Fig. 19.1(b)) the biomarker will be entirely insensitive to the drug's effects and indicate the drug has no effect. This figure also illustrates that a biomarker well suited to one specific therapeutic intervention (e.g. a specific drug class acting in accord with Fig. 19.1(a)) cannot be automatically generalized to other interventions (which might act as in Fig. 19.1(b)) without careful consideration, including regarding the pathophysiologic processes of the disease, the location of the biomarker within those processes, and the mechanism of the drug. Each drug development program will need to carefully consider the existing information on the drug mechanism and the disease processes to assess which, if any, biomarkers may be usefully employed in the development program.

The actual situation in MS is probably more complex than the ideal of a single sequential causal chain of processes. There may be multiple process chains acting in parallel with unequal amounts of influence upon the clinical outcome; one of many possible scenarios is illustrated in Fig. 19.1(c). The true biology may also be that some early processes influence both the biomarker and the clinical outcome, but there is no process leading from the surrogate to the clinical outcome (e.g. Fig. 19.1(c)) with process chain P2 of little or no importance) and the biomarker will fail as a surrogate efficacy end-point for drugs acting at P1. In this illustration of biological complexity, the biomarker may be well informative of drug effect upon the clinical outcome or entirely misleading, being either over- or under-sensitive. For example, if the drug intervention acts as illustrated in Fig. 19.1(c), then a marked effect upon the biomarker could be observed but the effect on the clinical outcome is dependent upon the relative strength of influence of the two alternative paths to the clinical outcome, P2 vs. P3. Alternatively, a drug acting upon the P3 process might provide worthwhile clinical benefits even though the biomarker is uninformative of this effect.

These considerations illustrate the importance of understanding the relationship between the biomarkers and the clinical outcomes of interest for each drug development program. Disadvantageous decisions can result from a true relationship being different than that assumed. The degree of quantitative precision to that understanding, beyond the qualitative level, should be part of the consideration. Biological processes in complex diseases such as MS are unlikely to yield a simple, linear relationship. The relationship is likely non-uniform; with most of the informative change-relationship in the two measures falling within a restricted portion of the possible values for at least one of the measures. How narrow the range of informativeness (i.e. how steep the relationship) and where within the range it is located determines whether the biomarker will be useful for the drug, dose, and MS population under study. For example, it may be that only biomarker changes within some modest portion of the full possible biomarker range will relate to the full range of the clinical measure, with floor and ceiling behavior of the clinical measure outside that range. If this is unrecognized and a more uniform relationship across the full range of biomarker values is assumed, critical decisions that need to be made (e.g. drugs, drug doses, MS population subset to study further, regulatory decisions) may be incorrect.

The potential for a drug-induced change in the biomarker–clinical status relationship is a potential difficulty in relying on a biomarker as a surrogate end-point. The source of knowledge of quantitative descriptions of the relationship, if known, is often from natural history studies. The selected biomarker may reflect the level of activity in only one pathway of multiple pathogenic process chains occurring in parallel (as discussed in relation to Fig. 19.1(c)). If the drug does not broadly affect all pathways similarly, the biomarker–clinical status quantitative relationship may differ in the presence of the drug treatment from the relationship existing in absence of the drug as the balance of influence shifts among the processes. Consequently, natural history studies alone will not be sufficient to ensure that a biomarker will predict the effect of a particular drug on the clinical outcome. Prior experience with the specific biomarker in clinical trials with other interventions, particularly drugs of the same class of mechanism, are can improve confidence that drug-related effects on the biomarker will predict drug-related effects on the clinical outcome.

Conclusions

Clinical development of new drugs for MS is complicated by the variability of the disease course. The practical difficulties of conducting large trials will further increase as laboratory research findings progress to suggest increasing numbers and diversity of products for clinical investigation. An important aspect of efficient and informative drug development programs is selection of appropriate endpoints for each study in the clinical development program. Identifying informative biomarkers has the potential to assist in this goal.

Each clinical trial within a development program needs to have the important objectives for that particular stage of the program clearly identified. Those objectives generally relate to the knowledge needed to enable study design choices for the next stage in development. The optimal endpoints of an individual trial are those that contribute to this incremental advancement of the overall drug development program.

True clinical efficacy end-points are necessary for the studies that are intended to definitively demonstrate the benefits of the product. These endpoints should be adequately validated for the manner in which they will be used within the clinical study. Clinical assessment methods not yet validated, as for inadequately validated surrogates, should be used with caution and largely in supportive roles. Validation of a new clinical assessment method cannot be expected from within a clinical trial relying upon it as a primary end-point. Instead, efficacy end-point validation can best be advanced in the framework of an end-point development program designed to evaluate the reliability and interpretability of the end-point, and conducted with regulatory agency consultation when intended to be a basis for critical regulatory decisions.

Biomarkers play an important role in clinical development and are often essential in early phases. This is because they can provide insight into the early pharmacologic processes in drug action and may reveal effects on biologic processes potentially involved in the disease pathophysiology. The appropriate biomarker end-points for each study should be selected to address the goals of the study with an understanding of the specific mechanism expected for the drug. Although surrogate end-points for use in Phase 3 studies have attraction, there are no biomarkers currently accepted as qualified for this use. The complexity of the disease will likely make justification for

any specific biomarker as a surrogate end-point for wide use across varied therapeutic approaches difficult to accomplish.

Since clinical efficacy always remains the ultimate goal, clarity regarding the strength of knowledge of the relationship between the biomarker and the intended clinical effect is important, and influences the ability to rely on the biomarker in making clinical development decisions. Misunderstanding the relationship can lead to erroneous expectations regarding the optimal manner of the drug's use and potentially lead to clinical trials which fail to demonstrate the drug's value. Nonetheless, appropriate application of biomarkers is an essential tool in development of new therapies for MS.

Disclaimer

The views expressed in this article are those of the author, and do not represent an official FDA position.

References

1. Biomarkers Definitions Working Group. Biomarkers and Surrogate Endpoints: Preferred Definitions and Conceptual Framework. *Clin Pharmacol Ther* 2001; 69: 89–95.

2. Frohman EM, Filippi M, Stuve O, *et al.* Characterizing the mechanisms of progression in multiple sclerosis. *Arch Neurol* 2005; 62: 1345–56.

3. Kurtzke JF. Rating neurologic impairment in multiple sclerosis: an expanded disability status score (EDSS). *Neurology* 1983; 33:1444–52.

4. Fischer JS, Rudick RA, Cutter GR, Reingold SC. The Multiple Sclerosis Functional Composite measure (MSFC): an integrated approach to MS clinical Outcome Assessment. *Mult Scler* 1999; 5: 244–50.

5. Cutter GR, Baier ML, Rudick RA, *et al.* Development of a multiple sclerosis functional composite as a clinical trial outcome measure. *Brain* 1999; 122: 871–82.

6. Rudick RA, Polman CH, Cohen JA. Assessing disability progression with the Multiple Sclerosis Functional Composite. *Mult Scler* 2009; 15: 984–97.

7. Balcer LJ, Baier ML, Cohen JA. Contrast letter acuity as a visual component for the Multiple Sclerosis Functional Composite. *Neurology* 2003; 61: 1367–73.

8. Balcer LJ, Galetta SL, Calabresi PA. Natalizumab reduces visual loss in patients with relapsing multiple sclerosis. *Neurology* 2007; 68: 1299–304.

9. Sartori E, Gilles E. Assessment of cognitive dysfunction in multiple sclerosis. *J Neurol Sci* 2006; 245: 169–75.

10. Huijbregts SCJ, Kalkers NF, de Sonneville LMJ, *et al.* Cognitive impairment and decline in different MS subtypes. *J Neurol Sci* 2006; 245: 187–94.

11. Brochet G, Deloire MSA, Bonnet M, *et al.* Should SDMT substitute for PASAT in MSFC? A 5-year longitudinal study. *Mult Scler* 2008; 14: 1242–9.

12. Drake AS, Weinstock-Guttman B, Morrow SA, *et al.* Psychometrics and normative data for the Multiple Sclerosis Functional Composite: replacing the PASAT with the Symbol Digit Modalities Test. *Mult Scler* 2010; 16: 228–37.

13. Morrow SA, O'Connor PW, Polman CH, *et al.* Evaluation of the symbol digit modalities test (SDMT) and the MS neuropsychological screening questionnaire (MSNQ) in natalizumab-treated MS patients over 48 weeks. *Mult Scler* 2010; 16: 1385–92.

14. Schwid SR, Goodman AD, McDermott MP, *et al.* Quantitative functional measures in MS: What is a reliable change? *Neurology* 2002; 58: 1294–6.

15. Kaufman M, Moyer D, Norton J. The significant change for the Timed 25-Foot Walk in the Multiple Sclerosis Functional Composite. *Mult Scler* 2000; 6: 286–90.

16. Bosma LVAE, Kragt JJ, Khaleli Z, *et al.* Progression on the Multiple Sclerosis Functional Composite in multiple sclerosis: what is the optimal cut-off for

the three components? *Mult Scler* 2010; 16: 862–67.

17. Kragt JJ, Van Der Linden FAH, Nielsen JM, *et al.* Clinical impact of 20% worsening on timed 25-foot Walk and 9-hole Peg Test in multiple sclerosis. *Mult Scler* 2006; 12: 594–8.

18. van Winsen LML, Kragt JJ, Hoogervorst ELJ, *et al.* Outcome measurement in multiple sclerosis: detection of clinically relevant improvement. *Mult Scler* 2010; 16: 604–10.

19. Owsley C. Contrast sensitivity. *Ophthalmol Clin N Am* 2003; 16: 171–7.

20. Mills RJ, Young CA, Pallant JF, *et al.* Development of a patient reported outcome scale for fatigue in multiple sclerosis: The Neurological Fatigue Index (NFI-MS). *Health Qual Life Outcomes* 2010; 8: 22.

21. Meads DM, Doward LC, McKenna SP, *et al.* The development and validation of the Unidimensional Fatigue Impact Scale (U-FIS). *Mult Scler* 2009; 15: 1228–8.

22. US Food and Drug Administration. Guidance for Industry. Patient-reported outcome measures: *Use in medical product development to support labeling claims.* 2009. http://www.fda.gov/ downloads/Drugs/Guidance ComplianceRegulatoryInformation/ Guidances/UCM193282.pdf. (Accessed October 10, 2010.)

23. Mehta LR, Schwid SR, Arnold DL, *et al.* Proof of concept studies for tissue-protective agents in multiple sclerosis. *Mult Scler* 2009; 15: 542–6.

24. Healy B, Valsasina P, Fillippi M, *et al.* Sample size requirements for treatment effects using gray matter, white matter and whole brain volume in relapsing–remitting multiple sclerosis. *J Neurol Neurosurg Psychiatry* 2009; 80: 1218–23.

25. Katz R. Biomarkers and Surrogate Markers: *An FDA Perspective. NeuroRx* 2004; 1: 189–95.

26. Fleming TR. Surrogate endpoints and FDA's accelerated approval process. *Health Affairs* 2005; 24: 67–78.

27. Prentice RL. Surrogate endpoints in clinical trials: Definition and Operational Criteria. *Stat Med* 1989; 8: 431–40.

28. Freedman LS, Graubard BI, Schatzkin A. Statistical validation of intermediate endpoints for chronic diseases. *Stat Med* 1992; 11: 167–78.

29. Lin DY, Fleming RT, De Gruttola V. Estimating the proportion of the treatment effect explained by a surrogate marker. *Stat Med* 1997; 16: 1515–27.

30. Molenberghs G, Burzykowski T, Alonso A, Buyse M. A perspective on surrogate endpoints in controlled clinical trials. *Stat Meth Med Res* 2004; 13: 177–206.

31. Fleming TR, DeMets DL. Surrogate end points in clinical trials: are we being misled? *Ann Intern Med* 1996; 125: 605–13.

32. Echt DS, Liebson PR, Mitchell LB, *et al.* Mortality and Morbidity in patients receiving encainide, flecainide, or placebo. *N Engl J Med* 1991; 324: 781–8.

33. Riggs BL, Hodgson ST, O'Fallon WM, *et. al.* Effect of fluoride treatment on the fracture rate in postmenopausal women with osteoporosis. *N Engl J Med* 1990; 322: 802–9.

34. International Chronic Granulomatous Disease Cooperative Study Group. A controlled trial of interferon gamma to prevent infection in chronic granulomatous disease. *N Engl J Med* 1991; 324: 509–16.

35. Temple R. Are surrogate markers adequate to assess cardiovascular disease drugs? *J Am Med Assoc* 1999; 282: 790–5.

Chapter

20

The challenge of demonstrating long-term benefit of disease-modifying therapies in multiple sclerosis

Maria Trojano

Introduction

Scientific advances in understanding multiple sclerosis (MS) pathogenesis have been extraordinary in the last 30 years. We have seen areas of basic scientific research burgeon and as a consequence, the treatment of MS has changed radically. Prior to the early 1990s, management of MS patients was limited to symptomatic treatment without any ability to alter the disease course; since the 1990s, disease-modifying therapies (DMTs) have been approved for patients with relapsing–remitting MS (RRMS) (Chapters 25–28, 30). Numerous randomized, placebo-controlled trials (RCTs) consistently demonstrated that these DMTs alter favorably the short-term course in patients with RRMS[1-7] and clinically isolated syndrome.[8-11] Although these RCTs typically evaluated relapses and brain lesions measured using magnetic resonance imaging (MRI), rather than disability outcomes, most studies also reported a trend toward risk reduction – ranging between 12 and 42% – in confirmed expanded disability status scale (EDSS) progression, after 2–5 years of treatment.[1-7,10] At present, the RCT design is considered the gold standard for providing evidence of short- and medium-term efficacy of preventive and therapeutic interventions in the clinical setting. However, MS is a lifelong, progressively disabling disease with a clinical course evolving over 30 years, and a highly variable prognosis. The vast majority of patients experience an initial RR phase, but, as the disease progresses, recovery tends to be incomplete, the level of disability begins to deteriorate steadily, even in the absence of relapses, and the disease transitions over a median time of about 20 years to the secondary progressive stage (SPMS). Median times from onset to irreversible limitation in ambulation (EDSS 4), unilateral aid required for walking (EDSS 6), and wheelchair-dependency (EDSS 7) were reported to be approximately 8, 20, and 30 years, respectively.[12,13] As a consequence, preventing or delaying development of long-term disability represents the most important goal of therapy. To date, there is no treatment that will reverse established neurological impairment, but there is hope that early treatment may alter the long-term course of MS. Despite the fact that interferon beta (IFNβ) products and glatiramer acetate (GA)

have been licensed for over 15 years, we have no definitive evidence on long-term efficacy, because a definitive method to determine the magnitude and duration of long-term treatment benefit has not been developed.[14] Several study designs, including long-term RCTs, extension trials of short-term RCTs, and non-randomized observational trials (NROTs) have been proposed, but none of them is free from criticisms.[15]

This chapter provides an overview of the range of study designs used to estimate long-term treatment effects of DMTs in MS. Their strengths and weaknesses, and remaining methodological challenges are highlighted and discussed.

Long-term RCTs

Long-term trials that remained randomized and blinded, using a well-matched, untreated control group, and retaining all patients randomized into the trial would provide a definitive answer to long-term efficacy of DMTs. The key principle of this study design is randomization, which reduces biases by making treatment and control groups "equal with respect to all features," except for the treatment assignment.[16] Randomization enhances the internal validity of a study, meaning that the observed difference in outcomes between the study groups can be attributed to the intervention rather than to other factors. This option is not practical, and many would argue not ethical. Long-term RCTs would require a large sample of patients followed for many years with consequent difficulties in maintaining blinding and with retention of patients in the assigned treatment arm. A RCT lasting for 10 years or more may also not be ethical, as the safety and efficacy of DMTs now available has already been demonstrated to the satisfaction of regulatory authorities. Patients who eventually fail treatment are likely to drop out, and the accumulating number of dropouts is likely to occur at different rates in the different trial arms. This will bias estimates of results. Therefore, an ideal RCT, with placebo or active comparator, can last for no more than 3–6 years, if that. The "time to EDSS 4" might be a feasible outcome, given this trials duration,[17] and this might be highly meaningful, given the predictability of disability progression after that milestone is reached.[18,19]

Multiple Sclerosis Therapeutics, Fourth Edition, ed. Jeffrey A. Cohen and Richard A. Rudick. Published by Cambridge University Press.
© Cambridge University Press 2011.

Long-term follow-up (LTFU) studies after RCTs

Open-label LTFU studies[20–23] of patients from the pivotal trials have been undertaken. In these studies, differences in clinical outcomes were compared in patients who received treatment from study inception with those who switched to the active drug 2–3 years later (i.e. patients originally randomized to placebo). As a whole, the results suggest that sustained early treatment in MS patients can delay progression to significant disability and these studies support the concept that early treatment with DMTs has long-lasting effects. However, LTFU studies have significant limitations, including loss of randomization and blinding, incomplete ascertainment, and the absence of an appropriate comparator. After the RCTs, patients were managed in clinical practice by physicians outside the context of a research protocol. For most of these studies[20–22] data were collected retrospectively, in an unblinded context, and after considerable intervals in which patients were not monitored and during which they may have discontinued therapy for long periods, switched therapy, or added other medications to the therapy under study. Moreover, despite efforts to retain study participants, ascertainment was often incomplete with retention rate between 40% and 80%.[20–23] Commonly, patients doing poorly were censored as "failures" or dropped out to seek other treatments. As a result, there is probably an inevitable selection bias favoring retention of "responders" in the long-term cohort remaining in the study. These methodological restrictions limit the interpretation of the results from LTFU studies.[24] Recommendations for the planning of future LTFU studies have recently been published.[19,25] The most important recommendation is that new RCTs include a plan for long-term data collection before the RCT is started. Selection of sites where routine follow-up occurs independently of the RCT, and with a better capacity to maintain long-term patient contact is strongly advised. RCTs must be sufficiently powered to detect differences in disability between the treatment groups over time. The choice of clinically significant, unequivocal outcomes such as the need for assistance to ambulate, are advised. Measures of cognitive function that best predict the medical, social, and economic impacts of MS should be included in the original RCT, so that long-term changes induced by treatment can be better evaluated. The running of high-quality LTFU trials demands a concentrated effort by a team, including trialists, information technology specialists, bioethicists, and clinicians.[26]

Long-term non-randomized observational trials (NROTs)

NROTs include a wide range of study designs, such as prospective and retrospective cohort studies, case-control studies, and cross-sectional studies, with the common feature that any intervention studied is determined by clinical practice and not by the protocol.[27]

Data derived from NROTs may be especially valuable for assessing drug effectiveness in subgroups not studied in RCTs,

Table 20.1. *Comparison between randomized controlled trials (RCTs) and non-randomized observational trials (NROTs)*

RCTs	NROTs
• Test efficacy in highly selected subgroups with the greatest potential for benefit	• Test effectiveness in typical patient population who might potentially benefit
• Randomization determines treatment allocation and addresses known and unknown confounding	• Clinical judgment determines treatment allocation
• Placebo or active drug as comparator	• Known factors can be controlled
• Treatment blinded.	• Usual care as comparator
• Short-term follow-up	• Open label
• Dosage regimen is inflexible	• Long-term follow-up
• One treatment for each patient enrolled	• Dosing is flexible
• Standardized measure of soft outcomes or surrogate outcomes	• Different treatments can be assigned to the same patient
• Extremely costly	• Outcomes are usually more robust and can include rare events
	• Relatively inexpensive

for detecting rare side effects of drugs and drug–drug interactions and for generating hypotheses, establishing questions, and providing indication of the effect sizes for future RCTs.[28] When RCTs are deemed not to be feasible or ethical, properly designed NROTs are an alternative for providing clinically relevant information about the long-term safety and efficacy. Some of the differences between RCTs and NROTs are summarized in Table 20.1. A major strength of NROTs is that they reflect daily clinical practice more closely than do RCTs, both in terms of the heterogeneous patient populations that are included, and the medical interventions that patients receive. This is a major advantage compared with RCTs, where the emphasis on internal validity through standardization and control reduces external validity (i.e. generalizability of conclusions to MS patients other than the original study population).[29] RCTs tend to gather accurate, detailed, and standardized information on highly selected subgroups of patients, treated with a particular drug, at a fixed dosage, with the greatest potential for benefit over a short time, but do not necessarily provide the best answer to drug effectiveness. Therefore, treatment effects under study conditions (efficacy) are demonstrated and a drug is approved by regulatory agencies; its clinical effectiveness in real-life should be tested by NROTs.[30] In this respect, the NROT is currently considered a research tool that provides information complementary to that provided by RCTs.[31]

Nevertheless, controversy sometimes surrounds NROTs, especially if they focus on the intended benefit of a therapy, because this trial design has inherent limitations in its susceptibility to bias and confounding.[32] Two meta-analyses demonstrated that NROTs did not overestimate the treatment effect observed in the corresponding RCTs,[33–34] but there are some examples where NROTs clearly failed to predict findings from RCTs.[35–38] Therefore, a clear understanding of the role of bias and confounding in the interpretation of NROTs and methods that can minimize these effects is important.[39] Failure to recognize the limitations of NROTs in assessing treatment effects can result in use of ineffective treatments, or inappropriate abandonment or limitation of effective treatments.[40–42]

Table 20.2. *Bias and confounding in NROTs*

- **Selection bias:** An error in choosing the individuals to take part in a study causing systematic differences between comparison groups in prognosis or responsiveness to treatment.
- **Recall bias:** Systematic error due to the differences in accuracy or completeness of recall of treatment exposure between comparison groups.
- **Recording bias:** information bias particularly common in administrative data.
- **Detection bias:** Systematic error that occurs when, because of the lack of blinding or related reasons, the measurement methods are consistently different between groups in the study.
- **Confounding:** Systematic error due to the failure to account for the effect of one or more variables that are related to both the causal factor being studied and the outcome, and are not distributed the same between the groups being studied. Confounding occurs when a factor is associated with the use (*confounding by indication*) or avoidance (*confounding by contraindication*) of the treatment, but independently, influences the risk of the outcome of interest.

Table 20.3. *Strategies for reducing selection bias and confounding in NROTs*

- **Matching:** a method to match individual cases (i.e. treated patients) with individual controls on measured background covariates that need to be adjusted for.
- **Stratification:** a method to group subjects into strata on measured background characteristics. Analysis is then performed on each subgroup separately.
- **Multivariate regression analysis:** a method to estimate the association of each independent variable (baseline characteristics and the intervention) with the dependent variable (outcome of interest) after adjusting for the effects of all the other variables.
- **Propensity score:** a measure of a patient's probability of being treated versus control as a function of his/her relevant observed background characteristics. It may be considered as a "balancing score" to reduce the impact of treatment selection bias.
- **Bayesian risk score:** a simple tool for the early prediction, at individual level, of the long-term disease evolution as a function of patient measured background characteristics. It may be used as a "corrective factor" when analyzing treatment effectiveness in observational data.
- **Instrumental variable:** a variable, related to the treatment, but not associated to the outcome, which may be used to create a pseudo-randomization reducing potential measured and unmeasured confounding.
- **Sensitivity analysis:** a method to provide, through simulations, direct estimates of the size and degree of imbalance of a potential unmeasured confounder (hidden bias) needed to negate the results of a study.

Sources of bias and confounding in NROTs

NROTs attempt to estimate the effect of a treatment between groups by comparing outcomes for non-randomized subjects. The principal criticism of this approach is that confounding factors, either known or unknown, may influence the measured association between the intervention of interest and a given outcome (Table 20.2). Differences in outcomes can be due to differences between the patient groups, differences in ascertainment of outcomes, unintended differences in other treatment factors, or to the treatment factor being studied.[40,43] Selection bias is the most frequent systematic error, due to design and execution errors in sampling, selection or allocation methods.[15] Treatment-by-indication bias may arise when patient characteristics influence drug prescription and, at the same time, also relate to outcome, therefore acting as confounders.[44] The reasons why certain patients received a treatment while others did not are often difficult to account for fully, and if these characteristics also affect the outcome, direct comparison of the groups is likely to produce biased conclusions. Patients receiving any treatment will tend to be seen by doctors or other health professionals more frequently than others will, and this may result in the earlier detection of a variety of outcomes.[45] Recall bias can be a problem in NROTs when there is a difference in the reliability of the data collected on treatment exposure between cases that have the disease of interest and controls that do not.[40,46] Finally, both missing data and information censoring can bias NROT results.

Methods to adjust for bias and confounding in NROTs

Several epidemiological and statistical methods are available to deal with confounding, in both design and analytical phases of NROTs (Table 20.3), although one must be aware that some bias may be insurmountable (i.e. absence of blinding is still the major weakness of all observational studies).

Each of these methods has its assumptions, advantages, and limitations.[47]

Within-subject methods (case-only designs) include self-controlled case-series method, case-crossover designs, and case-time-control designs.[15] In these methods, outcomes are compared between periods before and after treatment exposure within the same individuals. These methods are less susceptible to confounding by indication. In fact, in these studies the exposure history of each patient is used as his/her own control, thus eliminating between-person confounding.[48–49] Although within-subject methods may avoid biases resulting from differences between exposed and non-exposed patients, they may have time-trend biases,[50] in that disease severity or activity may change within individuals over time, which could influence the probability of exposure. Limited assessment and correction of this bias are possible by including time-trend controls.[51]

A pre–post-treatment analysis of EDSS change was applied in an observational, unrandomized study[52] in a cohort of 590 RRMS patients in Nova Scotia. Instead of an untreated control group, the authors used DMT-treated patients as their own self-controls. DMT effectiveness was examined by comparing estimated annual changes in EDSS score during the treatment years with those in the years preceding and following the treatment within individuals. The results showed a positive impact of DMTs on disability progression, and more rapid EDSS increase in the years following drug switches and treatment stops.

Matching is the simplest traditional statistical method for adjustment in NROTs. This allows individual cases (i.e. treated patients) to be matched with individual controls that have similar characteristics in order to reduce the effects of these confounding characteristics on the association being investigated. Patients can be matched on one factor (e.g. age), or on many factors. The major limitation of matching[39] is the difficulty finding exact matches between the two groups of patients. Problems finding exact matches increase with the number of factors chosen to match on, and "overmatching" can occur when patients are matched on variables that are associated with the exposure but not with the outcome. Overmatching can reduce the statistical power of a study and, in worst-case scenarios, create a new bias.[53] Matching is most commonly used in case-control studies when there is only a limited number of treated patients and a much larger number of untreated (or control) patients.

Another simple method is *stratification*, which consists of grouping subjects into strata determined by observed background characteristics that are believed to confound the analysis. Treated and control subjects in the same strata are compared directly. Stratification creates subgroups that are more balanced in terms of confounders than the total population and this can result in less biased estimates of the intervention effect.[47] Stratification may be appropriate when there are only one or two confounders that allow easy grouping. However, this method quickly becomes unwieldy if there are multiple confounders, each having multiple categories.[39] Stratification is often combined with regression techniques. Most regression models assume a constant relation between the outcome and intervention across all baseline characteristics, and stratification provides a technique for examining this assumption.[47]

The most common tool for reducing confounding in critical care research is *regression* (i.e. linear, logistic, and proportional hazard regression). Multivariate regression allows for models that include many confounders, which can make it a more appealing method than matching or stratification. After initially examining the relationship between the exposure of interest and the outcome (unadjusted result), variables that are known confounders are then added to the model to provide an effect that is adjusted for these known confounders.[39] Therefore, regression analyses estimate the association of each independent variable (baseline characteristics and the intervention) with the dependent variable (outcome of interest) after adjusting for the effects of all the other variables, so that they provide an adjusted estimate of the intervention effect.[47]

The choice of the exact method of regression analysis (e.g. linear, logistic, and proportional hazard regression) depends on the type of research question being asked and on the type of dependent variable (binary, continuous, or associated with time). If the outcome of interest is continuous, then linear regression is chosen,[54] if it is binary, a logistic regression modeling is most appropriate;[55] in contrast, if the outcome is the time to an event, then a proportional hazards model can be used.[56] It is noteworthy that in multicenter observational studies, involving data from multiple units and/or hospitals, the regression models may need multilevel modeling.[57]

A multivariate Cox proportional hazard model was used to assess gender differences for risk of relapses and disability progression in a cohort of 2570 IFNβ-treated RRMS patients prospectively followed in 15 Italian MS Centers.[58] To adjust for the imbalance of pre-treatment, demographic, and clinical features between the female and male groups, covariates as age, disease duration, EDSS score, and number of relapses in the last year were introduced in the model. The multivariate Cox regression analysis showed that, after adjusting for the effects of all these other variables, male patients had a significant ($P = 0.0097$) lower risk for first relapse and a trend for a higher risk to reach 1 point EDSS progression than female patients. Moreover, the analysis allowed us to demonstrate, also, a significant ($P < 0.001$) higher incidence in EDSS progression for older patients and for those with a longer disease duration at treatment initiation.

However, all the above-mentioned traditional methods of adjustment are limited when there is an extreme imbalance in the background characteristics, and by adjustment for only a finite number of covariates.[59]

These limitations are avoided with the *propensity score (PS) technique*, introduced by Rosenbaum and Rubin in 1983.[60] PS weightings provide a scalar summary measure of the covariate information, and is considered an alternative method for estimating treatment effects when treatment assignment is not random. It is often viewed as a balancing score that is used to reduce the impact of treatment selection bias through the above-mentioned adjustment methods. The PS is a patient's probability of being treated vs. control, as a function of all relevant observed covariates (e.g. age, disease severity) that may be related to post-treatment outcomes.[61] The PS can be derived from a multivariate logistic regression analysis that includes variables likely related to exposure and/or the outcome. PSs range from 0 to 1, with scores close to 1 indicating participant characteristics associated with a high probability of being exposed.[62] Treated and untreated subjects with the same propensity score will have the same distribution of measured baseline covariates. Matching, stratification, or regression adjustment using the PS can be used to produce relatively unbiased estimates of the treatment effects. The most common methods in medical and epidemiological literature are stratification on the PS.[61,63] PS matching,[61] covariate adjustment using the PS,[63,64] and inverse probability of treatment weighting (IPTW) using the PS.[66,67] With all four techniques, the PS is calculated the same way,[68] but once estimated, the PS is applied differently. In some of these methods, the PS is used in analyses as a weight or factor (regression adjustment, IPTW), whereas in others it is used to construct the appropriate comparisons (stratification or matching), but not in the analyses directly.[58] A comparison of the ability of different propensity score models to balance measured variables between treated and untreated subjects was recently performed.[69] The authors found that PS matching and IPTW removed systematic differences between treated and untreated subjects to a greater degree compared with stratification on the PS and covariate adjustment using the PS.

In recent years adjustment techniques based on PS have become increasingly popular and are being widely used in statistical analyses, particularly to test drug effects in many therapeutic areas[70-72] and also in MS[73-75] to evaluate long-term

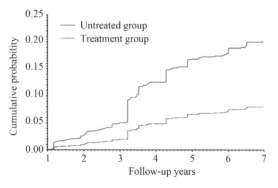

Fig. 20.1. Propensity score-adjusted survival curve for time from first visit to SPMS end-point. Seven-year cumulative probability of reaching the endpoint in never-treated and IFNβ-treated MS patient groups. Cumulative probability represents the estimated proportion of patients reaching the endpoint. (Reproduced with permission from: Trojano *et al. Ann Neurol* 2007.[74])

effectiveness of DMTs. The risk of long-term disability progression according to the length of exposure to IFNβ was assessed in a large cohort of 2090 MS patients prospectively collected by the Italian MS Database Network.[73] Cox proportional hazards regression models were adjusted for PS.[60,76] The analysis demonstrated that risk of one-point EDSS worsening, confirmed at the end of the 8.4-year treatment follow-up period, was reduced by 4–5-fold in patients exposed to IFNβ for more than four years, compared with patients exposed for up to two years.

The impact of IFNβ treatment for up to seven years on times from first visit (or from date of birth) to EDSS 4.0, 6.0, or SPMS, was prospectively evaluated[74] in a large cohort of untreated ($n = 401$) and IFNβ-treated ($n = 1103$) RRMS patients, using an IPTW-PS-adjusted Cox proportional hazards regression model.[77] In this study, the concurrent untreated control group consisted of RRMS patients who refused DMT treatment, planned a pregnancy, had concomitant diseases (i.e. neoplasm, psychiatric diseases, or severe depression) that prevented them from receiving DMTs, discontinued DMT treatment in the first three to six weeks because of clinical or hematological adverse events, or had low disease activity at first presentation. The results of this observational study demonstrated that patients selected to receive IFNβ treatment responded better than those who were untreated. The IFNβ-

treated group showed a highly significant reduction in the incidence of SPMS (Fig. 20.1), EDSS ≥ 4.0 and EDSS ≥ 6.0, compared with untreated patients. Time to SPMS, EDSS ≥ 4.0, and ≥ 6.0 were significantly delayed from first visit by 3.8, 1.7, and 2.2 years, respectively with IFNβ treatment.

More recently, the impact of early vs. delayed IFNβ treatment on disability course was evaluated in a cohort of 2570 RRMS, prospectively followed for up to seven years in 15 Italian MS Centers,[75] using a Cox proportional hazards regression model adjusted for PS quintiles.[61] The results showed early treatment initiation (within one year from disease onset) significantly reduced the risk of reaching the EDSS 4.0 milestone (Fig. 20.2(a)), and one-point worsening in EDSS score (Fig. 20.2(b)) in comparison to a delayed treatment.

There have also been some efforts to generate methods to infer causality from observational data using probabilistic networks such as *Bayesian or belief networks* that use computer modeling to identify plausible causal relationships.[78] A Bayesian risk estimate for multiple sclerosis (BREMS) score, obtained from the Bayesan modeling of the natural history of MS, was recently proposed as a simple tool for the early prediction, at the individual patient level, of the long-term evolution of MS.[79] The BREMS score might be useful to evaluate the effect of therapies in NROTs, facilitating an "a posteriori" subdivision of non-randomized patients on the basis of their different propensity to reach a poor end-point.

A Bayesian analysis was performed in an Irish observational study[80] to establish whether two-year IFNβ treatment delayed disability progression in a cohort of 175 RRMS patients in comparison with a cohort of untreated matched historical control subjects from the Sylvia Lawry Centre for MS. The results supported the use of IFNβ in RRMS even if a number of potential biases such as the use of a historical control group, a retrospective assessment of data and the exclusion of patients who stopped IFNβ during the first two years of treatment, lessened their relevance.

Finally, the *instrumental variable* analysis, an econometric method,[81] was recently used as a pseudo-randomization tool to remove the effects of both observed and hidden bias in NROTs. An instrumental variable is a factor that is related to treatment (e.g. the prescribing physician's preference), but unrelated to observed and unobserved patient risk factors,

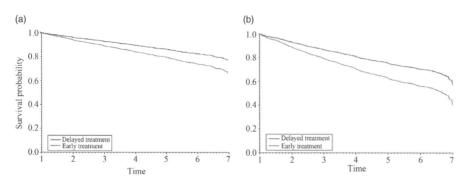

Fig. 20.2. Propensity score-adjusted survival curves for seven-year cumulative probability of reaching end-points in early vs. delayed treatment in MS patient groups. Survival probability represents the estimated proportion of patients who did not reach the end point. Top line indicates delayed treatment group; bottom line indicates early treatment group. (a) Survival curve for sustained EDSS ≥ 4.0; (b) Survival curve for confirmed 1-point worsening of EDSS score. (Reproduced with permission from: Trojano *et al. Ann Neurol* 2009.[75])

and also unrelated to the outcome.[82] The patients are divided according to the levels of this instrumental variable and the outcome is then analyzed. The instrumental variable may lead to an equal distribution of the characteristics in both exposed and non-exposed patients, simulating a random assignment of patients to the exposure of interest[39] and thus reducing potential confounding.[15] Although instrumental variable methods are just beginning to appear in medical literature, the first applications are promising. However, the ability to define an actual instrumental variable remains controversial.[83]

Hidden biases

For all methods, overt biases can be identified, and adjusted by the methods just described. The main limitation of observational studies is that these methods do little or nothing to address hidden biases due to unobserved or unrecorded differences between treated and control patients. Factors that have not been well measured or that are unknown to the investigator cannot be controlled in the design or analysis by any method, except indirectly to the extent that they are associated with the factors that are controlled. In an ideal RCT, randomization prevents hidden biases by equally allocating unmeasured differences equally to the treatment arms, although randomization is not a perfect solution for this problem either, because of potential biases from protocol violations, such as unbalanced withdrawals of patients from the treatment arms, non-adherence by patients, etc. In a non-randomized study, results could be heavily impacted by unknown or unmeasured confounders. Hidden biases may be addressed by *sensitivity analyses*,[84,85] which can be used to estimate the magnitude of a potential unmeasured confounder. Sensitivity analyses use simulations that provide direct estimates of the size and degree of imbalance of the unmeasured confounder needed to negate the results of a study.[74,75,86] A sensitivity analysis[75] was used to show that the positive effect of IFNβ treatment on time to SPMS remained significant under high, imbalanced scenarios because of a potential unmeasured confounder, whereas the end-points EDSS 4 and 6 appeared sensitive to small bias. A finding that could be sensitive to small unmeasured confounders should be interpreted with caution, but should not be dismissed on that basis.[76] Moreover sensitivity analysis does not show that the potential hidden bias is actually present. Finally, to test the sensitivity of results to missing observations in NROTs, the *multiple imputation method* may be used as proposed by Rubin and Schenker.[87]

Conclusions

Demonstration of long-term benefits from treatment in a chronic disease such as MS is still challenging, and the optimal methods are controversial. All study designs have flaws that can threaten external validity (i.e. whether or not the study results are generalizable to other populations) or internal validity (i.e. how the data are gathered and assigned).[88] RCTs remain the gold standard for inferring a "causal" association between

intervention and outcome, but they have significant limitations – they are resource intensive, last for no longer than 2–3 years, include small populations, and the inflexibility of treatment regimens may drive non-adherence or drop-out, which are major sources of error regarding exposure assessment.[89,90] NROTs are less expensive than RCTs, may be especially valuable for answering questions related to long-term or real-world effects, but they are more prone to bias than RCTs. When RCTs are unavailable, impratical, or unethical, NROTs are the only known alternative to ascertain the effects of therapeutic intervention. Therefore, rather than focusing on criticism of NROTs, we should optimize NROTs through more careful and rigorous approaches.[39,90–92]

Several factors should be considered when planning NROTs.[27] First, a careful characterization of the study population, based on a minimum set of inclusion/exclusion criteria, a rigorous choice of primary end-points, and the use of an appropriate concurrent comparator group are of paramount importance. There is consensus that historical controls may introduce an unacceptable risk of false-positive results since natural history studies published in the last 15 years[93,94] suggest that MS is progressing more slowly than previously thought, even if this is due to an apparent epidemiological paradox, known as the Will Rogers phenomenon[95] caused by earlier diagnosis through use of imaging in current diagnostic criteria.[96] Second, efforts should be made to minimize loss to follow-up by selecting sites with capacity to maximize the participants' retention. Third, a prospective, rigorous, prospectively defined protocol should be mandatory. High-quality databases, which eliminate many of the problems inherent in using clinical registries and institutional databases created for other purposes[97,98] should be implemented. Finally, proper statistical analyses, on an intention-to-treat basis,[27] aimed to reduce bias in treatment comparisons should be used. It is important that all relevant confounding factors be identified, measured, and adjusted for using the methods described in this chapter. PS-adjusted analyses, which can create groups of patients who have similar likelihood of receiving a therapy, and sensitivity analyses[60,82] are the most common methods currently used for this purpose.

RCTs and NROTs complement each other, and both are necessary to provide a comprehensive assessment of treatment benefit.[99] NROTs cannot replace RCTs, nor do RCTs make non-randomized studies unnecessary or undesirable.[89] Funding models for research should consider the substantially lower cost, the generalizability, and the timeliness of NROTs in comparison to RCTs.[43] Medical investigators, health authorities, and the pharmaceutical industry all have important roles to play in designing, approving, and performing high-quality long-term studies,[27] which are necessary to determine whether the early effects of a treatment persist and translate into meaningful long-term benefits for MS patients.[100] Importantly, as the MS field enters an era of more potent, but potentially less safe therapies, NROTs will provide crucial safety information that may not be identified by RCTs.

References

1. The IFNβ Multiple Sclerosis Study Group. Interferon beta-1b is effective in relapsing-remitting multiple sclerosis. I. Clinical results of a multicenter, randomized, double-blind, placebo controlled trial. *Neurology* 1993; 43: 655–61.

2. The IFNβ Multiple Sclerosis Study Group and The University of British Columbia MS/MRI Analysis Group. Interferon beta-1b in the treatment of multiple sclerosis: final outcome of the randomized controlled trial. *Neurology* 1995; 45:1277–85.

3. Jacobs LD, Cookfair DL, Rudick RA, et al. Intramuscular interferon beta-1a for disease progression in relapsing multiplesclerosis. *Ann Neurol* 1996; 39:285–94.

4. PRISMS (Prevention of Relapses and Disability by Interferon b-1a Subcutaneously in Multiple Sclerosis) Study Group. Randomised double-blind placebo-controlled study of interferonb-1a in relapsing/remitting multiple sclerosis. *Lancet* 1998; 352:1498–504.

5. PRISMS Study Group and the University of British Columbia MS/MRI Analysis Group. PRISMS-4: long-term efficacy of interferon-beta-1a in relapsing MS. *Neurology* 2001; 56: 1628–36.

6. Johnson KP, Brooks BR, Cohen JA, et al. Copolymer 1 reduces relapse rate and improves disability in relapsing remitting multiple sclerosis: results of a phase III multicenter, double-blind placebo-controlled trial. The Copolymer 1 Multiple Sclerosis Study Group. *Neurology* 1995; 45:1268–76.

7. Polman CH, O'Connor PW, Havrdova E, et al. AFFIRM Investigators. A randomized, placebo-controlled trial of natalizumab for relapsing multiple sclerosis. *N Engl J Med* 2006; 354: 899–910.

8. Jacobs LD, Beck RW, Simon JH et al. Intramuscular interferon beta-1a therapy initiated during a first demyelinating event in multiple sclerosis. CHAMPS Study Group. *N Engl J Med* 2000; 343:898–904.

9. Comi G, Filippi M, Barkhof F et al. Effect of early interferon treatment on conversion to definite multple sclerosis: a randomized study. *Lancet* 2001; 357:1576–82.

10. Kappos L, Polman CH, Freedman MS et al. Treatment with interferon beta-1b delays conversion to clinically definite and McDonald MS in patients with clinically isolated syndrome. *Neurology* 2006; 67:1242–9.

11. Kappos L, Freedman MS, Polman CH et al. Effect of early versus delayed interferon beta-1b treatment on disability after a first clinical event suggestive of multiple sclerosis: a 3-year follow-up analysis of the BENEFIT study. *Lancet* 2007; 370:389–97.

12. Weinshenker BG, Bass B, Rice GP, et al. The natural history of multiple sclerosis: a geographically based study. I. Clinical course and disability. *Brain* 1989; 112:133–46.

13. Confavreux C, Vukusic S, Moreau T et al. Relapses and progression of disability in multiple sclerosis. *N Engl J Med* 2000; 343:1430–8.

14. Noseworthy JH. The challenge of long term studies in multiple sclerosis: use of pooled data, historical controls and observational studies to determine efficacy. In Cohen JA, Rudick RA eds. *Multiple Sclerosis Therapeutics.* Cambridge, UK: Cambridge University Press, 2006; 319–30.

15. Lu CY. Observational studies: a review of study designs, challenges and strategies to reduce confounding. *Int J Clin Pract.* 2009; 63:691–7.

16. Collins R, MacMahon S. Reliable assessment of the effects of treatment on mortality and major morbidity, I. Clinical trials. *Lancet* 2001; 357: 373–80.

17. Carroll WM. Clinical trials of multiple sclerosis therapies: improvements to demonstrate long-term patient benefit. *Mult Scler* 2009; 15:951–8.

18. Confavreux, C, Vukusic, S. Natural history of multiple sclerosis: a unifying concept. *Brain* 2006; 129:606–16.

19. Kremenchutzky, M, Rice, GP, Baskerville, J, Wingerchuk, DM, Ebers, GC. The natural history of multiple sclerosis: a geographically based study 9: observations on the progressive phase of the disease. *Brain* 2006; 129:584–94.

20. Bermel RA, Weinstock-Guttman B, Bourdette D et al. Intramuscular interferon beta-1a therapy in patients with relapsing-remitting multiple sclerosis: a 15-year follow-up study. *Mult Scler* 2010; 16:588–96.

21. Kappos L, Traboulsee A, Constantinescu C et al. Long-term subcutaneous interferon beta-1a therapy in patients with relapsing–remitting MS. *Neurology* 2006; 67:944–53.

22. Ebers GC, Rice G, Konieczny A, et al. The interferon beta-1b 16-year long-term follow-up study: the final results. *Neurology* 2006; 66 (Suppl. 2):A32.

23. Ford C, Goodman AD, Johnson K et al. Continuous long-term immunomodulatory therapy in relapsing multiple sclerosis: results from the 15-year analysis of the US prospective open-label study of glatiramer acetate. *Mult Scler* 2010; 16:342–50.

24. Noseworthy JH. How much can we learn from long-term extension trials in multiple sclerosis? *Neurology* 2006 26; 67:930–1.

25. Ebers GC, Reder AT, Traboulsee A, et al. Investigators of the 16-Year Long-Term Follow-Up Study. Long-term follow-up of the original interferon-beta1b trial in multiple sclerosis: design and lessons from a 16-year observational study. *Clin Ther* 2009; 31:1724–36.

26. Nussenblatt RB, Meinert CL. The status of clinical trials: cause for concern. *J Transl Med* 2010; 8:65.

27. Yang W, Zilov A, Soewondo P, Bech OM, Sekkal F, Home PD. Observational studies: going beyond the boundaries of randomized controlled trials. *Diabetes Res Clin Pract* 2010; 88(Suppl 1):S3–9.

28. Noordzij M, Dekker FW, Zoccali C, Jager KJ. Study designs in clinical research. *Nephron Clin Pract* 2009; 113(3):c218–21.

29. Dekkers OM, von Elm E, Algra A, Romijn JA, Vandenbroucke JP. How to assess the external validity of therapeutic trials: a conceptual approach. *Int J Epidemiol* 2010; 39: 89–94.

30. Comber H, Perry IJ. Observational studies for intervention assessment. *Lancet* 2001; 357:2141–2.

31. McKee M, Britton A, Black N, McPherson K, Sanderson C, Bain C. Methods in health services research.

Interpreting the evidence: choosing between randomised and non-randomised studies. *BMJ* 1999; 319:312–15.

32. Rochon PA, Gurwitz JH, Sykora K, *et al.* Reader's guide to critical appraisal of cohort studies:1. Role and design. *BMJ* 2005; 330:895–7.

33. Benson K, Hartz AJ. A comparison of observational studies and randomized, controlled trials. *N Engl J Med* 2000; 342:1878–86.

34. Concato J, Shah N, Horwitz RI. Randomized, controlled trials, observational studies, and the hierarchy of research designs. *N Engl J Med* 2000; 342:1887–92.

35. Alpha-Tocopherol, Beta Carotene Cancer Prevention Study Group. The effect of vitamin E and beta carotene on the incidence of lung cancer and other cancers in male smokers. *N Engl J Med* 1994; 330:1029–35.

36. Yusuf S, Dagenais G, Pogue J, Bosch J, Sleight P. Vitamin E supplementation and cardiovascular events in high risk patients. The Heart Outcomes Prevention Evaluation Study Investigators. *N Engl J Med* 2000; 342:154–60.

37. Ray WA. Evaluating medication effects outside of clinical trials: new-user designs. *Am J Epidemiol* 2003; 158: 915–20.

38. Stampfer M. Commentary: hormones and heart disease: do trials and observational studies address different questions? *Int J Epidemiol* 2004; 33:454–5.

39. Wunsch H, Linde-Zwirbleb WT, Angus DC. Methods to adjust for bias and confounding in critical care health services research involving observational data. *J Crit Care* 2006; 21(1):1–7.

40. MacMahon S, Collins R. Reliable assessment of the effects of treatment on mortality and major morbidity, II: observational studies. *Lancet* 2001; 357:455–62.

41. Hennekens CH, Buring JE, Manson JE, *et al.* Lack of effect of long term supplementation with beta carotene on the incidence of malignant neoplasms and cardiovascular disease. *N Engl J Med* 1996; 334:1145–9.

42. Ad Hoc Subcommittee of the Liaison Committee of the World Health Organisation and the International Society of Hypertension. Effects of calcium antagonists on the risks of coronary heart disease, cancer and bleeding. *J Hypertens* 1997; 15: 105–15.

43. Wolfe RA. Observational studies are just as effective as randomized clinical trials. *Blood Purif* 2000; 18:323–6.

44. Reeves GK, Cox DR, Darby SC, Whitley E: Some aspects of measurement error in explanatory variables for continous and binary regression models. *Stat Med* 1988; 17:2157–77.

45. Bar-Oz B, Moretti ME, Mareels G, Van Tittelboom T, Koren G. Reporting bias in retrospective ascertainment of drug-induced embryopathy. *Lancet* 1999; 354:1700–1.

46. Swan SH, Shaw GM, Schulman J. Reporting and selection bias in case-control studies of congenital malformations. *Epidemiology* 1992; 3:356–63.

47. Normand SL, Sykora K, Li P, Mamdani M, Rochon PA, Anderson GM. Readers guide to critical appraisal of cohort studies: 3. Analytical strategies to reduce confounding. *BMJ* 2005; 330: 1021–3.

48. Maclure M. The case-crossover design: a method for studying transient effects on the risk of acute events. *Am J Epidemiol* 1991; 133:144–53.

49. Whitaker HJ, Farrington CP, Spiessens B, Musonda P. Tutorial in biostatistics: the self-controlled case series method. *Stat Med* 2006; 25:1768–97.

50. Schneeweiss S, Sturmer T, Maclure M. Case-crossover and case time-control designs as alternatives in pharmacoepidemiologic research. *Pharmacoepidemiol Drug Saf* 1997; 6 (Suppl. 3):S51–9.

51. Suissa S. The case–time–control design: further assumptions and conditions. *Epidemiology* 1998; 9:441–5.

52. Brown MG, Kirby S, Skedgel C *et al.* How effective are disease modifying drugs in delaying progression in relapsing-onset MS? *Neurology* 2007; 69:1498–507.

53. Day NE, Byar DP, Green SB. Over-adjustment in case-control studies. *Am J Epidemiol* 1980; 112: 696–706.

54. Schwann TA, Habib RH, Zacharias A, *et al.* Effects of body size on operative, intermediate, and long-term outcomes after coronary artery bypass operation. *Ann Thorac Surg* 2001; 71:521–31.

55. Milbrandt EB, Kersten A, Kong L, *et al.* Haloperidol use is associated with lower hospital mortality in mechanically ventilated patients. *Crit Care Med* 2005; 33:226–9.

56. Ely EW, Shintani A, Truman B, *et al.* Delirium as a predictor of mortality in mechanically ventilated patients in the intensive care unit. *J Am Med Assoc* 2004; 291:1753–62.

57. Goldstein H, Browne W, Rasbash J. Multilevel modelling of medical data. *Stat Med* 2002; 21:3291–315.

58. Trojano M, Pellegrini F, Paolicelli D, *et al.* Post-marketing of disease modifying drugs in multiple sclerosis: an exploratory analysis of gender effect in interferon beta treatment. *J Neurol Sci* 2009; 286:109–13.

59. D'Agostino RB Sr, Kwan H. Measuring effectiveness: what to expect without a randomized control group. *Med Care* 1995; 33(4 suppl):AS95–105.

60. Rosenbaum PR, Rubin DB. The central role of the propensity score in observational studies for causal effects. *Biometrika* 1983; 70:41–55.

61. D'Agostino RB Jr. Propensity score methods for bias reduction in the comparison of a treatment to a non-randomized control group. *Stat Med* 1998; 17:2265–81.

62. Rosenbaum PR. Propensity score. In Armitage P, Colton T, eds. *Encyclopedia of Biostatistics*. vol 5. New York: Wiley, 1998; 3551–5.

63. Rubin, D. B. Estimating causal effects from large data sets using propensity scores. *Ann InternMed* 127;1997 (Part 2):757–63.

64. Weitzen S, Lapane KL, Toledano AY, Hume AL, Mor V. Principles for modeling propensity scores in medical research: a systematic literature review. *Pharmacoepidemiol Drug Saf* 2004; 13:841–53.

65. Shah BR, Laupacis A, Hux JE, Austin PC. Propensity score methods give similar results to traditional regression modeling in observational studies: a systematic review. *J Clin Epidemiol* 2005; 58:550–559.

66. Rosenbaum PR. Model-based direct adjustment. *J Am Stat* 1987; 82:387–94.

67. Linden A, Adams JL. Evaluating health management programmes over time:

application of propensity score-based weighting to longitudinal data. *J Eval Clin Pract* 2010; 16:180–5.

68. Yanovitzky I, Zanutto E, Hornik R. Estimating causal effects of public health education campaigns using propensity score methodology. *Eval Prog Plann* 28, 2005; 209–20.

69. Austin PC. The relative ability of different propensity score methods to balance measured covariates between treated and untreated subjects in observational studies. *Med Decis Making* 2009; 29:661–77.

70. Glynn RJ, Schneeweiss S, Stürmer T. Indications for propensity scores and review of their use in pharmacoepidemiology. *Basic Clin Pharmacol Toxicol* 2006; 98:253–9.

71. Gum PA, Thamilarasan M, Watanabe J, Blackstone EH, Lauer MS. Aspirin use and all-cause mortality among patients being evaluated for known or suspected coronary artery disease: a propensity analysis. *J Am Med Assoc* 2001; 286:1187–94.

72. Ko DT, Chiu M, Austin PC, Bowen J, Cohen EA, Tu JV. Safety and effectiveness of drug-eluting stents among diabetic patients: A propensity analysis. *Am Heart J* 2008; 156:125–34.

73. Trojano M, Russo P, Fuiani A, et al. The Italian Multiple Sclerosis Database Network (MSDN): the risk of worsening according to IFNb exposure in multiple sclerosis. *Mult Scler* 2006; 12:1–8.

74. Trojano M, Pellegrini F, Fuiani A, et al. New natural history of Interferon-β-treated relapsing Multiple Sclerosis. *Ann Neurol* 2007; 61:300–6.

75. Trojano M, Pellegrini F, Paolicelli D, et al. Real-life impact of early interferonβ-therapy in relapsing multiple sclerosis. *Ann Neurol* 2009; 66:513–20.

76. Braitman LE, Rosenbaum PR. Rare outcomes, common treatments: analytic strategies using propensity scores. *Ann Intern Med* 2002; 137: 693–5.

77. Lunceford JK, Davidian M. Stratification and weighting via the propensity score in estimation of causal treatment effects: a comparative study. *Stat Med* 2004; 23:2937–60.

78. Cowell RG, Dawid AP, Lauritzen SL, Spiegelhalter DJ. *Probabilistic Networks and Expert Systems*. New York (NY): Springer-Verlag; 1999.

79. Bergamaschi R, Quaglini S, Trojano M, Amato MP et al. Early prediction of the long term evolution of multiple sclerosis: the Bayesian Risk estimate for Multiple Sclerosis (BREMS). *J Neurosurg Neurol Pscyhiatr* 2007; 78:757–9.

80. O'Rourke K, Walsh C, Hutchinson M. Outcome of beta-interferon treatment in relapsing-remitting multiple sclerosis: a Bayesian analysis. *J Neurol* 2007; 254:1547–54.

81. Greenland S. An introduction to instrumental variables for epidemiologists. *Int J Epidemiol* 2000; 29:722–9.

82. Brookhart MA, Wang PS, Solomon DH, Schneeweiss S. Evaluating short-term drug effects using a physician-specific prescribing preference as an instrumental variable. *Epidemiology* 2006; 17:268–75.

83. McClellan M, McNeil BJ, Newhouse JP. Does more intensive treatment of acute myocardial infarction in the elderly reduce mortality? Analysis using instrumental variables. *J Am Med Assoc* 1994; 272:859–66.

84. Rosenbaum PR. Discussing hidden bias in observational studies. *Ann Intern Med* 1991; 115:901–5.

85. Lin DY, Psaty BM, Krommal RA. Assessing the sensitivity of regression results to unmeasured confounders in observational studies. *Biometrics* 1998; 54:948–63.

86. Schneeweiss S, Wang PS. Association between SSRI use and hip fractures and the effect of residual confounding bias in claims database studies. *J Clin Psychopharmacol* 2004; 24:632–8.

87. Rubin DB, Schenker N. Multiple imputation in health-care databases: an overview and some applications. *Stat Med* 1991; 10:585–98.

88. Rubin DB. The design versus the analysis of observational studies for causal effects: parallels with the design of randomized studies. *Stat Med* 2007; 26:20–36.

89. Sørensen HT, Lash TL, Rothman KJ. Beyond randomized controlled trials: a

critical comparison of trials with nonrandomized studies. *Hepatology* 2006; 44:1075–82.

90. Black N. Why we need observational studies to evaluate the effectiveness of health care. *BMJ* 1996; 312:1215–18.

91. Horwitz RI, Viscoli CM, Clemens JD, Sadock RT. Developing improved observational methods for evaluating therapeutic effectiveness. *Am J Med* 1990; 89:630–8.

92. Vandenbroucke JP, von Elm E, Altman DG, et al. STROBE initiative. Strengthening the Reporting of Observational Studies in Epidemiology (STROBE): explanation and elaboration. *Ann Intern Med* 2007; 147:W163–94.

93. Sormani MP, Tintorè M, Rovaris M et al. Will Rogers phenomenon in multiple sclerosis. *Ann Neurol* 2008; 64:428–33.

94. Pittock SJ, Mayr WT, McClelland RL, et al. Disability profile of MS did not change over l0 years in a population-based prevalence cohort. *Neurology* 2004; 62:601–6.

95. Tremlett H, Paty D, Devonshire V. Disability progression in multiple sclerosis is slower than previously reported. *Neurology* 2006; 66:172–7.

96. McDonald WI, Compston A, Edan G, et al. Recommended diagnostic criteria for multiple sclerosis: guidelines from the International Panel on the Diagnosis of Multiple Sclerosis. *Ann Neurol* 2001; 50:121–7.

97. Padkin A, Rowan K, Black N. Using high quality clinical databases to complement the results of randomised controlled trials: the case of recombinant human activated protein C. *BMJ* 2001; 323:923–6.

98. Black N, Payne M. Improving the use of clinical databases. *BMJ* 2002; 324: 1194.

99. Dobre D, van Veldhuisen DJ, deJongste MJL, et al. The contribution of observational studies to the knowledge of drug effectiveness in heart failure. *Br J Clin Pharmacol* 2007 64:4 406–14.

100. Sormani MP, Bonzano L, Roccatagliata L, et al. Surrogate endpoints for EDSS worsening in multiple sclerosis. A meta-analytic approach. *Neurology* 2010; 75:302–9.

Chapter

21

The growing need for alternative clinical trial designs for multiple sclerosis

Stephen C. Reingold, Henry F. McFarland, and A. John Petkau

Introduction

Prior to the early 1980s, most multiple sclerosis (MS) clinical trials were observational, without appropriate controls and with little attention paid to the fluctuating natural history of MS. Consensus developed at a 1982 international conference on MS trials recommended that Phase 3 clinical trials for MS should be randomized, blinded, and placebo-controlled.[1] The relative benefits and safety of multiple agents for relapsing forms of MS, "worsening" disease, "clinically isolated syndromes," and symptomatic management have since been shown using such studies.

MS clinical trials follow a pattern that begins with mechanistic (including preclinical) studies, continues into toxicity and safety studies (Phase 1), through preliminary and proof-of-concept exploratory studies (Phase 2) and then into registration studies (Phase 3). Biological and imaging markers have become standard primary outcomes in Phase 1 and 2 studies but have been restricted to secondary or exploratory outcomes in Phase 3 studies, as regulatory agencies continue to require evidence based on clinical outcomes for pivotal studies.

The widespread use of disease-modifying treatments for MS since 1993 not only has changed short- and potentially long-term outcomes for people with MS, but has also altered the ability to undertake clinical trials using established approaches.[2] Use of approved therapies for individuals with active disease has led to recruitment of subjects with less severe disease into new trials, often resulting in subjects with less disease activity than in the past. This lower frequency of events in patients entered into contemporary clinical trials has rendered popular outcomes less sensitive to change over reasonable time-frames and thus has had an impact on the statistical power of studies.

Nonetheless, the incomplete control of disease by available agents, high cost, associated side effects and inconvenience, and the fact that many individuals with MS (advanced secondary progressive, primary progressive patients) remain without proven safe and effective therapy mean that new therapies must be developed. New paradigms are needed to make the therapeutic development process faster, more efficient, and more cost-effective, including trials that use new and more efficient designs and outcomes, are shorter in duration, use

fewer subjects, and reduce or eliminate the reliance on placebo-treated groups to demonstrate safety and efficacy.[3]

Alternative clinical trial design strategies for MS: a theoretical approach

Alternatives to traditional clinical trial designs in MS must be considered as theoretical since virtually none has been tested sufficiently, if at all, in MS, and there is no assurance a priori that any will prove to be practical or ethical, or convey advantages over current MS clinical trial designs. Most alternative approaches lack the endorsement of regulatory bodies anywhere in the world, although draft guidelines for adaptive designs have recently been circulated by the US Food and Drug Administration.[4] To move alternative design strategies forward, alternative designs need to be evaluated in Phase 2 exploratory trials, where less might be at stake for investigators and sponsors, and where new design approaches might be tested sufficiently to allow consideration for subsequent Phase 3 registration studies.

Designs that reduce reliance upon placebos

The placebo problem

A mainstay of current MS clinical trial conduct is the comparison of randomized groups of patients using experimental therapy and a placebo. Placebo-controlled trials can provide clear efficacy and safety outcomes for new agents and there has been little sympathy among regulatory agencies for relaxing the requirement for such studies, especially in pivotal studies.[5]

However, with the advent of multiple approved therapies, fewer patients (and physicians) are willing to participate in a study where there is a chance that subjects will receive placebo and thus remain untreated. For studies of relapsing forms of MS in populations where approved therapy is available, the problem is clearly demonstrated by the difficulty that recent placebo-controlled clinical trials have had to recruit subjects, particularly in large academically based clinical practices where there is increasing competition for subjects to fulfill obligations for multiple ongoing studies. The result is significantly longer

Multiple Sclerosis Therapeutics, Fourth Edition, ed. Jeffrey A. Cohen and Richard A. Rudick. Published by Cambridge University Press.
© Cambridge University Press 2011.

enrollment periods, with consequent added costs and significant drop-out rates as subjects seek available therapy rather than continue to participate in experimental protocols. Recruitment delays can lead to extended time on an inactive placebo treatment for some patients, if all patients remain on trial medication and blinded until the last patient enrolled completes the trial. Sponsors and investigators increasingly resort to aggressive advertising to find patients and there is an increasing trend to recruit clinical centers from locations around the world that have not traditionally participated in such studies. There may be regional or site-specific differences in the performance of clinical centers in global clinical trials that could compromise trial outcomes or the generalizability of results, and these need to be monitored and accounted for in trial conduct and interpretation of results.

Use of placebo-controlled trials when approved therapies are available have been considered to be unethical since the fifth revision of the Helsinki Declaration, because active therapy is generally withheld.[5,6] A Task Force of the US National Multiple Sclerosis Society suggested that studies using placebos could be done ethically if patients actively decline available therapy for whatever reason.[7,8] While partially successful in trials in recent years, this creates a special group of patients who may be enrolled – "active decliners" – that could make results not easily generalized to the larger MS population. Additionally, this approach has been questioned by some Institutional Review Boards, which do not accept the logic or ethics of requiring that patients actively decline available therapy to participate in a prospective trial.[3] An alternative strategy is to recruit patients who have failed approved therapies. Even if the criteria for failure can be clearly defined, the results from trials that recruit non-responders to approved therapies may not reflect the response in a population of treatment naive patients. Finally, some studies recruit for patients in regions of the world where approved therapies are not readily available, raising additional ethical issues.[7,8]

Unbalanced randomization and deferred treatment to reduce reliance upon placebo

If placebo must be used, it may be possible to limit the number of subjects exposed to placebo by unbalanced randomization, in which fewer subjects are randomized onto placebo than onto experimental therapy. Alternatively, in deferred treatment studies, after an intermediate pre-specified time-point, patients initially randomized to placebo can be re-randomized to active treatment arms thereby reducing the time of exposure to placebo. Such a design allows for a period of comparison between the experimental arms and placebo and increases the number of patients receiving experimental therapy, which can increase the likelihood of identifying treatment-related adverse events. Deferred treatment designs require that, at a predetermined intermediate time point, there is acceptable safety in the treatment arms and no signal that suggests patients on experimental therapy are demonstrating less efficacy than those on

placebo. As an additional benefit, information may be gained in a prospectively planned analysis of potential differences in efficacy from early treatment vs. delayed treatment with the experimental therapy. Usually such data are gathered only from Phase 4 post-approval studies in which there is often significant compromise of quality because of differential patient dropout after the completion of a Phase 3 study.

While such strategies could increase the practical ability to recruit subjects and reduce the ethical burden of placebo when approved therapies exist, there may still be concern that even abbreviated placebo use before initiating therapy may be harmful. Additionally, short-term placebo-controlled studies in MS will not necessarily reveal efficacy if the onset of treatment effect is delayed after therapy initiation and may not allow for adequate collection of safety data if safety is a function of duration of use or cumulative dosing.

Dose–response designs that eliminate a placebo group

It could, in theory, be possible to replace a placebo arm with a treatment arm in which patients are exposed to a considerably lower dose of active therapy that is not expected to be maximally effective, but is expected to show some benefit. If there is a statistically significant difference between outcomes for the low dose and higher dose arms, this provides data on dose-related toxicity and efficacy without a placebo population and can be informative for determining dosing to be used in subsequent registration studies. Dose-related information can also be obtained using three or more arms with low, intermediate, and full dose treatments. The efficacy assessment can be based on the data from all arms with a test for trend that provides a sensitive assessment for a dose–response relationship. However, if lower dose(s) lack efficacy, patients are still exposed to inactive therapy, as with placebo. If it can be determined early that lower dose(s) have therapeutic value, it might be ethical to dispense with placebo in further studies, especially if there is a need to assess risk/benefit of lower vs. higher doses.

Use of "virtual placebos"

Creating a "virtual placebo" cohort using extant data from natural history and placebo-controlled studies could reduce the need for, or even replace, placebo groups in future studies. A virtual placebo requires an adequate database of previous studies, the ability to conduct valid meta-analyses of individual datasets to create a useful virtual placebo model, and is dependent upon the assumption that patients to be treated in the planned trial will show similar disease outcomes as the patients treated in those past studies. Unfortunately, recent experience suggests that patient outcomes from past studies may be substantially different from outcomes in more contemporary studies and thus may be of limited value for designing virtual placebos or for accurate modeling of required sample sizes. Relapse rates at baseline in the first Phase 3 studies of new therapies for relapsing forms of MS were higher than they are currently for what seem to be the same patient phenotypes, making it difficult to predict placebo behavior in a new study based on past data. Even nearly simultaneous data collected from different locales may exhibit critical differences in placebo activity in what appear to be identical patient populations, as was exhibited by the baseline relapse rate in patients with secondary progressive disease from the parallel North America and European studies of interferon β-1b.[9] Because of the potentially misleading nature of historical compared with contemporary controls, it remains to be seen whether efforts to develop virtual placebos will help to reduce the reliance upon placebo groups in prospective trials. Despite the potential attractiveness of a virtual placebo group, it is unlikely that any database will contain sufficient data to allow the multiple variables of patients entering a prospective clinical trial to be controlled adequately.

Designs that use composite, multiple, or combined outcomes to reduce sample size and/or shorten studies

Most MS clinical trials have employed a single primary outcome measure, usually clinical in nature, for Phase 3 studies. Acceptable clinical outcomes depend on the validity of the measure(s) and the expected event rate over the course of the trial. An outcome with a low expected event rate is less likely to show differences between groups with any therapeutic intervention. Composite outcomes based on measures of multiple distinct clinical domains can increase the number of expected events in the course of a trial and could potentially reduce both sample size and study duration and could have advantages over single outcomes.[10,11] In fact, the Kurtzke Expanded Disability Status Scale (EDSS), a composite score measuring disability, has been used in numerous MS trials as a primary or secondary outcome measure.[12] The EDSS, however, overemphasizes ambulation, is non-linear and relatively insensitive to change over time, and thus has not been viewed as the most satisfactory of composite end-points for disability in MS trials. There is a need for better composite end-points if the goal of efficiency is to be met.

In a useful composite outcome, the contributing clinical domains need to be meaningful and a change in the composite should signal a meaningful change in clinical outcome. Individual domains that make up a composite should be weighted appropriately, since some contributing elements could have more clinical or statistical meaning than others.[13,14] Weighting can be done implicitly, as with the EDSS which is obtained from the functional system scores of the neurological examination, or explicitly, when a composite is obtained as a linear combination of the outcome measures describing the individual clinical domains, as with the Multiple Sclerosis Functional Composite (MSFC), an alternative composite measure for disability.[15,16] The MSFC was used as a primary outcome in a controlled clinical trial of interferon β-1a for secondary progressive MS, allowing a shorter trial duration than projected to be needed with

EDSS as the primary outcome.[17] The study showed a statistically significant impact of slowing of progression of disability of interferon ß-1a against placebo using the composite "z-score" of the MSFC, while there was no effect seen on change in disability measured by the EDSS over the same time period. However, the MSFC has not been accepted as valid by regulators, in part because of the view that the z-score from the MSFC in itself is not a clinically meaningful outcome,

Rather than using a pre-specified composite outcome such as the EDSS or the MSFC, information from multiple clinical outcomes can be combined into an overall assessment of efficacy. The simplest general approach is to compare each of the individual outcomes, controlling the Type I error with the Bonferroni or a more sophisticated multiple comparison procedure.[18,19] Alternatively, clinical judgment may allow a meaningful combined outcome to be defined. For example, in the Phase 2 trial of weekly low dose oral methotrexate in chronic progressive MS, "treatment failure" was defined by a specified change on any of the EDSS, the ambulation index, the box and block test, or the 9-hole peg test.[20] Similarly, "without disease activity," a combined outcome reflecting a combination of clinical and imaging outcomes, was shown in clinical studies of natalizumab in relapsing forms of MS to be statistically significantly impacted by therapy.[21]

Statistical strategies for creating combined outcomes may also be used. A simple method, only applicable if all the outcomes are continuous or ordinal, ranks each outcome across treatment groups and then sums the ranks for each patient across the outcomes to determine their combined (rank sum) score.[13,22] A more generally applicable approach combines z statistics comparing the treatment groups on the individual outcomes into a global test statistic. The "ordinary least squares method" uses the simple average of these z statistics, thus more heavily weighting outcomes with less variability across patients.[11,13,23] Studies of mitoxantone in "worsening MS" used such a combined outcome (based on five outcomes) and the results of these studies gained regulatory approval for the product.[24] Various generalizations of this global test statistic approach have been studied.[13,25,26] With this approach, if the null hypothesis of no therapeutic effect is rejected, one can then go on to identify individual outcomes (or collections of outcomes) that also exhibit a significant effect. Application of the "closed testing principle" provides a stepwise procedure for testing all the null hypotheses of possible interest while maintaining strong control of the overall Type 1 error [27] as was done in the mitoxantrone trial.[24]

Adaptive randomization schemes

In most traditional clinical trial designs, patients are randomized at a preset proportional rate between study arms, and this treatment allocation does not change during recruitment for the trial. However, randomization schemes that adapt to developing departures from the target allocation ("treatment-adaptive" randomization) or imbalances in prognostic baseline covariates ("covariate-adaptive" randomization) are sometimes employed. Less frequently used are schemes in which results seen early in a study that point to benefits between groups, lead to changes in the subsequent randomization allocation while the study is still enrolling patients ("response-adaptive" randomization).[28] Such schemes take advantage of early results in a clinical trial to allocate more patients than initially intended to the treatment that is performing better and may help address ethical concerns about long use of placebo controls.

Response-adaptive randomization

Response-adaptive randomization is most appropriate for studies in which the biological effect of the test agent is expected to have a relatively early impact on outcomes, so that there is adequate on-treatment data in hand from the early-enrolled subjects to make randomization decisions on a still-enrolling population. To implement this strategy, there must be an early analysis of data in an unblinded fashion, requiring that an independent Data Monitoring Committee (DMC) have access to unblinded data to make recommendations regarding randomization patterns while not unblinding study investigators and sponsors. Response-adaptive randomization is often used in Phase 1 and early Phase 2 studies, but is much less common in late Phase 2 and Phase 3, in part because many questions remain open about how to carry out statistical inferences for such designs.[29–31]

Deferred randomization

If high-quality, well-monitored "run-in" baseline data can be obtained from an untreated study population prior to randomization, it might be possible to reduce sample size because of a better understanding of the magnitude of expected treatment effect on the patients. This approach can also help to identify patients who may be expected to be more responsive to the experimental therapy based on pretreatment clinical, imaging, or biological activity, enriching the study population for patients expected to be high responders, increasing the study power and reducing the required sample size. Collecting more extensive "run-in" data also allows for more precise estimation of average changes over time and enhances covariate adjustment at the end of the study, leading to more sensitive assessments of the treatment effect.

Non-inferiority and superiority studies to provide direct comparison among therapies

Trials in which an experimental therapy is compared only with placebo do not permit an understanding of the value of new therapies relative to existing approved therapies, a comparison that is increasingly important to regulators and important to informed therapeutic decision-making. Comparison of the efficacy of therapies tested only in separate studies is often of little value. Modern MS clinical trials need to consider the inclusion of an approved therapy comparator arm, either in the course

of clinical development, or less desirably, in post-marketing Phase 4 trials.[32]

Head-to-head clinical studies can provide information on the relative performance to two agents. The EVIDENCE (evidence for interferon dose response: European–North American comparative efficacy) study used a superiority design successfully to compare efficacy and safety of two interferon ß-1a products in relapsing forms of MS.[33] This was done to facilitate United States regulatory approval for an agent that had been on the market in Europe but not in the USA, because of provisions related to the "orphan drug" regulations that prevented marketing of the agent in the USA in the absence of demonstration of superiority compared to an already-marketed agent.

However, this approach generally creates problems of sample size. The targeted magnitude of the difference in outcomes is likely to be much smaller for an experimental agent tested against a partially effective agent in a superiority study as opposed to an ineffective placebo, so an appropriate study power will require a much larger sample size. Non-inferiority studies may require even larger samples sizes and since there may be no formal evidence that the active "control" therapy in the trial in fact has significant therapeutic effect in the specific study population and environment – something that can usually only be determined in a placebo-controlled study – interpretation of a non-inferiority trial can be difficult. Thus, the benefits of active control studies might be outweighed by the problems of recruiting (and funding) an adequate study sample.

Use of surrogate end-points to shorten the duration and size of a clinical trial

MS therapeutic trial outcomes are largely clinical, relating to relapse parameters and progression of disability. Because of the relatively slow accumulation of events, especially those related to disability, trials must either be of long duration or have very large study cohorts. If biological surrogate end-points could validly predict treatment effects on longer-term clinical end-points, trials might be shorter, with reduced sample size.

A true surrogate is not the same as a biomarker for disease, which is simply a non-clinical adjunctive measure that correlates with clinical disease activity. For a surrogate to serve as a replacement for a clinical outcome of interest, it must predict change on that clinical outcome, must be impacted on by treatment through the same biological mechanisms that impact on that clinical outcome (Fig. 21.1) and must be applicable (and demonstrated) across classes of therapeutic intervention, not just a single agent or class of agents.[34,35]

There are no current validated surrogates for clinical outcomes for MS, even though this has been a major area of discussion for several years. However, most large-scale MS clinical trials are collecting a host of imaging, immunologic, and genetic

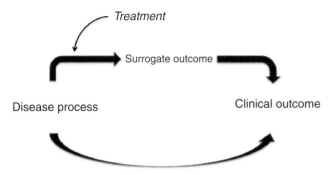

Fig. 21.1. Criteria for a valid surrogate outcome. For a valid surrogate outcome, a treatment will work via the surrogate in a way that is directly seen on the desired clinical outcome and a treatment-induced change in the surrogate will predict a change on the clinical outcome. No pathway of impact of treatment can exist on the clinical outcome that bypasses the surrogate. Formal validation of a surrogate outcome[34] requires that a treatment is effective on the surrogate outcome and on the desired clinical outcome, that the surrogate outcome is correlated significantly with the clinical outcome, and that adjustment for the surrogate outcome causes the impact of treatment on the clinical outcome to disappear. It should also be demonstrated that the surrogate is valid for different classes of therapeutic intervention and in a spectrum of trial settings; otherwise a surrogate may be considered valid only for a single agent and trial setting in which it has been demonstrated.

data in a rationally designed prospective fashion to allow exploration and validation of possible surrogate outcomes against clinical outcomes once the studies are completed.

Many investigators believe that the count of contrast-enhancing lesions in the brain detected by magnetic resonance imaging (MRI) is the most reasonable candidate as a surrogate for MS disease relapse. The current experimental paradigm for Phase 2 clinical trials for relapsing forms of MS often uses changes in contrast enhancing brain lesions as the primary outcome to demonstrate proof of principle. However, recent investigations of active MRI lesions as possible surrogate end-points based on data from the placebo arms of MS clinical trials that focused on "individual-level surrogacy" failed to find strong correlations between MRI outcomes and the clinical disease course.[36,37]

Arguably of greater relevance for clinical trials is "trial-level surrogacy": do the effects of treatment on MRI outcomes predict the effects of treatment on clinical end-points? A recent application of a meta-analytic approach to evaluate "trial-level surrogacy" based on data from randomized, placebo-controlled trials in relapsing-remitting MS (23 trials, 6591 patients) identified a strong correlation between the treatment effects on active MRI lesions and on relapses (adjusted $r^2 = 0.81$).[38] While this analysis did not take fully into account the variability of the estimated treatment effects, nevertheless, this result suggests that the effect of a treatment in reducing relapses can be reasonably well predicted by a decrease in active MRI lesions.[39–41]

In spite of the promise that surrogate outcomes offer to reduce duration and perhaps sample size in future studies, trials of relatively short duration using a surrogate endpoint will not provide mid-range to long-term safety data. Any studies that are

successful in demonstrating benefit of an experimental agent on surrogate outcomes will require longer-term confirmatory analyses for safety and efficacy.

Alternative statistical design and analysis
Statistical considerations for adaptive designs

Adaptive designs use accumulating data to modify aspects of an ongoing study. While the potential advantages of adaptive designs to describe the relationship between dose and a response on a biomarker, surrogate, or clinical outcome have been known for decades, fixed sample size designs, in which a predetermined number of patients are allocated to a relatively small number of doses and placebo without any adaptive possibilities have been more commonly used in drug development.

Recently, there has been a resurgence of interest in adaptive designs for Phase 1 dose-ranging toxicity studies where one objective is to identify a "maximum tolerated dose".[42,43] Here, an initial cohort of subjects (animals or patients) is first investigated at a low dose expected to lead to minimal toxicity, after which the next cohort will be studied at a lower, equal, or a higher dose depending on the prior cohort response. These studies aim to estimate features of the dose–response relationships, not to confirm hypotheses about the toxicity or the efficacy of the drug, and are thus exploratory in nature: the decision to be made at the end of these studies is which, if any, dose(s) to take forward to further testing in Phase 2b and Phase 3. Since the primary concern is to provide the information necessary to make good future decisions, strict control of the Type 1 error is not a major concern.

However, there has also been a great deal of recent interest in the potential for using adaptive designs in confirmatory Phase 2b and Phase 3 studies, where, particularly from the regulatory standpoint, strict control of the Type 1 error is essential. Group sequential designs, a simple form of adaptive design, are now commonly used.[44] Here, the only modification made once the trial is underway is to potentially stop the trial at an interim analysis if accumulated data clearly indicate the treatment is efficacious or that it is futile to continue the study. More dramatic adaptations can be considered,[45] including changing the planned size of the study to maintain power,[46–49] merging a dose-selection phase with a confirmatory phase into a "seamless Phase 2/3" trial,[50,51] and switching recruitment to focus on a sensitive patient sub-population ("enrichment" designs).[52,53]

A major impetus for increased interest in adaptive designs was the US FDA's 2006 *Critical Path Initiative Opportunity List*, where use of adaptive design methods was identified as a potential factor for improving the drug development process.[54] Statisticians have responded by developing innovative new adaptive designs and corresponding methods for appropriate statistical inferences described in overviews for clinical audiences[55,56] and in critical appraisals of these designs and methods.[46,57,58]

Regulatory concerns about the use of adaptive designs are detailed by the US Food and Drug Administration and the European Medicines Agency.[4,59] Of foremost concern is avoiding increased rates of false-positive results through strict control of the overall Type 1 error rate. Specialized methods based on the combination test approach or the conditional error function approach have been developed to achieve this.[60–63] The regulatory view is that all adaptations should be pre-planned but these approaches also apply even for unplanned adaptations, thereby allowing for the "rescue" of studies that turn out to have been planned on too optimistic a basis.

A second major regulatory concern is the possibility of bias, for which there are two main potential sources in adaptive designs. The first arises because the usual estimate of the treatment effect evaluated at the end of an adaptive study will typically be biased. Statisticians continue to develop methodologies to allow evaluation of appropriate estimates of treatment effects and corresponding confidence intervals.[64,65] The second potential source of bias is operational bias arising from the adaptation process itself. Most adaptations require use of unblinded data for decision-making, so control of the flow of that information is critical to ensuring the study integrity. For adaptations to be effective, they must be rapidly implementable, so an up-to-date and cleaned database must be promptly available. Logistical issues relating to drug supply may emerge and require careful advance consideration. In general, adaptive designs require much more detailed planning to ensure smooth study execution. Regulators indicate that adaptive designs cannot be used to avoid rigorous pre-planning of trials, but can be used to anticipate difficult experimental situations if documented and described in the study protocol.[4,59]

Adaptations are most effective when the response of interest is quickly observable (and recruitment is relatively slow) so that an adequate number of patients randomized will already have responded at the time of any planned adaptation. The feasibility of effective adaptations in a chronic disease like MS needs careful consideration, since times-to-response on outcomes of interest tend to be long. The impact of any planned adaptation on statistical properties of the proposed design must be thoroughly evaluated, often requiring extensive time-consuming simulation studies so that the implications are well understood in advance.

Bayesian design and analysis

Clinical trials in MS have traditionally been designed with a frequentist approach to statistical inference. For example, a superiority trial is designed so that a test of the null hypothesis with a given Type 1 error has a specified power for treatment effects that are of clinically meaningful magnitudes; confidence intervals and P-values describe the treatment effect.

An alternative statistical inference approach uses Bayesian procedures,[66,67] which require descriptions of uncertainty about all the unknown parameters (not only the treatment

effect) determined prior to the study initiation, based on knowledge of the disease natural history and treatment outcomes in prior studies. If such "prior distributions" are strong, this can reduce sample size in a proposed study, provided that new data are not in conflict with the prior distributions, since less new data will be needed to arrive at a conclusion. Data accumulating in the new study are used to revise the prior distributions into posterior distributions that update uncertainties about the parameters. The posterior distribution of the treatment effect is of particular interest as it will be the primary basis for decision-making in the ongoing study.

Blinded monitors use posterior distributions most appropriately to alter study design (duration, sample size, etc.) as a consequence of accumulating information. Such adaptive decision-making is easily accommodated in the Bayesian approach since, in contrast to the frequentist approach, adaptations create no serious complications for Bayesian inference.

Bayesian techniques have yet to be formally applied to MS trials. However, such approaches have been used in other disease areas in studies in the early stages of drug development and in later stage studies.[66–71]

Key to the Bayesian approach is the prior distribution assumptions that depend upon historical data that may not be relevant to patients in the current environment. Also, since the prior distribution assumptions are to a degree subjective in value and weighting, they may be weak. Weak priors can lead to a study that is no more efficient than a traditional frequentist approach. Finally, Bayesian approaches rely upon a parametric model for the likelihood function and thus may be more model dependent than frequentist approaches to statistical analyses and interim monitoring.

Regulatory authorities continue to insist on a comprehensive description of the frequentist properties of proposed confirmatory trial designs to ensure strict control of the Type I error as well as adequate power. Extensive modeling and simulation are required to obtain such descriptions for a Bayesian design. Thus, securing regulatory approval of a Bayesian design for a confirmatory trial is a major challenge.

Conclusions

Two decades of clinical trials in MS have led to the availability of multiple agents for relapsing forms of the disease and a vigorous academic and corporate effort to find safe and effective agents for all forms of disease. The success of the past years, however, has created a crisis in the conduct of clinical trials and traditional trial designs may no longer be viable. There is no consensus about which, if any, of possible design and analysis innovations might be appropriate alternatives to traditional MS clinical trials.[3] Nonetheless, alternative trial design and analysis approaches must be considered; detailed modeling of new designs is needed to determine if they could enhance the conduct of prospective trials for MS. This is an effort that requires the full attention of investigators, sponsors, and regulators.

References

1. Herndon R. Multiple sclerosis. Proceedings of the International Conference on Therapeutic Trials in Multiple Sclerosis. Grand Island, NY, April 23–24, 1982. *Arch Neurol* 1983; 40: 663–710.

2. Wolinsky JS, Reingold SC. When progress slows progress. *ACP Med* 2008; 31: 1–3.

3. McFarland HF, Reingold SC. The future of multiple sclerosis therapies: redesigning multiple sclerosis clinical trials in a new therapeutic era. *Mult Scler* 2005; 11: 669–76.

4. Food and Drug Administration. 2010. Adaptive design clinical trials for drugs and biologics. www.fda.gov/downloads/Drugs/Guidance ComplianceRegulatoryInformation/ Guidances/UCM201790. (Accessed September 19, 2010.)

5. Hollon T. FDA uneasy about placebo revision. *Nat Med* 2001; 7: 7.

6. Bland JM, Kerr D. Fifth revision of Declaration of Helsinki. Clause 29 forbids trails from using placebos when effective treatment exists. *BMJ* 2002; 324: 975.

7. Lublin FD, Reingold SC. Placebo-controlled clinical trials in multiple sclerosis: ethical considerations. National Multiple Sclerosis Society (USA) Task Force on Placebo-Controlled Clinical Trials in MS. *Ann Neurol* 2001; 49: 677–81.

8. Polman CH, Reingold SC, Barkhof F, *et al.* Ethics of placebo-controlled clinical trials in multiple sclerosis: a reassessment. *Neurology* 2008; 70: 1134–40.

9. Kappos LK, Weinshenker B, Pozzilli, C, *et al.* Interferon beta-1a in secondary progressive MS. *Neurology* 2004; 63: 1779–87.

10. Coste J, Fermanian J, Venot A. Methodological and statistical problems in the construction of composite measurement scales: a survey of six medical and epidemiological journals. *Stat Med* 1995; 331–45.

11. Petkau AJ. Statistical and design considerations for multiple sclerosis clinical trials. In Goodkin DE and Rudick RA, eds. *Multiple Sclerosis: Advances in Clinical Trials.* London: Springer-Verlag, 1996: 63–103.

12. Kurtzke JF. Rating neurological impairment in multiple sclerosis: an expanded disability status scale (EDSS). *Neurology* 1983; 33: 1444–52.

13. O'Brien PC. Procedures for comparing samples with multiple endpoints. *Biometrics* 1984; 40: 1079–87.

14. Pocock SJ, Geller NL, Tsiatis AA. The analysis of multiple endpoints in clinical trials. *Biometrics* 1987; 43: 487–98.

15. Rudick R, Antel J, Confavreux C, *et al.* Clinical outcomes assessment in multiple sclerosis. *Ann Neurol* 1996; 40: 469–79.

16. Rudick R, Antel J, Confavreux C, *et al.* Recommendations from the National Multiple Sclerosis Society Clinical Outcomes Assessment Task Force. *Ann Neurol* 1997; 42: 379–82.

17. Cohen JA, Cutter GR, Fischer JS, *et al.* Benefit of interferon beta-1a on MSFC progression in secondary progressive MS. *Neurology* 2002; 59: 679–87.

18. Hommel G. A stagewise rejective multiple test procedure based on modified Bonferroni test. *Biometrika* 1988; 75: 383–6.

19. Hochberg Y. A sharper Bonferroni procedure for multiple tests of significance. *Biometrika* 1988; 75: 800–2.

20. Goodkin DE, Rudick RA, VanderBrug Mendendorp S, *et al.* Low dose (7.5 mg) oral methotrexate reduces the rate of progression in chronic progressive multiple sclerosis. *Ann Neurol* 1995; 37: 30–40.

21. Havrdova E, Galetta S, Hutchinson M, *et al.* Effect of natalizumab on clinical and radiological disease activity in multiple sclerosis: retrospective analysis of the Natalizumab Safety and Efficacy in Relapsing–Remitting Multiple Sclerosis (AFFIRM) study. *Lancet Neurol* 2009; 8: 254–60.

22. Follmann D, Wittes J, Cutler JA. The use of subjective rankings in clinical trials with an application to cardiovascular disease. *Stat Med* 1992; 427–37.

23. Wei LJ, Lachin JM. Two-sample asymptotically distribution-free test for incomplete multivariate observations. *J Am Stat Assoc* 1984; 79: 653–61.

24. Hartung HP, Gonsette R, Konig N, *et al.* Mitoxantone in progressive

multiple sclerosis: a placebo-controlled, double-blind, randomized, multicentre trial. *Lancet* 2002; 360: 2018–25.

25. Tang D-I, Geller NL, Pocock SJ. On the design and analysis of randomized clinical trials with multiple endpoints. *Biometrics* 1993; 49: 23–30.

26. Follmann D. A simple multivariate test for one-sided alternatives. *J Am Stat Assoc* 1996: 91: 854–61.

27. Lehmacher W, Wassmer G, Reitmeir P. Procedures for two-sample comparisons with multiple endpoints controlling the experimentwise error rate. *Biometrics* 1991: 47: 511–21.

28. Rosenberger WF, Lachin JM. *Randomization in Clinical Trials: Theory and Practice.* New York, Wiley, 2002.

29. Hu F, Rosenberger WF. *The Theory of Response – Adaptive Randomization in Clinical Trials.* New York: Wiley, 2006.

30. Ware JH, Investigating therapies of potentially great benefit: ECMO. *Stat Sci* 1989; 4: 298–306.

31. Begg CB. On inferences from Wei's biased coin design for clinical trials. *Biometrika* 1990; 77: 73.

32. European Medicines Agency. Guideline on clinical investigation of medicinal products for the treatment of multiple sclerosis. 2006. http://www.ema. europa.eu/ema/index.jsp?curl=pages/ regulation/general/general_ content_000425.jsp&murl=menus/ regulations/regulations.jsp&mid= WC0b01ac0580034cf5. (Accessed September 19, 2010.)

33. Schwid SR, Thorpe J, Sharief M, *et al.* Enhanced benefit of increasing interferon beta-1a dose and frequency in relapsing multiple sclerosis: the EVIDENCE study. *Arch Neurol* 2005; 2: 785–92.

34. Prentice RL. Surrogate endpoints in clinical trials: definition and operational criteria. *Stat Med* 1989; 8: 431–40.

35. Fleming TR, DeMets DL. Surrogate endpoints in clinical trials: are we being misled? *Ann Intern Med* 1996; 125: 605–13.

36. Petkau J, Reingold SC, Held U, *et al.* Magnetic resonance imaging as a surrogate outcome for multiple sclerosis relapses. *Mult Scler* 1998; 14: 770–8.

37. Daumer M, Neuhaus, A, Morrissey S, *et al.* MRI as an outcome in multiple sclerosis clinical trials. *Neurology* 2009; 72: 705–11.

38. Sormani MP, Bonzano L, Roccatagliata L, *et al.* Magnetic resonance imaging as a potential surrogate for relapses in MS: a meta-analytic approach. *Ann Neurol* 2009; 65: 268–75.

39. Daniels MJ, Hughes MD. Meta-analysis for the evaluation of potential surrogate markers. *Stat Med* 1997: 16: 1965–82.

40. Korn EL, Albert PS, McShane LM. Assessing surrogates as trial endpoints using mixed models. *Stat Med* 2005: 24; 163–82.

41. Burzykowski T, Molenberghs G, Buyse M. *The Evaluation of Surrogate Endpoints.* New York, Springer, 2006.

42. Bornkamp B, Bretz F, Dmitrienko A, *et al.* Innovative approaches for designing and analyzing adaptive dose-ranging trials. *J Biopham Stat* 2007; 17: 965–95.

43. Bretz F, Hsu J, Pinheiro J, Liu Y. Dose finding – a challenge in statistics. *Biom J* 2008; 50: 480–504.

44. Jennison C, Turnbull BW. *Group Sequential Methods with Applications to Clinical Trials.* Boca Raton: Chapman & Hall/CRC, 2000.

45. Chow S-C, Chang M. *Adaptive Design: Methods in Clinical Trials.* Boca Raton, Chapman & Hall/CRC, 2007.

46. Jennison C, Turnbull BW. Mid-course sample size modification in clinical trials based on the observed treatment effect. *Stat Med* 2003; 23: 971–93.

47. Friede T, Kieser M. Sample size recalculation in internal pilot study designs: a review. *Biom J* 2006; 48: 537–55.

48. Prochan MA. Sample size re-estimation in clinical trials. *Biom J* 2009; 51: 348–57.

49. Friede T, Schmidli H. Blinded sample size reestimation with count data: methods and applications in multiple sclerosis. *Stat Med* 2010; 29: 1145–56.

50. Schmidli H, Bretz F, Racine A, Maurer W. Confirmatory seamless phase II/III clinical trials with hypotheses selection at interim: application and practical considerations. *Biom J* 2006; 48: 635–43.

51. Jennison C, Turnbull BW. Adaptive seamless designs: selection and prospective testing of hypotheses. *J Biopharm Stat* 2007; 17: 1135–61.

52. Wang SJ, Hung HM, O'Neill RT. Adaptive patient enrichment designs in therapeutic trials. *Biom J* 2009; 51: 358–74.

53. Brannath W, Zuber E, Branson M, *et al.* Confirmatory adaptive designs with Bayesian decision tools for a targeted therapy in oncology. *Stat Med* 2009; 28: 1445–63.

54. US Food and Drug Administration. Critical Path Initiative Opportunity List. 2006. http://www.fda.gov/ ScienceResearch/SpecialTopics/ CriticalPathInitiative/ CriticalPathOpportunitiesReports/ ucm077251.htm. (Accessed September 17, 2010.)

55. Mehta C, Gao P, Bhatt DL, *et al.* Optimizing trial design: sequential, adaptive and enrichment strategies. *Circulation* 2009; 119: 597–605.

56. Bretz F, Branson M, Burman C-F, *et al.* Adaptivity in drug discovery and development. *Drug Dev Res* 2009; 70: 169–90.

57. Jennison C, Turnbull BW. Adaptive and nonadaptive group sequential designs. *Biometrika* 2006; 93: 1–21.

58. Burman C-F, Sonesson C. Are flexible designs sound? *Biometrics* 2006: 62: 664–9.

59. European Medicines Agency. Reflection paper on methodological issues in confirmatory clinical trials planned with an adaptive design. 2006. www.ema.europa.eu/ema/pages/ includes/document/open_document. jsp?webContentId=WC500003616. (Accessed September 19, 2010.)

60. Bauer P, Köhne K. Evaluations of experiments with adaptive interim analyses. *Biometrics* 1994; 50: 1029–41.

61. Brannath W, Posch M, Bauer P. Recursive combination tests. *J Am Stat Assoc* 2002; 97: 236–44.

62. Prochan MA, Hunsberger SA. Designed extension of studies based on conditional power. *Biometrics* 1995; 51: 1315–24.

63. Müller H, Schäfer H. A general statistical principle for changing a design any time during the course of a trial. *Stat Med* 2004; 23: 2497–508.

64. Brannath W, Mehta CR, Posch M. Exact confidence bounds following adaptive group sequential tests. *Biometrics* 2009; 65: 539–46.

65. Wu SS, Wang W, Yang MCK. Interval estimation for drop-the-losers designs. *Biometrika* 2010; 97: 405–18.

66. Spiegelhalter DJ, Freedman LS, Parmar MK. *Bayesian Approaches to Clinical Trials and Health Care Evaluation.* New York: Wiley, 2004.

67. Carlin BP, Louis TA. *Bayesian Methods for Data Analysis, Third Edition.* New York: Chapman & Hall/CRC, 2008.

68. Thall PF, Russell KE. A strategy for dose-finding and safety monitoring based on efficacy and adverse outcomes in phase I/II clinical trials. *Biometrics* 1998; 54: 251–64.

69. Krams M, Lees KR, Hacke W, *et al.* Acute stroke therapy by inhibition of neutrophils (ASTIN): an adaptive dose-response study of UK-279,276 in acute ischemic stroke. *Stroke* 2003; 34; 2543–8.

70. Wilber DJ, Pappone C, Neuzil P, *et al.* Comparison of antiarrythmic drug therapy and radiofrequency catheter ablation in patients with paroxysmal atrial fibrillation: a randomized controlled trial. *J Am Med Assoc* 2010: 303: 333–40.

71. Berry SM, Carlin BP, Lee JJ, Müller P. *Bayesian Adaptive Methods for Clinical Trials.* New York: Chapman & Hall/CRC, 2010.

Chapter 22

Ethical considerations in multiple sclerosis clinical trials

Aaron E. Miller, Nada Gligorov, and Stephen C. Krieger

Progress in the development of strategies to prevent, treat, and ultimately cure multiple sclerosis (MS), and human disease in general, is critically dependent on the conduct of scientifically valid research. Indeed, scientists and physicians have an ethical mandate to pursue this goal, but to do so in a manner that conforms to the highest ethical standards. Research aimed at the target of successful treatment for MS invariably begins at the laboratory bench. In most instances, progress with in vitro studies leads to the next step of animal experimentation. Should the agent under investigation continue to look promising, research with human subjects begins. Each of these levels of investigations entails its own set of ethical controls. This chapter, however, will exclusively address ethical issues that relate specifically to the conduct of human investigation.

For centuries, humans have been the subjects of clinical experimentation, albeit only for decades has the process been regularly formalized into protocol-based clinical trials. As the sophistication of clinical trial science has evolved, pari passu has become the increasing recognition of the primacy of the protection of human subjects.

This chapter will present the general ethical requirements for clinical research; broadly review the pertinent criteria for the ethical conduct of placebo controlled trials including the concept of equipoise; and identify conditions for the ethical conduct of placebo-controlled trials specifically in multiple sclerosis.

General ethical requirements for clinical research

Research ethics guidelines were prompted by past research abuses, and each of the guidelines emphasizes particular aspects of protection of research subjects. The Nuremberg Code of 1947, responding to the egregious behavior of Nazi physicians, emphasized the need for consent and favorable risk–benefit ratios.[1] The Declaration of Helsinki of the World Medical Association was developed to correct weaknesses in the Nuremberg Code and specifically addressed the issue of physicians conducting research with patients, emphasizing favorable risk–benefit ratios and independent review. In 1978, the Belmont Report, issued by the National Commission for the Protection

of Human Subjects of Biomedical and Behavioral Research, in reaction to Tuskegee and Willowbrook, added a focus on informed consent and the protection of vulnerable populations.[2] The Council for International Organizations of Medical Sciences (CIOMS) issued its International Ethical Guidelines for Biomedical Research involving Human Subjects, which intended to apply the Declaration of Helsinki to research in developing countries, especially regarding large trials of vaccines and drugs.[3] Eventually, human research in the United States has become regulated in order to conform to the Code of Federal Regulations Title 45 Part 46, generally known as the Common Rule, which was issued in 1991; and by Good Clinical Practice: Consolidated Guidelines, produced in 1996 by the International Conference on Harmonization of Technical Requirements for Registration of Pharmaceuticals for Human Use.[4] Taken separately, none of these guidelines is able to specify universally applicable procedures; taken together they are sometimes contradictory.[5]

A more coherent approach to the ethical evaluation of clinical research trials has been provided by Emanuel *et al.* (2000),[1] see Table 22.1. The authors present a framework that applies generally to clinical research, and later in this chapter these guidelines will be applied to research trials in MS. Emanuel *at al.* (2000) have delineated seven requirements for determining whether a research trial is ethical, which combine the requirements often emphasized by other guidelines, such as informed consent and risk–benefit ratios. In addition, they highlight the requirement for scientific validity. Listed in chronological order from the conception of the research through its distribution, these elements include the list in Table 22.1.

Social and scientific value

Studies that lack social or **scientific value** are ipso facto unethical because they subject participants to risk without the potential for any significant benefit. This element is founded on the underlying ethical value of avoiding the waste of scarce resources and the non-exploitation of human subjects. Its application dictates that trials should not reduplicate clearly established results and should not be conducted if the results will not

Table 22.1. *Requirements for the ethical conduct of research*

Social or scientific value
Scientific validity
Fair subject selection
Favorable risk–benefit ratio
Independent review
Informed consent
Respect for potential and enrolled subjects

produce practical implementation, even if the treatment proves effective. It also requires that investigators consider the implication of both positive and negative trials. For example, is a very small, open-label MS trial likely to have meaningful implications? Will it provide enough useful information, beyond existing anecdotally driven impressions, to warrant a change in practice? Will the results enable the progression to a more scientifically reliable randomized clinical trial? Unfortunately, the answer to the last question sometimes depends on economic considerations. If the drug in question is available generically, for instance, the pharmaceutical industry will likely have little interest in funding a trial; or the population at risk may not be of sufficient interest to generate financial support from the National Institutes of Health (NIH), probably the only non-pharmaceutical source of funds (at least in the United States) sufficient to permit the conduct of a large-scale clinical trial in MS.

The principle of **social value** also requires dissemination of clinical trial results, whether positive or negative. Recent uproars over the suppression of negative clinical trial results, which has significant implications for clinical practice, has led to an outcry from both the academic community and the lay press, and a demand that trials be registered on readily accessible, reliable websites such as www.clinicaltrials.gov,[6] maintained by the NIH. The scientific editorial community has responded by agreeing that they will not publish the results of trials that are not registered.[7] Major pharmaceutical companies have expressed willingness to comply with these responsibilities and a recent visit to the clinicaltrials.gov website did reveal substantial compliance, in that most, if not all, current pharmaceutically funded clinical trials in MS were listed.

Scientific validity

The requirement for **scientific validity** requires little clarification or elaboration. A statement in the CIOMS guidelines tersely makes the point: "Scientifically unsound research on human subjects is ipso facto unethical in that it may expose subjects to risks or inconvenience to no purpose."[3] Of course, the study must be conducted with sound scientific principles and valid methodology. It is worth emphasizing that this includes the need to power the trial appropriately in order to adequately test its objectives. Furthermore, a trial that is likely to have great difficulty enrolling subjects may be unethical because it will

be unable to answer its questions and thereby cannot generate valid scientific information. The same ethical principles that justify the requirement for **social and scientific value**, i.e. scarce resources and non-exploitation, are operative here.

Fair subject selection

Fair subject selection is based on the ethical principle of justice. It aims to avoid the exploitation of vulnerable individuals as subjects for the trial. On the other hand, it requires that inclusion in the trial of an attractive agent does not favor those of wealth and station. Ideally, all members of the class of subjects eligible for the trial according to the protocol should have equal access. This may entail particular efforts to encourage inclusion of minorities. The trial should not exclude classes of patients for whom the drug, if it proves safe and effective, is likely to be prescribed. Inclusion of women in MS trials has not been an issue. However, many drugs developed for MS will be administered to adolescents and even to younger children. Therefore, the arbitrary exclusion of minors from MS clinical trials may be inappropriate. Of course, adequate safeguards for the prevention of undue risk to this vulnerable population must be assured. Applicable to this ethical requirement, an important debate has developed as to whether clinical trials should be conducted in developing countries where patients may not have access to existing therapies, and, in fact, many may not subsequently be able to attain the drug under investigation. This issue will be discussed further with specific regard to MS later in the chapter.

Favorable risk–benefit ratio

The principle of **favorable risk–benefit ratio** justifies the ethical values of non-maleficence and beneficence. The concept, which will be discussed in greater detail later in this chapter, requires that the investigator take every precaution to minimize risks to the subjects. The trial should be designed to enhance potential benefits, and recruit participants who have the best possibility of achieving benefit. Finally, it is important that the potential benefits to individual subjects and to society are appropriate to the risks involved. While this equation is difficult enough to balance in Phase 2 and 3 trials, it is even more problematic for Phase 1 trials, in which no potential direct benefit to the participant is anticipated. Here, the critical assessment, considered by Weijer (2003) as "the risk-knowledge calculus,"[8] is whether the knowledge gained from the study is likely to convey sufficient benefit for society to outweigh the risk to the subject. Determining this balance, in the absence of mathematical formulae, is difficult, but individuals make such decisions on a regular basis. In the setting of clinical research, the comparisons are made not only by the subjects and investigators, but also by members of the institutional review board (IRB). Legal scholar Paul Freund's comments are as applicable to patients accepting participation in Phase 1 studies as they are to those entering Phase 2 and 3 trials:

The dialectic in the law's solicitude for physical integrity is supplied by the concomitant ideal of free individual choice and self-assertion, within socially approved bounds. The concepts of assumption of risk, waiver consent, or voluntary participation, whether in playing football or tying oneself to a mountaineering guide, reflect the countervailing social legal value. This is, in turn, qualified by the reservation that consent to procedures that are negligent will not be binding, and that a fiduciary relationship imposes special obligations of disclosure and good judgment in accepting consent or participation.[9]

Independent review

The principle of **independent review** most obviously involves IRBs. These bodies, composed of scientific researchers, physicians, individuals with ethical knowledge, and lay people, are charged with assuring that a trial is ethically designed, has a favorable risk–potential benefit ratio, and does not unjustly benefit some members of society through the misuse of others. In addition, the IRB scrutinizes the trial to make sure that conflicts of interest – inevitable albeit often legitimate – have minimal impact. The IRB is not alone in providing independent oversight that helps guarantee the ethical conduct of a clinical trial. Granting agencies often conduct a first review. Today, virtually all Phase 2 and 3 trials have data and safety monitoring committees, composed of knowledgeable individuals and usually including a statistician, with access in an ongoing fashion, to aggregate or individual data, as needed. The committee is thus best situated to assess potential danger signals during the conduct of the trial, as well as to recommend, at times, early termination of a trial because it will be unable to achieve statistically significant results. This procedure thereby helps to prevent continued risk to subjects in the absence of potential benefit.

The existence and process of data safety and monitoring boards have their own ethical implications, as recently analyzed by Slutsky and Lavery (2004).[10] These authors contend that the study participants should be informed, as part of the formal consent process, "about the board, how it assesses risks, and how it makes its recommendations to the investigators through the course of the trial." They argue further that the behavior of the board "is directly relevant to potential subjects and must be conveyed in order to meet even the basic regulatory requirements of disclosure." In addition, the process by which board members reach their conclusions should be transparent and ought to be publicly disclosed at the conclusion of a trial.

Informed consent

Informed consent is a process of ensuring that "individuals control whether or not they enroll in clinical research and participate only when the research is consistent with their values, interests, and preferences."[1] This process embodies the ethical principle of respect for persons by allowing an individual to exercise autonomy in the decision-making process. Informed consent is a necessary, but hardly sufficient, requirement for assuring that a clinical trial is ethical, as evident from the discussions above and below. Some potential investigators may have the mistaken impression that informed consent is a

document, the simple signing of which allows the ethical enrollment and participation of the patient in the clinical trial. On the contrary, informed consent must be a dynamic process, which begins prior to the subject's enrollment and continues throughout the course of the trial (and sometimes even afterwards). Good clinical practice dictates that the investigator conduct a dialog with the potential subject in order that he or she gains a complete understanding of the trial before making an autonomous decision about whether or not to participate. Elements of the informed consent process include adequate, accurate, and complete explanation of the rationale for the trial, the methods of conduct, foreseeable risks, potential benefits, and alternatives to participation. It enables the potential subject to query the investigator about any points of confusion and to receive information about whom to contact should questions or concerns later arise. It also reminds the subject that participation is voluntary and that he or she may withdraw from the trial at any time without prejudice to his continuing care. Furthermore, the informed consent process continues throughout the trial, as the subject should always have the opportunity to ask questions as they arise. The investigator is, of course, obligated to inform the subject of any new information that may impact the decision to continue to participate, as well as to notify him of any relevant changes in the protocols. Often this exchange of information is done on an informal basis, but at times the importance of new information is considered critical enough to warrant more formal "re-consenting" of the subject.

Unfortunately, studies have consistently demonstrated inadequacies of the informed consent process. The term "therapeutic misconception," coined by Appelbaum *et al.*[11] recognizes the phenomenon that many patients believe that anything recommended by the physician (in the case of the clinical trial, the principal investigator) is intended for their benefit.[12] The misconception persisted even after subjects were properly consented for research and had received the information that trials were randomized and some participants were likely to be in the control group receiving no treatment. The phenomenon of therapeutic misconception makes salient that participants, even after consent, do not understand that a trial is not intended to provide benefit to a particular subject (patient), but has the purpose of answering an important scientific question and thus is most likely to provide direct benefit to future patients. An additional illustrative example is provided by the results of a survey conducted among 14 subjects who had very recently completed participation at the first author's site in a trial comparing two doses of oral glatiramer acetate vs. placebo in the treatment of RRMS, which proved to be negative (AM Miller, personal communication). Although the subjects were aware of the existence of the injectable immunomodulatory drugs and understood the concept of placebos, astonishingly only five recalled that they had been in a placebo-controlled trial and eight failed to recognize that they had been exposed to any health risk by participating (despite the fact that they were not receiving effective therapy for a potentially serious disease). Furthermore, only three patients correctly understood the likelihood that they were receiving glatiramer acetate. These studies taken together indicate that informed consent alone may not provide ethical justification for a trial.

Respect for potential and enrolled subjects

The final ethical requirement in the framework of Emanuel *et al.* is the respect for potential and enrolled subjects. This includes not only the elements of continued information transfer and dialogue, but also the necessity to protect the subject's privacy. In order to acknowledge and respect the importance of the subject's contribution to the advancement of medical knowledge by their participation in the trial, the investigator has the obligation to inform them of the results and implications of the research. Subjects in a blinded trial should have the opportunity to learn their treatment assignment once unblinding of the trial has occurred.

Clearly, designing and conducting a clinical trial in the most ethical manner is a complex and ongoing process that involves many individuals. At the nidus, however, is the relationship between the principal investigator and the potential or actual subject. This relationship should be frank and open, allowing for free communication throughout both the consent process and the subject's actual participation in the trial. Having explored the ethical requirements, in general, which are necessary for clinical research, we can now turn our attention to specific issues related particularly to placebo-controlled trials in MS.

Case discussion (See also Chapter 50)

In early 2009, Professor Paolo Zamboni described a condition he called "chronic cerebrospinal venous insufficiency" (CCSVI) in patients with MS. He operationally defined this condition based on observations using transcranial and extracranial color-coded Doppler ultrasound studies. A diagnosis of CCSVI was said to be present when at least two of five findings were present:

1. Reflux in the internal jugular veins or vertebral veins
2. Reflux in intracranial veins or sinuses
3. B-mode detection of stenoses in internal jugular veins
4. Absence of Doppler signal in internal jugular veins or vertebral veins
5. Cross-sectional area of the internal jugular veins greater in sitting position than in supine position

Using these criteria, Zamboni reported the presence of CCSVI in 100% of 65 MS patients, and in none of 235 control subjects. He postulated that impaired venous drainage of brain or spinal cord due to CCSVI led to breakdown of the blood–brain barrier, accumulation of iron in brain, and inflammation, resulting in MS.

In a subsequent paper, Zamboni reported the results of an uncontrolled, unblinded trial in which patients with CCSVI underwent venoplasty of the presumably abnormal veins. The procedure was termed the "liberation procedure." He reported that patients, mainly those with RRMS improved, and had fewer relapses and MRI abnormalities in the year after treatment

than they had experienced in the year prior to the procedure. Patients with more advanced, progressive disease did not appear to benefit from the procedure. However, 47% of patients who underwent the "liberation procedure" experienced restenosis of the internal jugular veins (IJV).

Following the Zamboni reports, the mainstream media – print, television, and the internet – touted the Italian results, asserting a breakthrough. This publicity occurred initially and extensively in Canada, but ultimately spread throughout the world. As a result, a surge of patient demand for the procedure occurred. Refusal of provincial governments in Canada to authorize venous angioplasty for MS spurred waves of anger and demands that the procedure be covered. Venomous communications were directed at both the Canadian MS Society and the National MS Society of the United States (NMSS). In addition, scores of blogs sprung up, including those in which patients lambasted the Canadian government and the MS "establishment," as well as others providing testimonials from those who had undergone the procedure. Facebook pages were established and the social media fanned the fires of hope and expectation. Searching the internet yields numerous medical "tourism" sites, providing the promise not only of "liberation," but also of flight arrangements and hotel accommodations.

Meanwhile, the "liberation procedure" caused some devastating complications. A death from intracerebral hemorrhage occurred following the procedure at Stanford University. Open heart surgery was required in a second patient from the same institution when a stent used in the procedure migrated to the heart. As a result of these complications, Stanford University halted the performance of the procedure at that institution. At least one additional death has been reported by the Canadian press of a patient who underwent venoplasty.

MS specialists and scientists were generally skeptical of the Zamboni observations. They cited the limitations of the ultrasound procedures, which are highly operator dependent and subjective; and the unblinded nature of the therapeutic trial. In addition, they raised a number of other issues that cast doubt on the validity of the observations. CCSVI has not previously been described, and the normal venous anatomy in humans is not well defined. Furthermore, the venous drainage of the brain is highly flexible and redundant, and is posture dependent. Other causes of blockage of the internal jugular veins have been long recognized, but are not associated with MS, and surgeons have regularly tied off one or both IJVs when performing head and neck surgery, particularly for cancer. In that setting, there are no known consequences of IJV ligation. Furthermore, MS patients have none of the clinical or radiological findings that one would ordinarily expect with increased pressure in the cerebral venous system. In addition, experts pointed out that, even if the findings on ultrasound were valid, they did not necessarily imply causation. CCSVI, if it exists, could be the result of the disease process, rather than its cause.

Faced with mounting discontent in the MS patient community and increasing numbers of patients seeking the procedure, the Canadian MS Society and NMSS reached the decision to fund research studies on CCSVI in an attempt to test the Zamboni findings. Proposals were sought and an international multidisciplinary panel was convened to review the submissions. After the deliberations of the panels, seven studies were funded in the amount of $2.4 million. The decision to spend research dollars on CCSVI was criticized by some prominent MS researchers who felt the expenditures were unwarranted because of what they considered to be the implausibility of the Zamboni observations.

Ethical considerations

1. Social value vs. scientific validity
2. Just allocation of scarce resources
3. Autonomy vs. justice

The CCSVI saga invokes many ethical issues, which are simply raised here for the reader's consideration, for neither can they be easily resolved nor adequately discussed in the limited space available in this chapter. First, the physician must respect the patient's autonomy and allow him or her to seek any legally available care that is desired. At the same time, the physician must uphold the principle of beneficence, and specifically nonmaleficence, in seeking to maximize a favorable risk–benefit ratio for the patient. Furthermore, the physician has an ethical mandate to assess all the available evidence about the potential risks and benefits of a procedure before offering his considered opinion. The physician must make clear to the patient that he will continue to provide care irrespective of the patient's decision about treatment.

Although the principle of autonomy remains primary, consideration of the concept of "fairness" does not require that society pay for medical procedures that do not have established effectiveness. In a society that provides medical care for its citizens, it seems ethically appropriate that medical and scientific experts should determine whether available evidence is sufficient to justify coverage.

To what extent should society invest money, energy, and intellectual capital in research on a particular subject, especially when experts believe the efforts are likely to be futile? This question evokes consideration of the concepts of justice. Allocation of scarce resources to one area, such as CCSVI, potentially deprives many individuals of the benefits of research that could be directed elsewhere. Similarly, when society decides to allocate financial resources to pay for a specific medical procedure that benefits few, it may divert capital from research that could benefit many.

What role should the patient community play in determining the allocation of resources either for health care itself or for health care research? Clearly, they have a large stake in the decision, but they may also lack the objectivity and scientific expertise to enable the wisest and most ethical resolution of the question.

The ethical complexities of a medical–social phenomenon such as CCSVI are enormous. The major ethical issues pertaining to patient care invoked by CCSVI stem from considerations that the research was not rigorous enough to reliably show benefit, and adequate to support migration to patient care. Utilizing Emanuel's framework, the research on CCSVI does not yet fulfill the requirement of scientific validity, underscoring the continued need for double-blind and placebo-controlled investigation.

Placebo-controlled trials

In testing drugs for MS, most late phase treatment trials have been conducted in a double-blind fashion, meaning that neither the patient nor the physician evaluating the patient is aware of the specific treatment assignment. Indeed, failure to blind a trial when circumstances could allow that process may potentially render the trial unethical because bias may influence study results, which degrades scientific validity. The need for blinding in MS clinical trials has led to the practice of utilizing both an *examining* and a *treating* physician. The former is charged with performing the critical evaluations that serve as the basis for the clinical end-points in the study. The latter, also usually blinded, has the responsibility of providing regular care and treatment for the patient. As this entails taking interval histories from the patient, as well as performing examinations, there is considerably greater potential for the treating physician to become unblinded. Indeed, in unusual circumstances, the treating physician may be deliberately unblinded in order to assure patient safety while maximizing the possibility of the patient's remaining in the trial.

The success of this approach has led to the approval of eight agents for the treatment of MS since 1993, including interferon beta,[13–15] glatiramer acetate,[16] mitoxantrone,[17] natalizumab,[18] and fingolimod.[19] The availability of these drugs, each only partially effective, has created a therapeutic environment in which the ethics of placebo-controlled clinical trials has been challenged.[20] Placebo-controlled trials face three important hurdles: ethical concerns regarding the use of placebo, when approved therapies are available; decreasing numbers of patients who qualify for studies, resulting in the utilization of potentially disadvantaged populations as study subjects; and limited applicability of placebo-controlled trial results given the availability of several effective agents.[21] A vortex of controversy continues to engulf the question of whether – and, if so, in what circumstances – placebo-controlled trials can be ethically undertaken in MS.

Equipoise

The ethical underpinnings of the randomized clinical trial (RCT) reflect the evolving concept of equipoise. This term in the construct of Miller and Weijer (2003) constitutes "the full set of answers to the question, "when may a physician legitimately offer randomized clinical trial enrollment to her patient?'"[22] When the physician Charles Fried originally described equipoise in his monograph,[23] he required that an *individual* researcher be genuinely uncertain about the relative merits of the treatment alternatives in a clinical trial before offering enrollment to a patient. Fried further argued that virtually all new information about a patient or the condition tilted the balance away from "genuine uncertainty." Though apparently not his intention, this conundrum dampened enthusiasm for randomizing patients into clinical trials because frequently the individual physician felt a bias – albeit often without scientific justification – toward a particular therapeutic option and thus did not meet the test of "genuine uncertainty" that would allow him/her, in good conscience, to enroll the patient in a RCT.[22] Attitudes changed after the landmark, widely cited paper by Freedman (1987), which established the concept of *clinical equipoise*.[24] For Freedman, the concept of equipoise did not rest in the lap of the individual physician. Rather, he defined clinical equipoise as a state in which "honest, professional disagreement among expert clinicians about the preferred treatment exists and motivates the design and conduct of a clinical trial "'with the aim of resolving this dispute'." To what extent must "honest, professional disagreement" exist to justify the trial? While Freedman does not specify the answer precisely, he clearly did not require a 50:50 split. Nor would he accept the outlier views of a rare curmudgeon to justify proceeding. Presumably, then, dissenting opinion of at least a substantial minority of bona fide expert clinicians would be sufficient. Both Fried and Freedman were acting in order to provide a sound moral framework. How then may these two seemingly disparate viewpoints be reconciled? In their scholarly discussion, Miller and Weijer[22] argue that Fried's equipoise and clinical equipoise are complementary. "Fried's equipoise provides a moral condition that satisfies the demands of the continuing fiduciary relationship between physician and patient (i.e. the duty to care), once individual patients have been identified, approached and asked for participation, and enrolled in a trial. Clinical equipoise, on the other hand, addresses the overarching need of the state to protect its citizens from harm and provides clear guidance to IRBs as to when a RCT may ethically proceed."

Equipoise could not only be influenced by a difference in expert opinion, but also by other factors. London (2000) argues that the concept of equipoise should be broadened to include social, cultural, and economic context.[25] Such a view of equipoise would make placebo-controlled trials acceptable in a wider variety of cases because standard of care would differ in their efficacy between populations or countries. Although there might be a standard of care accepted in the USA or Western Europe, that same standard of care might not be applicable in countries significantly different in their health care delivery. Clinical equipoise is disturbed if a treatment for a particular disease exists anywhere; but if the differences in health care delivery are considered, equipoise could still exist in places where the delivery of care would affect the efficacy of the treatment. Clinical equipoise could then be redefined to apply locally where the majority of experts agree that a treatment is effective relative to a particular population.

Can clinical trials continue to use placebo controls ethically?

Partial efficacy of the currently approved disease-modifying therapies creates a moral imperative that MS investigators work to find more effective treatments. This mandate is challenged by the ethical requirement to do so safely. So, can clinical trialists ethically continue to conduct placebo-controlled RCTs in multiple sclerosis?

Many organizations and authors have chimed in with statements relevant to the subject of placebo controls. The Declaration of Helsinki, a product of the World Medical Association, declared that "every medical patient – including those of a control group, if any – should be assured of the best proven…therapeutic method."[26] In a more specific statement, Declaration of Helsinki (Article 32) issued in October 2008 declared, "The benefits, risks, burdens and effectiveness of a new intervention must be tested against those of the best current proven intervention, except in the following circumstances: (a) the use of placebo, or no treatment, is acceptable in studies where no current proven intervention exists; or (b) where for compelling and scientifically sound methodological reasons the use of placebo is necessary to determine the efficacy or safety of an intervention and the patients who receive placebo or no treatment will not be subject to any risk of serious or irreversible harm. Extreme care must be taken to avoid abuse of this option."[27] It should noted, however, that the US Food and Drug Administration (FDA) strongly favors placebo-controlled studies and has stopped requiring that foreign studies comply with the Declaration of Helsinki. The FDA now requires that studies comply with the International Conference on Harmonization (ICH) Good Clinical Practice Guidance (GCP).[28]

Under ICH guidelines, placebo-controlled trials are justified with full informed consent from participants if the only harm to subjects is "discomfort." These statements are generally consistent with the position of Temple and Ellenberg (2000)[29] with which virtually all ethicists agree that, "Placebo controls are clearly inappropriate for conditions in which the delay or omission of available treatments would increase the mortality or serious morbidity in the population to be studied. For conditions in which foregoing therapy imposes no important risk, however, the participation of patients in placebo-controlled trials seems appropriate and ethical, as long as patients are fully informed."

Clinical equipoise in multiple sclerosis

With this background in mind, for the sake of further discussion the authors make the assumption that currently available immunomodulatory agents reduce the relapse rate in MS and are the standard of care for RRMS (this is clearly so, at least in the United States). The issue of the ethical use of placebo-controlled trials in RRMS thus depends, for the most part, on the consideration of whether withholding treatment would pose significant risk. Data support the conclusion that it does. Clearly, some attacks leave permanent residual disability and omitting a treatment that might have prevented such an attack is unduly risky. Lublin *et al.*[30] analyzed the placebo groups from several placebo-controlled RCTs and found that 42.4% had an increase of 0.5 points or more on the Expanded Disability Status Scale and 28.1% had an increase of 1 point or more at least 60 days after an attack. Therefore, clinical equipoise cannot exist for placebo-controlled trials in RRMS.

Table 22.2. *Requirements for the ethical conduct of placebo-controlled trials in MS*

1. If patients declined or refused available established effective therapy
2. If patients have not responded to an established effective therapy
3. In forms of MS for which there is no established effective therapy
4. In resource-restricted environments where access to established effective therapy is limited

The imperative to develop more effective medication for MS, however, persists. Even in the age of multiple approved disease-modifying therapies, these medications are all incompletely effective, none halts relapses or progression, and all have problematic side effect profiles that affect tolerability and adherence.[31] The number needed to treat (NNT) measure derived from published trials provides insight into the limitations of the current therapies: Noseworthy *et al.* calculated that in RRMS, nine patients have to receive interferon to prevent a single relapse at one year, and eight must be treated for two years to prevent one patient from worsening by a single EDSS point during this interval.[32] Despite success at reducing relapse rates, strategies addressing neurodegeneration remain a major unmet need, and clearly work remains to be done to discover and evaluate potentially better therapies.

National multiple sclerosis task force

In view of the availability of several partially effective immunomodulatory drugs for the treatment of MS, the NMSS convened an international task force in 2006 to deliberate the continued use of placebo-controlled trials. The task force, which included many MS investigators, as well as ethicists and regulatory officials, published their consensus opinion most recently in 2008, in which they concluded that offering participation in randomized, placebo-controlled trials for MS was ethical under certain circumstances (Table 22.2).[31]

Use of placebo-controlled trials is ethical for patients whose disease falls outside the regulatory or regionally accepted criteria for treatment with available agents. This category has been taken to include primary progressive MS, for which no treatment has been shown to be effective, and to some degree secondary progressive disease, for which there is limited consensus on the true risk–benefit ratio of the approved disease-modifying therapies.[33–37] Therefore, because many physicians are unwilling to prescribe mitoxantrone for some patients because of the drug's toxicity and because many patients do not wish to take it, ethical conduct of placebo-controlled trials in SPMS remains possible.

The Task Force's position on the ethical legitimacy of placebo-controlled trials if the patient declines available therapy warrants further discussion. An earlier 2001 Task Force stated that patients should "be fully informed of available treatment options and given the opportunity to partake of those prior to being considered as a potential trial participant." They went on to state, "When there is available therapy, the patient should first be offered and encouraged to undertake treatment with those therapies. If the patient declines therapy, participation in a placebo-controlled clinical trial may be considered."[36]

This position, in the authors' view, risked violating patient autonomy by potentially withholding information about available clinical trials that might influence the patient's decision. The implication of the task force recommendations is that information about novel therapies under investigation in placebo-controlled trials be withheld until the patient declines conventional therapy. Perhaps, however, this is too strict an interpretation of the position. If, indeed, they meant that, almost in the same breath, the patient is informed of the utility of currently approved treatments and the opportunity to use one of them, and then offered, in a non-coercive fashion, the possibility of the placebo-controlled trial, the ethical imperative of respect for persons is upheld. The 2008 Task Force report was somewhat less prescriptive in its statement that "placebo-controlled trials should not be presented as an alternative to prescribed established effective therapy (EET), but the best ways to present the differences between treatment with EET and a placebo-controlled clinical trial are uncertain."[31] The challenge, of course, remains to guarantee the presentation of information to the patient in a comprehensible, non-biased fashion. Recommendations to ensure rigorous informed consent include the separation of clinical and research responsibilities between two neurologists; the use of a study subject advocate separate from the research team to assist with the decision-making process; and re-consent after defined instances of disease worsening.[31]

Clearly, patients should not be deprived of the opportunity to participate in a placebo-controlled trial if they do not wish to use approved therapies. As Fost (2003) wrote, in considering osteoporosis trials, "It would be odd to hold the position that a competent informed patient may decide to forego any treatment at all…but should be prohibited from entering a trial where he has a 50% chance of receiving possibly effective therapy."[38] Of course, designing a placebo-controlled trial that would be unlikely to recruit enough subjects in a reasonable period of time would fail to satisfy the ethical requirements of social or scientific value.

Is it ethical to conduct placebo-controlled trials in countries where patients do not have access to interferons or glatiramer acetate?

If one does conclude that placebo-controlled trials for RRMS are no longer ethical in countries where disease-modifying therapy is readily available, what about the possibility of conducting such trials in regions in which MS patients do not have access to established effective therapy? This question remains at the fulcrum of intense debate. On the one hand, a series of papers in *The New England Journal of Medicine*, including an editorial by its then editor Marcia Angell (1997, 2000)[39,40] has taken up the banner of a universal standard of care and has argued that to provide less than that, even in the context of a clinical trial in a developing country, is ethically unacceptable. She argues that investigators are responsible for the welfare of their subjects irrespective of regional political and economic conditions.[39] Ruth Macklin has argued that not just individual but entire communities or countries could be considered vulnerable in the context of multinational research.[41] Given that vulnerable populations are often excluded from research to prevent exploitation, the ethical justification of placebo-controlled trials rests not just on the availability of standard treatment but on the vulnerability of the potential subjects and their ability to give true informed consent.

Addressing the issue of vulnerability, Carl H. Coleman distinguished between consent-based, risk-based, and justice-based vulnerability, where justice-based vulnerability applies to participants in developing countries. Coleman argues that such vulnerabilities can be rectified by extending the benefits of the study to the population from which the study participants were recruited, where the benefits to be conferred may be broadly construed.[42]

Indeed, a number of scientific bodies have taken a stance that justifies conducting placebo-controlled trials if the justice-based vulnerability is ameliorated. Shapiro and Meslin (2001), reflecting the deliberations of the National Bioethics Advisory Commission (NBAC) (United States), suggested that an exception to the use of a control group that receives less than "an established, effective treatment" might be acceptable "in a situation in which the only useful research design, from the host country's perspective, required a less effective intervention in the control group, if the condition being studied was not life-threatening and if the trial received approval from an ethics review committee in the host country as well as one in the United States."[43] In an accompanying editorial, Koski and Nightingale (2001) agree with the NBAC that the position stated in the Declaration of Helsinki, Oct. 2000 concerning placebo-controlled trials was too rigid and noted the position of the US Department of Health and Human Services "that a study should be responsive to the health needs of the host country," and "to be useful and ethical, the study should include a control group that is appropriate for the host country."[44] A report by the Nuffield Council on Bioethics agreed that participants in a control group should be offered a universal standard of care unless there were good reasons not to do so.[45] However, they recognized that circumstances exist where "it is not appropriate to offer a universal standard of care," and suggested that, in such situations, "the minimum standard of care that should be offered to the control group is the best intervention available for that disease as part of the national public health system."[46] Research under these conditions, the report suggests, should proceed because it might lead to improvements in the response to the health care needs of the local population. Citing the response of a number of national and international groups that have weighed in on the so-called standard of care debate, Lie *et al.* (2004) have concluded that these groups have agreed on three conditions that constitute "ethically acceptable exceptions to providing research participants the worldwide best standard of care."[47] As delineated by these authors the conditions are:

1. "Valid science: there must be a valid scientific reason for using a lower standard of care than that available elsewhere;
2. Social benefits: the research must provide a sufficient level of benefit for the host community, and
3. Favorable individual risk–benefit ratio: there must be an acceptable balance of risks and potential benefits for the participants in the trial."

In addressing the first point, the Council for International Organizations of Medical Sciences (CIOMS) has concluded that the scientific and ethical review committee "must be satisfied that the established effective intervention cannot be used as a comparator because its use would not yield scientifically reliable results that would be relevant to the health needs of the study population."[3] If one considers then the question, for example, of how a potential new oral drug treatment for MS should be tested in a country that does not have the health resources to make available the existing immunomodulatory agents, one can make a reasonable argument for comparing the drug to a placebo. Were it tested against the active comparator and failed to show superiority, nothing would have been gained and the study would not have met the criterion of scientific value. Furthermore, a trial seeking equivalence or "non-inferiority" to the current drugs, would run up against the criticisms pointed out by Ellenberg (2003)[48] concerning the use of "active controls", which are discussed below. With regard to social benefit, testing, for example, a novel oral drug might yield an agent that is of lower cost and more readily administered to the local population than existing treatment. Finally, the criterion of favorable individual risk–benefit ratio is no different from that required of any clinical trial.

Returning to the NMSS Task Force,[31] several recommendations were provided to ensure the ethical performance of placebo-controlled trials in resource-restricted environments where access to established effective MS therapy is limited. Efforts must be made to understand local availability of MS therapies and consider these in the informed consent process. Study sponsors must also anticipate post-trial access to the investigational product, both for the study subjects and for the region in which the trial is conducted.

Viewpoints about the ethical acceptability of conducting trials that omit the most effective treatment options continue to be polarized. Resolution is unlikely to come through written commentary. It is likely that decisions will be made on an ad hoc basis in respect to specific clinical trial scenarios, rather than through blanket policy.

Independent of the ethical issues, it has become increasingly difficult to recruit and retain patients for MS placebo-controlled trials. Many recent trials have recruited subjects from Eastern European and Asian countries where treatment availability is variable; this raises further concerns regarding the provision of MS therapy to the participants at the conclusion of these trials as discussed. In addition, in this competitive treatment era, placebo-controlled trials fail to provide increasingly important information about comparative efficacy among available agents.[49] Is it meaningful to know simply that a new agent is more effective than placebo when there are 8 agents already approved for the treatment of MS?[21]

Alternative clinical trial designs (Chapter 21)

The ethical issues and practical limitations governing placebo-controlled trials remain complex. What, then, are the alternatives? Can we use other clinical trial designs to obtain the required information? Particular focus has been placed on trials that either avoid the use of a placebo because of the ethical considerations or on designs that allow new therapies to be studied more rapidly or with fewer patients than would be needed in a conventional placebo-controlled trial.[49]

The use of historical controls has been widely considered unreliable, because with the passage of time too many variables that potentially impact the natural history of disease may have occurred. Some authors have argued that the requirement for placebo-controlled trials is based on an exaggerated concern about the inherent bias in non-randomized observational studies. They suggest that the results of modern observational studies seldom differ significantly from those of RCTs. (Benson and Hartz, 2000[50]; Concato et al., 2000[51]). However, in an accompanying editorial, Pocock and Elbourne (2000)[52] provide major criticism of this position. A related concept for an alternative study design has been to use a "virtual placebo" group. This requires computer modeling based on existing placebo data bases and is, in fact, a more modern version of the use of historical controls, which might perhaps be more reliable. Unfortunately, such models, including those developed at the Sylvia Lawry Centre for Multiple Sclerosis Research, have not thus far become widely adopted.

Other investigators have argued for the substitution of "active-control" trials, in which a new treatment is tested against an accepted therapy. The clinical design can aim either to demonstrate superiority of the new agent over the old or "non-inferiority" of the two treatments. Such active-control trials hold the attraction (at least for patients) that all subjects are receiving medication. Because the test medication is of unproved value, however, such trials do not fulfill the mandate of Declaration of Helsinki V, which required that "every patient be assured of the best proven … therapeutic method."[26] On the other hand, such active comparator studies would appear to satisfy the later iteration, in which Declaration of Helsinki VI stated, "The benefits, risks, burdens, and effectiveness of a new method should be tested against those of the best current prophylactic, diagnostic, and therapeutic methods."[27]

An important argument that has been raised against the use of active-control trials has been the issue of "assay sensitivity."[48] This contends that such trials may not be valid because in the particular trial the accepted treatment may not, in fact, be as effective as it was in some previous trials. (Furthermore, some earlier trials that produced negative results may not have been reported.) In other words, the active-control trial might demonstrate "non-inferiority," but neither agent might be effective. Active-control trials are associated with other problems as well. As placebo-controlled trials can be performed with smaller populations than active-comparator or add-on trials, they potentially could expose fewer patients to a novel agent of unknown risk and unclear benefit than the larger trials required to test an investigational drug against an existing treatment. It is notable, then, that as of 2010 the entire Phase 2 and Phase 3 alemtuzumab research program consists of active-comparator rather then placebo-controlled trials. The deaths of patients in recent MS clinical trials of alemtuzumab,[53] natalizumab,[54] and fingolimod[55] are humbling reminders that every patient who agrees to participate in a trial of an experimental medication assumes not just foreseeable risks and those risks associated with placebo, but unforeseeable risks associated with novel therapeutics as well.[21]

Another alternative to monotherapy placebo-controlled trials are add-on trials, in which the investigational agent or placebo is added on to an existing therapy to evaluate whether the investigational drug will confer increased efficacy. This is best suited for use when the two agents have different and potentially synergistic mechanisms of action. If not, a substantial possibility exists that a ceiling effect may be reached so that the combination therapy may fail to show a statistically significant advantage over treatment with the established drug plus placebo. This may obscure the fact that the new drug may be of value – perhaps even greater than the existing treatment – when used alone. Methodological issues arise owing to our often incomplete understanding of the drugs' molecular mechanisms of action, and consequent difficulty in predicting how the combination of agents will behave clinically, including unexpected antagonism. In addition, success of an agent in an add-on trial yields subsequent ethical and practical challenges when considering whether the new agent should be approved and prescribed as monotherapy if it was never tested in such a manner.[21]

A further strategy is a deferred treatment/crossover design, where after an initial randomization to placebo or active drug, the placebo patients are switched to active treatment either at a prespecified interval or after they reach a clinical end-point. This was the design of the BENEFIT trial of interferon beta-1b in CIS,[56] whereby at conversion to CDMS the CIS patients on placebo were switched to interferon. This design addressed the ethical concerns inherent in keeping patients who now met McDonald criteria off of an approved therapy, and allowed for a comparison between early- and delayed-treatment in the CIS population. If, however, one takes this study as incontrovertible evidence of the need for early treatment, it ethically precludes the further use of this placebo-controlled CIS design. This presents a paradigmatic example of the changing landscape of MS research: as existing treatments are shown to be superior to placebo in more numerous contexts, the study of new agents in the same manner is no longer ethically permissible.[21]

Conclusion

Clinical trialists clearly have a mandate to include ethical considerations in all aspects of the design, implementation, and conduct of clinical trials. The continued use of placebo-controlled randomized clinical trials in an era of partially effective therapy remains controversial, but should not be arbitrarily dismissed. Investigators seeking better treatments for MS must meet the challenge of developing new, scientifically valid study designs where placebo-controlled trials are deemed inappropriate. Both the utility and ethical conduct of placebo-controlled trials in MS are likely to continue to evolve as the MS therapeutic armamentarium grows increasingly refined.

References

1. Emanuel EJ, Wendler D, Grady C. What makes clinical research ethical? *J Am Med Assoc* 2000;283:2701–11.

2. The Belmont Report: Ethical Principles and Guidelines for the Protection of Human Subjects of Research. 1979. Available online at, http://www.fda.gov/oc/ohrt/IRBS/belmont.html

3. Council for International Organizations of Medical Sciences. *International Ethical Guidelines for Biomedical Research Involving Human Subjects.* Geneva, Switzerland: CIOMS; 1993.

4. International Conference on Harmonisation of Technical Requirements for Registration of Pharmaceuticals for Human Use (ICH). *Good clinical practice: consolidated guidance*, 62 Federal Register 25692 (1997).

5. Emanuel EJ, Miller FG. The ethics of placebo-controlled trials – a middle ground. *N Engl J Med* 2001;345: 915–19.

6. http://www.clinicaltrials.gov. *Accessed on November* 5, 2005.

7. DeAngelis CD, Drazen JM, Frizelle FA *et al.* Clinical trial registration: a statement from the International Committee of Medical Journal Editors. *J Am Med Assoc* 2004;292:1363–64.

8. Weijer C. The ethics of placebo-controlled trials. *J Bone Miner Res.* 2003;18:1150–3.

9. Freund PA. Legal frameworks for human experimentation. *Daedalus* 1969;98:314–24.

10. Slutsky AS, Lavery JV. Data safety and monitoring boards. *N Engl J Med* 2004;350:1143–7.

11. Appelbaum PS, Roth LH, Lidz CW. The therapeutic misconception: Informed consent in psychiatric research. *Int J Law Psychiatry* 1982;5:319–29.

12. Levine RJ. Placebo controls in clinical trials of new therapies for osteoporosis. *J Bone Mineral Res* 2003;18:1154–9.

13. The IFNB Multiple Sclerosis Study Group. Interferon beta-1b is effective in relapsing-remitting multiple sclerosis: I. Clinical results of a multicenter, randomized, double-blind, placebo-controlled trial. *Neurology* 1993;43:655–61.

14. Jacobs LD, Cookfair DL, Rudick RA, *et al.* Intramuscular interferon beta-1a for disease progression in relapsing multiple sclerosis. The Multiple Sclerosis Collaborative Research Group (MSCRG). *Ann Neurol* 1996;39:285–94.

15. PRISMS (Prevention of Relapses and Disability by Interferon beta-1a Subcutaneously in Multiple Sclerosis) Study Group. Randomised double-blind placebo-controlled study of interferon beta-1a in relapsing/remitting multiple sclerosis. *Lancet* 1998;352:1498–504.

16. Johnson KP, Brooks BR, Cohen JA, *et al.* Extended use of glatiramer acetate (Copaxone) is well tolerated and maintains its clinical effect on multiple sclerosis relapse rate and degree of disability. Copolymer 1 Multiple Sclerosis Study Group. *Neurology* 1998;50:701–8.

17. Hartung HP, Gonsette R, Konig N, *et al.* Mitoxantrone in progressive multiple sclerosis: a placebo-controlled, double-blind, randomized, multicentre trial. *Lancet* 2002;360:2018–25.

18. Polman CH, O'Connor PW, Havrdova E, *et al.* AFFIRM Investigators. A randomized, placebo-controlled trial of natalizumab for relapsing multiple sclerosis. *N Engl J Med* 2006 2;354(9): 899–910.

19. Kappos L, Radue EW, O'Connor P, *et al.* FREEDOMS Study Group. A placebo-controlled trial of oral fingolimod in relapsing multiple sclerosis. *N Engl J Med* 2010 4;362(5):387–401.

20. McFarland HF. Alemtuzumab versus interferon beta-1a: implications for pathology and trial design. *Lancet Neurol.* 2009;8(1):26–8.

21. Krieger, SC, Oynhausen, S, Miller, A. Clinical trials in multiple sclerosis. In Giésser BA (ed.) *Primer on Multiple Sclerosis*: New York: Oxford University Press, 2010 Chapter 29: 435–49.

22. Miller PB, Weijer C. Rehabilitating equipoise. Kennedy Inst. *Ethics J* 2003;13:93–118.

23. Fried C. *Medical Experimentation: Personal Integrity and Social Policy.* 1974. Amsterdam: North Holland.

24. Freedman B. Equipoise and the ethics of clinical research. *New Engl J Med* 1987;317:141–5.

25. London AJ. The Ambiguity and the Exigency: Clarifying 'Standard of Care' Arguments in International Research. *J Med Phil* 2000;25(4):379–97.

26. No Author Listed. World Medical Association Declaration of Helsinki: Ethical principles for medical research involving human subjects. *J Am Med Assoc* 2000;284:3043–5.

27. Declaration of Helsinki 2008 Available online at http://www.wma.net/en/30publications/10policies/b3/index.html. Accessed on October 4, 2010.

28. Macklin R. The Declaration of Helsinki: another revision. *Ind J Med Ethics* 2009;6(1): 2–4.

29. Temple R, Ellenberg SS. Placebo-controlled trials and active-control trials in the evaluation of new treatments. Part 1: Ethical and scientific issues. *Ann Int Med* 2000;133:455–63.

30. Lublin FD, Baier M, Cutter G. Effect of relapses on development of residual deficit in multiple sclerosis. *Neurology* 2003;61:1528–32.

31. Polman CH, Reingold SC, Barkhof F, *et al.* Ethics of placebo-controlled clinical trials in multiple sclerosis: a reassessment. *Neurology.* 2008;70(13, 2):1134–40.

32. Noseworthy JH, Miller D, Compston A. Disease modifying treatments in multiple sclerosis. In Compston A, McDonald IR, Noseworthy J, Lassmann H, eds. *McAlpine's Multiple Sclerosis*. London: Churchill Livingstone Elsevier, 2006: 729–802.

33. European Study Group on Interferon beta-1b in secondary progressive MS. Placebo-controlled multicentre randomised trial of interferon beta-1b in treatment of secondary progressive multiple sclerosis. *Lancet* 1998;352: 1491–7.

34. Secondary Progressive Efficacy Clinical Trial of Recombinant Interferon-beta-1a in MS (SPECTRIMS) Study Group. Randomized controlled trial of interferon- beta-1a in secondary progressive MS: Clinical results. *Neurology* 2001;56:1496–504.

35. Cohen JA, Cutter GR, Fischer HJS, *et al.* Benefit of interferon beta-1a on MSFC progression in secondary progressive MS. *Neurology* 2002;59:679–87.

36. The North American Study Group on Interferon beta-1b in Secondary Progressive MS. Interferon beta-1b in secondary progressive MS. Results from a 3-year controlled study. *Neurology* 2004;63:1788–95.

37. Lublin FD, Reingold SC, the National Multiple Sclerosis Society (USA) Task Force on Placebo-Controlled Clinical Trials in MS. Placebo-controlled clinical trials in multiple sclerosis: Ethical considerations. *Ann Neurol* 2001;49:677–81.

38. Fost N. Ethical issues in clinical research on fracture prevention in patients with osteoporosis. *J Bone Miner Res* 2003;18:1110–15.

39. Angell M. The ethics of clinical research in the third world. *N Engl J Med* 1997;337:847–9.

40. Angell M. Investigators' responsibilities for human subjects in developing countries. *N Engl J Med* 2000;342: 967–9.

41. Macklin R. Bioethics, Vulnerability, and Protection. *Bioethics* 2003: 17:472–86.

42. Coleman CH, Vulnerability as a regulatory category in human subject research. *J Law, Med Ethics* 2009: 12–18.

43. Shapiro HT, Meslin EM. Ethical issues in the design and conduct of clinical trials in developing countries. *N Engl J Med* 2001;345:139–42.

44. Koski G, Nightingale SL. Research involving human subjects in developing countries. *N Engl J Med* 2001;345: 136–38.

45. Nuffield Council on Bioethics. *The Ethics of Research Related to Health Care in Developing Countries*. London: Nuffield Council on Bioethics, 2002.

46. McMillan, Conlon C. The ethics of research related to health care in developing countries. *J Med Ethics* 2004;30:204–6.

47. Lie RK, Emanuel E, Grady C, *et al.* The standard of care debate: the Declaration of Helsinki versus the international consensus opinion. *J Med Ethics* 2004;30:190–3.

48. Ellenberg SS. Scientific and ethical issues in the use of placebo and active controls in clinical trials. *J Bone Mineral Res* 2003;18:1121–4.

49. McFarland HF, Reingold SC. The future of multiple sclerosis therapies: redesigning multiple sclerosis clinical trials in a new therapeutic era. *Mult Scler* 2005;11(6):669–76.

50. Benson K, Hartz AJ. A comparison of observational studies and randomized, controlled trials. *N Engl J Med* 2000;342:1878–86.

51. Concato J, Shah N, Horwitz RI. Randomized, controlled trials, observational studies, and the hierarchy of research designs. *N Engl J Med* 2000;342:1887–92.

52. Pocock SJ, Elbourne DR. Randomized trials or observational tribulations. *N Engl J Med* 2000;342:1907–9.

53. Coles AJ, Compston DA, Selmaj KW, *et al.* for the CAMMS223 Trial Investigators. Alemtuzumab vs. interferon beta-1a in early multiple sclerosis. *N Engl J Med* 2008;359(17): 1786–801.

54. Goodin DS, Cohen BA, O'Connor P, Kappos L, Stevens JC, Therapeutics and Technology Assessment Subcommittee of the American Academy of Neurology. Assessment: the use of natalizumab (Tysabri) for the treatment of multiple sclerosis (an evidence-based review): report of the Therapeutics and Technology Assessment Subcommittee of the American Academy of Neurology *Neurology* 2008;71(10):766–73.

55. Leypoldt F, Münchau A, Moeller F, Bester M, Gerloff C, Heesen C. Hemorrhaging focal encephalitis under fingolimod (FTY720) treatment: a case report. *Neurology* 2009;72(11):1022–4.

56. Kappos L, Polman CH, Freedman MS, *et al.* Treatment with interferon beta-1b delays conversion to clinically definite and McDonald MS in patients with clinically isolated syndromes. *Neurology* 2006;67(7):1242–9.

23

Pharmacogenomics and related discovery-driven approaches in multiple sclerosis

Paulo Fontoura and David Leppert

Introduction

This chapter covers research based on the concept of discovery-driven approaches using high-throughput technologies (DNA, RNA, protein, and metabolite analysis) in relation to drugs used to treat MS. In the prior edition of this book, this chapter was named "Pharmacogenetics and pharmacogenomics in multiple sclerosis." However, definitions of these terms have changed in official documents by the US[1] and European[2] regulatory agencies. Table 23.1 lists the earlier[3] and current[4,5] definition of pharmacogenetics and pharmacogenomics. In the literature, the two are often used interchangeably. In fact, they overlapped in the old nomenclature, as both referred to DNA analysis, while the difference was based on the number of genes analyzed, and implicitly the analytical technique used (Table 23.1). The most prominent change in terminology is the exclusion of "proteomics" and "metabolomics" from the generic term "pharmacogenomics."[1,2] Members of the Pharmacogenetics Working Group have raised concerns about the exclusion of proteomics and called these changes "unnecessary and confusing."[5] They suggested that DNA analysis be referred to as "pharmacogenetics," irrespective of the analytical technique, and "that 'pharmacogenomics' relates specifically to the analysis of gene expression (i.e. RNA) and its products (i.e. proteins, metabolites," definitions that we used in the prior edition of this book and elsewhere.[6] These suggestions have been rejected, and we use here the new definitions, but continue to cover research on all -omics platforms related to MS.

Pathogenesis of MS remains poorly understood. In particular, initiating events and molecular mechanisms underlying neurodegeneration at different disease stages are uncertain. Many presently undefined molecules may be involved in pathogenetic pathways (undefined referring to both novel genes and known genes whose involvement in MS has not been recognized so far). Therefore, novel approaches are required to complement standard hypothesis testing approaches. "*Discovery-driven research*" is one such novel approach.

Discovery-driven research involves simultaneous analysis of a large number of targets in an unbiased manner, which theoretically would lead to understanding of a comprehensive *matrix of interactions* between genes, biological factors, and clinical features.[6] "-Omics" techniques have provided flexible analytical platforms for discovery-driven research that enable detection of gene variation, and to quantify gene expression in a high-throughput fashion (Table 23.2). Hence, pharmacogenomics and related platforms are sister disciplines of genetics and genomics (Fig. 23.1), the distinction being that genetics and genomics (Chapter 4) are observational disciplines that relate to disease susceptibility, diagnosis and disease course; whereas pharmacogenomics relates the genome to drug effects – efficacy, dose–response, adverse events, tolerability, and the like. The technologies are identical: genotyping refers to elucidating DNA sequences; transcriptomics, proteomics, and metabolomics refer to measures of RNA, proteins, and metabolites, respectively.

The need for predictive biomarkers as a driver for pharmacogenomics research

Although the term pharmacogenomics entered the medical lexicon in the 1950s, when researchers became aware that drug metabolism was linked to a person's genetic make-up,[7–9] it took another 40 years for systematic application of this concept to research and clinical practice. In 1997, trastuzumab was the first drug approved for a specific form of breast cancer when tumor cells over express the HER2 receptor. Since HER2 receptor expression by tumor cells predicts response to trastuzumab, its use requires an immunohistochemical "eligibility" test. Since then over 50 drugs have specific genetic markers included in their product label, mainly related to safety aspects.[4] Clinical application of "personalized medicine," as in these examples is not the only 'end-product' of pharmacogenomics. There are specific reasons why pharmacogenomics and related

Both authors are employees of Roche and have stock ownership of this company. The subject matter and materials discussed in the manuscript are not linked to their corporate work, nor has Roche vested interests in the materials discussed here. No writing assistance was utilized in the production of this manuscript.

Table 23.1. *Comparison of old and new definitions of pharmacogenomics*

	"Pharmacogenetics"	"Pharmacogenomics"
2003[1]	"application of single gene sequences or a limited set of gene sequences, but *not* gene expression or genome-wide scans, ... to study variation of DNA sequences related to drug action and disposition observed"	"applications of genome-wide SNP scans and gene expression analysis to study variations that influence drug action" *abbreviation: Pgmx*
2006[4,5]	"The study of variation in DNA in DNA sequence as related to drug response"[a] *abbreviation: Pgt* "Pharmacogenetics (PGt) is a subset of pharmacogenomics (Pharmacogenomics)"	"The study of variation of DNA and RNA characteristics as related to drug response"[a] *abbreviation: Pharmacogenomics* "The definitions of Pharmacogenomics and PGt do *not* include other disciplines such as proteomics and metabolomics"

[a] "drug reponse" includes the processes of drug absorption and disposition (e.g. pharmacokinetics (PK)), and drug effects (e.g. pharmacodynamics, drug efficacy, and adverse effects of drugs). The term *drug* should be considered synonymous with investigational (medicinal) product, medicinal product, medicine, and pharmaceutical product (including vaccines and other biological products). The terms "Pharmacogenomics" and "Pgt" are applicable to activities such as drug discovery, drug development, and clinical practice.

Table 23.2. *High-throughput techniques (omics platforms)*

	Target	Analytical method	Conventional research equivalent
Genetics	DNA	microarrays ("gene chips")	Gene sequencing RLFP, others
Transcriptomics	RNA	microarrays ("gene chips") 5' nuclease assay (TaqMan)	Northern, RNase protection assay, others
Proteomics	protein	microarrays ("protein chips"), 2-dimensional electrophoresis, various spectroscopic techniques	Western, ELISA
Metabolomics	metabolites	NMR-spectroscopy, HPLC, cellular assays mass spectrometry	HPLC, cellular assays

technologies are likely to have significant impact on understanding of MS, and MS drug development:

1. The course of MS for individuals is largely unpredictable, as is response to standard and experimental treatments. Additionally, several compounds tested for MS have led to unanticipated severe side effects, or unexpectedly aggravated MS itself. Analogous to other therapeutic areas, pharmacogenomics could theoretically have allowed mechanistic understanding of the cause of those adverse events, minimizing risks for future development of novel therapeutic compounds.
2. MS is genetically complex (Chapter 4), and may not be a single nosologic entity, but a syndrome with shared clinical features, and heterogeneous pathophysiology.[10] This may partially explain individual variation in drug efficacy in MS patient groups. Molecular understanding of *endophenotypes* for drug response will be needed to optimize the benefit/risk ratio of candidate compounds and realize the promise of personalized medicine.
3. Current biomarkers for MS (e.g. CSF oligoclonal bands) are of diagnostic value, but lack prognostic value

regarding disease course or drug response. To a large extent, this also applies to imaging and neurophysiological tests.
4. The cost of MS therapies has become a concern for regulators and payers, especially given modest efficacy of current therapies, and uncertain long-term impact. It would be very helpful to target current treatments to individuals who are predicted to respond well to particular therapies, so that limited resources could be targeted more efficiently. In addition, development of natalizumab and fingolimod provide more effective drugs, but present more risk. Biomarkers that predict risk for these more effective therapies would be of enormous medical and economic value.

There is an obvious need for biomarkers that would predict future disease course (*prospective markers*) and drug response (*predictive markers*). Patients likely to have a benign course could be observed without treatment, and patients with a worse prognosis could be treated with more potent, but riskier drugs.

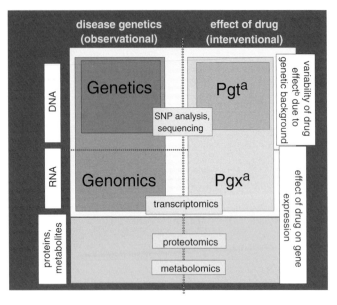

Fig. 23.1. Pharmacogenetics, pharmacogenomics, and their relationship to genetics, genomics, and "-omics" platforms
[a]Pgt (pharmacogenetics and Pgx (pharmacogenomics) as per new definitions[1,2]
[b]efficacy, safety, and tolerability

Table 23.3. *Pharmacogenomics and other -omics platforms vs. conventional biomarkers*

Approach	Pharmacogenomics/ proteomics/ metabolomics	Conventional biomarker
Strategic	discovery-driven (open platform, unbiased, inductive, "hypothesis-free")	hypothesis-driven deductive
Operational	integration of structure and expression of multiple genes	targeted analysis of single/few gene(s) or its regulation/function
read-out	matrix analysis, pathway analysis	mono-vectorial
Technical	'omics platforms	conventional assays
throughput	high	low
quantitative capacity	semi-quantitative (low dynamic measuring range)	high

"-omics" technologies and conventional methods are not exclusive alternatives, but mutually complementary approaches in the search for biomarkers.

Relation of pharmacogenomics to conventional biomarkers

The factors that differentiate pharmacogenomics from conventional biomarker research on a strategic, operational, and technical level are outlined in Table 23.3. Discovery-driven approaches are sometimes erroneously called "hypothesis-free," which insinuates that they are tools of researchers lacking a proper hypothesis. In fact, the hypothesis is that there are genes active in the pathogenesis of disease, whose involvement cannot be anticipated on the basis of current deductive knowledge, but which can be discovered by unbiased "open platform" technologies.[6] The most striking example is the detection of ApoE4 as a susceptibility gene for sporadic Alzheimer's disease, as well as a risk factor for progression in other neurodegenerative diseases, including MS.[11]

While genotyping data are discrete in character, gene expression delivers continuous data, i.e. variable both by interindividual cross-comparison and by intra-individual expression levels over time. Current open platform technologies have the important drawback of a relatively poor dynamic measuring range, and consequently little quantitative capacity. Hence, most "-omic" platform technologies are used for screening purposes and, once a target is identified, it must be validated by conventional, more quantitative measuring systems. Moreover, high-throughput technologies are relatively expensive for data acquisition, and evaluation (bioinformatics) as compared with conventional methods. Accordingly, genotyping may identify genetic regions that are *linked* to a specific drug response, but not necessarily the specific gene/allele *causing* it. For this, conventional sequencing methods must be used. In essence,

The role of "-omics" research in drug development

Current clinical trial end-points take considerable time, and are partly subjective, resulting in the need to run Phase 3 trials over the course of years. Since almost every patient with active relapsing MS will be treated with disease-modifying therapy in the future, the available patient pool to test candidate drugs will become increasingly limited. Except for early phase, brief trials, placebo-controlled trials have become increasingly impractical, and comparison of newer therapies with more effective new therapies (e.g. natalizumab, fingolimod) will inherently lead to smaller incremental treatment effects for new compounds. The end result will be that to demonstrate superior efficacy of a new drug, further increase in patient numbers per study, or longer study durations, or both will be required. The lack of *surrogate markers* that would allow demonstration of drug efficacy more reliably and at an earlier time point, compared to current clinical and imaging read-outs, may become a major logistical and financial road-block in the attempt to develop novel therapies for MS. Pharmacogenomics may be an essential approach to define such surrogate markers to improve the odds for successfully developing new therapies, and later to implement the paradigm of personalized medicine. Currently, the "raw material" for pharmacogenomics studies lies mostly in the hands of the pharmaceutical industry in the form of clinical trial cohorts. At the time of the previous edition of this book, it seemed that there was an interest in such studies as several companies had begun to initiate studies within or independent of Phase 3 studies. However, many of these projects have never been developed to result level, e.g.[12] In other study cohorts only genome-wide association with disease diagnosis has been performed, i.e. leaving out the drug response aspects.[13] In recent years the industry has largely stopped conducting pharmacogenomics programs, due to financial constraints, initial underestimation of resource needs, and the perceived slow pace of progress in this field.[14] A further reason may be that "individualized medicine" may be perceived as a commercial challenge due to "market fragmentation" (i.e. the prospect of drug approval only for a subgroup of "ideal responders," as opposed to a "fit-for-all" label).

Examples from other disease areas have shown that pharmacogenomics could also be a valuable way to identify patients prone to side effects based on their genetic fingerprint in early phases of drug development, which may prevent later stage compound attrition due to unexplained adverse events. The occurrence of progressive multifocal leukencephalopathy in 1 of 1000 patients treated with natalizumab is a prime example of a missed opportunity of identifying susceptibility markers for this side effect: no systematic sampling of DNA probes during Phase 3 trials or post marketing has been performed, and no gene expression profiling has been done to define molecular determinants of risk. Therefore, in future years, and as more potent drugs become available, the need to better identify the benefit–risk ratio for new therapies between patient groups, and during the patient's drug exposure period, will necessitate the identification of markers of both response to therapy, as well as for the development of side effects, especially those of low frequency and major clinical impact.

Pharmacogenomics studies in MS

The genetic component of MS risk has been the focus of study for a long time, and beyond the classic association with the MHC locus, seven genome-wide association studies (GWAS) reported in recent years have helped identify other candidate genes, such as the IL-7 and IL-2 receptors, and have supported the view that genetic risk is associated with several common allelic variants in multiple genes.[15] However, apart from the theoretical connection of IL-2R with daclizumab (Chapter 33), no other therapy insights have yet been generated through this approach.

Genomic expression studies in MS have variously looked at messenger RNA expression profiles in human peripheral blood mononuclear cells (PBMC) or brain tissue from post-mortem samples. Some study results have not been reproduced, but others have resulted in findings of therapeutic relevance, such as osteopontin,[16–18] or confirmed other suspected targets, such as matrix metalloproteinases.[19–21] More recently, genomic expression studies have been used to identify prognostic biomarkers for disease course. Corvol *et al.* evaluated expression profiles in CD4 T-cells from CIS patients at onset and one year later. They identified a gene expression pattern associated with markedly increased risk of conversion to MS.[22] The most underexpressed gene in patients converting to MS was *TOB1* (transducer of ERBB2), a transcriptional repressor known to play a major role in preventing proliferation of naïve T-cells.

Studies of micro RNA (miRNA) have become a hot topic in MS research. Micro RNAs are small[20–24] nucleotide RNA sequences that can bind to messenger RNA molecules and influence their expression. Micro RNAs have been implicated in the regulation of immune responses in several diseases, including MS.[23] Although a specific pharmacogenomic study of miRNA expression in MS has not been conducted, it has been shown that interferon beta (IFNβ) can modulate the expression of several miRNAs in hepatocytes, and that these molecules play an integral part in the antiviral effects of IFN.[24]

Predicting response to MS therapy is one of the major goals of current research, given the need for better prediction of the benefit–risk ratio on an individual basis.[25] Pharmacogenomics studies have multiple layers of evidence to offer for this goal: generating evidence for diagnostic and prognostic biomarkers of MS, identifying disease subtypes at risk of progression; identifying a "pharmacodynamic signature" of drug response, including hints into the mechanism of action of drugs; and validation of predictive biomarkers of response to therapy or susceptibility to adverse events.[26]

Most studies that we will review (see Table 23.4 and 23.5)[27] have focused on these last two categories, but there are several caveats that deserve notice. First, studies have mainly focused on the use of IFNβ, with relatively little attention being paid to other approved therapies. Second, there is no truly validated definition of responder at the individual patient level;[51] only recently has the approach of focusing on so-called "extreme phenotypes," defined as the absence of relapses and EDSS progression for a two-year period, and "non-response" as the presence of two or more relapses and 1 point progression on the EDSS become widely used for comparison of cohorts. Besides the known problems with the EDSS scale, it must be noted that, at this moment, it is not clear if the pathophysiological drivers behind relapses and progression are the same, and whether we may be defining a hybrid endophenotype of "response/non-response." Finally, the issue of neutralizing antibodies (NAbs), including their method of measurement and temporal dynamic, has continued to be a significant confounder for most of these studies. For IFNβ response studies, determination of NAb status should be an integral part of the dataset used for response comparison, given its potential role in determining clinical effectiveness.

Genotype-related studies of drug therapy response

In comparison with the previous edition of this chapter, in recent years there has been an increase in the number of studies conducted, mainly using a candidate-gene approach, although recently the first genome-wide association results have been published. It should be noted that for several of these studies, the sample size is relatively small and geographically contained, thereby raising concerns about the generalizability of the reported findings. A common limitation for these studies is the absence of reporting for neutralizing antibody (NAb)

Table 23.4. *DNA-based studies*

Pharmacogenetics/GWAS[a]	
SNPs modify response to IFN	
- HLA class II:	Fusco 2001[28]
	Villoslada 2002[29]
	Comabella 2009[30]
- IFNAR1/2:	Sriram 2002[31]
	Leyva 2004[32]
	Cunningham 2005[33]
	Comabella 2009[34]
	Byun 2008[35]
- intronic IFNγ polymorphisms:	Martinez 2005[36]
- MxA:	Cunningham 2005[33]
	Weinstock-Guttman 2007[37]
- Cathepsin S:	Cunningham 2005[33]
- IL10 promotor polymophisms:	Wergeland 2005[38]
- Glypican 5:	Byun 2008[35]
	Cénit 2009[39] (also a marker of MS predisposition: Cavanillas 2010[40])
- CD46	Alvarez-Fuente 2010[41] (see mRNA expression below)
- gene combinations differentiate responders from non-responders	O'Doherty 2009[42]
SNPSs modify response to GA	
- Cathepsin S:	Grossman 2007[43]
- HLA class II:	Fusco 2001[28]
	Grossman 2007[43]
- TCRbeta:	Grossman 2007[43]

[a] GWAS: genome-wide association studies.

Table 23.5. *RNA-based studies*

Pharmacogenomics PBMC	
Response to IFNβ	
Descriptive *:differential RNA expression*	
- Wandinger 2001:[44]	Th1 genes IL12Rbeta2, CCR↑
- Weinstock-Guttman 2003[45]	antiviral response, interferon signaling, lymphocyte activation
- Koike 2003[46]	↑ interferon-responsive genes (IRF7, ISG15IF 16–16)
- Hong 2004[47]	distinctive pattern compared to GA therapy
- Iglesias 2004:[48]	downregulation of E2F pathway targets
- Fernald 2007:[49]	first study using network analysis of gene regulation
- Cepok 2009:[50]	set of chemokines and CCR1↑
- Serrano-Fernandez 2010[51]	IFN regulated genes (EIF2AK2, IF16, IFI44)
- Bernal 2009:[19]	at base line: MMP-8/-9/-14/-19, TIMP-1/-2↑; TIMP-3↓ under IFN:MMP-8/-9/-11/-14/-19/-25↓, TIMP-1/-2/-3↓
- Goertsches 2010:[52]	CD20↓, CMPK2↑, FFAR2↑, FCER1A↓
- Hecker 2010:[53]	network analysis
Identification of clinical responders/non-responders:	
- Stürzebecher 2003:[54]	responders IL8↓
- Weinstock-Guttman 2008:[55]	responders IL8↓, IFNAR1↓, CASP10↓; MxA↑, IFNAR2↑, IL6↑, among other genes
- Baranzini 2005:[56]	sets gene triplet analysis at baseline predicts response with up to 86% accuracy (Caspase 2/10, FLIP); 6 genes show differential regulation between responders and non-responders (IRF2/4/6, Caspase 7/10, IL4Ralpha)
van Baarsen 2008:[57]	first report of correlation of responders with low expression on IFN response genes at baseline
- Comabella 2009:[58]	(a) expression pattern of 8 genes (IFIT3, RASGEF1B, IFIT1, OASL, IFI44, IFIT2, FADS1, after 24 m with 78% accuracy b) activated type I IFN-signalling pathway is associated with lack of response to IFN
- Alvarez-Fuente 2010:[41]	CD46↑ more frequent in responders
Response to GA	
Descriptive: *	
- Hong 2004:[47]	regulation of IFN response genes distinctive pattern compared to IFN therapy
- Valenzuela 2007:[59]	clinical response correlates with IFNγ ↓, IL4/IFNγ ↑
Clinical response to natalizumab	
Descriptive: *	
- Lindberg 2008:[60]	B-cell associated genes (↑BLK, ↑MS4A1, ↓IL6R, ↑CD24, ↑CD79) neutrophil associated genes (↓IL8R, ↓C5R1, ↑defensin α1and α4)

status in these patients. Assuming an average NAb positivity ratio of 10%–30%, this may mean that a significant proportion of patients may have been misclassified a priori as non-responders due to their NAb status.

Overall, for IFNβ, several polymorphic variants (SNPs) have been reported in association with therapeutic response, belonging both to IFN and immune-related categories, as well as more general neurotoxic and neuroprotective categories (for an updated list see Table 23.4).[62] Several studies focused on genes associated with the IFN receptor (the heterodimer IFNAR1/IFNAR2), its canonical signaling pathway through Jak/STAT, or genes possessing an interferon-stimulated response element (ISRE consensus sequence) in their promoter region. Initial studies evaluated the impact of eight SNPs and microsatellites in the non-promoter region of the genes for the two subunits of the IFN-receptor, and failed to find an effect on the response to IFNβ based on clinical and MRI criteria.[31,32] Later, Cunningham *et al.*,[33] looking at the promoter regions of 100 ISRE-containing genes identified four candidates associated with IFN response, including IFNAR1, as well as LMP7 (proteasome beta subunit), CTSS (cathepsin S) and MxA,[33] although this last one was not replicated in a subsequent study.[37] A SNP in the IFNAR2 gene has subsequently been identified in a genome-wide association study, although it failed to retain significance for multiple comparisons.[34] Downstream of the IFN receptor, no significant genetic polymorphism hits have been reported, although, as discussed later, there may be a relationship between TYK2 and JAK2 expression and response to therapy.[50] It is interesting that of the other genetic associations reported by Cunningham, both LMP7 and CTSS, may be related to the processing of self-antigens for presentation to T lymphocytes, and may therefore be implicated in the pathophysiology of the autoimmune response in MS.

Other genes that have been looked at relate to known relevant players in immune response regulation, such as the prototype Th1-Th2 cytokines, gamma interferon and IL-10. Four alleles of a polymorphic microsatellite in the first intron of the IFNγ gene were differentially associated with relapse frequency in RRMS patients being treated with IFNβ, but not before treatment.[36] Wergeland et al, analyzed three polymorphisms in the promoter region of IL-10 for their relationship to clinical and imaging response to IFNβ therapy in 63 RRMS patients. They found that, in the first 6 months of IFNβ therapy, two non-GCC polymorphisms (one of which, ATA, is linked to lower IL-10 levels and has been associated with better treatment response in hepatitis C) were associated with fewer new imaging lesions, but no difference in clinical disease activity.[38]

In another candidate-gene study, O'Doherty et al. screened for 61 polymorphisms in the 5'UTR promoter regions of 34 genes presumed to be associated with MS pathophysiology and interferon response (e.g. IFN signaling pathway, cytokines, apoptosis) in 255 Irish MS patients. Despite not finding any significant individual associations, several allelic combinations were associated with therapy response (JAK2-IL10-CASP3) and non-response (JAK2-IL10RB-GBP1-PIAS1), illustrating that response to interferon probably has a polygenic basis.[42]

"Hypothesis-free" pharmacogenomics genome-wide association studies (pharmacogenomics-GWAS) have been conducted to identify novel candidate target genes. In the first of these reports, Byun et al. studied 206 MS patients treated with IFNβ therapy for at least two years, focusing on extreme "responder/non-responder" phenotypes.[35] Results were filtered by statistical significance-based ranking and a haplotype-clustering algorithm, and gene ontology analysis was used to identify functional categories of genes. Interestingly, over-represented gene ontology categories that differentiated responder populations included ligand-gated ion channels for the neurotransmitters glutamate and GABA (e.g. GRIA1, GABRA2, GABRB1) and signal transduction pathways. In MS and experimental autoimmune encephalomyelitis (EAE), glutamate and GABA have been implicated both in excitotoxic damage of neurons and glia, as well as in the regulation of the immune response.[63–65] Responder-associated SNPs were identified in several genes that had not been reported before by a combination of significance and cluster ranking: these included SNPs located within the genes for glypican 5, hyaluronan proteoglycan link protein, calpastatin, neuronal PAS domain protein 3, and TAFA1. In contrast to previous studies, no association

with IFNAR, or with CTSS and LMP7 was found (although the relevant SNPs in the promoter region of CTSS or LMP7 were not present in the microarray used for the GWAS study).[35] Interestingly, SNPs in the glypican 5 gene have since been reported in a different Spanish population of 199 MS patients in association with IFN response,[39] and in a Norwegian population of 1355 patients,[66] and a Spanish population of 2863 patients[40] as a risk gene for the disease at the 13q31–32 locus. Glypicans are heparan sulfate proteoglycans implicated in synapse formation, axonal growth and guidance and may therefore play a role in neuroprotection.

Interestingly, in another recently reported pharmacogenomics-GWAS study in 106 patients using a higher density array (500K vs. 100K SNPs for the Byun et al. study), the strongest association was found with the GRIA3 gene, which codes for a glutamate (AMPA) receptor. Other significant associations were found in genes related to the IFN pathway, such as ADAR (RNA-specific adenosine deaminase) and IFNAR2, and in IL-6 pathway-associated genes.[34] The finding of another association of IFN responsiveness to genes in the glutamatergic system again points to the potential multiple effects this immunomodulator may have on the CNS, including neuroprotection effects.

In comparison with these studies, there have been few reports of genetic association with drug response for glatiramer acetate (GA) (Chapter 26). The HLA-DRB1*1501 haplotype, which is the most validated genetic susceptibility allele for MS, has been linked to a higher probability of response to GA, in contrast to IFNβ, where no such association was observed.[28] This finding is consistent with the proposed mode of action for GA, i.e. functioning as an altered peptide ligand for T-cells cross-reactive with myelin antigens, therefore interfering with the primary mechanism of auto-immune activation. In this capacity, GA would work as a molecular mimic for the same trimolecular complex of MHC-antigen-TCR for MBP reactive T-cells, and therefore, it is natural that it might share the same genetic association with a MHC molecule known to be highly specific for binding to MBP.[67] A second study confirmed the lack of HLA association with clinical response to IFNβ when patients were stratified according to HLA-DR2 (DRB1*1501, DQB1*0602) status.[29] Absence of association to HLA is in line with the concept that IFNβ acts on secondary mechanisms of MS pathogenesis (modulation of cytokine expression towards anti-inflammatory mediators, down-regulation of effector molecules of cell migration, such as matrix metalloproteinases (MMPs)).

A recent study in 174 MS patients culled from two randomized controlled trials of GA (containing 85 GA treated and 89 matched placebo MS patients) looked at SNPs in genes selected for their relevance to GA's mode of action, MS pathogenesis, general immune- or neurodegeneration-related processes; therapy response was defined according to the original clinical trial description, but generally corresponded to the "extreme phenotype" concept.[43] After correction for multiple comparisons, SNPs in TRB@ (TCR gene cluster) and CTSS (cathepsin S) were associated with response to GA in both patient populations, and other immune-related genes such as MBP, FAS, IL1R1, IL12RB2, and CD86 in patients from one clinical trial.[43] Interestingly, although an association with HLA DRB1*1501 was not confirmed, this study again points to elements associated with the trimolecular complex and the immunological synapse, such as the TCR beta chain, MBP, FAS and CD86, and the antigen-processing enzyme cathepsin, in accordance with the mode of action of GA.

Gene expression (RNA) studies of drug therapy response

The power of gene expression studies lies in the potential to establish a real-time relationship between continuous biological ("*real-world*") signals and a specific disease state of MS, and the potential to integrate results from different levels of expression (RNA, protein, and metabolite), helping determine the role of specific genes and their products.[68] Genomic expression markers in MS are expected to have wide variability across subjects and during time, which, together with their pleiotropic roles, makes it largely impossible to define a "normal range". Cross-sectional ascertainment of gene expression patterns typically yields little relevant information at the individual clinical level, or for population epidemiological purposes. Therefore, in order to capture relevant genomic changes relating to drug effect or disease pathology, *longitudinal, intra-individual* analysis becomes the focus. As was identified in the previous edition of this chapter, methodological shortcomings limit interpretation of published pharmacogenomics studies in MS. These include restriction to PMBC as a source for RNA, heterogeneity in sampling and technology platforms, poor correlation to imaging and clinical findings, and relatively small patient samples.

Development of individual biomarkers for monitoring drug response has generated strong interest, especially as concerns IFNβ as it relates to NAb.[69] Candidate markers should ideally be IFN-responsive and show close temporal correlation to the beginning of therapy, as well as sensitivity to loss of bioactivity due, for example, to the development of NAb. Among the genes studied, myxovirus resistance protein A (MxA) has generated the most interest, and loss of MxA expression by IFN therapy correlated with loss of bioactivity.[70] Pathophysiologically plausible markers, like TRAIL and XAF-1, which initially generated considerable interest, appear to be less sensitive than MxA,[20,71] and there is no evidence for prediction of response to therapy for either of these genes; MMPs and tissue inhibitors of metalloproteinases (TIMPs) expression continue to show promise, and have been shown to be more sensitive to NAb presence than MxA in at least one study,[72] and predictive for a more severe disease course.[21] However, given the remaining uncertainties in this field, recent recommendations have continued to stress the integration of clinical, imaging and gene expression data as a monitoring strategy for IFNβ in MS and for therapeutic decision guidance.[73]

Several genomic expression studies in MS have focused on the detection of a "pharmacodynamic" signature of drug action in PBMC. An initial longitudinal study by Wandinger et al. revealed a counter-intuitive upregulation in a number of pro-inflammatory mediators, like the chemokine receptor CCR5 and the IL-12Rβ2 chain in six relapsing MS patients treated with IFNβ.[44] In a follow-up study of IFNβ treatment[54] the same group identified 25 genes regulated ex vivo, and an additional 87 by in vitro stimulation, associated with cell migration, matrix degradation, cell cycle control, apoptosis, and chemokine/cytokine regulation. Similarly, another microarray profiling of PBMC from 17 relapsing MS patients highlighted the role of the E2F pathway in MS pathogenesis.[48] Several E2F1-dependent genes showed increased expression in MS PBMC, and two (E2F3, Ha/D) were negatively regulated in patients receiving IFNβ. In another study, the expression profiles of 34 genes selected based on their role in inflammation and their susceptibility to regulation by IFNβ and GA were compared in PBMC from 45 MS patients and nine healthy volunteers. The authors were able to identify a panel of genes differentially regulated by IFNβ or GA, in accordance with the different mode of action for these compounds.[47]

Further insight into the mechanism of action of IFNβ has emerged from studies looking at the expression of key molecules involved in the immune response such as cytokines and matrix metalloproteinases. Cepok et al. looked at the gene and protein expression of 14 chemokines and chemokine receptor pairs in 17 relapsing MS patients treated with intramuscular IFNβ, and reported that in NAb negative patients there was a clear up-regulation in several of these pro-inflammatory molecules (CCL1, 2, 7, CXCL10 and 11, CCR1), in comparison with NAb positive, untreated MS patients and healthy controls.[50] This surprising finding, although in line with the results of Wandinger et al.[44] may be partly reconciled with the known anti-inflammatory effects of IFNβ by postulating a loss of chemokine gradient between the periphery and the CNS, or alternatively by desensitization of immune system cells to high concentrations of these molecules. MMPs and their inhibitors TIMPs are considered to play a key role in the immunopathogenesis of MS, namely by regulating the penetration of immune cells into the CNS. The expression profile of MMPs and TIMPs can be influenced by IFNβ treatment. Initially, Galboiz et al. reported a reduction in MMP-7 and MMP-9 expression in treated MS patients,[74] and Gilli et al.,[72] found a suppression of MMP-2 and -9 in long-term IFNβ treated patients, and no effect on TIMP-1 and -2; the development of NAb led to a loss of this expression pattern. These findings were recently confirmed and expanded to include a bigger list of IFN-responding members of the family, including down-regulations of MMP-8, -9, -11, -14, -19, -25, TIMP-1, -2, and TIMP-3, in 14 MS patients treated with IFNβ for 6 months.[19] Loss or decrease in MMP suppression pattern has been associated with non-response to therapy. In a 2-year longitudinal study looking at 50 relapsing MS patients treated with IFNβ, a two-fold increase in the MMP-9/TIMP-1 expression ratio was correlated with the appearance of NAbs and a higher probability of relapse or, and was a better marker of bioactivity than the expression of MxA progression.[21]

Looking at the temporal dynamics of gene expression after IFNβ therapy, Koike et al. compared the profile of T and non-T-cells derived from 13 RRMS patients before and after treatment with IFNβ-1b at multiple time points. Twenty-one genes out of 1263 sequences tested had significantly altered expression patterns, but no correlation with clinical effectiveness was reported.[46] Weinstock-Guttman et al.[45] studied eight patients with active RRMS, looking at over 4000 genes before and at eight time points over seven days after a single IM injection, and found a specific and time-dependent expression profile upon start of therapy. They detected changes in genes implicated in the antiviral response, interferon signaling, and lymphocyte activation. Taking this approach one step further, Fernald et al. performed similar temporal expression profiling in two patients dosed with IM IFNβ-1a at as many as eight time-points post-dosing, and analyzed results using a relevance network (Relnet) method to detect mutual information relationships, i.e. networks of co-expressed genes.[49] Using this approach, together with gene ontological classification, the authors identified an expression profile enriched in genes related to cell adhesion, apoptosis and immune response, and were able to create a directional network of metagenes (transcripts with similar biological function and expression dynamics), which illustrated the potential mechanism of action of IFN. Finally, two studies from the same group have been recently published looking at the long-term temporal dynamics of gene expression. In these studies, a small cohort of patients treated with sc IFNβ were sampled two days, one month, one year and two years after initiation of therapy. In the first of these studies, a subset of 15 genes was identified, which showed a consistent expression pattern at these time-points, with modest upregulation at two days, marked increase at one month, then reduction after one year of therapy.[51] Regulated genes included mostly IFN-regulated genes (such as EIF2AK2, IFI6, IFI44) known to be involved in the antiviral response. The second study also applied a gene ontology network analysis, revealing that the most represented biological processes included antiviral response genes, immune effector and innate immunity responses, and apoptosis.[52] Novel findings were down-regulation in the B-cell associated marker CD20 observed at one month post-therapy, up-regulation of cytidine monophosphate kinase 2, CMPK2, free fatty acid receptor 2, and down-regulation of IgE Fc fragment FCER1A, findings that may generate further insight into the mode of action or IFNβ.

In comparison with IFNβ, there has been a paucity of studies looking at gene expression biosignatures of response to other MS therapies, such as GA or natalizumab. Besides the already cited study by Hong et al.,[47] a small study has associated ex vivo expression of IFNγ and IL-4 with response to GA;[59] recently, Achiron et al. performed gene microarray profiling in PBMCs of RRMS patients treated with GA and detected significant changes in 480 genes, mainly associated with antigen-activated apoptosis, inflammation, adhesion, and MHC class

I antigen presentation.[75] Finally, in a gene expression study looking at 11 natalizumab-treated RRMS patients, Lindberg et al. reported differential expression of several genes associated with immune response, signal transduction, protein synthesis, and metabolism.[60] Interestingly, the effects of natalizumab on gene expression were not limited to T-cell-associated genes, but extended to several genes involved in B-cell activation and differentiation (BLK, MS4A1, IL6R, CD24, CD79), and neutrophil-associated genes (C5R1, defensin a1).[4] This interesting finding illustrates the potential downstream immunomodulatory effects of therapies beyond their target, as neutrophils are not known to express the target integrin for natalizumab.

In conclusion, the above studies have been useful in establishing a gene expression signature for response therapy, and in a few cases, in providing further insight into the mechanism of action for these drugs. Applying the same strategy to identify biomarkers of response to therapy lagged behind, and only a few studies related to IFN response have been conducted. Initially, Stürzebecher et al. identified down-regulation of IL-8 expression in responders to IFNβ,[54] a finding that was later confirmed in a study of 22 RRMS patients treated with weekly IM IFNβ.[55] A correlation was found between good response and lower expression of IFNAR1, IL8, and CASP10, and higher expression of a few genes including MX1, IFNAR2, IL6, and TGFβ2.

In another longitudinal study, Baranzini et al. looked at a predefined set of 70 genes associated with IFN signaling pathways, cytokine receptors, apoptosis genes and transcription factors in 52 patients treated with IFNβ. The study used advanced bioinformatics analysis methods. Nine sets of gene triplets were identified whose expression before and during IFNβ therapy correlated with treatment response with up to 87% accuracy.[56] Notably, the genes in the top-scoring triplet coded for apoptosis-related molecules: Caspase-2, Caspase-10, and FLIP. Recently, Comabella et al. reported on a study in 47 RRMS treatment-naïve patients starting IFNβ therapy, for whom gene expression profiling was done at baseline and three months after start of therapy; clinical criteria of response were applied after two years of follow-up using the extreme phenotype approach. A pattern of over-expression of genes associated with type I IFN signaling pathway at baseline (with eight best predicting genes including IFIT1–3, IFI44, OASL), followed by lack induction of IFN-responsive genes after 3 months of therapy was associated with clinical non-response at the 2 years time-point, with a mean predictive accuracy of 78%.[58] This gene expression pattern was validated in the same study in a further cohort of 30 MS patients, and in vitro studies using IFNβ and innate system stimulation of PBMC support the conclusion that in IFN non-responders there is a higher state of activation of innate immune system myeloid dendritic cells related to higher endogenous type I IFN production and gene expression pattern, which is therefore unresponsive to exogenous IFNβ.[58] Should these findings be confirmed, it may be possible to select patients for IFNβ therapy based on simple tests of their immune function at baseline.

Proteomics and metabolomics studies in MS

Compared with DNA- and RNA-based analyses, proteomics and metabolomics are less advanced techniques and relatively few publications related to MS have appeared so far. The platforms rely on technologies (Table 23.2) that are not truly high-throughput and show a higher degree of technical variability. The higher complexity of factors modulating protein and metabolite levels in tissue compartments like brain, CSF, lymphocytes, plasma/serum, or urine, and their variation over time, are additional complexities that challenge the correlation between signals and disease mechanisms. Analogous to the definition of pharmacogenomics, we cover in Tables 23.6 and 23.7 not only *ex vivo* analyses of human biofluid and tissue samples based on open platforms (e.g. 2D-electrophoresis and mass spectroscopy), but also studies that are based on the analysis of larger sets of gene products via conventional methods (e.g. ELISA). Earlier publications on proteomics and metabolomics in MS are for the most part descriptive: findings were lists of targets that were differentially expressed between MS and reference samples (Table 23.6 and 23.7). Typically, results were not validated by standard quantitative tests and lacked confirmation by independent replication studies. Their value lies in the demonstration that sets of differentially regulated genes can be observed in different disease groups,[76–78] and endophenotypes related to drug response[82–85,88–90] can be identified by statistical pattern analysis, in some cases with specific values for sensitivity and specificity.[92–100,104,105] The field has progressed in recent years, and some targets identified by -omics methods have now been validated with quantitative assays[58,79–81,101,103,77,105] and differential expression of a number of gene products in MS is now confirmed in independent studies. The most prominent example for this is matrix metalloproteinase-9 (MMP-9) and its endogenous inhibitor TIMP-1, molecules modulating lymphocyte trafficking across the blood–brain barrier. MMP-9 has been found to be up-regulated in blood, CSF and brain tissue of MS,[90,91,94–96,98–101] and downregulated by IFNβ.[76,79,80,97,107] By analysis of several members of the MMP and TIMP molecule families, it is now established that (a) MMP-9 protein level is selectively increased in MS, (b) IFNβ therapy reverses this increase, and (c) IFNβ therapy upregulates TIMP-1.[108,109,76,79,80,97] These results confirm similar findings on the transcriptional level.[19] Accordingly, decrease MMP-9/TIMP-1 ratio is one established biomarker that separates IFNβ responders from non-responders,[82,94–96] while high serum MMP-9 and MMP-9/TIMP-1 ratio indicates abrogation of IFNβ effects, as seen with NAb.[22,72] Other examples of confirmed differential expression in MS are vitamin D binding protein (VDBP) and chitinase-3-like protein 1. Increased levels of VDBP were found in CSF of RRMS[100,101] and differentiate CIS patients who convert to definite MS from non-converters.[99] In the same patient group an increase of Chitinase-3-like protein 1 in CSF, a protein secreted by activated macrophages, was demonstrated to have the same predictive capacity,[99] while in SPMS its concentration is increased vs. controls.[101] Further

examples of confirmed differential protein expression in MS are clusterin,[78,95] Apo E,[94,101] and haptoglobin.[98,101] Fetuin A, however, is an example of seemingly conflicting results.[14,96] A further step ahead was the use of proteomic analysis in MS plaque tissue as a source of hypothesis generation and preclinical testing of disease modifying drug candidates.[87] The finding of protein C inhibitor and tissue factor increases in chronic plaques led to testing of hirudin and activated protein C, molecules with anticoagulant properties, in EAE.

Many tissue compartments and biofluids are relatively inaccessible, which may severely limit availability (e.g. brain tissue), or at least limit repeated sampling for longitudinal studies (e.g. CSF). Urine is readily available for longitudinal sampling, and may be the ideal biofluid source for potential metabolic biomarkers of disease and drug response. 't Hart *et al.*[102] pioneered the field of metabolomics in MS: they used proton nuclear magnetic resonance (1H-NMR) spectroscopy in combination with pattern recognition techniques to investigate the composition of organic compounds in urines from patients with MS and controls. They also showed that development of EAE in primates is associated with changes in the chemical composition of the urine. The composition of urine in MS was unambiguously different from controls. The concept that NMR spectroscopic profiling of urine in combination with statistical pattern recognition can be used to identify brain disease has been confirmed by Griffin *et al.* in a rodent EAE model,[110] who found that cerebral microinjection of cytokine producing adenovirises in rats led to a specific metabolite pattern in urine. Metabolomic analysis not only allowed differentiation of animals with focal inflammatory brain lesions from controls, but also distinguished TNFα and IL-1β induced lesions on the basis of a very limited number of metabolites. The first attempt to correlate metabolite analysis in serum of MS patients with clinical and MRI measures of neurodegeneration was undertaken by Weinstock-Guttman *et al.*[106] Here, lower levels of metabolites of the active form of Vitamin D were associated with higher MSSS and EDSS. Moreover, higher values of the $25(OH)VD_3$ to $24, 25(OH)2VD_3$ ratio were associated with higher MSSS and lower brain parenchymal fraction. On the background of the present interest on the role of Vitamin D in the pathogenesis of MS and the proteomic finding of increased Vitamin D binding protein expression in MS,[78,95,99–101] this work represents an excellent example for how "-omics" research can help expand understanding of MS pathophysiology. Currently, no pharmacometabolomic evaluation in the sense of discovery-driven research has been undertaken. However, a first step into this field was the analysis of neopterin and nitric oxide in urine in PPMS patients with and without IFN therapy. IFN treatment led to an increased neopterin/creatinin ratio, while levels of nitric oxide products decreased only with a higher dose of IFN.[103] Further, among IFN treated patients, the median neopterin/creatinin ratio was higher in clinically stable (no EDSS change) compared with progressive patients; in contrast, no correlation for nitric oxide product levels with disability measures was found. The same authors had earlier found

Table 23.6. *Proteomics-based studies*

Plasma/serum	
*Descriptive:**	
- Waubant 1999:[76]	rrMS: MMP-9↑ in rrMS vs. controls
	MMP-9↑, TIMP-1↓ correlates with occurrence of new Gd+ lesion
- Sakurai 2010:[77]	prevalence of anti-mtHSP70 Abs in MS ↑ vs. positive (Parkinson, multinfarction syndrome infectious meningoencephalitis) and negative controls (68% sensitivity, 74% specificity), no correlation with clinical course; alpha-PGAM-Ab↑ in MS; combination of both Abs ↑ (57% sensitivity, 93% specificity)
- Rithidech 2009:[78]	pediatric MS vs. controls: 12 differentially up-regulated genes predict MS vs. controls, e.g.Vit D binding protein, complement factor-I, hemopexin, clusterin
Identification of clinical responders/non-respondersto IFN:	
- Waubant 2003:[79]	SPMS: MMP-9↑ in patients who develop new Gd+ lesions
	MMP9↓ andTIMP-1↑under IFN; transient MMP-9/TIMP-1
	MMP-2 and TIMP-2 levels not affected by IFN
- Comabella 2009:[81]	TIMP-1↑ in IFN responders vs. non-responders;
	MMP-9↓; TIMP-1 and -2↑ by IFN
- Alexander 2010:[80]	decreased levels of MMP-8/MMP-9/IL12p40/Il17/IL23 decreased MMP-8, MMP-9, IL-12 and IL-23 levels were correlated with a decrease in the number of contrast-enhanced T2-weighted lesions
Blood cells, monocytes	
*Descriptive**	
- Kantor 2007:[82]	MMP-9↓ by IFN; further changes in multiple monocyte-associated cell
	surface molecules and monocyte related soluble factors due to IFN: HLA class II, CCR5, CD38, CD40, CD54, CD64, CD69, CD86, CD101, TLR2, TLR4, and MCP2.
- De Masi 2009:[83]	correlation of PBMC protein expression and brain atrophy in rrMS
Identification of differential protein expression due to IFN:	
- Comabella 2009:[58]	IFN non-responders characterized by increased STAT1 levels and IFN eceptor 1 expression in monocytes at base line; and increased monocyte type I IFN secretion
Brain tissue	
*Descriptive:**	
- Satoh 2009:[84]	comparison of proteome profile between chronic active vs. chronic plaques
- Fissolo 2009:[85]	characterization of CNS expressed MHC ligandome
- Dhaunchak 2010:[86]	comparison of myelin and axogliasomal fractions
Hypothesis generation and drug testing:	
- Han 2008:[110]	
	comparison of various stages of plaques from MS and controls: protein C inhibitor and tissue factor increased in chronic active plaques, in total 5 proteins related to coagulation differentially regulated; anticoagulative compounds hirudin and activated protein C down-regulate severity of EAE. This is the first proteomic study in humans to generate a hypothesis (dysregulation of coagulation-related molecules as pathogenetic factors) to be tested and confirmed in animal model of MS
CSF	
*Descriptive:**	
- Dumont 2004[88]	analysis of CSF from 5 MS patients, no controls
- Hammack 2004[89]	comparative analysis of pooled CSF from 3 MS patients and 3 patients with other inflanmmatory disorders (2 sarcoid, 1 viral meningitis)
- Noben 2006:[90]	comparison of analytical techniques, using pooled samples of rrMS and controls: identification of Cystatin A in MS, but not in control CSF; higher concentration of Cystatin A in serum, but not in CSF and serum validated by ELISA
- Lehmensiek 2007:[91]	comparison samples from rrMS, CIS,and normal controls, rrMS; vitamin D-binding protein isoforms, ApoE ↓ in CIS/rrMS vs. controls; ApoA1 ↑ in CIS and rrMS vs. controls validated by immunoblot
- Liu 2009:[92]	comparison of 2 proteomic technologies in MS vs. controls (OND): Cystatin C↓ in MS vs. controls, as detected with both techniques, and validated by ELISA

(cont.)

Table 23.6. (cont.)

- D'Aguanno 2008:[93]	comparison of Leber hereditary optic neuropathy with MS and controls
- Chiassirini 2008[94]	comparison of CI, rrMS and controls: IgG free kappa light chain ↑ in CIS and rrMS vs. controls (validated by Western), and ApoE and ApoA1 isoforms↑ in rrMS vs. CIS and controls.
- Stoop 2008[95]	comparison of MS, CIS, OIND, OBND: similar profiles between MS and CIS, significant diff. between them and OND: 3 proteins↑ in MS, CIS vs OND chromogranin A (validated by ELISA), clusterin and C3
- Tumani 2009[96]	Nine genes indentified that differentiate CIS patients who convert to rrMS from non-converters, Fetuin-A↑ in non-converters vs. converters validated
- Kuenz 2008[97]	comparison of cell profile with proteom inCIS, rrMS and cpMS, controls: levels of MMP9↑ in CIS and rrMS; MMP9↑ in relapse vs. remission or progression; MMP9↑ correlates with (a) Gd+ lesions, (b) specifically with B-cells/plasmablasts, but not other cell types.
- Bai 2009,[98]	NMO vs. normal controls: 4 genes increased, 7 genes decreased in NMO; Vitamin D binding protein↓ and haptoglobin↑ validated.
- Comabella 2010[99]	comparison of CIS converters to rrMS vs. non-converters: coeruloplasmin, Vit D binding protein, chitinase3-like protein 1↑ in CSF of non-converters; all 3 targets subjected to ELISA validation, only Chitinase3-like protein 1 validated and correlated with Gd+ and T2 lesions at base line, and were associated with shorter time to conversion
- Stoop 2010[100]	ppMS and rrMS proteome overlap to large extent; 2 proteins differentially regulated and validated by quantitative assays: (1) protein jagged-1 3x more abundant in rrMS, and (2) Vit D binding protein ca. 1.5x more abundant in rrMS.
Descriptive and natalizumab response	
- Ottervald 2010[101]	longitudinal effect of Natalizumab in CIS, spMS, rrMS, ppMS: largest and most refined proteomic study so far: statistical significant upregulation as per validating immounassays: alpha-1 chymotrypsin, alpha-1 macroglobulin, fibulin 1↑ in rrMS vs. controls; in spMS vs. controls in addition upregulation of contactin 1, fetuin A, Vit D binding protein and angiotensinogen;further increased expression (not statistically significant) in various types of MS: ceruloplasmin, chitinase 3-like protein 1, haptoglobin, ApoE effect of natalizumab: downregulation of alpha-1 chymotrypsin, alpha-1 macroglobulin, fibulin 1, Vit D binding protein

Apart from work using open platform technology, also studies covering several targets with conventional methodology simultaneously are included, in analogy to the definition of pharmacogenetics (Table 23.1).

Table 23.7. *Metabolomics based studies*

Urine

Descriptive:*
- 't Hart 2003[102]

IFN reponse in PPMS
- Rejdak 2010[103]:

Placebo patients had lower neopterin/creatinin ratio levels than IFN-treated patients, the latter had higher neopterin/creatinin ratios in patients without vs. patients with EDSS progression

Only higher dose of IFN decreased nitric oxide metabolites (NOx) excretion

CSF

Descriptive:*
- Rejdak 2008[104]:

increased levels of NOx, neurofilament heavy chain (NfH), S100B in rrMS during relapse vs. controls; NfH correlated with NOx, both targets corelated with change of EDSS in follow-up
- Sinclair 2010:[105]

MS, CVD, IIH, controls, OND: sensitivity and specificity of 80% to identify MS (study analyses as well as serum metabolomes)

Serum

Descriptive:*
- Weinstock-Guttman 2011[106]

lower levels of vitamin D metabolites correlated with higher brain atrophy, and clinical signs of disability (EDSS, MSSS)

compartment that is remote from the site of its generation and has inherently undergone metabolic modification.

Conclusions

Discovery-driven approaches to screen the entire genome and measure expression parameters (RNA, protein, metabolites) in large numbers, based on high-throughput measuring platforms ("-omics") have significantly advanced the molecular understanding of disease pathogenesis in MS. This has been paralleled recently by a relevant body of data relating genetic background to drug response, and relating drug effects to gene expression. Such data will be necessary for understanding variability of efficacy and safety of drugs in a disease whose pathogenesis appears to be markedly heterogeneous. The application of such data to clinical practice may allow the optimization of individual treatment regimens and the prospective identification of treatment response for a given compound. This capability would allow implementation of personalized medicine in MS.

Pharmacogenomics research is also expected to have important socio-economic impact. Better molecular understanding of drug mode of action should accelerate development of novel compounds for MS therapy, as well as use of specific therapies only in subgroups of MS patients who most profit from them, based on their genetic background. The challenge for the future is overlaying longitudinal pharmacogenomics and related "-omics" data onto phenotypically characterized patient cohorts, in order to establish a comprehensive and integrated matrix of genotype/phenotype interaction. The requirements for this are three-fold: (a) development of technologies for

that in untreated RRMS increased CSF levels of nitric oxide metabolites (nitrate, nitrite) at baseline correlate with increased EDSS over time.[104] This discrepancy may result from decreasing sensitivity and specificity for identifying markers in a fluid proteomics and metabolomics to the same level as genotyping and trancriptomics, so that results from these different methods can be combined and analyzed simultaneously; (b) development of bioinformatic tools to improve evaluation and interpretation of large data sets; and (c) development of longitudinally studied cohorts characterized using standardized, high-quality clinical and paraclinical (e.g. imaging, conventional biomarkers) methods, so that "-omics" results can be correlated with the disease characteristics. It is important to emphasize that the last point will be decisive for the long-term impact of pharmacogenomics on our understanding of disease pathophysiology, and for future improvement of MS patient therapy.

References

1. FDA. www.fda.gov/downloads/ RegulatoryInformation/Guidances/ ucm129296.

2. EMA.www.ema.europa.eu/docs/ en_GB/document_library/ Scientific_guideline /2009/09/WC500002880

3. Lesko LJ, Salerno RA, Spear BB, *et al.* Pharmacogenetics and pharmacogenomics in drug development and regulatory decision making: report of the first FDA-PWG-PhRMA-DruSafe Workshop. *J Clin pharmacol* 2003; 43:342–58.

4. FDA. Table of Valid Genomic Biomarkers in the Context of Drug Labels www.fda.gov/Drugs/ScienceResearch/ ResearchAreas/Pharmacogenetics/ ucm083378.htm.

5. FDA. www.fda.gov/ohrms/dockets/ dailys/04/feb04/021104/ 03D-0497_emc-000004-02.pdf.

6. Martin R, Leppert D. A plea for "omics" research in complex diseases such as multiple sclerosis – a change of mind is needed. *J Neurol Sci* 2004; 222:3–5.

7. Porter IH. Genetic basis of drug metabolism in man. *Toxicol Appl Pharmacol* 1964; 6:499–511.

8. Evans DA, Clarke CA. Pharmacogenetics. *Br Med Bull* 1961; 17:234–40.

9. Hughes HB, Biehl JP, Jones AP, Schmidt LH. Metabolism of isoniazid in man as related to the occurrence of peripheral neuritis. *Ame Rev Tuberculosis* 1954; 70:266–73.

10. Barcellos LF, Oksenberg JR, Green AJ, *et al.* Genetic basis for clinical expression in multiple sclerosis. *Brain* 2002; 125:150–8.

11. Fazekas F, Strasser-Fuchs S, Kollegger H, *et al.* Apolipoprotein E epsilon 4 is associated with rapid progression of multiple sclerosis. *Neurology* 2001; 57:853–7.

12. Kappos L, Achtnichts L, Durelli L, *et al.* BEST-PGx: design of a pharmacogenomic and pharmacogenetic study to identify criteria for prediction of treatment response to interferon-b-1b. *Mult Scler* 2005; 11: S245, abstract P592.

13. Baranzini SE, Galwey NW, Wang J, *et al.* Pathway and network-based analysis of genome-wide association studies in multiple sclerosis. *Hum Mol Genet* 2009; 18:2078–90.

14. Lesko LJ, Zineh I. DNA, drugs and chariots: on a decade of pharmacogenomics at the US FDA. *Pharmacogenomics* 2010; 11:507–12.

15. Oksenberg JR, Baranzini SE. Multiple sclerosis genetics–is the glass half full, or half empty? *Nat Rev Neurol* 2010; 6:429–37.

16. Hur EM, Youssef S, Haws ME, Zhang SY, Sobel RA, Steinman L. Osteopontin-induced relapse and progression of autoimmune brain disease through enhanced survival of activated T cells. *Nat Immunol* 2007; 8:74–83.

17. Chabas D, *et al.* The influence of the proinflammatory cytokine, osteopontin, on autoimmune demyelinating disease. *Science NY* 2001; 294:1731–5.

18. Lock C, Hermans G, Pedotti R, *et al* Gene-microarray analysis of multiple sclerosis lesions yields new targets validated in autoimmune encephalomyelitis. *Nat Med* 2002; 8:500–8.

19. Bernal F, Elias B, Hartung HP, Kieseier BC. Regulation of matrix metalloproteinases and their inhibitors by interferon-beta: a longitudinal study in multiple sclerosis patients. *Mult Scler* 2009; 15:721–7.

20. Gilli F, Marnetto F, Caldano M, *et al.* Biological markers of interferon-beta therapy: comparison among interferon-stimulated genes MxA, TRAIL and XAF-1. *Mult Scler* 2006; 12:47–57.

21. Garcia-Montojo M, Dominguez-Mozo MI, de las Heras V, *et al.* Neutralizing antibodies, MxA expression and MMP-9/TIMP-1 ratio as markers of bioavailability of interferon-beta treatment in multiple sclerosis patients: a two-year follow-up study. *Eur J Neurol* 2010; 17:470–8.

22. Corvol JC, Pelletier D, Henry RG, *et al.* Abrogation of T cell quiescence characterizes patients at high risk for multiple sclerosis after the initial neurological event. *Proc Natl Acad Sci USA* 2008; 105:11839–44.

23. Junker A, Hohlfeld R, Meinl E. The emerging role of microRNAs in multiple sclerosis. *Nat Rev Neurol* 2011; 7:56–9.

24. Pedersen IM, Cheng G, Wieland S, *et al.* Interferon modulation of cellular microRNAs as an antiviral mechanism. *Nature* 2007; 449:919–22.

25. Rio J, Comabella M, Montalban X. Predicting responders to therapies for multiple sclerosis. *Nat Rev Neurol* 2009; 5:553–60.

26. Pappas DJ, Oksenberg JR. Multiple sclerosis pharmacogenomics: maximizing efficacy of therapy. *Neurology* 2010; 74 (Suppl 1):S62–9.

27. Martinez-Forero I, Pelaez A, Villoslada P. Pharmacogenomics of multiple sclerosis: in search for a personalized therapy. *Expert Opin Pharmacother* 2008; 9:3053–67.

28. Fusco C, Andreone V, Coppola G, *et al.* HLA-DRB1*1501 and response to copolymer-1 therapy in relapsing-remitting multiple sclerosis. *Neurology* 2001; 57:1976–9.

29. Villoslada P, Barcellos LF, Rio J, Begovich AB, *et al.* The HLA locus and multiple sclerosis in Spain. Role in disease susceptibility, clinical course and response to interferon-beta. *J Neuroimmunol* 2002; 130:194–201.

30. Comabella M, Fernandez-Arquero M, Rio J, *et al.* HLA class I and II alleles and response to treatment with interferon-beta in relapsing–remitting multiple sclerosis. *J Neuroimmunol* 2009; 210:116–9.

31. Sriram U, Barcellos LF, Villoslada P, et al. Pharmacogenomic analysis of interferon receptor polymorphisms in multiple sclerosis. *Genes Immun* 2003; 4:147–52.

32. Leyva L, Fernandez O, Fedetz M, et al. IFNAR1 and IFNAR2 polymorphisms confer susceptibility to multiple sclerosis but not to interferon-beta treatment response. *J Neuroimmunol* 2005; 163:165–71.

33. Cunningham S, Graham C, Hutchinson M, et al. Pharmacogenomics of responsiveness to interferon IFN-beta treatment in multiple sclerosis: a genetic screen of 100 type I interferon-inducible genes. *Clin Pharmacol Ther* 2005; 78:635–46.

34. Comabella M, Craig DW, Morcillo-Suarez C, et al. Genome-wide scan of 500,000 single-nucleotide polymorphisms among responders and nonresponders to interferon beta therapy in multiple sclerosis. *Arch Neurol* 2009; 66:972–8.

35. Byun E, Caillier SJ, Montalban X, et al. Genome-wide pharmacogenomic analysis of the response to interferon beta therapy in multiple sclerosis. *Arch Neurol* 2008; 65:337–44.

36. Martínez, A, de las Heras V, Mas Fontao A, et al. An IFNG polymorphism is associated with interferon-beta response in Spanish MS patients. *J Neuroimmunol* 2006; 173:196–9.

37. Weinstock-Guttman B, Tamano-Blanco M, Bhasi K, Zivadinov R, Ramanathan M. Pharmacogenetics of MXA SNPs in interferon-beta treated multiple sclerosis patients. *J Neuroimmunol* 2007; 182:6–239.

38. Wergeland S, Beiske A, Nyland H, et al. IL-10 promoter haplotype influence on interferon treatment response in multiple sclerosis. *Eur J Neurol* 2005; 12:171–5.

39. Cenit MD, Blanco-Kelly F, de las Heras V, et al. Glypican 5 is an interferon-beta response gene: a replication study. *Mult Scler* 2009; 15:913–917.

40. Cavanillas ML, Fernandez O, Comabella M, et al. Replication of top markers of a genome-wide association study in multiple sclerosis in Spain. *Genes Immun* 2011;12(2):100–5.

41. Alvarez-Lafuente, R, Blanco-Kelly F, Garcia-Montojo M, et al. CD46 in a Spanish cohort of multiple sclerosis patients: genetics, mRNA expression and response to interferon-beta treatment. *Mult Scler* 2010.

42. O'Doherty C, Favorov A, Heggarty S, et al. Genetic polymorphisms, their allele combinations and IFN-beta treatment response in Irish multiple sclerosis patients. *Pharmacogenomics* 2009; 10:1177–86.

43. Grossman I, Avidan N, Singer C, Goldstaub D, Hayardeny L, et al. Pharmacogenetics of glatiramer acetate therapy for multiple sclerosis reveals drug-response markers. *Pharmacogenet Genom* 2007; 17:657–66.

44. Wandinger KP, Sturzebecher CS, Bielekova B, et al. Complex immunomodulatory effects of interferon-beta in multiple sclerosis include the upregulation of T helper 1-associated marker genes. *Ann Neurol* 2001; 50:349–57.

45. Weinstock-Guttman B, Badgett D, Patrick K, et al. Genomic effects of IFN-beta in multiple sclerosis patients. *J Immunol* 2003; 171: 2694–702.

46. Koike F, Satoh J, Miyake S, et al. Microarray analysis identifies interferon beta-regulated genes in multiple sclerosis. *J Neuroimmunol* 2003; 139:109–18.

47. Hong J, Zang YC, Hutton G, Rivera VM, Zhang JZ. Gene expression profiling of relevant biomarkers for treatment evaluation in multiple sclerosis. *J Neuroimmunol* 2004; 152:126–39.

48. Iglesias AH, Camelo S, Hwang D, Villanueva R, Stephanopoulos G, Dangond F. Microarray detection of E2F pathway activation and other targets in multiple sclerosis peripheral blood mononuclear cells. *J Neuroimmunol* 2004; 150:163–77.

49. Fernald GH, Knott S, Pachner A, et al. Genome-wide network analysis reveals the global properties of IFN-beta immediate transcriptional effects in humans. *J Immunol* 2007; 178: 5076–85.

50. Cepok S, Schreiber H, Hoffmann S, et al. Enhancement of chemokine expression by interferon beta therapy in patients with multiple sclerosis. *Arch Neurol* 2009; 66:1216–23.

51. Serrano-Fernandez P, Moller S, Goertsches R, et al. Time course transcriptomics of IFNB1b drug therapy in multiple sclerosis. *Autoimmunity* 2010; 43:172–8.

52. Goertsches RH, Hecker M, Koczan D, et al. Long-term genome-wide blood RNA expression profiles yield novel molecular response candidates for IFN-beta-1b treatment in relapsing remitting MS. *Pharmacogenomics* 2010; 11:147–61.

53. Hecker M, Goertsches RH, Fatum C, et al. Network analysis of transcriptional regulation in response to intramuscular interferon-beta-1a multiple sclerosis treatment. *Pharmacogenom J* 2010 Oct 19 [Epub ahead of print].

54. Sturzebecher S, Wandinger KP, Rosenwald A, et al. Expression profiling identifies responder and non-responder phenotypes to interferon-beta in multiple sclerosis. *Brain* 2003; 126:19–1429.

55. Weinstock-Guttman B, Bhasi K, Badgett D, et al. Genomic effects of once-weekly, intramuscular interferon-beta1a treatment after the first dose and on chronic dosing: Relationships to 5-year clinical outcomes in multiple sclerosis patients. *J Neuroimmunol* 2008; 205: 113–25.

56. Baranzini SE, Mousavi P, Rio J, et al. Transcription-based prediction of response to IFNbeta using supervised computational methods. *PLoS Biol* 2005; 3:e2.

57. van Baarsen LG, Vosslamber S, Tijssen M, et al. Pharmacogenomics of interferon-beta therapy in multiple sclerosis: baseline IFN signature determines pharmacological differences between patients. *PloS one* 2008; 3:e1927.

58. Comabella M, Lunemann JD, Rio J, et al. A type I interferon signature in monocytes is associated with poor response to interferon-beta in multiple sclerosis. *Brain* 2009; 132:3353–65.

59. Valenzuela RM, Costello K, Chen M, Said A, Johnson KP, Dhib-Jalbut S. Clinical response to glatiramer acetate correlates with modulation of IFN-gamma and IL-4 expression in multiple sclerosis. *Mult Scler* 2007; 13:754–62.

60. Lindberg RL, Achtnichts L, Hoffmann F, Kuhle J, Kappos L. Natalizumab alters transcriptional expression profiles of blood cell subpopulations of

multiple sclerosis patients. *J Neuroimmunol* 2008; 194:153–64.

61. Rudick RA, Polman CH. Current approaches to the identification and management of breakthrough disease in patients with multiple sclerosis. *Lancet Neurol* 2009; 8:545–59.

62. Vandenbroeck K, Comabella M. Single-nucleotide polymorphisms in response to interferon-beta therapy in multiple sclerosis. *J Interferon Cytokine Res* 2010; 30:727–32.

63. Bhat R, Axtell R, Mitra A, *et al.* Inhibitory role for GABA in autoimmune inflammation. *Proc Natl Acad Sci USA* 2010; 107: 2580–5.

64. Karadottir R, Cavelier P, Bergersen LH, and Attwell D. NMDA receptors are expressed in oligodendrocytes and activated in ischaemia. *Nature* 2005; 438:1162–6.

65. Smith T, Groom A, Zhu B, Turski L. Autoimmune encephalomyelitis ameliorated by AMPA antagonists. *Nat Med* 2000; 6:62–6.

66. Lorentzen AR, Melum E, Ellinghaus E, *et al.* Association to the Glypican-5 gene in multiple sclerosis. *J Neuroimmunol* 2010; 226:194–7.

67. Farina C, Weber MS, Meinl E, Wekerle H, Hohlfeld R. Glatiramer acetate in multiple sclerosis: update on potential mechanisms of action. *Lancet Neurol* 2005; 4:567–75.

68. Giallourakis C, Henson C, Reich M, Xie X, Mootha VK. Disease gene discovery through integrative genomics. *Ann Rev Genomi Hum Genet* 2005; 6:381–406.

69. Hemmer B, Stuve O, Kieseier B, Schellekens H, Hartung HP. 2005. Immune response to immunotherapy: the role of neutralising antibodies to interferon beta in the treatment of multiple sclerosis. *Lancet Neurol* 2005; 4:403–12.

70. Hesse D, Sellebjerg F, and Sorensen PS. Absence of MxA induction by interferon beta in patients with MS reflects complete loss of bioactivity. *Neurology* 2009; 73:372–77.

71. Wandinger KP, Lunemann JD, Wengert O, *et al.* TNF-related apoptosis inducing ligand (TRAIL) as a potential response marker for interferon-beta treatment in multiple sclerosis. *Lancet* 2003; 361:2036–43.

72. Gilli F, Bertolotto A, Sala A, *et al.* Neutralizing antibodies against IFN-beta in multiple sclerosis: antagonization of IFN-beta mediated suppression of MMPs. *Brain* 2004; 127:259–68.

73. Polman CH, Bertolotto A, Deisenhammer F, *et al.* Recommendations for clinical use of data on neutralising antibodies to interferon-beta therapy in multiple sclerosis. *Lancet Neurol* 2010; 9:740–50.

74. Galboiz Y, Shapiro S, Lahat N, Rawashdeh H, Miller A. Matrix metalloproteinases and their tissue inhibitors as markers of disease subtype and response to interferon-beta therapy in relapsing and secondary-progressive multiple sclerosis patients. *Ann Neurol* 2001; 50:443–51.

75. Achiron A, Feldman A, and Gurevich M. Molecular profiling of glatiramer acetate early treatment effects in multiple sclerosis. *Dis Markers* 2009; 27:63–73.

76. Waubant E, Goodkin DE, Gee L, *et al.* Serum MMP-9 and TIMP-1 levels are related to MRI activity in relapsing multiple sclerosis. *Neurology* 1999; 53:1397–401.

77. Sakurai T, Kimura A, Yamada M, *et al.* Identification of antibodies as biological markers in serum from multiple sclerosis patients by immunoproteomic approach. *J Neuroimmunol* 2011;233(1–2):175–80.

78. Rithidech, KN, Honikel L, Milazzo M, Madigan D, Troxell R, Krupp LB. Protein expression profiles in pediatric multiple sclerosis: potential biomarkers. *Mult Scler* 2009; 15:455–64.

79. Waubant E, Goodkin D, Bostrom A, *et al.* IFNbeta lowers MMP-9/TIMP-1 ratio, which predicts new enhancing lesions in patients with SPMS. *Neurology* 2003; 60:52–7.

80. Alexander JS, Harris MK, Wells SR, *et al.* Alterations in serum MMP-8, MMP-9, IL-12p40 and IL-23 in multiple sclerosis patients treated with interferon-beta1b. *Mult Scler* 2010; 16:801–9.

81. Comabella M, Rio J, Espejo C, *et al.* Changes in matrix metalloproteinases and their inhibitors during interferon-beta treatment in multiple sclerosis. *Clin Immunol* 2009; 130:145–50.

82. Kantor AB, Deng J, Waubant E. Identification of short-term pharmacodynamic effects of interferon-beta-1a in multiple sclerosis subjects with broad- based phenotypic profiling. *J Neuroimmunol* 2007; 188:103–16.

83. De Masi, R, Vergara D, Pasca S. PBMCs protein expression profile in relapsing IFN-treated multiple sclerosis: A pilot study on relation to clinical findings and brain atrophy. *J. Neuroimmunol* 2009; 210:80–6.

84. Satoh JI, Tabunoki H, Yamamura T. Molecular network of the comprehensive multiple sclerosis brain-lesion proteome. *Mult Scler* 2009; 15:531–41.

85. Fissolo N, Haag S, de Graaf KL, *et al.* Naturally presented peptides on major histocompatibility complex I and II molecules eluted from central nervous system of multiple sclerosis patients. *Mol Cell Proteomics* 2009; 8:2090–101.

86. Dhaunchak, AS, Huang JK, De Faria Junior O, *et al.* A proteome map of axoglial specializations isolated and purified from human central nervous system. *Glia* 2010; 58:1949–60.

87. Han MH, Hwang SI, Roy DB, *et al.* Proteomic analysis of active multiple sclerosis lesions reveals therapeutic targets. *Nature* 2008; 451:1076–81.

88. Dumont D, Noben JP, Raus J, Stinissen P, and Robben J. Proteomic analysis of cerebrospinal fluid from multiple sclerosis patients. *Proteomics* 2004; 4:2117–24.

89. Hammack BN, Fung KY, Hunsucker SW, *et al.* Proteomic analysis of multiple sclerosis cerebrospinal fluid. *Mult Scler* 2004; 10:245–60.

90. Noben JP, Dumont D, Kwasnikowska N, *et al.* Lumbar cerebrospinal fluid proteome in multiple sclerosis: characterization by ultrafiltration, liquid chromatography, and mass spectrometry. *J Proteome Res* 2006; 5:1647–57.

91. Lehmensiek V, Sussmuth SD, Tauscher G, *et al.* Cerebrospinal fluid proteome profile in multiple sclerosis. *Mult Scler* 2007; 13:840–9.

92. Liu S, Bai S, Qin Z, Yang Y, Cui Y, Qin Y. Quantitative proteomic analysis of the cerebrospinal fluid of patients with multiple sclerosis. *J Cell Mol Med* 2009; 13:1586–603.

93. D'Aguanno, S, Barassi A, Lupisella S, *et al.* Differential cerebro spinal fluid proteome investigation of Leber hereditary optic neuropathy (LHON) and multiple sclerosis. *J Neuroimmunol* 2008; 193:156–60.

94. Chiasserini, D, Di Filippo M, Candeliere A, *et al.* CSF proteome analysis in multiple sclerosis patients by two-dimensional electrophoresis. *Eur J Neurol* 2008; 15:998–1001.

95. Stoop, MP, Dekker LJ, Titulaer MK, *et al.* Multiple sclerosis-related proteins identified in cerebrospinal fluid by advanced mass spectrometry. *Proteomics* 2008; 8:1576–85.

96. Tumani H, Lehmensiek V, Rau D, *et al.* CSF proteome analysis in clinically isolated syndrome (CIS): candidate markers for conversion to definite multiple sclerosis. *Neurosci Lett* 2009; 452:214–7.

97. Kuenz B, Lutterotti A, Ehling R, *et al.* Cerebrospinal fluid B cells correlate with early brain inflammation in multiple sclerosis. *PloS one* 2008; 3:e2559.

98. Bai S, Liu S, Guo X, *et al.* Proteome analysis of biomarkers in the cerebrospinal fluid of neuromyelitis optica patients. *Molec Vision* 2009; 15:1638–48.

99. Comabella M, Fernandez M, Martin R, *et al.* Cerebrospinal fluid chitinase 3-like 1 levels are associated with conversion to multiple sclerosis. *Brain* 2010; 133:1082–93.

100. Stoop MP, Singh V, Dekker LJ, *et al.* Proteomics comparison of cerebrospinal fluid of relapsing remitting and primary progressive multiple sclerosis. *PloS one* 2010; 5:e12442.

101. Ottervald J, Franzen B, Nilsson K, *et al.* Multiple sclerosis: Identification and clinical evaluation of novel CSF biomarkers. *J Proteomics* 2010; 73:1117–32.

102. 't Hart BA, Vogels JT, Spijksma G, Brok HP, Polman C, van der Greef J. 1H-NMR spectroscopy combined with pattern recognition analysis reveals characteristic chemical patterns in urines of MS patients and non-human primates with MS-like disease. *J Neurol Sci* 2003; 212:21–30.

103. Rejdak K, Leary SM, Petzold A, Thompson AJ, Miller DH, Giovannoni G. Urinary neopterin and nitric oxide metabolites as markers of interferon beta-1a activity in primary progressive multiple sclerosis. *Mult Scler* 2010; 16:1066–72.

104. Rejdak K, Petzold A, Stelmasiak Z, Giovannoni G. Cerebrospinal fluid brain specific proteins in relation to nitric oxide metabolites during relapse of multiple sclerosis. *Mult Scler* 2008; 14:59–66.

105. Sinclair AJ, Viant MR, Ball AK, *et al.* NMR-based metabolomic analysis of cerebrospinal fluid and serum in neurological diseases–a diagnostic tool? *NMR Biomed* 2010; 23:123–32.

106. Weinstock-Guttman B, Zivadinov R, Qu J, *et al.* Vitamin D metabolites are associated with clinical and MRI outcomes in multiple sclerosis patients. *J Neurol Neurosurg Psychiatry* 2011; 82:189–95.

107. Lindberg, RL, De Groot CJ, Certa U, *et al.* Multiple sclerosis as a generalized CNS disease–comparative microarray analysis of normal appearing white matter and lesions in secondary progressive MS. *J Neuroimmunol* 2004; 152:154–67.

108. Leppert D, Waubant E, Burk MR, Oksenberg JR, Hauser SL. Interferon beta-1b inhibits gelatinase secretion and in vitro migration of human T cells: a possible mechanism for treatment efficacy in multiple sclerosis. *Ann Neurol* 1996; 40:846–52.

109. Stuve O, Dooley NP, Uhm JH, *et al.* Interferon beta-1b decreases the migration of T lymphocytes in vitro: effects on matrix metalloproteinase-9. *Ann Neurol* 1996; 40:853–63.

110. Griffin JL, Anthony DC, Campbell SJ, *et al.* Study of cytokine induced neuropathology by high resolution proton NMR spectroscopy of rat urine. *FEBS Lett* 2004; 568:49–54.

Chapter

24

Neutralizing antibodies directed against biologic agents to treat multiple sclerosis

Per Soelberg Sørensen

Introduction

All biopharmaceuticals produced by recombinant gene technologies are potentially immunogenic.

The mechanisms that underlie generation of antibodies to recombinant protein drugs are not well understood.[1] With IFNβ, the underlying mechanism is the breaking of immune tolerance, which typically exists to self-antigens, and is associated with presentation of the self-antigen in a repetitive way,[2] whereas antibodies against natalizumab may be IgE antibodies giving rise to type I allergic reactions early after institution of therapy or to delayed type III allergic reactions.[3]

The detrimental effects of neutralizing antibodies (NAbs) on the clinical response to IFNβ in multiple sclerosis (MS) patients have been recognized even from the first pivotal study of IFNβ-1b,[4] and it might therefore be hard to understand the long-lasting controversies about whether NAbs do neutralize the effect of IFNβ in MS.

Previously, differences of opinion were expressed between the European Guidelines on the use of anti-IFNβ antibody measurements in multiple sclerosis, produced by an European Federation of Neurological Societies Task Force,[5] and the American Academy of Neurology report on NAbs to IFNβ and assessment of their clinical and radiographic impact, produced by a working group under the Therapeutics and Technology Assessment Subcommittee.[6] Recently, a transatlantic consensus was reached concerning the most important issues about NAbs against IFNβ,[7] including how to integrate testing for NAbs into daily clinical practice.

The present chapter reviews our current knowledge about neutralizing antibodies directed against biologic agents to treat MS including the clinical consequences of NAbs and the importance of incorporating NAb measurements in daily practice.

Antibodies against IFNβ (see Chapter 25 for a review of data on IFNβ studies in MS and

Chapter 51 for review of the use of disease-modifying therapy in RRMS)

IFNβ immunogenicity

The explanation for the immunogenecity of IFNβ is not known in complete detail. Unlike the classic reaction to foreign proteins that produces an immune response after a single administration, antibodies against IFNβ are caused by a breakdown of the immune tolerance to self-antigens that normally exist. The self-antigen has to be presented to the immune system in a repetitive way during several months before the immune tolerance is broken.[2]

There are several factors that determine whether administration of a recombinant IFNβ human molecule causes development of NAbs to IFNβ.

Some important factors are patient linked: recent studies have shown a genetic HLA-based predisposition to development of NAbs to IFNβ.[8] A comparative study found that MS patients tended to have a higher incidence of IFNβ NAbs compared with cancer patients, suggesting that the immune response of MS patients may differ from that in patients with other disorders.[9] Further, a correlation was found between NAbs and CSF oligoclonal band positivity,[10] the presence of autoreactive antibodies, i.e. antiphospholipid antibodies and anti-thyroid peroxidase antibodies,[11] low plasma levels of apolipoprotein E, and tobacco smoking.[12]

Other factors are harbored in the IFNβ product: impurity and contamination originating from bacterial or mammalian cells used in the production are main causes of immunogenicity.[13] The amino acid sequence and the structure of the protein made by non-mammalian cells may differ from the human molecule and reveal foreign epitopes. Also, lack of glycosylation or differences in the glycoproteins can expose normally hidden epitopes or make the molecule less soluble. IFNβ-1b is produced in an *E. coli* cell line. The amino acid sequence differs from the human IFNβ; in IFNβ-1b cysteine at position 17 is substituted by serine and the N-terminal

Multiple Sclerosis Therapeutics, Fourth Edition, ed. Jeffrey A. Cohen and Richard A. Rudick. Published by Cambridge University Press.
© Cambridge University Press 2011.

methionine has been deleted. Further, IFNβ-1b is not glycosylated, because bacteria are unable to attach sugar molecules. IFNβ-1a engineered in a Chinese hamster ovary cell line has the full 166 amino acid sequence of the human IFNβ and is glycosylated, but not necessarily with the same pattern as human IFNβ.

Use of fetal bovine serum, addition of human albumin to the product, and properties of the container in which the product is stored may contribute to the formation of aggregates that is associated with induction of antibodies.[14] The relative potency in vivo of IFNβ-1b is only about 10% of that of IFNβ-1a. Therefore, IFNβ-1b is administered in approximately ten times higher doses to achieve an equivalent in vivo activity, and NAbs develop faster with IFNβ-1b, indicating that the protein load in the single injection seems to play a role.[15,16] Intramuscular administration is less immunogenic than subcutaneous injections,[17,18] and more frequent administration induces a higher incidence of antibodies.[15]

The effect of the size of the single dose is unclear, and studies have reported conflicting results.[4,19–21]

In vitro, two different classes of antibodies are recognized according to the assay used to identify them: binding antibodies (BAbs) and neutralizing antibodies (NAbs). BAbs bind to the IFNβ molecule and may or may not interfere with its functions, whereas NAbs interfere with functions of the IFNβ molecule in vitro, most likely by preventing the binding of IFNβ to the IFN receptor (IFNAR) on cells used in the assay. BAbs can be demonstrated in the majority of patients treated with an IFNβ preparation, but only a smaller proportion of patients develop NAbs.[15]

Early-appearing antibodies are generally low-affinity IgM and IgG antibodies, and the difference between BAbs and NAbs may be quantitative rather than qualitative, i.e. defined by differences in binding affinities rather than by differences in epitope specificities.[22] Interestingly, BAbs and in vitro neutralizing activity in the serum may be present already within 3 months after initiation of IFNβ therapy. These low-affinity NAbs bind reversibly and may protect the IFNβ molecule from degradation and/or consumption, and, thereby, prolong the half-life of IFNβ and enhance the effect of an IFNβ injection. With prolonged therapy, affinity maturation develops and the binding becomes irreversible and the anti-IFNβ antibodies become neutralizing.[23]

Approximately 4% of IFNβ-treated patients have a non-antibody mediated neutralizing activity caused by circulating soluble IFN receptors (sIFNAR), which competitively inhibits the bioactivity of IFNβ both in vitro and in vivo.[24] Using traditional assays these patients will be NAb-positive, but BAb-negative.[25]

It is generally agreed that the frequency of NAbs is significantly less with IFNβ-1a i.m. compared with IFNβ-1b s.c. or IFNβ-1a s.c.[15,18,26–29] A new formulation of IFNβ-1a s.c. has reduced the immunogenicity, although not to the levels seen with IFNβ-1a i.m.[30]

The NAb titers from IFNβ-1a-treated patients seem to be higher than those from IFNβ-1b-treated patients.[27,31]

Measurements of anti-IFNβ antibodies

Because assays for NAb detection usually are cumbersome, many laboratories use a simpler binding assay for screening purposes and only BAb-positive samples are analyzed by the NAb assay. The use of this practice will imply false negative tests in those 4% of patients, who have neutralizing activity caused by circulating sIFNAR.[24]

BAbs can be measured with ELISA, Western Blotting, and radio-immunoprecipitation or affinity chromatography assays. The ELISA methods comprise direct binding assays (dELISA), i.e. direct coating of test wells with IFNβ, and capture assays (cELISA), i.e. coating of test wells with a capture anti-IFNβ antibody.[32,33] The Western Blot method does not allow calculation of BAb titers.[34] A comparison of dELISA, cELISA, western blot, and a commercial immunoassay favored cELISA.[35] The advantage of affinity chromatography[36] and radio-immunoprecipitation assay[37] is that the antigen is in solution and, therefore, no epitopes are obscured or denatured by binding to a solid phase.

The principle in NAb in vitro assays is the utilization of cultured cell lines that are responsive to IFNβ. Test samples are incubated with IFNβ prior to addition of the cells. If the test samples contain NAbs, receptor activation is blocked. One type of assay measures the capacity of NAbs in the patient's serum to neutralize IFNβ's protective effect on cells challenged with virus, i.e. the cytopathic effect assay (CPE).[36,38–40] The MxA induction assay measures the ability of NAbs in the patients serum to reduce the IFNβ-induced expression of a specific IFNβ marker, MxA, either at the mRNA[41–43] or the protein level.[44–47] A comparison of the assays indicated that MxA mRNA is the most sensitive assay to detect lower concentrations of NAbs.[41,48]

Titers were three–five-fold higher[49] and positive samples were more frequently found[50] with use of IFNβ-1a than with use of IFNβ-1b for assaying the same samples, independently whether the neutralizing serum was obtained from patients on therapy with IFNβ-1a or IFNβ-1b. The sensitivity of the assay chosen for measurements of NAbs has profound influence on the proportion of patients that are classified as NAb-positive.[15] Not surprisingly, the reported frequencies and titres of anti-IFNβ antibodies therefore vary considerably from trial to trial (Fig. 24.1).[4,19,21,51–56]

Recently, a reporter gene luciferase assay that uses human fibrosarcoma cells, which have been stably transfected with a luciferase reporter gene cassette, has been introduced. When the IFNβ molecule binds to its receptor, it activates a transcellular signaling mechanism and causes transcription of the luciferase gene. The amount of luciferase induced can be quantified in terms of luminescent counts per second. In the presence of NAbs, the response is blocked. The luciferase assay appear to be reliable and sensitive and requires less time than other available NAb methods,[57] and NAb titers measured with a luciferase reporter gene assay correlated with NAb titers measured with an established cytopathic effect

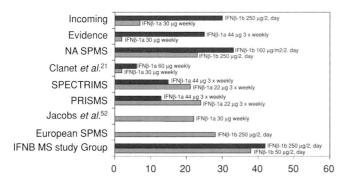

Fig. 24.1. Frequency of NAb-positive patients in controlled therapeutic trials of IFNβ.

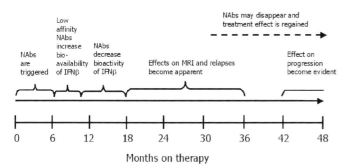

Fig. 24.2. Dynamics and clinical effects of NAbs by time during treatment with IFNβ.

assay when a number of samples were measured with both assays.[58]

Occurrence and disappearance of neutralizing antibodies

Low concentration of NAbs can be detected in vitro with sensitive assays after six months,[15,59] whereas NAbs with clinically negative effects usually develop between 9 and 18 months after start of IFNβ therapy (Fig. 24.2).

Patients who have been persistently NAb-negative during the first two years of IFNβ therapy only rarely become NAb-positive.[16] NAbs develop faster with IFNβ-1b than with IFNβ-1a, but after 12 months the proportions of NAb-positive patients treated with IFNβ-1b s.c. and IFNβ-1a s.c were similar.[15,59]

Add-on therapy with methylprednisolone administered monthly intravenously (i.v.) reduced the frequency of patients that had developed NAbs after 12 months by more than 50%.[60] Combination of IFNβ with an immunosuppressive agent have shown inconsistent results.[61,62]

In some NAb-positive patients, NAbs may subsequently disappear during continuous therapy with IFNβ. This happens in a significantly higher proportion of patients treated with IFNβ-1b than in patients treated with IFNβ-1a s.c.[16] Approximately 50% of all NAb-positive patients treated with IFNβ-1b had reverted to NAb-negative status 4 years after they had become

NAb-positive,[16] and after reversion to the NAb-negative state patients regained the full effect of IFNβ-1b therapy.[63]

Reversion of NAb status largely depends on the titer. Patients with low NAb titres are likely to revert to NAb negativity, whereas patients with high titers rarely become NAb-negative within a time span of 2 to 3 years.[64–69]

NAbs may persist for years after cessation of treatment. In a study of 29 IFNβ treated patients, who were NAb-positive at termination of therapy, only three patients (two of whom had a titer below 200 NU/ml) reverted to a NAb-negative status during a mean follow-up time of 22 months. The longest period that a patient maintained NAb positivity in the study was 59 months. In some patients the NAb titer even increased after cessation of IFNβ therapy.[70] One explanation for this phenomenon could be long-lived plasma cells, another that NAb-producing B-lymphocytes are activated by natural IFNβ, e.g. during viral infections.

Recently, a long-term study showed that 17 out of 71 patients were NAb-positive after a median interval of 25 months after cessation of IFNβ therapy. Persisting NAbs were associated with higher relapse rate and reduced time to progression to EDSS 6.0.[71]

When NAbs have developed, it is difficult to make patients revert to a NAb-negative state after cessation of IFNβ therapy. Treatment with monthly cycles of high-dose methylprednisolone did not significantly reduce NAb levels in the blood or restore IFNβ bioavailability,[72] and neither did a combination of azathioprine and monthly methylprednisolone cycles.[58]

A possible strategy to overcome loss of IFNβ bioactivity associated with NAbs could be i.v. injections of IFNβ-1b, but high-dose IFNβ i.v. did only restore the bioavailabilty of IFNβ transiently and did not seem to restore of tolerance and reversion to NAb-negative status.[73]

Measurement of the bioactivity of IFNβ

The bioactivity of IFNβ can be studied by measuring a number of IFNβ-induced gene products including the Myxovirus resistance protein (Mx) family (e.g. MxA and MxB),[42,74] β2-microglobulin,[75] neopterin,[76] 2–5′ oligoadenylate synthase 2,5 OAS),[42] major histocompatability complex (MHC) class I molecules, Stat-1,and tumor necrosis factor-related apoptosis-inducing ligand (TRAIL), among many others.[77–79]

In order to clearly reflect a response to IFNβ, the chosen biomarker needs to be specific for IFNβ and furthermore the induction needs to be of a certain magnitude. Among all tested IFNβ, induced genes so far, MxA has proven to be one of the most reliable markers of the in vivo bioactivity of IFNβ.[77,80] Up-regulation of MxA could be shown in all patients after the first IFNβ injection,[81] and several studies have reported that, in NAb-positive patients, especially those with high titers, the MxA response decreases to baseline levels indicating that NAbs abrogate the bioactivity of IFNβ.[42,46,79,82–84]

A study using Affymetrix GeneChip Human Genome Focus Array demonstrated that NAb-positive patients without an

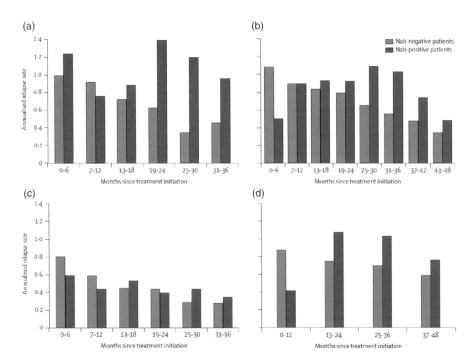

Fig. 24.3. Annualized relapse rates in Nab-negative patients and eventually Nab-positive patients in randomized placebo-controlled trial of IFNβ in MS. Reproduced with permission from Sorensen *et al.*[93]

MxA response did not express a differential expression in any of 1077 IFNβ-regulated genes identified in NAb-negative patients. Hence, lack of MxA in vivo response is a marker of a completely blocked biologic response to IFNβ.[85]

However, the blocking of IFNβ inducible genes by NAbs is not an all-or-nothing phenomenon. Already titres between 5 and 20 progressively attenuated in vivo induction of neopterin and β2-microglobulin.[86] Measurements of neopterin and β2-microglobulin blood levels showed that, whereas all NAb-negative patients had a biological response and all high-level NAb-positive patients had no response, the response in low-level NAb-positive patients varied: one third had a full response, one-third a partial, and one-third no response.[75]

Using an in vitro MxA induction assay to measure NAbs and mRNA MxA assessment of IFNβ bioactivity, it was found that patients with NAb titers of up to 150 TRU/ml still had retained IFNβ bioactivity, whereas profoundly reduced levels of IFNβ bioactivity were found in patients with NAbs of 150–600 TRU/ml, and titers above 600 TRU/ml were associated with loss of IFNβ bioactivity.[87]

Side effects to IFNβ was to some degree a biomarker for IFNβ bioactivity, significantly associated with NAb-negative status.[88]

Until recently, it was unknown whether the presence of NAbs had any implication on endogenous IFNβ. However, in vivo expression of the anti-inflammatory cytokine IL10 was found to be lower in NAb-positive patients than in untreated MS patients and normal controls, and ex vivo serum from NAb-positive MS patients blocked expression of IL10 induced by IFNβ in mononuclear blood cells.[89] Moreover, in vitro serum from NAb-positive patients induced neutralization of both recombinant and endogenous IFNβ bioactivity.[90] These observations suggest that persisting NAbs may impede the immune system.

Clinical implications of IFNβ neutralizing antibodies

There is emerging agreement that NAbs are correlated with reduced therapeutic efficacy of IFNβ.[91,92] Previous uncertainty can be ascribed to the fact that clinically relevant NAbs usually do not appear until 9–18 months after initiation of IFNβ therapy, and that early low-affinity NAbs present 6–12 months after start of therapy may even enhance the effect of IFNβ (Fig. 24.3) which increases the risk of overlooking the detrimental effect of NAbs, when data of only the two first years of treatment are analyzed.[93]

Also the definition of NAb positivity is of importance. Three different methods to determine when a patient can be considered NAb-positive are shown in Fig. 24.4. All three methods, however, will tend to underestimate the effects of NAbs.

It is a major problem that splitting patients into subgroups according to both their treatment arm and NAb status produces small patient groups, and lack the statistic power leads to false-negative results, i.e. a type-II error. If 30% of the treated patients are NAb positive and the original design power were 80%, then the power of the comparison of NAb-positive and NAb-negative subgroups is only 44% (Fig. 24.5).[7]

Overall, the duration of a trial is by far the most crucial criterion for deciding whether a study is suitable for evaluation of the clinical impact of NAbs, and only trials of sufficient duration (≥ 3 years) are suitable for evaluation of the clinical consequences of NAbs. Table 24.1 gives an overview of the large clinical trials of duration of 3 years or more.

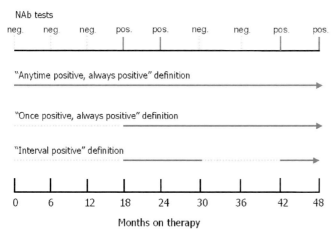

Fig. 24.4. Methods of defining NAb-status based on NAb testing in a hypothetical patient treated with IFNβ. NAb test were performed with 6-month intervals. "Anytime positive, always positive" method: the patient is classified as NAb-positive from the start of therapy and onwards. "Once positive, always positive" method: the patient is classified as NAb-negative from the start of treatment until month 18 and as NAb-positive from month 18 and onwards. "Interval positive" method: the patient is classified as NAb-negative from the start of treatment until month 18, as NAb-positive from month 18 until month 30, as NAb-negative from month 30 until month 42, and as NAb-positive from month 42 and onwards.

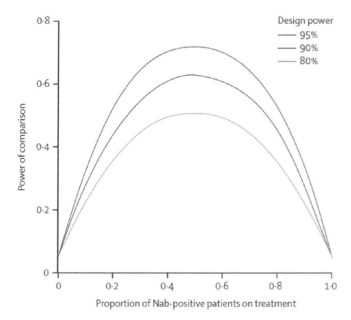

Fig. 24.5. Power of comparisons of NAb-positive and NAb-negative subgroups in compared with the original power of the trial. Reproduced with permission from Polman *et al.*[7]

Effect of NAbs on relapses

Applying the "anytime positive, always positive" method for defining NAb positivity 45% in the 8 MIU group developed NAbs in the pivotal trial of IFNβ-1b s.c.[4] The annual relapse rate was significantly higher in NAb-positive patients compared with NAb-negative patients ($P < 0.001$), and in the period from 13 to 36 months after start of treatment the relapse rates in

NAb-positive patients and placebo-treated patients were identical. A re-analysis of the study using both the "once positive, always positive" definition and the "interval analysis" method still showed higher relapse rates in the NAb-positive compared to the NAb-negative patients.[94,99]

In the pivotal Phase 3 placebo-controlled trial of IFNβ-1a i.m. 30 μg weekly for up to two years, there were no significant differences in relapse rate and progression between NAb-positive and NAb-negative patients.[86,100]

The PRISMS study compared IFNβ-1a 22 μg, 44 μg or placebo three times weekly for two years in 560 patients.[19] NAb-positive patients were defined using the "anytime positive, always positive" method. No significant differences in the relapse rate or progression were seen over the two years' study duration between NAb-positive and NAb-negative patients. However, in the extension phase of this study, PRISMS-4, NAbs caused a clear reduction in the efficacy on relapses in the third and the fourth year.[95] A re-analysis employing both the "any time positive, always positive" method and the "interval analysis" method confirmed the detrimental effects of NAbs.[101]

The European secondary progressive MS study comprised 718 patients treated for three years with either IFNβ-1b 8 MIU every other day or placebo. Using the "once positive, always positive" method NAb-positive patients had a significant 45% increase in relapse rates, but the increase was only borderline statistically significant when the "interval analysis" method was applied. Higher titres seemed to reduce the treatment effect more.[96]

The North American Placebo Control Randomized Study of IFNβ-1b in secondary progressive MS evaluated patients for three years and showed a significant higher relapse rate in NAb-positive patients.[54]

The SPECTRIMS study of IFNβ-1a s.c. was the only study in secondary progressive MS that did not show a statistically significant impact of NAbs on the relapse rate.[53]

A study comparing IFNβ-1a i.m. 30 μg and 60 μg once weekly for four years showed that NAb-positive patients had significantly higher relapse rate compared to NAb-negative patients ($P = 0.04$).[97]

An unselected comparative trial comprising a large sample of all Danish patients treated with an IFNβ preparation included 541 patients with relapsing–remitting MS followed for up to 60 months. Testing of NAbs was performed blindly and the effect of NAbs was assessed using the "interval analysis" method. In NAb-positive periods the annual relapse rate increased more than 50% compared with NAb-negative periods, and the time to the first relapse was significantly longer, and the proportion of relapse-free patients was significantly higher in NAb-negative patients.[26]

A retrospective study of 262 patients treated with an IFNβ preparation for more than three years showed that, whereas the relapse rate appeared to be unaffected by the subsequent NAb status in the first two years, it was significantly higher in NAb-positive patients than in NAb-negative patients in the third and fourth year.[98]

Table 24.1. *Effect of NAbs to IFNβ on clinical and MRI outcomes in large controlled therapeutic trials in relapsing–remitting and secondary progressive MS of more than 2 years' duration with blind evaluation of NAb testing. See text for definition of the different clinical and MRI outcomes*

Study	IFNβ product	Number of patients on IFNβ	Duration	Relapse rate	MRI activity	MRI severity	Disease progression
Placebo-controlled trials							
IFNB MS Study Group, 1996[94]	IFNβ-1b (Betaferon)	249	3 years	+ (*)	+ (ns)	+ (ns)	+ (ns)
PRISMS-4, 2001[95]	IFNβ-1a (s.c.) (Rebif) 44 μg	506	4 years	+ (**)	+ (***)	+ (***)	+ (*)
SPECTRIMS, 2001[53]	IFNβ-1a (s.c.) 44 μg	413	3 years	+ (ns)	ND	ND	- (ns)
European SPMS IFNβ-1b Study; Polman et al., 2003[96]	IFNβ-1b	360	3 years	+ (**)	ND	+ (**)	+ (ns)
North American SPMS IFNβ-1b Study Group; Panitch et al., 2004[54]	IFNβ-1b	631	3 years	+ (*)	ND	ND	ND
Comparative trials							
Danish National IFNβ Study; Sorensen et al., 2003[26]	IFNβ-1b / IFNβ-1a (IM)/IFNβ-1a (s.c.) (Betaferon/ Avonex/ Rebif)	541	5 years	+ (**)	ND	ND	+ (ns)
IFNβ-1a i.m. Dose Comparison Study; Kappos et al., 2005[97]	IFNβ-1a (IM) 30 μg/ 60 μg	802	4 years	+ (*)	+ (*)	+ (*)	+ (**)
Boz et al. 2007[98]	IFNβ-1b / IFNβ-1a (IM)	262	3 years	+ (*)	ND	ND	+ (ns)

+ = outcome worse in the NAb-positive group than in the NAb-negative group.
− = outcome better in the NAb-positive group than in the NAb-negative group.
ND = not done
Statistical significance is given in parentheses (ns = not significant; * = $P < 0.05$; ** = $P < 0.01$; *** = $P < 0.001$)

It has been claimed that NAbs induced by IFNβ-1b should not be associated with increased disease activity,[102] but recently it was shown that the clinical effect of NAbs was independent of the type of IFNβ that had induced NAbs.[103]

Effect of NAbs on disease progression

None of the pivotal trials in relapsing–remitting MS showed an effect of NAbs on disease progression and neither did any of the trials in secondary progressive MS (Table 24.1).[19,52,53,86,94,104] However, all the trials were underpowered to show an effect of NAbs because IFNβ by itself had no or only marginal effect on disease progression. Also the Danish study showed only a trend toward more progression in NAb-positive patients.[26]

The IFNβ-1a i.m 30 μg vs. 60 μg dose comparison study with four years duration showed a significant negative effect of NAbs on disease progression.[97]

In a study comparing IFNβ-1a i.m 30 μg weekly and IFNβ-1a s.c. 44 μg three times weekly for up to five years significantly more NAb-positive patients compared with NAb-negative patients had disability progression.[18]

The presence of NAbs was associated with a higher risk of developing disability during the subsequent five years in a long-term follow-up study of 68 patients receiving IFNβ,[105] and in a study of 78 patients followed for three years a higher proportion of persistently NAb-positive patients worsened one or more points on EDSS compared with NAb-negative patients.[106]

Effect of NAbs on disease activity measured on MRI

All large, randomized, placebo-controlled trials have shown an effect on disease activity measured on MRI and as gadolinium-positive lesions or new T2-lesions measured or severity as T2-lesion load (Table 24.1).[52,86,95,107,108]

The EVIDENCE trial comparing IFNβ-1a 44 μg s.c. with IFNβ-1a 30 μg i.m showed higher MRI activity in NAb-positive compared to NAb-negative patients,[55] and the comparative study of IFNβ-1a i.m. 30 μg and 60 μg once weekly for four years showed that disease activity measured on MRI either as gadolinium-positive lesions or new T2-lesions was negatively affected by NAbs.[100]

Implications for clinical practice

Today, it is generally acknowledged that NAbs reduce the biological and clinical efficacy of IFNβ. The ultimate goal to overcome the problems with NAbs would be development of IFNβ preparations with very low immunogenicity. However, an adequate follow-up of IFNβ treated patients with measurements of NAbs and in vivo IFNβ bioactivity and switching NAb positive patients without in vivo MxA response to effective therapy might prevent unnecessary disabling disease activity.

As virtually all eventually NAb-positive patients develop NAbs before 24 months on therapy, it seems reasonable to screen a patient for NAbs after 12 and 24 months' treatment with IFNβ.

It is not known exactly at which NAb titer antibody-mediated decreased bioactivity becomes significant and it is not known how much the bioactivity should be decreased before all beneficial effects of IFNβ are abrogated. However, there is substantial evidence indicating that titers >100 NU/ml with IFNβ-1a and >400 NU/ml with IFNβ-1a when IFNβ-1a is used in the assay are associated with reduction or abrogation of the effect of IFNβ. Persistent high titers should imply discontinuation of IFNβ therapy. At best, continued therapy is a waste of money and at worst, patients may experience a severely disabling relapse. The course of MS is unpredictable and even untreated patients may do well for long periods. Further, NAbs are only one among other causes of failure to IFNβ therapy. Some patients are constitutive non-responders and fail IFNβ therapy even with absence of NAbs. Hence, some patients with high titers of NAb will do well because they have a benign course while other NAb-negative patients will experience severe disease activity.[109] However, such observations do not change the fact that with high NAb titres the therapeutic response to IFNβ is abolished.

Another argument for continued IFNβ therapy in NAb-positive patients has been that patients may revert to the NAb-negative state during continued therapy with interferon beta. However, patient with high titers usually remain NAb-positive for several years, and apart from low NAb titers there are no predictors of reversion to NAb negative status.[16] As other therapies are available, patients with high NAb titers that are without protection from IFNβ therapy should be offered an alternative therapy.

For many reasons it is not possible to define a cut-off titer above which NAbs severely reduce or abolish the therapeutic effect of IFNβ. Low and medium titers are ambiguous and their relevance should be checked by measurement of the in vivo bioactivity of IFNβ.

Measurement of mRNA MxA induction after an IFNβ injection is a reliable method for determination of IFNβ bioactivity, and treatment decision should be guided by determination of mRNA MxA induction. If the IFNβ response is absent, the patient is prone to become an antibody-mediated non-responder, and the patient should be offered the possibility of change of therapy.

The recommendations of an international expert group with representatives from both sides of the Atlantic Ocean are summarized in Fig. 24.6.

Antibodies against natalizumab (see Chapter 27 for a review of natalizumab clinical trials)

Natalizumab is a monoclonal antibody directed against the α_4 component of the $\alpha_4\beta_1$ integrin (VLA4; CD49d) expressed on the surface of lymphocytes and monocytes.[110] By binding to $\alpha_4\beta_1$ integrin, which is a mediator of transendothelial leukocyte migration, natalizumab blocks the migration of T-cells

	Doing well	Intermediate disease activity	Doing poorly
Negative NAb titre			
Diagnostic recommendation	Repeat at 12 months	Repeat at 12 months	Do not repeat
Treatment recommendation	No change	Consider continuation of current therapy*	Switch therapy
Low NAb titre			
Diagnostic recommendation	Repeat at 3–6 months if low titer is persistent, consider MxA assay	Repeat at 3–6 months if low titer is persistent, consider MxA assay	Do not repeat May consider MxA assay for additional information
Treatment recommendation	If no MxA bioactivity, consider switch to non-interferon-beta therapy	If no MxA bioactivity, consider switch to non-interferon-beta therapy	Switch therapy
High NAb titre			
Diagnostic recommendation	Repeat at 3–6 months	Repeat at 3–6 months	Do not repeat
Treatment recommendation	if high titer is persistent, consider switch to non-interferon-beta therapy	if high titer is persistent, consider switch to non-interferon-beta therapy	Switch therapy

Definitions were applied by the panel as a starting point for their discussions (see panel 1, table 1). Diagnostic recommendations were for further diagnostic NAb testing (or MxA assay, if available). MxA assay-in-vivo bioactivity test (MxA mRNA). MxA=myxovirus resistance protein A, NAb=neutralising antibody, *Determination to switch therapy depends mainly on clinical and radiological situation.

Fig. 24.6. Diagnostic recommendations and treatment recommendations according to clinical disease activity and NAb titers measured 1–2 years after initiation of IFNβ therapy. Reproduced with permission from Polman et al.[7]

into the central nervous system.[111] Natalizumab was originally generated in mice, but humanized by grafting the antibody complementarity-determining regions into a human IgG4 antibody frame.

In the AFFIRM[112] and SENTINEL[113] trials binding anti-natalizumab antibodies were measured using a sandwich/bridging ELISA method.[114] Flow cytometric assay was used to detect natalizumab-blocking antibodies. The blocking assay detected the ability of natalizumab specific antibodies to block the binding of biotinylated natalizumab to its cognate α_4 receptor.[114] All patients exhibiting antibodies by ELISA were also antibody-positive in the blocking assay.[114]

About 6% of the patients were persistently antibody positive, defined as antibodies detected at two or more times with an interval of at least 42 days,[112–114] whereas about 3% were transiently antibody positive with disappearance of antibodies after a few months of treatment. The anti-natalizumab antibodies typically developed 12 weeks after initiation of treatment.[112–114]

The presence of antibodies was correlated with a reduction in trough serum concentrations of natalizumab, more pronounced in persistent than in transient positive patients.[114]

The presence of anti-natalizumab antibodies was related to both so-called acute infusion-related reactions that occurred in 76% of persistently positive patients, 25% of transiently positive patients, 20% of antibody-negative patients, and 18% of placebo-treated patients, and, in particular, hypersensitivity reactions that were experienced by 46% of persistently positive patients, 15% of transiently positive patients, and 0.7% of

antibody-negative patients.[114] In these cases NAb test is a keypoint, as the true IgE-mediated allergic reactions associated with antibody development, are not clinically distinguishable from the so-called infusion reactions that may be mediated by complement activation or Fc receptor with release of tumor necrosis factor-alpha.[3]

Infusion-related hypersensitivity occurs most frequently after the second infusion and has not been reported later than after the seventh infusion of natalizumab.[115]

One patient, however, developed a severe systemic hypersensitivity reaction with urticaria, dyspnea, abdominal pain, and fever eight days after the first infusion, and had anti-natalizumab antibodies on two analyses performed 20 and 60 days after the beginning of the symptoms.[116]

Delayed infusion reactions resembling serum sickness–type reactions (type III reaction) are commonly reported in other monoclonal antibody therapies (e.g. infliximab and rituximab), but have only rarely been observed in patients treated with natalizumab.[117,118] In one report, however, delayed infusion reactions occurred, however, in four out of 40 patients treated with natalizumab, of whom only two had developed anti-natalizumab antibodies.[3]

Post-marketing studies from several countries have shown frequencies of anti-natalizumab antibodies comparable to those reported in the AFFIRM study. In an Italian study of 285 patients anti-natalizumab antibodies had developed in 6.6% of patients six months after treatment start,[119] and a study from Switzerland reported a frequency of anti-natalizumab antibodies in 7.1% of the patients.[120]

Neutralizing antibodies against IFNβ do not predispose to antibodies against natalizumab.[121]

In the clinical trials the presence of anti-natalizumab antibodies resulted in abrogation of the therapeutic efficacy.[112–114] In permanent antibody-positive patients the relapse rate was similar to that seen in placebo-treated patients.[112]

Antibody testing in patients treated with natalizumab has been introduced in the majority of EU countries. Some recommend routine testing, while others have argued that antibody testing should be considered only in patients, who after six months of therapy continue to have clinical activity or persistent infusion reactions.[114] A positive test should always be repeated after 3 months to determine whether antibodies are transient or permanent.

Unlike the situation with IFNβ treatment, it has from the start been generally accepted that patients with confirmed persistent antibody positivity on retesting should be discontinued from natalizumab treatment, probably because the negative affect of antibodies can be easily observed on the background of strong therapeutic effect of natalizumab in antibody negative patients. Further, the time of occurrence of antibodies against natalizumab is more predictable than the occurrence of NAbs against IFNβ.[112–114]

Antibodies against other monoclonal antibodies (see also Chapter 32 – alemtuzumab; Chapter 33 – daclizumab; and Chapter 42 – rituximab)

Among the therapeutic monoclonal antibodies natalizumab, alemtuzumab, and daclizumab are humanized monoclonal antibodies, whereas rituximab is a mouse–human chimeric antibody. In the humanized monoclonal antibodies immunogenicity has been reduced via genetic engineering that combines regions of mouse immunoglobulin with human immunoglobulin sequences. The immunogenicity of alemtuzumab and daclizumab in MS patients has not been fully explored as yet. The prevalence of anti-monoclonal antibody therapeutic antibodies in MS patients has been reported, primarily based on results of binding (e.g. ELISA), and further exploration of the characteristics and dynamics of such binding antibodies is needed.

In the CAMMS study comparing annual cycles of alemtuzumab 12 mg or 24 mg/day with IFNβ-1a s.c. 44μ three times weekly, alemtuzumab-binding antibodies were detected in one

of 208 patients (0.5%) at 12 months and in 51 of 194 patients (26.3%) at 24 months. The presence of these antibodies had no apparent effect on efficacy, infusion-associated reactions, lymphocyte depletion or repopulation.[122]

In the CHOICE study of daclizumab as an add-on to IFNβ, 12 of 152 patients (8%) treated with daclizumab were positive for human anti-human (HAHA) neutralizing antibodies to daclizumab. The presence of neutralizing antibodies to daclizumab was associated with reduced serum daclizumab concentrations.[123]

Therapeutic mouse–human chimeric antibodies, such as rituximab, are associated with the development of human anti-chimeric antibodies (HACAs). In a Phase 2, double-blind, placebo-controlled 48-week study of rituximab in RRMS approximately one-fourth of 65 patients receiving rituximab developed HACAs. No effect on safety or efficacy was observed during the study.

Larger studies of extended duration in emerging monoclonal therapies are required to evaluate potential associations of antibody development with therapeutic efficacy and safety.

Conclusions

NAbs against IFNβ occur frequently, and routine measurements of NAbs using a standardized assay are recommended. NAbs are associated with reduction of the therapeutic effect of IFNβ, and patients with persistent high titers of NAbs should be switched to an alternative therapy. Patients with low or intermediate titers should have their IFNβ bioactivity measured with an in vivo mRNA MxA induction test. Patients with repeated abrogation of the mRNA MxA response to IFNβ injections should be switch to another therapy.

Anti-natalizumab antibodies that occur with a lower frequency than NAbs to IFNβ abrogate the therapeutic efficacy of natalizumab, and in patients with persistent antibodies natalizumab should be discontinued.

The frequency and clinical importance of antibodies against other therapeutic monoclonal antibodies have not yet been fully explored.

Acknowledgments

Economic support to the Danish Multiple Sclerosis Center was obtained from the Danish Multiple Sclerosis Society, the Warwara Larsen Foundation, and the Danish Medical Research Council.

References

1. Schellekens H, Casadevall N. Immunogenicity of recombinant human proteins: causes and consequences. *J Neurol* 2004;251 (Suppl 2):114–19.

2. Schellekens H. Bioequivalence and the immunogenicity of biopharmaceuticals.

Nat Rev Drug Discov 2002;1(6):457–62.

3. Hellwig K, Schimrigk S, Fischer M, *et al.* Allergic and nonallergic delayed infusion reactions during natalizumab therapy. *Arch Neurol* 2008;65(5): 656–8.

4. Duquette P, Girard M, Despault L, *et al.* Interferon Beta-1B is effective in relapsing–remitting multiple-sclerosis – clinical-results of a multicenter, randomized, double-blind, placebo-controlled trial. *Neurology* 1993;43(4):655–61.

5. Sorensen PS, Deisenhammer F, Duda P, *et al.* Guidelines on use of anti-interferon-beta antibody measurements in multiple sclerosis – Report of an EFNS Task Force on IFN-beta antibodies in multiple sclerosis. *Eur J Neurol* 2005;12(11):817–27.

6. Goodin DS, Frohman EM, Hurwitz B, *et al.* Neutralizing antibodies to interferon beta: assessment of their clinical and radiographic impact: an evidence report: report of the Therapeutics and Technology Assessment Subcommittee of the American Academy of Neurology. *Neurology* 2007;68(13):977–84.

7. Polman CH, Bertolotto A, Deisenhammer F, *et al.* Recommendations for clinical use of data on neutralising antibodies to interferon-beta therapy in multiple sclerosis. *Lancet Neurol* 2010;9(7):740–50.

8. Hoffmann S, Cepok S, Grummel V, *et al.* HLA-DRB1*0401 and HLA-DRB1*0408 are strongly associated with the development of antibodies against interferon-beta therapy in multiple sclerosis. *Am J Hum Genet* 2008;83(2):219–27.

9. Larocca AP, Leung SC, Marcus SG, Colby CB, Borden EC. Evaluation of neutralizing antibodies in patients treated with recombinant interferon-beta ser. *J Interferon Res* 1989;9 (Suppl 1):S51–60.

10. Lundkvist M, Greiner E, Hillert J, Fogdell-Hahn A. Multiple sclerosis patients lacking oligoclonal bands in the cerebrospinal fluid are less likely to develop neutralizing antibodies against interferon beta. *Mult Scler* 2010;16(7):796–800.

11. Garg N, Weinstock-Guttman B, Bhasi K, Locke J, Ramanathan M. An association between autoreactive antibodies and anti-interferon-beta antibodies in multiple sclerosis. *Mult Scler* 2007;13(7):895–9.

12. Sena A, Bendtzen K, Cascais MJ, Pedrosa R, Ferret-Sena V, Campos E. Influence of apolipoprotein E plasma levels and tobacco smoking on the induction of neutralising antibodies to interferon-beta. *J Neurol* 2010; 257: 1703–7.

13. Schellekens H. The immunogenicity of biopharmaceuticals. *Neurology* 2003;61(9 Suppl 5):S11–12.

14. Runkel L, Meier W, Pepinsky RB, *et al.* Structural and functional differences between glycosylated and non-glycosylated forms of human interferon-beta (IFN-beta). *Pharm Res* 1998;15(4):641–9.

15. Ross C, Clemmesen KM, Svenson M, *et al.* Immunogenicity of interferon-beta in multiple sclerosis patients: influence of preparation, dosage, dose frequency, and route of administration. Danish Multiple Sclerosis Study Group. *Ann Neurol* 2000;48(5):706–12.

16. Sorensen PS, Koch-Henriksen N, Ross C, Clemmesen KM, Bendtzen K. Appearance and disappearance of neutralizing antibodies during interferon-beta therapy. *Neurology* 2005;65(1):33–9.

17. Perini P, Facchinetti A, Bulian P, *et al.* Interferon-beta (INF-beta) antibodies in interferon-beta1a- and interferon-beta1b-treated multiple sclerosis patients. Prevalence, kinetics, cross-reactivity, and factors enhancing interferon-beta immunogenicity in vivo. *Eur Cytokine Netw* 2001;12(1):56–61.

18. Minagara A, Murray TJ. Efficacy and tolerability of intramuscular interferon beta-1a compared with subcutaneous interferon beta-1a in relapsing MS: results from PROOF. *Curr Med Res Opin* 2008;24(4):1049–55.

19. PRISMS (Prevention of Relapses and Disability by Interferon beta-1a Subcutaneously in Multiple Sclerosis) Study Group. Randomised double-blind placebo-controlled study of interferon beta-1a in relapsing/remitting multiple sclerosis. *Lancet* 1998;352(9139):1498–504.

20. Freedman MS, Francis GS, Sanders EA, *et al.* Randomized study of once-weekly interferon beta-1la therapy in relapsing multiple sclerosis: three-year data from the OWIMS study. *Mult Scler* 2005;11(1):41–5.

21. Clanet M, Radue EW, Kappos L, *et al.* A randomized, double-blind, dose-comparison study of weekly interferon beta-1a in relapsing MS. *Neurology* 2002;59(10):1507–17.

22. Bendtzen K. Anti-IFN BAb and NAb antibodies: a minireview. *Neurology* 2003;61(9 Suppl 5):S6–S10.

23. Gneiss C, Tripp P, Ehling R, *et al.* Interferon-beta antibodies have a higher affinity in patients with neutralizing antibodies compared to patients with non-neutralizing antibodies. *J Neuroimmunol* 2006;174(1–2):174–9.

24. Gilli F, Marnetto F, Caldano M, *et al.* Anti-interferon-beta neutralising activity is not entirely mediated by antibodies. *J Neuroimmunol* 2007;192(1–2):198–205.

25. Gilli F, Hoffmann F, Sala A, *et al.* Qualitative and quantitative analysis of antibody response against IFNbeta in patients with Multiple Sclerosis. *Mult Scler* 2006; 12(6), 738–46.

26. Sorensen PS, Ross C, Clemmesen KM, *et al.* Clinical importance of neutralising antibodies against interferon beta in patients with relapsing-remitting multiple sclerosis. *Lancet* 2003;362(9391):1184–91.

27. Sominanda A, Rot U, Suoniemi M, Deisenhammer F, Hillert J, Fogdell-Hahn A. Interferon beta preparations for the treatment of multiple sclerosis patients differ in neutralizing antibody seroprevalence and immunogenicity. *Mult Scler* 2007;13(2):208–14.

28. Prince HE, Lape-Nixon M, Audette C, Van HK. Identification of interferon-beta antibodies in a reference laboratory setting: Findings for 1144 consecutive sera. *J Neuroimmunol* 2007;190(1–2):165–9.

29. Pachner AR, Warth JD, Pace A, Goelz S. Effect of neutralizing antibodies on biomarker responses to interferon beta: the INSIGHT study. *Neurology* 2009;73(18):1493–500.

30. Giovannoni G, Barbarash O, Casset-Semanaz F, *et al.* Safety and immunogenicity of a new formulation of interferon {beta}-1a (Rebif(R) New Formulation) in a Phase IIIb study in patients with relapsing multiple sclerosis: 96-week results. *Mult Scler* 2008;15(2):219–28.

31. Gneiss C, Tripp P, Reichartseder F, *et al.* Differing immunogenic potentials of interferon beta preparations in multiple sclerosis patients. *Mult Scler* 2006;12(6):731–7.

32. Friedman JE, Zabriskie J, Bourganskaia E. A pilot study of pentoxifylline in multiple sclerosis [letter]. *Arch Neurol* 1996;53(10):956–7.

33. Smith DR, Balashov KE, Hafler DA, Khoury SJ, Weiner HL. Immune

deviation following pulse cyclophosphamide/methylprednisolone treatment of multiple sclerosis: increased interleukin-4 production and associated eosinophilia. *Ann Neurol* 1997;42(3):313–18.

34. Thompson AJ, Miller D, Youl B, *et al.* Serial gadolinium-enhanced MRI in relapsing/remitting multiple sclerosis of varying disease duration. *Neurology* 1992;42:60–3.

35. Gneiss C, Brugger M, Millonig A, *et al.* Comparative study of four different assays for the detection of binding antibodies against interferon-{beta}. *Mult Scler* 2008;14(6):830–6.

36. Wood NW, Sawcer SJ, Kellar Wood HF, *et al.* The T-cell receptor beta locus and susceptibility to multiple sclerosis. *Neurology* 1995;45(10):1859–63.

37. Freeman JA, Langdon DW, Hobart JC, Thompson AJ. The impact of inpatient rehabilitation on progressive multiple sclerosis. *Ann Neurol* 1997;42(2):236–44.

38. Bansil S, Singhal BS, Ahuja GK, *et al.* Comparison between multiple sclerosis in India and the United States: a case-control study. *Neurology* 1996;46(2):385–7.

39. Grossberg SE, Kawade Y, Kohase M, Klein JP. The neutralization of interferons by antibody. II. Neutralizing antibody unitage and its relationship to bioassay sensitivity: the tenfold reduction unit. *J Interferon Cytokine Res* 2001;21(9): 743–55.

40. Grossberg SE, Kawade Y, Kohase M, Yokoyama H, Finter N. The neutralization of interferons by antibody. I. Quantitative and theoretical analyses of the neutralization reaction in different bioassay systems. *J Interferon Cytokine Res* 2001;21(9):729–42.

41. Bertolotto A, Sala A, Caldano M, *et al.* Development and validation of a real time PCR-based bioassay for quantification of neutralizing antibodies against human interferon-beta. *J Immunol Methods* 2007;321(1–2):19–31.

42. Pachner A, Narayan K, Price N, Hurd M, Dail D. MxA Gene Expression Analysis as an Interferon-beta Bioactivity Measurement in Patients with Multiple Sclerosis and the Identification of Antibody-Mediated Decreased Bioactivity. *Mol Diagn* 2003;7(1):17–25.

43. Capra R, Sottini A, Cordioli C, *et al.* IFNbeta bioavailability in multiple sclerosis patients: MxA versus antibody-detecting assays. *J Neuroimmunol* 2007;189(1–2):102–10.

44. Pungor E, Jr., Files JG, Gabe JD, *et al.* A novel bioassay for the determination of neutralizing antibodies to IFN-beta1b. *J Interferon Cytokine Res* 1998;18(12): 1025–30.

45. Kob M, Harvey J, Schautzer F, *et al.* A novel and rapid assay for the detection of neutralizing antibodies against interferon-beta. *Mult Scler* 2003;9(1):32–5.

46. Deisenhammer F, Reindl M, Harvey J, Gasse T, Dilitz E, Berger T. Bioavailability of interferon beta 1b in MS patients with and without neutralizing antibodies. *Neurology* 1999;52(6):1239–43.

47. Aarskog NK, Maroy T, Myhr KM, Vedeler CA. Antibodies against interferon-beta in multiple sclerosis. *J Neuroimmunol* 2009;212(1–2):148–50.

48. McKay F, Schibeci S, Heard R, Stewart G, Booth D. Analysis of neutralizing antibodies to therapeutic interferon-beta in multiple sclerosis patients: a comparison of three methods in a large Australasian cohort. *J Immunol Methods* 2006;310(1–2): 20–9.

49. Files JG, Hargrove D, Delute L, Cantillon M. Measured neutralizing titers of IFN-beta neutralizing antibodies (NAbs) can depend on the preparations of IFN-beta used in the assay. *J Interferon Cytokine Res* 2007;27(8):637–42.

50. Massart C, Gibassier J, de SJ, *et al.* Determination of interferon beta neutralizing antibodies in multiple sclerosis: Improvement of clinical sensitivity of a cytopathic effect assay. *Clin Chim Acta* 2008;391(1–2):98–101.

51. European Study Group on interferon beta-1b in secondary progressive MS. Placebo-controlled multicentre randomised trial of interferon beta-1b in treatment of secondary progressive multiple sclerosis. *Lancet* 1998;352(9139):1491–7.

52. Jacobs LD, Cookfair DL, Rudick RA, *et al.* Intramuscular interferon beta-1a for disease progression in relapsing multiple sclerosis. The Multiple Sclerosis Collaborative Research Group (MSCRG). *Ann Neurol* 1996;39(3):285–94.

53. SPECTRIMS. Randomized controlled trial of interferon-beta-1a in secondary progressive MS: clinical results. *Neurology* 2001;56(11):1496–504.

54. Panitch H, Miller A, Paty D, Weinshenker B. Interferon beta-1b in secondary progressive MS: results from a 3-year controlled study. *Neurology* 2004;63(10):1788–95.

55. Panitch H, Goodin DS, Francis G, *et al.* Randomized, comparative study of interferon beta-1a treatment regimens in MS: The EVIDENCE Trial. *Neurology* 2002;59(10):1496–506.

56. Durelli L, Verdun E, Barbero P, *et al.* Every-other-day interferon beta-1b versus once-weekly interferon beta-1a for multiple sclerosis: results of a 2-year prospective randomised multicentre study (INCOMIN). *Lancet* 2002;359(9316):1453–60.

57. Lam R, Farrell R, Aziz T, *et al.* Validating parameters of a luciferase reporter gene assay to measure neutralizing antibodies to IFN[beta] in multiple sclerosis patients. *J Immunol Methods* 2008;336(2):113–18.

58. Ravnborg M, Bendtzen K, Christensen O, *et al.* Treatment with azathioprine and cyclic methylprednisolone has little or no effect on bioactivity in anti-interferon beta antibody-positive patients with multiple sclerosis. *Mult Scler* 2009;15(3):323–8.

59. Ross C, Svenson M, Clemmesen KM, Sorensen PS, Koch-Henriksen N, Bendtzen K. Measuring and evaluating interferon-beta-induced antibodies in patients with multiple sclerosis. *Mult Scler* 2006;12:39–46.

60. Pozzilli C, Antonini G, Bagnato F, *et al.* Monthly corticosteroids decrease neutralizing antibodies to IFNbeta1 b: a randomized trial in multiple sclerosis. *J Neurol* 2002;249(1):50–6.

61. Calabresi PA, Wilterdink JL, Rogg JM, Mills P, Webb A, Whartenby KA. An open-label trial of combination therapy with interferon beta-1a and oral methotrexate in MS. *Neurology* 2002;58(2):314–17.

62. Fernandez O, Guerrero M, Mayorga C, *et al.* Combination therapy with interferon beta-1b and azathioprine in secondary progressive multiple

sclerosis. A two-year pilot study. *J Neurol* 2002;249(8):1058–62.

63. Sorensen PS, Koch-Henriksen N, Flachs E, Bendtzen K. Is the treatment effect of IFN-{beta} restored after the disappearance of neutralizing antibodies? *Mult Scler* 2008;14(6):837–42.

64. Bellomi F, Scagnolari C, Tomassini V, *et al*. Fate of neutralizing and binding antibodies to IFN beta in MS patients treated with IFN beta for 6 years. *J Neurol Sci* 2003;215(1–2):3–8.

65. Gneiss C, Reindl M, Lutterotti A, *et al*. Interferon-beta: the neutralizing antibody (NAb) titre predicts reversion to NAb negativity. *Mult Scler* 2004;10(5):507–10.

66. Herndon RM, Rudick RA, Munschauer FE, III, *et al*. Eight-year immunogenicity and safety of interferon beta-1a-Avonex treatment in patients with multiple sclerosis. *Mult Scler* 2005;11(4):409–19.

67. Rice GP, Paszner B, Oger J, Lesaux J, Paty D, Ebers G. The evolution of neutralizing antibodies in multiple sclerosis patients treated with interferon beta-1b. *Neurology* 1999;52(6):1277–9.

68. Sominanda A, Hillert J, Fogdell-Hahn A. Neutralizing antibodies against interferon beta: fluctuation is modest and titre dependent. *Eur J Neurol* 2009; 18(1):21–8.

69. Malucchi S, Capobianco M, Gilli F, *et al*. Fate of multiple sclerosis patients positive for neutralising antibodies towards interferon beta shifted to alternative treatments. *Neurol Sci* 2005;26 Suppl 4:S213–14.

70. Petersen B, Bendtzen K, Koch-Henriksen N, Ravnborg M, Ross C, Sorensen PS. Persistence of neutralizing antibodies after discontinuation of IFNbeta therapy in patients with relapsing–remitting multiple sclerosis. *Mult Scler* 2006;12(3):247–52.

71. Van Der Voort LF, Gilli F, Bertolotto A, *et al*. Clinical effect of neutralizing antibodies to interferon beta that persist long after cessation of therapy for multiple sclerosis. *Arch Neurol* 2010;67(4):402–7.

72. Hesse D, Frederiksen JL, Koch-Henriksen N, *et al*. Methylprednisolone does not restore biological response in multiple sclerosis

patients with neutralizing antibodies against interferon-beta. *Eur J Neurol* 2009;16(1):43–7.

73. Millonig A, Rudzki D, Holzl M, *et al*. High-dose intravenous interferon beta in patients with neutralizing antibodies (HINABS): a pilot study. *Mult Scler* 2009;15(8):977–83.

74. Deisenhammer F, Mayringer I, Harvey J, *et al*. A comparative study of the relative bioavailability of different interferon beta preparations. *Neurology* 2000;54(11):2055–60.

75. Sorensen PS, Tscherning T, Mathiesen HK, *et al*. Neutralizing antibodies hamper IFNbeta bioactivity and treatment effect on MRI in patients with MS. *Neurology* 2006;67(9): 1681–3.

76. Cook SD, Quinless JR, Jotkowitz A, Beaton P. Serum IFN neutralizing antibodies and neopterin levels in a cross-section of MS patients. *Neurology* 2001;57(6):1080–4.

77. Gilli F, Marnetto F, Caldano M, *et al*. Biological markers of interferon-beta therapy: comparison among interferon-stimulated genes MxA, TRAIL and XAF-1. *Mult Scler* 2006;12(1):47–57.

78. Wandinger KP, Lunemann JD, Wengert O, *et al*. TNF-related apoptosis inducing ligand (TRAIL) as a potential response marker for interferon-beta treatment in multiple sclerosis. *Lancet* 2003;361(9374):2036–43.

79. Santos R, Weinstock-Guttman B, Tamano-Blanco M, *et al*. Dynamics of interferon-beta modulated mRNA biomarkers in multiple sclerosis patients with anti-interferon-beta neutralizing antibodies. *J Neuroimmunol* 2006;176(1–2):125–33.

80. Pachner A, Narayan K, Pak. Multiplex analysis of expression of three IFN-beta-induced genes in antibody-positive MS patients. *Neurology* 2006;66(3):444–6.

81. Gilli F, Marnetto F, Caldano M, *et al*. Biological responsiveness to first injections of interferon-beta in patients with multiple sclerosis. *J Neuroimmunol* 2005;158(1–2):195–203.

82. Bertolotto A, Gilli F, Sala A, *et al*. Persistent neutralizing antibodies abolish the interferon beta bioavailability in MS patients. *Neurology* 2003;60(4):634–9.

83. Pachner AR, Dail D, Pak E, Narayan K. The importance of measuring IFNbeta bioactivity: monitoring in MS patients and the effect of anti-IFNbeta antibodies. *J Neuroimmunol* 2005;166(1–2):180–8.

84. Vallittu AM, Eralinna JP, Ilonen J, Salmi AA, Waris M. MxA protein assay for optimal monitoring of IFN-beta bioactivity in the treatment of MS patients. *Acta Neurol Scand* 2007 118: 12–17.

85. Hesse D, Sellebjerg F, Sorensen PS. Absence of MxA induction by interferon beta in patients with MS reflects complete loss of bioactivity. *Neurology* 2009;73(5):372–7.

86. Rudick RA, Simonian NA, Alam JA, *et al*. Incidence and significance of neutralizing antibodies to interferon beta-1a in multiple sclerosis. Multiple Sclerosis Collaborative Research Group (MSCRG). *Neurology* 1998;50(5):1266–72.

87. Sominanda A, Hillert J, Fogdell-Hahn A. In vivo bioactivity of interferon-beta in multiple sclerosis patients with neutralising antibodies is titre-dependent. *J Neurol Neurosurg Psychiatry* 2008;79(1):57–62.

88. Farrell R, Kapoor R, Leary SM, *et al*. Neutralizing anti-interferon beta antibodies are associated with reduced side effects and delayed impact on efficacy of Interferon-beta. *Mult Scler* 2008;14(2):212–18.

89. Hesse D, Krakauer M, Lund H, *et al*. Disease protection and interleukin-10 induction by endogenous interferon-beta in multiple sclerosis? *Eur J Neurol* 2011; 18(2): 266–72.

90. Sominanda A, Lundkvist M, Fogdell-Hahn A, *et al*. Inhibition of endogenous interferon beta by neutralizing antibodies against recombinant interferon beta. *Arch Neurol* 2010;67(9):1095–101.

91. Giovannoni G, Goodman A. Neutralizing anti-IFN-beta antibodies: how much more evidence do we need to use them in practice? *Neurology* 2005;65(1):6–8.

92. Pachner AR, Bertolotto A, Deisenhammer F. Measurement of MxA mRNA or protein as a biomarker of IFNbeta bioactivity: detection of antibody-mediated decreased bioactivity (ADB). *Neurology* 2003;61(9 Suppl 5):S24–6.

93. Sorensen PS, Koch-Henriksen N, Bendtzen K. Are ex vivo neutralising antibodies against IFN-{beta} always detrimental to therapeutic efficacy in multiple sclerosis? *Mult Scler* 2007;13(5):616–21.

94. Duquette P, Girard M, Dubois R, *et al.* Neutralizing antibodies during treatment of multiple sclerosis with interferon beta-1b: Experience during the first three years. *Neurology* 1996;47(4):889–94.

95. PRISMS Study Group. PRISMS-4: Long-term efficacy of interferon-beta-1a in relapsing MS. *Neurology* 2001;56(12):1628–36.

96. Polman C, Kappos L, White R, *et al.* Neutralizing antibodies during treatment of secondary progressive MS with interferon beta-1b. *Neurology* 2003;60(1):37–43.

97. Kappos L, Clanet M, Sandberg-Wollheim M, *et al.* Neutralizing antibodies and efficacy of interferon beta-1a: a 4-year controlled study. *Neurology* 2005;65(1):40–7.

98. Boz C, Oger J, Gibbs E, Grossberg SE. Reduced effectiveness of long-term interferon-{beta} treatment on relapses in neutralizing antibody-positive multiple sclerosis patients: a Canadian multiple sclerosis clinic-based study. *Mult Scler* 2007;13(9):1127–37.

99. Petkau AJ, White RA, Ebers GC, *et al.* Longitudinal analyses of the effects of neutralizing antibodies on interferon beta-1b in relapsing–remitting multiple sclerosis. *Mult Scler* 2004;10(2):126–38.

100. Jacobs LD, Beck RW, Simon JH, *et al.* Intramuscular interferon beta-1a therapy initiated during a first demyelinating event in multiple sclerosis. CHAMPS Study Group. *N Engl J Med* 2000;343(13):898–904.

101. Francis GS, Rice GP, Alsop JC. Interferon beta-1a in MS: results following development of neutralizing antibodies in PRISMS. *Neurology* 2005;65(1):48–55.

102. Goodin DS, Hurwitz B, Noronha A. Neutralizing antibodies to interferon beta-1b are not associated with disease worsening in multiple sclerosis. *J Int Med Res* 2007;35(2):173–87.

103. Koch-Henriksen N, Sorensen P, Bendtzen K, Flachs E. The clinical effect of neutralizing antibodies against interferon-beta is independent of the type of interferon-beta used for patients with relapsing-remitting multiple sclerosis. *Mult Scler* 2009;15(5):601–5.

104. Polman CH, Kappos L, Petkau J, Thompson A. Neutralising antibodies to interferon beta during the treatment of multiple sclerosis. *J Neurol Neurosurg Psychiatry* 2003;74(8):1162–3.

105. Tomassini V, Paolillo A, Russo P, *et al.* Predictors of long-term clinical response to interferon beta therapy in relapsing multiple sclerosis. *J Neurol* 2006;253(3):287–93.

106. Malucchi S, Sala A, Gilli F, *et al.* Neutralizing antibodies reduce the efficacy of betaIFN during treatment of multiple sclerosis. *Neurology* 2004;62(11):2031–7.

107. Paty DW, Li DK. Interferon beta-1b is effective in relapsing-remitting multiple sclerosis. II. MRI analysis results of a multicenter, randomized, double-blind, placebo-controlled trial. UBC MS/MRI Study Group and the IFNB Multiple Sclerosis Study Group [see comments]. *Neurology* 1993;43(4):662–7.

108. Polman C, Kappos L, White R, *et al.* Neutralizing antibodies during treatment of secondary progressive MS with interferon beta-1b. *Neurology* 2003;60(1):37–43.

109. Chiu AW, Ehrmantraut M, Richert ND, *et al.* A case study on the effect of neutralizing antibodies to interferon beta 1b in multiple sclerosis patients followed for 3 years with monthly imaging. *Clin Exp Immunol* 2007;150(1):61–7.

110. Frenette PS, Wagner DD. Adhesion molecules–Part 1. *N Engl J Med* 1996;334(23):1526–9.

111. Rudick RA, Sandrock A. Natalizumab: alpha 4-integrin antagonist selective adhesion molecule inhibitors for MS. *Expert Rev Neurother* 2004;4(4):571–80.

112. Polman CH, O'Connor PW, Havrdova E, *et al.* A randomized, placebo-controlled trial of natalizumab for relapsing multiple sclerosis. *N Engl J Med* 2006;354(9):899–910.

113. Rudick RA, Stuart WH, Calabresi PA, *et al.* Natalizumab plus interferon beta-1a for relapsing multiple sclerosis. *N Engl J Med* 2006;354(9):911–23.

114. Calabresi PA, Giovannoni G, Confavreux C, *et al.* The incidence and significance of anti-natalizumab antibodies: results from AFFIRM and SENTINEL. *Neurology* 2007;69(14):1391–403.

115. Phillips JT, O'Connor PW, Havrdova E, *et al.* Infusion-related hypersensitivity reactions during natalizumab treatment. *Neurology* 2006;67(9):1717–18.

116. Cohen M, Rocher F, Vivinus S, Thomas P, Lebrun C. Giant urticaria and persistent neutralizing antibodies after the first natalizumab infusion. *Neurology* 2010;74(17):1394–5.

117. Krumbholz M, Pellkofer H, Gold R, Hoffmann LA, Hohlfeld R, Kumpfel T. Delayed allergic reaction to natalizumab associated with early formation of neutralizing antibodies. *Arch Neurol* 2007;64(9):1331–3.

118. Killestein J, Jasperse B, Liedorp M, Seewann A, Polman C. Very late delayed-allergic reaction to natalizumab not associated with neutralizing antibodies. *Mult Scler* 2009;15(4):525–6.

119. Sangalli F, Moiola L, Bucello S, *et al.* Efficacy and tolerability of natalizumab in relapsing-remitting multiple sclerosis patients: a post-marketing observational study. *Neurol Sci* 2011; **31** (Suppl 3): 299–302.

120. Putzki N, Yaldizli O, Buhler R, Schwegler G, Curtius D, Tettenborn B. Natalizumab reduces clinical and MRI activity in multiple sclerosis patients with high disease activity: results from a multicenter study in Switzerland. *Eur Neurol* 2010;63(2):101–6.

121. Sorensen PS, Koch-Henriksen N, Jensen. P.E.H. Neutralizing antibodies against interferon-beta do not predispose antibodies against natalizumab. *Neurology* 2011;76(8):759–60.

122. Somerfield J, Hill-Cawthorne GA, Lin A, *et al.* A novel strategy to reduce the immunogenicity of biological therapies. *J Immunol* 2010;185(1):763–8.

123. Wynn D, Kaufman M, Montalban X, *et al.* Daclizumab in active relapsing multiple sclerosis (CHOICE study): a phase 2, randomised, double-blind, placebo-controlled, add-on trial with interferon beta. *Lancet Neurol* 2010;9(4):381–90.

Chapter

25

Interferon beta to treat multiple sclerosis

Richard A. Rudick

History and overview

The first disease-modifying drug for relapsing remitting MS (RRMS) – subcutaneous (SC) interferon β-1b (IFNβ-1b) – was approved by the US FDA 18 years ago, in 1993. This landmark achievement followed 15 years of pioneering clinical studies using natural Type I IFN, derived from various cell sources.[1-5] The rationale for Type I IFN was based on its anti-viral properties, with the presumption that MS was caused by an unidentified virus. Trials of IFNα were abandoned because of side effects, and trials of IFNγ (a Type II IFN) were discontinued because IFNγ seemed to cause severe relapses in some MS patients.[6] However, early studies suggested that IFNβ reduced disease activity. On that basis, randomized, placebo-controlled registration trials were conducted, leading to approval of IFNβ-1b,[7] intramuscular IFNβ-1a (IFNβ-1a [IM]);[8] and subcutaneous IFNβ-1a (IFNβ-1a [SC]).[9] The IFNβ products were shown to significantly reduce the frequency of relapse and the occurrence of new brain lesions. Some studies demonstrated reduced frequency of EDSS worsening, and IFNβ-1a (IM) was reported to slow whole brain atrophy.[10] These findings were extended to patients with clinically isolated syndromes (CIS), where clinical and MRI benefits were slightly more robust. Results in progressive MS[11-14] were mixed, but generally disappointing. At the present time IFNβ is widely used as a first-line disease-modifying drug (DMD) for patients with CIS and RRMS. In clinical practice, effectiveness appears to vary. Some patients remain disease free for many years; other patients exhibit continued disease while on IFNβ, suggesting there are "responders" and "non-responders". For patients who seem to respond to IFNβ, treatment benefits persist for many years,[15-18] and serious toxicity with long-term use has not become evident.

This chapter will summarize IFNβ biological effects, its possible mechanisms of action, and the key studies in CIS, RRMS, and progressive MS. Dose-comparison studies, and studies comparing different IFNβ products, or comparing IFNβ with other therapies will be summarized, as will observational studies. The reader should consult recently published reviews of IFNβ for MS or the prior edition of this book for study details. Here we will summarize the effects of IFNβ, generalizing and drawing conclusions as appropriate, and will end with a listing of important unresolved issues requiring further research.

Biological effects of IFN and mechanisms of action

Biological effects of interferon

Interferons were first identified in 1957 as potent antiviral agents, and were subsequently found to be secreted proteins having properties that resulted in their classification as growth factors, differentiation factors, or cytokines. Currently, interferons are considered to be members of the cytokine family of proteins, and a key component of the innate immune system. Interferon β is a member of the Type I IFN family, which consists of IFNα, IFNτ, and IFNβ. Type I IFNs are relatively small (~15–25 kDa), single-chain polypeptides with similar structures: compact, ordered proteins with alpha helices and beta pleated sheets. Type I IFN binds to a heterodimeric receptor, which signals through JAK/STAT phosphorylation cascades, ultimately resulting in the transcriptional regulation of several hundred genes.[19-22]

In contrast to IFNα, where at least 12 functional subtypes have been identified, IFNβ is encoded by a single gene with no introns and hence, no splice variants, and no polymorphisms that have been identified. Although IFNβ was originally called fibroblast IFN – because fibroblasts could be induced to produce it in vitro – numerous other cell types can express IFNβ, including endothelial cells, epithelial cells, and various leukocytes.[23] The physiological source of IFNβ has not been identified. Endogenous IFNβ is not detected at significant levels in humans. Human IFNβ, expressed by fibroblasts in vitro, is glycosylated at one site with an N-linked complex carbohydrate, the exact structure of which can be influenced by growth conditions and the cell type producing the IFN.[24] While important for monomer stability, solubility and, perhaps biodistribution, the carbohydrate moiety is not required for receptor binding.[25]

The IFNβ receptor consists of a signaling chain (IFNAR1) and a binding chain (IFNAR2). Both IFNAR1 and IFNAR2 are constitutively expressed on the surface of virtually all cells. IFNβ can bind to IFNAR2 alone, but can bind to IFNAR1 only

Multiple Sclerosis Therapeutics, Fourth Edition, ed. Jeffrey A. Cohen and Richard A. Rudick. Published by Cambridge University Press.
© Cambridge University Press 2011.

in the presence of IFNAR2. Knockout experiments indicate that both IFNAR1 and IFNAR2 are required for IFNβ activity,[26,27] but it remains uncertain whether there are auxillary receptors or alternative receptor complexes in some cell types.[28,29]

IFNβ biological activity can be explained as follows: (1) IFN binds to the extracellular domain of IFNAR2; (2) IFNAR1 then engages with the IFNβ–IFNAR2 complex, allowing the intracellular domains of the two receptor chains and associated proteins to interact; (3) this interaction, which includes JAK1 associated with IFNAR2 and Tyk2 associated with IFNAR1, results in a cascade of phosphorylation events leading to activation of STATS; (4) activated STATS form a complex with other cytoplasmic proteins, then translocate into the nucleus to bind interferon sensitive response elements (ISRE), which are upstream of many IFN regulated genes; and 5) ISRE binding results in transcriptional regulation (both induction and inhibition) of >1000 genes.[30,31]

While the function of some of these genes is clear (e.g. the antiviral product MxA), the specific transcripts mediating the therapeutic benefit of IFNβ in MS are unknown. This is, in part, due to the complexity and heterogeneitiy of MS, but also because IFNβ is an agonist that can induce the expression not only of ISRE-regulated genes, but also through newly expressed transcription factors, can induce or inhibit subsequent waves of gene expression. In addition, some IFNβ-regulated proteins, which include cytokines and chemokines, can alter the level or function of particular cell populations. The resulting multifaceted biological response is in contrast to more specific therapies, such as monoclonal antibodies, that have a much more specific molecular target. Thus, IFNβ may exert its therapeutic effects in two distinct ways: (1) direct effects of IFNβ-regulated gene products; or (2) indirect effects of IFN-regulated gene products, via effects on other genes (e.g. transcription factors), or by altering populations or functions of cells including Type 2 dendritic cells, monocytes, regulatory T-cells, and CD56 bright NK cells.[32–36]

Mechanisms of action, and biomarkers

Because of its complexity, there is no simple way to capture the complete biological response to IFNβ injections. In Chapter 23, Fontoura and Leppert provide a comprehensive description of studies linking genetic polymorphisms in relevant genes (Class II MHC, IFN receptors, IL10, etc.) to IFNβ responsiveness; studies documenting gene expression patterns following IFNβ injections; and studies at the gene expression and protein level linking specific IFNβ responses to treatment response. Study detail will not be repeated here. Rather, this section provides an overview, and summary. There are now numerous reports of gene expression by peripheral blood cells in response to IFNβ injections.[37–43] RNA transcripts change within hours for primary IFNβ-regulated genes. The levels of these early transcripts generally peak within 8–12 hours then rapidly fall. No obvious gene expression pattern distinguishes good treatment response from poor response. Hesse

and colleagues documented preservation of gene induction by IFNβ in patients with a poor treatment response,[39] suggesting that loss over time of IFNβ-induced gene transcription doesn't explain poor treatment response. Individual variability in the response to IFNβ has been well documented.[40,43] Rani and colleagues confirmed individual heterogeneity and also documented that specific molecular responses were highly conserved within individual patients over time.[44] van Baarsen reported that pre-treatment expression of 15 IFN response genes correlated inversely with on-treatment responses,[43] suggesting that some MS patients may have up-regulated endogenous IFNβ activity prior to IFNβ treatment, and that these patients may have a weaker response to exogenous IFNβ. An interesting parallel was observed in chronic hepatitis C infection, in which viral clearance in response to IFNα and ribavarin was reduced in patients with exaggerated pre-treatment expression of IFN-induced genes in liver biopsies.[45] In general, gene expression studies have demonstrated consistent responses over time within individuals but great variability from one individual to another, and no clear relationship between gene expression patterns and treatment responsiveness. Simple attenuation of the general molecular response does not explain loss of therapeutic effect, except in the presence of neutralizing antibodies (NAb), when biological response at the gene expression level and beyond is abrogated.

Measures of specific IFNβ-induced products, such as oligoadenylate synthetase (OAS), β-2 microglobulin, or neopterin, have been useful in pharmacodynamic studies to determine the magnitude and duration of the IFNβ response, since serum levels of IFNβ are undetectable following injections. Protein studies have also been used in identifying biomarkers for the treatment benefits – both to monitor therapy and to understand mechanisms. Many such reports describe specific IFNβ-regulated products, including neopterin,[46] IL10,[47] IL17F,[48] matrix metalloproteases,[49] IL23,[49] IL12,[50] and soluble VCAM,[51] among many others. The CSF IL10 concentration increased in MS patients treated for 2 years with intramuscular IFNβ-1a but not placebo, and within the IFNβ-1a recipients, increased CSF IL-10 correlated with less disability progression.[52] Increased levels of soluble VCAM correlated with the effect of subcutaneous IFNβ-1b on gadolinium-enhancing brain lesions.[51]

Still other studies reported alterations in various cell populations with IFNβ treatment. Changes have been reported in cells from all parts of the immune system and include increases in T$_H$2 cells, T-reg cells, NK reg cells, Type 2 dendritic cells, and monocytes. Decreases are seen in CD8 and CD4 T-cells, B-cells, and NK cells.[36] While most of these observations suggest a decrease in inflammatory cell activity, IFNs also have proinflammatory effects. The balance between these pro- and anti-inflammatory effects of IFNβ may be affected by how IFNβ is administered (route, dose, and/or frequency).

Neutralizing antibodies develop in some patients taking IFNβ products. The frequency of NAb is highest for the subcutaneous IFNβ products (IFNβ-1b and IFNβ-1a SC) and

Table 25.1. *Overview of randomized, placebo-controlled clinical trials of IFNβ for patients with clinically isolated syndromes*

Study	Study design, duration, sample size,	Study results	References
CHAMPS Study	R, DB, PL-C, 3 years, n = 383 IFNβ-1a (IM) 30 μg qw vs. placebo	Reduced probability of CDMS – IFNβ, 35% vs. placebo, 50%; percent difference = 30% Positive effects on T2 lesions and Gd lesions; Free of new lesions at 18 months – IFN, 47%; placebo, 18%	Jacobs 2000[53]
ETOMS Study	R,DB,PL-C, 2 years, n = 309 IFNβ-1b (SC) 22 μg qw vs. placebo	Reduced proportion developing CDMS – IFNβ 34% vs. placebo 45%; Percent difference = 24%; positive effect on time to conversion to CDMS and relapse rate Positive effects on T2 lesions, and PBVC	Comi 2001[55] Filippi 2004[56]
BENEFIT Study	R,DB,PL-C, 2 years, n = 468 IFNβ-1b (SC) 250 μg qod vs. placebo	Reduced proportion developing CDMS – IFNβ, 26% vs. placebo, 44%; Percent difference = 41% Positive effect on T2 and Gd-enhancing lesions	Kappos 2006[57]

Abbreviations: n = number; R = randomized; DB = double blind; PL-C = placebo controlled; μg = micrograms; im = intramuscular; sc = subcutaneous; qw = weekly; qod = every other day; tiw = 3 times weekly; PBVC = percent brain volume change; CDMS = clinically definite multiple sclerosis; Gd = gadolinium.

Table 25.2. *Overview of randomized, placebo-controlled clinical trials of IFNβ for patients with RRMS*

Study	Study design, duration, sample size, treatments	Study results	References
IFNb RRMS Study	R,DB,PL-C, 3 years, n = 372; IFNβ-1b 50 μg qod vs. IFNβ-1b 250 μg qod vs. placebo	Annualized relapse rate reduced – IFNβ, 0.84 vs. placebo, 1.27; Percent difference = 35%; increased proportion relapse free; No effect on EDSS change Reduced T2 burden of disease	IFNB MS Study Group 1995[7] Paty 1993[67]
MSCRG Study	R,DB,PL-C, 2 years, n =301 IFNβ-1a (IM) 30 μg qw vs. placebo	Estimate of the proportion with 6 month sustained EDSS worsening reduced – IFNβ, 21.9%; placebo, 34.9%; Percent difference = 37%; 32% reduction in relapse rate in 2-year cohort; 18% in entire cohort Reduced new or enlarging T2 lesions, and Gd-enhancing lesions	Jacobs 1996[8] Simon 1998[68]
PRISMS	R,DB,PL-C, 2 years, n =560 IFNβ-1a 22 μg (SC) tiw vs. IFNβ-1a 44 μg (SC) tiw vs. placebo	Reduced relapse number over 2 years – IFNβ, 1.73 vs. placebo, 2.56; Percent difference = 32%; increased relapse-free, lower 3-month confirmed EDSS worsening Less T2 lesions and Gd-enhancing lesions	PRISMS Study Group 1998[9] Li 1999[69]
OWIMS Study	293; R,DB,PL-C, 1 year, n =293 IFN β-1a (SC) 22 μg qwk vs. IFN β-1a (SC) 44 μg qwk vs. placebo	Reduced relapse rate over 1 year – IFNβ, 0.87; placebo, 1.08; Percent difference = 19% Reduced new T2, Gd-enhancing, and combined unique lesions	OWIMS Study Group 1999[61]

Note: For studies with multiple IFNβ doses, results for the highest dose only are presented. See Table 25.4 for results from dose comparison studies

Abbreviations: as in Table 25.1.

lower for IFNβ-1a (IM). NAb induced by IFNβ are thoroughly reviewed in Chapter 24. Suffice it to say that development of NAb is a serious complication of IFNβ therapy because high-titer NAb block clinical and biological effects of IFNβ injections, are long-lived, and NAb that develop while a patient is taking one product will cross-react with all other IFNβ products. Further, it is not clear whether IFNβ NAb aggravate underlying disease severity by blocking endogenous IFNβ.

Efficacy of IFNβ in multiple sclerosis: clinical trials and beyond

Randomized, placebo-controlled, double-blind studies tested the efficacy and toxicity of IFNβ products in patients with CIS, RRMS, SPMS, and PPMS. Some of the pivotal trials

included multiple doses along with placebo, allowing the most meaningful dose comparisons; subsequent studies have further addressed issues surrounding the optimal dose, relative benefits of different IFNβ products, and benefits of IFNβ compared with non-IFNβ drugs. The effects of IFNβ over time have been reported in observational studies, including follow-up assessments of patients from the original clinical trials. Finally, longitudinal studies have identified correlates of the clinical response to IFNβ. These studies may allow more rational use of IFNβ at the individual patient level. Thus, 18 years after approval of the first IFNβ product, the MS IFNβ literature is mature and robust, although questions remain.

Tables 25.1–25.7 summarize key trials organized into the following categories: CIS studies (Table 25.1); RRMS studies (Table 25.2); progressive MS studies (Table 25.3); dose

Table 25.3. *Overview of randomized, placebo-controlled clinical trials of IFNβ for patients with progressive MS*

Study	Study design, duration, sample size, treatments	Study results	References
European SPMS Study	R,DB,PL-C, 3 years, n =718 IFNβ-1b 250 μg sc qod (Betaferon®) vs. placebo	Reduced 3-month confirmed EDSS worsening – IFNβ, 38.9% vs. placebo, 49.8%; percent difference = 22% Positive results on relapses, T2 lesions, and Gd-enhancing lesions	European Study Group 1998[14]
North American SPMS Study	R,DB,PL-C, 3 years, n = 939 IFNβ-1b 250 μg qod vs. IFNβ-1b 160 μg/m² qod vs. placebo	No difference in time to 6-month sustained EDSS worsening, EDSS change, or neuropsychological score Positive results on relapses, T2 lesions, and Gd-enhancing lesions	Panitch 2004[70]
SPECTRIMS	R,DB,PL-C, 3 years, n = 618 IFNβ-1a (SC) 22 μg tiw vs. IFNβ-1a (SC) 44 μg tiw vs. placebo	No differences in time to 3- month confirmed EDSS worsening Positive results for relapses, T2 lesions, and Gd-enhancing lesions	SPECTRIMS Study Group 2001[71] Li 2001[72]
IMPACT	R,DB,PL-C, n = 436 IFNβ-1a (IM) 60 μg qw vs. placebo	Positive results for MSFC z-score change IFNβ, −0.096 vs. placebo −0.161; percent difference = 40.4%; No benefit on confirmed EDSS worsening Positive effect on relapses, T2 lesions, Gd-enhancing lesions, and QOL	Cohen 2002[73]
NORDIC SPMS	R,DB,PL-C, n = 371 IFNβ-1a (SC) 22 μg qw vs. placebo	No effect on time to 3-month confirmed EDSS worsening, relapses, or RFSS	Andersen 2004[74]
PPMS IFNβ-1a (IM) Study	R,DB,PL-C, 2 years, n = 50 IFNβ-1a (IM) 30 μg qw vs. IFNβ-1a (IM) 60 μg qw vs. placebo	No effect on time to confirmed EDSS worsening, Less T2 lesion accrual with 30 μg dose; higher rate of ventricular enlargement with the 60 μg dose.	Leary, 2003[13]

Note: For studies with multiple IFNβ doses, results for the highest dose only are presented. See Table 25.4 for results from dose comparison studies.
Abbreviations: as in Table 25.1.

comparison studies (Table 25.4); head-to-head studies of different products (Table 25.5); observational studies (Table 25.6); and IFNβ response predictor studies (Table 25.7). In total, the tables summarize results from more than 30 separate studies, representing hundreds of thousands of patient-years of documented experience. No attempt will be made to describe all relevant details on these studies – the reader is referred to the original studies, to prior editions of this book, and to recent reviews of IFNβ. The purpose of this chapter will be to provide an overview of these studies, drawing conclusions when possible.

The reader is cautioned that comparison of *specific* results across trials (e.g. relapse rate reduction, percent relapse free, reduction of new lesions) is ill advised. Clinical outcome measures in MS are inherently imprecise; they are defined and used differently in separate clinical trials and probably differently at different sites within a given trial. MRI parameters have the same name, but differ in important details. For example, T2 lesion data vary depending on MRI equipment, slice thickness, magnet strength, and other acquisition parameters, and post-processing methods. Numbers generated by brain volume studies can not be directly compared when the methods differ. Most importantly, patients in the different trials are different, with distinct characteristics that may strongly influence results. This is best illustrated by two trials of IFNβ for SPMS, which yielded different results even though the IFNβ product was the same (IFNβ-1b), the category of MS was the same (SPMS), and the study designs were nearly identical. These trials are discussed in more detail below.

Clinically isolated syndromes (Table 25.1)

Three studies tested the effects of IFNβ initiated shortly after an initial MS episode (two studies of IFNβ-1a, and one IFNβ-1b). All the studies required patients to have multiple MRI lesions in addition to a typical inflammatory demyelinating event. The CHAMPS study[53] randomized 383 CIS patients to IFNβ-1a (IM) 30 μg weekly, or placebo. At three years, the proportion of patients developing a second relapse, which defined clinically definite MS (CDMS) in all the CIS studies, was reduced from 50% to 35%. IFNβ-1a treatment increased the proportion of patients without new lesions from 18% to 47%. The theme of a higher effect size for MRI lesion parameters compared with clinical benefits persists with nearly all IFNβ studies reviewed in this chapter. At the end of the trial, approximately 50% of the patients entered into long-term follow-up. At five years, the proportion of patients who had developed CDMS was still lower in patients initially randomized to IFNβ-1a (36%) than in patients randomized to placebo (49%), supporting early compared with delayed treatment.[54] The relatively low enrollment rate resulted from sites electing to not participate; characteristics of the follow-up cohort were representative of the full CHAMPS population.

The ETOMS study[55] randomized 309 patients with CIS to IFNβ-1a (SC) 22 μg weekly or placebo. CDMS developed in 24% fewer IFNβ recipients (34%) compared with placebo recipients (45%). The time for 30% of patients to convert to CDMS increased from 252 days in the placebo group to 569 days in the IFNβ-1a group. Benefits were observed on T2 hyperintense

Table 25.4. *Overview of randomized active arm comparison studies comparing different doses of the same IFNβ product*

Study	Design comparison (n)	Principal question length of F/U	Key outcomes	References
IFNb RRMS Study IFNβ-1b	R,DB,PL-C IFNβ-1b 50 μg qod (125) vs. IFNβ-1b 250 μg qod (124)	Comparison of two IFNβ-1b doses 3 years	Benefit of higher dose on ARR (1.17 vs. 0.84). Some dose effect on MRI parameters, but less significant than the dose effect on ARR. No difference between doses for % scans with active lesions, active lesion rate, or new lesion rate.	IFNb Study Group 1993[7] Paty 1993[67]
PRISMS Study IFNβ-1a (SC)	R,DB,PL-C IFNβ-1a (SC) 22 μg tiw (189) vs. IFNβ-1a (SC) 44 μg tiw (184)	Comparison of two IFNβ-1a doses 2 years	No significant differences for relapse rate, EDSS change, confirmed EDSS worsening, Trend toward benefit of higher dose on T2 volume change. Benefit of higher dose on MRI lesion activity.	PRISMS Study Group 1998[9] Li 1999[69]
OWIMS 3-yr f/u IFNβ-1a (SC)	R,DB,PL-C IFNβ-1a (SC) 22 μg qw (95) vs. IFNβ-1a (SC) 44 μg qw (98)	Comparison of two IFNβ-1a doses 3 years	No significant differences in relapse rate or MRI lesion activity.	Freedman 2005[75]
European Dose Comparison Study IFNβ-1a (IM)	R,DB IFNβ-1a (IM) 30 μg q wk (402) vs. IFNβ-1a (IM) 60 μg q wk (400)	Comparison of two IFNβ-1a doses 3 years	No significant differences in EDSS change, relapse rate MRI lesions, or brain atrophy. More side effects and higher proportion of Nab in high dose group.	Clanet 2002[65]
OPTIMS Study IFNβ-1b	R,SB IFNβ-1b 250 μg sc qod (40) vs. IFNβ-1b 375 μg sc qod (36)	Comparison of two doses of IFNβ-1b for patients with relapses on standard dose 6 months	Fewer patients had MRI activity with the higher dose.	Durelli 2008[76]
SPECTRIMS Study IFNβ-1a (SC)	R,DB,PL-C IFNβ-1a (SC) 22 μg tiw (209) vs. IFNβ01a (SC) 44 μg tiw (204)	Comparison of two IFNβ-1a doses 3 years	No significant differences in EDSS change, relapses, T2 lesion change, combined unique lesions	SPECTRIMS Study Group 2001[85] Li 2001[86]
North American SPMS Study IFNβ-1b	R,DB,PL-C IFNβ-1b 250 μg qod (317) vs. IFNβ-1b 160 5 μg/m² qod (314)	Comparison of two IFNβ-1b doses 3 years	No significant differences in EDSS change, relapses, MRI lesions.	Panitch 2004[67]

Abbreviations: as in Table 25.1, and: SB = single blind; ARR = annualized relapse rate.

lesions and on percent brain volume change.[56] Of note, brain atrophy in the IFNβ-1a patients was lower than in placebo patients in year 1, year 2, and for the combined years 0 through 2. The ETOMS study, which used IFNβ-1a (SC) 22 μg weekly, is the only IFNβ-1a (SC) trial to demonstrate benefits on brain atrophy.

The BENEFIT study[57] randomized 468 patients with CIS to IFNβ-1b SC 250 μg every other day (n = 292) or placebo (n = 176). After two years, 41% fewer IFNβ-1b recipients developed CDMS (26%) compared with placebo patients (44%). At three years, the effect of early compared with delayed treatment was evident,[58] in that 37% of the patients receiving IFNβ-1b had CDMS compared with 51% of those receiving placebo first. Also, by three years, 16% of the patients who had received IFNβ-1b first had confirmed EDSS worsening compared with 24% of the delayed-treatment group.

Although the three CIS studies tested different IFNβ products, they enrolled apparently similar patient populations, and results were similar. They independently demonstrated a benefit for IFNβ treatment beginning at the CIS stage, and follow-up studies have suggested that the benefits of early

compared with delayed treatment persists for three to five years. Several issues are unresolved. First, what markers at CIS presentation can be used to decide whether patients might be observed without therapy? Analysis of the BENEFIT study[59] indicated a higher risk of conversion to CDMS in patients with ≥9 T2 lesions or with Gd-enhancing lesions. These patients are at high risk of conversion, and very appropriate for early IFNβ therapy. Additional analysis indicated consistent treatment effects in groups stratified by the presence of multifocal vs. monofocal onset, and by baseline MRI disease severity. Subgroup analysis in the CHAMPS study also demonstrated similar IFNβ treatment effects in patients presenting with optic neuritis, brain stem-cerebellar, or spinal cord syndromes; and for subgroups defined by baseline MRI parameters.[60] Second, does treatment delayed until the second clinical episode significantly increase the risk of long-term disability? Follow-up studies from both the CHAMPS study (five years) and the BENEFIT study (three years) support long-term beneficial effects of early treatment, but these studies will not be definitive because patients in both studies were given the option of starting IFNβ when they converted to CDMS.

Table 25.5. *Overview of randomized, active arm comparison studies comparing IFNβ products or comparing IFNβ with other drugs*

Study	Design comparison (n)	Principal question length of F/U	Key outcomes	References
Danish IFNβ Study IFNβ-1b vs. IFNβ-1a (SC)	R,OL IFNβ-1b 250 μg qod (158) vs. IFNβ-1a (SC) 22 μg qw (143)	Comparison of two IFNβ-1a doses 2 years	No differences in relapse rate, time to first relapse, or confirmed EDSS progression.	Koch-Henriksen 2006[79]
EVIDENCE Study IFNβ-1a (IM) vs. IFNβ-1a (SC)	R,SB IFNβ-1a (IM) 30 μg q wk (338) vs. IFNβ-1a (SC) 44 μg tiw (339)	Comparison of IFNβ-1a (SC) and IFNβ-1a (IM) 1 year	Higher likelihood of relapse free after 6 months with IFNβ-1a (SC) vs. IFNβ-1a (IM) (74.9% vs. 63.3%); Less active MRI lesions per patient per scan at 6 months for IFNβ-1a (SC). No significant differences between IFNβ-1a (SC) and IFNβ1a (IM) after 6 months	Panitch 2002[80]
INCOMIN Study IFNβ-1a (IM) vs. IFNβ-1b	R,SB IFNβ-1a (IM) 30 μg q wk (92) vs. IFNβ-1b 250 μg qod (96)	Comparison of IFNβ-1b and IFNβ-1a (IM) 2 years	Higher proportion relapse free with IFNβ-1b (51% vs. 36%); higher proportion free of new MRI lesions with IFNβ-1b 55% vs. 26%	Durelli 2002[81]
BEYOND Study IFNβ-1b vs. GA	R,DB (for IFN arms),PL-C IFNβ-1b 250 μg qod (897) vs. IFNβ-1b 500 μg qod (899) vs. GA 20 mg sc qd (448)	Comparison of two IFNβ-1b doses, and glatiramer acetate 3 years	No differences in relapses, EDSS change, T1-hypointense lesions, or brain atrophy between groups	O'Connor 2009[66]
BECOME Study IFNβ-1b vs. GA	R,SB IFNβ-1b 250 μg qod (36) vs. GA 20 mg sc qd (39)	Comparison of MRI effects of IFNβ-1b vs. GA Up to 2 years	No difference between the number of combined unique MRI lesions (primary outcome) in year 1 (0.63 for IFN β-1b and 0.58 for GA). No differences in relapse rate over 2 years.	Cadavid 2009[82]
REGARD Study IFNβ-1a (SC) vs. GA	R,OL IFNβ-1a (SC) 44 μg tiw (386) vs. GA 20 mg sc qd (378	Comparison of sc IFNβ-1a (SC) and GA 2 years	No significant difference between groups in time to first relapse (primary outcome measure), or in the number of new T2 lesions or volume of Gd-enhancing lesions. Patients on IFN β-1a had fewer Gd-enhancing lesions per scan.	Mikol 2008[83]
TRANSFORMS IFNβ-1a (IM) vs. fingolimod	R,DB,PL-C IFNβ-1a (IM) 30 μg q wk (435) vs. fingolimod 0.5 mg po qd (431) vs. fingolimod 1.25 mg po qd (426)	Comparison of IFNβ-1a 30 μg qw with fingolimod 1 year	Patients on IFNβ-1a 30 μg im had higher relapse rates, more worsening on EDSS and MSFC, and more brain MRI lesions,	Cohen 2010[84]
CombiRx Study IFNβ-1a (IM) vs. GA vs. Both	R,DB IFNβ-1a (IM) 30 μg q wk (~250) vs. GA 20 mg sc qd (~250) vs. Both (~500)	Comparison of IFNβ-1a, GA, and both in combination All patients followed at least 3 years F/U 3–6 years	Comparison of relapse rate in each group (primary outcome). Key secondary outcomes MSFC, EDSS, MRI lesions, atrophy	ClinicalTrials. gov, Jan 2011

Abbreviations: As in Table 25.1 and 25.4, and: OL = open label, qd = every day, GA = glatiramer acetate.

Relapsing–remitting MS (see Table 25.2 for pivotal trials; Table 25.4 for dose comparison trials)

Randomized, placebo-controlled, double-blind trials with IFNβ-1b, IFNβ-1a (IM), and IFNβ-1a (SC) are listed in Table 25.2. For trials that included 2 IFNβ doses, only results for the higher dose are provided in this table. Comparisons between separate doses are made in Table 25.4. The OWIMS trial[61] was an exploratory one-year study to test weekly IFNβ-1a (SC). There was a 19% reduction in the relapse rate with IFNβ-1a (SC), 44 μg weekly, and a 54% reduction in new combined unique MRI lesions. The other studies in Table 25.2 were pivotal trials that formed the basis for registration and marketing of

the IFNβ drugs. All three products were found to be adequately safe and effective to achieve approval by regulatory agencies world-wide.

Patient characteristics for the pivotal trials in Table 25.2 were similar – established, active RRMS with disease duration of six to eight years, and mild to moderate disability at trial entry. As shown in Table 25.2, results were similar in these studies. The primary outcome measure for the IFNβ-1b and IFNβ-1a (SC) trials was based on relapse counts. The annualized relapse rate was reduced by 35% in the IFNβ-1b study, and the number of relapses per patient in two years was reduced by 32% in the IFNβ-1a (SC) study. For IFNβ-1a (IM) the primary outcome measure was "time to onset of a 1.0 point

Table 25.6. *Overview of key observational studies of IFNβ in MS: long-term impact of IFN*

Study	Sample size and duration of F/U	Primary outcome	Key references
MSCRG IFNβ-1a (IM) 30 μg q wk F/U	Observational after end of clinical trial 164 of 172 (93%) evaluated 8.1 years after randomization into clinical trial	Disability at outcome defined as EDSS ≥ 6.0. At follow-up 42% of original placebo recipients and 29.1% of the original IFNβ-1a recipients had significant disability.	Rudick 2001[87]
PRISMS IFNβ-1a (SC) tiw F/U	Standardized follow-up but observational after end of clinical trial 382 of 560 (68%) evaluated 7–8 years after randomization into clinical trial	72% of the cases were still using IFNβ-1a at f/u. Patients originally randomized to IFNβ-1a 44 μg sc tiw had less EDSS worsening, lower relapse rate, and lower T2 burden at f/u.	Kappos 2006[18]
IFNβ-1b 16 year F/U	Observational after end of clinical trial 260 of 372 (70%) evaluated an average of 16 years after randomization into clinical trial	No observed difference between original IFNβ-1b vs. original placebo at F/U on clinical or MRI variables Mortality rates by original randomization differed – 18.3% placebo; 8.3% 50 μg; 5.4% 250 μg	Ebers 2010[16]
BENEFIT 3 year F/U	Standardized follow-up but observational after end of clinical trial 392 of 468 (84%) evaluated at 3 years following randomization	After 3 years, 37% of the original IFNβ-1b 250 μg patients had CDMS compared with 51% of the delayed treatment group. After 3 years, 16% of the original IFNβ-1b 250 ug patients had confirmed EDSS worsening compared with 24% of the delayed treatment group.	Kappos 2007[58]
CHAMPIONS 5 year F/U	Open-label extension of the CHAMPS Study. 208 of 383 (53%) of the CHAMPS patients enrolled in CHAMPIONS (100 initial IFNβ; 103 delayed IFNβ)	Median delay in treatment for the initial placebo group was 29 months. At 5 years, probability of CDMS in the initial treatment group was 36%, and in the delayed treatment group 49%.	Kinkel, 2006[54]
Italian Study	Observational 2570 patients treated with IFNβ products with median follow-up 4.5 years	Compared early (within 1 year of diagnosis) with delayed treatment. Outcome was (propensity score adjusted) proportion of patients with EDSS worsening, EDSS ≥ 4.0, and EDSS ≥ 6.0. All analyses favored early IFNβ treatment.	Trojano 2009[88]

Abbreviations: As in Table 25.1 and CDMS = Clinically definite MS; F/U = follow-up.

Table 25.7. *Overview of key observational studies of IFNβ in MS: markers of IFNβ benefit*

Study	Sample	Duration of F/U	Key finding	Reference
MSCRG Study	172	2 years	≥ 3 new T2 lesions at 2 years were associated with more EDSS MSFC, and brain atrophy worsening over the same 2-year interval	Rudick 2004[92]
One-year MRI predicts	394 treated with IFNβ	4.8 years	New MRI lesions 1 year after starting IFNβ predicted confirmed EDSS worsening during the duration of follow-up	Prosperini 2009[91]
MRI and NAb predictors	147 treated with IFNβ	2 years	MRI lesions at 6 months, and NAb status predicted relapse or confirmed EDSS worsening in the next 18 months. These two factors were additive.	Durelli 2008[90]
Roman Study	68 treated with IFNβ	6 years	Gd+ lesions predicted relapse or disability (OR 7.9)	Tomassini 2006[93]
Barcelona Study	152 treated with IFNβ	2 years	2 active MRI lesions at 1 year were the primary factor predicting confirmed EDSS worsening (OR 8.3)	Rio 2008[94]

Abbreviations: As in Table 25.1 and NAb = neutralizing antibodies; OR = odds ratio.

worsening from baseline EDSS confirmed at the next visit, six months later." This became known as a "disability progression" end-point. Subsequent studies have employed this end-point in RRMS trials, although most studies have shortened the time until the confirmation visit to three months. Based on analysis of Kaplan–Meier curves, the probability of six-month confirmed EDSS worsening was reduced by 37% from 34.9% in placebo patients to 21.9% in IFNβ-1a (IM) patients. Effects of IFNβ on EDSS worsening in the IFNβ-1b and IFNβ-1a (SC) studies conflicted. There was a significant treatment effect

on three-month sustained EDSS worsening in the IFNβ-1a (SC) study, but no effect on EDSS in the IFNβ-1b study. These differences are likely due to different methods for applying the EDSS scale in the separate studies.

The relapse results from the IFNβ-1a (IM) trial have generated controversy. Initially, all patients were to be followed at least two years. However, with IFNβ-1b approval in July 2003 while the IFNβ-1a (IM) study was ongoing, a decision was made to terminate the study early. This was possible because the primary outcome measure was based on a survival analysis, not on activity during a pre-specified interval. As a result of this decision, 129 of the 301 patients who entered into the study were followed less than two years. The annualized relapse rate reduction for the 172-patient two-year cohort was 32%, but was 18% for the entire 301 patient cohort. It seems likely that this reflected higher relapse activity in patients who were entered into the study early, but there may have also been an effect of admixing data from a group of patients with short follow up.

Brain atrophy study results have also been conflicting and somewhat controversial. Brain atrophy studies were planned prospectively for the IFNβ-1a (IM) trial[62] using relatively crude methods available at the time. A newly developed analysis method to calculate brain parenchymal fraction (BPF), a normalized measure of whole brain parenchymal volume, was applied post-hoc to serial MRIs from the IFNβ-1a (IM) study. Post-hoc analyses of MRIs were also undertaken using MRIs from the IFNβ-1a (SC) study. The BPF study with IFNβ-1a (IM) showed increased volume loss in the first year in IFNβ patients compared with placebo patients – an event termed "pseudoatrophy" based on the hypothesis that more rapid volume loss represented resolution of edema from brain inflammation. This was followed by significantly reduced atrophy with IFNβ-1a (IM) in the second year, postulated to represent a neuroprotective effect.[10] BPF was also measured in the European Dose Comparison Study, which tested IFNβ-1a (IM) 30 μg every week vs. 60 μg IM every week. In that study, which used the same BPF software used in the Phase 3 RRMS trial, patterns were similar to the Phase 3 study. A more rapid decline in BPF was observed during the first four months, followed by atrophy slowing for the remainder of the three year trial.[63] Post-hoc studies were also conducted to determine the impact of IFNβ-1a (SC) on brain atrophy.[64] Using a normalized measure of whole brain parenchyma called the whole-brain ratio (WBR), the UBC MRI research group reported that WBR declined significantly during the two-year trial, without any evidence of a treatment effect. No brain atrophy reports have been published for IFNβ-1b in RRMS. The discrepancy between brain atrophy results in RRMS patients with IFNβ-1a (IM) and IFNβ-1a (SC) are unresolved, mainly because different techniques were used to quantify brain volume change. The beneficial atrophy result reported with IFNβ-1a (SC) 22 μg weekly in the ETOMS study[56] raises the possibility that beneficial effects on brain atrophy are only observed with lower or less frequent IFNβ dosing.

Regarding dosing, both the IFNβ-1b and IFNβ-1a (SC) Phase 3 trials included two IFNβ doses (Table 25.4). A dose effect in favor of IFNβ-1b (SC), 250 μg every other day, compared with 50 μg SC every other day, was observed on the relapse outcome, but the dose effect was more subtle with MRI outcomes. There was no dose effect for percent scans with active lesions, active lesion rate, or new lesion rate, but there was a trend toward a dose effect on T2 volume change, and a significant dose effect on MRI lesion activity. Because the IFNβ-1a (IM) study only included a single dose, a subsequent study, the European Dose Comparison Study,[65] tested 30 μg vs. 60 μg

IM weekly for 3 years. EDSS change, relapse rate, MRI lesions, or brain atrophy did not differ between doses. One aim of the BEYOND study[66] was to compare IFNβ-1b (SC) 250 μg every other day with IFNβ-1b (SC) 500 μg every other day (Table 25.5). There were no differences between the two IFNβ-1b doses on relapses, EDSS change, T1 hypointense lesions, or brain atrophy. In all of these studies, adverse events were more significant and NAb were more frequent at the higher doses. The studies suggest that the approved doses for the three IFNβ products are near or on the plateau of the dose–clinical response curve. This further suggests that increasing doses of IFNβ beyond the recommended doses are not likely to substantially improve efficacy, but may cause more side effects. Two areas of significant uncertainty remain. The first is whether the evidence favoring IFNβ-1a (SC) 44 μg over 22 μg is sufficient to routinely prescribe the higher dose, particularly given the increased cost and side effect burden. Another question is whether more frequent IFNβ-1a (IM) dosing might improve efficacy over weekly injections.

Progressive MS (Tables 25.3 and 25.4)

Studies presented in Tables 25.3 and 25.4 tested the benefits of all three IFNβ products in SPMS. One small trial tested IFNβ in PPMS.[13] Generally, the studies show benefits on MRI lesions and relapses, but there have been no consistent benefits on disability progression, as measured by EDSS. The European SPMS IFNβ-1b trial was the only study in SPMS that showed an IFNβ benefit on EDSS worsening.[14] Interestingly, results from that study conflicted with another trial – the North American IFNβ-1b study,[70] even though the two trials tested the same drug in the same disease category. Since SPECTRIMS, IMPACT, and the Nordic SPMS studies also failed to show benefits of IFNβ on EDSS worsening in SPMS, the consensus is that IFNβ is ineffective at that stage of the disease, and the US FDA has not agreed to include progressive MS in product labels, based on these studies.

As listed in Table 25.4, two of the SPMS studies included two IFNβ doses. SPECTRIMS failed to demonstrate significant differences between IFNβ-1a (SC) 22 μg and 44 μg three times weekly on EDSS change, relapses, T2 lesion change, or the number of combined unique lesions over 3 years. The North American SPMS study failed to show significant differences between IFNβ-1b 250 μg vs 160 μg/m² on EDSS change, relapses, or MRI lesions. These studies suggest that increasing the IFNβ dose is not likely to significantly augment benefits in SPMS.

The IFNβ SPMS studies raise two interesting issues. The first is why the findings differed in the North American and European IFNβ-1b SPMS studies. Subjects in the European study were younger, had shorter duration of disease, higher relapse rates both before and during the studies, and greater MRI activity than did the North American study subjects. For patients in both studies with at least one pre-study relapse or EDSS worsening ≥1 point, there were treatment benefits on time to sustained ESSS worsening (combined HR 0.72; 0.59–0.88).[12]

However, the North American study showed no EDSS benefit for patients without pre-study relapses or pre-study EDSS worsening. It seems likely that IFNβ has its primary effect at the level of inflammation, thereby reducing relapses and MRI lesion activity. As the duration of MS increases, and the role of inflammation in disease progression lessens, the effectiveness of IFNβ is less. The discrepant results could be explained by a higher proportion of patients in the European study with more inflammatory, earlier disease.

A second interesting finding comes from the IMPACT Study,[93] which tested IFNβ-1a (IM), 60 µg every week in patients with SPMS. The IMPACT study was the first MS clinical trial to use MSFC as the primary clinical end-point. An increased sensitivity of the MSFC relative to EDSS was specifically anticipated when the MSFC was proposed,[77] because the MSFC has high reproducibility, the advantages of a continuous measurement instrument, and includes measures of arm and cognitive function, which are not well represented by EDSS. The greater sensitivity of the MSFC compared with EDSS was directly demonstrated in the IMPACT study, which showed a statistically significant difference on MSFC change in favor of IFNβ-1a (IM), but no difference in EDSS. The positive MSFC results were supported by positive therapeutic effects on annualized relapse rate (reduced by 33%,), new and enlarging T2 lesions (reduced by 46%), and statistically significant benefits on 8 of 11 subscales of the MS Quality of Life Index.[73] Despite these positive findings, IFNβ-1a (IM) failed to achieve regulatory approval for SPMS based on the IMPACT study, because EDSS results were negative, and regulators were uncertain of the clinical significance of the MSFC benefits observed in the study. Interestingly, the MSFC results from IMPACT showed that the IFNβ benefit was driven mostly by arm function and, to a lesser extent cognition, suggesting that EDSS might be insensitive because the EDSS scale is relatively non-informative about these functions. A prior study of oral methotrexate for progressive MS[78] showed similar findings –treatment benefited upper extremity function and cognition but not ambulation. One interpretation of these observations is that EDSS is largely insensitive to treatment effects in SPMS trials both because the scale is relatively nonresponsive, and because progressive gait impairment is less responsive to treatment in SPMS. The EDSS may present too high a hurdle for studies of partially effective therapies in SPMS.

Active arm comparison studies (Table 25.5)

Even though many studies comparing various products have been presented at meetings or published in the literature, only randomized studies are considered here. Table 25.5 lists three studies comparing separate IFNβ products (the Danish IFNβ study, EVIDENCE, and INCOMIN), and five studies comparing IFNβ with other products (BEYOND, BECOME, REGARD, TRANSFORMS, and CombiRx). Only TRANSFORMS and CombiRx used placebo injections to double-mask treatment. In the other studies, patients were aware of their treatments.

This introduces of bias of various types. Expectation bias can be a particular problem in these studies. Expectation bias is the presumption on the part of the patient or the investigator (or both) that the assigned treatment is either superior or inferior. This can obviously influence the assessments and reporting, and has the clear potential to greatly influence the results of studies using single-blind or open-label designs.

In the Danish IFNβ study,[79] RRMS patients starting IFNβ were asked to participate in a randomized open-label observational study. Those who agreed were randomized to IFNβ-1a (SC) 22 µg every week ($n = 143$) or to IFNβ1b 250 µg every other day ($n = 160$). Patients who were unwilling to be randomized were treated with open-label IFNβ1b every other day ($n = 125$), possibly indicating an expectation bias in favor of IFNβ-1b. However, the randomized groups did not differ in annualized relapse rate after 24 months (0.70 for IFNβ-1a (SC) and 0.71 for IFNβ-1b). The non-randomized IFNβ-1b arm had more drop-outs. The open-label design and lack of MRI data make interpretation difficult.

In the EVIDENCE Study,[80] RRMS patients were randomized to IFNβ-1a (SC) 44 µg three times weekly ($n = 338$) or IFNβ-1a (IM) 30 µg once every week ($n = 339$). The study used a single-blind design, in which examining neurologists and MRI readers were masked to the treatment, but patients and treating neurologists were not. The primary observation period was 24 weeks, followed by a second 24-week extension study. At 24 weeks, relapse frequency significantly differed, favoring IFNβ-1a (SC), and this difference was also evident over the entire 48-week study period. However, all of the entire 48-week benefit was accounted for by the differences in the initial 24 weeks. The relapse count in the second 24 weeks was nearly identical in the treatment arms. IFNβ-1a (SC) also exerted benefit as assessed by MRI lesion activity, although this effect also was significantly attenuated in the second 24-week observation period. The EVIDENCE study has been criticized for various design limitations[85] that make interpretation somewhat difficult, and because the relative benefits of IFNβ-1a (SC) seemed limited to the initial 24 weeks. This study led to approval of IFNβ-1a (SC) in the United States, despite the orphan drug status of IFNβ-1a (IM). In a follow-on study, patients on the IFNβ-1a (IM) arm of the study were given the option of switching to IFNβ-1a (SC), and were then followed for an additional 32 weeks. Of 306 patients receiving IFNβ-1a (IM), 223 (73%) switched to IFNβ-1a (SC). Patients who switched had lower relapse rates and MRI lesion activity following the switch.[86] The extension study is also difficult to interpret, because study results were made public during the trial, and the decision whether to switch from IFNβ-1a (IM) to IFNβ-1a (SC) was made by the IFNβ-1a (IM) patients.

The INCOMIN study randomized patients to IFNβ-1b, 250 µg sc every other day or IFNβ-1a (IM) 30 µg every week and followed the patients over two years.[81] No effort was made to blind patients or the treating or evaluating neurologists, but MRI readers had no knowledge of treatment assignment. A higher proportion of patients was relapse free on IFNβ-1b (51%

vs. 36%), and a higher proportion was free of new MRI lesions (55% vs. 26%). Interpretation of the INCOMIN study is also limited because of the open-label design, and because MRI was done only on a selected subset of the patients. Also, the study may have been influenced by premature reporting of the first-year study results, while the trial was still ongoing.

Three studies in Table 25.5 were designed and sponsored by companies producing IFNβ in the belief that IFNβ was more effective than glatiramer acetate (GA). The BECOME study[82] was designed to compare the effects of IFNβ-1b with GA on MRI parameters. The study was randomized, and MRI readers were blinded to the treatment arm. Patients with RRMS were randomized to IFNβ-1b (SC), 250 μg every other day, (n = 36) or GA (SC) 20 mg every day (n = 39). Frequent MRI scans were obtained for up to two years. There was no significant difference in the number of combined unique MRI lesions in year 1 (0.63 for IFNβ-1b and 0.58 for GA), or in the relapse rate over two years. The larger BEYOND study[66] randomly allocated RRMS patients to IFNβ-1b (SC), 250 μg every other day (n = 897), IFNβ-1b (SC), 500 μg every other day (n = 899), or GA 20 mg every day (n = 448). Over three years, relapse rate, EDSS change, T1 hypointense lesions, or brain atrophy did not differ between any of the groups. Therefore, BECOME and BEYOND provide no evidence for the superiority of IFNβ-1b over GA, and no support for higher doses of IFNβ-1b.

The REGARD study compared IFNβ-1a (SC), 44 μg three times weekly, with GA, 20 mg every day. Patients were randomized to IFNβ-1a (SC) (n = 386) or GA (n = 378) and followed for two years. There were no significant differences in time to first relapse, the number of new T2 lesions, or the volume of Gd-enhancing lesions. Patients on IFNβ-1a (SC) had fewer Gd-enhancing lesions per scan, but the significance of this finding is not clear.

The TRANSFORMS study[84] randomized active RRMS patients (some of whom had disease activity while on IFNβ or GA) to IFNβ-1a (IM), 30 μg every week (n = 435), oral fingolimod, 0.5 mg every day (n = 431), or oral fingolimod 1.25 mg every day (n = 426). Unlike the head-to-head studies summarized so far, the TRANSFORMS study used a double-blind design, by providing placebo pills to IFNβ-1a (IM) recipients, and placebo injections to fingolimod patients, thus significantly overcoming expectation bias. Patients on IFNβ-1a (IM) had a higher relapse rate, more worsening on EDSS, more worsening on MSFC, and more MRI lesions compared with either fingolimod arm. This study suggests that the treatment benefits of fingolimod exceed IFNβ-1a (IM), and provides a rationale for switching patients who have breakthrough disease to fingolimod.

A large investigator-initiated study is ongoing – the NIH-sponsored, CombiRx study (ClinicalTrials.gov Identifier: NCT00211887). This is a randomized, double-blind, controlled trial comparing IFNβ-1a (IM), 30 ug weekly (approximately 250 patients), GA, 20 mg daily (approximately 250 patients), and both in combination (about 500 patients). Like the TRANSFORMS study, CombiRx is minimizing expectation bias by administering daily SC placebo injections to the IFNβ patients, and IM placebo injections to the patients receiving GA. In this ambitious protocol, patients will be followed in a double-blind protocol, and continued on their initial treatment allocation until the last patient has been followed for three years. Thus, the follow-up interval will range from three to about six years. While the primary outcome measure is relapse rate, the study will also analyze various clinical and MRI secondary outcome measures, and biological material is being stored so that biomarker development can proceed once the study is completed. The CombiRx study will be the first randomized, double-blind comparison of IFNβ-1a (IM) and GA, and the first to combine standard first-line agents. Study completion is expected in spring 2012.

Observational studies (Table 25.6)

The impact of IFNβ over the long course of MS is not known. It is presumed that by inhibiting CNS inflammation early in the disease, IFNβ will provide secondary neuroprotection, thereby reducing brain atrophy and disability. However, long-term placebo-controlled studies are impractical and unethical, so it will be difficult to determine the long-term impact of IFNβ with complete confidence. Several groups have reported follow-up assessments of patients who had participated in the pivotal clinical trials. The two biggest problems with these reports are the lack of an appropriate control group and the problem of informative censoring. Informative censoring is a problem in these studies because patients with more severe disease are generally less likely to be included in the follow-up assessment. This leaves less severely affected cases in the assessed cohort, which can have the effect of exaggerating presumed treatment benefits.

Because trials in RRMS were done first, the follow-up durations are longest for the RRMS trials. Patients from the original IFNβ-1a (IM) trial were evaluated eight years after randomization, when their average disease duration was 14 years. Only the 172-patient two-year cohort from this trial was included in the follow-up study because the original purpose was to determine the predictive value of two-year MSFC change as support for the planned use of MSFC in the IMPACT study.[87] Of the 172 patients, 164 (93%) were evaluated at follow-up. Clinically meaningful disability was defined as an EDSS ≥ 6.0 at follow-up (entry criteria into the original trial included an EDSS score of 1.0 to 3.5). Of the patients receiving placebo in the original IFNβ-1a (IM) trial, 42% reached the EDSS ≥ 6.0 milestone, compared with 29.1% of the original IFNβ patients. Patients were treated in an uncontrolled fashion by their individual neurologists between the end of the clinical trial and follow-up, and treatment did not differ significantly between the two original treatment arms. Therefore, results were interpreted as suggesting a persisting benefit for early vs. delayed treatment and as suggesting a long-term disability benefit for IFNβ-1a (IM). The original PRISMS IFNβ-1a (SC) study participants were systematically followed using standardized visits for 7–8 years after randomization into the PRISMS trial.[18] Of the 560 patients enrolled and randomized, 383 (68%) were evaluated at follow up, and 72% of these patients were still using IFNβ-1a (SC). Patients initially randomized to IFNβ-1a, 44 μg three times weekly, had less EDSS worsening, lower relapse rates, and lower T2 disease burden compared with placebo patients, but there were no significant differences between the original dose arms. Finally, the original IFNβ-1b patients were evaluated an average of 16 years after randomization.[16] As with the MSCRG eight-year follow-up, these patients were treated in an open-label fashion by their treating neurologists at the end of the original clinical trial. A total of 260 (70%) of the original trial patients were evaluated. No differences were observed between the original IFNβ and placebo arms, but mortality rates differed by original treatment – cases receiving placebo had an 18.3% rate; those receiving IFNβ-1b (SC), 50 μg. 8.3%; and those receiving IFNβ-1b (SC) 250 μg every other day had a 5.4% rate. While not definitive, this outcome is consistent with a long-term, significant benefit of early compared with delayed treatment with IFNβ.

Long-term follow-up of the original CIS cohorts has lagged a bit behind, because these studies were started later. CHAMPIONS was a long-term follow-up study of the original CHAMPS patients. While only 53% of the original CHAMPS patients were enrolled in CHAMPIONS, follow-up evaluation was consistent, with a benefit of early vs. delayed treatment.[54] Similarly, three-year follow-up of the BENEFIT study patients showed convincing evidence in favor of early treatment.[58] In this study, 84% of the original study patients were evaluated at three years; 37% of the initial IFNβ-1b patients had CDMS, compared with 51% of the delayed treatment group, and early treatment also was beneficial as assessed on confirmed EDSS worsening.

A consistent finding of follow-up studies from the three pivotal IFNβ RRMS trials and two CIS trials is that early treatment is beneficial compared with delayed treatment. These trials are similar to randomized delayed-start trials (see Chapter 21), where persisting benefit on disability-related outcomes with early vs. delayed treatment implies an effect on the disease course, as opposed to a short-term symptomatic benefit.

Studies of IFNβ treatment markers (Table 25.7)

IFNβ is partially effective in clinical trial groups. The two possible explanations for this are that the effect size is the same for each individual (e.g. 30% benefit), with response varying between patients only on the basis of disease severity; or that the treatment effect size between individuals varies (i.e., there are "responders" and "non-responders"). The latter possibility was suggested by studies in which EAE mice with disease driven by Th1 cells improved with IFNβ treatment, while mice with EAE driven by Th17 cells were worse.[48] Assuming that pathogenic mechanisms also differ between MS patients, it follows that some patients may respond favorably and some unfavorably to a complex cytokine therapy. In that regard, Sormani and colleagues[89] measured the effect of IFNβ on MRI lesions

in individual patients in the European SPMS IFNβ-1b study. Two separate statistical models suggested individual heterogeneity existed in the MRI response to treatment. For 65% of the patients, there was an indication of a strong treatment effect, defined as > 60% reduction in MRI lesions with treatment. But in 7% of the patients, no treatment effect or even increased lesions with treatment was observed. This study suggests there are individual responder patterns.

The studies in Table 25.7 are very consistent with the Sormani analysis. They report remarkably consistent findings that development of new T2 or Gd-enhancing lesions after starting IFNβ is associated with relatively poor long-term outcome in RRMS patients. A study by Durelli et al. suggests that an MRI scan as early as six months after starting IFNβ predicts subsequent relapse or confirmed EDSS worsening.[90] The study by Prosperini and colleagues shows a dose-response between the number of new MRI lesions at one year after starting IFNβ and the likelihood of confirmed EDSS worsening over the next four years. The greater the number of new lesions, the greater the relative risk of EDSS worsening.[91] These studies strongly suggest that a subset of IFNβ-treated patients (perhaps 20%, depending on the definition for MRI breakthrough disease), can be identified within one year of IFNβ treatment as having a relatively poor prognosis with continued IFNβ treatment. These patients would be good candidates for second-line therapy.

Clinical trials in MS: adverse events

Adverse effects of IFNβ have been well described in many prior publications, and will not be reviewed in detail here. Common adverse events – skin reactions for SC products, fever, myalgia, headache, fatigue and chills, and malaise – are generally tolerable but disabling to a variable degree. Several points have emerged from the IFNβ adverse event experience and the literature: (1) side effects tend to persist over time, but the severity lessens during the initial 3–6 months of treatment; (2) common side effects are dose dependent, as are some serious adverse events (e.g. liver toxicity, depression). In all dose comparison studies, side effect profiles and adverse event tables demonstrate dose-dependency; (3) side effects, like biological effects, disappear in the presence of significant NAb concentrations. A "poor man's" NAb assay is to inquire whether side effects have persisted; and (4) the underlying biological mechanisms of IFNβ side effects are unclear, but presumably relate to upregulation of inflammatory cytokines.

Remaining issues and future directions

Since approval 18 years ago of the first IFNβ product for RRMS, treatment effects of IFNβ at all stages of MS have become fairly clear. The development of IFNβ for MS has illustrated many of the challenges in developing treatments for MS.

- Mechanisms underlying therapeutic efficacy in MS patients remain uncertain.

- Biological markers to support personalized use of IFNβ are lacking, even though it is becoming apparent that MRI monitoring will be useful for treatment decisions in the individual patient.
- Despite enormous financial investment, there is still no clear consensus about the optimal IFNβ dose or product (e.g. is there a role for higher doses of IFNβ in patients who breakthrough on lower IFNβ doses?).
- The optimal treatment for patients with CIS or RRMS who "break through" standard IFNβ therapy is not known. With more potent, but potentially more risky drugs emerging (natalizumab and fingolimod, among others), what will be the optimal treatment algorithm?
- Are there patients with SPMS (or even PPMS), in whom treatment with IFNβ is justified? The studies in SPMS suggest that patients with relapses and MRI disease activity may benefit, despite an underlying progressive course, but the IFNβ products are not approved for use in patients with SPMS.

- Are there biological or other predictors of IFNβ NAb?
- Can long-term observational studies (as discussed in Chapter 20) ever determine unequivocally the effect of early treatment with IFNβ on clinically important disability?
- Development of IFNβ as a treatment for MS has taken a very long time, indeed. While it has been 18 years since the first product was approved, the earliest clinical trials of Type I IFN preceded that watershed event by an additional 15 years. Thus, the IFNβ clinical development timeline has exceeded 30 years! Undoubtedly, while development of IFNβ as an effective MS treatment has been one of the major success stories in all of MS research, the experience has highlighted many of the major clinical challenges described in Chapter 1 of this book. Hopefully, as our understanding of MS pathogenesis improves, and as cutting-edge MRI, pharmacogenetic, and biological studies are applied to MS, increasingly rational use of IFNβ for individual MS patients will become feasible.

References

1. Jacobs L, O'Malley J, Freeman A, Ekes R, OMalley J. Intrathecal interferon reduces exacerbations of multiple sclerosis. *Science* 1981;214:1026–8.
2. Knobler RL, Panitch HS, Braheny SL, *et al.* Clinical trial of natural alpha interferon in multiple sclerosis. *Ann N Y Acad Sci* 1984;436:382–8.
3. Jacobs L, Salazar AM, Herndon R, *et al.* Multicentre double-blind study of effect of intrathecally administered natural human fibroblast interferon on exacerbations of multiple sclerosis. *Lancet* 1986;2:1411–13.
4. Interferon-alpha and transfer factor in the treatment of multiple sclerosis: a double-blind, placebo-controlled trial. AUSTIMS Research Group. *J Neurol Neurosurg Psychiatry* 1989;52:566–74.
5. Kastrukoff LF, Oger JJ, Hashimoto SA, *et al.* Systemic lymphoblastoid interferon therapy in chronic progressive multiple sclerosis. I. Clinical and MRI evaluation. *Neurology* 1990;40(3, 1):479–86.
6. Panitch HS, Hirsch RL, Haley AS, Johnson KP. Exacerbations of multiple sclerosis in patients treated with gamma interferon. *Lancet* 1987;1(8538):893–5.
7. The IFNB Multiple Sclerosis Study Group, The University of British Columbia MS/MRI Analysis Group. Interferon beta-1b in the treatment of multiple sclerosis: final outcome of the randomized controlled trial. *Neurology* 1995;45:1277–85.
8. Jacobs LD, Cookfair DL, Rudick RA, Herndon RM, Richert JR, Salazar, *et al.* Intramuscular interferon beta-1a for disease progression in relapsing multiple sclerosis. The Multiple Sclerosis Collaborative Research Group (MSCRG). *Ann Neurol* 1996;39:285–94.
9. PRISMS Study Group. Randomised double-blind placebo-controlled study of interferon beta-1a in relapsing/remitting multiple sclerosis. PRISMS (Prevention of Relapses and Disability by Interferon beta-1a Subcutaneously in Multiple Sclerosis) Study Group. *Lancet* 1998;352:1498–504.
10. Rudick RA, Fisher E, Lee JC, Simon J, Jacobs L. Use of the brain parenchymal fraction to measure whole brain atrophy in relapsing-remitting MS. Multiple Sclerosis Collaborative Research Group. *Neurology* 1999;53:1698–704.
11. Cohen JA, Cutter GR, Fischer JS, *et al.* Use of the multiple sclerosis functional composite as an outcome measure in a phase 3 clinical trial. *Arch Neurol* 2001;58:961–7.
12. Kappos L, Weinshenker B, Pozzilli C, *et al.* Interferon beta-1b in secondary progressive MS: a combined analysis of the two trials. *Neurology* 2004;63:1779–87.
13. Leary SM, Miller DH, Stevenson VL, Brex PA, Chard DT, Thompson AJ. Interferon beta-1a in primary progressive MS: an exploratory, randomized, controlled trial. *Neurology* 2003;60:44–51.
14. European Study Group on Inteferon Beta-1b in Secondary Progressive MS. Placebo-controlled multicentre randomised trial of interferon beta-1b in treatment of secondary progressive multiple sclerosis. European Study Group on interferon beta-1b in secondary progressive MS. *Lancet* 1998;352:1491–7.
15. Rudick RA, Cutter G, Baier M, *et al.* Estimating effects of disease modifying therapy in patients with multiple sclerosis followed longitudinally after a controlled clinical trial. *Neurology* 2001;56:A353.
16. Ebers GC, Traboulsee A, Li D, Langdon D, Reder AT, Goodin DS, *et al.* Analysis of clinical outcomes according to original treatment groups 16 years after the pivotal IFNB-1b trial. *J Neurol Neurosurg Psychiatry* 2010;81:907–12.
17. PRISMS-4: Long-term efficacy of interferon-beta-1a in relapsing MS. *Neurology* 2001;56:1628–36.
18. Kappos L, Traboulsee A, Constantinescu C, *et al.* Long-term subcutaneous interferon beta-1a therapy in patients with relapsing-remitting MS. *Neurology* 2006;67:944–53.

19. Sen GC, Lengyel P. The interferon system. A bird's eye view of its biochemistry. *J Biol Chem* 1992;267:5017–20.

20. Tyring SK. Interferons: biochemistry and mechanisms of action. *Am J Obstet Gynecol* 1995;172(4 Pt 2):1350–3.

21. Peters M. Actions of cytokines on the immune response and viral interactions: an overview. *Hepatology* 1996;23:909–16.

22. van Boxel-Dezaire AH, Rani MR, Stark GR. Complex modulation of cell type-specific signaling in response to type I interferons. *Immunity* 2006;25:361–72.

23. Taniguchi T, Takaoka A. The interferon-alpha/beta system in antiviral responses: a multimodal machinery of gene regulation by the IRF family of transcription factors. *Curr Opin Immunol* 2002;14:111–16.

24. Kasama K, Utsumi J, Matsuo-Ogawa E, Nagahata T, Kagawa Y, Yamazaki S, *et al.* Pharmacokinetics and biologic activities of human native and asialointerferon-beta s. *J Interferon Cytokine Res* 1995;15:407–15.

25. Runkel L, Meier W, Pepinsky RB, *et al.* Structural and functional differences between glycosylated and non-glycosylated forms of human interferon-beta (IFN-beta). *Pharm Res* 1998;15:641–9.

26. Cleary CM, Donnelly RJ, Soh J, Mariano TM, Pestka S. Knockout and reconstitution of a functional human type I interferon receptor complex. *J Biol Chem* 1994;269:18747–9.

27. Kumaran J, Colamonici OR, Fish EN. Structure-function study of the extracellular domain of the human type I interferon receptor (IFNAR)-1 subunit. *J Interferon Cytokine Res* 2000;20:479–85.

28. Ghislain J, Sussman G, Goelz S, Ling LE, Fish EN. Configuration of the interferon-alpha/beta receptor complex determines the context of the biological response. *J Biol Chem* 1995;270: 21785–92.

29. Rani MR, Ransohoff RM. Alternative and accessory pathways in the regulation of IFN-beta-mediated gene expression. *J Interferon Cytokine Res* 2005;25:788–98.

30. Stark GR, Kerr IM, Williams BR, Silverman RH, Schreiber RD. How cells respond to interferons. *Annu Rev Biochem* 1998;67:227–64.

31. Prejean C, Colamonici OR. Role of the cytoplasmic domains of the type I interferon receptor subunits in signaling. *Semin Cancer Biol* 2000;10:83–92.

32. Huang YM, Hussien Y, Yarilin D, Xiao BG, Liu YJ, Link H. Interferon-beta induces the development of type 2 dendritic cells. *Cytokine* 2001;13:264–71.

33. Then BF, Dayyani F, Ziegler-Heitbrock L. Impact of type-I-interferon on monocyte subsets and their differentiation to dendritic cells. An in vivo and ex vivo study in multiple sclerosis patients treated with interferon-beta. *J Neuroimmunol* 2004;146(1–2):176–88.

34. Zang YC, Skinner SM, Robinson RR, *et al.* Regulation of differentiation and functional properties of monocytes and monocyte-derived dendritic cells by interferon beta in multiple sclerosis. *Mult Scler* 2004;10:499–506.

35. Vandenbark AA, Huan J, Agotsch M, *et al.* Interferon-beta-1a treatment increases CD56bright natural killer cells and CD4+CD25+ Foxp3 expression in subjects with multiple sclerosis. *J Neuroimmunol* 2009;215(1–2):125–8.

36. Kantor AB, Deng J, Waubant E, *et al.* Identification of short-term pharmacodynamic effects of interferon-beta-1a in multiple sclerosis subjects with broad- based phenotypic profiling. *J Neuroimmunol* 2007;188(1–2):103–16.

37. Deisenhammer F. Neutralizing antibodies to interferon-beta and other immunological treatments for multiple sclerosis: prevalence and impact on outcomes. *CNS Drugs* 2009;23:379–96.

38. Weinstock-Guttman B, Badgett D, Patrick K, *et al.* Genomic effects of IFN-beta in multiple sclerosis patients. *J Immunol* 2003;171:2694–702.

39. Hesse D, Krakauer M, Lund H, *et al.* Breakthrough disease during interferon-[beta] therapy in MS: No signs of impaired biologic response. *Neurology* 2010;74:1455–62.

40. Reder AT, Velichko S, Yamaguchi KD, *et al.* IFN-beta1b induces transient and variable gene expression in relapsing-remitting multiple sclerosis patients independent of neutralizing antibodies or changes in IFN receptor RNA expression. *J Interferon Cytokine Res* 2008;28:317–31.

41. Sellebjerg F, Datta P, Larsen J, *et al.* Gene expression analysis of interferon-beta treatment in multiple sclerosis. *Mult Scler* 2008;14:615–21.

42. Serrano-Fernandez P, Moller S, Goertsches R, *et al.* Time course transcriptomics of IFNB1b drug therapy in multiple sclerosis. *Autoimmunity* 2010;43:172–8.

43. van Baarsen LG, Vosslamber S, Tijssen M, *et al.* Pharmacogenomics of interferon-beta therapy in multiple sclerosis: baseline IFN signature determines pharmacological differences between patients. *PLoS One* 2008;3:e1927.

44. Rani MR, Xu Y, Lee JC, *et al.* Heterogeneous, longitudinally stable molecular signatures in response to interferon-beta. *Ann N Y Acad Sci* 2009;1182:58–68.

45. Chen L, Borozan I, Sun J, *et al.* Cell-type specific gene expression signature in liver underlies response to interferon therapy in chronic hepatitis C infection. *Gastroenterology* 2010;138:1123–33.

46. Rejdak K, Leary SM, Petzold A, Thompson AJ, Miller DH, Giovannoni G. Urinary neopterin and nitric oxide metabolites as markers of interferon beta-1a activity in primary progressive multiple sclerosis. *Mult Scler* 2010;16:1066–72.

47. Rudick RA, Ransohoff RM, Peppler R, VanderBrug MS, Lehmann P, Alam J. Interferon beta induces interleukin-10 expression: relevance to multiple sclerosis. *Ann Neurol* 1996;40:618–27.

48. Axtell RC, de Jong BA, Boniface K, *et al.* T helper type 1 and 17 cells determine efficacy of interferon-beta in multiple sclerosis and experimental encephalomyelitis. *Nat Med* 2010;16:406–12.

49. Alexander JS, Harris MK, Wells SR, *et al.* Alterations in serum MMP-8, MMP-9, IL-12p40 and IL-23 in multiple sclerosis patients treated with interferon-beta1b. *Mult Scler* 2010;16:801–9.

50. Bahner D, Klucke C, Kitze B, *et al.* Interferon-beta-1b increases serum interleukin-12 p40 levels in primary progressive multiple sclerosis patients. *Neurosci Lett* 2002;326:125–8.

51. Calabresi PA, Tranquill LR, Dambrosia JM, et al. Increases in soluble VCAM-1 correlate with a decrease in MRI lesions in multiple sclerosis treated with interferon b-1b. Ann Neurol 1997;41:669–74.

52. Rudick RA, Ransohoff RM, Peppler R, VanderBrug Medendorp S, Lehmann P, Alam J. Interferon beta induces interleukin-10 expression: Relevance to multiple sclerosis. Ann Neurol 1996;40:618–27.

53. Jacobs LD, Beck RW, Simon JH, et al. Intramuscular interferon beta-1a therapy initiated during a first demyelinating event in multiple sclerosis. CHAMPS Study Group. N Engl J Med 2000;343:898–904.

54. Kinkel RP, Kollman C, O'Connor P, et al. im interferon beta-1a delays definite multiple sclerosis 5 years after a first demyelinating event. Neurology 2006;66:678–84.

55. Comi G, Filippi M, Barkhof F, et al. Effect of early interferon treatment on conversion to definite multiple sclerosis: a randomised study. Lancet 2001;357:1576–82.

56. Filippi M, Rovaris M, Inglese M, et al. Interferon beta-1a for brain tissue loss in patients at presentation with syndromes suggestive of multiple sclerosis: a randomised, double-blind, placebo-controlled trial. Lancet 2004;364:1489–96.

57. Kappos L, Polman CH, Freedman MS, et al. Treatment with interferon beta-1b delays conversion to clinically definite and McDonald MS in patients with clinically isolated syndromes. Neurology 2006;67:1242–9.

58. Kappos L, Freedman MS, Polman CH, et al. Effect of early versus delayed interferon beta-1b treatment on disability after a first clinical event suggestive of multiple sclerosis: a 3-year follow-up analysis of the BENEFIT study. Lancet 2007;370:389–97.

59. Polman C, Kappos L, Freedman MS, et al. Subgroups of the BENEFIT study: risk of developing MS and treatment effect of interferon beta-1b. J Neurol 2008;255:480–7.

60. Beck RW, Chandler DL, Cole SR, et al. Interferon beta-1a for early multiple sclerosis: CHAMPS trial subgroup analyses. Ann Neurol 2002;51:481–90.

61. Evidence of interferon beta-1a dose response in relapsing-remitting MS: the OWIMS Study. The Once Weekly Interferon for MS Study Group. Neurology 1999;53:679–86.

62. Simon JH, Jacobs LD, Campion MK, et al. A longitudinal study of brain atrophy in relapsing multiple sclerosis. The Multiple Sclerosis Collaborative Research Group (MSCRG). Neurology 1999;53:139–48.

63. Hardmeier M, Wagenpfeil S, Freitag P, et al. Rate of brain atrophy in relapsing MS decreases during treatment with IFNbeta-1a. Neurology 2005;64:236–40.

64. Jones CK, Riddehough A, Li DKB, Zhao G, Paty DW. MRI cerebral atrophy in relapsing-remitting MS: Results from the PRISMS trial. Neurology 2001;56: A379.

65. Clanet M, Radue EW, Kappos L, et al. A randomized, double-blind, dose-comparison study of weekly interferon beta-1a in relapsing MS. Neurology 2002;59:1507–17.

66. O'Connor P, Filippi M, Arnason B, et al. 250 mug or 500 mug interferon beta-1b versus 20 mg glatiramer acetate in relapsing-remitting multiple sclerosis: a prospective, randomised, multicentre study. Lancet Neurol 2009;8:889–97.

67. Paty DW, Li DK, UBC MS/MRI Study Group, The IFNB Multiple Sclerosis Study Group. Interferon beta-1b is effective in relapsing-remitting multiple sclerosis. II. MRI analysis results of a multicenter, randomized, double-blind, placebo-controlled trial. Neurology 1993;43:662–7.

68. Simon JH, Jacobs LD, Campion M, et al. Magnetic resonance studies of intramuscular interferon beta-1a for relapsing multiple sclerosis. The Multiple Sclerosis Collaborative Research Group. Ann Neurol 1998;43:79–87.

69. Li DK, Paty DW. Magnetic resonance imaging results of the PRISMS trial: a randomized, double-blind, placebo-controlled study of interferon-beta1a in relapsing-remitting multiple sclerosis. Prevention of Relapses and Disability by Interferon-beta1a Subcutaneously in Multiple Sclerosis. Ann Neurol 1999;46:197–206.

70. Panitch H, Miller A, Paty D, Weinshenker B. Interferon beta-1b in secondary progressive MS: results from a 3-year controlled study. Neurology 2004;63:1788–95.

71. Secondary Progressive Efficacy Clinical Trial of Recombinant Interferon-beta-1a in MS (SPECTRIMS) Study Group. Randomized controlled trial of interferon-beta-1a in secondary progressive MS. Clinical results. Neurology 2001;56:1496–504.

72. Li DK, Zhao GJ, Paty DW. Randomized controlled trial of interferon-beta-1a in secondary progressive MS: MRI results. Neurology 2001;56:1505–13.

73. Cohen JA, Cutter GR, Fischer JS, et al. Benefit of interferon beta-1a on MSFC progression in secondary progressive MS. Neurology 2002;59:679–87.

74. Andersen O, Elovaara I, Farkkila M, et al. Multicentre, randomised, double blind, placebo controlled, phase III study of weekly, low dose, subcutaneous interferon beta-1a in secondary progressive multiple sclerosis. J Neurol Neurosurg Psychiatry 2004;75:706–10.

75. Freedman MS, Francis GS, Sanders EA, et al. Randomized study of once-weekly interferon beta-1la therapy in relapsing multiple sclerosis: three-year data from the OWIMS study. Mult Scler 2005;11:41–5.

76. Durelli L, Barbero P, Bergui M, et al. The OPTimization of interferon for MS study: 375 microg interferon beta-1b in suboptimal responders. J Neurol 2008;255:1315–23.

77. Rudick RA, Cutter G, Reingold S. The multiple sclerosis functional composite: a new clinical outcome measure for multiple sderosis trials. Mult Scler 2002;8:359–65.

78. Goodkin DE, Rudick RA, Medendorp SV, et al. Low-dose (7.5 mg) oral methotrexate reduces the rate of pregression in chronic progressive multiple sclerosis. Ann Neurol 1995;37:30–40.

79. Koch-Henriksen N, Sorensen PS, Christensen T, et al. A randomized study of two interferon-beta treatments in relapsing-remitting multiple sclerosis. Neurology 2006;66:1056–60.

80. Panitch H, Goodin DS, Francis G, et al. Randomized, comparative study of interferon beta-1a treatment regimens in MS: The EVIDENCE Trial. Neurology 2002;59:1496–506.

81. Durelli L, Verdun E, Barbero P, et al. Every-other-day interferon beta-1b versus once-weekly interferon beta-1a for multiple sclerosis: results of a 2-year prospective randomised multicentre

study (INCOMIN). *Lancet* 2002;359: 1453–60.

82. Cadavid D, Wolansky LJ, Skurnick J, *et al.* Efficacy of treatment of MS with IFNbeta-1b or glatiramer acetate by monthly brain MRI in the BECOME study. *Neurology* 2009;72:1976–83.

83. Mikol DD, Barkhof F, Chang P, *et al.* Comparison of subcutaneous interferon beta-1a with glatiramer acetate in patients with relapsing multiple sclerosis (the REbif vs Glatiramer Acetate in Relapsing MS Disease [REGARD] study): a multicentre, randomised, parallel, open-label trial. *Lancet Neurol* 2008;7:903–14.

84. Cohen JA, Barkhof F, Comi G, *et al.* Oral fingolimod or intramuscular interferon for relapsing multiple sclerosis. *N Engl J Med* 2010;362: 402–15.

85. Kieburtz K, McDermott M. Needed in MS: evidence, not EVIDENCE. *Neurology* 2002;59:1482–3.

86. Schwid SR, Thorpe J, Sharief M, *et al.* Enhanced benefit of increasing interferon beta-1a dose and frequency in relapsing multiple sclerosis: the EVIDENCE Study. *Arch Neurol* 2005;62:785–92.

87. Rudick RA, Cutter G, Baier M, *et al.* Use of the Multiple Sclerosis Functional Composite to predict disability in relapsing MS. *Neurology* 2001;56: 1324–30.

88. Trojano M, Pellegrini F, Paolicelli D, *et al.* Real-life impact of early interferon beta therapy in relapsing multiple sclerosis. *Ann Neurol* 2009; 66:513–20.

89. Sormani MP, Bruzzi P, Beckmann K, *et al.* The distribution of magnetic resonance imaging response to interferonbeta-1b in multiple sclerosis. *J Neurol* 2005;252:1455–8.

90. Durelli L, Barbero P, Bergui M, *et al.* MRI activity and neutralising antibody as predictors of response to interferon beta treatment in multiple sclerosis. *J Neurol Neurosurg Psychiatry* 2008;79: 646–51.

91. Prosperini L, Gallo V, Petsas N, Borriello G, Pozzilli C. One-year MRI scan predicts clinical response to interferon beta in multiple sclerosis. *Eur J Neurol* 2009;16:1202–9.

92. Rudick RA, Lee JC, Simon J, Ransohoff RM, Fisher E. Defining interferon beta response status in multiple sclerosis patients. *Ann Neurol* 2004;56:548–55.

93. Tomassini V, Paolillo A, Russo P, *et al.* Predictors of long-term clinical response to interferon beta therapy in relapsing multiple sclerosis. *J Neurol* 2006;253:287–93.

94. Rio J, Rovira A, Tintore M, *et al.* Relationship between MRI lesion activity and response to IFN-beta in relapsing-remitting multiple sclerosis patients. *Mult Scler* 2008;14: 479–84.

Chapter

26

Glatiramer acetate to treat multiple sclerosis

Jenny Guerre and Corey C. Ford

Introduction

Multiple sclerosis (MS) is a disease of the central nervous system (CNS) characterized by multifocal inflammation, demyelination, axonal injury, and brain atrophy secondary to neurodegenerative changes. The current concepts assume that MS occurs as a consequence of immune tolerance breakdown in genetically susceptible individuals under the influence of unknown environmental factors.[1] Small peptide fragments of microbial or viral components with amino acid sequences similar to antigenic segments of myelin proteins could induce a cross-reactive immune attack on self by a process of molecular mimicry.[2]

Important insights into the mechanisms of immune-mediated myelin damage have come from animal models. For example, immunizing an animal to antigenic myelin components or peptide fragments can trigger experimental autoimmune encephalomyelitis (EAE), a form of CNS demyelination. Effective antigens in EAE induction include the major myelin proteins, myelin basic protein (MBP), proteolipid protein (PLP), and myelin oligodendrocyte glycoprotein (MOG). It is known that both patients with MS and normal individuals have potentially autoreactive T-cells specific to these myelin antigens in their peripheral circulation.[3-8]

The possibility that MS is driven by similar immune mechanisms has led to numerous studies of antigen-specific immune-modulating strategies. Recognition that axonal injury and axonal transaction occur early in MS and may correlate with permanent neurological deficits has reinforced the motivation to find more effective treatments to slow or halt the disease process and limit axonal damage.[9] When the US Food and Drug Administration (FDA) approved copolymer 1 for relapsing-remitting MS (RRMS) in 1997, the generic name, glatiramer acetate (GA), was created. The trademark name of the drug is Copaxone®. The term GA will be used in this review.

History of glatiramer acetate (copolymer 1)

The development of GA is a fascinating story. As an immune-mediated CNS disease, MS presents inherent barriers for human research. The development of animal models of demyelination was an important step in unraveling the immune mechanisms underlying MS. One model, EAE is a T-cell mediated disease that can be induced in susceptible animals by inoculating them with CNS homogenates in complete Freund's adjuvant. Certain purified protein components of myelin, such as MBP, can also be encephalitogenic or capable of producing EAE when injected into susceptible animals.[10,11]

Some 40 years ago, Ruth Arnon and colleagues at the Weitzmann Institute in Israel were interested in the structural aspects of protein antigens in EAE induction. They synthesized a family of 11 different copolymers with amino acid compositions chosen to be similar to MBP (copolymers 1–11) as potential encephalitogens. None was capable of inducing EAE, but several had the ability to prevent development or reduce the severity of EAE in animals inoculated with MBP. Copolymer 1 (GA), composed of L-glutamate, L-lysine, L-alanine, and L-tyrosine, was the most potent, reducing the incidence of MBP-induced EAE in guinea pigs by 20%–75%.[12,13]

Cross-reactivity of GA and MBP was shown at both the T-cell and B-cell levels. The degree of cross-reactivity with MBP in assays of lymphocyte transformation, delayed hypersensitivity, and monoclonal antibody binding correlated well with the ability of GA to suppress EAE.[14] Furthermore, the immune modulating effect of GA seemed to be restricted to responses induced by myelin antigens, and was not due to general immunosuppressive properties.[15]

An important series of experiments showed that GA could suppress the development or reduce the severity of EAE in a variety of animals, including mice, rats, guinea pigs, rabbits, and primates.[16-20] Studies in primates were of particular relevance to the treatment of MS in humans. It was known that Rhesus monkeys and baboons were very sensitive to MBP-induced EAE and typically died of the disease within 2 weeks of symptom onset. GA treatment was found to reverse EAE in these animals after the appearance of symptoms. Toxicity testing in animals did not reveal mutagenic or other serious adverse effects, and the stage was set for GA to enter clinical testing in humans.

Multiple Sclerosis Therapeutics, Fourth Edition, ed. Jeffrey A. Cohen and Richard A. Rudick. Published by Cambridge University Press.
© Cambridge University Press 2011.

Mechanism of action

Immunomodulatory effects

The immune pathology in MS could, in part, be driven by specific T-cell responses to myelin antigens. Possible myelin autoantigens in MS include MBP, MOG, and PLP.[21] Evidence from animal models for a potential role of these antigenic proteins in demyelinating diseases like MS derives from their use as encephalitogens in the induction of EAE. In fact, the early interest in GA was related to its ability to suppress the induction of EAE by MBP, PLP, and MOG.[22–24] GA inhibits cell-mediated immune responses to MBP and cross-reacts with MBP at both the cellular and humoral levels.[14,25–27] GA seems to affect immune cells in an antigenic specific way, as the peptide mixture is applied over many years by daily injections and could be considered an example of a therapeutic vaccination, as opposed to the prophylactic vaccinations commonly used for infectious diseases.[28]

There are several proposed mechanisms of action by which GA might exert therapeutic benefit in MS:[29]

- Competitive binding to molecules of the major histocompatibility complex (MHC) expressed on antigen-presenting cells (APCs) in preference to myelin protein antigens.
- Preferred binding of GA-MHC complexes over MBP–MHC complexes to appropriate T-cell receptors (TCR).
- Induction of tolerance in MBP-specific T-cells; induction of GA-specific T-cells expressing Th2 anti-inflammatory cytokines.
- A neuroprotective effect by expressing neurotrophic factors such as brain-derived neurotrophic factor (BDNF)
- Stimulation of neurogenesis.[30–32]

The avid binding of GA to MHC class II sites on APCs interferes with antigen presentation to T-cells.[33,34] Binding of GA to MHC class II sites blocks interactions with MBP, PLP, and MOG.[24,35] However, D-GA made from D-isomer amino acids, also binds to MHC class II sites, but does not have significant effect in treating or preventing EAE.[27] This finding demonstrates that competition at MHC sites alone does not explain the therapeutic effects of GA in EAE or MS.

GA might have an antigen-specific T-cell interaction, since MHC binding of the drug does not seem to block immune responses to non-myelin antigens. TCR antagonism was suggested in a study showing that GA-MHC complexes could function as a competitive antagonist to MBP peptide p82–100-MHC complexes.[36] In this model, GA may be acting as an altered peptide ligand for MBP fragments. Another study using different T-cell clones found no partial agonist or antagonist activity associated with GA interactions with TCR.[37] This mechanism of action would require the presence of GA-MHC complexes in the same compartment where MBP fragment–MHC interactions with TCR occur and, thus, is considered unlikely.

Kim and colleagues reported that release of interleukin (IL)-10 from monocytes was significantly enhanced in GA-treated patients and the production of IL-12 was reduced.[38] These findings were consistent with an anti-inflammatory type 2 monocyte phenotype. The studies suggested a systemic effect of GA treatment on monocytes that promoted Th2 differentiation of T-cells in vivo.[39] Expression of transforming growth factor beta (TGFβ) and IL-10, which have anti-inflammatory actions, is increased by resident astrocytes and microglia in CNS with GA-specific T-cell infiltration.[28]

Chabot et al. demonstrated that in humans GA impairs effective interaction between activated T-cells and microglia (ex vivo), thus suppressing induction of several pro-inflammatory cytokines.[40] CNS infiltration of GA-specific T-cells might result in increased expression of anti-inflammatory cytokines, TGFβ and IL-10. The net result would be a non-inflammatory milieu within the CNS, which may help account for the amelioration of disease activity in MS patients on GA in spite of T-cell infiltration.

It is unclear by which pathway GA treatment alters APC and T-cell functions. Some evidence points to the APC and some to T-cells as the primary target of GA. The phenotype of an APC influences differentiation of T-cells and differentiated T-cells in turn modify APC functions. In vitro studies showed that GA exerted a direct effect on APC populations[38,39] and that GA treated APCs were capable of promoting development of Th2 cells when co-cultured with naïve (untreated) T-cells in the absence of GA.[41]

The frequency of GA-reactive Th2 cells in the peripheral blood of GA-treated MS patients is only 1 in 20 000, raising the question of whether the quantity of Th2 cytokines derived from these cells could be sufficient to mediate type 2 APC development. Strikingly, studies in genetically altered mice indicated that in vivo GA treatment can induce type 2 monocytes in the absence of T-cells.[42] A recent study by Allie et al.[43] demonstrated that Th2 differentiation occurred independent of antigen specificity in patients treated with GA. This study supported APCs as the primary target by demonstrating that Th2 deviation or induction of regulatory T-cells was not restricted to GA-reactive T-cells. The concept of an antigen-nonspecific effect of GA is further supported by the observation that GA treatment is beneficial in models of other autoimmune or inflammatory conditions, including arthritis, uveoretinitis, and inflammatory bowel disease.[44,45] However, another study[46] did not detect an antigen-independent Th2 deviation of established T-cell responses with GA treatment and supported the concept that Th2 deviation primarily occurred with GA-reactive T-cells. Further studies are needed to determine by which pathway GA alters APC and T-cell functions.

Patients treated with GA for a few months initially develop an increase frequency of GA-specific T-cells that decreases with continued drug administration.[47] Possible mechanisms for this reduction in GA-specific T-cells include the induction of anergy or apoptotic cell death.[37,48] Binding of GA-MHC complexes to the TCR of MBP-specific T-cells could lead to differential signaling and the induction of unresponsiveness in these cells. This mechanism of action would also have GA functioning as an altered peptide ligand and is appealing because the process could occur in the peripheral circulation.

GA-specific Th2-polarized T-cells appear to recognize myelin antigens in a non-specific way and possibly mediate bystander suppression. This mechanism of action was suggested in EAE studies.[49] Helper T-cell lines induced by MBP secrete cytokines with a pro-inflammatory, Th1 profile (IL-2, interferon-gamma [IFNγ]), but GA-induced T-cell lines progressively shift to a Th2 secretion profile.[26] When exposed to MBP, these GA-specific T-cells also secrete the Th2 cytokines (IL-4, IL-6, and IL-10). Adoptive transfer of the GA-specific T-cells suppressed the development of EAE induced by whole mouse spinal cord homogenate. Since this form of EAE includes MBP as a major encephalitogenic antigen, it was possible that the effect of GA was related more to suppression of the MBP antigen responses than to other antigenic components of myelin. A follow-up study demonstrated that GA-specific T-cells secreting Th2 cytokines suppressed EAE induced by antigens to which the cells did not cross-react.[50] Adoptive transfer of GA-specific T-cells improved EAE induced by whole PLP and the PLP peptides p139–151 (RR EAE) and p178–191 (chronic-progressive EAE).

Activated T-cells specific to any antigen are capable of crossing the blood–brain barrier.[51] GA-specific T-cells secreting a Th2 profile of cytokines have been demonstrated in the CNS of mice treated with GA.[52] In this study, highly reactive GA-specific T-cells secreting IL-4, IL-5, IL-6, IL-10, and TGFβ were isolated from the brains and spinal cords of SJL/J x BALB/c mice. Those cytokines not only might modulate the local milieu but also suppress the activity of encephalitogenic Th1 cells. This so-called bystander suppression appears to be an essential part of the mechanism of action of GA. Adoptively transferred, labeled GA-specific T-cells were found in brain sections 7 and 10 days after peripheral injection.[52] To the extent that the treatment effects of GA on EAE and MS are similar, this study supports the role of GA-specific Th2 suppressor cells, which can cross the blood–brain barrier and accumulate in the CNS. Stimulation of these cross-reacting cells by MBP or MBP fragments could then result in secretion of immunomodulatory Th2 cytokines in situ.

In a study of eight MS patients initiating therapy with GA, T-cell lines were categorized by their proliferative responses to GA and MBP antigens, and profiled according to cytokine production.[53] A high percentage of lymphocytes in the pre-treatment samples responded to GA. As in previous studies, continued treatment with GA resulted in a decrease in the number of responsive T-cell lines. Using the ratio of IFNγ / IL-5 as a measure of Th1-Th2 proclivity, GA-reactive lymphocytes had a significant Th2 bias compared to MBP-reactive cells. While IFNβ treatment reduces the expression of IFNγ by T-cells, GA-treated MS patients are not different in their T-cell expression of IFNγ compared to untreated subjects.[54] Another study showed that the CD4+ T-cell response to GA was similar in both MS

patients and normal controls. However, pre-treatment CD8+ T-cell responses were significantly lower in MS patients and increased to the normal range after GA therapy.[55] Thus, GA may have different effects on CD4+ and CD8+ T-cells, operating on each population in a separate but synergistic manner to alter the immunological pathways involved in MS.[56]

Untreated MS patients demonstrate impaired CD4+ T-cell apoptosis compared with healthy individuals.[57] A study by Rieks et al.[58] showed that GA treatment enhances CD4+ T-cell (T helper) apoptosis leading to T helper elimination which is accompanied by increased frequencies of activated T-cells and elevated numbers of IL-4-producing lymphocytes.

GA-specific T-cell lines isolated from three patients with MS and one control produced tumor necrosis factor-alpha (TNFα), IFNγ, IL-4, IL-6, and IL-10.[59] MBP-specific T-cells produced the same cytokine profile except for IL-6. The GA-specific cell lines also inhibited the proliferation of MBP-specific cell lines in co-culture experiments. GA injected daily could therefore interact with lymphocytes in regional lymph nodes and suppress autoreactive T-cell production.

A novel mechanism for GA action was suggested by Allie et al. in the study of ten patients with RRMS.[43] Therapy with GA caused reduction in the expression of chemokine receptors associated with Th1 cell homing to tissue sites of inflammation. Specifically, CXCR3 and CCR5, which have been demonstrated on pathogenic infiltrating T-cells in MS brain tissue, and CXCR6, which is expressed on Th1 cells in the periphery, were reduced on not only the GA-reactive T-cell lines but also the MBP-specific T-cell lines, suggesting that bystander modulation of cytokine receptors occurred in the peripheral blood compartment of GA-treated patients with MS. This effect was most notable in CD4+ T-cell subset.

Several studies have examined the production of antibodies to GA.[60,61] A group of 130 patients from GA clinical trials were studied for GA-induced humoral immune responses.[62] All patients developed GA-reactive antibodies peaking at three months of therapy, then declining to near baseline. IgG1 levels were two to three times higher than IgG2 levels, suggesting a Th2 response. GA-reactive antibody activity in sera of GA-treated patients does not seem to affect therapeutic benefit.[63,64] In vitro activities of GA were enhanced in some cases by sera containing anti-GA antibodies. In a murine model of demyelinating disease induced by Theiler's virus, remyelination of spinal cord was enhanced by GA antibodies.[65] These results support the hypothesis that the antibody responses in GA-treated patients are not detrimental and may be beneficial by facilitating repair of demyelinated lesions.

The migration properties of T-cells isolated from GA-treated MS patients were reduced compared to T-cells from untreated patients but not to the extent of patients treated with IFNβ.[66] Furthermore, in contrast to IFNβ, GA does not seem to inhibit expression of adhesion molecules on vascular endothelium.[67]

Thus, GA functions as an antigen and induces proliferation of T-cell lines from controls and patients with MS. Repeated daily injections result in loss of proliferative responses and induce the production of the Th2 cytokines.[47] GA induces a Th1-to-Th2 shift in cytokine expression and GA-treated T-cells could have a bystander suppression effect by expressing in-situ cytokines (IL-10, TGFβ, IL-4, IL-5) which are able to suppress the activity of encephalitogenic Th1 cells.[28] Up to 25% of GA-specific T-cell clones secrete IL-5 in response to MBP or MBP peptide fragments. The MBP antigens may function as partial agonists inducing the expression of Th2, immunoregulatory cytokines.[68] GA is the first known treatment of an autoimmune disease that functions by binding to the TCR. In addition, although the GA-induced Th1-to-Th2 shift seems to be GA-specific,[46] these results support bystander suppression as a potential mechanism of action of GA in the treatment of MS.

In transplantation systems, GA treatment inhibited secretion of Th1 inflammatory cytokines and induced Th2/3 anti-inflammatory responses. GA significantly suppressed the various manifestations of trinitrobenzene sulfonic acid-induced colitis, including mortality, weight loss, and macroscopic and microscopic colonic damage.[69] GA suppressed local lymphocyte proliferations and TNFα, and increased TGFβ. These results added to the concept of a Th1-to-Th2 shift in GA mode of action.

Potential neuroprotective effects

GA-specific T-cells demonstrated a neuroprotective effect in a rat optic nerve crush injury model.[70] Adoptive transfer of GA-specific T-cells also demonstrated the protective effect. One potential mechanisms would be elaboration of neurotrophic factors such as BDNF, one of the most potent factors supporting neuronal survival and regulating neurotransmitter release and dendritic growth. Studies by Ziemssen et al.[71] showed that locally activated GA-reactive Th2 cells produce not only protective Th2 cytokines but also the BDNF. They further indicated that GA-specific Th1 cells, which are reduced but still present in GA-treated patients, could also act as a local source of BDNF.

In an EAE model, GA-specific regulatory T-cells were adoptively transferred to mice. Brain sections demonstrated extensive amounts of BDNF and the anti-inflammatory cytokines IL-10 and TGFβ.[36] In contrast to the low expression in the corresponding brain region of EAE untreated mice, BDNF was elevated in brains of mice adoptively transferred with GA-reactive T-cells and in those that were injected daily with GA. The in vitro production of BDNF by GA-induced cells was shown at the protein and the messenger RNA levels. BDNF secretion in the brain of MS patient by reactive astrocytes and immune cells has been established by Stadelmann and others.[72–74] Reduced levels of BDNF in the serum and the cerebrospinal fluid of MS patients and reversal by GA treatment have been reported,[75] indicating that this effect of GA is relevant to human therapy as well. Secretion of two additional neurotrophic factors, NT3 and NT4, are also increased with GA treatment.[76]

Treatment with GA seemed to reduce axonal damage in MOG-induced chronic EAE mice.[77] Spinal cord examination showed less inflammation with better preservation of myelin sheaths, and less axonal damage in the areas of inflammation. In a study quantifying the concentration of the neuronal marker, N-acetylaspartate (NAA) by magnetic resonance spectroscopy, GA treatment led to a significant increase in NAA, suggesting axonal metabolic recovery and protection from sublethal axonal injury.[78,79] Similar effects on NAA have not been consistently reported IFNβ therapy,[78,80,81] although studies by Toprak et al.[82] and Narayanan et al.[83] suggested positive effects of IFNβ on metabolites within MS lesions and in axons.

Summary of mechanism of action

The picture emerges that GA peptides bind efficiently to MHC class II molecules on peripheral APCs and displace other potential myelin antigens. Subsequent interaction with T-cells and their specific receptors in a trimolecular complex leads to induction of GA-specific T-cells. These T-cells are suppressor in nature and cross the blood–brain barrier where they can be reactivated in situ by the cross-reacting antigens originating from myelin proteins. The reactivated Th2 cells secrete suppressor cytokines, producing bystander suppression of the immune response directed against myelin, and neurotrophic factors, possibly leading to a degree of neuroprotection and stimulation of neurogenesis. Studies in patients demonstrated that treatment with GA treatment reduces the formation of permanent T1-hypointense MRI lesions, so-called "T1 black holes," which are associated with irreversible neurologic disabilities.[84] Whereas MBP-specific T suppressor cells either maintain some Th1 properties or can shift back to a Th1 profile when reactivated in vivo, GA-specific Th2 cells appear to be confined to a suppressor profile. This mechanism may be critical in diseases like EAE and MS where epitope spreading has been demonstrated.[21,85]

Clinical trial data
Preliminary clinical studies

The first human use of GA was in three patients with acute disseminated encephalomyelitis and four in the terminal stages of MS.[86] A small, Phase 1, open-label clinical trial was then carried out by Bornstein and colleagues at the Einstein College of Medicine to begin assessing efficacy of GA in MS and to further study toxicity and safety.[87] GA was well tolerated, and no toxicities or adverse effects (AEs) were noted.

Pilot trial of GA in RRMS

The first randomized, double-blind study of GA in MS was also conducted by Bornstein and colleagues at the Albert Einstein College of Medicine.[88] The primary end-point of the pilot trial was the proportion of relapse-free patients on treatment. The trial was also designed to characterize toxicities and significant AEs. The study enrolled 48 patients in 24 pairs matched for age, gender and disability, stratified in three Disability Status Scale (DSS)[89] ranges, 0–2, 3–4, and 5–6. One member of each pair was randomly assigned to GA, the other to placebo. All patients had active RRMS defined as relapses in the previous two years and were between 20 and 35 years of age. After an initial visit at month 1, each patient was assessed every three months for a total period of two years.

There were a total of 16 relapses in the 25 patients on GA and 62 in the 23 receiving placebo. More patients on GA completed the trial relapse free, and placebo treated patients were more likely to have had three or more relapses. Each of these results reached statistical significance. Survival curves showed a marginally significant slowing of progression of disability ($P = 0.05$) at the end of 24 months defined as an increase of one full point on the DSS sustained for three months.

No abnormalities were noted in any laboratory measures during the study. Two patients had an unusual, transient post-injection reaction to GA consisting of flushing and chest tightness, sometimes accompanied by anxiety and dyspnea. The symptoms resolved in 5–30 minutes without sequelae.

Trial in chronic-progressive MS

An early clinical trial of GA was completed for patients with chronic-progressive MS.[90] Of 169 patients followed for six to 15 months, 106 showed progression and were entered into the study. The primary study end-point was the time to confirmed progression of one point on the Expanded Disability Status Scale (EDSS) for patients with baseline EDSS of 5.0 or greater and 1.5 points with entry EDSS of less than 5.0. There was a trend for less progression in the GA group compared to placebo (17.6% vs. 25.5%), which did not reach statistical significance.

US Phase 3 trial in RRMS

Following publication of the positive pilot study of GA in RRMS, there was great interest in confirming safety and efficacy of the drug in a larger, Phase 3 trial. The further development and testing of GA was assumed by Teva Pharmaceuticals, Ltd. of Petah Tikva, Israel, and considerable effort was put into standardizing manufacturing methods to provide the kilogram quantities of drug needed to conduct such a trial. The final product was approved by the FDA and consisted of random, synthetic polypeptide chains ranging in molecular weight from 4000 to 13000 daltons. The four amino acids L-alanine, L-glutamate, L-lysine, and L-tyrosine were combined in molar ratios of 4.2, 1.4, 3, 4, to 1.0.

The double-blind, placebo-controlled Phase 3 trial of daily subcutaneous injections of GA 20 mg or placebo began in October 1991 at eleven university-based MS centers in the USA.[91] The primary end-point of the study was the mean relapse rate. Relapses were defined as the appearance or reappearance of one or more neurological abnormalities persisting for at least 48 hours. A total of 251 patients were randomized to GA or placebo. The two groups were well matched for age, sex, duration of disease, mean relapse rate in the preceding two years,

EDSS, and ambulation index. The mean age of the subjects was 34 years and 73% were women. All had clinically definite or laboratory supported MS with EDSS scores ranging from 0 to 5.0.

There were 161 confirmed relapses in the GA treated group, and 210 in the placebo-treated group. The mean annualized relapse-rate was 0.59 per year for the GA treated patients and 0.84 per year for the placebo group, a 29% reduction ($P = 0.007$). Patients with EDSS scores between 0 and 2 at study entry had a reduction in relapse rate of 33%. Several secondary endpoints were designed to evaluate the effects of GA on progression of neurological disability. Mean EDSS change from baseline was significantly lower for the treatment group compared with placebo ($P = 0.023$). Changes in ambulation index and the number of progression-free patients, defined as an increase of one or more steps on the EDSS sustained for three months, showed little difference between groups. A categorical analysis of patients as the same, better or worse during the trial showed a statistical benefit for GA.

Treatment with GA was not associated with any hematologic, metabolic, urine, or cardiac abnormalities. Mild erythema, stinging, and induration at injection sites were the most common adverse events reported. The transient post-injection reaction, first observed in the pilot trial, occurred in 15% of GA-treated patients, usually within minutes of an injection. Variable combinations of flushing, chest tightness, sense of shortness of breath, palpitations and anxiety characterized the reaction. Typical episodes lasted between 30 seconds and 30 minutes, and no patient experienced serious sequelae.

This two-year pivotal trial confirmed that daily, subcutaneous injections of GA were effective in reducing the relapse rate in patients with RRMS. Secondary end-point analyses showed benefit for GA in slowing the progression of disability. On the basis of the 24-month trial data, the FDA approved GA (Copaxone) for use in RRMS in December 1997.

Extension of the Phase 3 trial

Early in the course of the Phase 3 trial, a decision was made to continue all patients on blinded study medication until the last patient enrolled in the trial completed 24-month follow-up. Thus, some patients were on blinded medication for up to 35 months resulting in an average of 5.5 months of additional double-blind study data. Conditions of the extension period of the study with respect to blinding and protocol were unchanged. The 24-month core study and extension phase data were combined in a second report of the safety and efficacy of GA.[92]

Approximately equal numbers of patients in the GA ($n = 19$) and placebo ($n = 17$) arms of the 24-month core study dropped out after nearly equal periods of time. Overall, 215 patients completed 24 months of the core study and were eligible to continue in the extension phase. Of these, 208 (96.7%) elected to enter the extension phase. Near the end of the 24-month core study period, IFNβ-1b (Betaseron) became the first FDA-approved drug to treat RRMS. All patients in the GA trial were notified of this development and signed a new informed consent to continue in the trial. The availability of IFNβ-1b was the most common reason patients gave for dropping out after the core study and not continuing in the extension phase.

Like the core study, mean relapse rate was the primary end-point of the extension phase. The core plus extension period data showed that the annualized mean relapse rate was 0.67 per year for the GA-treated cohort and 0.99 per year for the placebo group (32% relative reduction; $P = 0.002$). At the end of the extension phase of the trial, 24.6% of the placebo group and 33.6% of the GA group were relapse-free from study initiation ($P = 0.035$). Placebo-treated patients were more likely to have had multiple relapses ($P = 0.008$).

Compared to the 24-month core trial data, more of the secondary measures of progression of disability showed significant benefit with GA treatment. A categorical analysis based on change by ≥ 1.0 EDSS steps demonstrated that more GA-treated patients improved compared to placebo-treated patients, who were more likely to worsen ($P = 0.001$). Excluding any relapse interval, 21.6% of GA-treated patients worsened by ≥ 1.5 EDSS steps compared to 41.6% of the placebo-treated (representing a relative reduction of almost 50%; $P = 0.001$). At the end of the extended trial, 25 of 125 placebo patients and 16 of 125 GA patients were worse by ≥ 1.5 EDSS points.

PreCISe

The benefit of GA on conversion to clinically definite (CD) MS in patients with a clinically isolated syndrome (CIS) was investigated in PreCISe (early glatiramer acetate treatment in delaying conversion to clinically definite multiple sclerosis in subjects Presenting with a Clinically Isolated Syndrome), a randomized, double-blind, placebo-controlled parallel group, Phase 3 study.[93] The study included 481 patients between 18 and 45 years with one unifocal neurological event and a positive brain MRI (at least two lesions 6 mm in diameter). Subjects were randomized to either placebo ($n = 238$) or GA ($n = 243$). The primary end-point was time to conversion to CDMS, defined as a new relapse with symptoms accompanied by objective neurological changes and increase of at least 0.5 points on the EDSS.

Conversion to CDMS was significantly delayed in the GA group compared with the placebo group (from 336 days to 772 days) with a 45% reduction in the risk of developing CDMS. Secondary end-points included a significant reduction of 58% (0.7 in the GA group vs. 1.8 in the placebo group) in the number of new T2 lesions detected at last scan in favor of GA (relative risk [RR] 0.42; 95% confidence interval [CI] 0.29–0.61; $P < 0.0001$). Patient receiving GA had a significant reduction in the cumulative number of new T2-weighted lesions up to the last observed value (RR 0.47; 95% CI 0.37–0.61; $P < 0.0001$) and in the cumulative number of gadolinium (Gd) lesions (RR 0.40; 95% CI 0.30–0.55; $P < 0.0001$).

These results were obtained at a pre-determined interim analysis and the trial Data Safety Monitoring Committee unanimously recommended terminating the trial and offering the placebo patients the opportunity to receive active treatment in an open-label extension of the study for 2 years.

PROMISE

PROMISE was a Phase 3 three-year double-blind, placebo-controlled trial that enrolled 943 patients with primary progressive MS (PPMS).[94] The primary end-point was slowed accumulation of disability defined as 3-month sustained 1.0-point change in EDSS (entry EDSS 3.0–5.0) or 0.5 point EDSS increase (entry EDSS 5.5–6.5). A planned interim analysis revealed that no treatment effect was detectable and would not occur by study end. A non-significant delay in time to sustained disability was observed in GA-treated subjects compared with placebo ($P = 0.18$). In post-hoc analyses there was a significant decrease in Gd-enhancing lesions at year 1, and males treated with GA had a better survival curve than placebo-treated males (hazard ratio [HR] 0.71; $P = 0.02$). A consideration of why males appeared to respond favorably did not result in an obvious explanation.[95] It is possible that there is a gender difference in response to GA in PPMS patients but better studies are needed to prove a potential benefit.

Comparative trials
REGARD

REGARD (REbif vs. Glatiramer Acetate in Relapsing MS Disease) was a 96-week multicenter, randomized, parallel-group, open-label trial comparing subcutaneous IFNβ-1a ($n = 386$) vs. GA ($n = 378$) in treatment-naive patients meeting McDonald criteria for RRMS.[96] Baseline demographics were similar between the treatment groups with the exception that more patients in the GA group had two or more relapses in the prior two years and were more likely to have had steroids therapy in the previous six months.

The primary outcome measure, time to first relapse over 96 weeks expressed as a HR, showed no difference between treatments groups (HR 0.94; 95% CI 0.74–1.21; $P = 0.64$). The 30th percentile for time to first relapse was 495 days for the IFNβ-1a group and 432 days for the GA group. The mean number of new or enlarging T2 active lesions per patient per scan reached a plateau earlier in the IFNβ-1a group (24 weeks) than in the GA group (72 weeks). The mean number of Gd-enhancing lesions per patient per scan over 96 weeks was significantly less in the IFNβ-1a group than in the GA group ($P = 0.0002$).

BEYOND

The BEYOND trial (Betaseron Efficacy Yielding Outcome of a New Dose)[97] compared the efficacy, safety, and tolerability of 500 mcg IFNβ-1b with that of 250 mcg IFNβ-1b (the currently approved dose), and 20 mg daily GA. The study enrolled 2444 treatment-naive patients with RRMS and similar demographics in a 2:2:1 ratio (899 and 897 patients for the 500 mcg and 250 mcg IFNβ-1b groups, respectively, and 448 patients for the GA group). Patients were followed for at least two years with relapse risk as the primary outcome measure. Secondary outcomes included sustained EDSS progression and change in T1 hypointense lesion volume on MRI.

No differences were found among the three groups for the primary or secondary outcomes. Change in total MRI disease burden was significantly lower in both IFNβ-1b groups compared with the patients who received GA (high dose $P = 0.0008$; low dose $P = 0.0001$). The incidence of AEs and the rate of adherence were similar among the three groups.

Both the REGARD and BEYOND studies failed to show a difference in the primary clinical outcome measures of time to first relapse(REGARD) and relapse risk (BEYOND) between GA and approved IFNβ preparations. The point has been made that patients in both the BEYOND and REGARD trials had lower levels of on trial disease activity than expected, which might have compromised the ability to detect differences in efficacy. Nonetheless, on a practical level for clinical decision making, IFNβ and GA appear to have comparable clinical efficacy.[98]

MRI studies

MRI studies in the Phase 3 RRMS trial

The Phase 3 trial of GA in RRMS did not include study-wide, serial MRI data as secondary end-points of efficacy. Twenty-seven patients at one center underwent frequent MRI scans. A subsequent analysis of images from this site suggested a decrease in Gd-enhancing activity and reduced atrophy progression in GA-treated patients compared with placebo.[99]

Cross-sectional analysis of data from the extended, open-label follow-up of the US trial investigated the consequences of long-term GA treatment on several MRI markers of MS activity and disease burden.[100] Data from 135 patients (54% of the cohort of 251 patients originally enrolled) were analyzed. At the time of MRI follow-up, the mean duration of active drug exposure was 2433 days for patients originally randomized to GA and 1476 days for placebo group. Absolute and normalized CSF volumes were found to be significantly lower for the first group and the difference remained statistically significant after correcting for age, disability, and disease duration. This analysis suggested that long-term treatment with GA might prevent the loss of brain parenchyma in RRMS patients.

Italian MRI study

A small study followed monthly MRI changes in ten patients with RRMS.[101] Patients received monthly Gad-enhanced MRI scans for 9–27 months before starting GA therapy. Six of the subjects had scans for 25–27 months before initiation of treatment. Each patient then received monthly MRI for 10–14 additional months while on GA. The incidence of new Gd-enhancing lesions was decreased from 2.20 per month pre-treatment to 0.92 per month with GA treatment, presenting a non-significant ($P = 0.1$) 57% reduction.

European/Canadian MRI study

A randomized, double-blind, placebo-controlled MRI trial was conducted at 35 centers in Canada and Europe.[102] Patients were randomized to GA or placebo for nine months followed by an open-label phase for an additional nine months. MRI scans were performed monthly for the first nine months and every three months for the remaining nine months. Patients were required to have a diagnosis of RRMS with ≥1 relapses in the two years preceding enrollment and ≥1 Gd-enhancing lesion on a screening MRI scan. A total of 485 patients were screened, and 239 were enrolled in the study. The primary outcome measure was the number of Gd-enhancing lesions on T1-weighted images. Secondary endpoints included proportion of patients with Gd-enhancing lesions, Gd-enhancing lesion volume, number of new Gd-enhancing lesions, total number of lesions on T2-weighted images, number of new lesions on T2-weighted images, T1-hypointense lesion.

The nine-month double-blind data showed a 29% reduction in the mean number of Gd-enhancing lesions in the GA treated group (25.96) compared with placebo (36.8) ($P = 0.003$). The change in volume of Gd-enhancing lesions from baseline in the GA cohort was less than placebo ($P = 0.01$). Examined monthly, the cumulative Gd-enhancing lesion volume in GA-treated patients began to separate from the placebo group around month 5 and reached statistical significance in the third trimester. The mean number of new Gd-enhancing lesions was reduced by 33%, and the mean number of new T2 lesions was reduced by 33% ($P \leq 0.003$ for both) in the GA cohort. Change in total T2 lesion volume from baseline was lower for the GA patients ($P = 0.006$). The reduction in relapse rate was 33% ($P = 0.012$), consistent with the pivotal Phase 3 trial extension data. Although GA significantly reduced MRI disease activity and lesion burden, the effects appeared to take several months to develop and parallel the observed evolution of clinical effects.

An interesting analysis of MRI scans from the European/Canadian MRI Study[102] examined the proportion of new MS lesions evolving into T1 black holes.[84] In this study 1722 MRI lesions active at baseline in 239 patients were evaluated. Over the nine months of the double-blind phase, these lesions could be tracked for changes up to eight months from initial identification. GA-treated patients had fewer lesions evolving into black holes than placebo-treated patients at month 7 (18.9 vs. 26.3%; $P = 0.04$) and 8 (15.6 vs. 31.4%; $P = 0.002$). Typically, about 40% of new MS lesions result in persistent T1 black holes, which indicate more severe tissue destruction.[103–106]

Further analysis of data from the European/Canadian MRI Study assessed treatment effects on brain volume changes.[107] Image sets from 113 of 119 patients randomized to GA and 114 of 120 randomized to placebo were segmented for brain volume measurements from seven contiguous periventricular slices. Scans were analyzed at baseline, month 9, and month 18. Although a trend was observed for a treatment effect on slowing the progression of brain atrophy at 9 months,

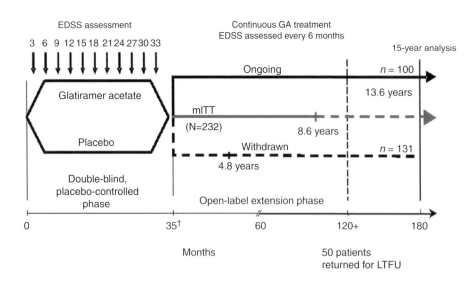

Fig. 26.1. Study design for the long-term study of patients who participated in the placebo-controlled study and were entered into the open-label study of GA. Patients on placebo in the placebo-controlled phase were switched to active treatment with GA in the open-label phase and those on GA in the placebo-controlled phase continued on it. At 15-year follow-up,[114] the mean durations of GA treatment were: ongoing cohort 13.6 years, modified intention-to-treat cohort 8.6 years, and withdrawn cohort 4.8 years. EDSS = Expanded Disability Status Scale, GA = glatiramer acetate, LTFU = long-term follow-up, MITT = modified intention-to-treat.

no statistically significant effects were noted. In a subsequent analysis, the images were re-assessed using a fully automated, normalized technique with whole brain coverage, the Structural Image Evaluation of Normalized Atrophy (SIENA) software.[108] A between-group difference favoring patients who had always been treated with GA was found to be significant over the entire study period.

Treatment effects on relapse rate and new MRI lesion activity are significant in this time frame,[101] and the lack of a significant effect on brain volume measures reinforces the possibility that control of inflammatory MS activity is only partly related to the subsequent development of brain atrophy.

BECOME

In the BECOME study (Betaseron vs. Copaxone in MS with Triple-Dose Gadolinium and 3-T MRI End-points), Cadavid *et al.* compared IFNβ-1b to GA using frequent 3T MRI, triple-dose Gd, and a 20–40 min delay to increase active lesion detection rate.[109] 75 treatment-naive patients with RRMS or CIS were randomized to every other day IFNβ-1b or daily GA subcutaneously and studied by monthly brain MRI for one year then optional monthly brain MRI during the second year. The primary endpoint was the number of combined active lesions (CALs), defined as the total of Gd-enhancing lesions plus new non-enhancing lesions on long repetition time scans that appeared since the most recent examination. New T2 lesions per subject in year 1 and through 2 years were secondary outcomes. MRI analysis was blinded to treatment. The sample size was selected to demonstrate superiority assuming a probability of 2/3 that a randomly chosen IFNβ-1b-treated patient would have fewer CALs than a randomly chosen GA patient based on prior monthly MRI studies. A sample size of 40 patients per arm was predicted to provide 74% power in two-sided testing at alpha = 0.05.

The primary and secondary outcomes were similar between the two groups. The CAL count per scan in months 1–12 was

0.63 for IFNβ-1b and 0.58 for GA (*P* = 0.58). The percentage of patients free of CALs during the first year showed no significant treatment difference. The number of new lesions showed a non-significant trend (*P* = 0.13) favoring GA (median 0.23 per month) compared to IFNβ-1b (0.46).

Using the BECOME data, Cadavid *et al.* studied new T1 black hole formation by examining every new Gd-enhancing lesion (NEL) for the corresponding acute black hole (ABH) and then following each ABH on all available MRI scans until they had resolved back to isointensity or to the last available scan.[110] The development of ABHs from NELs was similar with GA (65%) compared to IFNβ-1b (61%) (*P* = 0.21). The rate of conversion of ABHs to chronic black holes (CBHs) was 46% in the GA group and 37.5% with IFNβ-1b. The conversion rate of NELs to CBHs for the 849 NELs that had at least one year of follow-up was significantly lower with IFNβ-1b (47/480, 9.8%) than with GA (56/369, 15.2 %; *P* = 0.02).

Long-term studies
Open-label study of GA in MS over 15 years

At the end of the extension period of the Phase 3 trial of GA in RRMS, patients who had been on GA or placebo for up to 35 months were offered GA treatment in an open-label study, the design of which is shown in Fig. 26.1. Of the 251 patients enrolled in the core trial, 208 (82.8%) patients chose to continue. Data from this long-term treatment study at 6, 8, 10, and 15 years have been reported.[111–114] As of February 2008, 100 patients remained in the study for up to 15 years of therapy with only GA. These patients were followed at six-month intervals and reported to the study centers for evaluations of relapses, EDSS, and AEs. A total of 131 patients had left the study since inception.

This organized, prospective study is still ongoing, and all of the 11 original centers continue to participate. The 15-year follow-up data recently were reported.[114] The primary aim of

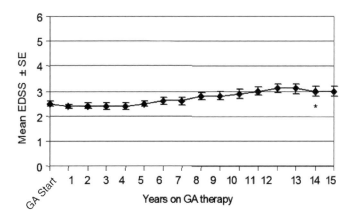

Fig. 26.2. Yearly mean Expanded Disability Status Scale (EDSS) scores for ongoing patients (*n* = 100) in the long-term glatiramer (GA) study at 15-year analysis.[114] The asterisk (*) indicates that yearly mean EDSS scores for years 14 and 15 are derived from scores of patients who were originally randomized to GA in the placebo-controlled phase of the study (*n* = 50).

this study was to determine the long-term effects of GA in carefully monitored patients who had received continuous GA for a mean of 13.6 years. A secondary goal was to gather information about patients who had withdrawn from the study. Patients were divided into several cohorts. The modified intention-to-treat (mITT) cohort included patients who had received at least one GA dose since study inception (*N* = 232). This cohort was subdivided into ongoing (continuing on GA) and withdrawn (those who left the study for any reason). At the time of the 15 year report, mean GA exposures were 8.6 ± 5.2, 4.81 ± 3.69, and 13.6 ± 1.3 years and mean disease durations were 17, 13, and 22 years for mITT, withdrawn and ongoing cohorts, respectively.

At the 15-year analysis, the ongoing cohort experienced a mean change in EDSS of 0.6 ± 2.0, the mITT 0.9 ± 1.8, and withdrawn 1.0 ± 0.7. While on GA, the percentages of patients who were improved or stable were similar in all groups 54% of the mITT, 57% of the ongoing, and 52% of the withdrawn.

Since EDSS scores and relapse rates were available for the 15-year follow-up, conversion to secondary progressive (SP) MS could be estimated. With a mean disease duration of 22 years, 35% of the ongoing cohort showed evidence of secondary progression, defined as an increase of >1.0 EDSS sustained for 12 months in the absence of relapses in that period.

Subjects were stratified into low (EDSS 0–2) and high (EDSS >2.0) disability strata at baseline and compared in a categorical analysis as stable or improved vs. worsened. At 15 years, the proportion of patients stable or improved in mITT cohort was 54.4 and 54.3 in the low and high EDSS strata, respectively. There were significant differences in the proportion of patients in these disability strata reaching landmark EDSS scores of 4, 6, and 8. In the low EDSS stratum of the mITT cohort, 25%, 9% and 1% reached EDSS thresholds of 4, 6, and 8 and in the high EDSS stratum, 61%, 34%, and 8% reached EDSS 4, 6, and 8, respectively. Overall, for this group of patients, there has been little change in disability over 15 years of therapy with GA. Yearly mean EDSS scores for the ongoing patient cohort out to year 15 are shown in Fig. 26.2. With 15 years of follow-up and neurological exams every 6 months, it was possible to construct life table, time to confirmed disability graphs. These showed that the time to reach EDSS 4, 6, and 8 is delayed in the ongoing cohort relative to the mITT cohort (Fig. 26.3).

The reasons given by patients for withdrawing from the study are summarized in Table 26.1. At an observational level, the patients on GA for up to 15 years had consistently low relapse rates and slow progression of disability. The alternative explanation to a long-term beneficial effect of GA for this group is that they were destined to have relatively mild MS. However, the baseline relapse rates and entry EDSS scores of the subjects in this study have been associated with significantly worse outcomes in natural history studies after more than 20 years with MS. Long-term safety assessments have not revealed any unusual or new concerns different from those reported in earlier studies. At the time of this review, the open-label trial was scheduled to end at 20 years in 2011.

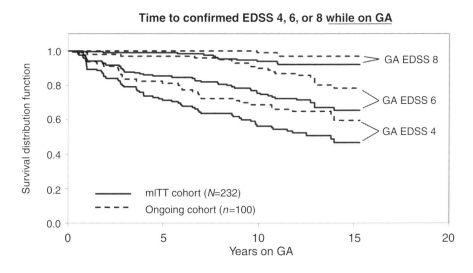

Fig. 26.3. Time to reach confirmed Expanded Disability Status Scale (EDSS) scores of 4, 6, or 8 for the modified intention-to-treat (mITT) and Ongoing cohorts while on GA therapy in the long-term glatiramer acetate study.[114] The mean disease durations at treatment initiation were: mITT cohort 8.3 years and for ongoing cohort 8.4 years.

Table 26.1. *Reasons for patient withdrawal from the long-term glatiramer acetate study.*[114]

Reason for withdrawal	N	Patient decision/ othersubcategories*	n
Total	132	Total	95
Lost-to-Follow-up	14	Patient perception of disease worsening	29
Adverse Event	23	Desire to switch or combine therapies	26
Patient Decision/Other	95	Difficulty, inability, or unwillingness to adhere to study protocol	32
		Pregnancy	8

* Patient decision/other subcategories were derived from written comments provided by withdrawn patients at their final visit.

This study is the longest continuous follow-up of any MS disease-modifying therapy and is unique in being prospectively designed and limited to subjects who have received only a single agent. It has inherent limitations, making it difficult to draw definitive conclusions about efficacy. Long-term studies cannot be performed with a control group and, with drop-outs over time, there is a selection bias favoring patients responding to the treatment and, thus, remaining in the study. A second limitation is the absence of a comparison group However, there is no practical or ethical way to obtain long-term efficacy data using a placebo group when effective treatments for a disease are available. Comparisons can be made to natural history data or to placebo groups from other clinical trials, but such comparisons are hazardous because studies are conducted differently, enroll diverse types of patients, and the outcome measures can be difficult to compare across trials. Despite inherent difficulties, carefully designed open-label studies remain the best alternative to placebo-controlled trials for obtaining long-term safety and efficacy data. This issue is discussed in detail elsewhere in this volume.

Long-term follow-up of the European/Canadian MRI trial

Clinical and MRI reappraisal of patients who completed the open-label extension phase of the European/Canadian MRI trial was conducted five years after study initiation.[115] The aim was to assess the potential impact of early treatment with GA in patients with active RRMS on the long-term evolution of clinical and imaging features of the disease.

After a mean of 5.8 years from trial initiation 142/224 (63.4%) patients who completed the original trial were evaluated. Age, disease duration, relapse rate in the prior two years, and EDSS score at baseline, and treatment disposition at follow-up did not differ between patients treated with GA and those treated with placebo during the core trial. There were 94 patients (66%) still treated with GA, 20 were taking IFNβ (mean

treatment duration 1.8 years), one patient was being treated with intravenous pulses of mitoxantrone, and the remaining seven were not taking any disease-modifying treatment for MS.

No significant difference was found for any MRI end-point comparing patients treated with GA or placebo during the double-blind phase of the trial. The frequency of patients who required walking aids was significantly lower in the group treated with GA from the beginning of the trial than in those randomized to placebo during the first nine months. This is partially counterbalanced by a modest trend for patient treated with GA from randomization to have a higher median EDSS score at follow-up and a greater likelihood of disability increase. Such contradictory findings indicate the need of further studies to ascertain the actual impact of an earlier treatment initiation on the long-term clinical prognosis of patients with active RRMS.[114]

Combination trials

Because GA has unique mechanisms of action, which differs from those of other MS disease therapies, use in combination with other agents might produce additive or synergistic therapeutic effects and better efficacy.[116,117] Since the recognition that both GA and the IFNβ have definite but partial efficacy in RRMS, the thought of combining the two drugs has been considered. Soos *et al.* tested GA and the IFNτ, a type I IFN, then GA and atorvastatin in combination in EAE mice models.[118] The combination of both therapy at suboptimal levels reconstituted clinical efficacy to a level comparable to that of the individual agents at optimal dose. A small in vitro study found that mitogen-induced T-cell activation was suppressed better by GA and IFNβ-1b together than by either drug alone.[119] However, in another study, CSJL/J F1 or SJL/J mice were given GA or saline before induction of EAE, and then treated with murine IFNα.[120] Mice receiving either GA or IFNα montherapy showed amelioration of EAE severity. Those receiving combination therapy developed EAE with a severity similar to untreated animals. A safety study showed that adding daily injections of GA to weekly IM IFNβ-1a was well tolerated, and no negative interactions were suggested by Gd-enhanced MRI data.[121] The National Institutes of Health and the National MS Society are currently funding CombiRx, the first large-scale multicenter clinical trial testing the combined use of intramuscular IFNβ-1a and GA in RRMS (discussed elsewhere in this volume).

GA is also being studied in combination with second-line MS disease-modifying drugs such as mitoxantrone in patients with very aggressive disease. The rationale of this combination is to promote transient immunosuppression with mitoxantrone and then allow reconstitution of the immune system in the presence of GA.[122–124] The treatment strategy involves initial use of a powerful immunosuppressant for as short a period as possible and once disease control is achieved, switch treatment to GA which has a better safety profile. Ramtahal and colleagues used mitoxantrone as an induction therapy followed by maintenance with GA in a non-randomized, uncontrolled observational case series and observed a 90% reduction in relapse rate.[125]

GA has been studied in combination with minocycline, an inhibitor matrix metalloproteinase-9 (MMP-9), which is believed to decrease the ability of leukocytes to cross the blood–brain barrier, in a 9-month multicenter, double–blind, placebo-controlled trial in 44 patients with RRMS.[126] Comparing GA plus minocycline vs. GA plus placebo, there was a 63% reduction in the total Gd-enhancing lesions at months 8 and 9 ($P = 0.08$), the primary end-point.

In a Phase 2 trial,[127] patients treated with GA for at least one year and who experienced at least one relapse in the previous year were randomized to receive either 300 mg of natalizumab monthly or placebo in addition to daily GA by subcutaneous injection. Combination therapy resulted in statistically significant fewer new active lesions and a lower mean number of new Gd-enhancing lesions over a 20-week period. The combination was well tolerated, and no significant adverse events were documented. However, with the emergence of cases of progressive multifocal leukoencephalopathy associated with use of natalizumab, the FDA recommended not to use it in combination with other MS disease modifying therapies.

Oral treatment with GA

The effects of oral GA were extensively studied in both rodents and primates in acute and chronic relapsing EAE models.[128–131] Teitelbaum *et al.* demonstrated that T-cells induced by either parenteral or oral GA administration were able to penetrate the CNS and function in situ as regulatory cells producing anti-inflammatory cytokines and neurotrophic factors.[131] However, a double-blind, placebo-controlled Phase 3 study of oral GA using 5 mg and 50 mg doses in RRMS patients yielded disappointing results, with no significant effect on the clinical and MRI outcomes.[132] Analysis of blood samples from these patients showed no changes expected with GA treatment, suggesting that orally administered GA either was not bioavailable to the systemic immune system or did not reach an effective bioactive dosage and was not effective clinically.

Conclusions

GA is one of the few drugs currently approved for use in MS that was directly derived from studies of EAE of the more than 100 compounds shown to prevent or ameliorate this animal model. It has proven therapeutic benefit in RRMS, based on a combination of immunodulatory effects. In vitro and animal studies also suggest GA may have neuroprotective effects. Although these findings are intriguing, more definitive evidence in humans is needed before a neuroprotective role of GA can be established. GA is well tolerated, a characteristic important for patients who typically require therapy for decades. The most common AE, injection site reactions, are typically minor and rarely a cause for discontinuing therapy. Transient post-injection reactions occur infrequently and have never been associated with serious sequelae. The demonstrated efficacy, tolerability, and safety of GA make it a legitimate first line drug choice for the treatment of RRMS. Its distinct mechanisms of action make it a reasonable option for patients with continued disease activity, intolerable side effects, or toxicity from other first-line therapies.

References

1. Gandhi R, Laroni A, Weiner HL. Role of the innate immune system in the pathogenesis of multiple sclerosis. *J Neuroimmunol* 2010;21:7–14.

2. Ewing C, Bernard CCA. Insights into the etiology and pathogenesis of multiple-sclerosis. *Immunol Cell Biol* 1998;76:47–54.

3. Allegretta M, Nicklas JA, Sriram S, Albertini RJ. T cells responsive to myelin basic protein in patients with multiple sclerosis. *Science* 1990;247:718–21.

4. Chou YK, Bourdette DN, Offner H, *et al.* Frequency of T cells specific for myelin basic protein and myelin proteolipid protein in blood and cerebrospinal fluid in multiple sclerosis. *J Neuroimmunol* 1992;38:105–14.

5. Hohlfeld R, Meinl E, Wever F, *et al.* The role of autoimmune T lymphocytes in the pathogenesis of multiple sclerosis. *Neurology* 1995;45:S33–8.

6. Jingwu Z, Medaer R, Hashim GA, *et al.* Myelin basic protein-specific T lymphocytes in multiple sclerosis and controls: precursor frequency, fine specificity, and cytotoxicity. *Ann Neurol* 1992;32:330–8.

7. Ota K, Matsui M, Milford EL, *et al.* T-cell recognition of an immunodominant myelin basic protein epitope in multiple sclerosis. *Nature* 1990;346:183–7.

8. Steinman L, Waisman A, Altmann D. Major T-cell responses in multiple sclerosis. *Molec Med Today* 1995;1:79–83.

9. Trapp BD, Peterson J, Ransohoff RM, Rudick R, Mork S, Bo L. Axonal transection in the lesions of multiple sclerosis. *N Engl J Med* 1998;338:278–85.

10. Bernard CCA, Mandel TE, MacKay IR. Experimental models of human autoimmune disease: overview and prototypes. In Rose NR, MacKay IR, eds. *The Autoimmune Diseases II.* San Diego: Academic Press, 1992:47–106.

11. Kerlero de Rosbo N, Mendel I, Ben-Nun A. Chronic relapsing experimental autoimmune encephalomyelitis with a delayed onset and an atypical clinical course, induced in PL/J mice by myelin oligodendrocyte glycoprotein (MOG)-derived peptide: preliminary analysis of MOG T cell epitopes. *Eur J Immunol* 1995;25:985–93.

12. Teitelbaum D, Meshorer A, Hirshfeld T, Arnon R, Sela M. Suppression of experimental allergic encephalomyelitis by a synthetic polypeptide. *Eur J Immunol* 1971;1:242–8.

13. Arnon R. The development of Cop 1 (Copaxone), an innovative drug for the treatment of multiple sclerosis: personal reflections. *Immunol Lett* 1996;50:1–15.

14. Teitelbaum D, Aharoni R, Sela M, Arnon R. Cross-reactions and specificities of monoclonal antibodies against myelin basic protein and against the synthetic copolymer 1. *Proc Natl Acad Sci USA* 1991;88:9528–32.

15. Einstein ER, Chao LP, Csejtey J, Kibler RF. Species specificity in response to tryptophan modified encephalitogen. *Immunochemistry* 1972;9:73–84.

16. Teitelbaum D, Meshorer A, Arnon R. Suppression of experimental allergic encephalomyelitis in baboons by Cop 1. *Isr J Med Sci* 1977;13:1038-.

17. Teitelbaum D, Webb C, Bree M, Meshorer A, Arnon R, Sela M. Suppression of experimental allergic encephalomyelitis in rhesus monkeys by a synthetic basic copolymer. *Clin Immunol Immunopathol* 1974;3: 256–62.

18. Lando Z, Teitelbaum D, Arnon R. Genetic control of susceptibility to experimental allergic encephalomyelitis in mice. *Immunogenetics* 1979;9:435–42.

19. Teitelbaum D, Webb C, Meshorer A, Arnon R, Sela M. Suppression by several synthetic polypeptides of experimental allergic encephalomyelitis induced in guinea pigs and rabbits with bovine and human basic encephalitogen. *Eur J Immunol* 1973;3:273–9.

20. Webb C, Teitelbaum D, Abramsky O, *et al.* Suppression of experimental allergic encephalomyelitis in Rhesus Monkeys by a synthetic basic copolymer [abstract]. *Isr J Med Sci* 1975;11:1388.

21. Bernard CCA, Kerlero de Rosbo N. Multiple sclerosis: an autoimmune disease of multifunctional etiology. *Curr Opin Immunol* 1992;4:760–5.

22. Teitelbaum D, Aharoni R, Arnon R, Sela M. Specific inhibition of the T-cell response to myelin basic protein by the synthetic copolymer Cop 1. *Proc Natl Acad Sci USA* 1988;85:9724–8.

23. Kerlero de Rosbo N, Mendel N, Milo R, Flechter S, Ben-Nun A. The autoimmune response to myelin oligodendrocyte glycoprotein (MOG) in multiple sclerosis and MOG-induced experimental autoimmune encephalomyelitis: effect of copolymer-1. *Eur J Neurol* 1996;3:57–8.

24. Teitelbaum D, Fridkis-Hareli M, Arnon R, Sela M. Copolymer 1 inhibits chronic relapsing experimental allergic encephalomyelitis induced by proteolipid protein (PLP) peptides in mice and interferes with PLP-specific T cell responses. *Neuroimmunology* 1996;64:209–17.

25. Arnon R, Sela M, Teitelbaum D. New insights into the mechanism of action of copolymer-1 in experimental allergic encephalomyelitis and multiple-sclerosis. *J Neurol* 1996;243(4/S1):S8-S13.

26. Aharoni R, Teitelbaum D, Sela M, Arnon R. Copolymer 1 induces T cells of the T helper type 2 that cross react with myelin basic protein and suppress experimental autoimmune encephalomyelitis. *Proc Natl Acad Sci USA* 1997;94:10821–6.

27. Webb C, Teitelbaum D, Herz A, Arnon R. Molecular requirements involved in suppression of EAE by synthetic basic copolymers of amino acids. *Immunochemistry* 1976;13:333–7.

28. Schrempf W, Ziemssen T. Glatiramer acetate: mechanisms of action in multiple sclerosis. *Autoimmun Rev* 2007;6:469–75.

29. Neuhaus O, Farina C, Wekerle H, Hohlfeld R. Mechanisms of action of glatiramer acetate in multiple sclerosis. *Neurology* 2001;56:702–8.

30. Arnon R, Aharoni R. Neuroprotection and neurogeneration in MS and its animal model EAE effected by glatiramer acetate. *J Neural Transm* 2009;116:1443–9.

31. Arnon R, Aharoni R. Neurogenesis and neuroprotection in the CNS–fundamental elements in the effect of glatiramer acetate on treatment of autoimmune neurological disorders. *Mol Neurobiol* 2007;36: 245–53.

32. Aharoni R, Arnon R, Eilam R. Neurogenesis and neuroprotection induced by peripheral immunomodulatory treatment of experimental autoimmune encephalomyelitis. *J Neurosci* 2005;25:8217–28.

33. Racke MK, Martin R, McFarland H, Fritz RB. Copolymer-1 induced inhibition of antigen-specific T cell activation: interference with antigen presentation. *Neuroimmunology* 1992;37:75–84.

34. Fridkis-Hareli M, Teitelbaum D, Gurevich E, *et al.* Direct binding of myelin basic-protein and synthetic copolymer-1 to class-II major histocompatibility complex-molecules on living antigen-presenting cells: specificity and promiscuity. *Proc Natl Acad Sci USA* 1994;91:4872–6.

35. Fridkis-Hareli M, Teitelbaum D, Rosbo K, Arnon R, Sela M. Synthetic copolymer 1 inhibits the binding of MBP, PLP and MOG peptides to class II major histocompatibility complex molecules on antigen-presenting cells. *J Neurochem* 1994;63(S1):S61.

36. Aharoni R, Teitelbaum D, Arnon R, Sela M. Copolymer 1 acts against the immunodominant epitope 82–100 of myelin basic protein by T cell receptor antagonism in addition to major histocompatibility complex blocking. *Proc Natl Acad Sci USA* 2005;96:634–639.

37. Gran B, Tranquill LR, Chen M. Mechanisms of immunomodulation by glatiramer acetate. *Neurology* 2000;55:1704–14.

38. Kim HJ, Ifergan I, Antel JP, *et al.* Type 2 monocyte and microglia differentiation mediated by glatiramer acetate therapy in patients with multiple sclerosis. *J Immunol* 2004;172:7144–53.

39. Weber MS, Hohlfeld R, Zamvil SS. Mechanism of action of glatiramer acetate in treatment of multiple sclerosis. *Neurotherapeutics* 2007;4:647–53.

40. Chabot S, Yong FP, Le DM, *et al.* Cytokine production in T lymphocyte-microglia interaction is attenuated by glatiramer acetate: a mechanism for therapeutic efficacy in multiple sclerosis. *Mult Scler* 2002;8:299–306.

41. Vieira PL, Heystek HC, Wormmeester J, Wierenga EA, Kapsenberg ML. Glatiramer acetate (copolymer-1, copaxone) promotes Th2 cell development and increased IL-10 production through modulation of dendritic cells. *J Immunol* 2003;170:4483–8.

42. Weber MS, Prod'homme T, Youssef S, *et al.* Type II monocytes modulate T cell-mediated central nervous system autoimmune disease. *Nat Med* 2007;13:935–43.

43. Allie R, Hu L, Mullen KM, Dhib-Jalbut S, Calabresi PA. Bystander Modulation of Chemokine Receptor Expression on Peripheral Blood T Lymphocytes Mediated by Glatiramer Acetate. *Arch Neurol* 2005;62:889–94.

44. Gur C, Karussis D, Golden E, Doron S, Ilan Y, Safadi R. Amelioration of experimental colitis by Copaxone is associated with class-II-restricted CD4

immune blocking. *Clin Immunol* 2006;118:307–16.

45. Zhang M, Chan CC, Vistica B, Hung V, Wiggert B, Gery I. Copolymer 1 inhibits experimental autoimmune uveoretinitis. *J Neuroimmunol* 2000;103:189–94.

46. Farina C, Then B.F., Albrecht H, *et al.* Treatment of multiple sclerosis with Copaxone (COP): Elispot assay detects COP-induced interleukin-4 and interferon-gamma response in blood cells. *Brain* 2001;124:705–19.

47. Duda PW, Schmied MC, Cook S.L., *et al.* Glatiramer acetate (Copaxone) induces degenerate, Th2-polarized immune responses in patients with multiple sclerosis. *J Exp Med* 2000;105:967–76.

48. Ragheb S, Abramczyk S, Lisak D, Lisak R. Long-term therapy with glatiramer acetate in multiple sclerosis: effect on T-cells. *Mult Scler* 2001;7:43–7.

49. Aharoni R, Teitelbaum D, Arnon R. T suppressor hybridomas and interleukin-2 dependent lines induced by copolymer 1 or by spinal cord homogenate down-regulate experimental allergic encephalomyelitis. *Eur J Immunol* 1993;23:17–25.

50. Aharoni R, Teitelbaum D, Sela M, Arnon R. Bystander suppression of experimental autoimmune encephalomyelitis by T-cell lines and clones of the Th2 type induced by copolymer-1. *J Neuroimmunol* 1998;91:135–46.

51. Wekerle H, Linington C, Lassmann H, Meyermann R. Cellular immune reactivity within the CNS. *Trend Neurosci* 1986;9:271–7.

52. Aharoni R., Teitelbaum D, Leitner O., *et al.* Specific Th2 cells accumulate in the central nervous system of mice protected against experimental autoimmune encephalomyelitis by copolymer 1. *Proc Natl Acad Sci USA* 2000;97:11472–7.

53. Qin Y, Zhang D, Prat A, Pouly S, Antel J. Characterization of T cell lines derived from glatiramer-acetate-treated multiple sclerosis patients. *J Neuroimmunol* 2000;108:201–6.

54. Becher B, Giacomini P, Pelletier D, *et al.* Interferon-gamma secretion by peripheral blood T-cell subsets in multiple sclerosis: Correlation with disease phase and interferon-beta

therapy. *Ann Neurol* 1999;45: 247–50.

55. Karandikar NJ, Crawford MP, Yan X. Glatiramer acetate (Copaxone) therapy induces CD8(+) T cell responses in patients with multiple sclerosis. *J Clin Invest* 2002;109:641–9.

56. Hafler DA. Degeneracy, as opposed to specificity, in immunotherapy. *J Clin Invest* 2002;109:581–4.

57. Aktas O, Ari N, Rieks M, *et al.* Multiple sclerosis: modulation of apoptosis susceptibility by glatiramer acetate. *Ann Neurol* 2001;104:266–70.

58. Rieks M, Hoffmann V, Aktas O, *et al.* Induction of apoptosis of CD4+ T cells by immunomodulatory therapy of multiple sclerosis by glatiramer acetate. *Eur Neurol* 2003;50:200–6.

59. Dabbert D., Rosner S, Kramer M, *et al.* Glatiramer acetate (copolymer-1)-specific, human T cell lines: cytokine profile and suppression of T cell lines reactive against myelin basic protein. *Neurosci Lett* 2000;289: 205–8.

60. Brenner T, Meiner Z, Abramsky O, *et al.* Humoral responses to copolymer-1 in multiple-sclerosis patients: preferential production of IgG1 over IgG2. *Ann Neurol* 1996;40:M111.

61. Teitelbaum D, Brenner T, Sela M, Arnon R. Antibodies to copolymer 1 do not interfere with its therapeutic effect (Abstract). *Eur J Neurol* 1996;3:134.

62. Brenner T, Arnon R, Sela M, *et al.* Humoral and cellular immune responses to Copolymer 1 in multiple sclerosis patients treated with Copaxone. *J Neuroimmunol* 2001;115:152–60.

63. Teitelbaum D, Brenner T, Abramsky O, *et al.* Antibodies to glatiramer acetate do not interfere with its biological functions and therapeutic efficacy. *Mult Scler* 2003;9:592–9.

64. Karussis D, Teitelbaum D, Sicsic C, Brenner T. Long-term treatment of multiple sclerosis with glatiramer acetate: natural history of the subtypes of anti-glatiramer acetate antibodies and their correlation with clinical efficacy. *J Neuroimmunol* 2010 Mar 30; 220:125–30.

65. Ure DR, Rodriguez M. Polyreactive antibodies to glatiramer acetate promote myelin repair in murine model of demyelinating disease. *FASEB J* 2002;16:1260–2.

66. Prat A. Lymphocyte migration and multiple sclerosis: relation with disease course and therapy. *Ann Neurol* 1999;46:253–6.

67. Dufour A, Corsini E, Gelati M, Massa G, Tarcic N, Salmaggi A. In vitro glatiramer acetate treatment of brain endothelium does not reduce adhesion phenomena. *Ann Neurol* 2000;47:680–2.

68. Chen M, Gran B, Costello K, *et al.* Glatiramer acetate induces a Th2-biased response and crossreactivity with myelin basic protein in patients with MS. *Mult Scler* 2001;7:209–19.

69. Arnon R, Aharoni R. Mechanism of action of glatiramer acetate in multiple sclerosis and its potential for the development of new applications. *Proc Natl Acad Sci USA* 2004;101(Suppl 2): 14593–8.

70. Kipnis J, Yoles E, Porat Z, *et al.* T cell immunity to copolymer 1 confers neuroprotection on the damaged optic nerve: possible therapy for optic neuropathies. *Proc Natl Acad Sci USA* 2000;97:7446–51.

71. Ziemssen T, Kumpfel T, Schneider H, Klinkert WEF, Neuhaus O, Hohlfeld R. Secretion of brain-derived neurotrophic factor by glatiramer acetate-reactive T-helper cell lines: Implications for multiple sclerosis therapy. *J Neurol Sci* 2005;233:109–12.

72. Stadelmann C, Kerschensteiner M, Misgeld T, Bruck W, Hohlfeld R, Lassmann H. BDNF and gp145trkB in multiple sclerosis brain lesions: neuroprotective interactions between immune and neuronal cells? *Brain* 2002;125:75–85.

73. Sarchielli P, Zaffaroni M, Floridi A, *et al.* Production of brain-derived neurotrophic factor by mononuclear cells of patients with multiple sclerosis treated with glatiramer acetate, interferon-beta 1a, and high doses of immunoglobulins. *Mult Scler* 2007;13:313–31.

74. Sarchielli P, Greco L, Stipa A, Floridi A, Gallai V. Brain-derived neurotrophic factor in patients with multiple sclerosis. *J Neuroimmunol* 2002;132:180–8.

75. Azoulay D, Vachapova V, Shihman B, Miler A, Karni A. Lower brain-derived neurotrophic factor in serum of relapsing remitting MS: reversal by

glatiramer acetate. *J Neuroimmunol* 2005;167:215–8.

76. Aharoni R, Eilam R, Domev H, *et al.* The immunomodulator glatiramer acetate augments the expression of neurotrophic factors in brains of experimental autoimmune encephalomyelitis mice. *Proc Natl Acad Sci USA* 2005;102:19045–50.

77. Gilgun-Sherki Y, Panet H, Holdengreber V, Mosberg-Galili R, Offen D. Axonal damage is reduced following glatiramer acetate treatment in C57/b1 mice with chronic-induced EAE. *Neurosci Res* 2003;47:201–7.

78. Khan O, Shen Y, Caon C, *et al.* Axonal metabolic recovery and potential neuroprotective effect of glatiramer acetate in relapsing-remitting multiple sclerosis. *Mult Scler* 2005;11:646–51.

79. Khan O, Shen Y, Bao F, *et al.* Long-term study of brain 1H-MRS study in multiple sclerosis: effect of glatiramer acetate therapy on axonal metabolic function and feasibility of long-Term H-MRS monitoring in multiple sclerosis. *J Neuroimaging* 2008;18:314–9.

80. Sarchielli P, Presciutti O, Tarducci R, *et al.* 1H-MRS in patients with multiple sclerosis undergoing treatment with interferon beta-1a: results of a preliminary study. *J Neurol Neurosurg Psychiatry* 1998;64:204–12.

81. Parry A, Corkill R, Blamire AM, *et al.* Beta-Interferon treatment does not always slow the progression of axonal injury in multiple sclerosis. *J Neurol* 2003;250:171–8.

82. Toprak MK, Cakir B, Ulu EM, *et al.* The effects of interferon beta-1a on proton MR spectroscopic imaging in patients with multiple sclerosis, a controlled study, preliminary results. *Int J Neurosci* 2008;118:1645–58.

83. Narayanan S, De SN, Francis GS, *et al.* Axonal metabolic recovery in multiple sclerosis patients treated with interferon beta-1b. *J Neurol* 2001;248:979–86.

84. Filippi M, Rovaris M, Rocca MA, *et al.* Glatiramer acetate reduces the proportion of new MS lesions evolving into "black holes". *Neurology* 2001;57:731–3.

85. McRae BL, Vanderlugt CL, Dal Canto MC, Miller SD. Functional evidence for epitope spreading in the relapsing pathology of experimental autoimmune encephalomyelitis. *J Exp Med* 1995;182:75–85.

86. Abramsky O, Teitelbaum D, Arnon R. Effect of a synthetic polypeptide (Cop 1) on patients with multiple sclerosis and with acute disseminated encephalomyelitis. *J Neurol Sci* 1977;31:433–8.

87. Bornstein MB, Miller AI, Teitelbaum D, Arnon R, Sela M. Multiple sclerosis: trial of a synthetic polypeptide. *Ann Neurol* 1982;11:317–19.

88. Bornstein MB, Miller AI, Slagle S, *et al.* A pilot trial of Cop 1 in exacerbating-remitting multiple sclerosis. *N Engl J Med* 1987;317:408–14.

89. Kurtzke JF. On the evaluation of disability in multiple sclerosis. *Neurology* 1961;11:686–94.

90. Bornstein MB, Miller AI, Slagle S. A placebo-controlled, double-blind, randomized, two-center, pilot trial of Cop 1 in chronic progressive multiple sclerosis. *Neurology* 1991;41:533–9.

91. Johnson KP, Brooks BR, Cohen JA, *et al.* Copolymer 1 reduces relapse rate and improves disability in relapsing-remitting multiple sclerosis: results of a phase III multicenter, double-blind, placebo-controlled trial. *Neurology* 1995;45:1268–76.

92. Johnson KP, Brooks BR, Cohen JA, *et al.* Extended use of glatiramer acetate (Copaxone) is well tolerated and maintains its clinical effect on multiple sclerosis relapse rate and degree of disability. *Neurology* 1998;50:701–8.

93. Comi G, Martinelli V, Rodegher, M, *et al.* Effect of glatiramer acetate on conversion to clinically definite multiple sclerosis in patients with clinically isolated syndrome (PreCISe study): a randomised, double-blind, placebo-controlled trial. *Lancet* 2009;374: 1503–1511.

94. Wolinsky JS, Narayana PA, O'Connor P, *et al.* Glatiramer acetate in primary progressive multiple sclerosis: results of a multinational, multicenter, double-blind, placebo-controlled trial. *Ann Neurol* 2007;61:14–24.

95. Wolinsky JS, Shochat T, Weiss S, Ladkani D. Glatiramer acetate treatment in PPMS: why males appear to respond favorably. *J Neurol Sci* 2009;286:92–8.

96. Mikol DD, Barkhof F, Chang P, *et al.* Comparison of subcutaneous interferon beta-1a with glatiramer acetate in patients with relapsing multiple sclerosis (the REbif vs Glatiramer Acetate in Relapsing MS Disease [REGARD] study): a multicentre, randomised, parallel, open-label trial. *Lancet Neurol* 2008;7:903–14.

97. O'Connor P, Filippi M, Arnason B, *et al.* 250 microg or 500 microg interferon beta-1b versus 20 mg glatiramer acetate in relapsing-remitting multiple sclerosis: a prospective, randomised, multicentre study. *Lancet Neurol* 2009;8:889–97.

98. Achiron A, Fredrikson S. Lessons from randomised direct comparative trials. *J Neurol Sci* 2009;277(Suppl 1):S19–S24.

99. Ge Y, Grossman RI, Udupa JK, *et al.* Glatiramer acetate (Copaxone) treatment in relapsing-remitting MS: quantitative MR assessment. *Neurology* 2000;54:813–7.

100. Wolinsky JS, Narayana P, Johnson KP, *et al.* US open-label glatiramer acetate extention trial for relapsing multiple sclerosis: MRI and clinical correlates. *Mult Scler* 2001;7:33–41.

101. Mancardi GL, Sardanelli F, Parodi RC. Effect of copolymer-1 on serial gadolinium-enhanced MRI in relapsing remitting multiple sclerosis. *Neurology* 1998;50:1127–33.

102. Comi G, Filippi M, Wolinsky JS, *et al.* European/Canadian multicenter, double-blind, randomized, placebo-controlled study of the effects of glatiramer acetate on magnetic resonance imaging–measured disease activity and burden in patients with relapsing multiple sclerosis. European/Canadian Glatiramer Acetate Study Group. *Ann Neurol* 2001;49:290–7.

103. van Walderveen MA, Barkhof F, Hommes OR, *et al.* Correlating MRI and clinical disease activity in multiple sclerosis: relevance of hypointense lesions on short-TR/short-TE (T1-weighted) spin-echo images. *Neurology* 1995;45:1684–90.

104. van Walderveen MA, Truyen L, van Oosten BW, *et al.* Development of hypointense lesions on T1-weighted spin-echo magnetic resonance images in multiple sclerosis: relation to inflammatory activity. *Arch Neurol* 1999;56:345–51.

105. van Walderveen MA, Kamphorst W, Scheltens P, *et al.* Histopathologic

correlate of hypointense lesions on T1-weighted spin-echo MRI in multiple sclerosis. *Neurology* 1998;50:1282–8.

106. Bruck W, Bitsch A, Kolenda H, *et al.* Inflammatory central nervous system demyelination: correlation of magnetic resonance imaging findings with lesion pathology. *Ann Neurol* 1997;42:783–93.

107. Rovaris M, Comi G, Rocca MA, *et al.* Short-term brain volume change in relapsing-remitting multiple sclerosis: effect of glatiramer acetate and implications. *Brain* 2001;124:1803–12.

108. Sormani M, Rovaris M, Valsasina P, Wolinsky JS, Comi G, Filippi M. Measurement error of two different techniques for brain atrophy assessment in multiple sclerosis. *Neurology* 2004;62:1432–4.

109. Cadavid D, Wolansky LJ, Skurnick J, *et al.* Efficacy of treatment of MS with IFNbeta-1b or glatiramer acetate by monthly brain MRI in the BECOME study. *Neurology* 2009;72:1976–83.

110. Cadavid D, Cheriyan J, Skurnick J, *et al.* New acute and chronic black holes in patients with multiple sclerosis randomised to interferon beta-1b or glatiramer acetate. *J Neurol Neurosurg Psychiatry* 2009;80:1337–43.

111. Ford CC, Johnson KP, Lisak RP, *et al.* A prospective open-label study glatiramer acetate: Over a decade of continuous use in MS patients. *Mult Scler* 2006;12:309–320.

112. Johnson KP, Brooks BR, Ford CC, *et al.* Sustained clinical benefits of glatiramer acetate in relapsing multiple sclerosis patients observed for 6 years. Copolymer 1 Multiple Sclerosis Study Group. *Mult Scler* 2000;6:255–66.

113. Johnson KP, Ford CC, Lisak RP, Wolinsky JS. Neurologic consequence of delaying glatiramer acetate therapy for multiple sclerosis: 8-year data. *Acta Neurol Scand* 2005;111:42–7.

114. Ford C, Goodman AD, Johnson K, *et al.* Continuous long-term immunomodulatory therapy in relapsing multiple sclerosis: results from the 15-year analysis of the US prospective open-label study of glatiramer acetate. *Mult Scler* 2010;16:342–50.

115. Rovaris M, Comi G, Rocca MA, *et al.* Long-term follow-up of patients treated with glatiramer acetate: a multicentre, multinational extension of the European/Canadian double-blind, placebo-controlled, MRI-monitored trial. *Mult Scler* 2007;13:502–8.

116. Costello F, Stuve O, Weber MS, Zamvil SS, Frohman E. Combination therapies for multiple sclerosis: scientific rationale, clinical trials, and clinical practice. *Curr Opin Neurol* 2007;20:281–5.

117. Tullman MJ, Lublin FD. Combination therapy in multiple sclerosis. *Curr Neurol Neurosci Rep* 2005;5:245–8.

118. Soos JM, Stuve O, Youssef S, *et al.* Cutting edge: oral type I IFN-tau promotes a Th2 bias and enhances suppression of autoimmune encephalomyelitis by oral glatiramer acetate. *J Immunol* 2002;169:2231–5.

119. Milo R, Panitch HS. Additive effects of copolymer-1 and interferon beta-1b on the immune responses to myelin basic protein. *J Neuroimmunol* 1995;61:185–93.

120. Brod SA, Lindsey JW, Wolinsky JS. Combination therapy with glatiramer acetate (copolymer-1) and a type I interferon (IFN-alpha) does not improve experimental autoimmune encephalomyelitis. *Ann Neurol* 2000;47:127–31.

121. Lublin F, Cutter G, Elfont R, *et al.* A trial to assess the safety of combining therapy with interferon beta-1a and glatiramer acetate in patients with relapsing MS. *Neurology* 2001;56(Suppl 3):A148.

122. Rieckmann P, Toyka KV, Bassetti C, *et al.* Escalating immunotherapy of multiple sclerosis–new aspects and practical application. *J Neurol* 2004;251:1329–39.

123. Maurer M, Rieckmann P. Relapsing–remitting multiple sclerosis: what is the potential for combination therapy? *BioDrugs* 2000;13:149–58.

124. Rieckmann P. Concepts of induction and escalation therapy in multiple sclerosis. *J Neurol Sci* 2009;277(Suppl 1):S42-S45.

125. Ramtahal J, Jacob A, Das K, Boggild M. Sequential maintenance treatment with glatiramer acetate after mitoxantrone is safe and can limit exposure to immunosuppression in very active, relapsing remitting multiple sclerosis. *J Neurol* 2006;253:1160–4.

126. Metz LM, Li D, Traboulsee A, *et al.* Glatiramer acetate in combination with minocycline in patients with relapsing–remitting multiple sclerosis: results of a Canadian, multicenter, double-blind, placebo-controlled trial. *Mult Scler* 2009;15:1183–94.

127. Goodman AD, Rossman H, Bar-Or A, *et al.* GLANCE: results of a phase 2, randomized, double-blind, placebo-controlled study. *Neurology* 2009;72:806–12.

128. Higgins PH, Weiner HL Suppression of experimental autoimmune encephalomyelitis by oral administration of myelin basic protein and its fragments. *J Immunol* 1998;140:440–5.

129. Al-Sabbagh, Miller A, Santos LM, Weiner HL. Antigen-driven tissue-specific suppression following oral tolerance: orally administered myelin basic protein suppresses proteolipid protein-induced experimental autoimmune encephalomyelitis in SJL mouse. *Eur J Immunol* 1994;24:2104–9.

130. Maron R, Slavin AJ, Hoffmann E, Komagata Y, Weiner HL. Oral tolerance to copolymer 1 in myelin basic protein (MBP) TCR transgenic mice: cross reactivity with MBP-specific TCR and differential induction of anti-inflammatory cytokines. *Int Immunol* 2002;14:131–8.

131. Teitelbaum D, Aharoni R, Klinger E, *et al.* Oral Glatiramer Acetate in Experimental Autoimmune Encephalomyelitis. *Ann NY Acad Sci* 2004;1029:239–49.

132. Filippi M, Wolinsky JS, Comi G. Effects of oral glatiramer acetate on clinical and MRI-monitored disease activity in patients with relapsing multiple sclerosis: a multicentre, double-blind, randomised, placebo-controlled study. *Lancet Neurol* 2006;5:213–20.

Chapter

27 Natalizumab to treat multiple sclerosis

Chris H. Polman, Joep Killestein, and Richard A. Rudick

Introduction

The inflammatory process that leads to demyelination and axonal injury in patients with relapsing multiple sclerosis (MS) has been shown to be closely linked to the infiltration of leukocytes into the central nervous system (CNS).[1–3] The accumulation of lymphocytes and monocytes in the CNS is a highly regulated process involving factors that promote migration across the blood–brain barrier and that support leukocyte proliferation and survival within the CNS.[3] The expression of activated adhesion molecules on the surface of lymphocytes and monocytes is required for migration across the blood–brain barrier. One such adhesion molecule is $\alpha4\beta1$ integrin, a glycoprotein expressed on the surface of activated lymphocytes, monocytes, mast cells, macrophages, basophils and eosinophils (but not neutrophils).[4] A major ligand for $\alpha4\beta1$ integrin is vascular cell adhesion molecule 1 (VCAM-1), which is expressed on the surface of vascular endothelial cells (including those of the brain and spinal cord blood vessels).[4,5] Expression of both $\alpha4\beta1$ integrin and VCAM-1 has been shown to be increased in chronic MS plaques.[5] Under the control of proinflammatory cytokines, activation of $\alpha4\beta1$ integrin and its interaction with VCAM-1 mediate the adhesion and passage of activated lymphocytes and monocytes into inflamed areas of the CNS.[4,6–8] The interaction of $\alpha4\beta1$ integrin with additional ligands, such as fibronectin[4] and osteopontin,[9] may modulate survival, priming or activation of leukocytes that have gained access to CNS parenchyma, further contributing to the inflammation cascade.

Natalizumab (Tysabri®; Biogen Idec, Cambridge, MA and Elan Pharmaceuticals, San Francisco, CA) is a recombinant humanized $\alpha4$ integrin antibody derived from a murine monoclonal antibody to human $\alpha4\beta1$ integrin, and is the first agent in a new class of selective adhesion molecule inhibitors for the treatment of relapsing MS.[10] Natalizumab (300 mg by intravenous (IV) infusion every 4 weeks) was approved in the United States in November 2004 for the treatment of patients with relapsing MS to reduce the frequency of clinical relapses.[10] In February 2005, marketing and clinical trial dosing of natalizumab were suspended by the manufacturers after they were notified of two cases of progressive multifocal leukoencephalopathy (PML) in patients with MS and a third

patient with Crohn's disease, all of whom had received natalizumab in clinical trials. Following an extensive safety evaluation, which found no new cases of PML in patients treated with natalizumab,[11] a Food and Drug Administration (FDA) advisory panel recommended in March 2006 that natalizumab again be approved for clinical use for the treatment of relapsing MS and it was subsequently approved for use in June 2006.

As of July 2011, PML has been confirmed in 145 MS patients on natalizumab, and the incidence of PML in MS patients who have had 24 or more natalizumab infusions was estimated to be at least one case per 1000 patients. Although the efficacy of natalizumab has revolutionized the management of MS patients, its widespread use is limited by the risk of PML. This is further complicated by the lack of accurate predictive markers for PML that can be used in the individual natalizumab-treated MS patient to guide therapy decisions. Therefore, use of natalizumab requires a careful risk–benefit analysis for each individual patient.

This chapter provides an overview of natalizumab, describes its pharmacokinetic and pharmacodynamic profile, and summarizes efficacy and safety results to date from clinical trials and post-marketing surveillance in MS, including the occurrence and management of PML.

Background on natalizumab

Natalizumab binds to the $\alpha4$ subunit of $\alpha4\beta1$ and $\alpha4\beta7$ integrins, blocking binding to their endothelial receptors (VCAM-1 and mucosal-addressing cell adhesion molecule 1, respectively) and attenuating inflammation by preventing the transmigration of lymphocytes across the endothelium into the parenchymal tissue. Although it is not fully known how natalizumab exerts its effects in relapsing MS, it may exert dual anti-inflammatory effects by both inhibiting trafficking of immune cells into inflamed tissue and suppressing existing inflammatory activity at the disease site.[12] The latter is achieved by three potential mechanisms of action. The first is through blockade of migration of lymphocytes into the CNS by inhibiting adhesion to endothelial cells and interaction with extracellular matrix proteins (e.g. fibronectin). The second is through blockade of

Multiple Sclerosis Therapeutics, Fourth Edition, ed. Jeffrey A. Cohen and Richard A. Rudick. Published by Cambridge University Press.
© Cambridge University Press 2011.

priming of lymphocytes in the parenchyma by inhibiting adhesion to osteopontin and VCAM-1 expressed on microglial cells and monocytes in situ. Finally, natalizumab may induce apoptosis of α4 integrin-expressing lymphocytes by blocking their interaction with extracellular matrix proteins (e.g. fibronectin).

Preclinical studies

Several preclinical studies evaluated the activity of α4β1 integrin antibody in preventing or reversing experimental autoimmune encephalomyelitis (EAE), the animal model of MS.[13,16] In a guinea-pig model, treatment with AN100226m, the mouse antibody against human α4 integrin, suppressed the pathological features of EAE during active disease in the brain and spinal cord, with rapid reductions in the degree of leukocyte infiltration into the CNS compared with control animals.[14] Importantly, demyelination was not observed in AN100226m-treated animals, although control animals showed early stages of demyelination with myelin damage in the white matter fasciculi.[14] In the first preclinical study to evaluate the activity of α4β1 integrin antibody using magnetic resonance imaging (MRI), treatment with AN100226m in a guinea-pig model was effective in decreasing the permeability of the blood–brain barrier (as evidenced by edema dissipation) and reversing MRI-detectable signs of EAE.[13] Together, these two studies indicated activity of AN100226m in decreasing the permeability of the blood–brain barrier, clearing edema and inflammatory cells from the lesion site, and preventing further damage to the CNS.

Given these promising preclinical findings, a humanized form of the antibody was developed to reduce antigenicity and allow chronic human treatment. Therefore, a separate in vitro analysis was conducted to establish whether the humanized form of AN100226m, AN100226, was as strong an inhibitor of α4β1 integrin as the murine antibody.[16] Indeed, both monoclonal antibodies produced nearly the exact inhibitory effects on α4β1 integrin-expressing cells. Further in vivo testing in guinea-pig models confirmed that humanized AN100226 was as active as AN100226m in reversing the clinical symptoms of active EAE and resulted in leukocyte clearance from the CNS.[16] These findings served as the basis for evaluating the safety and efficacy of humanized AN100226 (natalizumab) in clinical studies of patients with MS.

Pharmacokinetics and pharmacodynamics

The pharmacokinetics of a single i.v. dose of natalizumab were studied in a phase 1, dose-escalation study in 28 MS patients.[17] Serum drug concentrations indicated that the lowest two doses (0.03 mg/kg and 0.1 mg/kg) were insufficient to maintain therapeutic drug levels, with serum concentrations rapidly falling below detectable limits after the completion of drug infusion in these groups. Detectable serum drug concentrations were also only observed for one week in patients receiving the 0.3 mg/kg dose. In contrast, patients who received natalizumab 1.0 mg/kg or 3.0 mg/kg had detectable serum concentrations for 3–8

weeks. Serum concentrations of natalizumab showed a biphasic decline, with a rapid distribution phase followed by a prolonged terminal phase. Maximal plasma concentration and plasma elimination half-life were generally dose proportional. The mean plasma elimination half-life was 4.5 days (108.0 ± 30.1 hours) for the highest dose evaluated (3.0 mg/kg). Phase 2, repeat-dosing studies demonstrated minimal drug accumulation with repeated natalizumab dosing.[18,19] Natalizumab therapy does not appear to alter the pharmacokinetics of concomitantly administered interferon beta-1a (IFNβ-1a) and vice versa.[20]

The US prescribing information for natalizumab reports pharmacokinetic parameters following repeat administration of the approved dose (300 mg i.v. infusion) in patients with MS. The mean maximum observed serum concentration was 110 ± 52 μg/ml, and the mean average steady-state natalizumab concentrations over the dosing period ranged from 23 to 29 μg/ml. The observed time to steady stage was approximately 24 weeks after every 4 weeks of dosing. In addition, the mean plasma elimination half-life was 11 ± 4 days, with a clearance of 16 ± 5 ml/hour.

Maximal saturation (defined as > 80% saturation) of lymphocyte cell-surface α4 integrin receptors occurs 24 hours after the administration of single i.v. natalizumab doses of 1.0–6.0 mg/kg. Following a single natalizumab dose of 1.0, 3.0, or 6.0 mg/kg, receptor saturation is maintained for 1, 3–4 or 6 weeks, respectively. The infusion of 300 mg of natalizumab every 4 weeks resulted in sustained α4 integrin receptor saturation levels above 70% throughout a 116-week dosing period. The administration of natalizumab with IFNβ did not significantly alter receptor saturation.

Consistent with its mechanism of action, the administration of natalizumab increases the number of circulating leukocytes (except neutrophils) due to inhibition of their transmigration out of the vascular space. In MS patients treated with natalizumab 300 mg i.v. administered once every 4 weeks for 116 weeks, increases in lymphocytes, monocytes, eosinophils, and basophils were observed, without elevations in neutrophils. The mean total lymphocyte count in the natalizumab group was 3.44 × 10⁹/l at week 12, and continued to increase to 3.72 × 10⁹/l at week 24, after which time the mean count reached a plateau. The mean lymphocyte count remained within the normal range (0.91 × 10⁹ –4.28 × 10⁹/l) throughout the 116-week treatment period. In addition, transient increases in nucleated red blood cells were observed in a small number of patients. All changes were reversible, were without evident clinical effects and returned to baseline levels usually within 16 weeks after the last dose.[21]

Recently, an interesting though not yet completely understood phenomenon potentially related to the pharmacokinetics and dynamics of natalizumab was reported,[22] natalizumab exchanges Fab arms with endogenous human IgG4.[22] The ability of a therapeutic IgG4 antibody to engage with plasma IgG4 could have substantial biological consequences that may affect pharmacokinetics and pharmacodynamics. For

Table 27.1. *Efficacy results from Phase 2, randomized, double-blind, placebo-controlled studies of natalizumab in patients with relapsing multiple sclerosis*

Reference	Treatment	Assessment time-point	Mean no. new active lesions	Mean no. new Gd+ lesions	Patients with no new Gd+ lesions (%)	Patients with relapses (%)
Turbidy *et al.* 1999[18]	Natalizumab 3.0 mg/kg (n = 37)	12 weeks	1.8[‡]	1.6[†]	83.6[‡]	24
	Placebo (n = 35) (each administered at weeks 0 and 4)		3.6	3.3	73.1	30
Miller *et al.* 2003[19]	Natalizumab 3.0 mg/kg (n = 68)	24 weeks	0.8*	0.7*	75	19[†]
	Natalizumab 6.0 mg/kg (n = 74)		1.3*	1.1*	65	19[†]
	Placebo (n = 71) (each administered every 28 days x 6 months)		9.7	9.6	32	38

*P < 0.001 vs. placebo; [†] P ≤ 0.02 vs. placebo; [‡] P < 0.05 vs. placebo; Gd+, gadolinium-enhancing.

example, Fab arm exchange could offer an explanation for half-life discrepancies between manufacturers' claims (11 days as described above) and certain patient studies (4–5 days).[17,23] However, other mechanisms (e.g. assays used, antidrug antibodies) may also contribute to the observed differences. The clinical relevance of Fab-arm exchange should be further explored for natalizumab.[22]

Pre-registration studies

Phase 1 studies

As part of the clinical trial program to establish the pharmacokinetic/ pharmacodynamic and safety profiles of natalizumab, four Phase 1, dose-finding studies were conducted – one in healthy volunteers and the other three in patients with relapsing MS.[12] All of the Phase 1 studies evaluated natalizumab doses ranging from 0.03 to 6.0 mg/kg; the pharmacokinetic/ pharmacodynamic data from these trials are described in the previous section. These trials also provided important initial safety data for natalizumab in humans, showing natalizumab to be safe and well tolerated, with an adverse event profile similar to that with placebo. In addition, these studies helped to identify the most appropriate dose of natalizumab for clinical evaluation in Phase 2 studies.[12]

Phase 2 studies

Three randomized, double-blind, placebo-controlled Phase 2 studies were conducted.[18,19,24] The overall findings from the studies indicate that natalizumab is effective in reducing inflammatory lesions as visualized by MRI, and in decreasing the relapse rate compared with placebo in patients with relapsing MS (Table 27.1).

Turbidy *et al.* conducted a Phase 2 randomized, double-blind, parallel-group study that evaluated natalizumab in patients with relapsing–remitting or secondary progressive MS.[18] Patients received natalizumab 3.0 mg/kg (n = 37) or

placebo (n = 35) at weeks 0 and 4, and were followed up for 24 weeks with serial MRI and clinical assessment. The mean number of new active lesions (adjusted mean, 1.8 vs. 3.6; P = 0.042) and new enhancing lesions (adjusted mean, 1.6 vs. 3.3; P = 0.017) within the first 12 weeks of treatment (primary endpoint) were significantly lower in the natalizumab group.

In the next study, O'Connor *et al.* set out to determine whether natalizumab was useful in the setting of acute MS relapse.[24] In a randomized, double-blind, multicenter study, patients with relapsing–remitting or secondary progressive MS were randomly assigned to receive natalizumab 1.0 mg/kg (n = 57), natalizumab 3.0 mg/kg (n = 60), or placebo (n = 63), administered as a single IV infusion within 96 hours of the start of a relapse. Patients were followed for 14 weeks post-treatment. There was a reduction in the volume of gadolinium (Gd)-enhancing lesions in both natalizumab groups compared with the placebo group (P = 0.05).

A Phase 2b randomized, double-blind, multicenter study, conducted by Miller *et al.* evaluated the efficacy of six natalizumab infusions as compared with placebo in patients with relapsing–remitting or secondary progressive MS(19). Eligible patients were 18–65 years of age, had at least two relapses within the past 2 years, had an EDSS score of 2.0–6.5 and had at least three lesions on T2-weighted MRI scans of the brain. Patients were excluded if they had experienced a relapse within the preceding 30 days or had received immunosuppressants or immunomodulating treatments within the preceding 3 months. Eligible patients were randomly assigned to receive natalizumab 3.0 mg/kg (n = 68), 6.0 mg/kg (n = 74), or placebo (n = 71). Each infusion was administered every 28 days for 6 months. Baseline clinical and MRI characteristics were similar among groups. The number of new Gd-enhancing lesions per patient during the 6-month treatment period (primary endpoint) was significantly lower for both doses of natalizumab compared with placebo (natalizumab 3.0 mg/kg, 0.7; natalizumab 6.0 mg/kg, 1.1; placebo, 9.6) (P < 0.001 for both doses of natalizumab vs. placebo). Compared with the placebo group, patients treated with natalizumab had significantly fewer persistent Gd-enhancing lesions per patient (natalizumab 3.0 mg/kg, 0.8; natalizumab 6.0 mg/kg, 1.3; placebo, 3.6; $P \leq$ 0.005 for both doses of natalizumab vs. placebo), fewer new active lesions per patient (0.8, 1.3, and 9.7, respectively; $P <$ 0.001 vs. placebo) and a lower percentage of scans showing activity (9%, 11% and 39%, respectively; $P < 0.001$ vs. placebo). Nineteen per cent of patients in each natalizumab group experienced a relapse compared with 38% of placebo patients ($P = 0.02$ for both doses of natalizumab vs. placebo). This higher relapse rate in the placebo group resulted in a greater need for corticosteroid treatment in the placebo group (81% of the patients) compared with the natalizumab 3.0 mg/kg group (38% of the patients; $P < 0.001$) or the natalizumab 6.0 mg/kg group (50% of the patients; $P = 0.002$). Patients' well-being, as measured on a 100 mm visual analog scale, was significantly decreased from baseline in the placebo group (-1.38 mm), but significantly improved from baseline in the natalizumab 3.0 mg/kg group ($+9.49$ mm; $P = 0.04$) and the natalizumab 6.0 mg/kg group ($+6.21$ mm; $P = 0.03$). The Miller study included a six-month follow-up period to determine whether MS disease activity rebounded to a level higher than the control group following natalizumab discontinuation. There was no clear rebound disease activity on either clinical or MRI measures.

A subanalysis of the Miller *et al.* data suggested that natalizumab also suppressed evolution of new Gd-enhancing lesions to T1-hypointense lesions.[25] In this post-hoc analysis, which was conducted on data from a subset of patients who had at least one new Gd-enhancing lesion during the six-month study period, conversion of these lesions to new T1-hypointense lesions was assessed at month 12 of follow-up. Natalizumab produced significant decreases relative to placebo on the following measures: the proportion of patients with new Gd-enhancing lesions that evolved into T1-hypointense lesions (26% vs. 68%; $p < 0.01$); the proportion of patients developing large T1-hypointense lesions (5% vs. 40%; $P < 0.01$); the proportion of new Gd-enhancing lesions that became T1 hypointense (15% vs. 25%; $P = 0.045$); the mean proportion per patient of new Gd-enhancing lesions that converted to T1-hypointense lesions (0.15 vs. 0.28; $P = 0.005$); and the risk of converting from Gd-enhancing to T1-hypointense lesions (odds ratio 0.48, 95% confidence interval (CI) 0.24–0.94; $P = 0.031$).

Registration studies

Two large, Phase 3, randomized, double-blind, placebo-controlled studies of natalizumab in patients with relapsing MS were conducted.[21,26] The first was a study of natalizumab monotherapy[21] and the second was a study of natalizumab in combination with IFNβ-1a.[26] Both studies enrolled patients with relapsing MS who had experienced at least one clinical relapse during the prior year and had an EDSS score between 0 and 5.0. In both studies, neurological evaluations were performed every 12 weeks and at times of suspected relapse.

MRI evaluations for T1-weighted Gd-enhancing lesions and T2-hyperintense lesions were performed annually. Methodologies and key results from these major registration trials are presented in this section.

Monotherapy study

A Phase 3 randomized, double-blind, placebo controlled, parallel-group study was conducted to compare natalizumab to placebo in relapsing MS.[21] The AFFIRM study (Natalizumab Safety and Efficacy in Relapsing Remitting Multiple Sclerosis), enrolled 942 patients across 99 clinical centers in Europe, North America, Australia, and New Zealand. Eligible patients were 18–50 years old and had experienced at least one clinical relapse within the 12 months (but not within the 50 days) preceding study entry. Patients were excluded if they had received treatment with cyclophosphamide or mitoxantrone within the previous year, or had been treated with IFNβ, glatiramer acetate, cyclosporine, azathioprine, methotrexate or IV immunoglobulin within the previous six months. Patients also were excluded if they had received treatment with IFNβ or glatiramer acetate for > 6 months. Eligible patients were randomly assigned in a 2: 1 ratio to receive natalizumab 300 mg ($n = 627$) or placebo ($n = 315$) administered by i.v. infusion once every four weeks for up to 116 weeks. The primary end-point at one year was the annualized rate of clinical relapse; secondary end-points at one year included the number of new or enlarging T2-hypointense lesions, the number of Gd-enhancing lesions and the proportion of relapse-free patients during the study. The primary end-point after two years was the cumulative probability of sustained disability progression, defined as an increase of ≥ 1.0 on the EDSS from a baseline score of ≥ 1.0 or an increase of ≥ 1.5 from a baseline score of 0, sustained for 12 weeks. Secondary two-year end-points were the rate of clinical relapse, the volume of T2-hypointense lesions, the number of new T1-hypointense lesions and the progression of disability as measured by the Multiple Sclerosis Functional Composite (MSFC).

Patient demographics and baseline clinical characteristics were similar between groups. The mean age of patients was 36 years, and the majority were Caucasian (95%) and female (70%). The median disease duration was five years, and most patients (~90%) had experienced one or two relapses during the year prior to study entry. The mean EDSS score for all patients was 2.3. At two years, there was a 42% lower risk of disability progression in the natalizumab group compared to the placebo group (17% vs. 29%; hazard ratio (HR) 0.58, 95% CI 0.43–0.77; $P < 0.001$) (Fig. 27.1).

After one year of treatment, the annualized rate of relapse in the natalizumab group was reduced by 68% to 0.26 relapses per year compared with 0.81 relapses per year in the placebo group ($P < 0.001$). This 68% reduction in the annualized relapse rate was maintained at two years (0.23 vs. 0.73 relapses per year; $P < 0.001$).

Figure 27.2 shows Kaplan–Meier estimates of the cumulative probability of relapse in each treatment group. Over two

Table 27.2 *Magnetic resonance imaging (MRI) results from the AFFIRM study[21]*

MRI end-point	0–1 year		0–2 years	
	Natalizumab (n = 627)	Placebo (n = 315)	Natalizumab (n = 627)	Placebo (n = 315)
Patients with new or enlarging T2-hyperintense lesions [n (%)]				
0	382 (61)*	72 (23)	360 (57)*	46 (15)
1	112 (18)*	41 (13)	106 (17)*	32 (10)
2	40 (6)*	23 (7)	48 (8)*	24 (8)
≥ 3	93 (15)*	179 (57)	113 (18)*	213 (68)
Number of new or enlarging T2-hyperintense lesions				
Mean ± SD	1.2 ± 4.7	6.1 ± 9.0	1.9 ± 9.2	11.0 ± 15.7
Median (range)	0 (0–98)	3 (0–77)	0 (0–196)	5 (0–91)
Patients with Gd-enhancing lesions [n(%)]				
0	605 (96)*	213 (68)	608 (97)*	227 (72)
1	17 (3)*	42 (13)	12 (2)*	39 (12)
2	3 (<1)*	15 (5)	1 (<1)*	9 (3)
≥ 3	2 (<1)*	45 (14)	6 (<1)*	40 (13)
Number of Gd-enhancing lesions				
Mean ± SD	0.1 ± 1.3	1.3 ± 3.2	0.1 ± 1.4	1.2 ± 3.9
Median (range)	0 (0–32)	0 (0–33)	0 (0–32)	0 (0–48)

* $P < 0.001$ vs. placebo; Gd, gadolinium; SD, standard deviation.

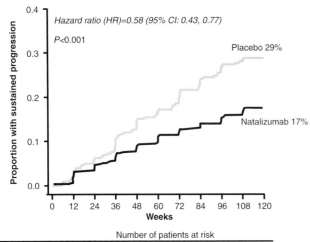

Fig. 27.1. Kaplan–Meier plots of the cumulative probability of sustained disability progression in the natalizumab and placebo groups from AFFIRM trial. With permission from Ref. 21 (*N Engl J Med* 2006;354:899–910).

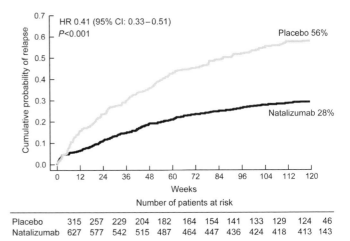

Fig. 27.2. Kaplan–Meier plots of the cumulative probability of relapse in the natalizumab and placebo groups from AFFIRM trial.

years, natalizumab treatment reduced the risk of relapse by 59% (HR 0.41, 95% CI 0.34–0.51; $P < 0.001$). Results for the one and two-year MRI end-points are presented in Table 27.2. Over two years, natalizumab reduced the mean number of new or enlarging T2-hyperintense lesions relative to placebo by 83% ($P < 0.001$). During this time period, there was no development of new or enlarging T2-hyperintense lesions in 57% of natalizumab-treated patients compared with 15% of placebo patients. In addition, only 18% of patients in the natalizumab group developed at least three new T2-hyperintense lesions compared with 68% of patients in the placebo group. The mean number of Gd-enhancing lesions was also reduced by 92% with

natalizumab compared with placebo both at one and two years ($P < 0.001$). The proportion of patients free of Gd-enhancing lesions at two years was significantly greater in the natalizumab group than in the placebo group (97% vs. 72%; $P < 0.001$).

Adverse events reported significantly more frequently in the natalizumab group than in the placebo group were fatigue (27% vs. 21%; $P = 0.048$) and allergic reaction (9% vs. 4%; $P = 0.012$). Adverse events leading to study drug discontinuation or early study withdrawal were uncommon, occurring in 6% and 3% of patients, respectively, in the natalizumab group and in 4% and 2% of patients, respectively, in the placebo group. The most common serious adverse events in the natalizumab and placebo groups, respectively, were MS relapse (6% and 13%; $P < 0.001$), cholelithiasis (<1% and <1%), and the need for rehabilitation therapy (<1% and <1%). Infections were generally mild to moderate and occurred in 79% of patients in each group. Serious infections occurred at a similar rate in both groups (3.2% in the natalizumab group and 2.6% in the placebo group). The rate of infusion reactions (defined as any adverse event occurring within two hours of infusion start) was higher in the natalizumab group than in the placebo group (24% vs. 18%; $P = 0.04$); the most common infusion reaction was headache (5% vs. 3%, respectively). Hypersensitivity reactions occurred in 4% of patients treated with natalizumab, with approximately 1% of patients developing serious hypersensitivity reactions.

A post-hoc analysis of this study examined the ability of natalizumab to achieve freedom from disease activity.[27] Clinically disease-free patients were defined as those who had no relapse and no progression of disability sustained for 12 weeks during the two-year study period. Radiologically disease-free patients were defined as those who had no Gd-enhancing lesions and no new or enlarging T2-hyperintense lesions during the two-year study period. Combined clinically and radiologically disease-free patients were defined as those who had no relapse, no progression of disability sustained for 12 weeks, no Gd-enhancing lesions, and no new or enlarging T2-hyperintense lesions during the two-year study period. Natalizumab significantly increased the proportion of patients who were free of disease activity according to the clinical, radiologic, and combined criteria over two years compared with placebo (Fig. 27.3 adapted from Havrdova et al., 2009).[27] Based on the composite of clinical and radiologic criteria, the proportion of patients who were free of disease activity over two years in the natalizumab group was five-fold greater than that in the placebo group (37% vs. 7%, $P < 0.0001$).[27]

In the AFFIRM study, the Short Form-36 (SF-36) and a subject global assessment visual analog scale were administered at baseline and weeks 24, 52, and 104. Natalizumab significantly improved the SF-36 physical component summary (PCS) and mental component summary (MCS) scores. Natalizumab-treated patients were more likely to experience clinically important improvement and less likely to experience clinically important deterioration on the SF-36 PCS. The visual analog scale also showed significantly improved HRQoL with natalizumab.[28]

Anti-natalizumab-binding antibodies were detected at least once during the AFFIRM study in 9% of patients, with persistent antibody positivity (at least two positive samples at least 42 days apart) in 6% of patients.[29] Approximately 90% of persistently positive patients developed detectable antibodies within 12 weeks of treatment. The presence of anti-natalizumab antibodies was associated with a reduction in serum natalizumab concentration; across both studies, the week-12 pre-infusion mean natalizumab serum concentration in antibody-negative patients was approximately 17 μg/ml, compared with <1 μg/ml in antibody-positive patients. Persistent antibody positivity also coincided with a decrease in natalizumab efficacy and an increase in infusion-related reactions.[29] Calabresi and colleagues concluded that patients with a suboptimal clinical response or persistent infusion-related adverse events should be considered for antibody testing.[29]

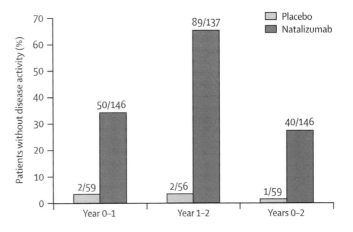

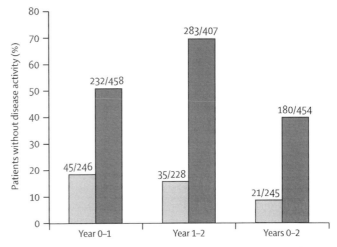

Fig. 27.3. Patients free of disease activity on the composite measure. Patients with highly active (top) and non-highly active disease (bottom) at baseline by study years. Absence of disease activity on combined clinical and radiological measures was defined as no relapse, no EDSS worsening (sustained for 12 weeks), no gadolinium enhancing lesions, and no new or enlarging T2-hyperintence lesions. Highly active disease was defined as at least 2 relapses in the year before study entry and at least one gadolinium-enhancing lesion at study entry; non-highly active disease was defined as fewer than two relapses or no gadolinium-enhancing lesions at study entry. $P < 0.0001$, natalizumab versus placebo, for both highly active and non-highly active subgroups. With permission from *Lancet Neurol* 2009;8:254–60.[27]

Combination therapy with IFNβ-1a

Currently available disease-modifying agents for the treatment of relapsing MS (e.g. IFNβ, glatiramer acetate) have been shown to be only partially effective, with many patients having breakthrough disease despite therapy with these agents.[30] Studies were conducted to determine whether the addition of natalizumab to these treatments may complement their mechanisms of action and result in improved efficacy. A Phase 2 open-label study of patients with relapsing MS found that a single i.v. dose of natalizumab co-administered during stable treatment with intramuscular IFNβ-1a was well tolerated, with no clinically relevant effects on the pharmacokinetics or pharmacodynamics compared with IFNβ-1a administered alone.[20] That study supported evaluation of combination

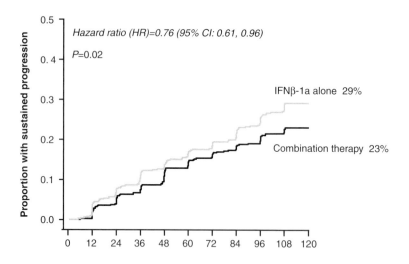

Fig. 27.4. Kaplan–Meier plots of the cumulative probability of sustained disability progression in the SENTINEL trial (IFNβ-1a plus natalizumab vs IFNβ-1a plus placebo). With permission from *N Engl J Med* 2006;354:911–23.[26]

Number of patients at risk											
IFNβ-1a alone	582	550	517	493	461	441	415	396	367	347	343
Combination therapy	589	569	543	520	494	479	459	438	421	399	395

therapy with natalizumab plus IFNβ-1a in larger controlled trials. Consequently, a Phase 3 randomized, double-blind, placebo-controlled, parallel-group study was conducted to determine whether adding natalizumab to IFNβ-1a therapy was more effective than IFNβ-1a monotherapy in patients with relapsing MS, who had one or more relapse despite IM IFNβ-1a treatment, and to also evaluate the safety of this combination regimen.[26] The SENTINEL study (Safety and Efficacy of Natalizumab in Combination with Interferon Beta-1a in Patients with Relapsing Remitting MS), enrolled 1196 patients at 124 clinical sites in Europe and the United States.

Eligible patients were 18–55 years old, had received treatment with IFNβ-1a for ≥12 months before randomization and had experienced at least one relapse within the 12 months (but not within the 50 days) preceding randomization. Patients were excluded if they had received treatment with any disease-modifying therapy other than IFNβ-1a within the 12 months preceding randomization. Patients were randomly assigned in a 1 : 1 ratio to receive natalizumab 300 mg or placebo by i.v. infusion every four weeks, each in combination with IFNβ-1a 30 μg intramuscularly once weekly, for up to 116 weeks. The primary end-point was the rate of clinical relapse at one year; secondary one-year end-points included the number of new or enlarging T2-hyperintense lesions the number of Gd-enhancing lesions and the proportion of relapse-free patients. The primary end-point at two years was the cumulative probability of sustained disability progression, defined as an increase of ≥1.0 on the EDSS from a baseline score of ≥1.0 or an increase of ≥1.5 from a baseline score of 0, sustained for 12 weeks. Secondary two-year end-points were the rate of clinical relapse, the volume of T2-hyperintense lesions, the number of new T1-hypointense lesions, and the progression of disability as measured by the MSFC.

Of 1196 patients randomized, data from 1171 patients ($n = 589$ combination therapy, $n = 582$ IFNβ-1a alone)

were analyzed, because a single center with 25 patients was excluded from the analysis due to data irregularities. The study was stopped approximately one month early because of two reports of PML. Patient demographics and baseline clinical characteristics of the 1171 patients evaluable for analysis were generally similar between groups. The mean age of patients was 38.9 years, with the majority being Caucasian (93%) and female (74%). Most patients (92%) experienced one or two relapses during the year prior to study entry, with a mean of 1.47 relapses. The mean EDSS score of all patients was 2.4, and the median duration of IFNβ-1a therapy before study initiation was 31 months. Patients treated with combination therapy had a 24% decrease in the risk of sustained disability progression relative to the IFNβ-1a alone group (HR 0.76; 95% CI 0.61–0.96; $P = 0.02$) (Fig. 27.4). The cumulative probability of sustained disability progression at two years was 23% with combination therapy and 29% with IFNβ-1a alone. Combination therapy also reduced the annualized rate of relapse at one year from 0.82 with IFNβ-1a alone to 0.38 with combination therapy (54% reduction) ($P < 0.001$). This reduction in the annualized relapse rate was also maintained at two years (0.34 vs. 0.75, respectively; $P < 0.001$). The overall proportion of patients remaining relapse-free after two years of treatment was 54% in the combination group versus 32% in the IFNβ-1a alone group ($P < 0.001$), representing a 50% reduction in the risk of relapse with combination therapy compared with IFNβ-1a therapy alone (HR 0.50; 95% CI 0.43–0.59; $P < 0.001$). Results for the one- and two-year MRI end-points are presented in Table 27.3. At the two-year assessment, the mean number of new or enlarging T2-hyperintense lesions was reduced by 83% from 5.4 with IFNβ-1a alone to 0.9 with combination therapy ($P < 0.001$). Further, the proportion of patients with no new or enlarging T2-hyperintense lesions was significantly higher in the combination therapy group than in the IFNβ-1a-alone group both

Table 27.3. *Magnetic resonance imaging (MRI) results from the SENTINEL study*[26]

MRI end-point	1 year		2 years	
	IFNβ-1a plus natalizumab (n = 589)	IFNβ-1a alone (n = 582)	IFNβ-1a plus natalizumab (n = 589)	IFNβ-1a alone (n = 582)
Patients with new or enlarging T2-hyperintense lesions [n (%)]				
0	422 (72)*	248 (43)	394 (67)[†]	176 (30)
1	108 (18)*	114 (20)	76 (13)[†]	55 (9)
2	32 (5)*	66 (11)	39 (7)[†]	59 (10)
≥ 3	27 (5)*	154 (26)	80 (14) [†]	292 (50)
Number of new or enlarging T2-hyperintense lesions				
Mean ± SD	0.5 ± 1.2	2.4 ± 4.1	0.9 ± 2.1	5.4 ± 8.7
Median (range)	0 (0–14)	1 (0–28)	0 (0–27)	3 (0–64)
Patients with Gd-enhancing lesions [n (%)]				
0	563 (96)*	436 (75)	568 (96) [†]	435 (75)
1	19 (3)*	73 (13)	13 (2) [†]	67 (12)
2	3 (<1)*	28 (5)	4 (<1)[†]	33 (6)
≥ 3	4 (<1)*	45 (8)	4 (<1)[†]	47 (8)
Number of Gd-enhancing lesions				
Mean ± SD	0.1 ± 0.4	0.8 ± 2.5	0.1 ± 0.6	0.9 ± 3.2
Median (range)	0 (0–4)	0 (0–43)	0 (0–12)	0 (0–43)

*$P < 0.001$ vs. IFNβ-1a alone; [†] $P < 0.001$ vs. IFNβ-1a alone; Gd, gadolinium; SD, standard deviation; IFN, interferon.

at one year (72% vs. 43%; $P < 0.001$) and at two years (67% vs. 30%; $P < 0.001$). The mean number of Gd-enhancing lesions at two years was also significantly reduced from 0.9 with IFNβ-1a alone to 0.1 with combination therapy (89% reduction; $P < 0.001$). The proportion of patients with no Gd-enhancing lesions was significantly higher in the combination therapy group than in the IFNβ-1a-alone group at one year (96% vs. 75%; $P < 0.001$) and two years (96% vs.75%; $P < 0.001$).

At least one adverse event was reported in >99% of patients in both groups. Adverse events leading to study drug discontinuation or early study withdrawal occurred in 8% and 3% of patients, respectively, in the combination therapy group and in 7% and 2% of patients, respectively, in the IFNβ-1a alone group. Adverse events with a significantly ($P \leq 0.05$) greater incidence in the combination therapy group than in the IFNβ-1a-alone group were anxiety (12% vs. 8%), pharyngitis (7% vs. 4%), sinus congestion (6% vs. 3%) and peripheral edema (5% vs. 1%). Serious adverse events occurred in 18% of patients in the combination therapy group, and 21% of patients in the IFNβ-1a group. One of the serious adverse events was a case of PML in a patient who received 29 doses of natalizumab in combination with IFNβ-1a; a second patient died from PML which developed while the patient was receiving natalizumab and IFNβ-1a after the SENTINEL study. Details of the cases of PML are described below. With the exception of the two PML cases, infections were generally mild to moderate in severity and occurred in 83% of patients in the combination therapy group and 81% of patients in the IFNβ-1a-alone group. The incidence of serious infections was low and similar in both groups (2.7% with combination therapy and 2.9% with IFNβ-1a alone). The incidence of infusion reactions was also not significantly different between groups, with headache being the most commonly reported infusion reaction. Hypersensitivity reactions were reported in 1.9% of patients in the combination therapy group and 0.3% of patients during placebo infusion in the IFNβ-1a-alone group. The percentage of persistently antibody-positive patients during natalizumab combination therapy was 6%.[29]

Combination therapy with glatiramer acetate

An additional Phase 2 study was conducted to evaluate the safety and efficacy of natalizumab in combination with glatiramer acetate (GA).[31] In this 6-month, double-blind, multicenter, parallel-group safety study, patients with relapsing MS were randomized to receive natalizumab 300 mg (n = 55) or placebo (n = 55) administered intravenously every four weeks along with GA 20 mg subcutaneously once daily. Eligible patients had received GA for ≥1 year and had experienced at least one relapse in the year prior to study entry. The primary objective of this safety study was to determine whether the addition of natalizumab to GA would lead to an increase in the number of new active lesions on cranial MRI scans compared with GA alone; new active lesions were defined as the sum of Gd-enhancing lesions and new or enlarging T2-hyperintense lesions. The secondary objective of the study was to determine whether combination therapy would increase the incidence or severity of adverse events (particularly hypersensitivity reactions). As such, the study was not powered on efficacy endpoints. The mean rate of development of new active lesions was 0.03 with combination therapy vs. 0.11 with GA alone ($P = 0.031$). Combination therapy resulted in lower mean numbers of new Gd-enhancing lesions (0.6 vs. 2.3 for GA alone, $P = 0.020$) and new/newly enlarging T2-hyperintense lesions (0.5

vs. 1.3, $P = 0.029$). The incidence of infection and infusion reactions was similar in both groups; no hypersensitivity reactions were observed. One serious adverse event occurred with combination therapy (elective hip surgery). With the exception of an increase in anti-natalizumab antibodies with combination therapy, laboratory data were consistent with previous clinical studies of natalizumab alone. Altogether, the combination of natalizumab and GA seemed safe and well tolerated during six months of therapy.[31]

Post-marketing observations

One of the recommendations of the therapeutics and technology assessment subcommittee of the AAN about the use of natalizumab was to carefully monitor patients receiving natalizumab to establish its long-term safety, i.e. the true risk of PML.[32] A large-scale postregistration study (TYGRIS) is underway to address this issue (start date January 2007). In addition to long-term safety, post-marketing studies also provide information on long-term efficacy, tolerability and drug adherence, especially in those patients who did not respond to first-line treatment with IFNβ or GA.

A Danish nation-wide observational study in 234 consecutive, natalizumab-treated MS patients,[33] with a median observation time of 11.3 months (range 3.0–21.5), showed a 73% reduction in annualized relapse rate from 2.53 pre-treatment to 0.68 post-treatment. Nine anaphylactoid reactions, two severe, were reported. Only seven out of 215 patients (3%) were persistently positive for antibodies to natalizumab.[33] Another post-marketing surveillance program, implemented in Sweden in August 2006 included (as of January 31, 2010) 1115 patients, of whom 363 were treated ≥24 months.[34] Dropout rate was 10%, mainly due to planned pregnancy. Serious adverse events were rare, but included three cases of PML (see below). Clinical outcome parameters showed significant improvements compared with baseline for patients exceeding 24 months of treatment (mean EDSS score at start of therapy was 3.86, which decreased to 3.38 at 12 months, and to 3.26 at 24 months). One of the smaller observational studies ($n = 45$) suggested that natalizumab not only decreased clinical and MRI disease activity in Relapsing-Remitting MS patients who had shown a high level of disease activity under first-line treatment, but also rapidly improved disability status during the first year of natalizumab.[35] Similar findings were reported by Putzki et al. in 97 MS patients on natalizumab after an initial insufficient response to first-line treatment.[36] These studies do not prove long-term efficacy, but provide useful hints of efficacy in those patients who did clearly not respond to first-line treatment.

Apart from the PML cases described below, several other remarkable case reports have been published on patients using natalizumab. These reports document infrequently observed, possibly drug-associated, adverse events, e.g., four cases of melanoma (one of which was observed during the AFFIRM trial)[21,37–39] and a case of primary CNS lymphoma in a subject receiving natalizumab.[40] The cases of melanoma highlight a potential long-term risk of natalizumab use, especially in patients with pre-existing skin moles. Despite the anecdotal reports, there is no evidence that indicates an increased risk of melanoma with natalizumab. Nevertheless, some clinicians recommend that MS patients with atypical moles or a family history of melanoma have dermatologist consultation before starting natalizumab and periodic visits with a dermatologist thereafter. Other case reports provide histories of ocular toxoplasmosis[41] and giant urticaria associated with persistent NAb titers.[42] As observed in the clinical trials, post-marketing observations confirm that the development of NAbs is associated with allergic reactions.[43]

Progressive multifocal leukoencephalopathy

Since reapproval in 2006, over 140 additional cases of PML have been reported in patients with relapsing forms of MS receiving natalizumab monotherapy. Clifford and colleagues recently reported a thorough overview of the first 28 confirmed cases.[44] The median treatment duration to onset of symptoms was 25 months (range 6–80 months). Initial signs and symptoms included changes in cognition, motor performance and seizures. Previous therapy with immunosuppressants seems to increase the risk. Clinical diagnosis is established by MRI and detection of JC virus in the CSF. In case of PML, plasma exchange (PLEX) or immunoabsorption is applied to hasten clearance of natalizumab.[45] Exacerbation of symptoms and enlargement of lesions on MRI have occurred within a few days to a few weeks after PLEX, indicative of immune reconstitution inflammatory syndrome (IRIS). IRIS seems to be more common and more severe in patients with natalizumab-associated PML than it is in patients with HIV-associated PML.[44]

So far, eight of 28 confirmed cases reviewed by Clifford were fatal. This survival rate is better than expected and might reflect early diagnosis and subsequent early immune reconstitution. However, the majority of the patients who survived had serious morbidity and/or permanent disability. It was suggested that prognosis is related to the location of lesions (more than absolute size), with the most serious consequences occurring when lesions affect crucial brain regions such as the brainstem. Higher JC viral titres in the cerebrospinal fluid (CSF) are generally associated with larger lesion size, but several deaths have occurred in patients who presented with low viral loads.[44]

PML is caused by infection of oligodendrocytes by the JC virus, a common DNA virus believed to infect the majority of healthy individuals at an early age. JC virus ordinarily remains in a latent state throughout a person's lifetime. Rarely, in the setting of immune compromise and through unknown activation mechanism, the JC virus infects oligodendroglia, causing PML. Cases were first described in the setting of hematological malignancy, but in recent times have been observed most commonly in patients with HIV infection and organ transplantation. For this reason, the first cases of PML reported in natalizumab-treated patients were completely unanticipated.[46–48]

Following discovery of the initial three PML cases, an extensive safety evaluation was conducted to evaluate patients with MS, crohns disease or rheumatoid arthritis (RA) who had received natalizumab.[11] In a safety study, all patients who had received natalizumab on clinical protocols were required to undergo a detailed medical history, a physical examination, a neurological evaluation, an MRI scan of the brain and, if possible, CSF testing for JC viral DNA. No additional cases of PML in natalizumab-treated patients were identified among these initial 3116 patients who had received natalizumab, despite an exhaustive search.[11]

Based on the first 65 000 patients with MS exposed to natalizumab, the incidence of confirmed PML cases in patients who have had 24 or more infusions of natalizumab is estimated to be a bit below one case of PML per 1000 patients (95% 0.73–1.0). Although the risk of PML seems to increase beyond 24 months, there is no indication of a further rise in incidence after month 36 so far, although it must be noted that available data beyond month 36 is limited.[44]

The mechanism by which PML occurs and how natalizumab influences this risk are not currently known. It is likely that the development of PML is a multi-step process that involves reactivation of the virus from sites of latency, DNA rearrangement of the viral genome, interactions with the host immune system and eventual migration from sites of latency into the CNS.[49] This idea has received support by the findings in a recent paper that JC virus DNA – but no viral proteins – are detectable in glial cells in brain tissue of healthy persons.[50] Natalizumab may intersect with the processes mentioned above at one or more points in the life cycle of the virus.[51] For example, it is possible that the inhibition of migration of mononuclear leukocytes may result in decreased immune surveillance within the CNS. A separate possibility is that mobilization of immature leukocytes harboring JC virus from bone marrow may occur following natalizumab treatment, leading to increased viral viremia and infection.

Although no randomized trial data is available, it are generally believed that immune reconstitution is the only effective therapy for PML at this time.[44] In all but one of the 28 reviewed cases mentioned above, either plasma exchange (PLEX) or immunoabsorption was used to rapidly remove natalizumab and to re-establish immune surveillance of the CNS. Recent reports suggest that the biologic half-life of natalizumab may be longer than its pharmacokinetics would suggest. Khatri and colleagues found that rapid elimination of natalizumab by plasma exchange leads to desaturation of the α_4-integrin and restoration of immune function in peripheral blood cells. The levels of natalizumab before and after plasma exchange and immunoabsorption support these findings. On the other hand, abrupt immune reconstitution may precipitate severe IRIS, a condition that is life threatening and that requires treatment of the inflammatory brain infiltrate that involves multinucleated cells and lymphocytes, as was recently shown by histopathological analysis of PML associated with HIV. Additional research is required to further establish whether the therapeutic algorithm using

rapid immune reconstitution is indeed superior to the natural course of reconstitution. It should be noted however, that delayed IRIS has been observed in a patient in which PML was detected very late and neither PLEX nor immunoabsorption was applied (Vennegoor et al., Neurology in press).

Other questions for further natalizumab-associated PML research should include: what are the effects of natalizumab on JC virus replication? And on anti-JC virus immunity? Pathogenic variants and host susceptibility factors (including evidence of previous JC virus infection) are also being sought.[52]

Jilek and colleagues assessed changes in viral replication and immune function over time in a small cohort of patients with multiple sclerosis who are treated with natalizumab ($n = 24$) in comparison with controls receiving IFNβ ($n = 16$). There were no changes in the measured variables. The investigators assessed anti-JC virus T-cell proliferation, T-cell cytokine (interferon γ) production, and anti-JC virus antibodies, as well as the presence of JC virus in the plasma, urine, and in blood-derived cells.[53] The findings were predominantly negative: there was no clear evidence for viral reactivation. The data from Jilek and colleagues are in line with recent data from Rinaldi et al., in 42 MS patients treated with natalizumab,[54] but are not in agreement with those reported by Chen and co-workers,[55] particularly with regard to the frequency of detection of JC virus in the urine, plasma, and blood cells of patients on natalizumab. The detailed methods used were different, with Chen and co-workers using a more sensitive assay for urine and plasma than Jilek and colleagues, but the assays used for blood cells in both studies had similar levels of detection. The two studies also differed in their assessment of the effects of natalizumab on anti-JC virus immunity, although the two methods were so different that comparisons are hazardous.

Recently, two more conclusive studies addressed the issue of JC virus measurement. Rudick and colleagues assessed a total of 12 850 blood and urine samples from nearly 1400 patients participating in natalizumab clinical trials and tested for JCV DNA using a commercially available quantitative polymerase chain reaction (qPCR) assay. A subset of these samples was also tested using a more sensitive qPCR assay developed at the National Institutes of Health (NIH). At the time natalizumab dosing was suspended, JCV DNA was detected in plasma by the commercial assay in 4 of 1397 (0.3%) patients; the NIH assay confirmed these positive samples and detected JCV DNA in an additional two of 205 (1%) patients who tested negative with the commercial assay. None of these six JCV DNA positive patients developed PML. In a 48-week study testing the safety of natalizumab redosing, JCV DNA was detected in plasma of six of 1094 (0.3%) patients, none of whom developed PML. Urine at baseline and week 48 was assessed in 224 patients; 58 (26%) were positive at baseline, and 55 (25%) were positive after 48 weeks of natalizumab, treatment. JCV DNA was not detected in peripheral blood mononuclear cells from any of these 1094 patients before or after natalizumab treatment. In five patients who developed PML, JCV DNA was not detected in blood at any time point before symptoms first occurred. Thus, measuring JCV DNA in blood or urine with currently available methods is unlikely to be useful for predicting PML risk in natalizumab-treated MS patients.[56]

Gorelik and co-workers used a two-step assay for detecting and confirming the presence of anti-JCV antibodies in human serum and plasma. The assay was used to determine the presence of anti-JCV antibodies in natalizumab-treated PML patients where serum samples were collected 16–180 months prior to the diagnosis of PML. 53.6% of natalizumab-treated MS patients tested positive for anti-JCV antibodies, with a 95% confidence interval of 49.9 to 57.3%. Importantly, they observed anti-JCV antibodies in all 17 available pre-PML serum samples, suggesting that the anti-JCV antibody assay appears promising as a tool for stratifying MS patients for higher or lower risk of developing PML.[57]

Altogether, natalizumab-associated PML is a severe, life-threatening adverse effect of natalizumab therapy. An early diagnosis, rapid wash-out of the drug and active treatment of the IRIS phase may improve prognosis.

Monitoring of natalizumab-treated patients

After the reintroduction of natalizumab in June 2006, Kappos and colleagues developed a diagnostic and management algorithm to monitor natalizumab-treated patients for PML and other opportunistic infections.[58] The algorithm includes strategies for clinical, MRI, and laboratory assessments. The European Medicines Agency began a new risk/benefit review of the drug in the autumn of 2009 in light of the first 23 PML cases reported after natalizumab's return.

The Agency's Committee for Medicinal Products for Human Use (CHMP) has concluded that the risk of developing PML increases after 2 years of use of natalizumab, although this risk remains low. The benefits of the medicine continue to outweigh its risks for patients with highly active relapsing-remitting MS, for whom there are few treatment options available. Because it is important that PML is detected early, the Committee recommended that a number of measures be put in place to ensure that patients and doctors are fully aware of the risks of PML. These include:

- an update of the product information to add information about the increase in the risk of PML after two years of treatment and additional advice on how to manage patients who show signs of PML;
- forms to be signed by patients at the beginning of treatment with natalizumab, and again after two years of treatment, after in-depth discussions about the risk of PML with their doctor.

A separate, somewhat controversial, monitoring issue is the recurrence of disease activity after cessation of natalizumab. In the context of a Phase 2 clinical trial, it was shown that as early as three months after discontinuation of natalizumab there was no difference between the treatment group and the placebo groups with regard to Gd-enhancing lesions.[19] Another

group of investigators showed an increase in T2-weighted lesion activity on cerebral MR images in a cohort of 21 patients 15 months after cessation of natalizumab therapy.[59] Thus, there is a concern that the discontinuation of natalizumab therapy may rapidly lead to a loss of its beneficial clinical effects, or even to a rebound phenomenon. Another longitudinal follow-up study in 23 patients who stopped natalizumab, however, did not support these concerns.[60] No worsening of radiographic or immunologic disease activity after cessation of natalizumab therapy was observed. It is important to point out that in contrast to the Phase 2 trial mentioned above, the vast majority of patients in this cohort received other pharmacotherapies while involved in the SENTINEL combination trial, as well as after discontinuing natalizumab.

It has been suggested that natalizumab-associated PML may be prevented by structured interruptions of treatment (drug holiday).[61] Recently, initial observations in 10 MS patients who responded well to natalizumab infusions, but decided to discontinue for a variety of reasons were reported.[62] Cumulatively, a combination of clinical relapse and new and/or enhancing lesions on MRI had occurred in seven of 10 patients. Others also found that natalizumab dosage interruption, which was retrospectively identified in medical records of 68 patients on natalizumab, was associated with clinical exacerbations and return of radiological disease activity. Some of the exacerbations were severe with a high number of active lesions.[63]

Although numbers were small, these data suggest that in patients who were switched to natalizumab because of disease activity despite first-line treatment, discontinuation of natalizumab as a drug holiday without reinstatement of alternate disease-modifying therapy should not be recommended.[62]

Remaining issues

Large Phase 3 trials of natalizumab alone or in combination with IFNβ-1a show that natalizumab reduces the progression of disability, and dramatically reduces the frequency of relapses and MRI lesion formation in patients with relapsing MS. In these studies, benefits were realized rapidly and persisted throughout the treatment period. Natalizumab was well tolerated in the vast majority of MS patients studied. These studies strongly suggest that natalizumab is a significant therapeutic advance over IFNβ or GA. Although no head-to-head comparisons have been performed, the magnitude of therapeutic effect on relapse rate seems to exceed that observed in multiple placebo-controlled clinical trials with other currently available drugs. Post-marketing data, although not from studies designed to prove efficacy, suggest continuation of the therapeutic effect on the longer term.

So far, several issues remain at least partially unresolved: which patients should use natalizumab? Should this be the first-line agent in patients at low risk of PML (e.g. JCV antibody negative patients)? Can patients use natalizumab in combination with immunomodulatory drugs? Its not recommended for use in combination with IFNβ (because of the SENTINEL results), but the risk of PML with monotherapy in the post-marketing arena raises questions about whether IFNβ actually has any impact on the risk of PML with natalizumab. Could it be used in combination with GA? Does early treatment with natalizumab stop progressive brain atrophy? What is the effect of natalizumab on gray matter pathology? Should natalizumab be directly compared with frequent dose IFNβ, fingolimod, or cladribine? How long should a patient stay on natalizumab? Does early and continuous use of natalizumab in Relapsing-Remitting MS prevent development of SPMS?

The occurrence of PML in natalizumab-treated patients indicates that the prominent beneficial effects will need to be balanced against the risk of a potentially life-threatening adverse event. Fortunately, PML is an active area of research. Management strategies have been proposed and promising studies focus on the pre-treatment identification of individuals who are at increased risk of PML, beyond those who have recently received potent immunosuppressive therapies. This will improve the selection of appropriate candidates for natalizumab treatment.

References

1. Duran I, Martinez-Caceres EM, Rio J, Barbera N, Marzo ME, Montalban X. Immunological profile of patients with primary progressive multiple sclerosis. Expression of adhesion molecules. *Brain* 1999;122 (12):2297–307.

2. Ffrench-Constant C. Pathogenesis of multiple sclerosis. *Lancet* 1994 29;343(8892):271–5.

3. Rice GP, Hartung HP, Calabresi PA. Anti-alpha4 integrin therapy for multiple sclerosis: mechanisms and rationale. *Neurology* 2005 26;64(8):1336–42.

4. Lobb RR, Hemler ME. The pathophysiologic role of alpha 4 integrins in vivo. *J Clin Invest* 1994;94(5):1722–8.

5. Cannella B, Raine CS. The adhesion molecule and cytokine profile of multiple sclerosis lesions. *Ann Neurol* 1995;37(4):424–35.

6. Baron JL, Madri JA, Ruddle NH, Hashim G, Janeway CA, Jr. Surface expression of alpha 4 integrin by CD4 T cells is required for their entry into brain parenchyma. *J Exp Med* 1993 1;177(1):57–68.

7. Carlos TM, Schwartz BR, Kovach NL, et al. Vascular cell adhesion molecule-1 mediates lymphocyte adherence to cytokine-activated cultured human endothelial cells. *Blood* 1990;76(5):965–70.

8. Elices MJ, Osborn L, Takada Y, et al. VCAM-1 on activated endothelium interacts with the leukocyte integrin VLA-4 at a site distinct from the VLA-4/fibronectin binding site. *Cell* 1990;60(4):577–84.

9. Bayless KJ, Meininger GA, Scholtz JM, Davis GE. Osteopontin is a ligand for the alpha4beta1 integrin. *J Cell Sci* 1998;111 (9):1165–74.

10. Tysabri (natalizumab) prescribing information. BiogenIdec, Cambridge, MA, November. 2004.

11. Yousry TA, Major EO, Ryschkewitsch C, et al. Evaluation of patients treated with natalizumab for progressive multifocal leukoencephalopathy. *N Engl J Med* 2006 2;354(9):924–933.

12. Rudick RA, Sandrock A. Natalizumab: alpha 4-integrin antagonist selective adhesion molecule inhibitors for MS. *Expert Rev Neurother* 2004;4(4):571–580.

13. Kent SJ, Karlik SJ, Rice GP, Horner HC. A monoclonal antibody to alpha 4-integrin reverses the MR-detectable signs of experimental allergic encephalomyelitis in the guinea pig. *J Magn Reson Imaging* 1995;5(5):535–540.

14. Yednock TA, Cannon C, Fritz LC, Sanchez-Madrid F, Steinman L, Karin N. Prevention of experimental autoimmune encephalomyelitis by antibodies against alpha 4 beta 1 integrin. *Nature* 1992 5; 356(6364):63–66.

15. Kent SJ, Karlik SJ, Cannon C, et al. A monoclonal antibody to alpha 4 integrin suppresses and reverses active experimental allergic encephalomyelitis. *J Neuroimmunol* 1995;58(1):1–10.

16. Leger OJ, Yednock TA, Tanner L, et al. Humanization of a mouse antibody against human alpha-4 integrin: a potential therapeutic for the treatment of multiple sclerosis. *Hum Antibodies* 1997;8(1):3–16.

17. Sheremata WA, Vollmer TL, Stone LA, Willmer-Hulme AJ, Koller M. A safety and pharmacokinetic study of intravenous natalizumab in patients with MS. *Neurology* 1999 23;52(5):1072–74.

18. Tubridy N, Behan PO, Capildeo R, et al. The effect of anti-alpha4 integrin antibody on brain lesion activity in MS. The UK Antegren Study Group. *Neurology* 1999 11;53(3):466–72.

19. Miller DH, Khan OA, Sheremata WA, et al. A controlled trial of natalizumab for relapsing multiple sclerosis. *N Engl J Med* 2003 2;348(1):15–23.

20. Vollmer TL, Phillips JT, Goodman AD, et al. An open-label safety and drug interaction study of natalizumab (Antegren) in combination with interferon-beta (Avonex) in patients with multiple sclerosis. *Mult Scler* 2004;10(5):511–20.

21. Polman CH, O'Connor PW, Havrdova E, et al. A randomized, placebo-controlled trial of natalizumab for relapsing multiple sclerosis. *N Engl J Med* 2006;354(9):899–910.

22. Labrijn AF, Buijsse AO, Van Den Bremer ET, et al. Therapeutic IgG4 antibodies engage in Fab-arm exchange with endogenous human IgG4 in vivo. *Nat Biotechnol* 2009;27(8):767–71.

23. Gordon FH, Lai CW, Hamilton MI, et al. A randomized placebo-controlled trial of a humanized monoclonal antibody to alpha4 integrin in active Crohn's disease. *Gastroenterology* 2001;121(2):268–74.

24. O'Connor PW, Goodman A, Willmer-Hulme AJ, et al. Randomized multicenter trial of natalizumab in acute MS relapses: clinical and MRI effects. *Neurology* 2004 8;62(11):2038–43.

25. Dalton CM, Miszkiel KA, Barker GJ, et al. Effect of natalizumab on conversion of gadolinium enhancing lesions to T1 hypointense lesions in

relapsing multiple sclerosis. *J Neurol* 2004;251(4):407–13.

26. Rudick RA, Stuart WH, Calabresi PA, *et al.* Natalizumab plus interferon beta-1a for relapsing multiple sclerosis. *N Engl J Med* 2006;354(9):911–23.

27. Havrdova E, Galetta S, Hutchinson M, *et al.* Effect of natalizumab on clinical and radiological disease activity in multiple sclerosis: a retrospective analysis of the Natalizumab Safety and Efficacy in Relapsing-Remitting Multiple Sclerosis (AFFIRM) study. *Lancet Neurol* 2009;8(3):254–60.

28. Rudick RA, Miller D, Hass S, *et al.* Health-related quality of life in multiple sclerosis: effects of natalizumab. *Ann Neurol* 2007;62(4):335–46.

29. Calabresi PA, Giovannoni G, Confavreux C, *et al.* The incidence and significance of anti-natalizumab antibodies: results from AFFIRM and SENTINEL. *Neurology* 2007;69(14):1391–1403.

30. Rudick RA, Polman CH. Current approaches to the identification and management of breakthrough disease in patients with multiple sclerosis. *Lancet Neurol* 2009;8(6):545–59.

31. Goodman AD, Rossman H, Bar-Or A, *et al.* GLANCE: results of a phase 2, randomized, double-blind, placebo-controlled study. *Neurology* 2009;72(9):806–12.

32. Goodin DS, Cohen BA, O'Connor P, Kappos L, Stevens JC. Assessment: the use of natalizumab (Tysabri) for the treatment of multiple sclerosis (an evidence-based review): report of the Therapeutics and Technology Assessment Subcommittee of the American Academy of Neurology. *Neurology* 2008;71(10):766–73.

33. Oturai AB, Koch-Henriksen N, Petersen T, Jensen PE, Sellebjerg F, Sorensen PS. Efficacy of natalizumab in multiple sclerosis patients with high disease activity: a Danish nationwide study. *Eur J Neurol* 2009;16(3):420–3.

34. Piehl F, Holmen C, Hillert J, Olsson T. Swedish natalizumab (Tysabri) multiple sclerosis surveillance study. *Neurol Sci* 2011;31 (Suppl 3):289–93.

35. Belachew S, Phan-Ba R, Bartholome E, *et al.* Natalizumab induces a rapid improvement of disability status and ambulation after failure of previous therapy in relapsing-remitting multiple sclerosis. *Eur J Neurol* 2011;18(2):240–5.

36. Putzki N, Yaldizli O, Maurer M, *et al.* Efficacy of natalizumab in second line therapy of relapsing-remitting multiple sclerosis: results from a multi-center study in German speaking countries. *Eur J Neurol* 2010;17(1):31–7.

37. Bergamaschi R, Montomoli C. Melanoma in multiple sclerosis treated with natalizumab: causal association or coincidence? *Mult Scler* 2009;15(12):1532–3.

38. Ismail A, Kemp J, Sharrack B. Melanoma complicating treatment with natalizumab (tysabri) for multiple sclerosis. *J Neurol* 2009;256(10):1771–2.

39. Mullen JT, Vartanian TK, Atkins MB. Melanoma complicating treatment with natalizumab for multiple sclerosis. *N Engl J Med* 2008;358(6):647–8.

40. Schweikert A, Kremer M, Ringel F, *et al.* Primary central nervous system lymphoma in a patient treated with natalizumab. *Ann Neurol* 2009;66(3):403–6.

41. Zecca C, Nessi F, Bernasconi E, Gobbi C. Ocular toxoplasmosis during natalizumab treatment. *Neurology* 2009;73(17):1418–19.

42. Cohen M, Rocher F, Vivinus S, Thomas P, Lebrun C. Giant urticaria and persistent neutralizing antibodies after the first natalizumab infusion. *Neurology* 2010;74(17):1394–5.

43. Sangalli F, Moiola L, Bucello S, *et al.* Efficacy and tolerability of natalizumab in relapsing-remitting multiple sclerosis patients: a post-marketing observational study. *Neurol Sci* 2011;31 (Suppl 3): 299–302.

44. Clifford DB, De LA, Simpson DM, Arendt G, Giovannoni G, Nath A. Natalizumab-associated progressive multifocal leukoencephalopathy in patients with multiple sclerosis: lessons from 28 cases. *Lancet Neurol* 2010;9(4):438–46.

45. Khatri BO, Man S, Giovannoni G, *et al.* Effect of plasma exchange in accelerating natalizumab clearance and restoring leukocyte function. *Neurology* 2009 Feb 3; 72(5):402–9.

46. Kleinschmidt-DeMasters BK, Tyler KL. Progressive multifocal leukoencephalopathy complicating treatment with natalizumab and interferon beta-1a for multiple sclerosis. *N Engl J Med* 2005;353(4):369–74.

47. Langer-Gould A, Atlas SW, Green AJ, Bollen AW, Pelletier D. Progressive multifocal leukoencephalopathy in a patient treated with natalizumab. *N Engl J Med* 2005;353(4):375–81.

48. Van AG, Van RM, Sciot R, *et al.* Progressive multifocal leukoencephalopathy after natalizumab therapy for Crohn's disease. *N Engl J Med* 2005;353(4):362–8.

49. Berger JR, Koralnik IJ. Progressive multifocal leukoencephalopathy and natalizumab–unforeseen consequences. *N Engl J Med* 2005;353(4):414–16.

50. Perez-Liz G, Del VL, Gentilella A, Croul S, Khalili K. Detection of JC virus DNA fragments but not proteins in normal brain tissue. *Ann Neurol* 2008;64(4):379–87.

51. Ransohoff RM. Natalizumab and PML. *Nat Neurosci* 2005;8(10):1275.

52. Ransohoff RM. PML risk and natalizumab: more questions than answers. *Lancet Neurol* 2010;9(3):231–3.

53. Jilek S, Jaquiery E, Hirsch HH, *et al.* Immune responses to JC virus in patients with multiple sclerosis treated with natalizumab: a cross-sectional and longitudinal study. *Lancet Neurol* 2010;9(3):264–72.

54. Rinaldi L, Rinaldi F, Perini P, *et al.* No evidence of JC virus reactivation in natalizumab treated multiple sclerosis patients: an 18 month follow-up study. *J Neurol Neurosurg Psychiatry* 2010;8(12):1345–50.

55. Chen Y, Bord E, Tompkins T, *et al.* Asymptomatic reactivation of JC virus in patients treated with natalizumab. *N Engl J Med* 2009;361(11):1067–1074.

56. Rudick RA, O'Connor PW, Polman CH, *et al.* Assessment of JC virus DNA in blood and urine from natalizumab-treated patients. *Ann Neurol* 2010;68(3):304–10.

57. Gorelik L, Lerner M, Bixler S, *et al.* Anti-JC virus antibodies: implications for PML risk stratification. *Ann Neurol* 2010;68(3):295–303.

58. Kappos L, Bates D, Hartung HP, *et al.* Natalizumab treatment for multiple sclerosis: recommendations for patient selection and monitoring. *Lancet Neurol* 2007;6(5):431–41.

59. Vellinga MM, Castelijns JA, Barkhof F, Uitdehaag BM, Polman CH. Postwithdrawal rebound increase in T2

lesional activity in natalizumab-treated MS patients. *Neurology* 2008;70(13, 2): 1150–1151.

60. Stuve O, Cravens PD, Frohman EM, *et al.* Immunologic, clinical, and radiologic status 14 months after cessation of natalizumab therapy. *Neurology* 2009;72(5):396–401.

61. Hauser SL, Johnston SC. Balancing risk and reward: the question of natalizumab. *Ann Neurol* 2009;66(3): A7–8.

62. Killestein J, Vennegoor A, Strijbis EM, *et al.* Natalizumab drug holiday in multiple sclerosis: poorly tolerated. *Ann Neurol* 2010;68(3): 392–5.

63. West TW, Cree BA. Natalizumab dosage suspension: are we helping or hurting? *Ann Neurol* 2010;68(3):395–9.

Chapter

28

Mitoxantrone to treat multiple sclerosis

Gilles Edan and Emmanuelle Le Page

Introduction

Mitoxantrone (1,4-dihydroxy-5,8-bis[[2-hydroxyethyl-ami-no]-ethyl]-amino]9,10 anthracendionehydrochloride; mitox), molecular weight 517 Da, is a synthetic antineoplastic agent first discovered in 1978. It has proven therapeutic efficacy in advanced breast cancer, non-Hodgkin's lymphoma, acute lymphoblastic leukemia, chronic myeloid leukemia, and liver and ovarian carcinomas.[1–5] Soon after its introduction as a cytotoxic agent in cancer chemotherapy, it was found to be immunosuppressive. Wang et al. showed that in vitro allore-activity was almost completely abrogated by mitox. The drug interfered only with lymphocytes capable of proliferating in response to newly presented antigens without affecting precursor populations. The effects were remarkably long-lasting.[6,7] This prompted the evaluation of mitox in experimental transplantation, where it was found to prolong greatly the survival of heterotopic cardiac transplants.[8] This evidence stimulated other investigators to examine whether mitox could modulate the course of experimental autoimmune encephalomyelitis (EAE), in which it suppressed both actively and passively induced EAE in mice and guinea-pigs.[9–12] At the same time, the contribution of macrophages in effecting myelin damage in EAE was established. Watson et al. demonstrated a blocking effect of mitox on in vitro myelin breakdown by macrophages retrieved from mice with EAE.[13] Mitox was first tested as a potential disease-modifying therapy in multiple sclerosis (MS) in 1990.[14] Benefit clinical and magnetic resonance imaging (MRI) parameters was initially shown in single-arm, unblinded trials.[14–17] Subsequently, on the basis of two controlled efficacy studies[18,19] and an open safety study,[20] the US Food and Drug Administration approved mitox for worsening relapsing–remitting (RR), secondary progressive (SP), and progressive relapsing (PR) MS in October 2000.

Mechanisms of action

Cytotoxic actions

Mitox has several cytotoxic activities. It arrests cell replication at the G2/M and S interphase. It has been shown to induce DNA protein cross-links and protein-concealed single- and double-strand breaks in DNA, but also non-protein-associated strand breaks.[1,21] Once cells are arrested in the G2 phase, they may enter cell-death pathways. Mitox induces programmed cell death of certain leukemia cells.[22,23] This evidence was corroborated by the demonstration that the natural resistance of acute myeloid leukemia cells is associated with a lack of apoptosis.[24] Mitox inhibits DNA topoisomerase II, an enzyme that promotes efficient condensation–decondensation of chromatin and segregation of replicated daughter chromosomes at cell division. Topoisomerase II changes the topology of DNA strands by the introduction of transient double-strand breaks through which an intact helix can pass. Topoisomerase II also engages in a non-covalent protein–DNA complex that equilibrates with a so-called "covalent–cleavable" complex.[25,26] The cleavable complex formed between DNA and topoisomerase II is stabilized by mitox, thereby preventing re-ligation of transient double-stranded DNA.[25,27] Mitox may induce aggregation and compaction of DNA by electrostatic cross-binding.[28] Mitox evokes the generation and release of highly reactive oxygen species to induce nonprotein-associated DNA strand breaks.[3,29] Metabolic oxidation of mitox to reactive 1,4-quinone and 5,8-diiminequinone intermediates may be an important mechanism of activation of this agent, and a prerequisite for its covalent binding to DNA.[28,30,31] Oxidation may take place in vivo through the action of nitrogen dioxide radicals.[30]

Immunosuppressive and immunomodulatory actions

In alloreactive mixed lymphocyte cultures, the proliferative response of lymphocytes to antigen is curtailed in the presence of mitox. It also abolishes the generation of cytotoxic T-cells.[6,7] Helper T-cell activity is diminished while suppressor T-cell function is enhanced.[32] Furthermore, mitox profoundly inhibits B-cell function and antibody secretion.[33] Mitox inhibits macrophage-mediated myelin degradation ex vivo.[13] Gonsette followed patients' lymphocyte subsets for three years in an open trial of mitox in MS,[34] and noted an immunosuppressive effect on CD4+ T-cells and an average reduction of the number of B-cells, human leukocyte antigen (HLA)-DR2+ and interleukin (IL)-2 receptor (+) cells by approximately 60%. This

Multiple Sclerosis Therapeutics, Fourth Edition, ed. Jeffrey A. Cohen and Richard A. Rudick. Published by Cambridge University Press.
© Cambridge University Press 2011.

reduction of the number of B-cells and the decreased CD4/CD8 ratio was maintained for the duration of mitox therapy. Similar effects have been observed by others.[35] More recently, several groups have reported that mitox induces apoptosis and necrosis of B-cells and monocytes,[23,36,37] probably in a dose-dependent manner.[37] Treatment with methylprednisolone (MP) and mitox modulates the expression of CXC chemokine receptors (CXCR1 and CXCR2) in peripheral blood mononuclear cells (PBMCs)[38] and reduces migration of leucocytes to the central nervous system via CCL5-related chemotaxis.[39] Putzki found that mitox does not influence Treg CD4+CD25+ cell frequency or function and seems to exhibit its efficacy mainly by a suppression of humoral immunity.[40] Mitox enhances the inducibility of Th2-type cytokines, IL-4 and IL-5, secretion by PBMCs and CD4+T-cells even further.[41]

Pharmacokinetics

Mitox is eliminated according to a three-compartment model, with successive half-lives of 6–12 min, 1.1–3.1 h, and 23–25 h. Mitox can be identified in high concentration in autopsy tissues obtained more than one month after drug administration.[42] These pharmacokinetic data provide a rational basis for an intermittent dosing schedule. Some 78% of the drug is bound to plasma proteins, and the relationship between the dose and the area under the curve is linear. Clearance of mitox is reduced in the setting of marked liver dysfunction.

Early clinical trials

Preliminary uncontrolled studies with mitox in MS

In a study by Gonsette and Demonty,[14] 16 patients with RRMS and six patients with SPMS with frequent and disabling relapses and progression of ≥ 1.0 Expanded Disability Status Scale (EDSS) points over one year were treated with infusions of 14 mg/m^2 mitox every three weeks for three cycles, and then infusions of 14 mg/m^2 every three months for up to two years. Of 20 patients were evaluable at two years, 16 (80%) were progression free. The mean annual relapse rate was reduced from 1.2 to 0.16. There were no serious adverse events, and treatment was generally well tolerated. Amenorrhea was observed in 15% of female patients. There were no instances of clinically significant cardiac dysfunction. Similar results were observed in 20 of 21 patients followed for three years. Kappos et al.[15] treated 14 patients with rapidly progressing MS with mitox 10 mg/m^2 every three weeks (for three to five courses). Three of eight patients who were followed for longer than three months improved, and five remained stable. MRI activity decreased from 139 gadolinium (Gd)-enhancing lesions at baseline to four Gd-enhancing lesions at month 6. Mauch et al.[16] treated ten patients (six RR, four SP) with mitox 12 mg/m^2 every three months. All patients had experienced rapid deterioration by at least one point on the EDSS over the 12 months preceding therapy. Eight of nine patients were followed for one year and showed an improvement in disability. The total number of

Gd-enhancing lesions was 169 at baseline and declined to three lesions at month 3, five at month 6, one at month 9, ten at month 12 and five at month 24. Noseworthy et al.[17] treated 13 patients with progressive MS with mitox 8 mg/m^2 every three weeks, for a total of seven infusions. Only three of 13 patients showed an increase of >0.5 EDSS steps after 18 months. The authors felt that this level of progression was consistent with the natural history of the disease. On Gd-enhanced MRI, 43 new lesions were observed before treatment, one new lesion at month 6 and six new lesions at month 18.

The Phase 2 Italian multicenter controlled trial of mitox in RRMS

This randomized, single-blinded, placebo-controlled trial conducted in eight Italian centers,[43] evaluated the efficacy of mitox over two years in a group of 51 patients with RRMS. Entry criteria included an EDSS score of 2.0–5.0 and two or more relapses in the previous two years. Patients were randomly assigned to monthly treatment with mitox (8 mg/m^2) or placebo for 12 months. Baseline clinical characteristics were similar for the groups. Patients were evaluated before treatment and at 12 and 24 months by an unblinded treating neurologist and a blinded evaluating physician who determined an EDSS score at each visit. Relapses were documented by the treating neurologist. T2-weighted MRIs were performed at months 0, 12, and 24. The primary end-point of the study was the proportion of patients with a progression of one or more EDSS points. Over two years, nine of 24 (37%) placebo patients and two of 27 (7%) mitox recipients worsened by one point or more on the EDSS ($P = 0.02$). Benefit also was observed on secondary end-points, including annual relapses ($P < 0.001$) and the proportion of relapse-free patients ($P < 0.01$). The mean EDSS score worsened in placebo recipients from baseline to month 24 (from 3.5 to 4.2, $P < 0.01$). In contrast, mitox recipients evidenced no change in EDSS (3.6 vs. 3.5, $P = NS$). Twenty-three mitox and 19 placebo recipients completed the annual MRI for two years. There was a 52% reduction in new T2 lesions in the mitox group compared with the placebo group (7.3 vs. 3.5, $P = 0.05$). There was no difference in the number of enlarging lesions between treatment groups. The most common adverse event was nausea, which was generally mild and easily controlled with antiemetics. Five of 17 women developed amenorrhea that resolved rapidly after cessation of therapy. There were no signs of cardiotoxicity on electrocardiogram or echocardiogram, no serious infections, no moderate or severe alopecia, and no severe hematological adverse reactions.

Trials supporting regulatory approval of mitoxantrone to treat multiple sclerosis

The Phase 2 French and British multicenter controlled trial of mitox in RRMS or SPMS

Forty-two patients with RRMS and SPMS, two relapses with sequelae, or progression of ≥ 2 EDSS points in the preceding

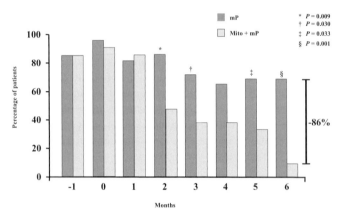

Fig. 28.1. French–British mitoxantrone trial: percentage of patients with new gadolinium-enhancing MRI lesions (primary end-point).[18]

12 months were enrolled in this trial.[18] All patients initially received three-monthly infusions of MP 1 g and had three-monthly Gd-enhanced MRI scans. Patients who had at least one new active lesion, on the baseline scans were randomly assigned to therapy, mitox 20 mg plus MP 1 g or MP 1 g alone, monthly for six months. Patients who initiated therapy completed monthly Gd-enhanced and T2-weighted scans. Lesion activity was evaluated by radiologists who were blinded to treatment assignment. Monthly clinical evaluations were performed by physicians who were aware of treatment assignment.

Baseline clinical characteristics were similar in both groups. Six patients in the control group and four patients in the mitox group had SPMS. Five MP recipients discontinued treatment. These five patients experienced progression of EDSS and active disease as evidenced by MRI. No mitox + MP recipient discontinued treatment. A significant treatment effect was observed on the primary endpoint, the proportion of patients by treatment group without new Gd-enhancing MRI lesions (Fig. 28.1). Treatment benefits were also observed on secondary end-points, the mean number of new Gd-enhancing lesions at month 6 ($P < 0.01$), and the mean number of new T2 lesions from baseline to the end of treatment ($P < 0.01$). Globally, there was an 85% reduction of new lesions in the mitox + MP group. Unblinded clinical assessments of the patients showed a benefit for mitox recipients. Improvements in mean EDSS scores from month 0 to months 2–6 were significant for mitox recipients (all $P < 0.005$). In contrast, the MP recipients generally deteriorated. During the two-month baseline period, the mitox +MP and MP recipients had annualized relapse rates of 3.1 and 2.9, respectively. These rates were similar for the 12 months preceding therapy (3.1 vs. 2.4). During the treatment period, there were fewer relapses in the mitox + MP group as compared with the MP group (seven vs. 31 relapses). This effect was even more pronounced during the last four months of treatment (one vs. 19 relapses). During the treatment period, the proportion of exacerbation-free patients was 67% in the mitox + MP group and 33% in the MP group.

Minor and transient alopecia occurred in seven patients (seven mitox + MP, zero MP). Eight of 15 women (eight mitox

+ MP, zero MP) developed amenorrhea between month 2 and 6. Amenorrhea was transient for seven women, and persistent for one woman aged 44. As expected, all patients in the mitox + MP group experienced pronounced neutropenia beginning two weeks after injection, but resolving within a few days. At the next monthly injection, minor leukopenia was noted in four patients and did not require a dose adjustment. Nine patients received concomitant treatment for nausea. There was no evidence of cardiotoxicity or serious side effects

The Phase 3 randomized, double-blind, placebo-controlled, multicenter trial of mitox in progressive MS

In the Mitoxantrone in Multiple Sclerosis (MIMS) study,[19] 194 patients were enrolled between 1993 and 1997 at 17 centers in Belgium, Germany, Hungary, and Poland, and randomly assigned to treatment with mitox 12 mg/m^2 ($n = 63$) or 5 mg/m^2 ($n = 66$) or placebo ($n = 65$), administered intravenously every three months for 24 months. One hundred and ninety-one patients received at least one dose, and 188 patients completed at least one clinical evaluation and were available for efficacy analyses. All patients met the following entry criteria: age 18–55 years, documentation of stepwise progression (worsening RRMS) or gradual progression of disability with or without superimposed relapses (SPMS), EDSS 3.0–6.0, worsening of ≥ 1.0 EDSS point over 18 months prior to enrollment, no clinical relapse or treatment with glucocorticoids within eight weeks of enrollment. Severe relapses were prospectively defined as the occurrence of new symptoms lasting for more than 48 hours, with a change in functional system (FS) score of more than two points or a deterioration of existing symptoms with a change of more than one point in at least one of the four following systems: pyramidal, brain, stem, cerebellar, or visual systems. EDSS, ambulation index (AI) and standardized neurologic status (SNS) scores were determined at each scheduled and unscheduled visit by a neurologist who was blinded to treatment assignment (assessing physician). A separate treating physician, not blinded to treatment assignment, performed all medical evaluations, reviewed laboratory data, adjusted the dose of study drug according to protocol, provided symptomatic therapies and diagnosed and graded the severity of clinical relapses. Baseline clinical and MRI characteristics were similar for evaluable patients across treatment groups.

A significant treatment effect ($P < 0.0001$) was detected with the primary efficacy outcome, a multivariate comparison of 12 mg/m^2 vs. placebo on five clinical measures tested in one combined hypothesis of stochastic ordered alternatives (Table 28.1). The pre-planned ordered analyses of each of the five components of the composite outcome showed significant treatment effects for change in EDSS, change in AI, number of relapses treated with corticosteroids, time to first severe relapse (treated with corticosteroids), and change in SNS. Time to first severe relapse differed significantly between the placebo and

Table 28.1. *MIMS study primary efficacy end-points[19]*

Variable	Mann–Whitney difference (95% confidence interval)	P-value of global test
Change in expanded disability status scale	0.2393 (0.0414, 0.4373)	
Change in ambulation index	0.2107 (0.0240, 0.3974)	
Number of treated relapses	0.3849 (0.1801, 0.5897)	
Years to first treated relapse	0.4821 (0.2077, 0.7565)	
Change in standardized neurological status	0.2302 (0.0299, 0.4305)	
Global difference	0.3094 (0.1721, 0.4468)	<0.0001 *

* Two-sided global test result is given (SmarTest software).
$P < 0.0001$ for one-side test as specified in protocol.

12 mg/m^2 mitox groups ($P = 0.0004$, log rank test). The median time to the first severe relapse was 14.2 months for the placebo group, but was not reached in 24 months by either mitox group. A highly significant difference ($P = 0.005$) was also demonstrated for the 5 mg/m^2 group as compared with placebo with the multivariate efficacy analysis. One hundred and thirty-eight of 188 patients (73%) who were included in the intent-to-treat analysis of efficacy at 24 months (24-month cohort) completed an additional clinical evaluation at 36 months (36-month cohort) for safety assessment. Comparing disability levels at 36 months relative to baseline, the mean EDSS change was 0.10 (SD = 1.22) in the 12-mg/m^2 group and 0.46 in placebo recipients. Six of 42 (16.2%) 12 mg/m^2 recipients and 16 of 40 (42.1%) placebo recipients deteriorated by at least one point on the EDSS. Similarly, the mean change in AI was 0.61 (± 1.78) in the 12 mg/m^2 and 1.13 (± 1.64) in the placebo group. The mean change in SNS was 0.19 (± 10.00) and 3.28 (± 9.08), respectively. The number of severe relapses decreased from 66 in placebo to 26 in 12 mg/m^2 recipients. Significant treatment effects were observed for most of the pre-planned secondary outcomes of efficacy. Treatment effects for the 5 mg/m^2 recipients were generally intermediate between those observed in 12 mg/m^2 and placebo recipients. The difference between groups in EDSS change at 24 months reflected fewer patients demonstrating deterioration of at least one point (25% for placebo and 8% for 12 mg/m^2, $P = 0.03$). Over 24 months, confirmed neurological progression was observed in significantly fewer patients receiving 12 mg/m^2 relative to placebo (5 (8.3%) vs. 14 (22%), $P = 0.04$). Patients in the 12 mg/m^2 mitox group showed a significant advantage in the analysis of time to confirmed EDSS deterioration at 3 months ($P = 0.027$) and 6 months ($P = 0.034$). Annualized relapse rates were significantly lower in the 12-mg/m^2 group relative to placebo at year 1 (0.42 vs. 1.15, $P < 0.0001$) and year 2 (0.27 vs. 0.85, $P = 0.0001$), a reduction by 63% and 68%, respectively. Moreover, significantly more patients in the 12 mg/m^2 group did not experience any relapse over 24 months relative to the placebo group (34

(57%) vs. 23 (36%), $P = 0.021$). Significantly more patients in the placebo group were hospitalized for reasons other than administration of study medication. Only 15 patients showed progression that required the use of a wheelchair (corresponding to an EDSS of 7.0). No significant difference between groups was apparent, but fewer 12 mg/m^2 recipients than placebo recipients progressed to EDSS 7.0 (3 (5%) vs. 7 (11%), $P = 0.23$). Quality of life assessment was conducted with the validated Stanford Health Assessment Questionnaire (HAQ). The placebo group mean score increased (0.26), with significantly less change observed in the 12 mg/m^2 mitox group (0.09; $P = 0.024$). Moreover, significantly more patients in the placebo group ($n = 41$) showed deterioration in HAQ index relative to the 12-mg/m^2 mitox group ($n = 25$, $P = 0.012$).

MRI scans were performed in a non-randomly selected subgroup of 110 patients (36 on placebo, 40 on 5 mg/m^2, and 34 on 12 mg/m^2 mitox) at eight centers to evaluate the influence of mitox treatment on the number of patients with Gd-enhancing lesions, number of Gd-enhancing lesions, number of active lesions, and the change in T2-weighted lesions from baseline to months 12 and 24.[44] Demographics and clinical features of this subgroup were similar to those of the total study population at baseline. These studies were performed 1.0 or 1.5 T systems. Using 5 mm slice thickness and a 256 × 256 matrix, double spin-echo sequences were performed with TR (repetition time) of 2500 ms and TE (echo time) of 40 ms and 90 ms. Lesion load was estimated using a scoring system described previously, with two experienced readers being blinded to treatment assignment. The pre-planned primary MRI outcome measure was the total number of MRI scans with positive Gd-enhancement, comparing mitox (12 and 5 mg/m^2) vs. placebo without baseline adjustment. Both doses of mitox (12 and 5 mg/m^2) failed to reach a statistically significant difference from placebo at months 12 and 24. There were a number of pre-planned secondary MRI measures. The number of T2-hyperintense lesions per scan showed a trend favoring 12 mg/m^2 mitox over placebo at month 12 ($P = 0.069$), and became statistically significant different from placebo at month 24 ($P = 0.027$). At month 12, the mean change from baseline of new T2-weighted lesions was 0.24 new lesions in the 12-mg/m^2 mitox group versus 1.17 new lesions for placebo, and at month 24 in the same group there were 0.29 new lesions vs. 1.94 in the placebo group. For the number of active lesions, in the 12 mg/m^2 mitox group only, a strong trend was detected at month 24 ($P = 0.054$).

Cardiac monitoring, electrocardiography (ECG), and left ventricular ejection fraction (LVEF) assessed by echocardiography or radionuclide scan, was performed before treatment and at months 12, 24, and 36.[19] Study drug administration was discontinued if LVEF decreased by 10% or more compared with baseline, or if the measured value was less than 50%. No significant differences in the numbers of patients who experienced reduced LVEF were detected between the mitox patients and the placebo group at the end of the first, second, or third year of the study. Over three years, LVEF decreased to less than 50% in one patient in the 5 mg/m^2 group, and two patients in the 12 mg/m^2

group. No congestive heart failure or other clinically significant cardiac dysfunction occurred. Mitox was generally well tolerated as administered during this study. Nausea, urinary tract infections, menstrual disorders, amenorrhea, and mild thinning of hair were observed more frequently in mitox recipients. The severity of these adverse events was usually graded as mild or moderate. There were no deaths or serious drug-related adverse events. One 5 mg/m^2 recipient developed renal cell carcinoma, believed to be unrelated to the study drug. The drug was discontinued as a result of an adverse event in five 12 mg/m^2 recipients (leukopenia, depression, decreased LVEF, bone pain, emesis, repeated urinary tract infections, and hydronephrosis), in none of the 5-mg/m^2, and in two placebo recipients (hepatitis and myocardial infarction). Leukopenia was observed in 19% of the 12 mg/m^2 patients and 9% of the 5 mg/m^2 patients, but in no patient of the placebo group. Elevated γ-glutamyl transpeptidase was noted in 15% of the 12 mg/m^2 patients, 3% of the 5 mg/m^2 patients, and 3% of the placebo recipients. Changes in other hematological and chemical parameters were not different between groups. At the 36-month evaluation, no significant differences in clinical or laboratory safety parameters, including alopecia, urinary tract infection, amenorrhea, nausea, and leukopenia, were observed between groups for the 138 patients followed up for one year after dosing completion. Two of 27 female patients receiving 5 mg/m^2 and seven of 25 patients on 12 mg/m^2 experienced secondary amenorrhea (cessation of menses for $\geq$6 months) during therapy. One year later, amenorrhea persisted in none of the 27 recipients of 5 mg/m^2 and five of 25 12 mg/m^2 recipients.

Post-approval studies of mitoxantrone in MS
Clinical follow-up of 304 patients with MS three years after mitox treatment

This study[45] assessed the benefit of mitox after three years of follow-up and the benefit of disease-modifying treatment (DMT) after stopping mitox. Patients with relapsing MS received six infusion of mitox (20 mg i.v. combined with 1 g MP per month) and patients with progressive MS (primary or secondary MS) received a mean of nine infusions of 12 mg/m^2 i.v. every three months for 24 months. A retrospective analysis was performed on 304 patients with active RR ($n = 141$) or progressive ($n = 163$) MS who were treated with mitox. After mitox therapy, 202 patients received DMT, interferon-beta (IFNβ), or glatiramer acetate (GA), while 102 patients did not. Before starting mitox, demographic and clinical parameters of predictive disability were not significantly different between patients who received DMT or not after mitox. The mean EDSS scores at starting mitox and three years after stopping mitox respectively, were: 3.3 ($\pm$ 1.3) and 3.2 ($\pm$ 1.7) for the RRMS patients and 5.9 ($\pm$ 1.2) and 6.4 ($\pm$ 1.4) for the progressive patients. The variation of EDSS between time of stopping mitox and three years later was significantly different for patients with RRMS who had not received DMT during the three

years following mitox compared with those who had received DMT in the same period (+0.9 vs. +0.3; $P = 0.03$). In this observational study, mitox treatment induced stable disease up to two years after discontinuation of mitox therapy. In the third year, patients without DMT deteriorated.

Mitox as induction treatment in aggressive RRMS: treatment response factors in a five-year follow-up observational study of 100 consecutive patients

This observational single-center study[46] reported 100 consecutive patients with aggressive RRMS who received mitox i.v. 20 mg combined with MP i.v. 1 g monthly for six months. Relapses, EDSS, and drug safety were assessed every six months for up to at least five years. Within six months after induction, 73 patients received maintenance therapy (mitox every three months ($n = 21$) IFNβ ($n = 25$), azathioprine ($n = 15$), methotrexate ($n = 7$), GA ($n = 5$)). During the 12 months following initiation of mitox, the annualized relapse rate (ARR) was reduced by 91%, 78% of patients remained relapse free, MRI activity was reduced by 89%, the mean EDSS decreased by 1.2 points ($P < 0.0001$), and 64% of patients improved by 1 point or more on the EDSS (Table 28.2). In the longer term, the ARR reduction was sustained (0.29–0.42 for up to five years), the median time to the first relapse was 2.8 years, and disability remained improved after five years. Younger age and lower EDSS score at the start of mitox treatment predicted better treatment response. Three patients presented with an asymptomatic decrease in LEVF to less than 50% (one reversible). One patient was diagnosed with acute myeloid leukemia (remission eight years after diagnosis). In this study, mitox monthly for six months as induction therapy followed by maintenance treatment showed sustained clinical benefit for up to five years with an acceptable adverse events profile in patients with aggressive RRMS.

Use of mitox in early MS with malignant disease course. Observational study in 30 patients with clinical and MRI outcomes after one year

This observational multicenter study[47] retrospectively analyzed 30 patients with malignant MS treated with mitox the year following the first neurological event. The 30 patients were selected according to Weinshenker criteria of malignant MS (either a "catastrophic" relapse or aggressive course). Clinical and MRI findings the year before were compared with these parameters collected the year following mitox onset. A total of 87 relapses were observed in the 5.7 months before and 10 during the year following onset of mitox treatment. The ARR decreased by 95% (6.0 $\pm$ 2 before and 0.3 $\pm$ 0.7 after). Twenty-four patients (80%) were relapse-free one year after onset of mitox treatment. The EDSS score improved in 87% of MS patients and the mean EDSS decreased by 1.9. Ninety-seven percent had at least one Gd-enhancing lesion before the start of mitox treatment as

Table 28.2. *Observational study of 100 patients with aggressive relapsing–remitting multiple sclerosis treated with mitoxantrone 20 mg and methylprednisolone 1 g for 6 months[46]*

	From M-12 to M0	At 1 Y	At 2 Y	At 3 Y	At 4 Y	At 5 Y
Number of patients	100	100	100	98	98	97
ARR	3.29	0.30[a]	0.39[a]	0.42[a]	0.38[a]	0.39[a]
RRR of relapse frequency		−91%	−88%	−87%	088%	−88%
Relapse-free patients (%)		78	62	42.5	39	32
Median time to first relaspe	2.72 Y, 95% confidence interval 1.7 to 5.2 Y					
Mean EDSS	4.1 ± 1 at M0	2.9 ± 1	3.1 ± 2	3.3 ± 2	3.5 ± 2	3.6 ± 2
P-value vs. M0 on paired samples		$<10^{-5}$	$<10^{-5}$	$<10^{-5}$	$<10^{-5}$	<0.008
Patients worsened (%)[b]	88	5	14	29	36	40
Patient not worsened (%)[c]	12	95	86	71	64	60
Improved (%)		64	−84%	−67%	−59%	−54%
Stable (%)		31%				
RRR of worsening		−94%				
Patients with Gd-enhancing lesions[d]	65/76 (85.5%)	7/76 (9%)[e]				
RRR of having Gd-enhancing lesions[d]		−89.5%				

[a] $P < 10^{-6}$ compared with M−12 to M0.
[b] Worsened was defined as a confirmed 1−point EDSS change (or 0.5-point for EDSS > 5.5) 3 months after start of a relapse.
[c] Not worsened was defined as patients who did not experience any new EDSS increase of 1 point or more (0.5-point for EDSS > 5.5) confired at 3 months, since the end of mitoxantrone induction.
[d] MRI with Gd performed within 12 months preceding mitoxantrone start and within 6 months following mitoxantrone withdrawal.
[e] Chi square of McNemar significant.
ARR = annualized relapse rate, EDSS = Expanded Disability Status Scale, g = gram, Gd = gadolinium, M = month, mg = milligram, RRR = relative risk reduction (compared with M−12 to M0), Y = year.

compared with 17% after. This study showed that mitox had a rapid and strong impact on malignant MS with short disease duration, suggesting that in this MS subgroup, mitox should be considered as an early treatment option.

GA after induction therapy with mitox in relapsing MS

In this controlled study,[48] 40 relapsing MS patients with 1–15 Gd-enhancing lesions on screening brain MRI and EDSS score 0–6.5 were randomized to receive short-term induction therapy with mitox (three monthly 12 mg/m^2 infusions) followed by 12 months of daily GA therapy 20 mg/day subcutaneously for a total of 15 months (M-GA, n =21) or daily GA 20 mg/day for 15 months (GA, n = 19). MRI scans were performed at months 6, 9, 12, and 15. The primary measure of outcome was the incidence of adverse events; secondary measures included number of Gd-enhancing lesions, confirmed relapses, and EDSS change. Except age, baseline demographic characteristics were well matched in the two treatment arms. Both treatments were safe and well tolerated. M-GA induction produced an 89% greater reduction (relative risk 0.11, 95% confidence interval (CI) 0.04–0.36, P = 0.0001) in the number of Gd-enhancing lesions at months 6 and 9 and a 70% reduction (relative risk 0.30, 95% CI 0.11–0.86, P = 0.0147) at months 12 and 15 vs. GA alone. Mean relapse rates were 0.16 and 0.32 in

the M-GA and GA groups, respectively. Short-term immunosuppression with mitox followed by daily GA for up to 15 months was found to be safe and effective with an early and sustained decrease in MRI disease activity.

Comparative study of mitox efficacy profile in RRMS and SPMS

This observational study[49] evaluated the clinical and neuroradiological response to mitox (treatment regimen was 10 mg/m^2 of mitox monthly for three months, followed by 10 mg/m^2 every two months) in patients with RRMS ($n = 79$) or SPMS ($n = 210$). Significant reduction ($P < 0.001$) in the number of relapses was observed during mitox treatment and in the year after in both RR and SP patients. There was significant improvement of EDSS during the mitox treatment ($P < 0.001$) and in the year after ($P < 0.001$) for the RR patients but continuous, mild worsening of disability in the SP patients ($P < 0.001$). Finally, in a subgroup of 224 patients, the number of Gd-enhancing lesions and of new Gd-enhancing lesions in both the RR and SP patients, before and after the mitox treatment were significantly reduced ($P < 0.001$).

Tolerability of mitoxantrone

Substantial tolerability data are available from oncology studies in which mitox was generally used in combination with cyclophosphamide, fluorouracil, mitomycin, methotrexate, and radiotherapy for leukemia, non-Hodgkin's lymphoma and solid tumors, and from MS studies in which mitox was used as monotherapy.

Cardiotoxicity

Cardiotoxicity has been reported in cancer patients who received mitox as a cytotoxic agent.[50–54] In these studies, mitox was typically administered in combination with cyclophosphamide, fluorouracil, mitomycin, methotrexate, or radiotherapy. In such studies, mitox-associated cardiotoxicity became evident by changes in ECG, indicating possible tachycardia and arrhythmia, an asymptomatic decrease in measures of LVEF, or symptomatic congestive heart failure (CHF). Histological endomyocardial changes associated with mitox administration include dilatation of the sarcoplasmic reticulum with vacuole formation and myofibrillar drop-out.[55] The increased risk of cardiotoxicity is associated with higher cumulative doses of mitox, prior treatment with anthracyclines, prior mediastinal radiotherapy, and pre-existing cardiovascular diseases.[50] The mechanisms of mitox-associated cardiotoxicity are not completely understood but potentially include the formation of free radicals,[56] increased oxidative stress,[57] lipid peroxidation,[58] alterations of adrenergic function,[59] alterations in sarcolemmal calcium transport,[60] and effects of tumor necrosis factor alpha and IL-2.[61] At least two mechanisms have been identified via which anthracyclines and anthracendiones, including mitox, could initiate the formation of reactive oxygen species. First, by chelating iron, mitox produces highly reactive hydroxyl radicals.[62] Second, by a redox-cycling process, mitox may produce hydrogen peroxide that promotes the formation of hydroxyl radicals. Hydrogen peroxide is inactivated by two enzymes, catalase and glutathione peroxidase. While the former is (virtually) lacking in the heart muscle, the latter enzyme is inhibited by mitox.[63]

The risk of cardiac toxicity after single-agent mitox therapy for MS has been assessed in retrospective and prospective studies. Ghalie et al.[64] reviewed the records of 1378 patients from three clinical trials of mitox in MS for signs and symptoms of cardiac dysfunction and LVEF results with median follow-up of 29 months (4084 patient–years). No patient experienced clinically significant cardiac dysfunction before treatment. Cumulative mitox doses ranged from 2 to 183 mg/m^2 (mean 60.2 mg/m^2, median 61.5 mg/m^2), and 141 patients received more than 100 mg/m^2. Two of 1378 patients experienced CHF after initiating mitox therapy. The incidence proportion of CHF in this cohort was 0.15% (95% CI = 0.02%-0.52%). Of 1378 patients, 779 completed baseline and scheduled follow-up LVEF testing. Baseline LVEF was >50% in all 779 patients. Seventeen of 779 patients with follow-up LVEF tests experienced asymptomatic LVEF <50% (incidence proportion 2.18%, 95% CI = 1.28–3.47%). Asymptomatic decrease in the LVEF <50% tended to be higher when the cumulative dose of mitox was ≥100 mg/m^2 (5%) vs. <100 mg/m^2 (1.8%).

Marriott et al.[65] reported a pooled analysis of Class III studies documenting cardiac toxicity in mitox-treated MS patients. Estimated risks of 3/716 (0.4%) for CHF and 83/716(12%) for decreased LVEF (either a reduction of LVEF >10% or LVEF value <50%) were reported, although the reported frequency, severity, and time course of cardiac complications varied markedly between studies.

Two prospective studies assessed the risk of cardiac toxicity of mitox in MS patients. The French consortium prospective study[66] followed 802 MS patients treated with mitox (mean cumulative dose of 70 mg/m^2) for at least five years. All the 802 patients had clinically healthy cardiac condition before the first course of mitox. Within the five years following mitox treatment, asymptomatic decrease of the LVEF under 50% was recorded in 39 patients (4.9%), at the end of mitox administration in 18 patients, and later in 21 patients (1.3 to 7 years after they started mitox). The abnormality was transient in 27 patients (69%) (returned to normal on the last scan), persistent in 11 patients (28%),and only observed on the last scan in one patient remaining clinically asymptomatic up to five years of follow-up (without additional control). Only one, a 54-year old woman with PPMS, presented with an acute heart failure (0.1%). This case was published as a case report.[67] The patient was previously treated with cyclophosphamide (cumulative dose 8.4 g) and was given mitox at a cumulative dose of 121 mg/m^2 (induction treatment followed by maintenance courses every three months). Her pre-treatment LVEF was 70% on radionuclide ventriculography and the LVEF decreased to 49% prior to her last course. A few days after her last course of mitox, she developed acute signs of heart failure with a LVEF of 29%. She improved under appropriate treatment but presented a new cardiac episode three years later due to a coronary and mitral valvular disease unrelated to mitox. In the RENEW study,[68] a Phase 4 study of mitox involving 509 US patients treated with mitox since 2001 and followed at least five years (last update 2009), an asymptomatic decrease in the LVEF <50% was observed in 5% of MS patients. Ten cases of CHF occurred (2%). This American population might have more cardiovascular risk factors than the French cohort where only one case of acute CHF (0.1%) was observed.

The definition of cardiotoxicity by a decrease of the LVEF was inconsistent between studies reporting mitox cardiac toxicity. An absolute reduction >10% between two evaluations has been considered by some authors,[65,69] leading to estimate the risk of cardiotoxicity at about 12% of the treated population, but this estimation might be uncertain because of the possible variations of the measure, especially when the LVEF is greater than 50%. Indeed, in the RENEW study,[68] among the 509 patients regularly monitored during treatment, a decrease of the LVEF by 10% was observed in 10% of patients but an increase by 10% of the LVEF was observed in 8.4% of patients. A decrease of the LVEF under 50% might be the best red flag to indicate the risk of cardiac side effect. Current recommendations to monitor LVEF include a MUGA (multiple gated acquisition) scan or echocardiogram at baseline and before

Table 28.3. *Summary of mitoxantrone safety profile in 802 multiple sclerosis patients over 5 years*[66]

Adverse effect		Frequency: N (%)
Cardiac	Symptomatic cardiac failure	1/802 (0.1%)
	Decrease in LVEF <50%	39/794
	Transitory decrease of LVEF	27/39 (69%)
	Persistent decrease of LVEF	11/39 (28%)
Hematological	Acute leukemia	2/802 (0.25%)
Reproduction dysfunction	Amenorrhea, age ≤35 years	9/167 (5.4%)
	Amenorrhea, age >35 years	46/150 (30.7%)
	Teratogenicity	0/52 births
Death attributed to mitoxantrone	Leukemia	1/802 (0.1%)

LVEF = left ventricular ejection fraction.

each infusion. We also recommend repeating this cardiac assessment yearly for the five years after mitox treatment.

Risk of therapy-related acute myeloid leukemia

The risk of therapy-related acute myeloid leukemia (t-AML) when using mitox was observed in oncology where mitox was administered as combination therapy with other chemotherapeutic agents with or without radiotherapy, making it difficult to estimate its precise contribution to the risk. In this context, Ghalie et al.[70] pooled the data on 2973 patients from seven independent oncological studies. In total, 31 patients (1.0%) developed a t-AML within four years after starting on mitox. Since 1995, sporadic cases of mitox-related t-AML were reported in MS.[71-90] Marriott et al.[65] pooled data from sporadic and retrospective studies and calculated an incidence of 33/4076 (about 0.8%). Martinelli et al.[91] reported a retrospective study of 3220 MS patients from 40 Italian MS centers and found an incidence of t-AMP of 0.9% and a mortality rate of 36%.

Only prospective long-term follow-up studies allow an accurate evaluation of the hematologic risk's magnitude. In the prospective study of the 802 French MS cohort followed at least five years after mitox withdrawal,[66] two cases of t-AML occurred, representing an incidence of 0.25% (95% CI 0.07–0.90%) (Table 28.3). The first patient was a 28-year old woman with early active SPMS who was given mitox as induction treatment for six months (cumulative dose: 70 mg/m^2) with a good clinical response (EDSS decreased from 6 to 4; relapse free). Twenty months after the first course of mitox, she developed night sweats, fever, gingival bleeding, and hepatosplenomegaly. Blood test showed hyperleukocytosis (41.5 x 10^9/L) with 30% blast cells, and bone marrow aspirate showed increased cellularity with 80% blast cells. The diagnosis of type 5 AML was made with a karyotype 46 XX, t(9;11) (p22;q23) [17]/47 XX t(9;11) (p22;q23), tri8 [2]/46 XX[1]. Despite specific chemotherapy, she died at the age of 30. The second patient was a 35-year-old woman with early and very active RRMS (despite treatment with IFNβ for 18 months she had four relapses and Gd-enhancing lesions on MRI within the preceding 12 months).

She was given mitox as an induction treatment for six months (cumulative dose 70 mg/m^2) with a good clinical response (EDSS decreased from 5 to 4; relapse free) but 20 months after starting on mitox, a systematic blood test showed hyperleukocytosis (11.3 × 10^9/L), and bone marrow aspirate showed increased cellularity with 60% blast cells. The diagnosis of type 4 AML was made. She had a normal white blood count (WBC) count on a systematic blood test performed three months earlier. She relapsed after a standard chemotherapy and was treated by bone marrow transplantation in May 2003. At the last contact in October 2010 (8 years after t-AML diagnosis), the hematologic remission was confirmed.

In the final results from the US registry to evaluate mitox safety (RENEW),[68] 509 MS patients were prospectively assessed for at least five years after the initiation of mitox. In this US cohort that received a mean of six infusions of 12 mg/m^2, two t-AL (0.4%) and one chronic myeloid leukemia case were reported. Interestingly, the second case of t-AML in the French cohort was diagnosed less than three months after the appearance of blood abnormalities allowing treatment of the patient very early on with a favorable outcome that was still confirmed eight years after the diagnosis. This point underlines the importance of performing WBC frequently to detect and treat potential leukemia as early as possible. This is all the more important since there is no myelodysplastic syndrome preceding the blast's detection. The association between the hematologic risk and the cumulative dose of mitox administered is unclear, but a higher risk at a cumulative dose of more than 60 mg/m^2 was reported.[89] One study[90] reported an accumulated incidence of mitox-t-AML of 2.8% among 142 MS patients in the community of Valencia and an accumulated incidence of t-AML 2.2% among 88 MS patients in the Catalonian cohort. This observed higher risk raises the possibility of specific genetic susceptibility to therapy-related AL in some communities.[92]

Gonadal dysfunction

Although rigorous studies of fertility have not been performed, secondary amenorrhea can be a delayed side effect of chemotherapy.[93] The frequency of mitox-induced amenorrhea (chemotherapy-induced amenorrhea, CIA) is clearly an age-dependent and a cumulative dose risk. This is well known in oncologic literature.[94,95] This possibility should be discussed with women considering mitox therapy for MS. This risk was evaluated in two MS cohorts. In the French prospective study[66] of 802 MS patients, the information about occurrence of transient or persistent amenorrhea was obtained in 317/391 (81%) of women starting mitox at 45 years old or younger. Transient CIA (duration several months) was reported in 27% and persistent CIA in 17.3%. The frequency of persistent CIA increased with increasing age at treatment start. Persistent CIA was not observed in women treated before the age of 25 years old (0/54 MS women) and in few women <30 years old (2/99). So, in women <35 years old, the global risk of persistent CIA (9/167, 5.4%) was much lower than the in women >35 years old (46/150, 30.7 %). Furthermore, 27 women gave birth to 32 normal babies (66% were females), between one and seven years after their last course of mitox. Fifteen men fathered 20 normal babies (50% were females). The FEMIMS[96] study reported a cohort of 189 MS women (mean age 37 years old), followed for a median period of 26 months after mitox administration, a global CIA risk of 26% that varied with dose, age, and estro-progestinic (EP) treatment. The probability of CIA increased by 2% for each increase of 1 mg/m^2 cumulative dose and by 18% for each year of age. Interestingly, EP treatment exerted a protective effect against CIA (protecting effect on oocytes by inhibition of ovarian cycle). At the age of 35 years, EP decreased the risk of permanent amenorrhea from 20% to 7% at the cumulative dose of 60 mg/m^2, from 36% to 15% at the cumulative dose of 100 mg/m^2, and from 46% to 21% at the cumulative dose of 120 mg/m^2. Compared with the French cohort of 317 women aged <45 years at mitox start, the global relative risk of persistent amenorrhea was higher (17.3% in the French study vs. 26 % in the FEMIMS study) for at least three reasons: a lower mean age at which mitox treatment was started in the French cohort (34 years old vs. 37 years old in the FEMIMS cohort), the duration of mean follow-up period after mitox administration (about 80 months in the French cohort vs. 26 months in the FEMIMS study), and presumably the potential protective effect of EP treatment that was systematically recommended in the French guidelines for the use of mitox in MS and the rather low rate of its use in the FEMIMS cohort (44% during mitox administration). These data emphasize the importance of EP treatment during mitox administration.

In men treated for Hodgkin's disease, mitox in combination with other chemotherapeutic agents (vincristine, vinblastine, prednisone) caused significant decreases in sperm counts and motility, but these parameters usually recovered within 3–4 months after completion of chemotherapy.[97] In contrast to other regimens with alkylating agents (e.g. cyclophosphamide), after cessation of mitox there is generally complete recovery of sperm production without morphological changes in vitro or genotoxic effects on germinal cells in vivo.[98]

Bone marrow suppression

Bone marrow suppression is the most common acute dose-limiting toxic side effect of mitox. Generally, granulocytopenia develops 8–14 days after a single large dose and persists for 4–10 days. Full recovery generally occurs by day 24 after drug administration.[99] Hemoglobin level, WBC, and platelet count should be performed 3–5 days before each course of mitox. Generally, prior to infusion, the absolute neutrophil count should exceed 1500/mm^3 and the platelet count should exceed 100 000/mm^3. In the French consortium study,[66] during mitox treatment six of 802 patients presented with signs of infection including fever and neutropenia (<500/mm^3). In a few cases, mild full-blood count abnormalities persisted for more than 3 months after the cessation of mitox.

Other acute side effects

Nausea or vomiting may occur in up to 60% of mitox recipients. This side effect is usually mild or moderate, and rarely requires cessation of therapy. Alopecia is infrequent and generally mild.

Discussion

Data from Phase 2 and 3 clinical trials,[18,19] indicate consistently that mitox is an effective and generally well-tolerated disease-modifying therapy for patients with MS. Benefit has been shown for relapse rate, progression of disability, and MRI activity in controlled clinical trials[18,19,43,48] and in observational studies.[44–47,49] Nonetheless, several important questions remain concerning the safety and use of mitox in MS.

What is the long-term safety profile of mitox in MS?

Although mitox is generally well tolerated, and the risk of clinically significant cardiac dysfunction and t-AL have been low in open-label studies, the long-term risk of these potential drug-related side effects needs to be considered before its use. Such long-term data data were collected in two prospective studies that started in 2001, one study from 802 MS patients in an open-label study conducted by the consortium of French MS centers[66] and a US registry study[68] from 504 MS patients followed for five years. They gave the magnitude of the risks (Table 28.3) and helped to determine the risk/benefit ratio of the drug that should be compared with other long-term DMT drugs.

What is the role of mitox in primary progressive MS patients?

Today, there are no robust data to recommend the use of mitox in PPMS. A Phase 2 study demonstrated no apparent benefit in any of the outcomes studied.[101]

What is the role of mitox for patients with SPMS without recent relapses?

The potential relationship between inflammatory aspects of MS pathology and disease-modifying treatment effects was not appreciated when the MIMS trial[19] was designed. It is possible that the demonstrated benefit reflected the clinical characteristics of patients enrolled in the MIMS trial. Not surprisingly, compared with the four clinical trials of IFNβ in SPMS, using IFNβ-1b,[102,103] subcutaneous IFNβ-1a,[104] and intramuscular IFNβ-1a,[105] patients in the MIMS trial most closely resembled patients in the European IFNβ-1b trial, the only one with positive results.[102] At baseline, the mean age of placebo recipients in the MIMS study was 40 years and in the European IFNβ-1b trial 41 years, mean EDSS scores were 4.7 and 5.2, and the proportions of patients who were free of relapses for 1–2 years prior to enrollment were 25.5% and 28.2%, respectively. We believe that the relative efficacy of mitox in progressive patients who do and do not experience superimposed relapses can only be answered definitively by a study which is designated to answer that question.

What is the role of mitox in rapidly worsening MS patients?

The important issue of treating rapidly worsening MS patients (e.g. two or more clinical relapses with sequelae or progression of more than two EDSS points and Gd-enhancing MRI lesions) with mitox was addressed by the French and British trial[18] and subsequently in open-label studies.[46,47] The prominent and rapid reduction in the inflammatory manifestations observed with the monthly combination of mitox (20 mg/month) and MP (1 g per month) for six months suggests a potential role for this regimen in treating patients with rapidly worsening MS.

What is the role of mitox as "rescue" therapy for patients who fail first-line agents?

Mitox may provide a new treatment option for patients with RRMS who experience a suboptimal treatment response to IFNβ or GA. Two studies showed dramatic dramatic benefit.[46,106] However, only limited data are available to support this notion at this time.

Mitox as an induction therapy

In recent years, the concept of induction treatment followed by a long-term maintenance treatment has been considered for treating autoimmune diseases, such as MS.[46,107] This approach seems particularly appropriate for patients with aggressive disease. A consortium of Italian and French academic neurologists conducted a trial[108] aiming to determine whether a treatment strategy combining induction treatment with mitox prior to IFNβ-1b can delay disability progression over three year as compared with IFNβ-1b alone in patients with aggressive RRMS. Overall, 109 patients with ≥ 2 relapses in prior 12 months and ≥ 1 Gd-enhancing MRI lesion were randomized into two groups: 54 patients received mitox (12 mg/m^2; maximum 20 mg) combined with MP (1 g) monthly for six months followed by IFNβ-1b for the last 27 months and 55 patients received IFNβ-1b monthly for three years combined with MP

(1 g) monthly for the first six months. The time to worsen by at least one EDSS point confirmed at 3 months (primary endpoint) was delayed in the mitox group compared with the IFNβ-1b group ($P < 0.008$). The percentage of worsened patients was reduced by 64.9% in the mitox group relative to the IFNβ-1b group (5/55 vs. 14/54 patients; odd ratio 0.29; 95% CI = 0.10–0.86; $P < 0.021$). Compared with the IFNβ-1b group, mitox patients had a reduced relapse rate by 61.7%, a reduced number of Gd enhancing lesions at month 9, and a slower accumulation of new T2 lesions at each time point. This study demonstrates the usefulness of mitox prior to IFNβ-1b as an induction therapy in aggressive RRMS patients.

Can the useful life-span of mitox be extended with dexrazoxane or an alternative treatment protocol?

Over the past several years, efforts have been made to reduce or prevent cardiotoxicity associated with mitox therapy. One promising approach is the use of liposomal agents that permit more specific organ-targeting of mitox and prolong the half-life of the drug.[90] Second, cardiotoxicity may be diminished by chelation agents that remove iron to prevent the formation of mitox–iron complexes, which catalyze the generation of extremely reactive hydroxyl radicals. One chelating agent, dexrazoxane, a member of the bisdioxopiperazine family, has shown encouraging results in reducing the incidence of anthracycline-related cardiotoxicity in adult cancer patients.[109] Bernitsas et al.[110] performed an open-label study to evaluate possible subclinical cardiotoxicity in 47 MS patients treated quarterly with mitox (48 mg/m^2 cumulative), with ($n = 28$) or without ($n = 19$) concomitant dexrazoxane. Patients receiving dexrazoxane, exhibited a significantly decreased decline in LVEF (mean change: -3.80% vs. – 8.55%, $P < 0.001$) on blinded serial radionucleide ventriculography.

Conclusions

The available data from studies in patients with MS suggest that mitox may have a role to play in the management of aggressive disease,[111] particularly as an induction therapy. As pointed out by Vollmer,[112] the key remaining question is whether cytotoxic agents offer real advantages over therapies that have more specific, targeted effects on the immune system.

References

1. Alberts DS, Peng YM, Bowden GT, et al. Pharmacology of mitoxantrone: mode of action and pharmacokinetics. *Invest New Drugs* 1985;3:101–7.

2. Faulds D, Balfour JA, Chrisp P, Langtry HD. Mitoxantrone: a review of its pharmacodynamic and pharmacokinetic properties, and therapeutic potential in the chemotherapy of cancer. *Drugs* 1991;41:400–99.

3. Lenk H, Müller U, Tanneberger S. Mitoxantrone: mechanisms of action, antitumor activity, pharmacokinetics, efficacy in the treatment of solid tumors and lymphomas, and toxicity. *Anticancer Res* 1987;7:1257–64.

4. Koeller J, Eble M. Mitoxantrone: a novel anthracycline derivative. *Clin Pharm* 1998;7:574–81.

5. Shenkenberg TD, Von Hoff D. Mitoxantrone: a new anticancer drug

with significant clinical activity. *Ann Intern Med* 1986;105:67–81.

6. Wang BS, Murdock KC, Lumanglas AL, et al. Relationship of chemical structures of anthraquinones with their effects on the suppression of immune responses. *Int J Immunopharm* 1987;9:733–9.

7. Wang BS, Lumaglas AL, Ruszala-Mallon VM, et al. Induction of alloreactive immuno-suppression by

1,4-bis [(2-aminoethyl)amino]-5,8-dihydroxy-9,10- anthracenedione dihydrochloride (CL 232,468). *Int J Immunopharmacol* 1984;6:475–82.

8. Schneider T, Kupiec-Weglinski J, Towpik E, *et al.* Mitoxantrone: an immunosuppressive agent potentially useful in organ transplantation. *Fed Proc* 1985;44:1681.

9. Bisteau M, Devos G, Brucher JM, Gonsette RE. Prevention of subacute experimental allergic encephalomyelitis in guinea-pigs with desferrioxamine, isoprinosine and mitoxantrone. In Gonsette RE, Delmotte P, eds. *Recent Advances in Multiple Sclerosis Therapy. International Congress Series.* Amsterdam: Elsevier Science Publishers, 1989;863:299–300.

10. Levine S, Saltzman A. Regional suppression therapy after onset and prevention of relapses in experimental allergic encephalomyelitis by mitoxantrone. *J Neuroimmunol* 1986;13:175–81.

11. Lublin FD, Lavasa M, Viti C, Knobler RL. Suppression of acute and relapsing experimental allergic encephalomyelitis with mitoxantrone. *Clin Immunol Immunopathol* 1987;45:122–8.

12. Ridge SC, Sloboda AE, McReynolds RA, *et al.* Suppression of experimental allergic encephalomyelitis by mitoxantrone. *Clin Immunol Immunopathol* 1985;35:35–42.

13. Watson CM, Davison AN, Baker D, *et al.* Suppression of demyelination by mitoxantrone. *Int J Immunopharmacol* 1991;13:923–30.

14. Gonsette RE, Demonty L. Immunosuppression with mitoxantrone in multiple sclerosis: a pilot study for 2 years in 22 patients (P573). *Neurology* 1990;40(Suppl 1):261.

15. Kappos L, Gold R, Künstler E, *et al.* Mitoxantrone in the treatment of rapidly progressive MS: a pilot study with serial gadolinium-enhanced MRI (P539). *Neurology* 1990;40(Suppl 1):261.

16. Mauch E, Kornhuber HH, Krapf H, *et al.* Treatment of multiple sclerosis with mitoxantrone. *Eur Arch Psych Clin Neurosci* 1992;242:96–102.

17. Noseworthy JH, Hopkins MB, Vandervoort MK, *et al.* An open-trial evaluation of mitoxantrone in the treatment of progressive MS. *Neurology* 1993;43:1401–6.

18. Edan G, Miller D, Clanet M, *et al.* Therapeutic effect of mitoxantrone combined with methylprednisolone in multiple sclerosis: a randomised multicentre study of active disease using MRI and clinical criteria. *J Neurol Neurosurg Psychiatry* 1997;62:112–18.

19. Hartung HP, Gonsette R, König N, *et al.* Mitoxantrone in progressive multiple sclerosis: a placebo-controlled, double-blind, randomised, multicentre trial. *Lancet* 2002;360:2018–25.

20. Mauch E, Eisenmann S, Hahn A, *et al.* Mitoxantrone in the treatment of patients with multiple sclerosis: a large single center experience. *Mult Scler* 1999;5(Supp 1):P366.

21. Bowden GT, Roberts R, Alberts DS, *et al.* Comparative molecular pharmacology in leukemic L1210 cells of the anthracene anticancer drugs mitoxantrone and bisantrene. *Cancer Res* 1985;45:4915–20.

22. Bhalla K, Ibrado AM, Tourkina E, *et al.* High-dose mitoxantrone induces programmed cell death or apoptosis in human myeloid leukemia cells. *Blood* 1993;82:3133–40.

23. Bellosillo B, Colomer D, Pons G, Gil J. Mitoxantrone, a topoisomerase II inhibitor, induces apoptosis of B chronic lymphocytic leukaemia cells. *Br J Haematol* 1998;100:142–6.

24. Bailly JD, Skladanowski A, Bettaieb A, *et al.* Natural resistance of acute myeloid leukemia cell lines to mitoxantrone is associated with lack of apoptosis. *Leukemia* 1997;11:1523–32.

25. Holden JA. Human deoxyribonucleic acid topoisomerases: molecular targets of anticancer drugs. *Ann Clin Lab Sci* 1997;27:402–12.

26. Smith PJ, Blunt NJ, Desnoyers R, *et al.* DNA topoisomerase II-dependent cytotoxicity of alkylaminoanthraquinones and their N-oxides. *Cancer Chemother Pharmacol* 1997;39:455–61.

27. Fox ME, Smith PJ. Long-term inhibition of DNA synthesis and persistence of trapped topoisomerase II complexes in determining the toxicity of the antitumor DNA intercalators mAMSA and mitoxantrone. *Cancer* 1990;50:5813–18.

28. Fisher GR, Patterson LH. DNA strand breakage by peroxidase-activated mitoxantrone. *J Pharm Pharmacol* 1990;43:65–8.

29. Basra J, Wolf CR, Brown JR, Patterson LH. Evidence for human liver mediated free-radical formation by doxorubicin and mitoxantrone. *Anticancer Drug Design* 1985;1:45–52.

30. Reszka KJ, Matuszak Z, Chignell CF. Lactoperioxidase- catalyzed oxidation of the anticancer agent mitoxantrone by nitrogen dioxide (NO$_2$*) radicals. *Chem Res Toxicol* 1997;10:1325–30.

31. Panousis C, Kettle AJ, Phillips DR. Neutrophil-mediated activation of mitoxantrone to metabolites which form adducts with DNA. *Cancer Lett* 1997;113:173–8.

32. Fidler JM, Quinn DeJoy S, Gibbons JJ Jr. Selective immunomodulation by the anti-neoplastic agent mitoxantrone. I. Suppression of B lymphocyte function. *J Immunol* 1986;137:727–32.

33. Fidler JM, Quinn DeJoy S, Smith FR, Gibbons JJ Jr. Selective immunomodulation by the antineoplastic agent mitoxantrone. II. Nonspecific adherent suppressor cells derived from mitoxantrone-treated mice. *J Immunol* 1986;136:2747–54.

34. Gonsette RE. Mitoxantrone immunotherapy in multiple sclerosis. *Mult Scler* 1996;1:329–32.

35. Zaffaroni M, Ghezzi A, Baldini SM, Zibetti A. *Effetti immunosuppressori del mitoxantrone nella sclerosi multipla cronica-progressiva.* In Ghezzi A, *et al.*, eds. La Ricerca sulla Sclerosi Multipla in Italia. Salerno: Momento Medico, 1995:112–14.

36. Chan A, Weilbach FX, Toyka KV, Gold R. Mitoxantrone induces cell death in peripheral blood leucocytes of multiple sclerosis patients. *Clin Exp Immunol* 2005;139:152–8.

37. Neuhaus O, Wiendl H, Kieseier BC, *et al.* Multiple sclerosis: immunological effects of mitoxantrone in vitro reveal antigen-presenting cells as major targets [Abstract]. *Eur J Neurol* 2002;9(Suppl 2):130.

38. Bielecki B, Mazurek A, Wolinski P, Glabinski A. Treatment of multiple sclerosis with methylprednisolone and mitoxantrone modulates the expression of CTC chemokine receptors in PBMC. *J Clin Immunol* 2008;28:122–130.

39. Jalosinski M, Karolczak K, Mazurek A, Glabinski A. The effects of methylprednisolone and mitoxantrone

40. Putzki N, Kreuzfelder E, Grosse-Wilde H et al. Mitoxantrone does not restore the impaired suppressive function of natural regulatory T-cells in patients suffering multiple sclerosis. A longitudinal ex vivo and in vitro study. *Eur Neurol.* 2009;61:27–32.

41. Vogelgesang A, Rosenberg S, Skrzipek S et al. Mioxantrone treatment in multiple sclerosis induces Th2-type cytokines. *Acta Neurol Scand* 2010;122:237–243.

42. Stewart DJ, Green RM, Mikhael NZ, et al. Human autopsy tissue concentrations of mitoxantrone. *Cancer Treat Rep* 1986;70:1255–61.

43. Millefiorini E, Gasperini C, Pozzilli C, et al. Randomised placebo-controlled trial of mitoxantrone in relapsing–remitting multiple sclerosis: a 24-month clinical and MRI outcome. *J Neurol* 1997;244:153–9.

44. Krapf H, Morrissey SP, Zenker O, et al. Effect of mitoxantrone on MRI in progressive MS: results of the MIMS trial. *Neurology* 2005;65:690–6.

45. Debouverie M, L Taillandier, Pittion-Vouyovitch S et al. Clinical follow-up of 304 patients with multiple sclerosis three years after mitoxantrone treatment. *Mult Scler* 2006;12:1–6.

46. Le Page E, Leray E, Taurin G, et al. Mitoxantrone as induction treatment in aggressive relapsing remitting multiple sclerosis: treatment response factors in a 5 year follow-up observational study of 100 consecutive patients. *J Neurol Neurosurg Psychiatry* 2008;79:52–6.

47. Ory S, Debouverie M, Le Page E, et al. Use of mitoxantrone in early multiple sclerosis with malignant disease course. Observational study in 30 patients with clinical and MRI outcomes after one year. *Rev Neurol (Paris)* 2008;164:1028–34.

48. Vollmer T, Panitch H, Bar-Or A, et al. Glatiramer acetate after induction therapy with mitoxantrone in relapsing multiple sclerosis. *Mult Scler* 2008;14:663–670.

49. Esposito F, Radaelli M, Martinelli V et al. Comparative study of mitoxantrone efficacy profile in patients with relapsing-remitting and secondary progressive multiple sclerosis. *Mult Scler* 2010;16:1490–9.

50. Dukart G, Barone JS. An overview of cardiac episodes following mitoxantrone administration. *Cancer Treat Symp* 1984;3:35–41.

51. Gams RA, Wesler MJ. Mitoxantrone cardiotoxicity: results from Southeastern Cancer Study Group. *Cancer Treat Symp* 1984;3:31–3.

52. Foster BJ, Lev L, Bergemann C, et al. Cardiac events in phase II trials with mitoxantrone. *Cancer Treat Symp* 1984;3:43–6.

53. Posner LE, Dukart G, Goldberg J, et al. Mitoxantrone: an overview of safety and toxicity. *Invest New Drugs* 1985;3:123–32.

54. Fountzilas G, Afthonidis D, Geleris P, et al. Cardiotoxicity evaluation in patients treated with a mitoxantrone combination as adjuvant chemotherapy for breast cancer. *Anticancer Res* 1992;12:231–4.

55. Herman EH, Zhang J, Hasinoff BB, et al. Comparison of the structural changes induced by doxorubicin and mitoxantrone in the heart, kidney and intestine and characterization of the Fe(III)–mitoxantrone complex. *J Mol Cell Cardiol* 1997;29:2415–30.

56. Doroshow JH. Anthracycline antibiotic-stimulated superoxide, hydrogen peroxide, and hydroxyl radical production by NADH dehydrogenase. *Cancer Res* 1983;43:4543–51.

57. Singal PK, Deally CM, Weinberg LE. Subcellular effects of adriamycin in the heart: a concise review. *J Mol Cell Cardiol* 1987;19:817–28.

58. Myers CE, McGuire WP, Liss RH, et al. Adriamycin: the role of lipid peroxidation in cardiac toxicity and tumor response. *Science* 1977;197:165–7.

59. Robison TW, Giri SN. Effects of chronic administration of doxorubicin on myocardial beta adrenergic receptors. *Life Sci* 1986;39:731–6.

60. Singal PK, Pierce GN. Adriamycin stimulates lowaffinity Ca2+ binding and lipid peroxidation but depresses myocardial function. *Am J Physiol* 1986;250:419–25.

61. Ehrke MJ, Maccubbin D, Ryoyama K, et al. Correlation between adriamycin-induced augmentation of interleukin 2 production and of cell-mediated cytotoxicity in mice. *Cancer Res* 1986;46:54–60.

62. Hasinoff BB. Chemistry of dexrazoxane and analogues. *Semin Oncol* 1998;25(Suppl 10):3–9.

63. Doroshow JH, Locker GY, Myers CE. Enzymatic defenses of the mouse heart against reactive oxygen metabolites: alterations produced by doxorubicin. *J Clin Invest* 1980;65:128–35.

64. Ghalie RG, Edan G, Laurent M, et al. Cardiac adverse effects associated with mitoxantrone (Novantrone) therapy in patients with MS. *Neurology* 2002;59:909–13.

65. Marriott JJ, Miyasaki JM, Gronseth G, O'Connor PW. Evidence Report: The efficacy and safety of mitoxantrone (Novantrone) in the treatment of multiple sclerosis: Report of the Therapeutics and Technology Assessment Subcommittee of the American Academy of Neurology. *Neurology* 2010;74:1463–70.

66. Le Page E, Leray E, Edan G, et al. Long-term safety profile of Mitoxantrone in a French cohort of 802 multiple sclerosis patients: a 5-year prospective study. *Mult Scler* 2011;17:867–75.

67. Feuillet L, Guedj E, Eusebio A, et al. Acute heart failure in a patient treated by mitoxantrone for multiple sclerosis. *Rev Neurol* 2003;159:1169–72.

68. Rivera V, Weinstock-Guttman B, Beagan J, et al. Final results from Registry to Evaluate Novantrone Effects in Worsening Multiple sclerosis study (RENEW). *Mult Scler* 2009;15:S254.

69. Kingwell E, Koch M, Leung B, Isserow S, Geddes J, Rieckmann P, Tremlet. H Cardiotoxicity and other adverse events associated with mitoxantrone treatment for MS. *Neurology* 2010;74:1822–6.

70. Ghalie RG, Mauch E, Edan G, et al. A study of therapy-related acute leukaemia after mitoxantrone therapy for multiple sclerosis. *Mult Scler* 2002;8:441–5.

71. Brassat D, Recher C, Waubant E, et al. Therapy-related acute myeloblastic leukemia after mitoxantrone treatment in a patient with MS. *Neurology.* 2002;59:954–5.

72. Capobianco M, Malucchi S, Ulisciani S, et al. Acute myeloid leukemia induced by mitoxantrone treatment for aggressive multiple sclerosis. *Neurol Sci.* 2008;29:185–7.

73. Ramkumar B, Chadha MK, Barcos M, et al. Acute promyelocytic leukemia

on CCL5-induced migration of lymphocytes in multiple sclerosis. *Acta Neurol Scand* 2008;118:120–125.

after mitoxantrone therapy for multiple sclerosis. *Cancer Genet Cytogenet.* 2008 Apr 15; 182:126–9.

74. Sumrall A, Dreiling B. Therapy-related acute nonlymphoblastic leukemia following mitoxantrone therapy in a patient with multiple sclerosis. *J Miss State Med Assoc* 2007;48:206–7.

75. Cartwright MS, Jeffery DR, Lewis ZT et al. Mitoxantrone for multiple sclerosis causing acute lymphoblastic leukaemia. *Neurology* 2007;68:1630–1631.

76. Ledda A, Caocci G, Spinicci G, Cocco E, Mamusa E, La Nasa G. Two new cases of acute promyelocytic leukemia following mitoxantrone treatment in patients with multiple sclerosis. *Leukemia* 2006;20:2217–8.

77. Nollet S, Berger E, Deconinck E, et al. Acute leukaemia in two multiple sclerosis patients treated with mitoxantrone. *Rev Neurol (Paris)* 2006;162:195–9.

78. Arruda WO, Montú MB, de Oliveira Mde S, Ramina R. Acute myeloid leukaemia induced by mitoxantrone: case report. *Arq Neuropsiquiatr* 2005;63:327–9.

79. Voltz R, Starck M, Zingler V, et al. Mitoxantrone therapy in multiple sclerosis and acute leukaemia: a case report out of 644 treated patients. *Mult Scler* 2004;10:472–4.

80. Tanasescu R, Debouverie M, Pittion S, Anxionnat R, Vespignani H. Acute myeloid leukaemia induced by mitoxantrone in a multiple sclerosis patient. *J Neurol* 2004;251:762–3.

81. Novoselac AV, Reddy S, Sanmugarajah J. Acute promyelocytic leukemia in a patient with multiple sclerosis following treatment with mitoxantrone. *Leukemia* 2004;18:1561–2.

82. Delisse B, de Seze J, Mackowiak A, et al. Therapy related acute myeloblastic leukaemia after mitoxantrone treatment in a patient with multiple sclerosis. *Mult Scler* 2004;10:92.

83. Cattaneo C, Almici C, Borlenghi E, et al. A case of acute promyelocytic leukaemia following mitoxantrone treatment of multiple sclerosis. *Leukemia* 2003;17:985–6.

84. Heesen C, Bruegmann M, Gbdamosi J, et al. Therapy-related acute myelogenous leukaemia (t-AML) in a patient with multiple sclerosis treated

with mitoxantrone. *Mult Scler* 2003;9:213–4.

85. Jaster JH, Niell HB, Dohan FC Jr, Smith TW. Therapy-related acute myeloblastic leukemia after mitoxantrone treatment in a patient with MS. *Neurology* 2003;60:1399–400.

86. Vicari AM, Ciceri F, Folli F, et al. Acute promyelocytic leukemia following mitoxantrone as single agent for the treatment of multiple sclerosis. *Leukemia* 1998;12:441–2.

87. Pielen A, Goffette S, Van Pesch V, et al. Mitoxantrone-related acute leukemia in two MS patients. *Acta Neurol Belg* 2008;108:99–102.

88. Ellis R, Boggild M. Therapy-related acute leukaemia with mitoxantrone: what is the risk and can we minimise it? *Mult Scler* 2009;15:505–8.

89. Bosca I, Pascual AM, Casanova B, et al. Four new cases of therapy-related acute promyelocytic leukemia after mitoxantrone. *Neurology* 2008;71:457–8

90. Pascual AM, Bosca I, Belenguer A, et al. Revisions of the risk of secondary leukemia after mitoxantrone in multiple sclerosis populations is required. *Mult Scler* 2009;15:1303–10.

91. Martinelli V, Bergamaschi R, Bellantonio P, et al. Incidence rate of acute myeloid leukaemia and related mortality in Italian MS patients treated with mitoxantrone (P480). *Mult Scler* 2010(Suppl 10): 16: S160–1.

92. Knight JA, Skol AD, Shinde A, et al. Genome-wide association study to identify novel loci associated with therapy-related myeloid leukemia susceptibility. *Blood* 2009;113:5575–82.

93. Bines J, Oleske DM, Cobleigh MA. Ovarian function in premenopausal women treated with adjuvant chemotherapy for breast cancer. *J Clin Oncol* 1996;14:1718–29.

94. Blumenfeld Z, Dann E, Avivi I, et al. Fertility after treatment for Hodgkin's disease. *Ann Oncol.* 2002;13:138–47.

95. Walshe JM, Denduluri N, Swain SM. Amenorrhea in premenopausal woman after adjuvant chemotherapy for breast cancer. *J Clin Oncol* 2006;24:5769–79.

96. Cocco E, Sardu C, Gallo P, et al. Frequency and risk factors of mitoxantrone induced amenorrhea in multiple sclerosis: the FEMIMS study. *Mult Scler* 2008;14:1225–33.

97. Meistrich ML, Wilson G, Mathur K, et al. Rapid recovery of spermatogenesis after mitoxantrone, vincristine, vinblastine, and prednisone chemotherapy for Hodgkin's disease. *J Clin Oncol* 1997;15:3488–95.

98. Manandhar M, Cheng M, Iatropoulos MJ, Noble JF. Genetic toxicology profile of the new antineoplastic drug mitoxantrone in the mammalian test systems. *Arzneimittelforschung* 1986;36:1375–9.

99. Crossley RJ. Clinical safety and tolerance of mitoxantrone. *Semin Oncol* 1984;11(Suppl 1):54–8.

100. Fox EJ. Management of worsening multiple sclerosis with mitoxantrone: a review. *Clin Ther* 2006;28:461–74.

101. Kita M, Cohen JA, Fox RJ, et al. A phase II trial of mitoxantrone in patients with primary progressive multiple sclerosis (S12.004). *Neurology* 2004;62(Suppl 5):A99.

102. European Study Group on Interferon beta-1b in secondary progressive MS. Placebo-controlled multicentre randomised trial of interferon beta-1b in treatment of secondary progressive multiple sclerosis. *Lancet* 1998;352:1491–7.

103. Panitch H, Miller A, Paty D, et al. Interferon beta-1b in secondary progressive MS: results from a 3-year controlled study. *Neurology* 2004;63:1788–95.

104. Secondary Progressive Efficacy Clinical Trial of Recombinant Interferon-beta-1a in MS (SPECTRIMS) Study Group. Randomized controlled trial of interferon-beta-1a in secondary progressive MS: clinical results. *Neurology* 2001;56:1496–504.

105. Cohen JA, Cutter GR, Fischer JS, et al. Benefit of interferon beta 1a on MSFC progression in secondary progressive MS. *Neurology* 2002;59:679–88.

106. Correale J, Rush C, Amengual A, Goicochea MT. Mitoxantrone as rescue therapy in worsening relapsing–remitting MS patients receiving IFN-b. *J Neuroimmunol* 2005;162:173–83.

107. Bar-Or A, Oger J, Gibbs E, et al. Serial combination therapy: is immune modulation in multiple sclerosis enhanced by initial immune suppression? *Mult Scler* 2009;15:959–64.

108. Edan G, Comi G, Le Page E, *et al.* Mitoxantrone prior to interferon beta-1b in aggressive relapsing multiple sclerosis a 3-year randomized trial. *J Neurol Neurosurg Psychiatry* 2011 March 24 [Epub ahead of print].

109. Swan SM. Adult multicenter trials using dexrazoxane to protect against cardiac toxicity. *Semin Oncol* 1998;25: 43–7.

110. Bernitsas E, Wei W, Mikol D. Suppression of mitoxantrone cardiotoxicity in multiple sclerosis patients by dexrazoxane. *Ann Neurol* 2006;59:206–20.

111. Boster A, Edan G, Frohman E, *et al.* Intense immunossuppression in patients with rapidly worsening multiple sclerosis: treatment guidelines for the clinician. *Lancet Neurol* 2008;7;1723–183.

112. Vollmer T, Stewart T, Baxter N. Mitoxantrone and cytotoxic drugs. Mechanisms of action. *Neurology* 2010;74(Suppl 1):S41-6.

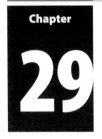

Chapter

Cladribine to treat multiple sclerosis

29

Gavin Giovannoni and Stuart D. Cook

Introduction

Multiple sclerosis (MS) is a chronic inflammatory autoimmune disorder of the central nervous system (CNS) characterized by inflammation, demyelination, and variable degrees of axonal loss and gliosis. Inflammation is considered to be a pivotal component of MS pathology and involves both T- and B-cells.[1–4] Targeted reduction of lymphocyte subtypes is a potential therapeutic strategy.[5,6] Cladribine is a synthetic small molecule that depletes lymphocytes, which acts both in the periphery and within the CNS.[5,7–9]

Cladribine, a synthetic purine nucleoside analog, is a prodrug that is resistant to deamination by the enzyme adenosine deaminase, but which undergoes intracellular phosphorylation by deoxycytidine kinase (DCK). Its active metabolite, cladribine triphosphate, accumulates within the cell, resulting in disruption of cellular metabolism, DNA damage, and subsequent apoptosis.[10] Cladribine preferentially targets lymphocytes due to their relatively high ratio of DCK to 5′-nucleotidase (5′-NT), producing rapid and sustained reductions in CD4+ and CD8+ T-cells and rapid, though more transient, effects on CD19+ B-cells. Cladribine is relatively sparing of other immune cells.[10,11] Cladribine was developed as a result of the understanding of the molecular basis of the genetic disease adenosine deaminase (ADA) deficiency. In this condition, children experience severe immunodeficiency resulting from accumulation of toxic deoxyadenosine nucleotides in lymphocytes.[5,10] The effects of cladribine mimic the intracellular process that occurs in ADA deficiency. Cladribine is licensed for the treatment of active hairy cell leukemia; extensive clinical experience with cladribine in oncology has been accumulated over more than two decades.

Cladribine's mechanism of action provided the rationale for its development as a potential agent for the treatment of MS. In clinical trials, cladribine has been found to be active in patients with relapsing–remitting (RR) forms of MS.[7,12,13] Reductions in lymphocyte counts are accompanied by reductions in proinflammatory cytokines, serum and chemokine levels, adhesion molecule expression, and mononuclear cell migration.[14–17]

Following the encouraging results with short treatment courses of parenteral cladribine in patients with MS,[7,12,13] an oral tablet formulation was developed. The efficacy and safety of cladribine tablets were investigated in a 96-week, double-blind, placebo-controlled, multicenter Phase 3 trial in RRMS: the CLARITY (CLAdRIbine tablets Treating multiple sclerosis orallY) study; clinicaltrials.gov identifier: NCT00213135, EudraCT number: 2004–005148–28.[18] Cladribine tablets differ from currently available MS treatments because they are given as short-course orally, requiring only 8 to 20 days of treatment per 48-week cycle.

This chapter will review the mechanism of action of cladribine, summarize data from clinical trials in patients with MS, and provide guidance on the management of these patients in clinical practice.

Mechanism of action

The cladribine molecule (2-chlorodeoxyadenosine, 2-CdA) is an adenosine analog, which enters cells via specific nucleoside transporter proteins. Cladribine acts as a prodrug; its activity is dependent on the intracellular accumulation of its active triphosphate, which occurs preferentially in certain cell types.[19] Three intracellular enzymes play a key role in determining the availability of its active form, 2-CdATP (Fig. 29.1):

1. Deoxycytidine kinase (DCK) – catalyzes the first of the three phosphorylation steps required to convert cladribine into its biologically active nucleotide triphosphate, 2-CdATP.

2. 5′-nucleotidase (5′-NTase) – catalyzes the re-conversion of phosphorylated cladribine to the cladribine nucleoside.

3. Adenosine deaminase (ADA) – in addition to dephosphorylation by 5′-NTase, deamination by ADA can also remove phosphorylated nucleotides via deamination by ADA. However, cladribine is resistant to deamination by ADA due to the substitution of a hydrogen atom with a chlorine atom.

The accumulation of the active 2-CdATP compound is dependent on the ratio of DCK, which creates it, to 5′-NTases, which break it down.[19] This ratio varies between different cell types. Data from messenger RNA profiling studies in the public domain (BioGPS Database)[20,21] show that levels of DCK and

Multiple Sclerosis Therapeutics, Fourth Edition, ed. Jeffrey A. Cohen and Richard A. Rudick. Published by Cambridge University Press.
© Cambridge University Press 2011.

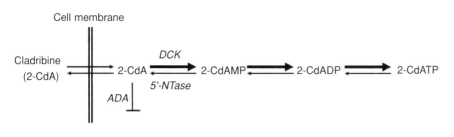

Fig. 29.1. Cladribine activation and intracellular metabolism.

2-CdAMP, 2-chlorodeoxyadenosine monophosphate
2-CdADP, 2-chlorodeoxyadenosine diphosphate
2-CdATP, 2-chlorodeoxyadenosine trisphosphate
5'-NTase, 5'-nucleotidase
ADA, adenosine deaminase
DCK, deoxycytodine kinase

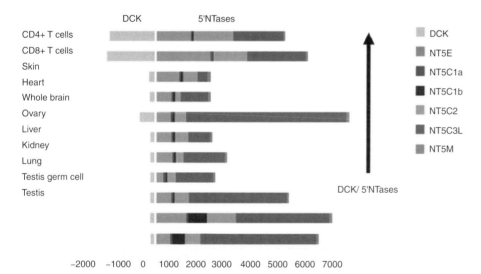

Fig. 29.2. The ratio of DCK to 5′-NTases contributes to the preferential reduction in lymphocytes by cladribine [BioGPS Database]. 5′-NT=5′-nucleotidase, DCK=deoxycytidine kinase.

the ratio of DCK: 5′-NTases are high in T-cells (both CD4+ and CD8+ subsets), B-cells, and dendritic cells (Fig. 29.2). In contrast, ratios are very low in numerous non-hematological cell types, including liver, heart, skin, brain, lung, kidney, ovarian, testicular, and germ cells. This results in selective accumulation of 2-CdATP in lymphocytes, allowing cladribine to preferentially target these cells.[22,23] As the active compound 2-CdATP builds up within lymphocytes, it results in inhibition of DNA synthesis and repair, disruption of cellular proliferation in actively dividing lymphocytes, and apoptosis and/or autophagy of quiescent lymphocytes through the accumulation of DNA strand breaks.[9,22,24,25] Alteration of cytokine patterns that includes induction of interleukin-4 and -5, interferon-gamma, and tumor necrosis factor, may also contribute to the sustained effects of cladribine tablets seen in clinical trials.[26]

Early studies

Cladribine has been used extensively in a variety of hematological disorders.[27,28] Parenteral cladribine is the treatment of choice for hairy cell leukemia.[22] Cladribine has been investigated in several other autoimmune disorders, including rheumatoid arthritis and systemic lupus erythematosus-associated glomerulonephritis.[29–31]

In early studies studies, parenteral cladribine was evaluated in both relapsing and progressive forms of MS. Three randomized, double-blind, parallel-group, placebo-controlled, Phase 2 trials were conducted; MS-001 was multicenter,[11] and Scripps-C and MS-Scripps were conducted at the Scripps Research Institute.[12,13] In the placebo-controlled phases of these studies, 183 patients received intravenous or subcutaneous cladribine at doses of 0.7 to 2.8 mg/kg, administered in monthly 5-7-day courses for two to six months, and were followed for up to 24 months.[12] In all studies, parenteral cladribine was associated with a statistically significant improvement in MRI measures of disease activity regardless of dosing regimen or route of administration.[12]

In the 18-month Scripps-C study, patients with RRMS received cladribine 2.1 mg/kg by subcutaneous injection or placebo and were followed for an additional 12 months.[13] Treatment with cladribine led to a significant reduction in the number of gadolinium (Gd)-enhancing lesions at 12 months compared with placebo ($P = 0.0001$), which remained significantly lower at 18 months ($P = 0.002$). There was a significant reduction in a combined measure of the frequency and severity of relapses in patients receiving cladribine compared with those receiving placebo from months 7 to 12 ($P = 0.021$), which was maintained at month 18 ($P = 0.010$).

The potential benefit of cladribine in patients with progressive forms of MS was examined in the 12-month multicenter MS-001 study.[11] Cladribine (0.7 or 2.1 mg/kg) administered by subcutaneous injection reduced the number and volume of Gd-enhancing lesions ($P < 0.003$).[11] However, there was no benefit on mean Expanded Disability Status Scale (EDSS) score change, the primary outcome, or on time to EDSS progression or mean change in the Scripps Neurologic Rating Scale.

The 24-month MS-Scripps study[12] also assessed the benefit of cladribine in progressive forms of MS, using a crossover design. Prior to treatment crossover at month 12, significantly fewer patients receiving cladribine (2.8 mg/kg) than placebo had Gd-enhancing lesions: two of 24 patients receiving cladribine vs. 12 of 24 receiving placebo ($P < 0.001$). Furthermore, disability and neurological performance scores were significantly better in patients receiving cladribine than in those receiving placebo ($P < 0.01$ and $P < 0.001$, respectively). It is somewhat difficult to compare the results of MS-001 and MS-Scripps studies as they had different designs and enrolled different admixtures of patients with secondary and primary progressive MS.

Pharmacokinetics and pharmacodynamics

These studies of parenteral cladribine showed encouraging results, which lead to the development of an oral tablet formulation. Cladribine is rapidly absorbed with C_{max} within 30–50 minutes after oral administration.[32] Oral bioavailability is between 37% and 51%, and food intake does not significantly affect absorption.[32,33] Up to 20% of cladribine is plasma protein bound.[32] The metabolism is not extensive; after oral administration 25% $\pm$ 21% of a dose is excreted unchanged in urine and 3.8 $\pm$ 1.9% as a metabolite.[33] Importantly in the context of MS, cladribine is able to cross the blood–brain barrier, reaching a concentration in cerebrospinal fluid (CSF) of approximately 25% of that in the periphery. This should allow lymphocyte levels to be reduced at sites of focal inflammation in the brain, as well as in the periphery.[33] Cladribine has preferential and sustained activity in lymphocytes, reducing the circulating populations, most notably for CD4+ and CD8+ T-cells, and B-cells, with effects sustained for ≥10 months following the last dose of either parenteral[11,12,34] or oral cladribine,[35] which is likely due to cladribine's effect on both resting and actively dividing lymphocytes, including quiescent progenitor cells.[5,8,22] This prolonged recovery of lymphocyte populations allows for infrequent dosing and underpins the strategy of using an annual short-course treatment schedule. Cladribine has comparatively mild, transient effects on innate immune cells such as neutrophils following parenteral administration,[11] an effect which has also observed in the subsequent clinical trial of cladribine tablets.[35] This should allow, at least theoretically, a relative preservation of an immunocompetent state.[6]

The Phase 3 CLARITY study
Design and patient population

CLARITY, a 96-week, placebo-controlled Phase 3 study of cladribine tablets as an annual short-course oral monotherapy in RRMS, was recently completed and the principal results published.[18] The results summarized below are from that publication unless otherwise specified. Patients were assigned 1:1:1 to receive a cumulative dose over the 96-week study of either cladribine 5.25 mg/kg or 3.5 mg/kg, or placebo. Each treatment course consisted of once-daily dosing for 4–5 days. Patients received two or four short courses at 28-day intervals at the start of each 48-week treatment period. Eligible patients had RRMS according to the McDonald criteria,[36] lesions consistent with MS confirmed on pre-treatment MRI scans according to the Fazekas criteria,[37] at least one relapse within 12 months of study entry, and EDSS score of 0–5.5. The primary endpoint was annualized relapse rate (ARR) over 96 weeks. Secondary endpoints included proportion of patients who were relapse free, time to sustained progression of disability, time to first relapse, proportion of patients receiving rescue therapy, MRI end-points, and safety assessments.

1326 patients were enrolled, 1184 completed the full 96 weeks of study, and 1165 completed treatment. Demographics and baseline characteristics (Table 29.1) were generally well balanced between groups, although mean duration of disease was shorter in patients in the cladribine 3.5 mg/kg group ($P < 0.05$ for the overall comparison across treatment groups). Approximately 70% of patients had not received prior disease therapy. Of 456, 433, and 437 patients randomized to 5.25 or 3.5 mg/kg cladribine doses, or placebo, respectively, 87.0%–91.9% completed the 96-week study and 86.2%–91.2% completed full-course treatment to week 52. The rates of treatment compliance (i.e. the number of tablets taken relative to the number of tablets expected to be taken) were 99.7%–99.9%. The median time on study was longer with cladribine 5.25 mg/kg (41.2 weeks) and 3.5 mg/kg (43.0 weeks) than placebo (36.1 weeks).[38]

Clinical efficacy

Benefit of both doses of cladribine over placebo was demonstrated for a variety of clinical and imaging end-points (Table 29.2). ARR at 96 weeks was significantly reduced in both cladribine groups compared to placebo (5.25 mg/kg: 0.15, relative reduction 54.5%; 3.5 mg/kg: 0.14, 57.6%; placebo 0.33; each $P < 0.001$ vs. placebo). Early benefit of treatment effect was seen, with significantly lower relapse rates in both cladribine arms vs. placebo by 16 weeks. The advantage of cladribine over placebo in reducing ARR was seen across a range of clinically important patient subgroups in post-hoc analyses, when patients were stratified by factors including age, sex, prior disease-modifying treatment, and baseline disease severity.[39] A significantly higher percentage of patients remained relapse-free at 96 weeks in both cladribine groups

Table 29.1. *Baseline patient demographics and disease characteristics (intent-to-treat population) from the CLARITY study* (reproduced with permission from the *N Engl J Med*)[18]

	Placebo (N = 437)	Cladribine 3.5 mg/kg (N = 433)	Cladribine 5.25 mg/kg (N = 456)
Age (yr)			
Mean ± SD	38.7 ± 9.9	37.9 ± 10.3	39.1 ± 9.9
Range	18–64	18–65	18–65
Gender, N female (%)	288 (65.9)	298 (68.8)	312 (68.4)
Weight, mean ± SD (kg)	70.3 ± 15.4	68.1 ± 14.6	69.3 ± 14.8
Race, N (%)			
White	429 (98.2)	425 (98.2)	446 (97.8)
Black	1 (0.2)	2 (0.5)	4 (0.9)
Other	7 (1.6)	6 (1.4)	6 (1.3)
Prior treatment with any disease-modifying drug*, N (%)	142 (32.5)	113 (26.1)	147 (32.2)
Disease duration from first attack, years			
Mean ± SD	8.9 ± 7.4	7.9 ± 7.2[†]	9.3 ± 7.6
Range	0.4–39.5	0.3–42.3	0.4–35.2
EDSS category, N (%)			
0	13 (3.0)	12 (2.8)	11 (2.4)
1	70 (16.0)	75 (17.3)	80 (17.5)
2	127 (29.1)	133 (30.7)	119 (26.1)
3	96 (22.0)	108 (24.9)	108 (23.7)
4	83 (19.0)	71 (16.4)	84 (18.4)
≥5	48 (11.0)	34 (7.9)	54 (11.8)
Mean ± SD	2.9 ± 1.3	2.8 ± 1.2	3.0 ± 1.4
T1 gadolinium-enhancing lesions			
Patients with lesions, N (%)	128 (29.3)	138 (31.9)	147 (32.2)
Number of lesions, mean ± SD	0.8 ± 2.1	1.0 ± 2.7	1.0 ± 2.3
T2 lesion volume, mm^3			
Mean ± SD	14 287.6 ± 13104.8	14 828.0 ± 16266.8	17 202.1 ± 17467.7

EDSS = Expanded Disability Status Scale; SD = standard deviation

* Most commonly: intramuscular interferon beta-1a (Avonex, 11.2%), subcutaneous interferon beta-1b (Betaseron, 10.6%), subcutaneous interferon beta-1a (Rebif, 9.4%) and subcutaneous glatiramer acetate (Copaxone, 6.5%)

[†] $P = 0.005$

vs. placebo (5.25 mg/kg: 78.9%, 3.5 mg/kg: 79.7%, placebo 60.9%; each $P < 0.001$ vs. placebo). Time to first relapse was significantly longer in both the cladribine groups compared with placebo (each $P < 0.001$). In the placebo group, the 15th percentile of time to event was 4.6 months, compared with 13.3 months (hazard ratio [HR] 0.46) in the 5.25 mg/kg group and 13.4 months (HR 0.44) in the 3.5 mg/kg group. Significantly more patients in the placebo group (6.2%) required rescue therapy than those receiving cladribine treatment: 2.0% in the cladribine 5.25 mg/kg group; $P = 0.003$ and 2.5% in the cladribine 3.5 mg/kg group; $P < 0.001$. The time from last dose to rescue therapy was similar across groups: median 178 (range −4 to 678) days for 5.25 mg/kg, 131 (range 60 to 300) days for 3.5 mg/kg, and 163 (range 31 to 592) days for placebo.[38] Time to three-month sustained change in EDSS score was significantly longer in patients receiving cladribine treatment (13.6 months in both cladribine arms vs. 10.8 months with placebo: HR 0.69,

$P = 0.03$ in the 5.25 mg/kg group and HR 0.67, $P = 0.02$ in the 3.5 mg/kg group). The odds of remaining free of three-month disability progression were increased in both cladribine treatment groups compared with placebo: odds ratio (OR) 1.46, $P = 0.03$ in the 5.25 mg/kg group and OR 1.55, $P = 0.02$ in the 3.5 mg/kg group.

MRI analyses at 96 weeks showed relative reductions in Gd-enhancing lesions with cladribine of 87.9% in the 5.25 mg/kg group and 85.7% in the 3.5 mg/kg group compared to placebo (both $P < 0.001$).[18,40] Relative reductions in active T2-hyperintense lesions were observed with cladribine of 76.9% in the 5.25 mg/kg group and 73.4% in the 3.5 mg/kg group vs. placebo (both $P < 0.001$). Relative reductions of 77.9% and 74.4% in combined unique lesions were observed with cladribine in the 5.25 and 3.5 mg/kg groups, respectively, vs. placebo (both $P < 0.001$). Significant improvements in MRI outcomes were consistently observed in clinically relevant patient

Table 29.2. *Clinical and MRI efficacy outcomes over 96 weeks (intent-to-treat population) from the CLARITY study (reproduced with permission from the* N Engl J Med*)*[18]

End-point	Placebo (N = 437)	Cladribine 3.5 mg/kg (N = 433)	Cladribine 5.25 mg/kg (N = 456)
Relapse rate – primary end point			
Annualized relapse rate (95% confidence interval)	0.33 (0.29, 0.38)	0.14 (0.12, 0.17)	0.15 (0.12, 0.17)
Relative reduction in annualized relapse rate for cladribine vs. placebo[a]		57.6%	54.5%
P-value[b]		< 0.001	< 0.001
Relapse-free rate, N (%)	266 (60.9%)	345 (79.7%)	360 (78.9%)
Odds ratio for cladribine vs. placebo, point estimate (95% confidence interval)[c]		2.53 (1.87, 3.43)	2.43 (1.81, 3.27)
P-value[d]		< 0.001	< 0.001
Number of relapses over 96 weeks, N patients (%)			
0	266 (60.9)	345 (79.7)	360 (78.9)
1	109 (24.9)	69 (15.9)	77 (16.9)
2	44 (10.1)	13 (3.0)	13 (2.9)
3	15 (3.4)	5 (1.2)	5 (1.1)
>4	3 (0.7)	1 (0.2)	1 (0.2)
P-value[e]		< 0.001	< 0.001
Patients receiving rescue therapy, N (%)	27 (6.2)	11 (2.5)	9 (2.0)
Odds ratio for cladribine vs. placebo, point estimate (95% confidence interval)[c]		0.40 (0.19, 0.81)	0.31 (0.14, 0.66)
P-value[d]		0.01	0.003
Time to first relapse, 15th percentile in days (months)[f]	141 (4.6)	408 (13.4)	406 (13.3)
Hazard ratio for cladribine vs. placebo, point estimate (95% confidence interval)[g]		0.44 (0.34, 0.58)	0.46 (0.36, 0.60)
P-value[g]		< 0.001	< 0.001
Time to 3-month sustained change in EDSS score, 10th percentile in days (months) [f]	330 (10.8)	414 (13.6)	414 (13.6)
Hazard ratio for cladribine vs. placebo, point estimate (95% confidence interval)[g]		0.67 (0.48, 0.93)	0.69 (0.49, 0.96)
P-value[g]		0.02	0.03
Patients without a 3-month sustained change in EDSS score, N (%)	347 (79.4)	371 (85.7)	387 (84.9)
Odds ratio for cladribine vs. placebo, point estimate (95% confidence interval) [c]		1.55 (1.09, 2.22)	1.46 (1.03, 2.07)
P-value[d]		0.02	0.03
Lesion activity on brain MRI			
T1 gadolinium-enhancing lesions, mean Relative reduction in T1 gadolinium-enhancing lesions	0.91	0.12 85.7%	0.11 87.9%
Active T2 lesions, mean relative reduction in active T2 lesions	1.43	0.38 73.4%	0.33 76.9%
Combined unique lesions, mean Relative reduction in combined unique lesions	1.72	0.43 74.4%	0.38 77.9%
P-value[h]		< 0.001	< 0.001

EDSS = Expanded Disability Status Scale; SD = standard deviation.
[a] Calculated as the ratio of the difference in annualized relapse rate (placebo – cladribine) relative to the annualized relapse rate in the placebo group.
[b] P-value based on Wald Chi-square test from analysis of number of relapses using a Poisson regression model with fixed effects for treatment and region, and using log time on study as an offset variable.
[c] Odds ratio and associated 95% confidence intervals were estimated using a logistic regression model with fixed effects for treatment group and region.
[d] P-value based on Wald Chi-square test from analysis of end-point using a logistic regression model with fixed effects for treatment group and region.
[e] P-value from Cochran-Mantel-Haenszel row means score differ test, adjusted for baseline number of relapses.
[f] The 10th and 15th percentile values are estimated from the Kaplan–Meier survival curve.
[g] The hazard ratio, 95% confidence intervals and P-values were estimated using Cox proportional hazards model with fixed effects for treatment group and region.
[h] P-value based on non-parametric ANCOVA model on ranked data with fixed effects for treatment group and region and baseline T1 gadolinium-enhancing lesions as a covariate.

Table 29.3. *Safety overview from the CLARITY study* (reproduced with permission from *Multiple Sclerosis*)[42]

Patients, N (%)	Placebo (N = 435)	Cladribine 3.5 mg/kg (N = 430)	Cladribine 5.25 mg/kg (N = 454)	Cladribine overall (N = 884)
Any AE	319 (73.3)	347 (80.7)	381 (83.9)	728 (82.4)
Most common AEs[a]				
Headache	75 (17.2)	104 (24.2)	94 (20.7)	198 (22.4)
Lymphopenia	8 (1.8)	93 (21.6)	143 (31.5)	236 (26.7)
Nasopharyngitis	56 (12.9)	62 (14.4)	58 (12.8)	120 (13.6)
URTI	42 (9.7)	54 (12.6)	52 (11.5)	106 (12.0)
Nausea	39 (9.0)	43 (10.0)	50 (11.0)	93 (10.5)
AEs leading to treatment discontinuation	9 (2.1)	15 (3.5)	36 (7.9)	51 (5.8)
AEs leading to study withdrawal	5 (1.1)	5 (1.2)	10 (2.2)	15 (1.7)
Serious AEs	28 (6.4)	36 (8.4)	41 (9.0)	77 (8.7)
Deaths	2 (0.5)	2 (0.5)	2 (0.4)	4 (0.4)
Events, n (%)	(n = 1958)	(n = 2514)	(n = 2712)	(n = 5226)
Any AE	1958 (100)	2514 (100)	2712 (100)	5226 (100)
Most common AEs				
Headache	189 (9.7)	264 (10.5)	265 (9.8)	529 (10.1)
Lymphopenia	11 (0.6)	123 (4.9)	195 (7.2)	318 (6.1)
Nasopharyngitis	95 (4.9)	107 (4.3)	91 (3.4)	198 (3.8)
URTI	80 (4.1)	118 (4.7)	100 (3.7)	218 (4.2)
Nausea	49 (2.5)	74 (2.9)	69 (2.5)	143 (2.7)

AE = adverse event; URTI = upper respiratory tract infection.
[a] Reported by ≥10% of patients in any group.

subgroups stratified according to baseline disease severity.[40] When stratified by baseline relapse rate, the relative reductions in combined unique lesions/patient/scan for the 5.25 and 3.5 mg/kg groups were 75.5 % and 74.8% (≤1 relapse), 86.7% and 83.1% (2 relapses), and 90.0% and 76.7% (≥3 relapses), respectively (all $P < 0.001$). Similarly, relative reductions for the 5.25 mg/kg and 3.5 mg/kg groups were 75.2% and 73.5% for patients without Gd-enhancing lesions at baseline, and 84.9% and 80.8% for patients with ≥1 Gd-enhancing lesion(s) at baseline, respectively (all $P < 0.001$).[40]

Disease activity-free status, a composite measure of efficacy, was analyzed post-hoc and confirmed the efficacy findings.[41] In the cladribine 5.25 and 3.5 mg/kg vs. placebo groups, respectively, 69.7% and 67.3% vs. 38.9% of patients were disease activity free over 24 weeks; 56.1% and 54.2% vs. 23.9% over 48 weeks; and 46.0% and 44.2% vs. 15.8% over the entire 96-week study (all $P < 0.001$ for cladribine vs. placebo).[41] Significant differences between cladribine and placebo disease activity free status were seen across patient subgroups, including patients who had received prior disease-modifying therapy (42.9% and 37.2% on cladribine 5.25 and 3.5 mg/kg, respectively vs. 16.2% on placebo) and treatment-naive patients (45.0% for cladribine doses vs. 15.9% on placebo); patients with baseline disease-duration < 3 years (46.5% and 38.1% vs. 8.2%), 3–10 years (40.3% and 47.0% vs. 15.5%), and >10 years (47.8% and 41.8% vs. 22.1%) (all $P < 0.001$ for active

treatments vs. placebo).[41] OR (95% confidence interval [CI]) for patients remaining disease activity-free were 4.24 (3.09–5.82) with cladribine 5.25 mg/kg and 3.99 (2.89–5.49) with 3.5 mg/kg vs. placebo (each $P < 0.001$).[41]

Safety

The most common adverse events (AEs) were lymphopenia, headache, nasopharyngitis, and upper respiratory tract infections (URTI) (Tables 29.3 and 29.4).[18,42] Lymphopenia occurred more frequently in the cladribine treatment groups, which is expected due to cladribine's mechanism of action. The rates of infections were cladribine 5.25 mg/kg (48.9%) and 3.5 mg/kg (47.7%) vs. 42.5% in the placebo group; most cases were mild to moderate. Herpes zoster infections occurred in 2% of patients receiving cladribine; all cases were restricted and dermatomal in nature. AEs infrequently led to treatment delay/interruption (5.6% and 9.5% for cladribine 5.25 and 3.5 mg/kg, and 3.2% for placebo) or study discontinuation (1.2% and 2.0% for cladribine 5.25 and 3.5 mg/kg, and 1.1% for placebo).[38] AEs led to treatment discontinuation in 3.5%, 7.9%, and 2.1% of patients receiving cladribine 5.25 mg/kg, 3.5 mg/kg, and placebo groups, respectively. The incidence of serious AEs was 9.0% and 8.4% in the cladribine 5.25 and 3.5 mg/kg groups vs. 6.4% in the placebo group.

Table 29.4. *Adverse events reported in ≥1% patients in any treatment group that show two-fold treatment differences in the CLARITY study[a] (reproduced with permission from* Multiple Sclerosis*).[42]*

System organ class Preferred term,[b] N (%)	Placebo (N = 435)	Cladribine 3.5 mg/kg (N = 430)	Cladribine 5.25 mg/kg (N = 454)	Cladribine overall (N = 884)
Blood and lymphatic system disorders				
Lymphopenia	8 (1.8)	93 (21.6)	143 (31.5)	236 (26.7)
Leukopenia	3 (0.7)	24 (5.6)	39 (8.6)	63 (7.1)
Neutropenia	2 (0.5)	8 (1.9)	10 (2.2)	18 (2.0)
Anemia	2 (0.5)	5 (1.2)	5 (1.1)	10 (1.1)
Investigations				
Lymphocyte count decreased	0	13 (3.0)	26 (5.7)	39 (4.4)
White blood cell count decreased	0	3 (0.7)	7 (1.5)	10 (1.1)
Body temperature increased	5 (1.1)	2 (0.5)	2 (0.4)	4 (0.5)
Ear and labyrinth disorders				
Vertigo	11 (2.5)	14 (3.3)	23 (5.1)	37 (4.2)
Tinnitus	2 (0.5)	2 (0.5)	10 (2.2)	12 (1.4)
General disorders and administration site conditions				
Pyrexia	8 (1.8)	14 (3.3)	18 (4.0)	32 (3.6)
Gait disturbance	2 (0.5)	2 (0.5)	5 (1.1)	7 (0.8)
Hyperthermia	2 (0.5)	5 (1.2)	1 (0.2)	6 (0.7)
Pain	5 (1.1)	2 (0.5)	3 (0.7)	5 (0.6)
Skin and subcutaneous tissue disorders				
Alopecia	5 (1.1)	15 (3.5)	14 (3.1)	29 (3.3)
Rash	5 (1.1)	10 (2.3)	11 (2.4)	21 (2.4)
Dermatitis allergic	3 (0.7)	12 (2.8)	6 (1.3)	18 (2.0)
Acne	2 (0.5)	7 (1.6)	2 (0.4)	9 (1.0)
Infections and infestations				
Viral upper respiratory tract infection	5 (1.1)	13 (3.0)	7 (1.5)	20 (2.3)
Herpes zoster[c]	0	8 (1.9)	12 (2.6)	20 (2.3)
Vaginal infection	1 (0.2)	8 (1.9)	5 (1.1)	13 (1.5)
Viral infection	2 (0.5)	6 (1.4)	6 (1.3)	12 (1.4)
Respiratory tract infection viral	2 (0.5)	6 (1.4)	5 (1.1)	11 (1.2)
Vulvovaginal mycotic infection	2 (0.5)	1 (0.2)	6 (1.3)	7 (0.8)
Tooth abscess	3 (0.7)	1 (0.2)	5 (1.1)	6 (0.7)
Tonsillitis	6 (1.4)	0	4 (0.9)	4 (0.5)
Injury, poisoning and procedural complications				
Contusion	3 (0.7)	6 (1.4)	9 (2.0)	15 (1.7)
Ankle fracture	5 (1.1)	4 (0.9)	2 (0.4)	6 (0.7)
Joint sprain	6 (1.4)	3 (0.7)	1 (0.2)	4 (0.5)
Procedural pain	7 (1.6)	0	2 (0.4)	2 (0.2)
Nervous system disorders				
Hypesthesia	4 (0.9)	2 (0.5)	9 (2.0)	11 (1.2)
Syncope	3 (0.7)	6 (1.4)	5 (1.1)	11 (1.2)
Somnolence	6 (1.4)	3 (0.7)	6 (1.3)	9 (1.0)
Paraesthesia	2 (0.5)	4 (0.9)	5 (1.1)	9 (1.0)
Migraine	8 (1.8)	4 (0.9)	4 (0.9)	8 (0.9)
Radiculopathy	5 (1.1)	0	0	0
Reproductive system and breast disorders				
Dysmenorrhea	3 (0.7)	7 (1.6)	4 (0.9)	11 (1.2)
Metrorrhagia	1 (0.2)	1 (0.2)	5 (1.1)	6 (0.7)
Cardiac disorders				
Angina pectoris	3 (0.7)	6 (1.4)	5 (1.1)	11 (1.2)
Gastrointestinal disorders				
Dry mouth	1 (0.2)	4 (0.9)	6 (1.3)	10 (1.1)
Gastritis	9 (2.1)	3 (0.7)	5 (1.1)	8 (0.9)

Table 29.4. (cont.)

System organ class Preferred term,[b] N (%)	Placebo (N = 435)	Cladribine 3.5 mg/kg (N = 430)	Cladribine 5.25 mg/kg (N = 454)	Cladribine overall (N = 884)
Periodontitis	3 (0.7)	6 (1.4)	2 (0.4)	8 (0.9)
Flatulence	1 (0.2)	2 (0.5)	5 (1.1)	7 (0.8)
Gastritis erosive	5 (1.1)	1 (0.2)	1 (0.2)	2 (0.2)
Respiratory, thoracic, and mediastinal disorders				
Dyspnea	4 (0.9)	1 (0.2)	8 (1.8)	9 (1.0)
Rhinorrhea	2 (0.5)	3 (0.7)	6 (1.3)	9 (1.0)
Eye disorders				
Conjunctivitis	2 (0.5)	3 (0.7)	6 (1.3)	9 (1.0)
Vision blurred	2 (0.5)	5 (1.2)	0	5 (0.6)
Renal and urinary disorders				
Dysuria	2 (0.5)	4 (0.9)	5 (1.1)	9 (1.0)
Neoplasms benign, malignant, and unspecified (including cysts and polyps)				
Uterine leiomyoma	1 (0.2)	5 (1.2)	4 (0.9)	9 (1.0)
Musculoskeletal and connective tissue disorders				
Muscle spasms	5 (1.1)	2 (0.5)	6 (1.3)	8 (0.9)
Vascular disorders				
Hot flush	1 (0.2)	1 (0.2)	5 (1.1)	6 (0.7)

[a] AEs for which the percentage of patients in one active treatment group is ≥2 x the percentage of patients in the placebo group, or the percentage of patients in the placebo group is ≥2 x the percentage of patients in the active treatment group.
[b] Medical Dictionary for Regulatory Activities (MedDRA) v11.0 terminology.
[c] Includes one case of herpes zoster oticus (Ramsay-Hunt syndrome) reported in the cladribine 5.25 mg/kg group.

Table 29.5. *Serious adverse events from the CLARITY study* (reproduced with permission from *Multiple Sclerosis*)[42]

Patients, n (%)	Placebo (N = 435)	Cladribine 3.5 mg/kg (N = 430)	Cladribine 5.25 mg/kg (N = 454)	Cladribine overall (N = 884)
Any SAE	28 (6.4)	36 (8.4)	41 (9.0)	77 (8.7)
Most common[a] SAEs that show treatment differences[b] by system organ class				
Neoplasms – benign, malignant, and unspecified	0	6 (1.4)	4 (0.9)	10 (1.1)
Gastrointestinal disorders	2 (0.5)	4 (0.9)	5 (1.1)	9 (1.0)
Injury, poisoning, and procedural complications	2 (0.5)	9 (2.1)	0	9 (1.0)
Most common[c] SAEs that show treatment differences[b] by preferred term				
Uterine leiomyoma	0	3 (0.7)	2 (0.4)	5 (0.6)
Lymphopenia	0	3 (0.7)	1 (0.1)	4 (0.5)
Events, n (%)	**(n = 1958)**	**(n = 2514)**	**(n = 2712)**	**(n = 5226)**
Any SAE	44 (2.2)	61 (2.4)	80 (2.9)	141 (2.7)
Most common[a] SAEs that show treatment differences[b] by system organ class				
Neoplasms – benign, malignant, and unspecified	0	6 (0.2)	4 (0.1)	10 (0.2)
Gastrointestinal disorders	4 (0.2)	5 (0.2)	7 (0.3)	12 (0.2)
Injury, poisoning, and procedural complications	3 (0.2)	17 (0.7)	0	17 (0.3)
Most common[c] SAEs that show treatment differences[b] by preferred term				
Uterine leiomyoma	0	3 (0.1)	2 (0.1)	5 (0.1)
Lymphopenia	0	3 (0.1)	1 (<0.1)	4 (0.1)

SAE = serious adverse event.
[a] Reported in >1% of patients in any treatment group.
[b] The percentage of patients in one active treatment group is ≥2 x the percentage of patients in the placebo group, or the percentage of patients in the placebo group is ≥2 x the percentage of patients in the active treatment group.
[c] Reported in >0.5% of patients in any treatment group.

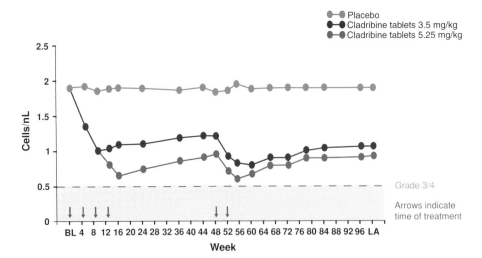

Fig. 29.3. Change in lymphocyte count over time in the CLARITY study. The shaded area indicates the cut-off for grade 3/4 severity. Adapted from Giovannoni et al.[18]

Malignancies reported in cladribine tablets groups of the CLARITY study were isolated cases across different organ systems, and comparable to the incidence in the general population (Table 29.5).[42] Three cases were reported during the study – a melanoma, pancreatic carcinoma, and ovarian carcinoma – and one case of malignant cervical carcinoma in situ. One case of choriocarcinoma was reported post-study. Due to the low number of malignancies, it is not currently possible to determine with certainty whether there is any increased risk of malignancy associated with the use of cladribine tablets. However, due to the prolonged immunosuppression and the genotoxic potential of cladribine, a risk for development of malignancy cannot be excluded. Safety registries have been set up to collect information on malignancies and other safety end-points in patients treated with cladribine.[43]

The follow-up of 979 patients treated with cladribine for hairy cell leukemia, for a median of 5.1 years, reported an observed to expected frequency of secondary tumors of 1.50 (95% CI, 1.14 to 1.93), indicating a significant ($P < 0.05$) increase in risk for patients treated with cladribine compared with a normal population.[44] The 61 malignancies were most commonly lymphoma (13 patients), prostate (16), gastrointestinal (6), breast (5), bladder (3) and lung (3) but CNS, stomach, ovary, melanoma, sarcoma, testicular, and myeloid leukemias also were observed. However, these values are consistent with the increase already associated with hairy cell leukemia, which led to the conclusion that cladribine can be administered to patients with hairy cell leukemia without a significantly increased risk of secondary malignancies.

Despite instruction in the CLARITY study protocol on the use of contraception, 25 pregnancies were reported (12 in 5.25 mg/kg group, 7 in the 3.5 mg/kg group, and 6 in the placebo group).[42] Six conceptions occurred during study treatment periods (2, 1, and 3 in the 5.25 mg/kg, 3.5 mg/kg, and placebo groups, respectively), 18 during study off-treatment periods (9, 6, and 3 in the 5.25 mg/kg, 3.5 mg/kg, and placebo groups,

respectively), and one occurred post-study (in the 5.25 mg/kg group). These resulted in four miscarriages (two, one, and one in the 5.25 mg/kg, 3.5 mg/kg, and placebo groups, respectively), 14 elective abortions (seven, five, and two in the 5.25 mg/kg, 3.5 mg/kg, and placebo groups, respectively), six normal-term live births (3, 0, and 3 in the 5.25 mg/kg, 3.5 mg/kg, and placebo groups, respectively), and one ectopic pregnancy (in the 3.5 mg/kg group).

Rapid decreases in leukocyte counts were observed following oral cladribine administration in CLARITY, mainly driven by reductions in lymphocytes, which reached a first nadir at weeks 16 and nine in the 5.25 mg/kg and 3.5 mg/kg groups, respectively, and a second nadir at weeks 55 and 60 in the 5.25 mg/kg and 3.5 mg/kg groups, respectively (Fig. 29.3).[18,35] At the first nadir, though some individual patients had reductions in leukocytes that reached common terminology criteria for adverse events grade 3/4 levels, on average, levels were less than grade 3/4 severity. The first nadir was followed by a period of recovery until the second short-course dosing at week 48. Compared with lymphocytes, there was a relative preservation of neutrophils and other immune cells. Rapid and sustained decreases in CD3+, CD4+, and CD8+ T-cell counts were seen,[35] with levels remaining fairly consistent from week 16 onwards, even after redosing at week 48. Decreases in CD19+ B-cell counts were pronounced and both reduction and recovery occurred faster than for T-cell changes.

There were four deaths during the study and two deaths after patients were withdrawn from study (withdrawals had been due to AEs); the six deaths were equally distributed across the three treatment groups (Table 29.3).[42] Causes of death during the study were suicide (placebo), hemorrhagic stroke (placebo), acute myocardial infarction (cladribine 3.5 mg/kg), and drowning (cladribine 5.25 mg/kg). Causes of death following study withdrawal were metastatic pancreatic carcinoma (cladribine 3.5 mg/kg group), and acute cardiopulmonary arrest in a patient with tuberculosis (cladribine 5.25 mg/kg).

The patient who died from metastatic carcinoma was a 61-year-old woman in the 3.5 mg/kg group who was discontinued from the study following her week 72 visit due to gastrointestinal and constitutional symptoms. She was subsequently diagnosed with metastatic pancreatic carcinoma and initiated chemotherapy, but died about three months after diagnosis.

The acute cardiopulmonary arrest was considered to be related to an exacerbation of pre-existing tuberculosis. A 21-year-old woman in the 5.25 mg/kg group received a single treatment course of cladribine tablets (0.875 mg/kg). Approximately one week after her last dose of cladribine, she developed pancytopenia after which she was permanently withdrawn from treatment. A second episode of pancytopenia occurred approximately two months after the end of cladribine treatment. A chest X-ray at this stage showed bilateral alveolar-interstitial infiltrates, and a bone marrow biopsy performed six days later showed "slight myelodysplasia." At approximately five months after the last dose of cladribine, the patient experienced a third episode of pancytopenia. A chest X-ray showed recurrent bilateral alveolar–interstitial lung infiltrates. Repeat bone marrow examination revealed an apparent myelodysplastic syndrome. The patient died from an acute cardiopulmonary arrest approximately six months after receiving a single 0.875 mg/kg treatment course of cladribine. The diagnosis of tuberculosis was obtained post-mortem, and the chronic pathological nature of lesions in the liver and lungs, together with the temporal relationship between treatment and acute onset of symptoms, suggested that the tuberculosis was long-standing and present prior to cladribine treatment. Cladribine therapy is likely to have contributed to the worsening of the tuberculosis infection. The myelodysplasia-like condition was probably reactive bone marrow changes caused by the chronic tuberculosis infection. Upon review, this was determined not to be a case of bona fide myelodysplastic syndrome as there were no cytogenetic abnormalities, and its presentation was not consistent with the natural history of myelodysplasia.

Considerations for patient management

The efficacy and safety findings in the CLARITY study were associated with additional benefits in reducing health care resource utilization.[45] In a comparison of resource use across treatment arms, the outcomes observed during the CLARITY study were associated with a reduced consumption of health care resources and a decreased need for medical and societal support, suggesting a potential economic benefit of treatment with cladribine tablets. Compared with placebo, the mean number of hospital days per patient over 96 weeks was 1.92 days fewer in the cladribine 5.25 mg/kg group and 3.90 days fewer in the 3.5 mg/kg group, both $P < 0.01$. The numbers of emergency room visits, clinic visits, and missed work days also were significantly lower for both cladribine treatment arms compared to placebo. Additionally, corticosteroid use was lower amongst patients in the cladribine groups than in the placebo group (mainly due to fewer relapses).

Follow-on studies

Currently, cladribine tablets are being studied as monotherapy and in combination with other disease-modifying therapies.[46] A 96-week CLARITY extension study is in progress, which will build on the data of the 96-week core Phase 3 study to give efficacy and safety data for up to four years of treatment. Phase 2 ONWARD (Oral cladribine added **ON** to Rebif new formulation in patients **W**ith **A**ctive **R**elapsing **D**isease) and ONWARD EXTENSION trials are evaluating cladribine tablets as add-on therapy to interferon-beta in RRMS.[46] A Phase 3 ORACLE MS (**ORA**l **CL**adribine in **E**arly **MS**) trial is also in progress in subjects with a first clinical event who are at high risk of converting to MS.[46] To provide long-term safety data all patients who have participated in clinical trials of oral cladribine are eligible for the PREMIERE study (the **PR**ospective observational long-term saf**E**ty registry of **MS** pat**IE**nts who have participated in clinical trials with clad**R**ibin**E** tablets).[43,46]

Conclusions

CLARITY demonstrated cladribine tablets to have potent efficacy on relapses, EDSS progression, and MRI lesion activity in RRMS. Its oral route of administration, need for infrequent dosing, and generally good tolerability make it an attractive MS treatment option. However, as of the time this writing, cladribine has not yet received regulatory approval in North America or the European Union. Like other emerging therapies in MS, some potential safety issues have been noted, and the overall experience with its use in MS, particularly long-term use, is limited. It is anticipated that ongoing studies will further elucidate cladribine's benefit risk relationship, including where to place it in the MS treatment algorithm.

References

1. Chitnis T. The role of CD4 T cells in the pathogenesis of multiple sclerosis. *Int Rev Neurobiol* 2007;79:43–72.

2. Owens GP, Bennett JL, Gilden DH, Burgoon MP. The B cell response in multiple sclerosis. *Neurol Res* 2006;28:236–44.

3. Delgado S, Sheremata WA. The role of CD4+ T-cells in the development of MS. *Neurol Res* 2006;28:245–9.

4. Weber MS, Hemmer B. Cooperation of B cells and T cells in the pathogenesis of multiple sclerosis. *Results Probl Cell Differ* 2010;51:115–26.

5. Sipe JC. Cladribine for multiple sclerosis: review and current status. *Expert Rev Neurother* 2005;5:721–7.

6. Leist TP, Vermersch P. The potential role for cladribine in the treatment of multiple sclerosis: clinical experience and development of an oral tablet

formulation. *Curr Med Res Opin* 2007;23:2667–76.

7. Sipe JC, Romine JS, Koziol JA, *et al.* Cladribine in treatment of chronic progressive multiple sclerosis. *Lancet* 1994;344:9–13.

8. Carson DA, Wasson DB, Taetle R, Yu A. Specific toxicity of 2-chlorodeoxyadenosine toward resting and proliferating human lymphocytes. *Blood* 1983;62:737–43.

9. Laugel B, Challier JA, *et al.* The mechanism of action behind the lymphocyte-depleting and immunomodulatory effects of cladribine (P01.108). *Neurology* 2009; 72(Suppl 3):A35.

10. Beutler E. Cladribine (2-chlorodeoxyadenosine). *Lancet* 1992;340:952–6.

11. Rice GP, for the Cladribine Clinical Study Group, Filippi M, Comi G, for the Cladribine MRI Study Group. Cladribine and progressive MS: clinical and MRI outcomes of a multicenter controlled trial. *Neurology* 2000;54: 1145–55.

12. Beutler E, Sipe JC, Romine JS, *et al.* The treatment of chronic progressive multiple sclerosis with cladribine. *Proc Natl Acad Sci USA* 1996;93: 1716–20.

13. Romine JS, Sipe JC, Koziol JA, Zyroff J, Beutler E. A double-blind, placebo-controlled, randomized trial of cladribine in relapsing-remitting multiple sclerosis. *Proc Assoc Am Physicians* 1999;111:35–44.

14. Bartosik-Psujek H, Belniak E, Mitosek-Szewczyk K, Dobosz B, Stelmasiak Z. Interleukin-8 and RANTES levels in patients with relapsing-remitting multiple sclerosis (RR-MS) treated with cladribine. *Acta Neurol Scand* 2004;109:390–2.

15. Janiec K, Wajgt A, Kondera-Anasz Z. Effect of immunosuppressive cladribine treatment on serum leucocytes system in two-year clinical trial in patients with chronic progressive multiple sclerosis. *Med Sci Monit* 2001;7:93–8.

16. Kopadze T, Dobert M, Leussink VI, Dehmel T, Kieseier BC. Cladribine impedes in vitro migration of mononuclear cells: a possible implication for treating multiple sclerosis. *Eur J Neurol* 2009;16:409–12.

17. Niezgoda A, Losy J, Mehta PD. Effect of cladribine treatment on beta-2

microglobulin and soluble intercellular adhesion molecule 1 (ICAM-1) in patients with multiple sclerosis. *Folia Morphol (Warsz)* 2001;60:225–8.

18. Giovannoni G, Comi G, Cook S, *et al.* A placebo-controlled trial of oral cladribine for relapsing multiple sclerosis. *N Engl J Med* 2010;362: 416–26.

19. Kawasaki H, Carrera CJ, Piro LD, *et al.* Relationship of deoxycytidine kinase and cytoplasmic 5'-nucleotidase to the chemotherapeutic efficacy of 2-chlorodeoxyadenosine. *Blood* 1993; 81:597–601.

20. Wu C, Orozco C, Boyer J, *et al.* BioGPS: an extensible and customizable portal for querying and organizing gene annotation resources. *Genome Biol* 2009;10:R130.

21. Su A, Orozco C, Wu C, Leglise M, MacLeod I. BioGPS: the gene portal hub. 2011 [updated 2011; cited]; Available from: http://biogps.gnf.org/ #goto=welcome.

22. Saven A, Piro LD. 2-Chlorodeoxyadenosine: a newer purine analog active in the treatment of indolent lymphoid malignancies. *Ann Intern Med* 1994;120:784–91.

23. Salvat C, Curchod ML, Guedj E, *et al.* Cellular expression profiling of genes involved in the cladribine metabolic pathway: insights into mechanism of action in multiple sclerosis (P280). *Mult Scler* 2009;15(Suppl 2):S74.

24. Griffig J, Koob R, Blakley RL. Mechanisms of inhibition of DNA synthesis by 2-chlorodeoxyadenosine in human lymphoblastic cells. *Cancer Res* 1989;49:6923–8.

25. Hentosh P, Peffley DM. The cladribine conundrum: deciphering the drug's mechanism of action. *Expert Opin Drug Metab Toxicol* 2010;6:75–81.

26. Korsen M, Broker B, Dressel A. Cladribine-induced alterations in cytokine patterns of peripheral blood mononuclear cells (P838). *Mult Scler* 2010;16(Suppl 10):S293.

27. Juliusson G, Christiansen I, Hansen MM, *et al.* Oral cladribine as primary therapy for patients with B-cell chronic lymphocytic leukemia. *J Clin Oncol* 1996;14:2160–6.

28. Ogura M, Morishima Y, Kobayashi Y, *et al.* Durable response but prolonged cytopenia after cladribine treatment in relapsed patients with indolent

non-Hodgkin's lymphomas: results of a Japanese phase II study. *Int J Hematol* 2004;80:267–77.

29. Schirmer M, Mur E, Pfeiffer KP, Thaler J, Konwalinka G. The safety profile of low-dose cladribine in refractory rheumatoid arthritis. A pilot trial. *Scand J Rheumatol* 1997;26:376–9.

30. Davis JC, Jr., Austin H, 3rd, Boumpas D, *et al.* A pilot study of 2-chloro-2'-deoxyadenosine in the treatment of systemic lupus erythematosus-associated glomerulonephritis. *Arthritis Rheum* 1998;41:335–43.

31. Beutler E, Sipe J, Romine J, *et al.* Treatment of multiple sclerosis and other autoimmune diseases with cladribine. *Semin Hematol* 1996;33(Suppl 1):45–52.

32. Sipe JC. Cladribine tablets: a potential new short-course annual treatment for relapsing multiple sclerosis. *Expert Rev Neurother* 2010;10:365–75.

33. Liliemark J. The clinical pharmacokinetics of cladribine. *Clin Pharmacokinet* 1997;32:120–31.

34. Guarnaccia JB, Rinder H, Smith B. Preferential effects of cladribine on lymphocyte subpopulations (P55). *Mult Scler* 2008;14(Suppl 1):S45.

35. Sorensen PS, Comi G, Cook S, *et al.* Effects of cladribine tablets on haematological profiles in patients with relapsing-remitting multiple sclerosis in the 96-week, phase III, double-blind, placebo-controlled CLARITY study (P472). *Mult Scler* 2009;15(Suppl 2): S137.

36. McDonald WI, Compston A, Edan G, *et al.* Recommended diagnostic criteria for multiple sclerosis: guidelines from the International Panel on the diagnosis of multiple sclerosis. *Ann Neurol* 2001;50:121–7.

37. Fazekas F, Barkhof F, Filippi M, *et al.* The contribution of magnetic resonance imaging to the diagnosis of multiple sclerosis. *Neurology* 1999;53:448–56.

38. Vermersch P, Comi G, Cook S, *et al.* Tolerability and retention on treatment with cladribine tablets for relapsing–remitting multiple sclerosis over 96 weeks in the phase III, double-blind, placebo-controlled CLARITY study (P852). *Mult Scler* 2010;16(Suppl 10):S298–9.

39. Rammohan K, Comi G, Cook S, *et al.* Consistent efficacy of short-course

cladribine tablets therapy across differing prognostic indicators for relapsing–remitting multiple sclerosis: results from the phase III, double-blind, placebo-controlled, 96-week CLARITY study (P441). *Mult Scler* 2010 (Suppl 10); 16:S146.

40. Comi G, Cook S, Giovannoni G, *et al.* Consistent MRI benefits with short-course cladribine tablets therapy across the range of patients with relapsing–remitting multiple sclerosis in the double-blind, placebo controlled, 96-week CLARITY study (P403). *Mult Scler* 2010;16(Suppl 10): S131–2.

41. Giovannoni G, Comi G, Cook S, *et al.* Analysis of sustained disease activity-free status in patients with relapsing–remitting multiple sclerosis treated with cladribine tablets, in the double-blind, 96-week CLARITY study (P825). *Mult Scler* 2010;16(Suppl 10): S288.

42. Cook S, Vermersch P, Comi G, *et al.* Safety and tolerability of cladribine tablets in multiple sclerosis: the CLARITY (CLAdRIbine Tablets treating multiple sclerosis orallY) study. *Mult Scler* 2011;17:578–93.

43. Miret M, Weiner J, Gedney L, Greenberg S, Alteri E. Evaluation of the long-term safety of cladribine tablets in multiple sclerosis: design of PREMIERE, a prospective, observational 8-year safety registry (P444). *J Neurol* 2010;257(Suppl 1): S144.

44. Cheson BD, Vena DA, Barrett J, Freidlin B. Second malignancies as a consequence of nucleoside analog therapy for chronic lymphoid leukemias. *J Clin Oncol* 1999;17: 2454–60.

45. Joyeux A, Ali S, Comi G, *et al.* Reduced healthcare resource utilization with cladribine tablets in patients with relapsing-remitting multiple sclerosis in the double-blind 96-week CLARITY study (P232). *Mult Scler* 2010;16 (Suppl 10):S70–1.

46. Viglietta V, Greenberg S, Mikol D, *et al.* Late stage clinical development plan for cladribine tablets in the treatment of multiple sclerosis (P443). *J Neurol* 2010;257(Suppl 1): S143.

Fingolimod to treat multiple sclerosis

Jeffrey A. Cohen

Introduction

Until recently, a key limitation of all the approved medications to treat relapsing–remitting (RR) MS – four forms of interferon beta (IFNβ), glatiramer acetate, mitoxantrone, and natalizumab – was their parenteral administration route. Fingolimod (FTY720, Gilenya®, Novartis AG), a sphingosine 1-phosphate receptor (S1PR) modulator, was approved by the United States Food and Drug Administration (FDA) in September 2010 as the first oral disease therapy for MS. Fingolimod's efficacy in RRMS is supported by a 6-month, placebo-controlled Phase 2 study,[1] a 2-year, placebo-controlled Phase 3 study,[2] a 1-year, active comparator Phase 3 study,[3] and a >4 year Phase 2 extension (see Table 30.1).[4] The prevailing theory is that fingolimod's efficacy in MS results from inhibiting egress of autoreactive lymphocytes from lymph nodes (LN) and preventing their recirculation to the central nervous system (CNS). Other immune effects and direct CNS actions may also contribute. Interaction of fingolimod with S1PRs in a variety of other tissues accounts for many of its adverse effects (AEs).

Lymphocyte recirculation

An important aspect of adaptive immunity is recirculation of T-cells and B-cells between secondary lymphoid organs and tissues. Although it is estimated that 73% of the body's lymphocytes are in lymphoid tissue and 2% in the blood, ~500 × 10^9 (equal to the total body number) traffic between blood and lymphoid tissues daily.[10] Naive T-cells enter LNs from the blood in search of antigen presented by dendritic cells. If activated, they proliferate, differentiate to effector cells, and migrate to B-cell areas in LN or leave the LN to enter inflamed tissues. A fraction of primed T-cells become circulating memory cells that persist for years to confer protection, and, upon secondary challenge, give a qualitatively different and enhanced response. It is presumed there is a comparable dependence on autoreactive T-cell recirculation between blood, CNS, and LNs to perpetuate the abnormal autoimmune response in MS.[11]

Biology of sphingosine 1-phosphate

Sources of sphingosine 1-phosphate

Sphingosine 1-phosphate (S1P) is a bioactive lysophospholipid that mediates diverse biological functions. It is generated from sphingomyelin by sequential reactions catalyzed by sphingomyelinase, ceramidase, and sphingosine kinase (SphK) (see Fig. 30.1). Two SphK isozymes have been identified, SphK1 and SphK2, with different kinetic properties, tissue distribution, developmental expression pattern, and regulation.[12,13] Erythrocytes are a main source of plasma S1P, which is also produced by platelets during activation and thrombotic processes. Other sources include mast cells, vascular and lymphatic endothelial cells, and fibroblasts. Neurons are one of the potential sources of S1P in the CNS.[14,15] Sphk activity in neurons and S1P production are stimulated by nerve growth factor, fibroblast growth factor, phorbol esters, dibutyryl cAMP, and forskolin.[16,17] Cultured astrocytes also secrete S1P, stimulated by phorbol esters, fibroblast growth factor, and tumor necrosis factor.[15,18,19] S1P levels increase in spinal cord following traumatic injury[14] and in association with inflammation in experimental autoimmune encephalomyelitis (EAE).[20]

Tissue S1P concentration is tightly regulated by a balance between synthesis, release, degradation, and binding and ranges between 0.5 and 6 pmol/mg wet weight.[17] The lowest levels are in heart and testes, and the highest are in brain, spleen, and eye. The concentration of S1P is relatively high in blood and lymph, but low in LNs. This concentration gradient plays a major role in lymphocyte trafficking.

S1P regulates diverse cellular responses, including proliferation, differentiation, survival, cytoskeletal reorganization, process extension, chemoattraction and motility, and cell–cell adherence and tight junction formation. As a result, S1P is involved in numerous physiologic processes, including immunity; vascular and pulmonary smooth muscle tone; endothelial barrier function; and morphogenesis of the cardiac, vascular, and nervous systems.

Multiple Sclerosis Therapeutics, Fourth Edition, ed. Jeffrey A. Cohen and Richard A. Rudick. Published by Cambridge University Press.
© Cambridge University Press 2011.

Table 30.1. *Fingolimod Phase 2 and 3 multiple sclerosis development program*

Study	Design	Population	Number of Participants	Comparator	Status
2201[1,4]	6-month Phase 2 then long-term open-label extension	Relapsing MS	281	Placebo	Core study completed, ongoing extension
FREEDOMS[2]	2-year Phase 3 then long-term open-label extension	RRMS	1272	Placebo	Core study completed, ongoing extension
TRANSFORMS[3,5]	1-year Phase 3 then long-term open-label extension	RRMS	1292	IM IFNβ-1a	Core study completed, ongoing extension
FREEDOMS II[6,7]	2-year Phase 3 then long-term open-label extension	RRMS	1088	Placebo	Ongoing
INFORMS[8]	Phase III	PPMS	~650	Placebo	Ongoing
1201 (Japan)[9]	6-month Phase 2 then extension	Relapsing MS	~165	Placebo	Ongoing

IFNβ-1a = interferon beta-1a, IM = intramuscular, MS = multiple sclerosis, RR = relapsing–remitting.

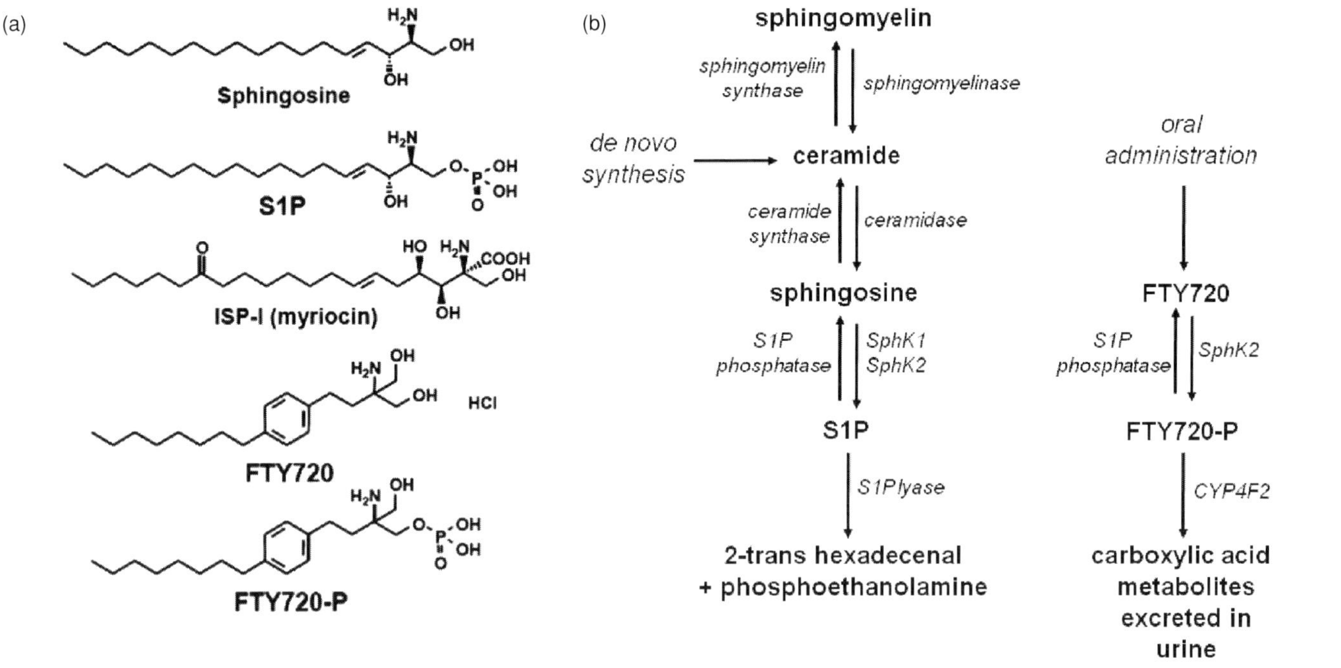

Fig. 30.1. Structure (a) and metabolism (b) of sphingosine, fingolimod (FTY720), and related compounds.

Sphingosine 1-phosphate receptors

Extracellular S1P functions in both a paracrine and autocrine fashion by binding to S1PRs, five members of a widely expressed, developmentally regulated family of G protein-coupled receptors with seven transmembrane domains.[12,21–24] Subtypes S1P1, S1P2, S1P3 are ubiquitously expressed. S1P4 is primarily expressed by lymphoid cells. S1P5 is expressed in spleen and CNS white matter. Differential cell-specific S1PR expression, changes related to cellular history, exposure to other mediators, differential coupling to G proteins and downstream signaling pathways, and cross-talk with other receptors provide for a wide dynamic range of S1P/S1PR-mediated actions.

Signaling is terminated by cell surface phosphohydrolase-mediated dephosphorylation of S1P to sphingosine and by receptor phosphorylation, uncoupling from G proteins, and internalization (see Fig. 30.2). After internalization, ligand and receptor dissociate, and the receptor is reinserted into the cell membrane.

There is evidence that S1P also can serve as an intracellular second messenger.[12,22,25–27] Intracellular levels are low and tightly regulated in a spatial and temporal manner by balance between synthesis and degradation. Transient increases in intracellular S1P have been demonstrated following treatment with hormones (e.g. vitamin D), growth

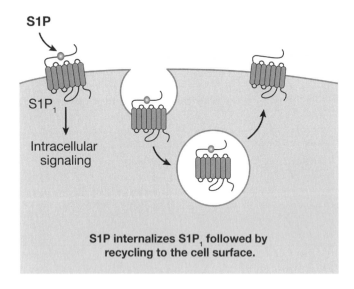

S1P

S1P₁

Intracellular
signaling

**S1P internalizes S1P₁ followed by
recycling to the cell surface.**

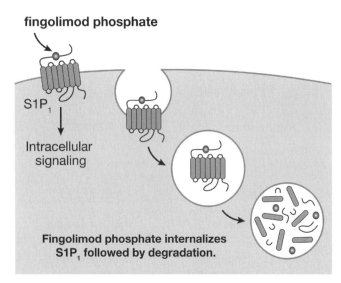

fingolimod phosphate

S1P₁

Intracellular
signaling

**Fingolimod phosphate internalizes
S1P₁ followed by degradation.**

Fig. 30.2. Interaction of sphingosine 1-phosphate (S1P) and fingolimod-phosphate with S1P1. Reprinted by permission.[158]

factors (e.g. platelet-derived growth factor, nerve growth factor), neurotransmitters (e.g. muscarinic acetylcholine agonists), tumor promoters (e.g. phorbol 12-myristate 13-acetate), cytokines (e.g. interleukin-1, tumor necrosis factor), and cross-linking of immunoglobulin receptors. The "receptors" or downstream mediators of intracellular S1P are, as yet, unidentified, but one possibility is mobilization of intracellular calcium.

Sphingosine 1-phosphate receptor expression by immune cells

Resting T-cells and B-cells express S1P1 and lower levels of S1P4 and S1P3.[28,29] The S1PR profile is similar for CD4[+], CD8[+], and CD4[+] CD25[+] subsets. S1P–S1P1 interaction plays a key role in lymphocyte trafficking, including egress from LNs. During lymphocyte recirculation, there is cyclical expression of S1P1 by lymphocytes.[30] The concentration of S1P is relatively high in blood and lymph, so blood lymphocyte S1PRs are normally down-regulated. After a few days in the LNs where the concentration of S1P is low, T-cells re-express S1PRs. If after entering the LN, T-cells fail to encounter their cognate antigen in the appropriate context to lead to activation, they exit to the efferent lymphatics in response to an S1P concentration gradient.[31] Antigen-induced activation leads to transient down-regulation of S1P1 expression and initial retention of activated T-cells in LNs. After proliferation and differentiation, S1P1 up-regulation re-establishes responsiveness to the LN-lymphatic S1P gradient allowing egress.

Expression of sphingosine 1-phosphate receptors in the central nervous system

S1PR subtype gene expression has been reported in virtually every CNS cell type under culture conditions.[32] The relevance of these culture data to the normal adult CNS are unclear, and reports in the prior literature of gene expression patterns in the absence of validated antibodies that can distinguish native proteins require cautious interpretation. S1P5 is particularly abundant in the CNS, mainly on oligodendrocytes.[33–35] Widespread S1P1 gene expression in the CNS also has been reported. However, recent in situ hybridization data suggest that most of the specific signal comes from astrocytes.[20] Similarly, recent functional data utilizing conditional knockout mice for S1P1 strongly implicated astrocytes as a major CNS target of fingolimod activity in neuroinflammation.[20] Removal of S1P1 from astrocytes using two independent Cre-drivers indicated that astrocytes are the major if not the only CNS locus of normal S1P1 gene expression (at least in mice), contrasting with prior reports using cell culture or low-resolution histological techniques.[32] This observation highlights possible astrocyte-mediated effects that S1P1 modulation by fingolimod could have in MS.

Pharmacology of fingolimod

Myriocin (ISP-1, thermozymocidin) is an immunosuppressant agent isolated from *Isaria sinclairii*, one of the entomopathogenic fungi known as "vegetable wasps and plant worms" used in traditional Chinese herbal medicine.[36] Fingolimod (2-amino-2-(2-[4-octylphenyl]ethyl)-1,3-propanediol hydrochloride, also known as FTY720) was first synthesized in the early 1990s as part of an extensive program of chemical derivatization of myriocin, with the goal of creating a novel immunosuppressant that would be more potent and less toxic in vivo (see Fig. 30.1).[36]

After oral administration in man, fingolimod gradually reaches a peak concentration 8–36 hours post-dose.[37–39] Oral bioavailability is good, approximately 93%, and the extent and rate of absorption are not affected by food.[37,39] Therefore, fingolimod can be taken without regard to meals. Blood levels are nearly linearly dose-related in the range 0.125–5 mg/day with low inter-individual variability,[37,38,40–42] so blood concentration monitoring is not necessary. Fingolimod is a prodrug and is reversibly phosphorylated to fingolimod-phosphate (fingolimod-P), the active moiety,[43,44] predominantly by SphK2 rather than SphK1.[45–49]

Fingolimod is greater than 99% protein bound in blood. Consistent with the molecule's amphipathic characteristics, fingolimod has a large volume of distribution and is extensively distributed to tissues, including brain.[39,42,50,51] It is presumed that because fingolimod-P is polar, it does not readily penetrate the intact blood–brain barrier (BBB). Rather, fingolimod crosses the BBB and is phosphorylated by endogenous SphKs in the CNS.[45,51]

Fingolimod-P is dephosphorylated to fingolimod by sphingosine phosphatase. Fingolimod is irreversibly metabolized by cytochrome P450 enzymes, primarily CYP4F2 with minor contributions from CYP2D6, 2E1, 3A4, 4F12, to inactive carboxylic acid metabolites then excreted in urine. The elimination half-life averages 8.8 days.[37,38] As predicted by the half-life, steady-state levels are reached after 4–8 weeks.[42,52] Pharmacokinetics are not affected by ethnicity, gender, and mild–moderate hepatic impairment.[37] Dose adjustment may be needed with severe hepatic impairment. Impaired renal function is not associated with accumulation of fingolimod, but 81% of the dose is excreted in urine as fingolimod metabolites, which may increase up to 13-fold with severe renal impairment. Fingolimod is predicted to have few interactions with other drugs. Potential drug–drug interactions are summarized in Table 30.2.

Fingolimod interactions with sphingosine 1-phosphate receptors

Fingolimod-P binds with high affinity to four of five S1PR subtypes: S1P1, S1P3, S1P4, and S1P5 but not S1P2.[43] As shown in Fig. 30.2, binding initially causes S1P1 agonist effects followed by aberrant phosphorylation, long-lasting internalization, ubiquitination, and proteosomal receptor degradation, leading to a pharmacologic null state ("functional antagonism").[54] Following fingolimod-P binding, internalized S1P1 receptors may maintain an active conformational state with persistent signaling via adenylyl cyclase inhibition and extracellular-signal regulated kinase (ERK) phosphorylation, and resultant cellular responses.[55] S1P does not have this action. Thus, the functional consequences of fingolimod-P interaction with S1P1 are a complex mixture of agonistic and functional antagonistic effects. Functional aspects of fingolimod-P interactions with other S1PR subtypes have been less well studied.

Potential mechanisms of fingolimod's efficacy in MS

Fingolimod's mechanism of action in MS is not known with certainty. The predominant view is that immunologic effects, specifically inhibition of lymphocyte egress from LNs and interruption of recirculation of autoreactive T-cells and B-cells to the CNS, account for the benefits in MS. This most directly results in reduced infiltration of blood-borne inflammatory cells into the CNS with reduced relapses and MRI lesion activity. Slowed disability progression and brain volume loss indicate tissue preservation, but it is unclear whether this represents secondary neuroprotection from reduced inflammation, direct neuroprotection, augmented repair, or a combination. Several observations, discussed below and summarized in Table 30.3, suggest that direct CNS actions may contribute. It is noteworthy that, in human renal transplantation trials, fingolimod showed modest efficacy,[56–58] suggesting it not a potent immunosuppressant.

Inhibition of lymphocyte recirculation

Down-modulation of lymphocyte S1P1 by fingolimod renders them unresponsive to the LN-efferent lymphatic S1P gradient required for egress, rapidly reducing lymphocyte counts in thoracic duct, peripheral blood, and spleen.[59] Redistribution of lymphocytes from blood to LNs does not produce lymphadenopathy, since the total number of lymphocytes in blood represents only about 2% of the total lymphocyte count in the body.[10]

In Phase 2 and Phase 3 MS studies, fingolimod treatment reduced peripheral blood lymphocyte counts within hours of the first dose, reaching 20%–30% of baseline (mean = 500–600/mm^3) in several weeks.[1–3] The degree of lymphopenia and persistence after drug discontinuation were dose dependent, though the relationships were not linear.[40,41] A dose of 5 mg per day produced a near-maximal lymphopenic reduction of 88%, 1.25 mg produced 70–80% reduction, and 0.5 mg produced an approximately half-maximal response.[1–3,38,52] Lymphopenia remained largely stable with continued treatment.[41,42] Because fingolimod causes lymphocyte redistribution rather than depletion, lymphopenia is reversible. When fingolimod was discontinued in a Phase 3 study, mean lymphocyte counts rose within several days and reached the normal range (0.8×10^9/l) within 6 weeks.[60] By three months, mean lymphocyte count was 80% of baseline (vs. 94% in the placebo group).

Fingolimod reduces both T-cells and B-cells but not granulocytes, monocytes, eosinophils, erythrocytes, or platelets.[40,41] T-cells (including CD3$^+$, CD4$^+$, CD8$^+$, CD45RA$^+$ naive T-cells, and CD45RO$^+$ memory T-cells) are more affected than B-cells.[40,41] CD4$^+$ T-cells are affected more than CD8$^+$ T-cells, decreasing the blood CD4/CD8 ratio.[40,61] Fingolimod preferentially impairs recirculation of T-cells expressing the LN homing receptors CCR7 and CD62L, naive T-cells and central memory

Table 30.2. *FDA Recommendations related to use of fingolimod*[53]

Administration	• The approved dose is 0.5 mg by mouth once per day. • Bioavailability after oral administration is unaffected by food, so it can be taken with regard to meals[37,39]. • The elimination half-life averages 8.8 days.[37,38] Steady-state levels are reached after 4–8 weeks.[42,52] Pharmacokinetics are not affected by ethnicity, gender, and mild–moderate hepatic or renal impairment.[37]
Drug–drug interactions	• Fingolimod does not interact significantly with other drugs used to treat MS, including fluoxetine, paroxetine, carbamazepine, baclofen, gabapentin, oxybutinin, amantadine, modafanil, amitryptyline, pregabalin, and corticosteroids. • Ketaconazole, a potent inhibitor of CYP3A and CYP4F increases fingolimod and fingolimod-P exposure up to 70%. • At present, there are no data concerning the safety and utility of combining fingolimod with other immunomodulatory or immunosuppressive medications. • Patients on Class Ia or Class III antiarrhythmic drugs, beta blockers, calcium channel blockers should be monitored for accentuated cardiac effects at initiation of fingolimod therapy.
Immunizations	• Live attenuated vaccines should be avoided during and for two months after stopping fingolimod therapy.
Hepatic abnormalities	• Elevations of liver enzymes may occur in patients receiving fingolimod, and patients with pre-existing liver disease may be at increased risk. • Recent transaminase and bilirubin levels should be checked prior to treatment. • No specific monitoring schedule is indicated once fingolimod is initiated, but hepatic function tests should be assessed in patients who develop symptoms suggestive of hepatic dysfunction. • Fingolimod should be discontinued in patients who develop significant liver injury. • Fingolimod exposure is increased with severe hepatic impairment and should be used with caution in this setting.
Cardiac effects	• Patients receiving Class Ia (e.g. quinidine, procainamide) or Class III (e.g. amiodarone, sotalol) anti-arrhythmic drugs, beta blockers, and calcium channel blockers; with a baseline low heart rate; or with a history of syncope, sick sinus syndrome, second-degree or higher AV conduction block, ischemic heart disease, or congestive heart failure may be at increased risk. • Patients should have a electrocardiogram prior to treatment. • All patients should be monitored for signs and symptoms of bradycardia for six hours after the first dose of fingolimod. Bradycardia or AV conduction slowing may require treatment with isoproterenol or atropine. • If fingolimod is discontinued for more than two weeks, the effects on heart rate and AV conduction may recur on reintroduction, so the same precautions apply.
Macular edema	• Ophthalmological exam should be performed before starting fingolimod and 3–4 months after treatment initiation. • Visual symptoms and acuity should be monitored at routine evaluations. If a patient reports visual disturbance at any time during treatment, additional ophthalmological evaluation should be undertaken. • Patients with diabetes mellitus and uveitis are at increased risk of macular edema and should have regular ophthalmologic evaluations. • In patients who develop macular edema, the risk of continuation of fingolimod or re-challenge is uncertain.
Blood pressure	• Blood pressure should be monitored during fingolimod treatment.
Pulmonary effects	• Routine pulmonary function testing is not needed prior to or during fingolimod treatment, but should be considered if clinically indicated.
Infection	• Patients should have a recent complete blood count prior to initiation of fingolimod. • Patients without a history of chicken pox or varicella-zoster virus vaccination should undergo serologic testing for varicella antibodies. Vaccination of antibody-negative patients should be considered prior to initiation of therapy, and therapy should be postponed for one month. • Fingolimod therapy should not be started in patients with acute or chronic infections. • Patients should be monitored for signs and symptoms of infection during fingolimod therapy and for two months after discontinuation. • Consider suspending fingolimod treatment if a patient develops a serious infection. • Concomitant use of fingolimod with antineoplastic, immunosuppressive, and immunomodulatory agents would be expected to increase the risk of immunosuppression.
Malignancy	• No special monitoring for cancer during fingolimod treatment is recommended.

AV = atrioventricular, FDA = Food and Drug Administration, fingolimod-P = fingolimod phosphate, MS = multiple sclerosis.

T-cells (TCM).[61–63] In humans, approximately 30% of circulating T-cells are resistant to the LN trapping effect of fingolimod over the dose range tested in MS clinical trials.[1–3] It is likely that this population predominantly is composed of CD8+ effector memory T-cells (TEM),[64,65] which lack expression of the LN homing receptors and, therefore, do not regularly recirculate through LNs. Thus, there is a pool of long-lived TEM in tissues that may provide at least partial immunologic memory and protection against pathogenic infections.

Fingolimod also inhibits B-cell trafficking. Mice treated with fingolimod have decreased IgG plasma cell and germinal center responses due to decreased egress from spleen.[66]

In mice treated with fingolimod, or that lack S1P1 in B-cells, IgG-secreting cells still can be induced and localize normally in secondary lymphoid organs but are reduced in number in blood and bone marrow.[66] Thus, fingolimod could reduce auto-aggressive B-cell activities by trapping them in LNs not draining auto-antigens from the CNS or by preventing B-cell trafficking into the CNS.

Abundant evidence indicates that fingolimod effects on lymphocyte recirculation are mediated by S1P1.[43,59,67] Two mechanisms for fingolimod inhibition of lymphocyte egress from LNs have been proposed. The "gatekeeper" hypothesis postulates that fingolimod initially acts as an agonist for S1P1 on

Table 30.3. *Observations that suggest mechanisms other than interference with lymphocyte recirculation may contribute to fingolimod's efficacy in MS*

- Between 0.5 and 5 mg, there is a dose effect for lymphopenia but lack of consistent dose effect on clinical or MRI efficacy measures.
- Slowed disability progression and brain volume loss indicate preservation of CNS tissue.
- Fingolimod readily enters the CNS and is phosphorylated in situ.
- S1P is produced in the CNS.
- S1PRs are expressed by neural cells.
- S1P and fingolimod have multiple effects neural cell growth and function in vitro.
- Benefit of fingolimod has been shown in animal models in which peripheral immune and direct CNS effects can be distinguished.
- Deletion of S1P1 from CNS cells, particularly astrocytes, reduces EAE severity and fingolimod efficacy.

CNS = central nervous system, EAE = experimental autoimmune encephalomyelitis, MS = multiple sclerosis, S1P = sphingosine 1-phosphate, S1PR = S1P receptor, S1P1 = S1PR subtype 1.

lymphatic endothelial cells causing cytoskeletal organization and increased barrier function, closing stromal gates.[68–70] In the alternative theory, fingolimod-P acts as a "functional antagonist" causing internalizing and degradation of S1P1 on lymphocytes making them unresponsive to the S1P gradient necessary for egress.[59] Although these two models are not mutually exclusive, most genetic and pharmacologic studies support the latter as the mechanism of long-term fingolimod-induced lymphopenia (summarized by Brinkmann[65]).

Immunological effects other than altered recirculation

Many studies indicate that fingolimod at therapeutically relevant concentrations modulates T-cell and B-cell trafficking rather than altering function. Although peripheral blood lymphocytes expressing a variety of surface markers, including chemokine and adhesion receptors, are reduced, mean expression levels are unaltered.[61] Fingolimod does not inhibit T-cell activation, proliferation, differentiation to an effector phenotype, or cytokine production, or antibody production by B-cells.[71–73]

Several immunologic actions of fingolimod in addition to interference with recirculation have been reported, including induction of CD4+ CD25+ Treg-cells in blood and spleen,[74] altered dendritic cell migration and/or antigen presentation,[75–79] and inhibition of cytosolic phospholipase A2.[80] These effects required higher fingolimod concentrations than those expected with doses used in MS studies. Several studies showed fingolimod therapy reduced vascular permeability in animal tissue injury models.[81–84] Similarly, augmented endothelial barrier function conceivably could contribute to improved BBB integrity demonstrated with fingolimod treatment of EAE[85] and MS.[1–3] However, at present, there is no evidence that S1PRs regulate BBB function or that fingolimod directly affects it.[86]

Potential direct central nervous system effects of fingolimod

Astrocytes mainly express S1P1 and S1P3; other subtypes are expressed at low or undetectable levels.[87–92] Immunohistochemical studies demonstrated a marked increase in S1P1 and S1P3 by reactive astrocytes in active and chronic MS lesions.[93] S1P stimulates proliferation of cultured astrocytes[19,87,89] and may contribute to fibroblast growth factor-induced proliferation.[94] Treatment of cultured human astrocytes with fingolimod-P inhibits production of inflammatory cytokines.[93]

CNS S1P5 mRNA and protein expression is predominantly by oligodendrocytes.[95,96] Cultured progenitor cells and mature oligodendrocytes also express S1P1 and, in some studies, low levels of S1P3 and S1P2.[95–102] Platelet-derived growth factor treatment of rat oligodendrocyte precursor cells up-regulated S1P1 and down-regulated S1P5.[98] S1P has a number of effects on oligodendrocyte lineage cell differentiation, migration, and survival that vary depending on developmental stage.[96,98] Several effects of fingolimod-P on cultured oligodendrocyte lineage cells have been seen at concentrations measured in brain and CSF of treated animals,[52] that also differ with developmental stage. Fingolimod-P stimulates differentiation of oligodendrocyte precursor cells into oligodendrocytes at low concentrations,[98] but high concentrations inhibit progenitor migration and differentiation.[98,99,101] Fingolimod-P protects oligodendrocyte progenitor cells from apoptosis induced by growth factor deprivation, inflammatory cytokines, or microglial activation.[101,103] Fingolimod-P also improves survival of cultured oligodendrocytes inhibiting apoptosis during serum withdrawal and glucose deprivation.[98,100] In progenitors but not mature oligodendrocytes, this effect was mimicked by the selective S1P1 agonist SEW2871. Fingolimod-P also stimulated membrane elaboration and process extension by mature oligodendrocytes cultured from adult human brain in a time- and dose-dependent manner.[100]

There is abundant evidence that sphingolipids, including ceramide, sphingosine, and S1P play important roles in the regulation of neuronal growth, differentiation, survival, and function.[104] Neural progenitor cells and neurons mainly express S1P1, S1P3, and, to lesser extent, S1P2.[33,105,106] Genetic constitutive deletion of S1P1 or combined deletion of SphK1 and SphK2 in mice severely disrupted neurogenesis, with increased apoptosis and decreased proliferation of neuroblasts, ultimately leading to neural tube defects,[107] suggesting S1P signaling is important during embryonic CNS development and growth. Studies of cultured neurons and neuron-like cell lines have identified a number of S1P effects, including cytoskeletal reorganization and morphological changes,[108–110] cytoprotection,[111,112] and electrophysiologic changes.[113] S1P/S1P1 mediates migration of neural stem cells to the site of spinal cord injury[14] and neural stem cell proliferation.[105] There have been very few studies of direct neuronal effects of fingolimod. Fingolimod-P treatment of primary cortical neuron cultures and embryonic stem cell derived neuron-like cells produced dose-dependent increase in phosphorylation of ERK1/2 and transcription of the CREB transcription factor followed by increased brain-derived neurotrophic factor mRNA.[114]

Fingolimod activity in experimental autoimmune encephalomyelitis

In a number of EAE variants in both mice and rats, fingolimod prevented development of clinical and pathologic features when given prophylactically[115–118] and reversed manifestations when started after disease onset.[115–119] Clinical benefit was accompanied by decreased electrophysiological abnormalities,[115] demyelination,[118,120] and axonal loss.[118,120] In single-cell recordings in brain slices from mice with severe motor deficits in chronic relapsing EAE, there was a dramatic decrease in the sensitivity of striatal neurons to the cannabinoid CB1 receptor agonist HU210. In Golgi preparations, there was marked reduction in dendritic spines on striatal neurons.[121] Prophylactic treatment with fingolimod prevented both these manifestations, indicating preservation of synaptic function and dendritic structure.

Although fingolimod's therapeutic effects and lymphopenia in EAE both are dose dependent and correlate somewhat,[119] several lines of evidence support direct CNS actions. First, mouse EAE induced by adoptive transfer of LN cells was ameliorated by fingolimod.[119] Second, intraventricular fingolimod administration two weeks after disease onset in acute EAE in DA rats lessened clinical features, demyelination, and axonal damage without producing lymphopenia.[122] Most critically, studies of EAE in CNS-cell-specific conditional S1P1 knockout mice strongly suggested a role for S1P1 expressed by astrocytes in EAE pathogenesis and fingolimod efficacy.[20] Conditional deletion of S1P1 in neuronal cell lineages (synapsin-cre) had no effect on EAE severity or fingolimod efficacy. In mice with pan-neural S1P1 deletion (nestin-cre), EAE was reduced in severity and fingolimod efficacy was abrogated. Astrogliosis also was reduced in nestin-cre mice and with fingolimod treatment in wild-type mice. Strikingly, the immunologic effects of fingolimod remained intact in all CNS mutants. Conversely, mice with selective deletion of S1P1 from T-cells exhibited similar EAE induction and therapeutic response to fingolimod compared to controls.

Fingolimod activity in other animal models of CNS pathology

In a rat traumatic brain injury model, fingolimod treatment reduced infiltration of macrophages and microglia.[123] Similarly, in rat spinal cord injury, fingolimod treatment improved functional recovery improved.[124] To determine whether fingolimod can effectively treat a delayed-type hypersensitivity (DTH) inflammatory response within the CNS behind an intact BBB, Lewis rats were injected stereotactically in the striatum with heat-killed bacillus Calmette–Guerin (BCG).[125]

Four weeks later, after the initial inflammatory response had resolved, intradermal injection of BCG produced a focal DTH lesion in the CNS with self-limited BBB disruption. Fingolimod treatment 19–31 days after intradermal injection, when the transient BBB disruption had resolved, still reduced the CNS inflammatory response and resultant demyelination.

Fingolimod clinical trials
Transplant trials

Fingolimod was initially developed to prevent allograft rejection after demonstration that it was effective in a variety of animal transplantation models, including kidney,[126,127] heart,[128–131] liver,[132] pancreatic islet cells,[133] and skin.[71,134–136] A Phase 2a multicenter, open-label, dose-finding study compared varying doses of fingolimod vs. mycophenolate mofetil, both combined with cyclosporine A, to prevent acute renal transplant rejection.[56] Fingolimod was as effective as mycophenolate mofetil. However, two Phase 3 trials,[57,58] completed enrollment but were discontinued because of AEs and worse graft function compared to mycophenolate mofetil.

Phase 2 study in MS

A randomized, double-blind, placebo-controlled Phase 2 trial[1] enrolled 281 participants with clinically and radiologically active relapsing MS. Participants were randomized to receive oral fingolimod 5 mg ($n = 77$) or 1.25 mg ($n = 93$), or placebo ($n = 92$) once daily. Overall, 255 (90.7%) participants completed the six-month core study on assigned treatment. Baseline characteristics were well-matched across groups: mean age 37–38 years, 69%–75% female sex, mean disease duration 8.4–9.5 years, 87%–90% RRMS and 10%–13% secondary progressive MS, mean of 1.2–1.3 relapses in the prior year, mean Expanded Disability Status Scale (EDSS) score 2.5–2.7, mean of 2.8–3.4 gadolinium (Gd)-enhancing MRI lesions.

The primary end-point, mean total cumulative number of Gd-enhancing MRI lesions on six monthly scans, was reduced compared with placebo (14.8) in both fingolimod groups: 5 mg (5.7, $P = 0.006$) and 1.25 mg (8.4, $P < 0.001$). Other MRI endpoints also favored fingolimod, including number of Gd-enhancing lesions at month 6, proportion of participants free of Gd-enhancing lesions over 6 months, total cumulative volume of Gd-enhancing lesions, Gd-enhancing lesion volume at month 6, total cumulative number of new T2 lesions, and change in T2 lesion volume at month 6 compared with baseline (non-significant trend in 1.25 mg group). Annualized relapse rate also was reduced: fingolimod 5 mg (0.36, 53% relative reduction, $P = 0.01$) and 1.25 mg (0.35, 55% relative reduction, $P = 0.009$) vs. placebo (0.77). Time to first relapse was prolonged in both fingolimod groups. There were no significant differences in mean or categorical Expanded Disability Status Scale (EDSS) score change from baseline.

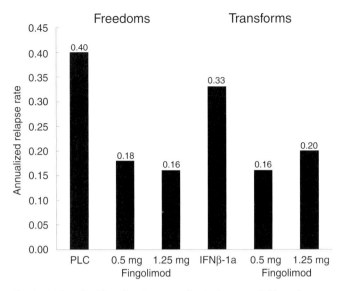

Fig. 30.3. Benefit of fingolimod on annualized relapse rate in Phase 3 multiple sclerosis trials. IFNβ-1a = interferon beta-1a, plc = placebo.

A total of 241 participants entered a long-term extension study in which those receiving fingolimod in the core study initially continued the previous dose and those receiving placebo were randomized to one of the fingolimod doses.[4] The clinical and MRI benefits of fingolimod treatment were maintained in the extension study and the crossover participants exhibited reduced MRI lesion activity and annualized relapse rate after converting to fingolimod treatment.

Freedoms

Two Phase 3 studies of fingolimod in RRMS have been published. FREEDOMS (FTY720 Research Evaluating Effects of Daily oral therapy in Multiple Sclerosis[2]) was a randomized, double-blind, placebo-controlled, two-year trial that enrolled 1272 participants with clinically active RRMS and randomized them oral fingolimod 1.25 mg ($n = 429$) or 0.5 mg ($n = 425$), or placebo ($n = 418$). Overall, 1033 (81.2%) participants completed 24-month follow-up, 945 (74.3%) on assigned treatment. Baseline characteristics were similar across treatment groups: mean age 37 years, 68%–71% female sex, mean disease duration 8.0–8.4 years, 57%–60% treatment-naive, 1.4–1.5 relapses in the prior year, mean EDSS 2.3–2.5, and 37%–39% with Gd-enhancing MRI lesions.

The primary end-point, annualized relapse rate, was reduced in both fingolimod groups compared with placebo (0.40): fingolimod 1.25 mg (0.16, 60% relative reduction, $P < 0.001$) and 0.5 mg (0.18, 54% relative reduction, $P < 0.001$) (see Fig. 30.3) Time to first relapse and proportion of participants remaining relapse free both significantly favored the fingolimod groups. The magnitude of benefit on relapses was comparable in treatment-naive and previously treated participants. The fingolimod vs. placebo hazard ratio for three-month sustained EDSS progression was 0.68 for fingolimod 1.25 mg (P

< 0.001) and 0.70 for 0.5 mg. Small mean changes in the MS functional composite z-score also favored fingolimod 1.25 mg (0.05, $P = 0.02$) and 0.5 mg (0.07, $P = 0.01$) vs. placebo (−0.01).

At 24 months, the mean number of Gd-enhancing lesions was 1.1 in the placebo group, and 0.2 in both fingolimod groups ($P < 0.001$ vs. placebo for both comparisons). Significant benefits for both fingolimod doses vs. placebo were seen on proportion of participants free of Gd-enhancing lesions, number of new or enlarged T2 lesions, and proportion of participants free of new or enlarged T2 lesions at month 24 ($P < 0.001$ for all comparisons). Change in total volumes of T2-hyperintense and T1-hypointense lesions were reduced in both fingolimod groups vs. placebo. Percent reduction of normalized brain parenchymal volume measured by structural image evaluation Using Normalization of Atrophy (SIENA)[137] was significantly less in both fingolimod groups vs. placebo at month 6 (fingolimod 1.25 mg −0.12, $P = 0.003$; fingolimod 0.5 mg −0.14, $P = 0.006$, placebo −0.34), month 12 (fingolimod 1.25 mg −0.44, $P = 0.001$; fingolimod 0.5 mg −0.50, $P = 0.03$, placebo −0.65), and month 24 (fingolimod 1.25 mg −0.89, $p < 0.001$; fingolimod 0.5 mg −0.84, $P < 0.001$, placebo −1.31) (see Fig. 30.4). A striking aspect of the benefit of fingolimod on slowing brain volume loss was the lack of initial acceleration, the "pseudo-atrophy" effect seen with other anti-inflammatory treatments in MS. As discussed in Chapter 11, the cause of this pseudoatrophy effect and the reason it is absent with fingolimod need further study.

Transforms

The second Phase 3 trial, TRANSFORMS (Trial Assessing Injectable Interferon versus FTY720 Oral in Relapsing-Remitting Multiple Sclerosis [TRANSFORMS]),[3] was a randomized, double-blind, double-dummy, active-comparator 1-year study. The eligibility criteria were identical to FREEDOMS, except there was no required washout for prior IFNβ or glatiramer acetate. A total of 1292 participants were randomized to daily oral fingolimod 1.25 mg ($n = 426$) or 0.5 mg ($n = 431$), or IFNβ-1a by weekly intramuscular injection ($n = 435$). A total of 1153 (89%) participants completed the study, 1123 (87%) on assigned treatment. Baseline characteristics were similar across treatment groups: mean age 36–37 years, 65%–69% female sex, mean disease duration 7.3–7.5 years, 41%–45% treatment-naïve, 1.5 relapses in the prior year, mean EDSS 2.2, and 33%–37% with Gd-enhancing MRI lesions.

The primary end-point, annualized relapse rate, was reduced in both fingolimod groups compared with IFNβ-1a (0.33): fingolimod 1.25 mg (0.20, 38% relative reduction, $P < 0.001$) and 0.5 mg (0.16, 52% relative reduction, $P < 0.001$) (see Fig. 30.3). Time to first relapse and proportion of participants remaining relapse free both significantly favored the fingolimod groups. The magnitude of benefit on relapses was comparable in treatment-naive and previously treated participants. There

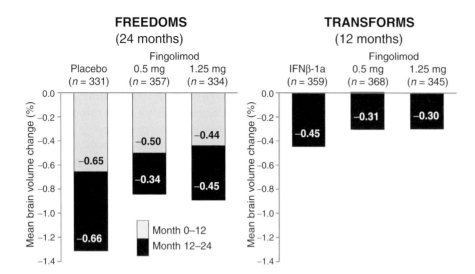

Fig. 30.4. Benefit of fingolimod on normalized brain parenchymal volume loss in Phase 3 multiple sclerosis trials. Percent change in normalized brain parenchymal volume was measured by Structural Image Evaluation Using Normalization of Atrophy (SIENA)[131] in both trials. IFNβ-1a = interferon beta-1a.

were no significant differences among treatment arms for confirmed EDSS progression, but small mean changes from baseline in EDSS and MSFC scores significantly favored the fingolimod groups.

At 12 months, the mean number of new or enlarged T2 lesions was 1.5 in the fingolimod 1.25 mg group ($P < 0.001$) and 1.7 in the 0.5 mg group ($P = 0.004$) compared to 2.6 in the IFNβ-1a group. The mean numbers of Gd-enhancing lesions were: fingolimod 1.25 mg 0.14, 0.5 mg 0.23, and IFNβ-1a 0.51 ($P < 0.001$ vs. IFNβ-1a for both comparisons). Significant benefit for both fingolimod doses vs. placebo was seen at month 12 on proportion of participants free of new or enlarged T2 lesions, volume of Gd-enhancing lesions, and percent change from baseline in normalized brain volume measured by SIENA (see Fig. 30.4).

In summary, these studies all demonstrated significant benefit of fingolimod on relapses and MRI lesion activity. FREEDOMS showed slowing of disability progression, and both Phase 3 studies showed reduced brain volume loss. There was no clear-cut dose effect for clinical or MRI outcomes comparing 1.25 mg vs. 5 mg in the Phase 2 study or 0.5 mg vs. 1.25 mg in the Phase 3 studies.

Safety and tolerability of fingolimod

General points

The overall MS safety experience at the time of FDA approval comprised more than 2600 patients and approximately 4600 patient–years of exposure.[138] Fingolimod was generally well tolerated, as evidenced by the low proportions of patients discontinuing medication or study participation due to a AE or abnormal test result (4%–10% in fingolimod groups in the Phase 3 trials).[2,3] The overall safety profile was better for 0.5 mg than 1.25 mg. Given that the efficacy advantages of the two fingolimod doses over placebo and IFNβ-1a were similar, 0.5 mg appeared to have a better benefit-to-risk profile. In

FREEDOMS, the risks of any AE, serious AE, or AE leading to drug discontinuation were similar between fingolimod 0.5 mg and placebo.[2] Five deaths occurred during FREEDOMS and TRANSFORMS: two in the placebo arms and three in the fingolimod 1.25 mg arms, with no deaths in the fingolimod 0.5-mg group of either trial.[2,3] Specific AEs associated with fingolimod included headache, influenza, diarrhea, back pain, cough, dyspnea, lower respiratory tract infection, elevation of liver enzymes, transient bradycardia and slowed atrioventricular (AV) conduction on treatment initiation, blood pressure effects, and macular edema.[1–3,53,138] These AEs typically were mild in severity and non-serious. Fingolimod's interaction with S1PRs in a variety of tissues and known pharmacodynamic effects largely account for the reported AEs. For others, the mechanism is uncertain. FDA recommendations related to fingolimod use are summarized in Table 30.2.[53]

Hepatic effects

After lymphopenia, increased alanine aminotransferase (ALT) was the most common laboratory abnormality. Increases in aspartate transaminase or bilirubin were uncommon. The abnormalities generally were mild and asymptomatic with no cases of symptomatic liver injury or a pattern/severity indicative of significant hepatocellular damage. The abnormalities were reversible, returning to normal with discontinuation of treatment. Like other AEs, risk of hepatic abnormalities was dose-dependent. In an integrated analysis of all patients in MS trials, ALT ≥3X upper limit of normal (ULN) occurred in 94/1172 (8.0%) of patients treated with fingolimod 0.5 mg and elevation ≥10X ULN occurred in 2/1172 (0.2%) patients.[138] After fingolimod discontinuation, median time to recovery of ALT to >ULN but ≤2X ULN was 64 days.[138]

Cardiac effects

S1P regulates heart rate and conduction.[139] S1P1, S1P2, S1P3 are the dominant receptors in the cardiovascular system,[140]

including atrial myocytes.[141] Fingolimod binding to S1PRs on atrial myocytes initially leads to activation of G protein-gated cholinergic potassium channels (IKACh) eliciting an inward rectifying potassium current, membrane hyperpolarization, reduced cell excitability, and decreased firing rate.[142] Receptor desensitization makes this effect self-limited. This phenomenon is mediated by S1P3 in rodents and rabbits,[67,68,143] but by S1P1 in humans.[143]

In clinical trials, fingolimod induced a transient, dose-dependent, usually mild negative chronotropic effect, reaching a maximum 4–5 hours after the first dose and attenuating over time, despite continued dosing and increasing blood levels, returning to baseline within one month.[144] In a pooled analysis of FREEDOMS and TRANSFORMS, there were mean reductions of ~8 bpm at nadir with 0.5 mg and ~11 bpm with 1.25 mg.[145] The decrease in heart rate usually was asymptomatic; in the Phase 3 trials, dizziness, fatigue, chest discomfort, palpitations were reported in <1% of fingolimod-treated patients, and there were no cases of syncope. Symptoms were self-limited and usually resolved spontaneously without intervention and despite continued fingolimod treatment. No cases of symptomatic bradycardia developed beyond 24 hours.

Fingolimod also can cause dose-dependent slowing of AV conduction. In a pooled analysis of FREEDOMS and TRANSFORMS,[145] first-degree AV block was the most common abnormality with mean PR prolongation of 4.5 ms with 0.5 mg and 11.3 ms with 1.25 mg. Second-degree block (Mobitz type I and type 2:1) was rare and also more frequent with 1.25 mg. Mobitz type II and higher degree of block were not seen. The incidence of electrocardiographic abnormalities was comparable across treatment groups at one month.

Vascular effects

S1P and fingolimod have complex effects on endothelial barrier function, vascular tone, blood flow, and blood pressure.[139] Vascular and lymphatic endothelial cells express high levels of S1P1 and lower levels of S1P2, and S1P3.[32,146,147] The effects of S1P and fingolimod on endothelial cells are heterogeneous, augmenting tight junction and barrier function in some vascular beds and increasing permeability in other tissues.[81,83,86,148] The direct effects of S1P on vascular smooth muscle cells are mainly via S1P3 which tends to cause vasoconstriction.[149] However, S1P and fingolimod induce endothelial nitric oxide synthase expression and nitric oxide production by endothelial cells via S1P3, indirectly producing vasodilation.[150,151]

Macular edema

In MS clinical trials, macular edema developed in 0.3% of patients treated with fingolimod 0.5 mg and 1.1% of patients on 1.25 mg.[138] Most cases occurred in the first 3–4 months of treatment. Approximately half were symptomatic (blurred vision), and the remaining cases were identified by ophthalmological examination. Most cases improved or resolved with fingolimod

discontinuation. The pathogenesis of fingolimod-related macular edema is unknown, but may relate to effects on endothelial barrier function.

Blood pressure

In Phase 3 MS trials, patients treated with fingolimod 0.5 mg had a mild increase in blood pressure (~2 mm Hg increase in systolic blood pressure and ~1 mm Hg increase in diastolic blood pressure) over the first 6 months of treatment, which persisted but did not increase further with continued treatment.[2,152] Blood pressure elevation may relate to effects on vascular smooth muscle.

Miscellaneous vascular events

Rare or single cases of ischemic and hemorrhagic stroke, peripheral arterial occlusive disease, and posterior reversible encephalopathy syndrome were reported in patients treated with fingolimod 1.25 or 5 mg but not 0.5 mg.[1–3] It is possible these vascular phenomena relate to effects on vascular endothelial or smooth muscle cells.

Pulmonary effects

S1PRs are expressed by airway smooth muscle cells and S1P may mediate airway hyper-responsiveness in some pathologic conditions.[153–155] Alveolar epithelium expresses S1P3, and S1P administered in the airways disrupts alveolar epithelial barrier function.[83] In the Phase 3 MS trials, cough was reported as an AE in 5%–10% of fingolimod-treated patients vs. 4%–8% of control patients, and dyspnea was reported as an AE in 2%–7% of fingolimod-treated patients vs. 2%–5% of controls.[2,3] Several patients discontinued fingolimod because of unexplained dyspnea. In a combined analysis of FREEDOMS and TRANSFORMS,[138] minor fingolimod dose-dependent decreases in forced expiratory volume at 1 second (FEV1) and diffusing capacity for carbon monoxide (DLCO) were seen at one month and were stable thereafter. At month 24 in FREEDOMS, the mean reduction from baseline in percentage of predicted FEV1 was 3.1% for fingolimod 0.5 mg and 2.0% for placebo. Reductions from baseline in DLCO were 3.8% with fingolimod 0.5 mg and 2.7% with placebo. FEV1 effects reversed following fingolimod discontinuation. At present, there are insufficient data to determine the reversibility of decreased DLCO or whether asthma, chronic obstructive pulmonary disease, or pulmonary hypertension increase the risk of fingolimod-related pulmonary AEs.

Infection

Because fingolimod is a potent immunomodulator, increased susceptibility to infection, including opportunistic infections, would not be unexpected. However, several factors may mitigate this risk. Fingolimod-induced lymphopenia reflects redistribution to LNs, not depletion. Fingolimod specifically retains only those T cells that regularly recirculate through LNs (i.e. naive T cells, TCM, and Th17 T-cells), not effector T-cells and TEM, which are important for immune surveillance and memory immune responses in the peripheral tissues.[64] Many aspects of immune function are preserved with fingolimod therapy, including lymphocyte numbers in LNs and tissues, function of LN and circulating lymphocytes, ability to generate antibodies, and innate immune mechanisms. However, due to effects on naïve T-cells and TCM, local immune responses can be reduced or delayed.[156] Normal volunteers treated with fingolimod for one month could mount an IgG responses to both T-cell-dependent (keyhole limpet hemocyanin) and independent (pneumococcal polysaccharide vaccine, PPV-23) novel antigens, although the responses were reduced and delayed.[157]

The proportions of patients with infection AEs, severe infections, and serious infections were similar in the treatment groups in FREEDOMS and in an integrated analysis of all MS studies, aside from increased lower respiratory tract infections (mainly bronchitis).[138] Overall, herpes virus infections were diagnosed in 2%–9% of patients. In TRANSFORMS, they occurred in more patients in the fingolimod 1.25 mg group, 5.5% compared with 2.1% in the 0.5 mg group and 2.8% with IFNβ-1a.[3] The incidence was similar across treatments in FREEDOMS[2] and the integrated analysis.[138] Most herpes infections were mild. A total of 11 herpes virus infection-related serious AEs were seen, including one case of fatal disseminated primary varicella zoster and one case of fatal herpes simplex encephalitis in TRANSFORMS. Both cases had complicating factors, but a role of fingolimod cannot be ruled out. There have been no other opportunistic infections and no cases of progressive multifocal leukoencephalopathy with fingolimod.

There was no clear-cut relation between the level of lymphopenia and infection risk in a pooled analysis of FREEDOMS and TRANSFORMS.[60] When fingolimod-treated patients were grouped based on nadir lymphocyte count: 156/206 (76%) of patients with a nadir of <0.2 $10^9/l$ had an infection of any type compared to 344/475 (72%) with nadir 0.2–0.4 $10^9/l$ 344/475 (72%), 97 of 168 (58%) with nadir >0.4 $10^9/l$, and 301/418 (72%) of placebo-treated patients. There was no clear-cut relationship between lymphocyte count and rates of any infection per patient-year, lower respiratory tract infection, or herpes infection.

There were no consistent AEs associated with short-term course of corticosteroids for fingolimod-treated patients in trials experiencing an MS relapse. However, the two patients who died of herpes-related infections in TRANSFORMS had recently received corticosteroids.[3] At present, there are no data concerning the safety and utility of combining fingolimod with other immunomodulatory or immunosuppressive medications, but the combination would be expected to increase risk of infection.

Malignancy

Like infection, because of fingolimod's immunomodulatory and cell growth effects, there is a potential for increased risk of malignancy. There was a suggestion of increased malignancies in TRANSFORMS in fingolimod-treated patients compared to IFNβ-1a.[3] In contrast, the rare malignancies in FREEDOMS were less common with fingolimod compared with placebo.[2] In the integrated safety analysis, skin cancers and all malignant neoplasms were reported in similar proportions across treatment groups.[138]

Target population for fingolimod therapy

Fingolimod was approved by the FDA to reduce relapses and disability progression in relapsing forms of MS.[139] Both FREEDOMS and TRANSFORMS showed that fingolimod is efficacious in both treatment-naive and previously treated patients.[2,3] For patients with an inadequate response to previously available agents and/or intolerable side effects, fingolimod is a reasonable alternative. For patients not currently on treatment, fingolimod was approved by the FDA as a first-line agent, i.e. patients are not required to fail other agents prior to initiating fingolimod. For patients currently receiving an approved MS treatment with effective disease control and good tolerability, although the oral route of administration is understandably attractive, it seems prudent not to switch therapy routinely until there is greater long-term experience with fingolimod in clinical practice. There are no published data concerning the safety and efficacy of fingolimod as combination therapy in MS.

Completed clinical trials of fingolimod in MS were restricted to patients with a relapsing course, the type of MS for which it was FDA approved. There are no published data concerning use in progressive MS or neuromyelitis optic. A 3-year Phase 3 trial in primary progressive MS is ongoing.[8] The Phase 2 study enrolled patients age 18–60[1] and the Phase 3 studies enrolled patients age 18–55.[2,3] Thus, the safety and efficacy of fingolimod in pediatric and elderly patients are not established. There have been no controlled studies of safety in pregnant women. Because studies in rats and rabbits demonstrated fetal development toxicity, including teratogenicity and embryo lethality,[139] fingolimod is Pregnancy Category C, and women of child-bearing potential should use effective contraception during and for 2 months after fingolimod treatment. Fingolimod is excreted in the milk of rats. It is not known if it is excreted in milk in humans.[139]

Conclusions

A Phase 2 and two Phase 3 MS trials confirmed fingolimod's benefit on relapses, disability progression, MRI lesion activity, and brain volume loss. Its generally good safety profile and tolerability, including oral route of administration, make fingolimod an attractive treatment option for patients with relapsing forms of MS. Interaction with S1PRs on T-cells and B-cells, inhibition of egress from LNs, and reduced recirculation of autoreactive cells to the CNS is the best characterized mechanism of efficacy in EAE and MS. Other potential immunologic effects and direct effects in the CNS may contribute. In addition, direct effects on neural cells may have neuroprotective and/or reparative effects. As there are no currently available treatments for MS demonstrated to directly limit damage or improve repair, there is a major unmet need in this regard, particularly for purely progressive forms of MS.

Further studies are needed to determine whether fingolimod meets this need. Interaction of fingolimod with S1PRs in a variety of tissues accounts for many of its off-target AEs. Thus, better delineation of the mechanisms leading to both the beneficial and adverse effects of fingolimod will be necessary to develop more effective and better-tolerated compounds.

References

1. Kappos L, Antel J, Comi G, *et al.* Oral fingolimod (FTY720) for relapsing multiple sclerosis. *N Engl J Med* 2006;355:1124–40.

2. Kappos L, Radue E-W, O'Connor P, *et al.* A placebo-controlled trial of oral fingolimod in relapsing multiple sclerosis. *N Engl J Med* 2010;362:387–401.

3. Cohen JA, Barkhof F, Comi G, *et al.* Oral fingolimod or intramuscular interferon for relapsing multiple sclerosis. *N Engl J Med* 2010;362:402–15.

4. Montalban X, O'Connor P, Antel J, *et al.* Oral fingolimod (FTY720) shows sustained low rates of clinical and MRI disease activity in patients with relapsing multiple sclerosis: four-year results from a phase II extension (P06.128). *Neurology* 2009;72(Suppl 3):A313. abstract.

5. Khatri B, Barkhof F, Comi G, *et al.* 24-month efficacy and safety from the TRANSFORMS extension study of oral fingolimod (FTY720) in patients with relapsing-remitting multiple sclerosis (P03.125). *Neurology* 2010;74 (Suppl 2):A239.

6. Calabresi PA, Goodin D, Jeffery D, *et al.* Oral fingolimod (FTY720) in relapsing-remitting multiple sclerosis: baseline patient demographics and disease characteristics from a 2-year Phase III trial (FREEDOMS II) (P05.038). *Neurology* 2010;74(Suppl 2):A416–A7.

7. Novartis. Efficacy and safety of fingolimod (FTY720) in patients with relapsing-remitting multiple sclerosis (FREEDOMS II). NCT00355134. [cited Aug 31, 2010]; Available from: http://clinicaltrials.gov/ct2/show/NCT00355134.

8. Novartis. FTY720 in patients with primary progressive multiple sclerosis (INFORMS). NCT00731692. [cited Aug 31, 2010]; Available from: http://clinicaltrials.gov/ct2/show/NCT00731692.

9. Novartis and Mitsubishi Tanabe Pharma. Efficacy and safety of FTY720 in patients with relapsing multiple sclerosis (MS). NCT00537082. [cited Aug 31, 2010]; Available from: http://clinicaltrials.gov/ct2/show/NCT00537082.

10. Westermann J, Pabst R. Distribution of lymphocyte subsets and natural killer cells in the human body. *Clin Investig* 1992;70:539–44.

11. Massberg S, Von Andrian UH. Fingolimod and sphingosine-1-phosphate – modifiers of lymphocyte migration. *N Engl J Med* 2006;355:1088–91.

12. Spiegel S, Milstien S. Sphingosine-1-phosphate: an enigmatic signalling lipid. *Nat Rev Mol Cell Biol* 2003;4:397–407.

13. Le Stunff HL, Milstien S, Spiegel S. Generation and metabolism of bioactive sphingosine-1-phosphate. *J Cell Biochem* 2004;92:882–99.

14. Kimura A, Ohmori T, Ohkawa R, *et al.* Essential roles of sphingosine 1-phosphate/S1P1 receptor axis in the migration of neural stem cells toward a site of spinal cord injury. *Stem Cells* 2007;25:115–24.

15. Anelli V, Bassi R, Tettamanti G, Viani P, Riboni L. Extracellular release of newly synthesized sphingosine-1-phosphate by cerebellar granule cells and astrocytes. *J Neurochem* 2005;92:1204–15.

16. Rius RA, Edsall LC, Spiegel S. Activation of sphingosine kinase in pheochromocytoma PC12 neuronal cells in response to trophic factors. *FEBS Lett* 1997;417:173–6.

17. Edsall LC, Spiegel S. Enzymatic measurement of sphingosine 1-phosphate. *Anal Biochem* 1999;272:80–6.

18. Riboni L, Viani P, Bassi R, Giussani P, Tettamanti G. Cultured granule cells and astrocytes from cerebellum differ in metabolizing sphingosine. *J Neurochem* 2000;75:503–10.

19. Bassi R, Anelli V, Giussani P, *et al.* Sphingosine-1-phosphate is released by cerebellar astrocytes in response to bFGF and induces astrocyte proliferation through G1-protein-coupled receptors. *Glia* 2006;53:621–30.

20. Choi JW, Gardell SE, herr DR, *et al.* FTY720 (fingolimod) efficacy in an animal model of multiple sclerosis requires astrocyte sphingosine 1-phosphate receptor (S1P1) modulation. *Proc Natl Acad Sci USA* 2011;108:751–6.

21. Fukushima N, Ishii I, Contos JJA, Weiner JA, Chun J. Lysophospholipid receptors. *Annu Rev Pharmacol Toxicol* 2001;41:507–34.

22. Hla T. Signaling and biological actions of sphingosine-1-phosphate. *Pharmacol Res* 2003;47:401–7.

23. Ishii I, Fukushima N, Ye X, Chun J. Lysophospholipid receptors: signaling and biology. *Annu Rev Biochem* 2004;73:321–54.

24. Chun J, Hla T, Lynch KR, Spiegel S, Moolenaar WH. International union of basic and clinical pharmacology. LXXVIII. Lysophospholipd receptor nomenclature. *Pharmacol Rev* 2010;2010:579–87.

25. Young KW, Nahorski SR. Intracellular sphingosine 1-phosphate production: a novel pathway for Ca2+ release. *Semin Cell Dev Biol* 2001;12:19–25.

26. Toman RA, Spiegel S. Lysophospholipid receptors in the nervous system. *Neurochem Res* 2002;27:619–27.

27. Chalfant CE, Spiegel S. Sphingosine 1-phosphate and ceramide 1-phosphate: expanding roles in cell signaling. *J Cell Sci* 2005;118:4605–12.

28. Graeler M, Goetzl EJ. Activation-regulated expression and chemotactic function of sphingosine 1-phosphate receptors in mouse splenic T cells. *FASEB J* 2002;16:1874–8.

29. Graler MH, Goetzl EJ. The immunosuppressant FTY720 down-regulates sphingosine 1-phosphate G-protein-coupled receptors. *FASEB J* 2004;18:551–3.

30. Lo CG, Xu Y, Proia RL, Cyster JG. Cyclical modulation of sphingosine-1-phosphate receptor 1 surface expression during lymphocyte recirculation and relationship to lymphoid organ transit. *J Exp Med* 2005;201:291–301.

31. Schwab SR, Pereira JP, Matloubian M, *et al*. Lymphocyte sequestration through S1P lyase inhbition and disruption of S1P gradients. *Science* 2005;309:1735–9.

32. Chae S-S, Proia RL, Hla T. Constitutive expression of the S1P1 receptor in adult tissues. *Prostaglandins Other Lipid Mediat* 2004;73:141–50.

33. Glickman M, Malek RL, Kwitek-Black AE, Jacob HJ, Lee NH. Molecular cloning, tissue-specific expression, and chromosomal localization of a novel nerve growth factor-regulated G-protein-coupled receptor, nrg-1. *Molec Cell Neurosci* 1999;14:141–52.

34. Im D-S, Heise CE, Ancellin N, *et al*. Characterization of a novel sphingosine 1-phosphate receptor, Edg-8. *J Biol Chem* 2000;275:14281–6.

35. Dev KK, Mullershausen F, Mattes H, *et al*. Brain sphingosine-1-phosphate receptors: Implications for FTY720 in the treatment of multiple sclerosis. *Pharmacol Ther* 2008;117:77–93.

36. Im D-S. Linking Chinese medicine and G-protein-coupled receptors. *Trends Pharmacol Sci* 2003;24:2–4.

37. Kovarik JM, Schmouder R, Barilla D, Wang Y, Kraus G. Single-dose FTY720 pharmacokinetics, food effect, and pharmacological responses in healthy subjects. *Br J Clin Pharmacol* 2004;57:586–91.

38. Kovarik JM, Schmouder R, Barilla D, *et al*. Multiple-dose FTY720: tolerability, pharmacokinetics, and lymphocyte responses in healthy subjects. *J Clin Pharmacol* 2004;44:532–7.

39. Kovarik JM, Hartmann S, Bartlett M, *et al*. Oral-intravenous crossover study of fingolimod pharmacokinetics, lymphocyte responses and cardiac effects. *Biopharm Drug Dispos* 2007;28:97–104.

40. Budde K, Schmouder R, Nashan B, *et al*. Pharmacodynamics of single doses of the novel immunosuppressant FTY720 in stable renal transplant patients. *Am J Transpl* 2003;3:846–54.

41. Kahan BD, Karlix JL, Ferguson RM, *et al*. Pharmacodynamics, pharmacokinetics, and safety of multiple doses of FTY720 in stable renal transplant patients: a multicenter, randomized, placebo-controlled, Phase I study. *Transplantation* 2003;76:1079–84.

42. Skerjanec A, Tedesco H, Neumayer HH, *et al*. FTY720, a novel immunomodulator in de novo kidney transplant patients: pharmacokinetics and exposure–response relationship. *J Clin Pharmacol* 2005;45:1268–78.

43. Brinkmann V, Davis MD, Heise CE, *et al*. The immune modulator FTY720 targets sphingosine 1-phosphate receptors. *J Biol Chem* 2002;277:21453–7.

44. Mandala S, Hajdu R, Bergstrom J, *et al*. Alteration of lymphocyte trafficking by sphingosine-1-phosphate receptor agonists. *Science* 2002;296:346–9.

45. Billich A, Bonrnancin F, Devay P, *et al*. Phosphorylation of the immunomodulatory drug FTY720 by sphingosine kinases. *J Biol Chem* 2003;278:47408–15.

46. Paugh SW, Payne SG, Barbour SE, Milstien S, Spiegel S. The immunosuppressant FTY720 is phosphorylated by sphingosine kinase type 2. *FEBS Lett* 2003;554:189–93.

47. Allende ML, Sasaki T, Kawai H, *et al*. Mice deficient in sphingosine kinase 1 are rendered lymphopenic by FTY720. *J Biol Chem* 2004;279:52487–92.

48. Kharel Y, Lee S, Snyder AH, *et al*. Sphingosine kinase 2 is required for modulation of lymphocyte traffic by FTY720. *J Biol Chem* 2005;280:36865–72.

49. Zemann B, Kinzel B, Muller M, *et al*. Sphingosine kinase type 2 is essential for lymphopenia induced by the immunomodulatory drug FTY720. *Blood* 2006;107:1454–8.

50. Meno-Tetang GML, Li H, Mis S, *et al*. Physiologically based pharmacokinetic modeling of FTY720 (2-amino-2[2-(-4-octylphenyl)ethyl]propane-1,3-diol hydrochloride) in rats after oral and intravenous doses. *Drug Metab Dispos* 2006;34:1480–7.

51. Foster CA, Howard LM, Schweitzer A, *et al*. Brain penetration of the oral immunomodulatory drug FTY720 and its phosphorylation in the central nervous system during experimental autoimmune encephalomyelitis: consequences for mode of action in multiple sclerosis. *J Pharmacol Exp Ther* 2007;323:469–75.

52. Park SI, Felipe CR, Machado PG, *et al*. Pharmacokinetic/pharmacodynamic relationships of FTY720 in kidney transplant recipients. *Braz J Med Biol Res* 2005;38:683–94.

53. NDA 02257 FDA Approved Labeling Text for Gilenya (fingolimod) capsules. September 21, 2010.

54. Oo ML, Thangada S, Wu M-T, *et al*. Immunosuppressive and anti-angiogenic sphingosine 1-phosphate receptor-1 agonists induce ubiquitinylation and proteosomal degradation of the receptor. *J Biol Chem* 2007;282(9082–9089).

55. Mullershausen F, Zecri F, Cetin C, *et al*. Persistent signaling induced by FTY720-phosphate is mediated by internalized S1P1 receptors. *Nature Chem Biol* 2009;5:428–34.

56. Tedesco-Silva H, Mourad G, Kahan BD, *et al*. FTY720, a novel immunomodulator: efficacy and safety results from the first Phase 2A study in de novo renal transplantation. *Transplantation* 2005;79:1553–60.

57. Salvadori M, Budde K, Charpentier B, *et al*. FTY720 versus MMP with cyclosporine in de novo renal tansplantation: a 1-year, randomized controlled trial in Europe and Australasia. *Am J Transpl* 2006;6:2912–21.

58. Tedesco-Silva H, Pescovitz MD, Cibrik D, *et al*. Randomized controlled trial of FTY720 versus MMF in de novo renal transplantation. *Transplantation* 2006;82:1689–97.

59. Matloubian M, Lo CG, Cinamon G, *et al*. Lymphocyte egress from thymus and peripheral lymphoid organs is dependent on S1P receptor 1. *Nature* 2004;427:355–60.

60. Francis G, Kappos L, O'Connor P, *et al*. Lymphocytes and fingolimod –

temporal pattern and relationship with infections (P442). *Mult Scler* 2010;16(Suppl 10):S146–7.

61. Bohler T, Waiser J, Schuetz M, Neumayer HH, Budde K. FTY720 exerts differential effects on CD4+ and CD8+ T-lymphocyte subpopulations expressing chemokine and adhesion receptors. *Nephrol Dial Transpl* 2004;19:702–13.

62. Yanagawa Y, Masubuchi Y, Chiba K. FTY720, a novel immunosuppressant, induces sequestration of circulating mature lymphocytes by acceleration of lymphocyte homing in rats, III. Increase in frequency of CD62L-positive T cells in Peyer's patches by FTY720-induced lymphocyte homing. *Immunology* 1998;95:591–4.

63. Hofmann M, Brinkmann V, Zerwes H-G. FTY720 preferentially depletes naive T cells from peripheral and lymphoid organs. *Int Immunopharmacol* 2006;6:1902–10.

64. Mehling M, Brinkmann V, Antel J, et al. FTY720 therapy exerts differential effects on T cell subsets in multiple sclerosis. *Neurology* 2008;71:1261–7.

65. Brinkmann V. FTY720 (fingolimod) in multiple sclerosis: therapeutic effects in the immune and the central nervous system. *Br J Pharmacol* 2009;158:1173–82.

66. Kabashima K, haynes NM, Xu Y, et al. Plasma cell S1P1 expression determines secondary lymphoid organ retention versus bone marrow tropism. *J Exp Med* 2006;203:2683–90.

67. Sanna MG, Liao J, Jo E, et al. Sphingosine 1-phosphate (S1P) receptor subtypes S1P1 and S1P3, respectively, regulate lymphocyte recirculation and heart rate. *J Biol Chem* 2004;279:13839–48.

68. Forrest M, Sun S-Y, Hajdu R, et al. Immune cell regulation and cardiovascular effects of sphingosine 1-phosphate receptor agonists in rodents are mediated by distinct receptor subtypes. *J Pharmacol Exp Ther* 2004;309:758–68.

69. Wei SH, Rosen H, Matheu MP, et al. Sphingosine 1-phosphate type 1 receptor antagonism inhibits transendothelial migration of medullary T cells to lymphatic sinuses. *Nature Immunol* 2005;6:1228–35.

70. Sanna MG, Wang S-K, Gonzalez-Cabrera PJ, et al. Enhancement of capillary leakage and restoration of lymphocyte egress by a chiral S1P1 antagonist *in vivo*. *Nature Chem Biol* 2006;2:434–41.

71. Chiba K, Yanagawa Y, Masubuchi Y, et al. FTY720, a novel immunosuppressant, induces sequestration of circulating mature lymphocytes by acceleration of lymphocytre homng in rats. I. FTY720 selectively decreases the number of circulating mature lymphocytes by acceleration of lymphocyte homing. *J Immunol* 1998;160:5037–44.

72. Brinkmann V, Chen S, Feng L, et al. FTY720 alters lymphocyte homing and protects allografts without inducing general immunosuppression. *Transpl Proc* 2001;33:530–1.

73. Xie JH, Nomura N, Koprak SL, et al. Sphoingosine-1-phosphate receptor agonism impairs the efficiency of the local immune response by altering trafficking of naive and antigen-activated CD4+ T cells. *J Immunol* 2003;170:3662–70.

74. Sawicka E, Dubois G, Jarai G, et al. The sphingosine 1-phosphate receptor agonist FTY720 differentially affects the sequestration of CD4+/CD25+ T-regulatory cells and enhances their functional activity. *J Immunol* 2005;175:7973–80.

75. Idzko M, Panther E, Corinti S, et al. Sphingosine 1-phosphate induces chemotaxis of immature and modulates cytokine-release in mature human dendritic cells for emergence of Th2 immune responses. *FASEB J* 2002;16:625–7.

76. Czeloth N, Bernhardt G, Hofmann F, Genth H, Forster R. Sphingosine-1-phosphate mediates migration of mature dendritic cells. *J Immunol* 2005;175:2960–7.

77. Muller H, Hofer S, Kaneider N, et al. The immunomodulator FTY720 interferes with effector functions of human monocyte-derived dendritic cells. *Eur J Immunol* 2005;35:533–45.

78. Lan YY, De Creus A, Colvin BL, et al. The sphingosine-1-phosphate receptor agonist FTY720 modulates dendritic cell trafficking in vivo. *Am J Transpl* 2005;5:2649–59.

79. Lan YY, Tokita D, Wang Z, et al. Sphingosine-1-phosphate receptor agonism impairs skin dendritic cell migration and homing to secondary lymphoid tissue: Association with prolonged allograft survival. *Transpl Immunol* 2008;20:88–94.

80. Payne SG, Oskeritzian CA, Griffiths R, et al. The immunosuppressant drug FTY720 inhibits cytosolic phospholipase A2 independently of sphingosine-1-phosphate receptors. *Blood* 2007;109:1077–85.

81. McVerry BJ, Garcia GN. Endothelial cell barrier regulation by sphingosine 1-phosphate. *J Cell Biochem* 2004;92:1075–85.

82. Peng X, Hassoun PM, Sammani S, et al. Protective effects of sphingosine 1-phosphate in murine endotoxin-induced inflammatory lung damage. *Am J Respir Crit Care Med* 2004;169:1245–51.

83. Brinkmann V, Baumruker T. Pulmonary and vascular pharmacology of sphingosine 1-phosphate. *Curr Opin Pharmacol* 2006;6:244–50.

84. Brinkmann V. Sphingosine 1-phosphate receptors in health and disease: mechanistic insights from gene deletion studies and reverse pharmacology. *Pharmacol Ther* 2007;115:84–105.

85. Rausch M, Hiestand P, Foster CA, et al. Predictability of FTY720 efficacy in experimental autoimmune encephalomyelitis by in vivo macrophage tracking: clinical implications for ultrasmall superparamagnetic iron oxide-enhanced magnetic resonance imaging. *J Magn Reson Imaging* 2004;20:16–24.

86. Marsolais D, Rosen H. Chemical modulators of sphingosine-1-phosphate receptors as barrier-oriented therapeutic molecules. *Nature Rev Drug Discovery* 2009;8:297–307.

87. Pebay A, Toutant M, Premont J, et al. Antiproliferative properties of sphingosine-1-phosphate in human hepatic myofibroblasts. *Eur J Neurosci* 2001;13:2067–76.

88. Malchinkhuu E, Sato K, Muraki T, et al. Assessment of the role of sphingosine 1-phosphate and its receptors in high-density lipoprotein-induced stimulation of astroglial function. *Biochem J* 2003;370:817–27.

89. Sorensen SD, Nicole O, Peavy RD, *et al.* Common signaling pathways link activation of murine PAR-1, LPA, and S1P receptors to proliferation of astrocytes. *Mol Pharmacol* 2003;64:1199–209.

90. Rao TS, Lariosa-Willingham KD, Lin F-F, Palfreyman EL. Pharmacological characterization of lysophospholipid receptor signal transduction pathways in rat cerebrocortical astrocytes. *Brain Res* 2003;990:182–94.

91. Rao TS, Lariosa-Willingham KD, Lin F-F, *et al.* Growth factor pre-treatment differentially regulates phosphoinositide turnover downstream of lysophospholipid receptor and metabotropic glutamate receptors in cultured rat cerebrocortical astrocytes. *Int J Dev Neurosci* 2004;22:131–5.

92. Mullershausen F, Craveiro LM, Shin Y, *et al.* Phosphorylated FTY702 promotes astrocyte migration through sphingosine-1-phosphate receptors. *J Neurochem* 2007;102:1151–61.

93. van Doorn R, van Horssen J, Verziji D, *et al.* Sphingosine 1-phosphate receptors 1 and 3 are upregulated in multiple sclerosis lesions (P662). *Mult Scler* 2010;16(Suppl 10):S228.

94. Riboni L, Viani P, Bassi R, Giussani P, Tettamanti G. Basic fibroblast growth factor-induced proliferation of primary astrocytes. *J Biol Chem* 2001;276:12797–804.

95. Terai K, Soga T, Takahashi M, *et al.* Edg-8 receptors are preferentially expressed in oligodendrocyte lineage cells of the rat CNS. *Neuroscience* 2003;116:1053–62.

96. Jaillard C, Harrison S, Stankoff B, *et al.* Edg8/S1P5: an oligodendroglial receptor with dual function on process retraction and cell survival. *J Neurosci* 2005;25:1459–69.

97. Yu N, Lariosa-Willingham KD, Lin F-F, Webb M, Rao TS. Characterization of the lysophosphatidic acid and sphingosine-1-phosphate-mediated signal transduction in rat cortical oligodendrocytes. *Glia* 2004;45:17–27.

98. Jung CG, Kim HJ, Miron VE, *et al.* Functional consequences of S1P receptor modulation in rat oligodendroglial lineage cells. *Glia* 2007;55:1656–67.

99. Novgorodov AS, El-Alwani M, Bielawski J, Obeid LM, Gudz TI. Activation of sphingosine-1-phosphate receptor S1P5 inhibits oligodendrocyte progenitor migration. *FASEB J* 2007;21:1503–14.

100. Miron VE, Hall JA, Kennedy TE, Soliven B, Antel JP. Cyclical and dose-dependent responses of adult human muture oligodendrocytes to fingolimod. *Am J Pathol* 2008;173:1143–52.

101. Miron VE, Jung CG, Kim HJ, *et al.* FTY720 modulates human oligodendrocyte progenitor process extension and survival. *Ann Neurol* 2008;63:61–71.

102. Miron VE, Schubart A, Antel JP. Central nervous system-directed effects of FTY720 (fingolimod). *J Neurol Sci* 2008;274:13–7.

103. Coelho RP, Payne SG, Bittman R, Speigel S, Sato-Bigbee C. The immunomodulator FTY720 has a direct effect cytoprotective effect in oligodendrocyte progenitors. *J Pharmacol Exp Ther* 2007;323:626–35.

104. Bucciliero R, Futerman AH. The roles of ceramide and complex sphingolipids in neuronal function. *Pharmacol Res* 2003;47:409–19.

105. Harada J, Foley M, Moskowitz MA, Waeber C. Sphingosine-1-phosphate induces proliferation and morphological changes of neural progenitor cells. *J Neurochem* 2004;88:1026–39.

106. McGiffert C, Contos JJA, Friedman B, Chun J. Embryonic brain expression analysis of lysophospholipid receptor genes suggest roles for s1p1 in neurogenesis and s1p1–3 in angiogenesis. *FEBS Lett* 2002;531:103–8.

107. Mizugishi K, Yamashita T, Olivera A, *et al.* Essential role for sphingosine kinases in neural and vascular development. *Mol Cell Biol* 2005;25:11113–21.

108. Postma FR, Jalink K, Hengeveld T, Moolenaar WH. Sphingosine-1-phosphate rapidly induces rho-dependent neurite retraction: action through a specific cell surface receptor. *EMBO J* 1996;15:2388–95.

109. Sato K, Tomura H, Igarashi Y, Ui M, Okajima F. Exogenous sphingosine 1-phosphate induces neurite retraction possibly through a cell surface receptor in PC12 cells. *Biochem Biophys Res Commun* 1997;240:329–34.

110. Van Brocklyn JR, Tu Z, Edsall LC, Schmidt RR, Spiegel S. Sphingosine 1-phosphate-induced cell rounding and neurite retraction are mediated by the G protein-coupled receptor H218. *J Biol Chem* 1999;274:4626–32.

111. Edsall LC, Pirianov GG, Spiegel S. Involvement of sphingosine 1-phosphate in nerve growth factor-mediated neuronal survival and differentiation. *J Neurosci* 1997;17:6952–60.

112. Culmsee C, Gerling N, Lehmann M, *et al.* Nerve growth factor survival signaling in cultured hippocampal neurons is mediated through TRKA and requires the common neurotrophin receptor P75. *Neuroscience* 2002;115:1089–108.

113. Kajimoto T, Okada T, Yu H, *et al.* Involvement of sphingosine-1-phosphate in glutamate secretion in hippocampal neurons. *Mol Cell Biol* 2007;27:3429–40.

114. Deogracias R, Klein C, Matsumoto T, *et al.* Expression of brain-derived neurotrophic factor is regulated by fingolimod (FTY720) in cultured neurons (P728). *Mult Scler* 2008;14(Suppl 1):S243.

115. Kataoka H, Sugahara K, Shimano K, *et al.* FTY720, sphingosine 1-phosphate receptor modulator, ameliorates experimental autoimmune encephalomyelitis by inhibition of T cell infiltration. *Cell Mol Immunol* 2005;2:439–48.

116. Balatoni B, Storch MK, Swoboda E-M, *et al.* FTY720 sustains and restores neuronal function in the DA rat model of MOG-induced experimental autoimmune encephalomyelitis. *Brain Res Bull* 2007;74:307–16.

117. Pryce G, Al-Izki S, Baker D, Giovannoni G. Control of chronic relapsing progressive EAE with fingolimod (P01.092). *Neurology* 2008;70(Suppl 1):A29.

118. Papadopoulos D, Rundle J, Patel R, *et al.* FTY720 ameliorates MOG-induced experimental autoimmune encephalomyelitis by suppressing both cellular and humoral immune responses. *J Neurosci Res* 2010;88:346–59.

119. Webb M, Tham C-S, Lin F-F, *et al.* Sphingosine 1-phosphate receptor agonists attenuate relapsing-remitting

experimental autoimmune encephalitis in SJL mice. *J Neuroimmunol* 2004;153:108–21.

120. Schubart AS, Howard L, Seabrook T, *et al*. FTY720 suppresses ongoing EAE and promotes a remyelinating environment preventing axonal degeneration within the CNS (P06.166). *Neurology* 2008;70(Suppl 1):A339.

121. Rossi S, De Chiara V, Motta C, *et al*. Fingolimod treatment prevents the clinical, synaptic and dendritic abnormalities of experimental autoimmune encephalomyelitis (P880). *Mult Scler* 2010;16(Suppl 10):S309–S10.

122. Schubart A, Seabrook T, Rausch M, *et al*. CNS mediated effects of FTY720 (fingolimod) (P07.101). *Neurology* 2007;68(Suppl 1):A315.

123. Zhang Z, Zhang Z, Fauser U, *et al*. FTY720 attenuates accumulation of EMAP-II+ and MHC-II+ monocytes in early lesions of rat traumatic brain injury. *J Cell Mol Med* 2007;11: 307–14.

124. Zhang J, Zhang A, Sun Y, Cao X, Zhing N. Treatment with immunosuppressants FTY720 and tacrolimus promotes functional recovery after spinal cord injury in rats. *Tohoku J Exp Med* 2009;219:295–302.

125. Anthony DC, Sibson NR, Leppert D, Piani Meier D. Fingolimod (FTY720) therapy reduces demyelination and microglial activation in a focal delayed-type hypersensitivity model of multiple sclerosis during the remission phase (P814). *Mult Scler* 2010;16(Suppl 10):S283–S4.

126. Kawaguchi T, Hoshino Y, Rahman F, *et al*. FTY720, a novel immunosuppressant possessing unique mechanisms. III. Synergistic prolongation of canine renal allograft survival in combination with Cycosporine A. *Transplant Proc* 1996;28:1062–3.

127. Schuurman H-J, Menninger K, Audet M, *et al*. Oral efficacy of the new immunomodulator FTY720 in cynomolgus monkey kidney allotransplantation, given alone or in combination with cyclosporine or RAD. *Transplantation* 2002;74: 951–60.

128. Hoshino Y, Suzuki C, Ohtsuki M, *et al*. FTY720, a novel immunosuppressant possessing unique mechanisms. II. Long-term graft survival induction in rat heterotopic cardiac allografts and synergistic effect in combination with Cyclosporine A. *Transplant Proc* 1996;28:1060–1.

129. Hwang M-W, Matsumori A, Furukawa Y, *et al*. FTY720, a new immunosuppressant, promotes long-term graft survival and inhibits progression of graft coronary artery disease in a murine model of cardiac transplantation. *Circulation* 1999;100:1322–1329.

130. Nikolova Z, Hof A, Rudin M, *et al*. Prevention of graft vessel disease by combined FTY720/Cyclopsporine A treatment in a rat carotid artery transplantation model. *Transplantation* 2000;69:2525–30.

131. Nikolova Z, Hof A, Baumlin Y, Hof RP. Efficacy of SDZ RAD compared with CsA monotherapy and combined RAD/FTY720 treatment in a murine cardiac allotransplantation model. *Transpl Immunol* 2001;9:43–9.

132. Anselmo DM, Amersi FF, Shen X-D, *et al*. FTY720 pretreatment reduces warm hepatic ischemia reperfusion injury through inhibition of T-lymphocyte infiltration. *Am J Transpl* 2002;2:843–9.

133. Fu F, Hu S, Deleo J, *et al*. Long-term islet graft survival in streptozotocin- and autoimmune-induced diabetes models by immunosuppressive and potential insulinotropic agent FTY720. *Transplantation* 2002;73: 1425–30.

134. Chiba K, Hoshino Y, Suzuki C, *et al*. FTY720, a novel immunosuppressant possessing unique mechanisms. I. Prolongation of skin allograft survival and synergistic effect in combination with Cyclopsporine in rats. *Transplant Proc* 1996;28:1056–9.

135. Yanagawa Y, Sugahara K, Kataoka H, *et al*. FTY720, a novel immunosuppressant, induces sequestration of circulating mature lymphocytes by acceleration of lymphocyte homing in rats. II. FTY720 prolongs skin allograft suvival by decreasing T cell infiltration into grafts but not cytokine production in vivo. *J Immunol* 1998;160:5493–9.

136. del Rio M, Pabst O, Ramirez P, *et al*. The thymus is required for the ability of FTY720 to prolong skin allograft survival across different histocompatibility MHC barriers. *Transpl Int* 2007;20:895–903.

137. Smith SM, Zhang Y, Jenkinson M, *et al*. Accurate, robust, and automated longitudinal and cross-sectional brain change analysis. *Neuroimage* 2002;17:479–89.

138. Collins W, Cohen J, O'Connor P, *et al*. Long-term safety of oral fingolimod (FTY720) in relapsing multiple sclerosis: integrated analyses of phase 1 and 3 studies (P843). *Mult Scler* 2010;16(Suppl 10):S295.

139. Peters SLM, Alewijnse AE. Sphingosine-1-phosphate signaling in the cardiovascular system. *Curr Opin Pharmacol* 2007;7:186–92.

140. Mazurais D, Roberts P, Gout B, *et al*. Cell type-specific localization of human cardiac S1P receptors. *J Histochem Cytochem* 2002;50:661–9.

141. Liliom K, Sun G, Bunemann M, *et al*. Sphingosylphosphocholine is a naturally occurring lipid mediator in blood plasma: a possible role in regulating cardiac function via sphingolipid receptors. *Biochem J* 2001;355:189–97.

142. Koyrakh L, Roman MI, Brinkmann V, Wickman K. The heart rate decrease caused by acute FTY720 administration is mediated by the G protein-gated potassium channel IKACh. *Am J Transplant* 2005;5:529–36.

143. Gergely P, Wallstrom E, Nuesslein-Hildesheim B, *et al*. Phase I study with the selective S1P1/S1P5 receptor modulator BAF312 indicates that S1P1 rather than S1P3 mediates transient heart rate reduction in humans (P437). *Mult Scler* 2009;15(Suppl 2):S125–6.

144. Schmouder R, Serra D, Wang Y, *et al*. FTY720: placebo-controlled study of the effect on cardiac rate and rhythm in healthy subjects. *J Clin Pharmacol* 2006;46:895–904.

145. DiMarco JP, O'Connor P, Cohen JA, *et al*. First-dose effect of fingolimod: pooled safety data from two phase 3 studies (TRANSFORMS and FREEDOMS) (P830). *Mult Scler* 2010;16(Suppl 10):S290.

146. Liu Y, Wada R, Yamashita T, *et al*. Edg-1, the G protein-coupled receptor for sphingosine-1-phosphate, is essential for vascular maturation. *J Clin Invest* 2000;106:951–61.

147. Singer II, Tian M, Wickham LA, *et al*. Sphingosine-1-phosphate agonists increase macrophage homing,

lymphocyte contacts, and endothelial junctional complex formation in murine lymph nodes. *J Immunol* 2005;175:7151–61.

148. Brinkmann V, Cyster JG, Hla T. FTY720: sphingosine 1-phosphate receptor-1 in the control of lymphocyte egress and endothelial barrier function. *Am J Transpl* 2004;4:1019–25.

149. Salomone S, Yoshimura S-i, Reuter U, *et al.* S1P3 receptors mediate the potent constriction of cerebral arteries by sphingosine 1-phosphate. *Eur J Pharmacol* 2003;469:125–34.

150. Rosen H, Goetzl EJ. Sphingosine 1-phosphate and its receptors: an autocrine and paracrine network. *Nature Reviews Immunology* 2005;5:560–70.

151. Tolle M, Levkau B, Keul P, *et al.* Immunomodulator FTY720 induces eNOS-dependent arterial vasodilatation via the lysophospholipid receptor S1P3. *Circ Res* 2005;96: 913–20.

152. Cohen JA. Supplement to: Oral fingolimod or intramuscular interferon for relapsing multiple sclerosis. *New Engl J Med* 2010;10. 1056/NEJMoa0907839.

153. Pfaff M, Powaga N, Akinci S, *et al.* Activation of the SPHK/S1P signalling pathway is coupled to muscarinic receptor-mediated regulation of peripheral airways. *Resp Res* 2005;6: 48.

154. Kume H, Takeda N, Oguma T, *et al.* Sphingosine 1-phosphate causes airway hyper-reactivity by rho-mediated myosin phosphatase inactivation. *J Pharmacol Exp Ther* 2007;320: 766–73.

155. Roviezzo F, Di Lorenzo A, Bucci M, *et al.* Sphingosine-1-phosphate/ sphingosine kinase pathway is involved in mouse airway hyperresponsiveness. *Am J Respir Cell Mol Biol.* 2007.

156. Pinschewer DD, Ochsenbein AF, Odermatt B, *et al.* FTY720 immunosuppression impairs effector T cell peripheral homing without affecting induction, expansion, and memory. *J Immunol* 2000;164: 5761–70.

157. Schmouder R, Boulton C, Wang N, David OJ. Effects of fingolimod on antibody response following steady-state dosing in healthy volunteers: a 4-week randomised, placebo-controlled study (P412). *Mult Scler* 2010;16(Suppl 10): S135.

158. Cohen JA, Chun J. Mechanisms of fingolimod's efficacy and adverse effects in multiple sclerosis. *Ann Neurol* 2011;69:759–777.

Dimethyl fumarate to treat multiple sclerosis

Robert J. Fox and Ralf Gold

Unmet need for multiple sclerosis therapies

For over 15 years, approved multiple sclerosis (MS) disease-modifying therapies were limited to parenteral routes of administration – subcutaneous, intramuscular, and intravenous modalities. These routes are not only unpleasant for patients because of needle-stick pain, but also lead to skin reactions such as rubor, pruritus, lipoatrophy, and rarely infection. Intravenous administrations are inconvenient because they require routine visits to an infusion center or with a home care nurse.

The US Food and Drug Administration approval of fingolimod in 2010 marked the beginning of a new period of oral MS treatment. In addition to fingolimod, at least four additional oral long-term MS disease-modifying therapies were in late Phase III trials in 2010. These oral therapies promise to lead to dramatic shifts in treatment patterns for relapsing forms of MS. As in any therapeutic area, a successful oral therapy will need to demonstrate convincing efficacy, reasonable safety, and convenience in administration. An emerging additional consideration for MS disease modifying therapies is their potential neuroprotective effects. MS is thought to be not only a neuroinflammatory disease, but also a superimposed neurodegenerative disease. The detailed interplay between these two pathophysiologies is not well understood, but one potential model is that neuroinflammation in the early years sets up a cascade of accelerated neurodegeneration in later years. Whatever the cause, a gradually progressive clinical disorder becomes manifest in the later years of the MS course, and this stage of MS has been uniformly recalcitrant to currently available immunotherapies. If new anti-inflammatory therapies are also effective against the neurodegenerative component of MS, they would meet a hitherto unmet need in MS therapeutics. Dimethyl fumarate is an oral therapy in development for MS which may meet these needs.

History of fumaric acid

Fumaric acid is the common name of an unsaturated dicarbonic acid (Fig. 31.1). In turn, the salts of this acid are named fumarate. In the Krebs cycle, succinate is converted via a specific dehydrogenase into fumarate, which subsequently is

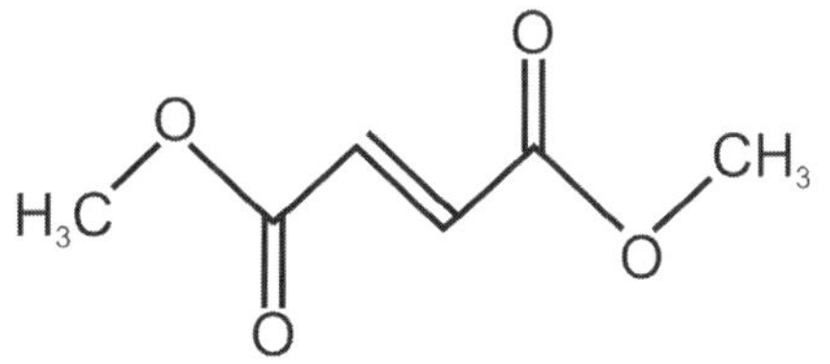

Fig. 31.1. Molecular structure of dimethyl fumarate.

metabolized to maleate. To date, there is no known disease which arises from inborn errors of this pathway.

In the late 1950s, the German chemist Walter Schweckendiek postulated that the pathogenesis of psoriasis vulgaris was due, at least in part, to a disturbed Krebs cycle. Thus, he aimed at modulating this pathway by exogenous administration of fumaric acid. He first used fumaric acid on his own psoriatic skin and preferred application as an ointment of fumaric ester. He continued studies on himself by swallowing fumaric esters and published its success in 1959.[1] Later, he used a combination of monomethyl fumarate and dimethyl fumarate (DMF), and by changing the galenic pharmacological formulation and adding a tablet coating, he achieved delayed release in the duodenum, leading to reduced side effects (Table 31.1). Further systematic studies demonstrated the efficacy of fumaric acids for the treatment of psoriasis.[2,3] The Swiss company Fumaderm obtained German regulatory approval in 1994 for this fumaric acid formulation (called Fumaderm) for treatment of severe psoriasis. Since then, Fumaderm is the preferred systemic treatment of severe psoriasis in German-speaking countries.[4] Thus, more than 100 000 patient–years of experience have accumulated with minimal serious complications. The mixture of these fumarate esters has been found safe for long-term therapy.

Table 31.1. Constituents of fumaric acid preparations

	Fumaderm	BG00012
Dimethyl fumarate	120 mg	120 mg
Ethylhydrogen fumarate Ca-salt	87 mg	
Ethylhydrogen fumarate Mg-salt	5 mg	
Ethylhydrogen fumarate Zn-salt	3 mg	

Multiple Sclerosis Therapeutics, Fourth Edition, ed. Jeffrey A. Cohen and Richard A. Rudick. Published by Cambridge University Press.
© Cambridge University Press 2011.

The successful use of fumaric acid in dermatology eventually led to its translational use in neurology. Since it was postulated that fumarates induce a so-called Th$_2$-shift,[5] Peter Altmeyer, dermatology chair at the Ruhr University of Bochum, inspired Horst Przuntek, his neurologist colleague, to test fumaric acids in active relapsing MS. From this study, the first small systematic observation on ten patients was published (see below), ultimately leading to a successful Phase 2 trial, the acquisition of Fumapharm by Biogen Idec, and finally the subsequent MS Phase 3 studies described below.[6]

Mechanism of action of fumaric acid

Immunomodulation

In the past, dermatological investigators performed a wide array of studies focusing on the adaptive immune system. During clinical trials a reduction of peripheral blood leukocytes, mainly CD4+ T-cells (up to 90%) and CD8+ T-cells (up to 53%), was observed as a putative consequence of apoptosis.[7] In addition, a shift from Th$_1$ to Th$_2$ cytokine production was also detected.[5] While levels of pro-inflammatory cytokines, tumor necrosis factor-alpha (TNFα) and interferon-gamma (IFNγ), levels were reduced, the levels of anti-inflammatory Th$_2$ type cytokines, namely interleukin (IL)-4, IL-5 and IL-10, were markedly increased.

In vitro experiments showed that an increased secretion of Th$_2$ cytokines up to ten-fold over normal was observed in CD45R0+ T-cells.[5] In addition, other blood cells were modulated. For example, dendritic cells, which play a central role in regulation of inflammatory processes, were down-regulated and secreted less IL-12. Apoptosis was also detected in dendritic cells.[5] Immunological effects of DMF were also observed in keratinocytes where major histocompatability complex class II gene products and the adhesion molecule, ICAM-1, were found to be down-regulated.[8,9] The immunomodulatory effects of DMF were shown to be functionally relevant in a rat model of organ transplantation, where transplant rejection was successfully modulated by fumarates.[10] Fumaric esters were shown to inhibit acute and chronic rejection in rat kidney transplantation models, providing further evidence of its immunosuppressant properties.[11]

Nonetheless, the molecular mechanisms of DMF have not been fully unraveled. In vitro studies in human endothelial cells have shown that DMF acts via transcriptional downregulation of TNF-induced genes as well as inhibition of TNF-induced nuclear entry of nuclear factor kappa B (NFκB).[12] DMF inhibits NFκB-dependent chemokines such as CXCL8, CXCL9 and CXCL10. Most studies involving the molecular effects of fumaric esters have focused on T-cells, and there is very little information available on their effects on B-cells.

Neuroprotection

Recently, novel potentially neuroprotective effects of DMF were observed in rodent glial cells and neurons, both in vitro and in vivo.[13] Since an oral formulation of DMF had demonstrated beneficial effects on MRI markers of axonal destruction in a Phase 2 MS trial,[14] one of us (RG)[15] studied immune effects and potential axonal protection in experimental autoimmune encephalomyelitis (EAE) induced by immunization with myelin oligodendrocyte glycoprotein peptide.[16] In C57BL/6 mice, preventive DMF treatment given twice a day by oral gavage, afforded a significant beneficial effect on the EAE disease course and a strongly reduced macrophage inflammation in the spinal cord as revealed by histology.[17] Multiparameter cytokine analysis from blood detected an increase of IL-10, an anti-inflammatory cytokine, in the treated animals. Thus, the underlying biological activity of DMF in EAE appears to be complex.

We then studied chronic EAE using the same C57BL/6 mouse EAE model.[13] Treatment with DMF improved preservation of myelin, axons, and neurons (Fig. 31.2). In vitro, the application of fumarates increased neuronal survival and protected human astrocytes against oxidative stress. Additional studies evaluated the functional pathway of fumarates and found that application of fumarates led to direct modification of a protein called Kelch-like ECH-associated protein 1 (Keap-1) which is an inhibitor of nuclear-factor- E2-related factor-2 (Nrf2). This modification of Keap-1 caused stabilization of Nrf2, activation of Nrf2-dependent transcription, and a concomitant accumulation of prototypical Nrf2 target proteins. In turn, there was induction of several substances which enhance cellular resistance to free radicals such as glutathione and NAD(P)H dehydrogenate quinine 1 (NQO1). DMF treatment resulted in increased Nrf2 immunoreactivity in neuronal subpopulations, oligodendrocytes, and astrocytes. These DMF-mediated beneficial effects were completely abolished in Nrf2 deficient mice. Human autopsy studies have observed up-regulation of Nrf2 in MS lesions within the spinal cord lesions, suggesting that the Nrf2 pathway may be activated through the body's endogenous protective mechanisms. Altogether, these observations suggest that DMF treatment may be effective in tissue preservation and protection in MS. The ability of DMF to activate Nrf2 may thus offer a novel cytoprotective modality that is not known to be targeted by other MS therapies. Fig. 31.3 illustrates the putative mechanism through which DMF may exert immunomodulating and neuroprotective effects.

Phase 1 clinical trial

Fumaric acids were first studied in MS in a Phase 1, open-label, baseline-controlled trial using the combination fumaric acid ester preparation Fumaderm. Ten patients with relapsing remitting (RR) MS and at least one relapse within the prior year were enrolled in the study. A 6-week untreated baseline phase was followed by an 18-week treatment phase, then a 4-week washout phase, and finally a second 48-week treatment phase. With each treatment phase, fumaric acid esters were titrated over 9 weeks. Primary efficacy outcome was the number and volume of triple-dose (0.3 mmol/kg body weight) gadolinium (Gd)-enhancing lesions.

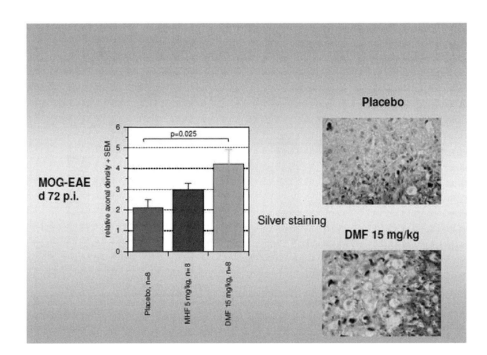

Fig. 31.2. Quantification of axonal density in EAE lesions of carrier-fed mice ("placebo"), or recipients of MHF or DMF. As illustrated in the Bielschowsky stain (right side) there are more black axonal profiles preserved under DMF treatment (see also color plate section).

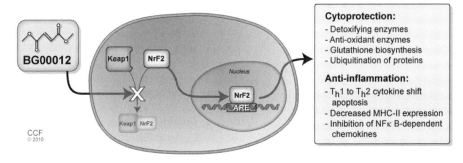

Fig. 31.3. Illustration of how dimethyl fumarate may exert both immunomodulatory and neuroprotective effects.

Of the ten patients enrolled, six completed the study. One patient each stopped because of unplanned pregnancy, gastrointestinal side effects, lack of compliance, and loss to follow-up. The most common adverse events were flushing and gastrointestinal symptoms (diarrhea, nausea, cramps), which were reported by almost all patients during the initial phase of the study. In general, symptoms improved over 6 weeks.

After 18 weeks of treatment, a significant reduction in Gd-enhancing lesions was observed. There were a mean of 11.3 Gd-enhancing lesions per patient at baseline, which decreased to 1.5 per patient at 18 weeks. Gd-enhancing lesions reduced further during the second treatment period, decreasing to a mean of 0.28 per scan per subject. The volume of Gd-enhancing lesions also decreased from 245 mm^3 at baseline, to 26.1 mm^3 at 18 weeks, to 2.1 mm^3 at 70 weeks. Clinical scores showed modest, non-significant improvements over the course of the study, including Expanded Disability Status Scale (EDSS), Ambulation Index, and nind-hole peg test. Two relapses were observed – one at week 18 and one at week 46. Immunologic studies on peripheral blood of these patients during the first 28 weeks showed similar findings to that from dermatology: an increase in IL-10 from CD4+ T-cells during treatment, as well as a transient increase in apoptosis of CD4+ T-cells. No change in IFNγ was observed over the course of treatment.

Phase 2 clinical trial

Based upon the encouraging Phase 1 results, Fumapharm partnered with Biogen Idec to conduct a Phase 2 trial of DMF in RRMS. To improve gastrointestinal tolerability, they used only dimethyl fumaric acid (rather than the multiple fumaric acid esters which constitute Fumaderm) and employed enteric-coated microtablets. This preparation of DMF is currently designated BG00012.

The Phase 2, multicentered, placebo-controlled clinical trial was performed to provide proof-of-concept evidence of DMF's efficacy in relapsing MS.[14] In this trial, 257 RRMS patients were enrolled and randomized to one of four treatment groups: 120 mg BG00012 once daily (and matching placebo twice daily), 120 mg BG00012 thrice daily (360 mg daily dose), 240 mg BG00012 thrice daily (720 mg daily dose), and placebo thrice daily. One patient did not receive treatment, so all results were based upon 256 patients. The high-dose group was titrated to full dose by taking 120 mg thrice daily for one week. Dosage reduction was allowed for one month for patients unable to tolerate the standard dose or for abnormal liver, renal, and hematology tests. Separate study personnel were assigned to perform neurologic assessments (blinded examining neurologist) and treat patients (treating neurologist and nurse). To help prevent potential unblinding of study personnel, patients were asked to not take their study medication within four hours of their study visit. MRI was performed monthly from baseline through week 24. Each MRI study included a dual echo fast (turbo) spin echo sequence for proton density and T2-weighted images and a conventional spin echo before and after standard-dose Gd contrast. Images were read centrally.

The primary outcome of the Phase 2 trial was the total number of new Gd-enhancing lesions on monthly scans from weeks 12–24. Secondary imaging outcomes included cumulative number of new Gd-enhancing lesions from weeks 4 to 24, the number of new or enlarging T2 lesions, and new T1-hypointense lesions (T1 holes) at week 24. The effect on relapse rate, disability progression, safety, and tolerability were also assessed.

Over the 24 weeks of the study, 21 (8.2%) of 256 patients who received study drug withdrew from the study. Another 30 patients (11.7%) discontinued treatment but completed follow-up. More patients receiving the higher two doses discontinued treatment than the other two groups.

The study met its primary outcome: patients receiving 720 mg/d of BG00012 had a 69% reduction in the number of new Gd-enhancing lesions compared to placebo patients (1.4 vs. 4.5, $P < 0.0001$; Fig. 31.4). A sensitivity analysis of the intention-to-treat population showed similar results ($P < 0.0001$). In contrast, the primary outcome was not met with either of the lower two dose groups. However, the middle (240 mg/d) dose group had a 76% higher mean number of Gd-enhancing lesions at baseline, which may have obscured a treatment effect. If the primary outcome is re-displayed as % reduction from each group's baseline enhancing lesion activity, a dose–response becomes more apparent (Fig. 31.4).

Secondary imaging outcomes were also met in the 720 mg/d group. Compared with placebo, there was a 44% reduction in Gd-enhancing lesions from week 4 to 24 ($P = 0.002$), a 48% reduction in number of new or enlarging T2 lesions over 24 weeks ($P = 0.0006$), and a 53% reduction in the number of T1 holes ($P = 0.014$). No significant difference was observed in either of the lower dose groups compared to placebo. The annualized relapse rate in the 720 mg/d group was 32% lower than the placebo group, although this was not statistically significant. As with many Phase 2 trials in relapsing MS, this study was not powered to detect a significant effect of treatment on relapses.

Additional analyses evaluated conversion of Gd-enhancing lesions to T1 holes. A subset of Gd-enhancing lesions will later become T1 hypointense lesions (T1 holes), and this type of lesion is thought to represent more significant tissue injury than lesions that do not develop into T1 holes. Imaging data from several clinical trials have evaluated the effect of different ther-

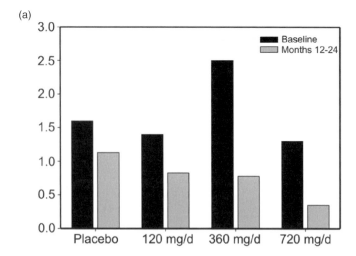

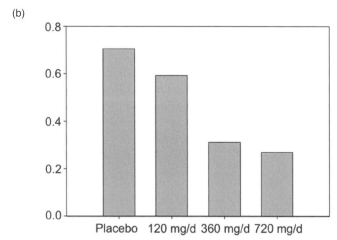

Fig. 31.4. Gadolinium-enhancing lesion outcome from the Phase 2 clinical trial in relapsing MS:[14] (a) mean enhancing lesions per subject per scan at baseline and averaged over weeks 12, 16, 20, and 24; (b) percent reduction in enhancing lesions at weeks 12–24, compared with baseline.

apies on the evolution of enhancing lesions into T1 holes.[18,19] T1 hole conversion is an imaging measure that is thought to reflect the potential neuroprotective effect of a therapy, beyond anti-inflammatory effects measured by new enhancing lesions and T2 lesions. A post hoc analysis of the BG00012 Phase 2 trial was performed to evaluate the evolution of new Gd-enhancing lesions into T1 holes.[20] New lesions that developed between weeks 4 and 12 were evaluated at week 24 to identify the proportion that evolved into T1 holes. The odds ratio (OR) for the evolution of new Gd-enhancing lesions into T1 holes in the 720 mg/d BG00012 group compared to placebo group was 0.51 ($P < 0.0001$). After adjusting for baseline Gd-enhancing lesions, years since disease onset, and relapses in the previous 3 years, the OR decreased to 0.40. The treatment effect was greater for smaller lesions (OR 0.30) than large lesions (OR 0.62). Analysis of the lower dose BG00012 groups was not reported, since they did not show a significant reduction in Gd-enhancing lesions.

The most common adverse events reported in the BG00012 treatment groups were flushing, headache, and gastrointestinal symptoms (nausea, diarrhea, abdominal pain). Flushing typically started within 30 minutes of dosing and resolved by 90 minutes. The frequency of flushing and gastrointestinal adverse events decreased markedly after 1 month. Flushing was reported in 66% of patients during month 1, but only 5% during month 6. Gastrointestinal adverse events were reported in 52% of patients during month 1, but only 4% during month 6.[14]

The frequency of infections was generally similar between treatment groups. One case of pelvic inflammatory disease was the only serious infection reported in the study. Adverse events that led to drug discontinuation included flushing (two patients), nausea (two patients), vomiting (two patients), diarrhea (two patients), and increased alanine aminotransferase (one patient). No clinically meaningful trends in laboratory tests were observed over the course of the study. A mild, dose-related increase in transaminase levels were observed, with most less than twice the upper limit of normal. None were associated with increase in bilirubin or other evidence of impaired hepatic function and no patients reported symptoms of hepatitis. In all cases, laboratory abnormalities resolved upon discontinuation of BG00012 and some patients tolerated later re-treatment without recurrent increase in transaminases. There were no clinically significant shifts in hematology profiles, anemia, or neutropenia.

Subjects who successfully completed the 24-week placebo-controlled study were offered enrollment into an open-label, dose-blinded, 24-week extension study.[14] Those on BG00012 in the first half of the study remained on the same dose of BG00012, while those on placebo were transitioned to 240 mg thrice daily (720 mg/d) of BG00012. 225 patients enrolled in open-label extension study. The profile of adverse events in the open-label study was similar to that seen in the placebo-controlled phase, with no new safety issues.

Phase 3 clinical trials

Following the successful Phase 2 clinical trial, BG0012 was further evaluated in two large, placebo-controlled Phase 3 clinical trials in relapsing remitting MS – the DEFINE and CONFIRM trials. Both trials were two years in duration and compared two doses of BG00012 with placebo. In addition to the 240 mg thrice daily (720 mg/d) dose found beneficial in the Phase 2 trial, 240 mg twice daily (480 mg/d, plus placebo capsules once a day) was also evaluated. This 480 mg/d dose is between the high (720 mg/d) and middle (360 mg/d) doses evaluated in the Phase 2 trial. The 480 mg/d dosing regimen also utilized twice daily dosing, which is more desired by patients than the thrice daily dosing of the 720mg/d dosing regimen. In addition, the CONFIRM trial has glatiramer acetate as an additional, fourth arm. This "tracking" arm is a requirement of some regulatory agencies, providing a comparator to an established, available relapsing MS therapy. The glatiramer acetate arm is open-label to the patients and treating neurologist (i.e. there are no placebo capsules for this group and no placebo injections for the oral

BG00012 and placebo groups), but blinded for the examining neurologists and image analysis team. Randomization was equal among each treatment arm.

Clinical assessments included clinical relapses and EDSS progression, as well as Multiple Sclerosis Functional Composite (MSFC) and visual contrast sensitivity test. A subset of patients were offered enrollment in an optional MRI sub-study. Analysis for the MRI sub-study included new Gd-enhancing lesions, new or enlarging T2 lesions, and atrophy. In addition, magnetization transfer ratio (MTR) imaging is included as an exploratory neuroprotection outcome. Safety assessments included laboratory studies and electrocardiographs. Rescue therapy is allowed for patients with clinical disease activity (relapses or progressive disability on EDSS).

The primary outcomes of the two trials were slightly different. The primary outcome of the DEFINE trial was the proportion of patients relapsing, while the primary outcome of the CONFIRM trial was the annualized relapse rate. Secondary outcomes were slightly different between the two studies, but included rate of disability progression at two years, reduction in new or newly enlarging T2 lesions, Gd-enhancing lesions, and T1 holes.

Both studies completed enrollment in 2009, with DEFINE enrolling 1239 subjects and CONFIRM enrolling 1431 subjects. Both are expected to complete two years of follow-up and report results in 2011. Preliminary, top-line results from the CONFIRM trial are very encouraging. Compared with placebo, MS patients treated with 240 mg twice daily (480 mg/d) had a 49% reduction in the proportion with relapses (the primary outcome), 53% reduction in annualized relapse rate, 85% reduction in new or enlarging T2 lesions, 90% reduction in Gd-enhancing lesions at 2 years, and 38% reduction in sustained progression of disability. No new significant safety issues were found.

Summary

The use of DMF in autoimmune diseases arose from a personal view of the immune system, whereby autoimmunity is caused by disruption in the Krebs's cycle. Despite the incorrect reason, it appears that DMF does indeed have immunomodulatory properties in both animals and humans. Perhaps equally important, laboratory evidence and preliminary imaging evidence from human clinical trials suggests that DMF may have neuroprotective properties via antioxidative mechanisms. A Phase 2 trial found that 720 mg/d of BG00012 both reduced active inflammation (Gd-enhancing lesions and T2 lesions) as well as conversion of Gd-enhancing lesions to T1 holes. BG00012 showed a favorable safety profile, with the main side effects being flushing and gastrointestinal symptoms. Phase 3 trials will provide pivotal and definitive evidence regarding the safety and efficacy of BG00012 in MS. Ongoing laboratory studies and advanced imaging studies in the Phase 3 trials are evaluating the potential neuroprotective effects of BG00012. Fumaric acids such as BG00012 are an exciting new class of potential MS treatment.

References

1. Schweckendiek W. [Treatment of psoriasis vulgaris]. *Med Monatsschr.* 1959;13:103–4.

2. Balasubramaniam P, Stevenson O, Berth-Jones J. Fumaric acid esters in severe psoriasis, including experience of use in combination with other systemic modalities. *Br J Dermatol* 2004;150:741–746.

3. Ormerod AD, Mrowietz U. Fumaric acid esters, their place in the treatment of psoriasis. *Br J Dermatol* 2004;150:630–2.

4. Altmeyer PJ, Matthes U, Pawlak F, *et al.* Antipsoriatic effect of fumaric acid derivatives. Results of a multicenter double-blind study in 100 patients. *J Am Acad Dermatol* 1994;30:977–81.

5. de Jong R, Bezemer AC, Zomerdijk TP, van de Pouw-Kraan T, Ottenhoff TH, Nibbering PH. Selective stimulation of T helper 2 cytokine responses by the anti-psoriasis agent monomethylfumarate. *Eur J Immunol* 1996;26:2067–74.

6. Schimrigk S, Brune N, Hellwig K, *et al.* Oral fumaric acid esters for the treatment of active multiple sclerosis: an open-label, baseline-controlled pilot study. *Eur J Neurol* 2006;13:604–10.

7. Treumer F, Zhu K, Glaser R, Mrowietz U. Dimethylfumarate is a potent inducer of apoptosis in human T cells. *J Invest Dermatol* 2003;121:1383–8.

8. Sebok B, Bonnekoh B, Geisel J, Mahrle G. Antiproliferative and cytotoxic profiles of antipsoriatic fumaric acid derivatives in keratinocyte cultures. *Eur J Pharmacol* 1994;270:79–87.

9. Sebok B, Bonnekoh B, Vetter R, Schneider I, Gollnick H, Mahrle G. The antipsoriatic dimethyl-fumarate suppresses interferon-gamma -induced ICAM-1 and HLA-DR expression on hyperproliferative keratinocytes. Quantification by a culture plate-directed APAAP-ELISA technique. *Eur J Dermatol* 1998;8:29–32.

10. Risch K, Strebel HP, Joshi RK, *et al.* Methyl hydrogen fumarate inhibits acute and chronic rejection in rat kidney transplantation models. *Transpl Proc* 2001;33:545–6.

11. Lehmann M, Risch K, Nizze H, *et al.* Fumaric acid esters are potent immunosuppressants: inhibition of acute and chronic rejection in rat kidney transplantation models by methyl hydrogen fumarate. *Arch Dermatol Res* 2002;294:399–404.

12. Loewe R, Holnthoner W, Groger M, *et al.* Dimethylfumarate inhibits TNF-induced nuclear entry of NF-kappa B/p65 in human endothelial cells. *J Immunol* 2002;168:4781–7.

13. Linker RA, Lee DH, Ryan S, *et al.* Fumaric acid esters exert neuroprotective effects in neuroinflammation via activation of the Nrf2 antioxidant pathway. *Brain* 2011;134:678–92.

14. Kappos L, Gold R, Miller DH, *et al.* Efficacy and safety of oral fumarate in patients with relapsing-remitting multiple sclerosis: a multicentre, randomised, double-blind, placebo-controlled phase IIb study. *Lancet* 2008;372:1463–72.

15. Stoof TJ, Flier J, Sampat S, Nieboer C, Tensen CP, Boorsma DM. The antipsoriatic drug dimethylfumarate strongly suppresses chemokine production in human keratinocytes and peripheral blood mononuclear cells. *Br J Dermatol* 2001;144:1114–20.

16. Gold R, Linington C, Lassmann H. Understanding pathogenesis and therapy of multiple sclerosis via animal models: 70 years of merits and culprits in experimental autoimmune encephalomyelitis research. *Brain* 2006;129:1953–71.

17. Schilling S, Goelz S, Linker R, Luehder F, Gold R. Fumaric acid esters are effective in chronic experimental autoimmune encephalomyelitis and suppress macrophage infiltration. *Clin Exp Immunol* 2006;145:101–7.

18. Filippi M, Cercignani M, Inglese M, Horsfield MA, Comi G. Diffusion tensor magnetic resonance imaging in multiple sclerosis. *Neurology* 2001;56:304–11.

19. Dalton CM, Miszkiel KA, Barker GJ, MacManus DG, Pepple TI, Panzara M, *et al.* Effect of natalizumab on conversion of gadolinium enhancing lesions to T1 hypointense lesions in relapsing multiple sclerosis. *J Neurol* 2004;251:407–13.

20. Macmanus DG, Miller DH, Kappos L, *et al.* BG-12 reduces evolution of new enhancing lesions to T1-hypointense lesions in patients with multiple sclerosis. *J Neurol* 2010 Epub Oct 21.

Chapter

32

Alemtuzumab to treat multiple sclerosis

Orla Tuohy and Alasdair J. Coles

Introduction

Alemtuzumab is emerging as one of the most effective treatments of multiple sclerosis (MS), albeit with significant safety concerns. Yet its route to Phase 3 trials has been slow and tortuous, with many years when its development was largely driven by academic interests rather than commercial sponsorship. Here we review its history, biology, efficacy, and safety as a treatment of MS. We propose that it is best understood as a drug which profoundly modulates, rather than suppresses, the immune response that underlies MS.

History and development of alemtuzumab

The discovery for which Kohler and Milstein won the Nobel Prize was the technique, published in 1975, to generate a permanent tissue culture cell line producing a continuous supply of a monoclonal antibody of defined specificity.[1] Milstein's students, Herman Waldmann and Geoff Hale, used their technology to generate the first monoclonal antibody to be used as a human therapy: a rat-derived IgM antibody that lysed human T-cells. Working in the Cambridge Pathology laboratory, they called this antibody Campath-1M.[2] One of its first clinical uses was in a patient undergoing allogenic bone marrow transplantation from a non-sibling donor for aplastic anemia.[3] Further use in the field of bone-marrow transplantation, which involved pre-treatment of donor marrow, in-vitro, with Campath-1M, prevented graft vs. host disease by removing potentially reactive T-cells from the donor marrow.[4] However, this reduction in the incidence of graft-vs.-host disease seen with alemtuzumab in bone marrow transplantation, was offset by an increased rate of graft rejection.[5] The team went on to generate a rat antibody of identical antigen specificity, but of IgG2b isotype, Campath-1G, which proved more effective at antibody-mediated and complement-mediated lysis of human T-cells.[6] In 1989, Campath-1G was given to a patient with pro-lymphocytic transformation of chronic lymphocytic leukemia (CLL).[7] The response was a marked clearance of peripheral blood and bone marrow malignant cells, although the patient subsequently died from a central nervous system relapse of their underlying disease. Another Cambridge academic, Greg

Winter, developed the technique of humanization of antibodies, where all but the antigen-binding fragments of the rat antibody are replaced by a human immunoglobulin backbone. The first antibody to be humanized was Campath-1G, to produce Campath-1H. This was first used in a patient in the leukemic phase of non-Hodgkin's lymphoma with a dramatic reduction in blood and bone marrow tumor cells.[8] Success in subsequent trials of Campath-1H in B-cell CLL,[9] led in 2001 to US Food and Drug Administration (FDA) licensing for the treatment of refractory B-cell CLL, and in 2007 to a license for first-line treatment. It is also been used increasingly, off-indication, in prevention of chronic rejection in solid organ transplantation.[10]

In the 1980s and 1990s, a handful of physicians in Cambridge, UK, explored the utility of Campath-1H as a treatment of autoimmune disease, especially systemic vasculitis,[11] but also rheumatoid arthritis, Wegner's granulomatosis, auto-immune cytopenias, and uveitis (and much more recently chronic inflammatory demyelinating polyneuropathy, and inclusion body myositis).[12-16] Success in these conditions, and a corridor conversation with Herman Waldmann, led Alastair Compston to propose a small study of Campath-1H in MS, which started in 1991. Experience of using Campath-1H has grown since then, leading to insights into the pathogenesis of MS and emergence as an exciting new therapy. More recently, Campath-1H has been renamed alemtuzumab; Genyme has proposed the trade name Lemtrada if it becomes licensed as a treatment of MS.

The biology of alemtuzumab

Alemtuzumab targets the antigen CD52, which is found densely on the surface of lymphocytes, monocytes, macrophages, natural killer (NK) cells, eosinophils, and mature sperm cells. This small glycoprotein, of just 12 amino acids,[17] is attached to the cell surface by a glycosylphosphatidylinositol anchor. Recent studies in a transgenic mouse model expressing human CD52 showed that lymphocyte depletion by alemtuzumab is mainly by antibody-dependent cytotoxicity, rather than complement mediated cytotoxicity.[18] The function of CD52 is not yet known. The glycosylphosphatidylinositol anchor structure lends itself to signal transduction, often following linkage of receptors, as

Multiple Sclerosis Therapeutics, Fourth Edition, ed. Jeffrey A. Cohen and Richard A. Rudick. Published by Cambridge University Press.
© Cambridge University Press 2011.

seen in other GPI-linked cell surface proteins such as CD59 and CD24. It has been postulated that CD52 plays a role, through signal transduction, in T-cell activation and proliferation. However, its ligand has not been identified. Other authors have suggested a more basic role in modifying the "stickiness" of the cell membrane. In the male reproductive tract, CD52 has been suggested as a "maturation-associated antigen" of sperm cells. The manufacture of CD52 was localized to the epididymal epithelial cells, following which CD52 was transferred to the surface of sperm cells on transit through the epididymal ductal system.

In the Phase 3 trials of alemtuzumab in MS, alemtuzumab is administered intravenously at a dose of 12 mg/day. The first cycle is given daily for 5 consecutive days, followed 12 months later by a second cycle of 3 days. Pre-medication with steroids, analgesics, and anti-histamines reduce cytokine-mediated, infusion-related side effects.[19] Lymphodepletion is rapid, with no detectable peripheral CD52-positive cells after infusion of only 3 mg alemtuzumab, and it is persistent; after one cycle of alemtuzumab it takes a median of three years for mean CD4+ T-cells to reach the lower limit of the normal range, and at least five years to return to baseline.[20] The mechanism for such prolonged lymphopenia is not clear because hematological precursors are not depleted by alemtuzumab.[21] In patients with rheumatoid arthritis, slow T-cell repopulation after autologous bone marrow transplantation is attributed to reduced response by the homeostatic cytokine, interleukin (IL)-7,[22] but this is not the case after alemtuzumab treatment of MS.[23]

The initial rationale for the early use of alemtuzumab to treat autoimmune disease was based on this profound and prolonged depletion of CD4+ T-cells. It was thought that removal of such a key orchestrator of the immune response would abrogate all inflammation and would bring any autoimmune process to a halt. The cost, it was anticipated, would be frequent opportunistic infections. It turns out that these assumptions were incorrect. First, as discussed in full below, the rate of infection after alemtuzumab is surprisingly low and, second, the main adverse effect is secondary autoimmunity. This autoimmunity is not expressed as a return of MS disease activity, but is directed against systemic organs, notably the thyroid gland or blood components.

We propose that the efficacy of alemtuzumab arises not from lymphocyte depletion but from the profound alterations in the immune repertoire induced by the homeostatic response to the lymphopenia induced by alemtuzumab. In summary, for six months after alemtuzumab, the depleted lymphocyte pool is dominated by regulatory T-cells, other memory T-cells[23] and recent bone marrow-derived B-cells.[24] For the next six months, there is some return of naive T-cells and memory B-cells, but the proportions of these cell types never return to baseline. Throughout this time, endogenous secretion by lymphocytes of cytokines of all classes (Th1, Th2, Th17) is lower than baseline (McCarthy, personal communication). When challenged with a panel of antigens, reconstituting lymphocytes have increased proliferative responses to auto-antigens after alemtuzumab.[25] In response to myelin basic protein, peripheral lymphocytes secrete neurotrophins, such as brain-derived neurotrophic factor (BDNF), which have the capacity to promote neuronal and oligodendrocyte culture in vitro.[25] We argue that these lymphocytes may enter the brain, after alemtuzumab, and contribute to the improvement in disability seen with early treatment in trials of alemtuzumab.

Efficacy of alemtuzumab treatment of multiple sclerosis

Open-label experience of alemtuzumab treatment of multiple sclerosis

Initial use of alemtuzumab in MS was in patients with secondary progressive disease.[26] From 1991, when alemtuzumab was first used in MS, until 1999, 36 such patients with progressive disease received treatment. The results were mixed. On one hand, alemtuzumab profoundly reduced the formation of new lesions on MRI scans and the number of relapses experienced by all patients, both makers of cerebral inflammation.[26,27] Indeed, when followed up radiologically, roughly seven years after the last alemtuzumab treatment, still no new lesions were evident.[20] On the other hand, most patients experienced continued progression of disability.[27] We noted that those patients who had continued progression were also those with the highest inflammatory load and lowest brain volume at the time of treatment.[27]

As a result of this experience, we were amongst the first to point out the dissociation between reduction in inflammation and continued progression in patients with established progressive MS.[27] We hypothesized that MS is a disease of two phases: that relapsing–remitting (RR) disease is inflammatory and sets up, through demyelination, the conditions for a second phase of non-inflammatory (or perhaps better "post-inflammatory") neurodegeneration. The corollary of this hypothesis is that, for anti-inflammatory treatments to be effective, they have to be given early in the course of the disease.

For that reason, in 1999, we shifted to using alemtuzumab in patients with early RRMS. The first 22 patients treated open-label as part of this strategy were those who seemed likely to develop an aggressive disease course due to a high early relapse rate or a failure to respond to currently licensed treatment with interferon-beta (IFNβ).[20] This cohort had disease duration of an average of 2.7 years, during which they had experienced a mean of 2.2 relapses per year and had acquired a mean Expanded Disability Status Scale (EDSS) score of 4.8. As in the progressive cohort, there was an impressive reduction in relapse rate, by 91% during a mean of 29 months follow-up. However, in contrast to our previous experience, and in line with our hypothesis, the cohort did not experience a progressive worsening of disability. Not only did their disability not worsen, but, unexpectedly, their disability improved by −1.4 EDSS points at 12 months. We used these data to promote our concept of a "window of therapeutic opportunity" in MS[20] for anti-inflammatory treatments: early on in the RR phase and before the conditions have set in which preconfigure neurodegeneration.

This experience was acquired in open-label studies, with limited financial support and largely independent of the commercial development of alemtuzumab as a treatment of MS, which had not been proceeding straightforwardly. What was required at this stage was significant investment to conduct a controlled trial. After some false starts, with the sponsorship of Ilex Oncology and then Genzyme, this was at last realized.

Controlled studies of alemtuzumab in relapsing–remitting multiple sclerosis

"CAMMS223" was a randomized, single-blinded, Phase 2 trial comparing alemtuzumab with a current standard therapy, IFNβ-1a (Rebif).[28] It began recruitment in 2003 and was reported in 2008. For a Phase 2 trial, it was unusually large (>300 patients) and prolonged (three years) and – uniquely – had as its primary outcome, a change in fixed disability (as opposed to relapse rate or MRI markers). Key inclusion criteria, framed on the basis of the "window of therapeutic opportunity" hypothesis were: disease onset had to be within the previous 36 months and patients were required to be free of significant disability (EDSS score less than 3.5). We selected for "active" MS, by requiring at least two relapses in the preceding two years, and a gadolinium (Gd)-enhancing lesion on MRI within the four months prior to enrollment. Patients were randomly assigned either IFNβ-1a ($n = 111$), or one of two alemtuzumab doses, 12 mg/day ($n = 112$), or 24 mg/day ($n = 110$). Alemtuzumab was administered over five days, with a schedule for repeat courses to be administered annually, for the three-year duration of the study. In 2005, there was a fatality from an unexpected adverse effect, immune thrombocytopenia (see below), which led to a voluntary suspension of dosing of alemtuzumab within the trial (a decision later endorsed by the FDA). By this date, all but two trial patients had received the planned second cycle of alemtuzumab, but only 25% had received a third cycle; so the efficacy outcomes are predominantly those of a three-year follow up to two cycles of alemtuzumab, at months 0 and 12.

The results of CAMMS223 confirmed the open-label studies. Alemtuzumab significantly reduced the risk of a relapse, in comparison with IFNβ-1a, by 74% over three years. And, in this cohort of people with early, active disease, who had not yet acquired disability, alemtuzumab reduced the risk of sustained accumulation of disability (by 1 EDSS point, confirmed at six months – or 1.5 EDSS points if the starting EDSS was 0) by 71% compared with IFNβ-1a. Furthermore, most patients who received alemtuzumab actually experienced an improvement in disability over three years: mean EDSS improved by 0.39 point in the alemtuzumab group and worsened by 0.38 point in the IFNβ-1a group ($P < 0.001$).[28] A recent analysis, not yet published but presented at ECTRIMS 2010, confirmed that alemtuzumab's superior efficacy over IFNβ-1a was maintained at five years, despite the fact that most alemtuzumab-treated patients had not received any further treatment.

There are several possible mechanisms for this improvement in disability, including plasticity,[29] remyelination,[30] and preservation of axons. Given that MRI measures of brain volume actually increase between months 12 to 36 (+0.9% in alemtuzumab group vs. atrophy of −2% in IFNβ-1a group), we propose that there is restoration of tissue underlying the disability improvement.[28] By post-hoc subgroup analyses of the CAMMS223 trial,[25] we have shown disability improves after alemtuzumab even amongst people with no clinical disease activity immediately before treatment, or any clinical or radiological disease activity on-trial, suggesting that it is mediated through a mechanism unrelated to its anti-inflammatory effect.

We hypothesized that lymphocytes, reconstituting after alemtuzumab, may permit or promote brain repair, providing so-called "neuroprotective autoimmunity." To investigate this, we studied peripheral blood mononuclear cells (PBMCs) from our patients. We showed that, after alemtuzumab, PBMCs stimulated with myelin basic protein secrete more BDNF, platelet-derived growth factor, ciliary neurotrophic factor, and fibroblast growth factor. We then cultured the PBMCs in "minimal medium," which barely supports survival of neurons and then put rat neurons and oligodendrocyte precursors in this "conditioned medium." There was enhanced neuronal survival and axonal growth, as well as oligodendrocyte maturation and survival. This supports the idea that alemtuzumab modulates the immune repertoire to include expanding cells, which release neurotrophins in response to myelin basic protein. If these were to cross the blood–brain barrier, they could potentially deliver neurotrophins to the central nervous system.[25]

Patients in the CAMMS223 trial have been offered the chance for further follow-up within a formal "extension trial." Also Phase 3 trials of alemtuzumab are now under way (http://www.care-ms.co.uk/) in patients with relatively early RRMS. CARE-MS I explores the efficacy and safety of two cycles of alemtuzumab, 12 mg/day, compared to IFNβ-1a over two years, in greater than 500 patients with treatment-naive MS. CARE-MS II investigates the same alemtuzumab regime in over 800 patients who have had at least one relapse whilst on a standard disease-modifying therapy. Both should be completed in 2011.

Safety of alemtuzumab as a treatment of multiple sclerosis

Just as the efficacy experience of alemtuzumab generated some novel concepts of MS biology, such as the possibility of "neuroprotective autoimmunity,"[25] so too has exploration of its adverse effects. Our expectation, when we started treating patients with alemtuzumab, was that opportunistic infections would be frequent. In fact, they are rare. The most significant adverse effect of alemtuzumab is, counter-intuitively, autoimmunity.

Infusion-associated symptoms of alemtuzumab

Administration of alemtuzumab is associated with the development of an infusion reaction characterized by fever, rigors, headache, and an urticarial skin rash. This is rather similar to that seen with many depleting antibodies, such as OKT3. It appears to be due to cross-linking of NK cells causing programmed release of cytokines.[31] In addition, a worsening of underlying neurological deficits, or a re-emergence of symptoms of a prior relapse, occurred after the administration of alemtuzumab in patients with MS.[27] We hypothesized that whatever mediated the infusion reaction might be causing conduction block at sites of previous demyelination. We showed that alemtuzumab's infusion reaction is accompanied by a rise in serum cytokines IL-6, tumor necrosis factor-alpha (TNFα), and IFNγ. Pre-administration of corticosteroids, but not soluble TNF receptor, significantly suppresses this syndrome, suggesting that it is caused by a cytokine other than TNFα. On the basis of Ken Smith's experimental work, we suspect soluble nitric oxide.[32] Intravenous methylprednisolone is now routinely administered prior to alemtuzumab in MS patients.

Infections

Despite the profound lymphopenia induced by alemtuzumab, the rate of serious infections after alemtuzumab remains low. It has been suggested that patients treated with alemtuzumab maintain immunocompetence through the relative sparing of lymphocytes sequestered in peripheral lymphoid organs from the cytotoxic effects of the drug. During 316 patient–years of follow-up for the first 58 patients with MS who received alemtuzumab, eight infections occurred that could be attributed to alemtuzumab.[20] In the CAMMS223 trial, mild-to-moderate infections, most commonly respiratory tract infections, were seen more frequently after alemtuzumab.[28] There have been no reports to date of any of the serious opportunistic infections, such as cytomegaolvirus, pneumocystis jirovecii, or progressive multifocal leukoencephalopathy, after alemtuzumab treatment of MS.

Neoplasia

To date, there is no signal that alemtuzumab causes neoplasia. Only one case raises this possibility: that of a woman who developed Epstein–Barr virus-negative Burkitt's lymphoma two years after her third cycle of treatment in the CAMMS223 trial.[28] The Phase 3 trials should provide further information on this important point.

Autoimmunity

The most significant adverse effect of alemtuzumab is "secondary autoimmunity," by which is meant autoimmunity that arises in the months or years after alemtuzumab. We now attribute it to faulty reconstitution of lymphocytes. Understanding its mechanism has allowed the possibility that people at risk of this adverse effect may be identified before treatment.

The main manifestation of autoimmunity, seen in 25% of people treated with alemtuzumab, is against the thyroid gland, usually autoimmune hyperthyroidism (Graves' disease)[33] compared with a prevalence in untreated patients with MS of 1%–3%.[34,35] Autoimmune thyroid disease after alemtuzumab can be detected presymptomatically by screening biochemical thyroid function every three months, and it appears to respond as well to treatment as the regular disease. The next most common form of autoimmunity after alemtuzumab is immune thrombocytopenic purpura (ITP), which has affected 3% of people treated to date.[28] The index case was not expected and, tragically, died after two weeks of symptoms of bleeding went unrecognized, due to an intracranial hemorrhage. This was doubly sad because ITP is normally manageable. Since that time, the sponsoring company, Genzyme, has developed a risk management plan, in collaboration with the regulatory authorities. In its current form in the Phase 3 trials, this requires patients to have a monthly blood count, and fill out a monthly survey reminding them of the early symptoms or easy bleeding. Five patients with ITP after alemtuzumab were identified with this monitoring in the CAMMS223 trial, and all are now well off treatment (which had been steroids or rituximab) with normal platelet counts. There have been other autoimmune diseases noted after alemtuzumab, occurring at lower frequency. Three patients have developed anti-glomerular basement membrane disease (Goodpasture's syndrome).[36] There have been single cases of autoimmune disease against neutrophils, lymphocytes, and red blood cells.

Autoimmunity after alemtuzumab presents a significant challenge to its future use to treat MS. All of the autoimmune conditions seen to date can be treated successfully, or cured, if identified early. So, the task is to develop a monitoring scheme that achieves early detection efficiently, whilst not overburdening patients and their physicians with excessive frequent tests.

The biology of autoimmunity arising during reconstitution of a depleted immune system is fascinating. It is seen following highly active anti-retroviral therapy treatment of human immunodeficiency virus infection[37] and on recovery from hemopoietic stem cell transplantation.[38] In patients with MS who develop autoimmunity after alemtuzumab, there is greater T-cell apoptosis and cell cycling. This is driven by higher circulating levels of IL-21. Indeed, blood samples taken before treatment from patients who subsequently went on to develop secondary autoimmunity had more than two-fold greater levels of serum IL-21 than the non-autoimmune group. We suggest that serum IL-21 may, therefore, serve as a biomarker for the risk of developing autoimmunity.[39] This will improve counseling of patients prior to alemtuzumab therapy. And it will direct patients who are treated into a "high-risk" or "low-risk" monitoring program.

Anti-alemtuzumab antibodies

Despite the humanization of alemtuzumab, it is immunogenic. One month after one cycle of alemtuzumab, 30% of patients have detectable antibodies against the antibody; this increases to 70% one month after the second cycle. However, the level of these antibodies has largely waned by the time of the next cycle of treatment: in the CAMMS223 trial significant anti-alemtuzumab antibodies were present in 0.5% of patients 12 months after treatment and 26.3% of patients at 24 months. There was no evidence, however, of any reduction in treatment efficacy or of an increased rate of adverse events in patients with elevated anti-alemtuzumab antibody levels at the time of treatment.

Nonetheless, we have explored a novel strategy to reduce the immunogenicity of a biological like alemtuzumab. Herman Waldmann and colleagues in Oxford have made a non-binding variant of alemtuzumab called SM3, which can be given in high concentration and so allows generation of "high zone tolerance." In a study that involved 20 alemtuzumab-treated patients with RRMS, pre-treatment with SM3 reduced the proportion of patients developing anti-alemtuzumab antibodies to 21% compared with 74% in the control group of CAMMS223 alemtuzumab-treated patients.[40] Thus, a mechanism exists for reducing the immunogenicity of alemtuzumab, despite the uncertainty surrounding the clinical significance of anti-alemtuzumab antibodies.

Conclusions

A straightforward conclusion from our experience of using alemtuzumab, both open-label and within trials, is that it has the potential to be one of the most efficacious treatments of MS to date. Enthusiasm for its use must be tempered by its significant adverse effects; to date, the most concerning of these is the risk of secondary autoimmune disease. The results of the Phase 3 trials should provide a comprehensive picture of alemtuzumab's safety profile. Understanding the biology of this complication has identified a pre-treatment biomarker, serum IL-21, of autoimmunity after alemtuzumab. The remaining challenge is to frame a monitoring scheme that efficiently and rapidly identifies autoimmunity early enough for treatment to be effective, but is not excessively onerous.

A key lesson from the history of alemtuzumab treatment of MS has been that the disease is only vulnerable to such anti-inflammatory treatments early in its course, before the conditions that predispose to neurodegeneration, and secondary progression, have been set up. This raises the difficult issue of identifying features in the early disease course that suggest sufficiently aggressive disease to justify the risks of alemtuzumab.

The finding of disability improvement after alemtuzumab suggests a new treatment paradigm in MS, where drugs are judged not by whether they arrest disease, but how much they reverse apparently fixed damage. And the finding of increased lymphocytic neurotrophin secretion after alemtuzumab raises the prospect that "neuroprotective autoimmunity" is a real and useful entity in MS.[25]

References

1. Kohler G, Milstein C. Continuous cultures of fused cells secreting antibody of predefined specificity. *Nature* 1975;256:495–7.

2. Hale G, Bright S, Chumbley G, *et al.* Removal of T cells from bone marrow for transplantation: a monoclonal antilymphocyte antibody that fixes human complement. *Blood* 1983;62:873–82.

3. Hale GaWH. From laboratory to clinic the story of CAMPATH-1. A.J. T George CEU, (ed.). New Jersey: Humana Press; 2000.

4. Waldmann H, Polliak A, Hale G, *et al.* Elimination of graft-versus-host disease by in-vitro depletion of alloreactive lymphocytes with a monoclonal rat anti-human lymphocyte antibody (CAMPATH-1). *Lancet* 1984;2:483–6.

5. Hale G, Cobbold S, Waldmann H. T cell depletion with CAMPATH-1 in allogeneic bone marrow transplantation. *Transplantation* 1988;45:753–9.

6. Hale G, Clark M, Waldmann H. Therapeutic potential of rat monoclonal antibodies: isotype specificity of antibody-dependent cell-mediated cytotoxicity with human lymphocytes. *J Immunol* 1985;134:3056–61.

7. Dyer MJ, Hale G, Hayhoe FG, Waldmann H. Effects of CAMPATH-1 antibodies in vivo in patients with lymphoid malignancies: influence of antibody isotype. *Blood* 1989;73:1431–9.

8. Hale G, Dyer MJ, Clark MR, *et al.* Remission induction in non-Hodgkin lymphoma with reshaped human monoclonal antibody CAMPATH-1H. *Lancet* 1988;2:1394–9.

9. Keating MJ, Flinn I, Jain V, *et al.* Therapeutic role of alemtuzumab (Campath-1H) in patients who have failed fludarabine: results of a large international study. *Blood* 2002;99:3554–61.

10. Barth RN, Janus CA, Lillesand CA, *et al.* Outcomes at 3 years of a prospective pilot study of Campath-1H and sirolimus immunosuppression for renal transplantation. *Transpl Int* 2006;19:885–92.

11. Lockwood CM, Thiru S, Isaacs JD, Hale G, Waldmann H. Long-term remission of intractable systemic vasculitis with monoclonal antibody therapy. *Lancet* 1993;341:1620–2.

12. Lockwood CM, Thiru S, Stewart S, *et al.* Treatment of refractory Wegener's granulomatosis with humanized monoclonal antibodies. *Quart J Med* 1996;89:903–12.

13. Lim SH, Hale G, Marcus RE, Waldmann H, Baglin TP. CAMPATH-1 monoclonal antibody therapy in severe refractory autoimmune thrombocytopenic purpura. *Br J Haematol* 1993;84:542–4.

14. Isaacs JD, Hale G, Waldmann H, Dick AD, *et al.* Monoclonal antibody therapy of chronic intraocular inflammation using Campath-1H. *Br J Ophthalmol* 1995;79:1054–5.

15. Marsh EA, Hirst CL, Llewelyn JG, *et al.* Alemtuzumab in the treatment of IVIG-dependent chronic inflammatory demyelinating polyneuropathy. *J Neurol* 2010;257:913–19.

16. Dalakas MC, Rakocevic G, Schmidt J, *et al.* Effect of Alemtuzumab (CAMPATH 1-H) in patients with

inclusion-body myositis. *Brain* 2009;132:1536–44.

17. Xia MQ, Tone M, Packman L, Hale G, Waldmann H. Characterization of the CAMPATH-1 (CDw52) antigen: biochemical analysis and cDNA cloning reveal an unusually small peptide backbone. *Eur J Immunol* 1991;21:1677–84.

18. Hu Y, Turner MJ, Shields J, *et al.* Investigation of the mechanism of action of alemtuzumab in a human CD52 transgenic mouse model. *Immunology* 2009;128:260–70.

19. Moreau T, Coles A, Wing M, *et al.* Transient increase in symptoms associated with cytokine release in patients with multiple sclerosis. *Brain* 1996;119:225–37.

20. Coles AJ, Cox A, Le Page E, *et al.* The window of therapeutic opportunity in multiple sclerosis: evidence from monoclonal antibody therapy. *J Neurol* 2006;253:98–108.

21. Gilleece MH, Dexter TM. Effect of Campath-1H antibody on human hematopoietic progenitors in vitro. *Blood* 1993;82:807–12.

22. Ponchel F, Verburg RJ, Bingham SJ, *et al.* Interleukin-7 deficiency in rheumatoid arthritis: consequences for therapy-induced lymphopenia. *Arthritis Res Ther* 2005;7:R80–92.

23. Cox AL, Thompson SA, Jones JL, *et al.* Lymphocyte homeostasis following therapeutic lymphocyte depletion in multiple sclerosis. *Eur J Immunol* 2005;35:3332–42.

24. Thompson SA, Jones JL, Cox AL, Compston DA, Coles AJ. B-cell reconstitution and BAFF after

alemtuzumab (Campath-1H) treatment of multiple sclerosis. *J Clin Immunol* 2010;30:99–105.

25. Jones JL, Anderson JM, Phuah CL, *et al.* Improvement in disability after alemtuzumab treatment of multiple sclerosis is associated with neuroprotective autoimmunity. *Brain* 2010;133:2232–47.

26. Moreau T, Thorpe J, Miller D, *et al.* Preliminary evidence from magnetic resonance imaging for reduction in disease activity after lymphocyte depletion in multiple sclerosis. *Lancet* 1994;344:298–301.

27. Coles AJ, Wing MG, Molyneux P, *et al.* Monoclonal antibody treatment exposes three mechanisms underlying the clinical course of multiple sclerosis. *Ann Neurol* 1999;46: 296–304.

28. Coles AJ, Compston DA, Selmaj KW, *et al.* Alemtuzumab vs. interferon beta-1a in early multiple sclerosis. *N Engl J Med* 2008;359:1786–801.

29. Pantano P, Mainero C, Caramia F. Functional brain reorganization in multiple sclerosis: evidence from fMRI studies. *J Neuroimaging* 2006;16:104–14.

30. Franklin RJ, Kotter MR. The biology of CNS remyelination: the key to therapeutic advances. *J Neurol* 2008;255(Suppl 1):19–25.

31. Wing MG, Moreau T, Greenwood J,, *et al.* Mechanism of first-dose cytokine-release syndrome by CAMPATH 1-H: involvement of CD16 (FcgammaRIII) and CD11a/CD18 (LFA-1) on NK cells. *J Clin Invest* 1996;98:2819–26.

32. Redford EJ, Kapoor R, Smith KJ. Nitric oxide donors reversibly block axonal conduction: demyelinated axons are especially susceptible. *Brain* 1997;120:2149–57.

33. Coles AJ, Wing M, Smith S, *et al.* Pulsed monoclonal antibody treatment and autoimmune thyroid disease in multiple sclerosis. *Lancet* 1999;354:1691–5.

34. Sloka JS, Phillips PW, Stefanelli M, Joyce C. Co-occurrence of autoimmune thyroid disease in a multiple sclerosis cohort. *J Autoimmune Dis* 2005;2:9.

35. De Keyser J. Autoimmunity in multiple sclerosis. *Neurology* 1988;38:371–4.

36. Clatworthy MR, Wallin EF, Jayne DR. Anti-glomerular basement membrane disease after alemtuzumab. *N Engl J Med* 2008;359:768–9.

37. Krupica T, Jr., Fry TJ, Mackall CL. Autoimmunity during lymphopenia: a two-hit model. *Clin Immunol* 2006;120:121–8.

38. Loh Y, Oyama Y, Statkute L, *et al.* Development of a secondary autoimmune disorder after hematopoietic stem cell transplantation for autoimmune diseases: role of conditioning regimen used. *Blood* 2007;109:2643–548.

39. Jones JL, Phuah CL, Cox AL, *et al.* IL-21 drives secondary autoimmunity in patients with multiple sclerosis, following therapeutic lymphocyte depletion with alemtuzumab (Campath-1H). *J Clin Invest* 2009;119:2052–61.

40. Somerfield J, Hill-Cawthorne GA, Lin A, *et al.* A novel strategy to reduce the immunogenicity of biological therapies. *J Immunol* 2010;185:763–8.

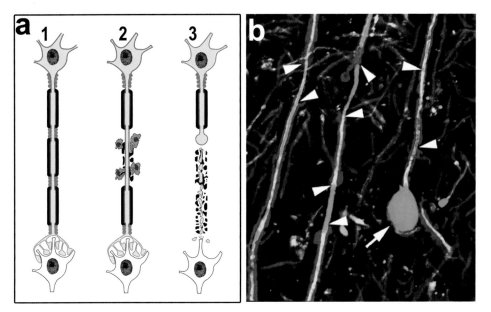

Fig. 2.1. Axons are transected during inflammatory demyelination. (*a*) Schematic summary of axonal response during and following transection. 1. Normal appearing myelinated axon. 2. Demyelination is an immune-mediated or immune cell-assisted process. 3. As many as 11 000 axons/mm³ of lesion area are transected during the demyelinating process. The distal end of the transected axon rapidly degenerates while the proximal end connected to the neuronal cell body survives. Following transection, the neuron continues to transport molecules and organelles down the axon, and they accumulate at the proximal site of the transection. These axon retraction bulbs are transient structures that eventually "die back" to the neuronal perikarya or degenerate. Transected axons were detected in confocal images of an actively demyelinating MS lesion stained for myelin protein (*red*) and axons (*green*). The three vertically oriented axons have areas of demyelination (*arrowheads*), which is mediated by microglia and hematogenous monocytes. The axon on the right ends in a large swelling (*arrowhead*), or axonal retraction bulb, which is the hallmark of the proximal end of a transected axon. Quantification of axonal retraction bulbs has established significant axonal transection in demyelinating lesions of MS. Reproduced from Trapp and Nave, 2008,² (Panel a), and Trapp *et al.*, 1998.¹⁵ (Panel b) with permission.

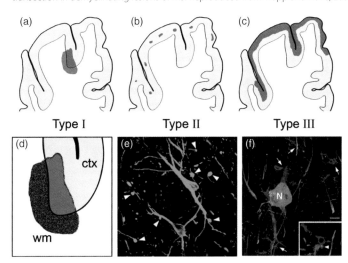

Fig. 2.2. Cortical pathology in multiple sclerosis: three types of cortical lesions were identified in MS. Type I lesions affect subcortical white matter and cortex (a). Type II lesions are small, circular intracortical lesions, often centered on vessels (b). Type III lesions extend from the pial surface into the cortex and often involve multiple gyri (c). Cortex is light gray, white matter is white, and orange represent areas of demyelination. (d) Cortical demyelination occurs without significant infiltration of hematogenous leukocytes, which is schematically depicted in a Type I lesion (ctx, cortex; wm, white matter). (e) Axons and dendrites are transected (white arrowheads) during cortical demyelination. (f) Stellate-shaped microglia were identified in close apposition to neuronal perikarya and extending processes to and around neurofilament-positive neurites (arrows). (Inset) High-magnification image of microglial process (red, arrowhead) ensheathing a branch of an apical dendrite (green). N, neuron. (Adapted from Trapp and Nave, 2008,² Peterson *et al.*, 2001,⁴⁴ with permission.).

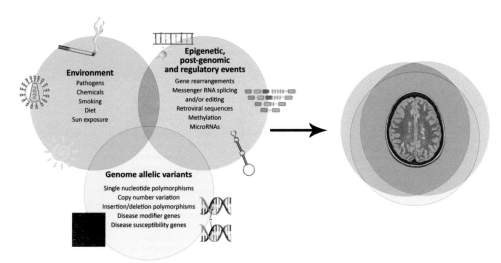

Fig. 4.2. Multiple sclerosis as a complex disease. MS is a complex genetic disease, characterized by a polygenic heritable component, epigenetic changes, and multifaceted interactions with environmental factors. The full roster of disease genes (susceptibility and modifiers) and environmental triggers in MS remains incomplete, whereas the study of epigenetic and other regulatory mechanisms linked to MS susceptibility is only beginning to emerge.

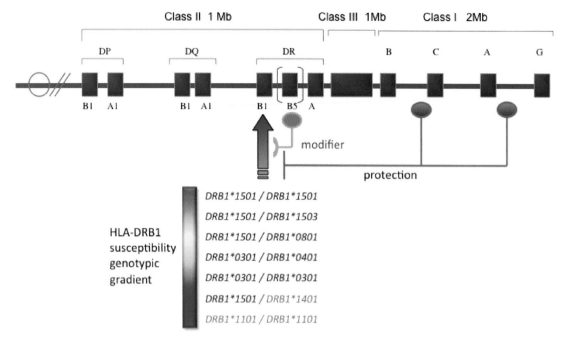

Fig. 4.3. The HLA system in MS. The human leukocyte antigen (*HLA*) gene complex is located on the short arm of chromosome 6 at p21.3, spanning almost 4000 KB of DNA. The full sequence of the region was completed and reported in 1999. From 224 identified loci, 128 are predicted to be expressed and about 40% to have immune-response functions. There are two major classes of HLA-encoding genes involved in antigen presentation. The telomeric stretch contains the *class I* genes, whereas the centromere proximal region encodes *HLA-class II* genes. The *HLA-class II* gene *DRB5* (in brackets) is only present in the DR51 haplotypic group (*DRB1* 15* and ** 16* alleles). *HLA class I* and *class II* encoded molecules are cell surface glycoproteins whose primary role in an immune response is to display and present short antigenic peptide fragments to peptide/MHC-specific T cells, which can then become activated by a second stimulatory signal and initiate an immune response. In addition, HLA molecules are present on stromal cells on the thymus during development helping to determine the specificity of the mature T cell repertoire. A third group of genes collectively known as *class III*, cluster between the *class I* and *II* regions and include genes coding for complement proteins, 21a-hydroxylase, tumor necrosis factor, and heat shock proteins. This super-locus contains at least one gene (*HLA-DRB1*) that strongly influences susceptibility to MS. *HLA-DRB1* allelic copy number and *cis/trans* effects have been detected, and suggest a disease association gradient, ranging from high vulnerability (*DRB1* 15* homozygotes and *DRB1* 15/08* heterozygotes) to moderate susceptibility (*DRB1* 03* homozygotes and heterozygotes) and resistance (*DRB1* 15/* 14* heterozygotes; in this genotypic configuration, the presence of *DRB1* 14:01* neutralizes the susceptibility effect of *DRB1* 15:01*). Modified from Figure 1, Oksenberg JR et al. Nature Reviews Genetics 9:516–526, 2008.

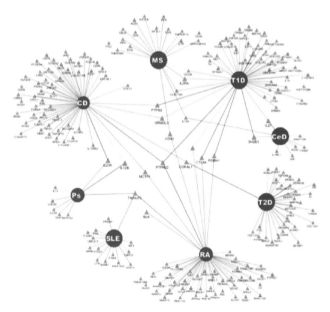

Fig. 4.4. Autoimmune disease-gene network. From the top genetic associations in 7 autoimmune diseases and Type 2 diabetes, the most significant SNP per gene was selected. Only associations with significance of at least $P < 10^{-7}$ are visualized. If a given gene was identified in more than one disease, multiple lines connecting it with each disease were drawn. Lines are colored using a "heat" scheme according to the evidence for association. Thus "hot" edges (e.g. red, orange) represent more significant associations than "cold" edges (e.g. purple, blue). Diseases are depicted by circles of size proportional to the number of associated genes, non-MHC genes by gray triangles, and genes in the MHC region are shown as red diamonds.

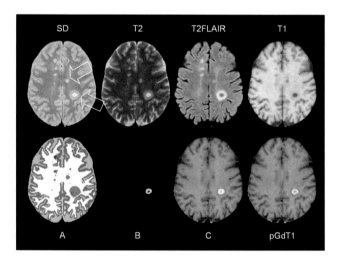

Fig. 9.7. Marked lesion heterogeneity is evident across these conventional 3 mm images obtained at 1.5 Tesla as part of a clinical trial. Illustrated are spin density (SD), T2-weighted without (T2) and with fluid attenuation by inversion recovery (T2FLAIR), and pre- (T1) and post-gadolinium T1-weighted (pGd T1) images, together with a segmented image (a) where gray matter is color coded as gray, white matter as white, T2-weighted lesion component as pink, and T1-hypointense non-enhanced tissue component as red; a threshold image (b) of the enhanced tissue volume, and (c) a localization of the enhanced tissue region on the pGd T1 image. The upper arrow points to a subcortical lesion that is not enhanced; the lower to a ring enhanced lesion. In this case, the total T2 lesion volume was 13.9 ml, the total T1-hypointense lesion volume 2.44 ml; while the enhanced lesion contributed 7.3 ml to the total lesion burden and 0.74 ml of the enhanced tissue. The amount of cerebrospinal fluid accounted for 324 with the non-CSF intracranial contents accounting for 1002 ml of total intracranial volume.

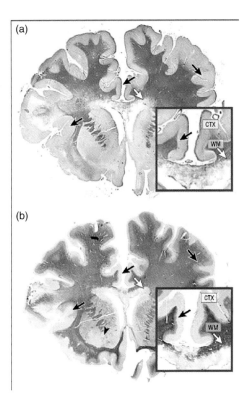

Fig. 13.1. Adjacent paraffin sections obtained from a MS patient with diffuse cortical subpial demyelination. The section is stained for myelin using Luxol fast-blue technique (a) and immunohistochemically for proteolipid protein (PLP) (b). Demyelination of the white matter such as the periventricular white matter and the corpus callosum is easily detectable (white arrows); cortical myelin is largely unstained. White matter lesions are also sharply delineated on the PLP stained specimen (green arrow). In the cortical gray matter, all areas show a superficial subpial myelin loss (black arrows). Please note also loss of myelin in deep gray matter structures such as the putamen (arrowhead). On higher magnification, a well delineated cortical lesion border (cingulate gyrus) is visible by PLP immunohistochemistry (b; inset, black arrow); the border not well detectable on the adjacent Luxol fast-blue stained section (a; inset, black arrow). Reproduced from Bö et al.,[2] with permission from the American Medical Association.

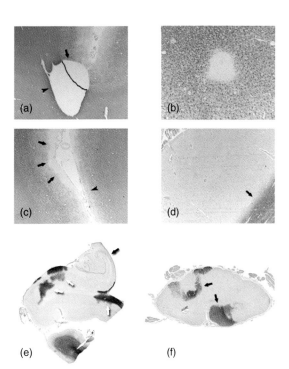

Fig. 13.2. Different types of cortical gray matter lesions on myelin immunohistochemistry, (proteolipid protein). Figures (a)–(d) show the different types of cortical according to the Bö classification. Type I lesion (a) represents mixed white matter–gray matter lesions. The black line represents the border between the cortex and the subcortical white matter. The gray matter part of the lesion is indicated by the arrow, the white matter part of the lesion is indicated by the arrow head. Type II (b) pure intracortical lesion surrounds a blood vessel. Type III (c) cortical lesion represents a subpial lesion (arrows), the adjacent cortex is not affected (arrowhead). Type IV (d) cortical lesion involves the entire width of the cortex. Arrow indicates the gray matter–white matter interface. Hippocampal lesions (e) can be frequently observed and involve most often the gray and white matter. The black arrow indicated the demyelinated areas and the white arrows indicate areas with preserved myelin. Spinal cord section (F) with a large demyelinated area and small areas with intact myelin (arrows). Reproduced from Geurts et al.,[10] and Geurts and Barkhof[1] with permission from Lippencott Williams and Wilkins and Elsevier.

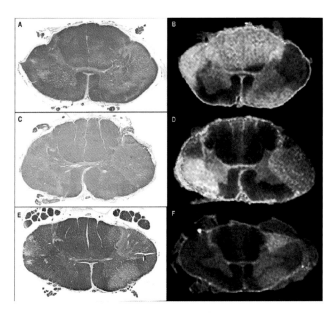

Fig. 13.8. Axial paraffin spinal cord sections of MS patients stained with immunohistochemically anti-myelin basic protein antibodies (a), (c), (e) and the corresponding proton-density-weighted MRI sections (b), (d), (f) at 4.7 T. Demyelinated lesions affect the white matter as well as the spinal cord gray matter. Reproduced from Gilmore et al., 2009[60] with permission from SAGE publications.

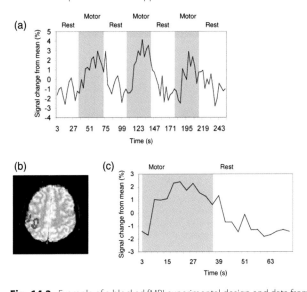

Fig. 14.2. Example of a blocked fMRI experimental design and data from a normal control subject. (a) BOLD signal changes in the most active voxel during a finger tapping motor paradigm. Gray background regions indicate motor task performance (36 s); white regions are rest (36 s). (b) The left hemisphere cortical region activated by performing the task in the right hand. (c) Average signal change in the same voxel as (a), over 3 cycles of the task. Data analysis was done using FEAT (FMRI Expert Analysis Tool) Version 5.1, part of FSL (FMRIB's Software Library, www.fmrib.ox.ac.uk/fsl).[19] Time series statistical analysis was carried out using FILM (FMRIB's Improved Linear Model).[20] Z statistic images were thresholded using voxel clusters determined by Z > 3.0 and a cluster significance threshold of P = 0.01.[21] Registration to standard images was carried out using FLIRT.[22]

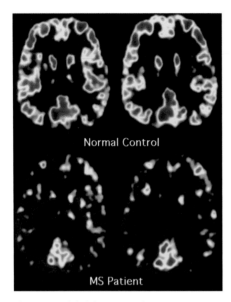

Fig. 14.3. Global decreases in brain activity in MS detected with FDG PET. Images from two slice locations in a normal control (top row) and a patient with MS (bottom row) displayed using the same scale. The MS patient scan demonstrates widespread reductions in cerebral glucose metabolism compared with the control scan. (From Bakshi et al.[37] used with permission).

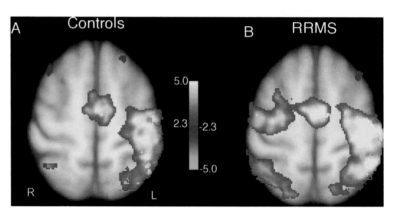

Fig. 14.4. Activated regions revealed by fMRI of healthy controls and MS patients performing a right-hand finger tapping motor task. Average fMRI activation (t-values) from one slice location in a group of 16 healthy controls (a) and a group of 24 early RRMS patients (EDSS < 3) (b), displayed using the same scale. A relative increase in cortical recruitment is evident in the MS group, demonstrated by extended activations in the left ipsilateral premotor, motor, and parietal cortices, as well as greater intensity activations in the right contralateral sensorimotor cortex and supplementary motor area.

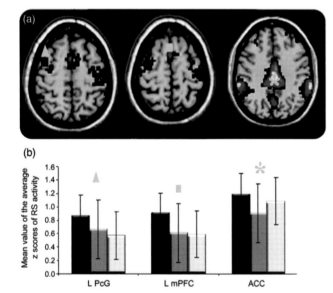

Fig. 14.6. Differences in default mode network (DMN) activity in progressive multiple sclerosis patients relative to healthy controls. Panel (a) shows three axial images demonstrating DMN activity measured by resting state fMRI activity in multiple sclerosis patients relative to healthy controls. Patterns of resting state activity differed significantly in the left precentral gyrus (triangle), medial prefrontal cortex (square), and anterior cingulate cortex (asterisk). Panel (b) shows averaged resting state activity in graphical form across the three groups studied. (Black bars = controls, dark gray bars = primary progressive MS, light gray = secondary progressive MS). (From Rocca et al., 2010,[78] used with permission.)

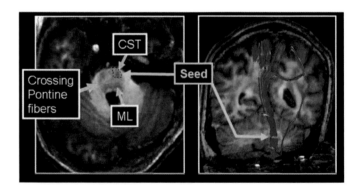

Fig. 15.1. Example of deterministic fiber tracking derived from DTI imaging data. The left panel shows an axial section of a colorized FA map through the level of the brainstem. The bilateral corticospinal tracks (CST) are visualized as purple regions in the anterior pons (the left CST is outlined by dashed lines, and forms an ROI for the "seeding" of fibertracks). Also seen are the crossing pontine fibers (orange) and the medial longitudinal fasciculus (purple). The right panel shows fiber tracks generated using the left CST ROI, using an anterior coronal 3D view. Several features are noteworthy: deterministic tracking of the CST always fails to find tracks extending to the lateral margins of the brain, secondary to strong effects of crossing fibers in the corona radiata; aberrant tracks are included that are not anatomic (for example crossing to contralateral side); while coarse features of tracks are anatomically reasonable, numerous details of the tracks are highly variable (not shown) and very sensitive to specified user input values.

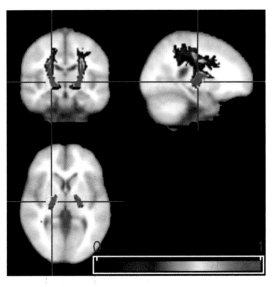

Fig. 15.5. A fiber probability map formed from deterministic fiber tracking on a group of normal humans. These tracts can then be co-registered in MS patients to allow identification of the track in the presence of disease (Reproduced with permission from Pagani, *et al.*, 2005).

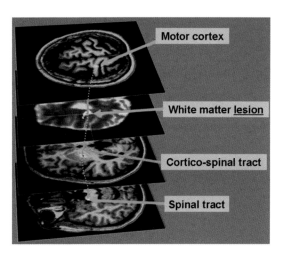

Fig. 15.6. Example of probabilistic fiber tracking through a lesion in an MS patient. A seed region was placed in the corticospinal tract, with a target region in the contralateral motor strip. The resulting tract density map correctly followed the expected anatomic course of the CST, and intersected a known white matter lesion in the corona radiata. Tract-based values using this path showed significant DTI differences compared to a symmetrical control path on the contralateral side, reflecting the long-range influence of the white matter lesion to diffusion properties along the entire associated tract.

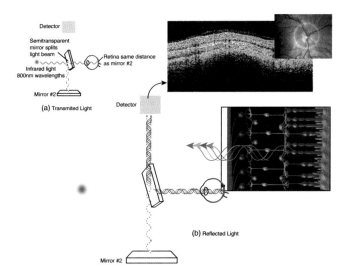

Fig. 17.1. Images of the internal retinal structure taken with optical coherence tomography (OCT), demonstrating the processes involved in using this technology. (a) Low-coherence infrared light is transmitted into the eye through use of an interoferometer. (b) The infrared light is transmitted through the pupil and then penetrates through the transparent nine layers of the retina. Subsequently, the light backscatters and returns through the pupil, where detectors can analyze the interference of light returning from the layers of the retina compared with light traveling a reference path (mirror #2). An algorithm mathematically uses this information to construct a gray-scale or false-color image representing the anatomy of the retina (shown in the upper right portion of the figure). (From Frohman EM *et al. Nat Clin Pract Neurol* 2008,[5] with permission.)

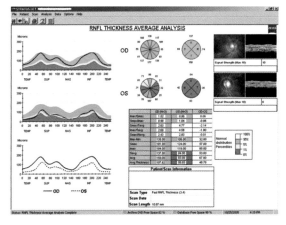

Fig. 17.2. A typical optical coherence tomography (OCT) report from a patient with MS, generated by Zeiss Stratus OCT3TM with software 4.0 (Carl Zeiss Meditec, Inc). On the upper left, retinal nerve fiber layer (RNFL) thickness is plotted (Y axis) with respect to a circumferential retinal map on the X axis (temporal-superior-nasal-inferior-temporal (TSNIT) quadrants of the RNFL). Note the normal 'double-hump' appearance of the topographic map of the right eye (OD), signifying the thicker RNFL measures derived from the superior and inferior retina compared with the nasal and temporal regions. Also note the quadrant and clockface sector measures of RNFL thickness (upper middle illustration). The table (lower middle) compiles the quantitative data, including the average RNFL thickness (bottom row). This patient experienced an episode of left optic neuritis 6 months before this study. Note the marked reduction in RNFL thickness across all quadrants (red region denoting values below 1% of what would be expected when compared with a reference population), multiple sectors, and with respect to the average RNFL thickness (bottom row of table). Abbreviations: OD, right eye; OS, left eye. (From Frohman EM *et al. Nat Clin Pract Neurol* 2008,[5] with permission.)

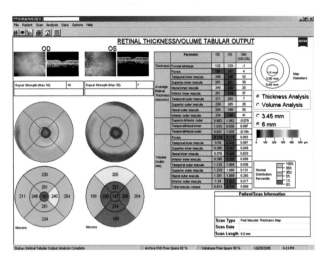

Fig. 17.3. An optical coherence tomography (OCT) report for the macular region of the retina from the same MS patient shown in Fig. 17.2. Note the volume reductions in the foveola (central macula) and the parafoveal quadrants on the left of the report. Whereas the reductions in retinal nerve fiber layer thickness implicate loss of ganglion cell axons, macular changes implicate losses of the ganglion cell neurons themselves. While the patient has had no history of optic neuritis in the right eye, there are some subtle macular changes on that side, suggesting occult involvement of this eye as well. Abbreviations: OD, right eye; OS, left eye. (From Frohman EM et al. Nat Clin Pract Neurol 2008,[5] with permission.)

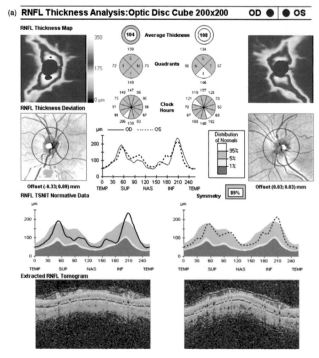

Fig. 17.4. (a) Example of a high-resolution, Fourier domain optical coherence tomography (OCT) report from a patient with neuromyelitis (NMO), generated by Zeiss Stratus Cirrus high-resolution Fourier domain OCT (Carl Zeiss Meditec, Inc.). The patient had bilateral mild disc hyperemia and edema in the setting of subacute visual loss.

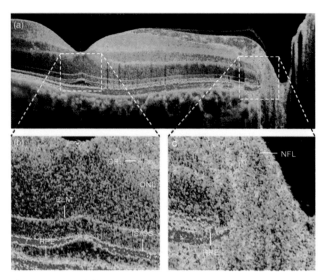

Fig. 17.5. High-definition, ultra-high-resolution optical coherence tomography (OCT) scans. The high data acquisition speeds available with spectral domain detection enable the acquisition of high-definition images with large numbers of transverse pixels. (a) A 10 000 axial scans per second image of the papillomacular axis acquired in 0.6 s. The axial image resolution is approximately 3 μm. The image may be zoomed in the (b) foveal or (c) optic disc regions to visualize details of internal retinal morphology. OCT has been termed "optical biopsy," and ultra-high-resolution OCT imaging can provide excellent visualization of retinal architecture. Abbreviations: ELM, external limiting membrane; IS/OS, junction between inner and outer photoreceptor segments; NFL, nerve fiber layer; ONL, outer nuclear layer; OPL, outer plexiform layer; RPE, retinal pigment epithelium. (Figure adapted from Drexler W and Fujimoto JG. Prog Retin Eye Res 2008;27:45–88,[42] published by Elsevier Ltd.)

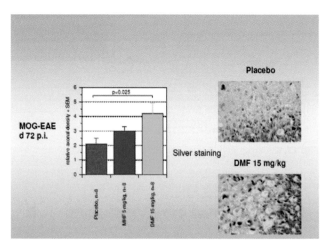

Fig. 31.2. Quantification of axonal density in EAE lesions of carrier-fed mice ('placebo'), or recipients of MHF or DMF. As illustrated in the Bielschowsky stain (right side) there are more black axonal profiles preserved under DMF treatment.

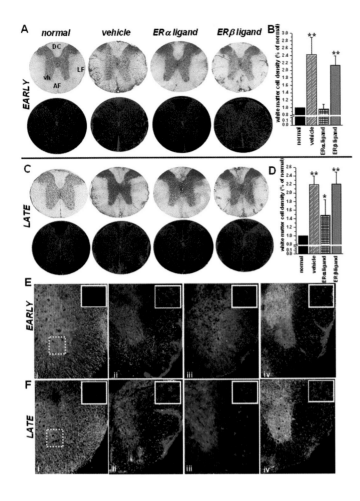

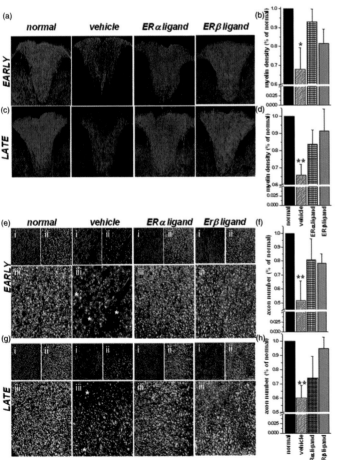

Fig. 43.2. Treatment with an ERα ligand, not an ERβ ligand, reduced inflammation in spinal cords of mice with EAE. (a) Representative H&E-stained and DAPI-stained thoracic spinal cord sections (4X magnification) from normal (healthy control), as well as vehicle-, ERα ligand PPT-treated, and ERβ ligand (DPN)-treated EAE mice all sacrificed at day 19 (early) post-disease induction. Compared to normal controls and PPT-treated spinal cords, vehicle-treated EAE spinal cord shows multifocal to coalescing areas of inflammation in the leptomeninges and white matter, around blood vessels, and in the parenchyma of the white matter. (b) The increase in total number of infiltrating cells after induction of EAE was quantified by counting DAPI[+] cells in the entire delineated white matter (including dorsal, lateral, and ventral funiculi) and presented as percent of normal. Vehicle-treated and DPN-treated EAE mice had a significant increase in white matter cell density compared to healthy normal control, while the ERα ligand PPT-treated groups did not. (c) At day 40 (late) after disease induction, representative H&E-stained and DAPI-stained vehicle, DPN-treated, and PPT-treated EAE thoracic spinal cord sections showed significantly increased inflammation compared to controls. (d) Total number of infiltrating cells after induction of EAE quantified by counting DAPI[+] cells as in (B). Number of mice = 3 per treatment group, number of T1–T5 sections per mouse = 6, total number of sections per treatment group = 18. Statistically significant compared with normals (*P<0.05; **P<0.001), 1 x 4 ANOVAs. Consecutive thoracic spinal cord sections were also co-immunostained with NF200 (green) and CD45 (red) at 10X magnification. Shown are partial images (lateral funiculus, a portion of anterior funiculus and gray matter) from normal control, vehicle-treated EAE, PPT-treated EAE, and DPN-treated EAE mice at day 19 (e) and day 40 (f) after disease induction. Vehicle-treated EAE cords had large areas of CD45+ cells associated with reduced NF200 axonal staining in white matter as compared to the normal control, while PPT-treated EAE mice had only occasional CD45 positivity, with intact NF200 axonal staining. ERβ ligand DPN-treated EAE mice had large areas of CD45+ cells with normal NF200 axonal staining. Consecutive sections from the same mice were also scanned at 40X magnification (within the section of the ventral horn designated by the dotted line square area in normal panel confocal microscopy) to show the morphology of CD45+ cells in the gray matter.[61] AF = anterior funniculus, ANOVA = analysis of variance, DAPI-4′,6-diamidino-2-phenylindole, DC = dorsal column, DPN = diarylpropionitrile, EAE = experimental autoimmune encephalomyelitis, ER = estrogen receptor, H&E = hematoxylin and eosin, LF = lateral funiculus, PPT = propyl pyrazole triol, vh = ventral horn.

Fig. 43.3. Treatment with an ERα ligand and an ERβ ligand each preserved MBP immunoreactivity and spared axonal pathology in white matter of spinal cords of mice with EAE. Dorsal columns of thoracic spinal cord sections were imaged at 10X magnification from mice in Fig. 43.2 that were immunostained with anti-MBP (red). At day 19 (a) and day 40 (c) after disease induction, vehicle-treated mice had reduced MBP immunoreactivity as compared to normal controls, while PPT-treated EAE and DPN-treated EAE mice showed relatively preserved MBP staining. Upon quantification (b, d), MBP immunoreactivity in dorsal column was significantly lower in vehicle-treated EAE mice as compared to normal mice, while PPT-treated and DPN-treated EAE mice demonstrated no significant decreases. Myelin density is presented as percent of normal. Statistically significant compared with normal (*P < 0.01; **P < 0.005), 1 x 4 ANOVAs. Part of the anterior funiculus of thoracic spinal cord sections was imaged at 40X magnification from mice in Fig. 43.2 that were co-immunostained with anti-NF200 (green, i) and anti-MBP (red, ii). Merged images of smaller (i) and (ii) panels are shown in (iii). Distinct green axonal centers surrounded by red myelin sheaths can be seen in normal controls, PPT-treated, and DPN-treated EAE mice from 19 day (e) and 40 day (g) after disease induction. Vehicle-treated mice show reduced axonal numbers and myelin, along with focal demyelination (white stars) and loss of axons. Upon quantification (f, h), neurofilament-stained axon numbers in white matter were significantly lower in vehicle-treated EAE mice as compared to normal mice, while PPT-treated and DPN-treated EAE mice demonstrated no significant reduction in axon numbers. Axon number is presented as percent of normal. Statistically significant compared with normal (*P < 0.01; **P < 0.005), 1 x 4 ANOVAs.[61] ANOVA = analysis of variance, DPN = diarylpropionitrile, EAE = experimental autoimmune encephalomyelitis, ER = estrogen receptor, MBP = myelin basic protein, PPT = propyl pyrazole triol.

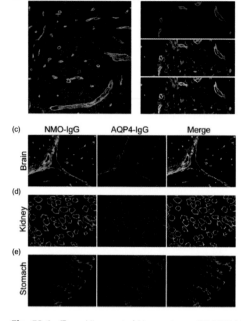

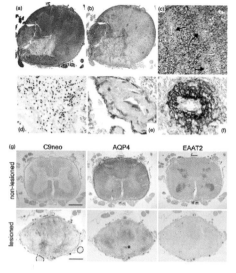

Fig. 53.1. (From Hinson *et al.* Neuroscience 2010;168:1009–18 with permission).

Pattern of NMO–IgG binding to mouse tissues. Dual immunofluorescence staining of mouse tissues. (a) Spinal cord: NMO–IgG (green) in a patient's serum binds to the abluminal face of microvessels; endothelium binds rabbit-IgG-specific for factor VIII (red) (× 400). (b) Cerebellar cortex: NMO–IgG (green) colocalizes with extracellular matrix protein laminin (red) around microvessels (i.e. at the blood–brain barrier), and also binds to astrocytic mesh in the granular layer (Lennon *et al.*, 2004[8]). Colocalization of NMO–IgG (green) and AQP4 (red) in brain (c), in distal renal collecting tubules (d) and gastric parietal cells (e) (Lennon *et al.*, 2005[6]).

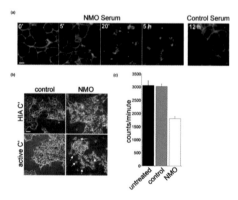

Fig. 53.3. (a) and (b) from Hinson *et al.*, Neurology 69:2221–2231, 2007[42] with permission; C provided by Hinson and Lennon, Mayo Clinic (same image submitted for article in Continuum: Lifelong Learning in Neurology series on Autoimmune Myelopathy). Functional effects of NMO-IgG binding to the extracellular domain of AQP4 in living cell membranes. (a) Time-Lapse imaging of GFP tagged AQP4 in transfected HEK293 cells during 12 hours of exposure to NMO serum reveals reorganization and internalization, but not in control serum where AQP4 remains linear on the membrane. (b) Complement activation by NMO-IgG binding to AQP4 expressing HEK293 cells. Cells expressing GFP-AQP4 are shown in green. Untransfected (AQP4 deficient) cells are shown in gray. In the presence of control or NMO serum and heat-inactivated complement (HIA C'), cells remain in a monolayer. Addition of active complement (active C') in the presence of NMO, but not control, serum induces cell death indicated by rounding up and floating morphology (arrows). Only cells that express the GFP-AQP4 (green) are killed by NMO-IgG and complement. (c) Glutamate uptake is reduced in primary astrocytes after treatment with NMO patient serum. Untreated (black bar) and control (gray bar) treated cells uptake radiolabelled glutamate at approximately 3000 counts/minute. Treating the cells with NMO serum reduces glutamate uptake by approximately 50% (white bar).

Fig. 53.2. (from Hinson *et al.* Neuroscience 2010;168:1009–18 with permission).[28] Histopathological characteristics of NMO lesions. (a) Spinal cord cross-sections demonstrate extensive demyelination involving both grey and white matter (Luxol fast blue and PAS myelin stain, mag 10 ×) and (b) infiltration of macrophages (KiM1p, pan-macrophage stain). (c) Thickened hyalinized blood vessels are prominent. (d) Eosinophils are prominent in the inflammatory infiltrate (haematoxylin-eosin, mag 100 ×). The terminal membrane attack complex of complement (C9neo antigen) is deposited around blood vessels in a "rim" (e) and "rosette" (f) pattern (Lucchinetti *et al.*, 2002[29]; Roemer *et al.*, 2007[59]). (g) Spinal cord sections from a single NMO–IgG-positive patient. Above: non-lesioned tissue, lumbar cord. Note lack of complement deposition (C9neo) and prominent AQP4 (brown stain) in both gray and white matter. EAAT2 (brown stain) is highly expressed in gray matter. Below: lesioned tissue, thoracic cord. Note prominence of C9neo deposition (brick red) in gray matter, corresponding to regions of AQP4 and EAAT2 loss in adjacent sections (Hinson *et al.*, 2008[48]). Asterisk indicates central canal. Scale bar = 200 μm.

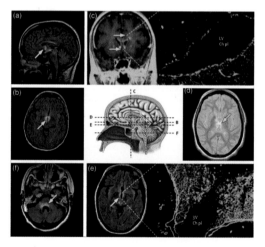

Fig. 53.5. NMO typical brain lesions (Wingerchuk *et al.*, 2007[7] with permission) NMO typical brain lesions localize at the sites of high aquaporin 4 expression (white dots on centre picture). In center picture dashed black lines show the anatomical level of MRI in the diagram; arrows show abnormality on fluid-attenuated inversion recovery (FLAIR), T2-weighted signal or after being given gadolinium Patient 1: FLAIR signal abnormality around the 3rd ventricle [image (a) (sagittal) and image (b) (axial)] with extension into the hypothalamus. Patient 2: Post-contrast T1-weighted image has subependymal enhancement along the frontal horns bilaterally and in the adjacent white matter [image C (coronal)]. The immunofluorescence photomicrograph linked to image (c) shows the binding pattern of the serum IgG from a patient with NMO in a mouse brain (400x). Intense immunoreactivity of basolateral ependymal cell membranes lining the lateral ventricle (LV) and extending into the subependymal astrocytic mesh coincides with aquaporin 4 immunoreactivity; the choroid plexus (Ch pl) is unstained. Patient 3 has contiguous signal abnormality throughout the periventricular tissues: diencephalon (image (d); axial T2-weighted), third ventricle (image (e); axial, FLAIR), and 4th ventricle (image (f); axial FLAIR). Immunofluorescence photomicrograph linked to image (e) shows the binding pattern of the serum IgG from a patient with neuromyelitis optica in a mouse brain (400x), with intense staining of periventricular tissues (third ventricle, 3V); choroid plexus (Ch pl) is unstained.

Chapter

33

Daclizumab to treat multiple sclerosis

Jaume Sastre-Garriga and Xavier Montalban

Background and mechanism of action

Daclizumab is a humanized monoclonal antibody, which binds to the interleukin-2 receptor (IL-2R). It was originally developed at the National Institutes of Health (NIH) in the early 1980s to be initially tested on adult T-cell leukemia and later in a number of inflammatory and autoimmune conditions, including prevention of renal allograft rejection and the treatment of non-infectious uveitis, tropical spastic paraparesis, psoriasis, pure red cell aplasia, and aplastic anemia.[1,2] It was approved by the US Food and Drug Administration (FDA) in December 1997 for "the prophylaxis of acute organ rejection in patients receiving renal transplants, to be used as a part of an immunosuppressive regimen including cyclosporine and corticosteroids." In July 2002 it was approved for its use in children. Beyond such indications, its "efficacy for the prophylaxis of acute rejection in recipients of other solid organ allografts has not been demonstrated" (FDA webpage for more info: www.fda.gov). Soon after, in 1999, under the name of Zenapax®, the European Commission granted daclizumab a marketing authorization "for the prophylaxis of acute organ rejection in de novo allogeneic renal transplantation and used concomitantly with an immunosuppressive regimen, including cyclosporine and corticosteroids in patients not highly immunized." In January 2009, the European Medicines Agency (EMA), following voluntary decision by the marketing authorization holder, Roche Registration Limited, withdrew this marketing authorization. This withdrawal was due to commercial reasons and not related to any safety concerns (EMA webpage for more info: www.ema.europa.eu). Daclizumab is an IgG1 humanized monoclonal antibody. A chimeric version, basiliximab (Simulect®), was approved in December 1998 for the same indication as daclizumab.

Daclizumab binds to the alpha chain subunit of the IL-2R (CD25, Tac) (Fig. 33.1).[3] IL-2 is a pro-inflammatory cytokine, which is crucial for the clonal expansion of autoreactive CD4+ T-cells; although recent evidence suggests a more complex bivalent role.[4] Accordingly, in vitro studies showed that daclizumab binding to CD25 decreases T-cell proliferation in culture, and this inhibition is overcome by the addition of exogenous IL-2.[5] By mechanisms that are not fully understood, daclizumab does not trigger relevant complement- or antibody-dependent cellular cytotoxicity, so targeted cells are not destroyed and absolute lymphocyte counts in vivo remain unaltered by daclizumab administration.[7,8] Daclizumab does not entirely modulate CD25, the number of CD25 molecules on the lymphocyte surface is altered only to a limited extent.[8] The other two subunits from which the full IL-2R is formed (beta and gamma) join to the alpha subunit to create the high-affinity IL-2R. Intermediate and low-affinity variants of the IL-2R arise from the union of beta and gamma (intermediate) and alpha alone (low) subunits.[9] Thus, daclizumab binding to the alpha subunit (CD25) specifically blocks the high-affinity IL-2R, leaving the intermediate-affinity IL-2R (which does not contain the alpha subunit) still available for IL-2 signal transduction.[3] Interestingly, a recent genome-wide study identified the IL-2R alpha chain gene as one of three heritable risk factors for multiple sclerosis (MS), together with IL-7 receptor alpha chain gene and the HLA locus.[10] Very importantly, It has been shown that low level IL-2 signaling through the intermediate affinity IL-2R is sufficient for many key aspects of regulatory T-cells.[11] Daclizumab therapy has been associated with significant expansion of CD56[bright] natural killer (NK) cells,[7,8,12] the magnitude of which correlates with clinical response to the drug.[8,12] Such increases in NK regulatory cells go beyond those observed during interferon beta (IFNβ) monotherapy.[7,12] This observation suggests that the benefit of daclizumab in MS is mediated not only via a direct inhibition of CD4+ T-cell responses, but also by up-regulation of a subset of regulatory NK cells. Conversely, the regulatory subset of T-cells (CD4+CD25+FoxP3+) has been shown to be significantly decreased on daclizumab therapy both in cancer patients (where it is used to induce cancer immunity)[13] and in patients with MS.[14] Such decrease in tolerance levels outside the central nervous system may be the explanation for daclizumab-associated autoimmunity, particularly cutaneous.[4,14]

Evidence on efficacy from clinical trials

Efficacy data from clinical trials are summarized in Table 33.1. Initial evidence of efficacy comes from three small open-label studies not listed on www.clinicaltrials.gov.[15–17] The initial,

Multiple Sclerosis Therapeutics, Fourth Edition, ed. Jeffrey A. Cohen and Richard A. Rudick. Published by Cambridge University Press.
© Cambridge University Press 2011.

Table 33.1. *Summary of design features for all daclizumab clinical trials published to date or presently on a recruiting stage*

Trial	Status	Design	n	MS forms	Regimen	Dose	Duration
Bielekova et al.[15]	Published	Open-label	11	RRMS/SPMS	Add-on – i.v. – monthly[a]	1 mg/kg	5.5 mo
Rose et al.[16]	Published	Open-label	21	RRMS/SPMS	Add-on/Monotherapy – i.v. – monthly[a]	0.8 to 1.9 mg/kg	25 mo
Rose et al.[17]	Published	Open-label	11	RRMS	Add-on/Monotherapy – i.v. – monthly[a]	1 to 1.5 mg/kg	27.5 mo
Bielekova et al.[12]	Published	Open-label	15	RRMS/SPMS	Add-on/Monotherapy – i.v. – monthly[a]	1 to 2 mg/kg	5.5 mo
CHOICE[7]	Published	RCT	230	RRMS/SPMS	Add-on – s.c. – eow or monthly	1 to 2 mg/kg	44 w
ZAPMS	Ongoing	Open-label	16	RRMS	Monotherapy – i.v. -monthly	1 mg/kg	30 w
NCT01143441	Ongoing	Open-label	31	RRMS/SPMS	Monotherapy – s.c. – monthly	150 mg	3 y
DECIDE	Ongoing	RCT	1500	RRMS	Monotherapy[b] – s.c. – monthly	150 mg	144 w
SELECT	Ongoing	RCT	600	RRMS/SPMS	Monotherapy – s.c. – monthly	150/300 mg	52 w

Eow = every other week, i.v. = intravenous, mo = months, MS = multiple sclerosis, N = number of subjects, RCT = randomized controlled trial, RR = relapsing–remitting, s.c. = subcutaneous, SP = secondary progressive, w = weeks, y = years.
[a] first two doses are only 15 days apart.
[b] with comparator arm.

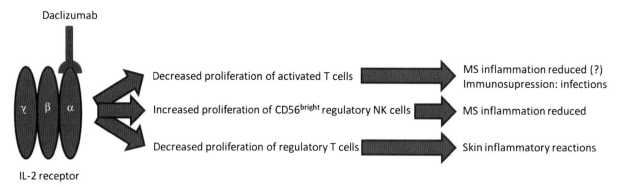

Fig. 33.1. Schematic representation of daclizumab clinical effects (modified from Bielekova and Becker).[4]

NIH-sponsored study[15] enrolled 11 patients (10 patients in the final analysis) with relapsing–remitting (RR) or secondary progressive (SP) MS and a suboptimal response to standard first line therapies, defined as sustained 1.0-point Expanded Disability Status Scale (EDSS) progression or ≥1 clinical relapse in the previous 18 months. Patients also were required to have a certain level of inflammatory activity (mean of new gadolinium (Gd)-enhancing lesions per month greater than 0.67 on monthly MRI scans performed during a four-month run-in period). All patients were kept on their standard doses of first-line therapies and intravenous daclizumab was added at a dose of 1 mg/kg on days 0 and 14 and thereafter every four weeks to complete a total of seven infusions. The primary outcome measure was the number of new and total Gd-enhancing lesions at follow-up compared with baseline. A number of clinical and MRI secondary outcomes also were assessed. There were significant decreases in the number of new Gd-enhancing lesions (1.38 vs. 0.75, 78% relative reduction, $P = 0.004$) and total number of Gd-enhancing lesions (1.50 vs. 1.00, 70% relative reduction, $P = 0.002$). This decrease was not immediate, but could be observed from the second month onwards. Statistically significant decreases during combination therapy were also observed

for the volume of Gd-enhancing lesions, relapse rate, Scripps scale, and nine-hole peg test.

In the first of two studies reported by Rose and coworkers,[16] 21 patients with RR or SPMS (17 of whom were deemed non-responders to first-line therapy) were initiated on daclizumab with the same dose of the previous study.[15] Follow-up data up to 25 months were reported for 19 patients. Sixteen patients were immediately converted to monotherapy with daclizumab; two were kept on IFNβ for six months and then were treated only with daclizumab, and one received monthly infusions of methylprednisolone. Daclizumab dosage was adjusted from 0.8 mg/kg to 1.9 mg/kg according to clinical response. There were no pre-established primary or secondary outcome measures, but patients were followed clinically and by MRI. All 19 patients were free of EDSS progression for the duration of the study; ten showed an improvement in their EDSS scores. Significant improvement in the mean EDSS was observed (post–pre = −1.5; $P = 0.0004$). Those patients with shorter disease duration were more likely to show an improvement in their EDSS score (7.7 vs. 19.0 years; $P < 0.008$). A positive effect on relapses was also observed (annualized relapse rate of 1.23 pre-daclizumab vs. 0.32 during daclizumab). Positive MRI outcomes were also reported for Gd-enhancing lesions and active scans.

A second study by Rose and coworkers[17] investigated again the clinical and MRI effects of daclizumab administered at the same dose and regimen as the previous two studies. Patients with RRMS were included if they had failed to respond to IFNβ therapy (minimum of six months of treatment) defined as the presence of ≥2 Gd-enhancing lesions on one of four baseline MRI scans, and ≥1 relapses in the previous year while on IFNβ therapy. Response initially was reassessed after 5.5 months of daclizumab therapy. In patients with cessation of Gd-enhancement on MRI scans, IFNβ was suspended and daclizumab administered as a monotherapy for a further period of 10 months. If Gd-enhancement reappeared, IFNβ was restarted, and the dose of daclizumab increased to 1.5 mg/kg. Maximum duration of therapy allowed was 27.5 months. The primary outcome measures were the number of new and total Gd-enhancing lesions (>3 mm) at follow-up compared with baseline. A number of clinical and MRI secondary outcomes also were evaluated. A total of 11 patients were recruited and nine completed the study (27.5 months). Three patients developed new Gd-enhancing lesions during daclizumab monotherapy and were restarted on IFNβ and had their daclizumab doses increased. A significant reduction in total and new Gd-enhancing lesions was observed ($P < 0.001$). Significant improvements in relapse number, EDSS score, and other clinical measures were observed. The main value of this study was to show efficacy over a two-year period treatment.

As of November 2010, there are eight clinical trials listed on www.clinicaltrials.gov testing daclizumab in patients with MS. Three studies have been completed (NCT00001934, NCT00109161, and NCT00071838). Results from trial NCT00001934 were recently published.[12] Of note, four out of 15 patients enrolled in this study had been reported already as part of previous trials by the same group of authors.[15] This was a Phase 2 open-label (baseline vs. treatment) add-on trial of intravenous daclizumab in patients with MS and suboptimal response to IFNβ. Main inclusion criteria were: (a) one relapse or a sustained 1.0-point increase of EDSS in the previous 12 months despite IFNβ treatment); (b) mean of at least 0.67 Gd-enhancing lesions in the three MRI scans performed monthly in the three months prior to baseline visit. Combination therapy was initially maintained for 5.5 months (total of seven daclizumab infusions – two initial fortnightly infusions followed by five monthly infusions). The number of Gd-enhancing lesions was analyzed after seven infusions to determine whether IFNβ could be withdrawn (more than 75% reduction in Gd-enhancing lesion count was required). In patients with a reduction in Gd-enhancing lesion count of 75% or less, IFNβ therapy was maintained and daclizumab dosage was doubled to 2 mg/kg per monthly infusion. In addition to Gd-enhancing lesion count, a number of clinical and immunological parameters were assessed. After seven daclizumab infusions, only one patient failed to show a 75% reduction in Gd-enhancing lesion counts; the other 14 patients

were changed to daclizumab monotherapy. In three of those patients, therapy with IFNβ had to be reinstated because of increasing numbers of Gd-enhancing lesions on daclizumab monotherapy. Statistically significant improvements were observed for the EDSS, Multiple Sclerosis Functional Composite MSFC, and Scripps outcome measures. T1 lesion volumes and brain volume significantly worsened during the combination therapy period then stabilized on daclizumab monotherapy, likely reflecting a pseudoatrophy effect.[18] No benefit on T2 lesion load was observed.

The CHOICE study (NCT00109161) was an international, double-blind, randomized, placebo-controlled, multicenter trial involving 230 patients with relapsing MS (92% RR and 8% SP).[7] Patients were randomized to receive add-on subcutaneous daclizumab 2 mg/kg every two weeks, daclizumab 1 mg/kg every 4 weeks, or placebo for 24 weeks. All patients received verum IFNβ (any kind) during the trial and had done so for an immediately previous period of a minimum of six months before randomization. Patients had to be active while on IFNβ therapy; active breakthrough disease was defined as: at least one relapse or at least one Gd-enhancing lesion while on a stable IFNβ regimen in the year before enrollment. The primary end-point was total number of new or enlarged Gd-enhancing lesions on brain MRI scans performed every four weeks between weeks 8 and 24. A number of clinical, MRI, and immunological secondary outcomes were also evaluated. After daclizumab/placebo discontinuation, there was a further 24-month clinical and MRI follow-up period. At baseline, the percentage of patients with Gd-enhancing lesions was slightly different between trial arms (36% in placebo vs. 46% in low-dose daclizumab vs. 30% in high dose daclizumab); this also resulted in patients in the low-dose group having a higher mean number of Gd-enhancing lesions at baseline (2.7) than those in the placebo (1.1) or high-dose groups (0.8). A total of 93% of patients completed the initial 24 weeks of the trial. Analysis of reasons for discontinuation did not yield any remarkable results. The result of the primary outcome showed positive results for the high-dose arm and did not find significant differences between the placebo and the low-dose arm: 4.75 for placebo, 1.32 for high-dose (difference 72%; $P = 0.004$) and 3.58 for low-dose (difference 25%; $P = 0.51$) (Fig. 33.2). The results at week 24 for T2 lesions were comparable: mean number of new or enlarged T2 lesions was 3.4 in the placebo group compared with 1.1 high-dose group ($P = 0.007$) and 2.2 in the low-dose group ($P = 0.60$). No statistically significant results were observed for T1 hypointensities on MRI scans or for any clinical parameter (relapses, EDSS, MSFC). After treatment discontinuation, the mean number of new Gd-enhancing lesions on MRI scans done at weeks 34 and 44 returned to pre-trial levels: 2.3 in placebo, 1.8 in high-dose ($P = 0.49$) and 3.5 in low-dose group ($P = 0.21$) (results were adjusted for the number of Gd-enhancing lesions at baseline, which were different between trial arms). Eight percent of patients treated with daclizumab developed neutralizing antibodies to daclizumab. In patients developing antibodies during the daclizumab therapy period,

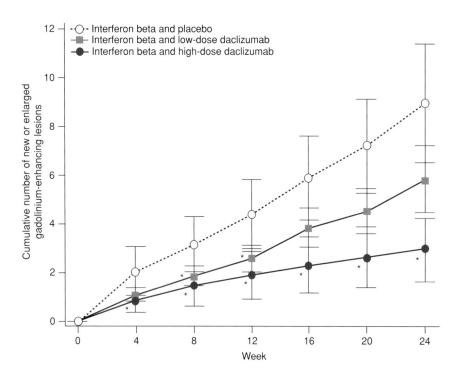

Fig. 33.2. Graphical representation of CHOICE trial main outcome measure. Lines represent cumulative number of new or enlarged gadolinium-enhancing lesions by visit. Bars = standard error. *$P < 0.05$ vs. interferon beta and placebo.

their presence was associated with a reduction in daclizumab concentrations.

In trial NCT00071838 – ZAPMS (sponsored by the National Institute of Neurological Disorders and Stroke), the authors investigated the efficacy of intravenous daclizumab monotherapy in patients with RRMS. This Phase 2 trial, led by B. Bielekova, was designed as a single-center, open-label, baseline to treatment cross-over study. Daclizumab was administered intravenously at a dose of 1 mg/kg. The primary outcome measure was reduction in the mean number of new Gd-enhancing lesions in the treatment phase (Weeks 18 to 30) vs. baseline (Weeks −12 to 0). To be allowed into the study, candidate patients needed to be non-eligible to receive standard therapies or have failed or opted not to start or continue on these therapies and must have at least two new Gd-enhancing lesions at baseline period. Data are still under analysis and the results are not yet available.

Safety

The safety experience with daclizumab is summarized in Table 33.2. The three small initial open-label studies performed by Bielekova and coworkers[15] and Rose and coworkers[16,17] share a number of similarities in terms of dosage and duration of daclizumab therapy. Bielekova *et al.* observed an increase in the number of mild urinary and upper respiratory tract infections and two transient elevations of liver function tests and bilirubin during daclizumab therapy.[15] In their trial published in 2004, Rose and coworkers[16] also observed one instance of upper respiratory tract infection and one instance of increase of liver enzymes. More notably, they reported four cases (out of 21 patients) of skin rash which responded to therapy with topic steroids. The second study by Rose and coworkers[17]

Table 33.2. *Summary of main adverse events reported on daclizumab clinical.studies*

Study	Adverse events
Bielekova et al.[15]	Increased number of mild urinary and upper respiratory tract infections Two instances of transient elevation of liver function tests
Rose et al.[16]	One instance of increased liver enzymes Four cases of skin rash responding to topic steroids
Rose et al.[17]	One case of transient thrombocytopenia Two cases of skin rashes A case of post-therapy febrile reaction One patient presented two respiratory tract infections and lymphadenopathy
Bielekova et al.[12]	Two cases of systemic immune responses One case of lymphopenia One case of lymphadenopathy One transient increase in bilirubin levels
Oh et al.[14]	Three patients presenting with dermatitis (one photodermatitis and two sebopsoriasis) One patient with palindromic rheumatism
CHOICE[7]	Cutaneous events: 24% in daclizumab arms vs. 6% in placebo arm Serious adverse events: 13% in daclizumab arms vs. 5% in placebo Most frequent adverse events: infections 5% in daclizumab arms vs. 1% in placebo No opportunistic infections or deaths Two malignancies (probably non-related)

incorporated a longer therapy period of up to 27.5 months for a total number of 253 daclizumab intravenous infusions in all patients. The authors reported a case of transient thrombocytopenia, two patients with skin rashes, and a case of post-therapy febrile reaction. One patient had two upper respiratory tract infections with fever and a lung infiltrate (diagnosed as pneumonia and treated with antibiotics) and concomitantly developed lymphadenopathy, which showed nonspecific changes on biopsy and resolved after protocol termination.

Bielekova *et al.*, in their trial published in 2009,[12] reported two patients developing systemic immune responses. These patients presented with mouth ulcers, photosensitive rash, transient formation of autoantibodies, and atypical serum sickness in one case, and with mouth ulcers, photosensitive rash, and delayed viral myositis in a second case. There was also one instance of lymphopenia, one instance of lymphadenopathy, and one case of transient increase in bilirubin levels.

Safety data coming from the CHOICE trial indicated an overall good safety and tolerability of daclizumab.[7] Two cases of malignancy were observed: one patient treated with daclizumab and with a family history of breast cancer who developed a ductal carcinoma in situ of the breast, and a further patient had a relapse of pre-existing *Pseudomyxoma peritonei*. Although general infections and infestations were more frequent in the daclizumab-treated arms, no opportunistic infections were observed. The incidence of rashes and other cutaneous adverse events was higher in the treated arms. Daclizumab subcutaneous injections displayed similar levels of tolerability as compared with IFNβ.

Oh and coworkers[14] reported three patients out of 15 presenting with dermatitis (one case of photodermatitis and two cases of sebopsoriasis) and one patient developing palindromic rheumatism during daclizumab therapy. Skin inflammatory reactions were thought to be related to a daclizumab-induced decrease in CD4+CD25+ regulatory T-cells.

Bearing in mind that, in this context, daclizumab is used over a very short period of time, safety data coming from daclizumab's regulatory-approved indication in renal transplantation suggest that the drug is overall safe and well tolerated.[19] However, safety data from other off-label indications, such as uveitis, seem to confirm safety concerns regarding a mild increase in infection rate as well as skin reactions.[20,21]

Clinical development plan

Four studies testing daclizumab in MS patients, out of eight listed on www.clinicaltrials.gov, have their recruitments ongoing as of November 2010 (NCT01143441, NCT01064401, NCT00390221, and NCT00870740), and one additional study is awaiting recruitment onset (NCT01051349).

One of the studies presently in the recruitment stage (NCT01143441) is a NIH-sponsored Phase 1 single arm trial to investigate the long-term safety and the mechanism of action of daclizumab high yield process (DAC-HYP) in highly inflammatory MS. The planned enrollment is 31 patients with completion in December 2015.

The DECIDE study (NCT01064401) is an industry-sponsored Phase 3 multicenter, double-blind, randomized, parallel-group, monotherapy, active-comparator trial, which aims to determine whether DAC HYP 150 mg administered subcutaneously every 4 weeks for 96 to 144 weeks is superior to intramuscular IFN β-1a (Avonex®) in patients with relapsing MS. It is in the recruitment phase with planned enrollment of 1500 patients.

Recruiting studies NCT00390221 (205-MS-201) and NCT00870740 (205-MS-202 – SELECT) are the core (52 weeks' duration) and initial extension (52 weeks' duration) stages, respectively, of a Phase 2, double-blind, randomized, placebo-controlled, dose-ranging trial to determine the effect of two doses of DAC-HYP (150 mg vs. 300 mg) administered subcutaneously every 4 weeks on relapse reduction in subjects with RRMS. The enrollment target is 600 patients. A further open-label extension (NCT01051349 – SELECTION study) of both studies is pre-planned, but not yet recruiting.

Conclusions

Daclizumab is a novel and promising therapy for MS patients now being tested as monotherapy (subcutaneous monthly administrations) in a large Phase 3 trial using an active comparator arm. Previous clinical evidence comes mostly from a number of small open-label studies (using intravenous monthly administrations of daclizumab) and from a rigorous double-blind, randomized placebo-controlled trial which investigated the efficacy of daclizumab (administered subcutaneously every 15 days) as an add-on therapy to IFNβ. Based on these studies, daclizumab appears to be effective in patients not responding to IFNβ.

Daclizumab's mechanism of action is not fully understood, but an increase in regulatory immune cells (CD56^bright NK cells) has been related to clinical response and is now thought to play a more important role than direct anti-inflammatory effects derived from IL-2 blockade.

Safety concerns include skin autoimmunity, which may be related to a decrease in the CD4+CD25+FoxP3+ regulatory T-cell subset, and a higher risk of infections. Results from ongoing trials are eagerly awaited to obtain conclusive data on the efficacy and safety of daclizumab.[22]

References

1. Schippling DS, Martin R. Spotlight on anti-CD25: daclizumab in MS. *Int MS J* 2008;15:94–98.

2. Waldmann TA. Anti-Tac (daclizumab, Zenapax) in the treatment of leukemia, autoimmune diseases, and in the prevention of allograft rejection: a 25-year personal odyssey. *J Clin Immunol* 2007;27:1–18.

3. Yang H, Wang J, Du J, *et al.* Structural basis of immunosuppression by the therapeutic antibody daclizumab. *Cell Res* 2010;20:1361–71.

4. Bielekova B, Becker BL. Monoclonal antibodies in MS: mechanisms of action. *Neurology* 2010 Jan 5;74(Suppl 1):S31–40.

5. Nelson BH. Interleukin-2 signaling and the maintenance of self-tolerance. *Curr Dir Autoimmun* 2002;5:92–112.

6. Kircher B, Latzer K, Gastl G, Nachbaur D. Comparative in vitro study of the immunomodulatory activity of humanized and chimeric anti-CD25 monoclonal antibodies. *Clin Exp Immunol* 2003;134: 426–30.

7. Wynn D, Kaufman M, Montalban X, *et al.* Daclizumab in active relapsing multiple sclerosis (CHOICE study): a phase 2, randomised, double-blind, placebo-controlled, add-on trial with interferon beta. *Lancet Neurol* 2010; 9:381–90.

8. Bielekova B, Catalfamo M, Reichert-Scrivner S, *et al.* Regulatory CD56(bright) natural killer cells mediate immunomodulatory effects of IL-2Ralpha-targeted therapy (daclizumab) in multiple sclerosis. *Proc Natl Acad Sci USA* 2006;103:5941–6.

9. Gaffen SL. Signaling domains of the interleukin 2 receptor. *Cytokine* 2001;14:63–77.

10. Hafler DA, Compston A, Sawcer S, *et al.* Risk alleles for multiple sclerosis identified by a genomewide study. *N Engl J Med* 2007;357:851–62.

11. Malek TR, Castro I. Interleukin-2 receptor signaling: at the interface between tolerance and immunity. *Immunity* 2010;33:153–65.

12. Bielekova B, Howard T, Packer AN, *et al.* Effect of anti-CD25 antibody daclizumab in the inhibition of inflammation and stabilization of disease progression in multiple sclerosis. *Arch Neurol* 2009;66: 483–9.

13. Rech AJ, Vonderheide RH. Clinical use of anti-CD25 antibody daclizumab to enhance immune responses to tumor antigen vaccination by targeting regulatory T-cells. *Ann NY Acad Sci* 2009;1174:99–106.

14. Oh U, Blevins G, Griffith C, *et al.* Regulatory T-cells are reduced during anti-CD25 antibody treatment of multiple sclerosis. *Arch Neurol* 2009; 66:471–9.

15. Bielekova B, Richert N, Howard T, *et al.* Humanized anti-CD25 (daclizumab) inhibits disease activity in multiple sclerosis patients failing to respond to interferon beta. *Proc Natl Acad Sci USA* 2004;101:8705–8.

16. Rose JW, Watt HE, White AT, Carlson NG. Treatment of multiple sclerosis with an anti-interleukin-2 receptor monoclonal antibody. *Ann Neurol* 2004;56:864–7.

17. Rose JW, Burns JB, Bjorklund J, Klein J, Watt HE, Carlson NG. Daclizumab phase II trial in relapsing and remitting multiple sclerosis: MRI and clinical results. *Neurology* 2007; 69:785–9.

18. Zivadinov R, Reder AT, Filippi M, *et al.* Mechanisms of action of disease-modifying agents and brain volume changes in multiple sclerosis. *Neurology* 2008;71:136–44.

19. Sageshima J, Ciancio G, Chen L, Burke GW, III. Anti-interleukin-2 receptor antibodies-basiliximab and daclizumab-for the prevention of acute rejection in renal transplantation. *Biologics* 2009;3:319–36.

20. Sen HN, Levy-Clarke G, Faia LJ, *et al.* High-dose daclizumab for the treatment of juvenile idiopathic arthritis-associated active anterior uveitis. *Am J Ophthalmol* 2009;148: 696–703.

21. Yeh S, Wroblewski K, Buggage R, *et al.* High-dose humanized anti-IL-2 receptor alpha antibody (daclizumab) for the treatment of active, non-infectious uveitis. *J Autoimmun* 2008;31:91–7.

22. Liu J, Wang L, Zhan S, Tan J, Xia Y. Daclizumab for relapsing remitting multiple sclerosis. *Cochrane Database Syst Rev* 2010;CD008127.

Chapter

34

Laquinimod to treat multiple sclerosis

Douglas R. Jeffery

Introduction

Laquinimod is a novel oral immunomodulatory agent in development for the treatment of relapsing forms of multiple sclerosis (MS). It is a derivative of roquinimex (linomide), which showed potent anti-inflammatory effects in acute and chronic experimental autoimmune encephalomyelitis (EAE) and in Phase 2 trials in MS. Unfortunately, in a Phase 3 trial, roquinimex caused a number of inflammatory toxicities including arthritis, pericarditis, pleuritis, pancreatitis, and coronary vasculitis resulting in several fatal myocardial infarctions.[1] As a result, its development was stopped.

Studies on structure–activity relationships with roqiuinmix led to the development of laquinimod. Laquinimod is a quinoline 3-carboxamide derivative that was selected from over 60 different quinoline carboxamide derivatives. On the basis of structure–activity relationships maximized to increase safety and efficacy in EAE, laquinimod was superior.[2] Numerous different compounds from this class were systematically evaluated to obtain a compound with maximal efficacy in EAE and an absence of proinflammatory effects in Beagle dogs. The type and position of the quinoline ring was the major determinant of efficacy, whereas the N-carboxyamide substitution appeared to be the major factor determining safety. Laquinimod had the best overall safety and efficacy profile of all the compounds tested.

Mechanism of action

Initial studies with laquinimod demonstrated that it ameliorated neurologic deficits in both acute and chronic relapsing EAE.[3–6] In acute EAE in SJL/N mice disease severity was decreased in a dose-dependent fashion and it was 20 times more potent than roquinimex.[4] In the Lewis rat model of EAE, laquinimod brought about a dose-dependent decrease in EAE severity and was more potent than interferon-beta (IFNβ), suggesting that it affected a biologically relevant target in inflammatory disease of the central nervous system (CNS). Its administration resulted in a decrease in the infiltration of CD4+ T-cells and macrophages into brain and spinal cord and this effect was more robust than that seen with the parent compound, roquinimex.[5] There was down-regulation of

pro-inflammatory cytokines, tumor necrosis factor alpha (TNFα) and interleukin (IL)-12, and up-regulation of anti-inflammatory cytokines, transforming growth factor-beta (TGFβ), IL-4, and IL-10, consistent with the hypothesis that it may act as a broad spectrum immunomodulating agent with an ability to shift the cytokine milieu from a pro-inflammatory to anti-inflammatory profile.

In chronic relapsing EAE generated by immunization with the encephalitogenic peptide fragment of myelin basic protein (MBP 89–101), laquinimod decreased disease severity and the number of relapses in a dose-dependent manner.[5] The administration of laquinimod following the onset of EAE significantly decreased the severity compared with vehicle-treated animals. There was also a marked reduction in the infiltration of T-cells and macrophages into the tissue.[4,6] There was a marked decrease in the severity of tissue damage in the form of demyelination and axonal injury in laquinimod-treated animals. The beneficial effects of laquinimod in different varieties of EAE suggest that laquinimod could be an effective therapy to reduce inflammatory disease activity MS.

Laquinimod has a complex mechanism of action that is incompletely understood. It has effects on variety of immne function, including antigen presentation,[7] dendritic cells,[8] monocytes,[9] B-cells,[10] T-cells,[11] microglial activation,[12] and elaboration of brain-derived neurotrophic factor (BDNF).[13] Of considerable importance, laquinimod does not appear to be a non-specific immunosuppressive agent. In acute EAE, B-cell and T-cell numbers or proliferative capacity were not decreased, and in IFNβ knock-out mice there was no reduction in laquinimod's effect suggesting its effects were independent of IFNβ.[6] It had no broad effect on cytokine production and there was no effect on heart allograft rejection in rats or on KLH-induced antibody response, suggesting that laquinimod modulates rather than suppresses the immune response.[14]

Laquinimod administration in the Lewis rat model of EAE brought about a shift from a proinflammatory Th1 cytokine profile to a Th2/Th3 "antinflammatory" profile.[5] The frequency of MBP-reactive Th1 cells secreting TNFα and IL-12 were reduced in laquinimod treated animals. Laquinimod also brought about an up-regulation of MBP-specific IL-4, IL-10,

Multiple Sclerosis Therapeutics, Fourth Edition, ed. Jeffrey A. Cohen and Richard A. Rudick. Published by Cambridge University Press.
© Cambridge University Press 2011.

and TGFβ expressing cells.[5] In the myelin oligodendrocyte glycoprotein (MOG) model of EAE, laquinimod reduced inflammatory infiltrates as well as axonal loss in treated animals.[6] In C57BL/6 mice with MOG-induced EAE, laquinimod significantly reduced the extent of demyelination and axonal damage by preventive and therapeutic treatment, and there was a marked reduction in macrophage and T-cell infiltration in lesions.[15]

In addition to its ability to decrease the infiltration of inflammatory cells, laquinimod also decreased the expression of major histocompatibility complex (MHC) class II antigens required for antigen presentation.[12] Laquinimod brought about a decrease in chemokine signaling molecules CCL11, CCL12, CCR1, and CCR2, integrin and other related adhesion molecules. This may also contribute to the down-regulation of CNS inflammation. Laquinimod was effective in decreasing the severity of experimental allergic neuritis (EAN).[3] Its administration decreased the production of TNFα and IFNγ and increased IL-4[5] and brought about a reduction in the disease specific T-cell response. Since laquinimod has effects in both EAE and EAN, it may affect a pivotal pathway involved in autoimmunity.

In murine EAE, laquinimod brought about a profound down-regulation of the dendritic cell compartment in suggesting that some of its effects could be operating through this mechanism.[7] There was a shift in the balance towards a CD8+ dendritic cells and a reduction in plasmacytoid dendritic cells. These effects are also consistent with a down-regulation of inflammatory disease activity. Laquinimod decreased the activity of CD 19+ B-cells and natural killer (NK) cells consistent with a down-regulation of inflammation.[10] In cells cultured from patients with relapsing–remitting (RR) MS, laquinimod activated IL-4 signaling in CD4+ T-cells. This led to the suppression of MHC class II molecules. In CD8+ cells and B-cells, laquinimod activated death receptor signaling and mitochondrial dysfunction promoting apoptosis. Metabolic activity in NK cells and CD 14+ macrophages was suppressed and this too, is consistent with a down-regulation of the immune response.[16]

In MOG immunized mice, laquinimod inhibited ability of CCL21 to stimulate very late antigen 4 (VLA-4) adhesiveness to vascular cell adhesion molecule 1 (VCAM-1). In doing so, laquinimod might decrease T-cell trafficking from the periphery into the CNS.[17] Another factor that might contribute to the immunomodulatory effects of laquinimod is its ability to down-regulate cytokine release from activated microglia and its ability to decrease microglial activation.[12] In cultured microglia stimulated with lipopolysaccharide, there is a marked increase in microglial size that is accompanied by the release of TNFα, IL-1, and matrix metalloproteinase (MMP)-9. Cytokine release was decreased when the cultures were treated with laquinimod and there was a concentration-dependent decrease in cell size. In humans participating in a clinical trial of laquinimod on RR MS, laquinimod significantly increased plasma concentrations of BDNF.[13] There was an 11-fold increase in the concentration of BDNF three months after treatment in the laquinimod-treated group compared with the placebo-treated patients. In studies of MOG-induced EAE with mice with a conditional deficiency of BDNF (LLF mice), those treated with laquinimod had a lesser effect than wild-type mice, suggesting that some degree of laquinimod effect may be mediated via release of BDNF.[18] The finding that levels of BDNF are increased and that a portion of its effect may be mediated by BDNF release could suggest a neuroprotective effect.

In summary, laquinimod appears to have a very broad spectrum of immunomodulatory effects. It down-regulates pro-inflammatory cytokines, up-regulates anti-inflammatory cytokines, promotes a Th1 to Th2/th3 shift, down-regulates MHC class II functions, inhibits antigen presentation, decreases microglial activation, and stimulates the production of BDNF. This is consistent with a broad spectrum immunomodulatory effect and suggests that this agent could be effective in MS.

Pharmacology

Laquinimod is rapidly absorbed following oral administration with bioavailability of 82%–95%; peak plasma concentration occurs within one hour.[19] The half-life is approximately 80 hours. The volume of distribution is approximately 10 liters. It is largely protein bound with only 1.4% free in plasma. Once steady-state is reached, there are small fluctuations between Cmin and Cmax and there is no accumulation of the drug. Brain penetration is low with a blood to brain ratio of 0.01 to 0.08, suggesting that its anti-inflammatory effects in EAE and MS are mediated by its effects on the immune system in the periphery.

Laquinimod is extensively metabolized prior to elimination with only about 10% of the parent compound excreted unchanged. The main metabolic pathway is glucuronidation of both the parent compound and its hydroxylated metabolites. Laquinimod is metabolized in the liver by the cytochrome P-450 enzyme system. The CYP3A4 isoenzyme is the predominant P-450 enzyme responsible for the metabolism.[20] While there may be a minor contribution from other P-450 isoenzynmes, CYP3A4 is predominant. As a result, laquinimod may interact with other agents metabolized by CYP3A4. This is clinically important because many symptomatic therapies used in MS are metabolized by the CYP3A4 isoenzyme. Significant interactions could occur with fluoxetine, fluvoxamine, sertraline, floxin antibiotics, erythromycin, and antifungal agents such as fluconazole. Interactions may also occur with amiodarone and calcium blockers. Dose adjustment of some symptomatic therapies might be necessary in laquinimod-treated patients.

Phase 2 clinical trials

Two Phase 2 clinical trials were conducted with laquinimod. Both demonstrated a reduction in the frequency of gadolinium (Gd)-enhancing lesions and relapses in patients with RR and secondary progressive (SP) MS. The first trial[21] compared laquinimod 0.1 mg and 0.3 mg vs. placebo in patients with RR or SP MS ages 18 to 65. Patients were dosed once daily for 24 weeks and then monitored for 8 weeks following the cessation of treatment. The inclusion criteria required that patients have at least one relapse in the year prior to study entry and at least nine T2 weighted lesions or at least three T2 weighted lesions and one Gd-enhancing lesion. This was done in order to recruit patients with more active disease. All MRI scans were done using triple dose Gd contrast to improve the detection of active lesions. The primary outcome measure was the reduction in the cumulative number of Gd-enhancing lesions during the 24-week treatment period.

At week 24, there was a statistically significant reduction in the cumulative number of Gd-enhancing lesions treated with the 0.3 mg dose. In the intent to treat the group there was a 42% reduction at 24 weeks ($P = 0.0498$). In a subgroup of patients with active lesions at baseline and with no protocol deviations, there was a 52% reduction in the cumulative number of active lesions ($P = 0.005$). There was a 64% reduction in Gd-enhancing lesion volume in this subgroup. After the cessation of treatment, lesion frequency increased further, suggesting a therapeutic effect of laquinimod. The study was not powered to detect an effect on relapse rate, and a significant effect on relapse rates was not detected. The results of this initial trial suggested that laquinimod might be an effective agent. Since it was well tolerated with few adverse events, a higher dose was studied in the second Phase 2 study.

In the second Phase 2 trial,[22] 306 patients with either RR or SP MS were randomized to treatment with placebo, 0.3 mg, or 0.6 mg of laquinimod. The inclusion criteria required that patients have at least one Gd-enhancing lesion on a baseline MRI and at least one relapse in the year prior to study entry. Because a single enhancing lesion is associated with a higher relapse frequency, a greater increase in T2 lesion burden, a greater rate of cerebral atrophy, and a higher frequency of enhancing lesions,[23] this criterion selects a group of patients with more aggressive disease. The duration of the study was 36 weeks with a planned extension. The primary outcome measure was the cumulative number of enhancing lesions at weeks 24, 28, 32, and 36. Secondary outcome measures included the number of Gd-enhancing lesions at 4-week intervals starting at week 12, cumulative number of new T2 lesions at week 24, 28, 32, and 36, and the total number of confirmed relapses.

Seven hundred and twenty patients were screened with 306 eventually being randomized. In the lower dose (0.3 mg) group, there was a trend toward a reduction in lesion frequency, while in the 0.6 mg group there was a 60% reduction in the median cumulative number of Gd-enhancing lesions. In the 0.6 mg group there was a significant decrease in the number of new T2 lesions (44%, $P = 0.0013$), new T1 hypointense lesions (50%, $P = 0.0064$), and a trend towards slowing the decrease in brain volume ($P = 0.07$). The reduction in relapse rate was a 33%. This did not reach statistical significance because the study was not powered to detect an effect on relapse rate.

Following the completion of the trial, an extension was carried out in which patients in the placebo group were randomized to treatment with either 0.3 or 0.6 mg of laquinimod.[24] Dosing was carried out for an additional 36 weeks. One hundred and thirty eight patients were assigned to 0.3 mg group and 118 patients to the 0.6 mg group. Ninety one percent of patients completed the extension in the 0.3 mg group and 94.9% completed treatment in the 0.6 mg group. The effect of laquinimod on MRI measures of disease activity was reproduced. In those switched from placebo to 0.3 mg, Gd-enhancing lesions decreased by approximately 33% and in those switched to 0.6 mg Gd-enhancing lesions decreased by approximately 55%. For those initially randomized to active treatment, the effect of laquinimod was persistent throughout the study with no increase in lesions frequency suggesting the effect was stable and did attenuate over time.

The results of the Phase 2 clinical trials suggest that laquimod has antinflammatory effects in MS. The results consistently showed there were significant reductions in Gd-enhancing lesions, new T2 lesions, new T1 hypointense lesions, and a trend toward decreasing the rate of cerebral volume loss. The effects were sustained in the extension phase of the trial and the effect on relapse rate, while not statistically significant, was of a magnitude comparable to that observed with first-line agents currently in use in RR MS.

Safety and tolerability

Laquinimod was well tolerated in both Phase 2 trials with few side effects. There was no difference in the overall number of adverse events (AEs) or serious adverse events (SAEs) between the placebo and laquinimod groups.[21] In the initial Phase 2 trial there was one SAE in the placebo group, one in the 0.1 mg group, and four in the 0.3 mg group. In the 0.3 mg dose group, one patient developed iritis. The erythrocyte sedimentation rate (ESR) was increased on at least one assessment in 6% of the placebo, 13.2% of the 0.1 mg group, and in 17.6% of the 0.3 mg patients. C-reactive protein (CRP) was elevated on at least one assessment in 34% of the placebo group, 25% of the 0.1 mg group, and 34% of the 0.3 mg dose group. There was no other indication of a pro-inflammatory effect. Elevations of liver function tests occurred on at least one occasion in 34% of the placebo group, 34% of the 0.1 mg group, and in 47% of the 0.6 mg group. There were no associated elevations of bilirubin or other findings suggesting hepatocellular injury. Elevations of liver function enzymes were generally mild and transient and not considered clinically significant.

In the second Phase 2 trial using the 0.6 mg dose, laquinimod showed a similar safety profile.[22] The frequency of early termination due to AEs was higher in the placebo group. There were five SAEs in the placebo group, five in the 0.3 mg group, and three in the 0.6 mg group. One of each was assessed as possibly study drug related. In the 0.3 mg group there were two early terminations due to liver functions tests abnormalities, one because of a respiratory tract infection, and one because of gastrointestinal difficulties. In the 0.6 mg group there was an early termination because an elevated CRP in the setting of a throat infection that was felt not to be drug related. A second patient developed fever and eosinophilia accompanied by an elevation of liver enzymes and was diagnosed with Budd–Chiari Syndrome (hepatic vein thrombosis). The patient recovered fully following treatment with anticoagulants and was found to have a factor V Leiden deficiency, which may have predisposed this patient to thrombotic events. Elevations of alanine transaminase were noted but most normalized while on therapy. There were no associated increases in bilirubin, again suggesting an absence of hepatocellular injury. CRP was elevated to a greater extent in the placebo than in the laquinimod 0.6 mg group (17.6% vs. 13.2%). Transient elevations of fibrinogen occurred in 29.4% of the placebo group, 32.6% of the 0.3 mg group, and 44.4% of the 0.6 mg group.[23] Again, there was no clinical evidence of a pro-inflammatory effect. All elevations of fibrinogen were reversible. Some patients developed mild arthralgias, arthritis, and edema, but all resolved spontaneously without intervention. There were no instances of leukopenia and no increased risk of infection.

An open-label study evaluated the safety and tolerability of laquinimod at a dose of 0.9 mg for 48 weeks in 22 patients with RR or SPMS.[25] Three patients withdrew and two patients required a reduction in dose to 0.6 mg, while seventeen patients completed the study. The events associated with dose reduction or early termination included nausea, abdominal pain, vomiting, and edema associated with joint pain. There were also transient elevations of liver function tests that were mild, reversible, and not associated with elevations of bilirubin.

To summarize the Phase 2 trial safety results, laquinimod had a good safety profile and was not associated with an increased risk of infection. There was no clearcut evidence of a pro-inflammatory effect as noted with the parent compound, roquinimex. The initial concerns regarding the safety of this agent centered on elevation of liver functions tests and pro-inflammatory effects. There was no indication of either toxicitytoxicity in the Phase 2 trials.

Phase 3 clinical trials

At the time of this writing, the first Phase 3 trial of laquinimod in RR MS has been completed. The ALLEGRO trial was a randomized, double-blind, placebo-controlled trial of laquinimod in RRMS. Inclusion criteria required that patients have at least one relapse in the year prior to study entry, two relapses in the prior 2 years, or one relapse between month 12 and 24 and one Gd-enhancing lesion in the year prior to study entry. The primary outcome measure was the annualized relapse rate. The main secondary outcome measure was disability progression as measure by the worsening on the Expanded Disability Status Scale sustained for three months. The duration of the study was two years and it enrolled 1100 MS patients. While the full results have not yet been reported, the initial press release reported that laquinimod brought about a statistically significant decrease in relapse rate and also decreased the proportion of patients with sustained disability progression.

A second trial Phase 3 trial, BRAVO, is currently ongoing. This is a global, randomized, rater-blinded, three arm trial comparing placebo, laquinimod 0.6 mg, and IFNβ-1a 30 mcg once weekly. The inclusion criteria for this trial are the same as those for the ALLEGRO Trial, and the trial is fully enrolled. The primary outcome measure is annualized relapse rate over two years.

Summary

Laquinimod is a novel, oral agent with a broad range of immunomodulatory effect. It effectively ameliorates both acute and chronic EAE decreasing both demyelination and axonal loss. It may have protective effects on axonal integrity beyond that associated with decreased inflammation. It has no immunosuppressive effects in animal models or in human studies and does not decrease the ability of animals to mount a cellular or humeral immune response. In animal models it decreases microglial activation, antigen presentation, and MHC class II expression. It may also decrease the activation of Th-17 cells and promotes a cytokine shift from a Th1 stance to an antinflammatory Th2/Th3 profile. In Phase 2 studies, laquinimod brought about reductions in Gd-enhancing lesion number and volume, decreased relapse rate, and showed a trend toward a reduction in the progression of brain volume loss. It was well tolerated with few SAEs and there was no definite pro-inflammatory effect as seen with its parent compound, roquinimex. There were mild elevations of liver function tests not associated with elevations of bilirubin most of which normalized while on therapy. In general, the safety profile appears quite favorable.

The results of the first Phase 3 clinical trial (ALLEGRO) have recently been made public in the form of a press release. Laquinimod brought about a statistically significant reduction in relapse rates and decreased disability progression thus meeting both its primary and main secondary outcome measures. While further results are not available at the time of this writing, laquinimod shows promise as a potential first-line oral agent for the treatment of RR MS.

References

1. Noseworthy JH, Wolinsky JR, Lublin FD, *et al*. Linomide in relapsing and secondary progressive MS: Part I: Trial design and clinical results. *Neurology* 2000;54:1726–33.

2. Jonsson S, Andersson G, Fex T, *et al*. Synthesis and biological evaluation of new 1,2-dihydro-4-hydroxy-2-oxo-3 quinolinecarboxamides for treatment of autoimmune disorders: structure-activity relationship. *J Med Chem* 2004;47:2075–88.

3. Zou L, Abbas N, Volkman I, *et al*. Suppression of experimental autoimmune neuritis by ABR-215062 is associated with altered Th1/Th2 balance and inhibited migration of inflammatory cells into peripheral nervous tissue. *Neuropharmacology* 2002;42: 731–9.

4. Brunmark C, Runstrom A, Ohlsson L, *et al*. The new orally active immunoregulator laquinimod (ABR-215062) effectively inhibits development and relapses of experimental autoimmune encephalomyelitis. *J Neuroimmunol* 2002;130:163–72.

5. Yang J-S, Xu LY, Xiao BG, Hedlund G, Link H. Laquinimod (ABR-215062) suppresses the development of experimental autoimmune encephalomyelitis, modulates the Th1/Th2 balance and induces the Th3 cytokine TGF-β in Lewis rats. *J Neuroimmunol* 2004:156;3–9.

6. Runstrom A, Leanderson T, Ohlsson L, Axelsson B. Inhibition of the development of chronic experimental autoimmune encephalomyelitis by laquinimod (ABR- 215062) in IFN-beta k.o. and wild type mice. *J Neuroimmunol* 2006;173:69–78.

7. Or Bach r, Sonis P, Gurevich, Achiron A. Down regulation of antigen presentation and inflammatory pathways by laquinimod in cultured peripheral blood mononuclear cells of untreated multiple sclerosis patients and healthy controls (P01.120). *Neurology* 2009;72 (Suppl 3):A38.

8. Birnberg T, Jung S. Effect of laquinimod on the dendritic cell compartment (P01.113). *Neurology* 2009;72(Suppl 3):A36.

9. Birnberg T, Jung S. The effect of laquinimod on the distribution of monocyte subsets (P808). *Mult Scler* 2009;15 (Suppl 2):S246.

10. Nussbaum S, Snir A, Hhayardeny L, *et al*. The immunoregulatory properties of laquinimod on human B-cells. *Neurology* 2010;74 (Suppl 2):P05.053.

11. Tarcic N, Raymond E, Kaye J. Laquinimod inhibits MOG-induced experimental encephalomyelitis (EAE)

in CD4+CD25+ regulatory T-cell depleted mice (P08.051). *Neurology* 2009;72(Suppl 3):A378–79.

12. Wang J, Silva C, Sloka S, *et al*. The activation of microglia and macrophages is attenuated by laquinimod (P04.222). *Neurology* 2010;74(Suppl 2):A373.

13. Linker R, Thone J, Comi G, *et al*. Laquinimod induces up-regulation of neurotrophins in serum of patients with relapsing-remitting multiple sclerosis (P783). *Mult Scler* 2009;15 (Suppl 2):S237.

14. Kaye J. Laquinimod does not result in prolongation of heart survival in a model of allogeneic heterotopic rat heart transplants. Study No.HeartTx/Teva- LQ/Jun 2006.

15. Wegner C, Stadelman C, Raymond E, *et al*. Axonal protection effect of laquinimod appears partially independent of its inhibitory effect on inflammation and demyelination in experimental autoimmune encephalomyelitis (P06.208). *Neurology* 2010;74(Suppl 2):A561.

16. Gurevich M, Gritzman T, Orbach R, *et al*. Laquinimod suppresses antigen presentation in relapsing-remitting multiple sclerosis: in vitro, high throughput gene expression study. *J Neuroimmunol* 2010;221:87–94.

17. Hayardeny L, Feigelson S, Grabovsky V, *et al*. The effect of Laquinimod on Lymphocyte VLA-4 properties under shear flow conditions (P628). *Mult Scler* 2009;15(Suppl 2):S188.

18. Thone J, Lee D, Seubert S, *et al*. Laquinimod ameliorates experimental autoimmune encephalomyelitis via BDNF-dependent mechanisms (P881). *Mult Scler* 2010;16(Suppl 10):S310.

19. Tuvesson H, Hallin I, Ellman M, *et al*. In vitro metabolism and *in vivo* pharmacokinetics in quinoline

3-carboxamide derivatives in various species. *Xenobiotica* 2005;35:295–304.

20. Tuvesson H, Hallin I, Persson R, *et al*. Cytochrome P450 3A4 is the major enzyme responsible for the metabolism of laquinimod, a novel immunomodulator. *Drug Metab Dispos* 2005;33:866–72.

21. Polman C, Barkof F, Sandberg-Wollheim M, *et al*. Laquinimod in Relapsing MS Study Group. Treatment with laquinimod reduces development of active MRI lesions in relapsing MS. *Neurology* 2005;64:987–9l.

22. Comi, G, Pulizzi A, Rovaris M, *et al*. Effect of laquinimod on MRI-monitored disease activity in relapsing-remitting multiple sclerosis: A multicentre, randomised, double-blind, placebo-controlled phase IIb study. *Lancet* 2008;317:2085–92.

23. Jeffery, DR. Early Interventions with Immunodulatory agents in the Treatment of multiple sclerosis. *J Neurol Sci* 2002;197:1–8.

24. Comi G, Abramsky T, Arbizu A, *et al*. Long-term open extension of oral laquinimod in patients with relapsing multiple sclerosis shows favourable safety and sustained low relapse rate and MRI activity (P443). *Mult Scler* 2009;15(Suppl 2):S127–8.

25. Sandberg-Wollheim M, Nederman T, Linde A. 48-week open safety study with a high dose oral laquinimod in MS patients (P587). *Mult Scler* 2005;11(Suppl 1):S154–5.

26. Comi G, Jeffery D, Kappos L, *et al*. Baseline demographics of a placebo-controlled, double-blind, randomised study of oral laquinimod 0.6 mg in treating relapsing-remitting multiple sclerosis: the ALLEGRO study (P442). *Mult Scler* 2009;15(Suppl 2):S127.

Chapter

35

Teriflunomide to treat multiple sclerosis

Paul W. O'Connor

Introduction

Since disease-modifying therapies (DMTs) for multiple sclerosis (MS) first became available in the early 1990s, the field of MS treatment has changed considerably. DMTs impede the activation, proliferation, and migration of inflammatory cells across the blood–brain barrier (BBB).[1] These treatments have been shown to reduce the frequency and severity of disease exacerbations and have a positive impact on lesion load as shown by MRI, with the two main groups of DMTs – the beta interferons (IFNβ) and glatiramer acetate (GA) – now considered first-line treatment for relapsing remitting MS (RRMS) in the US and Europe.[2]

Currently available DMTs are not without limitations. Crucially, they fail to prevent tissue damage accumulation and clinical disability in patients with long-standing, progressive phase MS, and to date there is an absence of effective treatments for MS that address the progressive phase of disease.[3] The requirement for parenteral administration also limits long-term adherence and impacts on opportunities for early treatment intervention that may prevent long-term tissue damage. Consequently, significant unmet medical needs persist in MS treatment.[3] The need for new DMTs to address these issues has, in recent years, driven the development of drugs with novel modes of action and non-parenteral routes of administration, and with improved efficacy and safety.

Teriflunomide is a novel oral DMT that targets the neuroimmunological basis of MS and is one of five orally administered DMTs in clinical development, all with differing mechanism of actions and efficacy and safety profiles.[4] Clinical data for teriflunomide show predictable pharmacokinetics, promising effects on disease activity when given either as monotherapy or as adjunctive therapy to conventional DMTs, and a favorable safety profile.[5–8]

Teriflunomide: mechanism of action

Teriflunomide [(Z)-2-cyano-3-hydroxy-but-2-enoic acid-(4′-trifluromethylphenyl)-amide] (Fig. 35.1) has both antiproliferative and anti-inflammatory activities.[4] Although the exact mechanism of action of teriflunomide remains unclear, it is known to be a potent (IC_{50} = 1.3 μM), non-competitive,

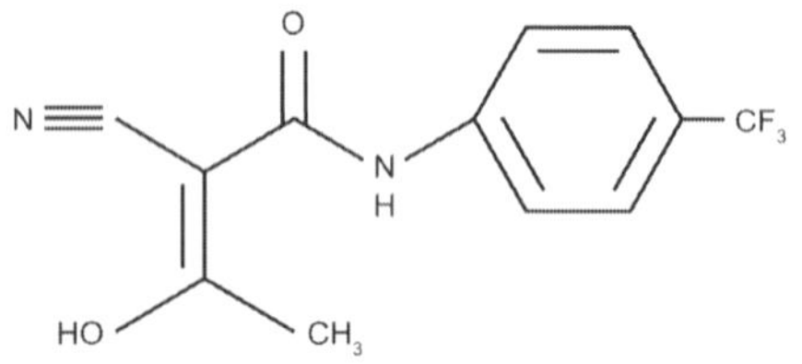

Fig. 35.1. Chemical structure of teriflunomide.

selective, and reversible inhibitor of the mitochondrial enzyme dihydro-orotate dehydrogenase (DH-ODH), required for de novo synthesis of pyrimidines.[9,10] This inhibition prevents expansion of the pyrimidine pool[10] thereby arresting proliferation of activated lymphocytes in response to autoantigens (Fig. 35.2), with no apparent cytotoxicity.[11,12] Salvage pathways appear to be spared; slowly dividing cells that rely on such DH-ODH-independent pathways to sustain pyrimidine synthesis, such as resting T- and B-cells (including memory T-cells), cells comprising the hematopoietic system and cells of the gastrointestinal lining, are largely unaffected by teriflunomide's antiproliferative effects.[13] Thus, the potential for significant leukocytopenia is reduced.[13] It has also been proposed that the reduced availability of pyrimidines could, in turn, lead to reduced phospholipid synthesis and protein glycosylation, thereby impairing the generation of lipid messengers and the function of surface cell molecules in activated immune cells. Interestingly, T-cell differentiation might be regulated at the level of de novo pyrimidine biosynthesis, restriction of which leads to inhibition of proinflammatory Th1 effector cell generation, promoting the differentiation of immunomodulatory Th2 cells from naïve T-cells in vivo and in vitro.[14]

Other mechanisms may also contribute to teriflunomide's effects and are under further investigation. In vitro experiments have shown that teriflunomide may inhibit protein tyrosine kinase (PTK) activity,[13] specifically the *Src* family of LCK and Fyn tyrosine kinases,[13,15–20] reducing T-cell proliferation and activation, and the production of cytokines. However, the concentration of teriflunomide needed to inhibit tyrosine kinase is considerably higher than that required for DH-ODH inhibition. Thus, it is less likely that inhibition of tyrosine kinase is a major contributor to the activity of teriflunomide. It has been also suggested that teriflunomide may interfere with the

Multiple Sclerosis Therapeutics, Fourth Edition, ed. Jeffrey A. Cohen and Richard A. Rudick. Published by Cambridge University Press.
© Cambridge University Press 2011.

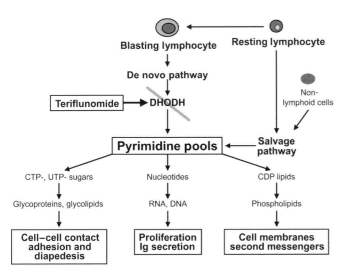

Fig. 35.2. Proposed mechanism of action of teriflunomide. Teriflunomide blocks the *de novo* pyrimidine synthesis pathway via non-competitive and reversible inhibition of the mitochondrial enzyme, dihydro-orotate dehydrogenase (DH-ODH). The resulting reduction of the pyrimidine pool leads to the inhibition of the proliferation of active T- and B-cells and the suppression of peripheral antibody production. Reproduced with kind permission from Gold & Wolinsky.[4]

interaction between T-cells and antigen presenting cells (APC), crucial for T-cell immune responses,[21] likely as a consequence of impaired function of cell surface molecules.

Teriflunomide: preclinical pharmacology/discovery data

The development of animal models of demyelination has been an important step in identifying the immune mechanisms that underlie MS pathophysiology. Experimental autoimmune encephalomyelitis (EAE) is a T-cell mediated, inflammatory, demyelinating disease of the central nervous system (CNS) that can be induced in susceptible animals and is widely studied as an animal model of MS.[22]

Teriflunomide has demonstrated both prophylactic and therapeutic effects in the Dark Agouti (DA) rat model of EAE.[23–25] This animal model shows progressive, sustained demyelination and associated axonal loss and is believed to more closely mimic and reflect the clinical course of human RRMS than acute monophasic rodent EAE models.[22]

When oral teriflunomide 1, 3 or 10 mg/kg was administered once daily prophylactically (i.e. beginning 1 day after disease induction) or therapeutically (i.e. at onset or during disease remission), in a chronic RR model of EAE in DA rats, dose-dependent delays in disease onset and reductions in disease severity were observed. When given prophylactically, 3 mg/kg teriflunomide delayed the time to disease onset by seven days, while animals receiving 10 mg/kg showed no signs of disease onset for the entire 36-day study. In addition, 3 or 10 mg/kg teriflunomide significantly inhibited overall disease severity as reflected in cumulative and maximal disease

scores. Although therapeutic administration of teriflunomide at onset of disease did not delay the first attack, both 3 and 10 mg/kg teriflunomide promoted a more rapid recovery, significantly reducing maximal disease scores and cumulative scores compared with those of vehicle-treated rats. Teriflunomide administered therapeutically during disease remission was also able to reduce neurological deficits, although the 10 mg/kg dose was more effective at eliminating further relapses than the 3 mg/kg dose. The same study demonstrated that teriflunomide inhibited the inflammation, demyelination and axonal loss associated with functional deficits.[25] Spinal cord histological assessments showed that teriflunomide, 3 or 10 mg/kg, administered prophylactically or therapeutically, significantly reduced demyelination and axonal loss by up to 90% in the gracile fascicle.[23,25] Teriflunomide also significantly reduced inflammation in the CNS; a marked decrease in the number of B-cells, T-cells and macrophage infiltrates was observed.[24] Prophylactic treatment with teriflunomide, 10 mg/kg, significantly improved the number of surviving oligodendrocytes (as shown by glutathione S-transferase placental form [GST-Pi] immunostaining) in the gracile fascicle.[24] Treatment with teriflunomide also improved several electrophysiological criteria as assessed by electrophysiological somatosensory-evoked potential (SSEP). Physiological defects in SSEP waveform parameters coincided with the point at which the study animals experienced significant inflammation, demyelination, and axonal loss in the gracile fascicle. When teriflunomide was administered at disease onset, a decrease in waveform amplitude was prevented and an increase in latency to waveform initiation was observed compared with vehicle-treated animals. Therapeutic dosing at disease remission improved evoked potential amplitude, decreased latency, and enhanced recovery time in the CNS. Whether this change is as direct or indirect consequence of prevention of inflammation, and therefore demyelination, is under investigation. Finally, MRI assessments using gadolinium (Gd)-enhanced T1 MRI, demonstrated a decrease in MRI lesion load that is indicative of preservation of BBB integrity in teriflunomide-treated animals. When dosed at 3 mg/kg, teriflunomide led to a decrease in lesion load and a delay in BBB disruption compared with vehicle-treated animals, while the 10 mg/kg dose virtually eliminated Gd-enhanced lesions.[23,25]

Additional studies are in progress to further investigate the biological effects of teriflunomide, including extensions to the animal studies already conducted and in vitro studies to investigate the effects of teriflunomide on immune cell subpopulations.

Teriflunomide: pharmacokinetic profile

The pharmacokinetic (PK) profile of teriflunomide was established in 11 studies of 260 healthy volunteers and one Phase 2 study of 179 MS patients with relapses. This information has been further supplemented with data from in vitro studies.[7,8]

The pharmacokinetic profile of teriflunomide after oral administration was characterized by rapid absorption (median peak plasma concentrations at 1 to 2 hours post-dose) and high bioavailability ($\sim$ 100%), with limited distribution and high (>99%) but non-saturable plasma protein binding, mainly to albumin. In vivo, teriflunomide was moderately metabolized. Unchanged teriflunomide was the only component detected in plasma. In urine, the predominant component was 4-trifluoro-methylaniline (TFMA) oxanilic acid, and in faeces it was unchanged teriflunomide. The primary biotransformation pathway for teriflunomide is hydrolysis, with oxidation being a minor pathway. Secondary pathways involved oxidation, *N*-acetylation and sulfate conjugation.

Teriflunomide is excreted via faeces (37.5%) and urine (22.6%). Teriflunomide $t_{1/2}$ was 10–12 days in healthy volunteers, thus allowing once-daily dosing. Dose proportionality in terms of trough concentrations of teriflunomide was observed after 7 and 14 mg multiple oral dosing in MS patients.[7] In vivo, teriflunomide was a weak inhibitor of CYP3A (27% increase in midazolam exposure), but not of CYP2C9 (based on S-warfarin).[7,26] Elimination of teriflunomide can be accelerated by activated charcoal or cholestyramine, most likely by interfering with enterohepatic recycling. Therefore, treatment with teriflunomide offers flexibility to address specific situations when it is desired by the patient to reduce teriflunomide plasma concentration or in situations such as overdose or emerging toxicity.[27]

There was no significant difference in pharmacokinetic profile when teriflunomide was taken with a high fat meal. Mild or moderate hepatic impairment, age, and gender did not appear to affect teriflunomide pharmacokinetics.[7]

Teriflunomide: clinical profile

Teriflunomide is being investigated in a comprehensive program of clinical trials in patients with MS with relapses and in patients with a clinically isolated syndrome (CIS). This program is evaluating the efficacy and safety of teriflunomide on a range of clinical and MRI end-points when administered either as monotherapy or as an adjunctive therapy to ongoing treatment with conventional DMTs.

Teriflunomide monotherapy

In 2006, the first "proof of concept", randomized, double-blind, placebo-controlled Phase 2 study to assess the efficacy and safety of oral teriflunomide in MS patients with relapses, was published.[8] Teriflunomide was evaluated over a 36-week double-blind treatment phase. Eligible patients were aged 18–65 years and were required to have clinically confirmed MS, an Expanded Disability Status Scale (EDSS) score $\leq$6.0, two documented relapses in the previous three years, and one clinical relapse during the preceding year. Patients who had received other immunosuppressant or immunomodulatory drugs within four months prior to the trial (with the exception of corticosteroids) were excluded. One hundred and seventy nine MS patients with relapses – including 157 patients

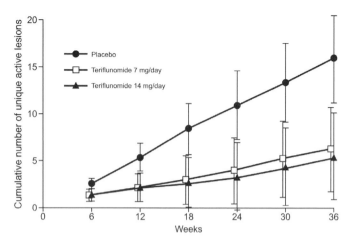

Fig. 35.3. Cumulative number of combined unique active lesions* with teriflunomide.

*Data adjusted for baseline activity.

Reproduced with kind permission O'Connor *et al.*[8]

with RRMS and 22 patients with secondary progressive MS (SPMS) with relapses – were randomized (1:1:1) to receive once-daily placebo ($n = 61$), teriflunomide 7 mg ($n = 61$), or teriflunomide 14 mg ($n = 57$). MRI scans were performed every six weeks throughout the 36-week treatment phase of the study, and disease activity was measured by pre- and post gadolinium (Gd)-enhanced T1 and T2/proton density sequences. The primary efficacy variable was the number of combined unique (CU) active lesions per scan – a combination of Gd-enhanced T1 and T2/proton density lesions. Additional MRI and clinical measures, including the number of patients experiencing MS relapse, annualized relapse rate (ARR), and disability progression, were also assessed.

The study demonstrated that patients receiving oral teriflunomide 7 mg or 14 mg one-daily had significant reductions in the number of CU active lesions per scan; the mean number of lesions after 36 weeks of treatment was 2.25, 0.87, and 0.86 with placebo, teriflunomide 7 mg, and teriflunomide 14 mg, respectively. The relative risk reduction (RRR) in MRI activity was over 61% for both teriflunomide doses ($P < 0.03$ and $P < 0.01$ for teriflunomide 7 and 14 mg vs. placebo, respectively). CU lesions were decreased in teriflunomide-treated patients as early as 6 weeks and had reached statistical significance at 12 weeks, with reductions maintained throughout the course of the study (Fig. 35.3). A significant reduction in the number of new or enlarging T2 lesions and fewer Gd-enhancing T1 lesions was also reported. There was also a trend towards lower ARRs with teriflunomide compared with placebo (0.81, 0.58, 0.55 for placebo, teriflunomide 7 mg/day, and 14 mg/day, respectively; relative risk reductions: 28% and 32%). Although the differences did not reach statistical significance, there was also a trend towards more patients being relapse-free in the 14 mg/day teriflunomide group compared with placebo (77% vs. 62%; $P = 0.098$). Fewer patients in the 14 mg/day group than in the placebo group had relapses that required steroid treatment (14% vs. 23%, respectively). The proportion of patients with progression in disability (i.e. an increase of at least 1 point if baseline EDSS was no more than 5.5, or an increase of at least 0.5 if greater) was also significantly lower in the 14 mg/day group compared with placebo-treated patients (7.4% vs 21.3% respectively; $P < 0.04$). These data support the efficacy of teriflunomide in treatment of patients with MS, and led to the initiation of an ongoing program of Phase 3 studies to further evaluate the utility of teriflunomide in this patient population.

Following completion of the 36-week placebo-controlled phase of the study, 147 patients (teriflunomide 7 mg: $n = 81$; teriflunomide 14 mg: $n = 66$) entered an open-label extension[28,29]. Patients originally allocated to teriflunomide continued in the same treatment dose as allocated at randomization into the placebo-controlled study, while those allocated placebo were re-randomized to receive teriflunomide 7 or 14 mg/day. MRI scans were performed and EDSS scores recorded every 24 weeks from the beginning of the extension study. The extension phase revealed a numerically lower reduction in cerebral volume (percentage change from baseline) in the 14 mg groups compared with the 7 mg groups, with a trend for the greatest reduction in patients who received placebo during the 36-week double-blind phase followed by teriflunomide 7 mg in the open-label extension. The number of newly active T2 lesions was lower in the 14 mg group compared with the 7 mg group regardless of treatment allocation during the 36-week double-blind phase. At week 372, the increase in T2 burden of disease was also numerically lower in the 14 mg group compared with the 7 mg group, with a trend for the greatest increase again occurring in the placebo followed by 7 mg group. ARRs decreased over the 372-week evaluation period in both teriflunomide dose groups, and the number of relapses was numerically lower in the combined 14 mg group compared with the combined 7 mg group over the course of the study. For MS patients who completed treatment with teriflunomide over 7 years, there was a moderate decline in their physical health-related quality of life (HRQoL), consistent with a small observed increase in EDSS, but patient-reported fatigue and mental HRQoL remained stable.[30] Given the non-comparative nature of the data, it is difficult to draw firm conclusions, but this long-term observation of patient-reported outcomes is encouraging. In summary, these observations suggest that longer-term exposure to teriflunomide has sustained effects on MRI, clinical end-points, and patient-reported outcomes, and indicate a possible trend towards a dose-dependent benefit with teriflunomide over a period of 7 years.

Data from the first pivotal Phase 3 study of teriflunomide (TEMSO; Teriflunomide Multiple Sclerosis Oral trial) were recently disclosed at the Congress of the European Committee for Treatment and Research in Multiple Sclerosis (ECTRIMS) held in Gothenburg, Sweden, from October 13 to 16 2010.[31,32] TEMSO, a randomized, double-blind, placebo-controlled, parallel-group study, enrolled 1088 MS patients with relapses. Patients were aged 18–55 years with EDSS scores ≤5.5, and had at least one relapse in the previous year or at least two

in the previous two years. Patients were randomized (1:1:1) to receive once-daily oral placebo or teriflunomide, 7 mg or 14 mg, for 108 weeks. The primary end-point was ARR and the key secondary endpoint was 12-week confirmed disability progression. Safety and tolerability was assessed by investigator- and subject-reported treatment emergent adverse events (TEAEs), physical examinations, vital signs, and laboratory investigations. Treatment effects on a variety of brain MRI markers of disease activity were also evaluated, with scans performed at baseline, and at weeks 24, 48, 72, and 108. Both doses of teriflunomide significantly reduced ARR (0.539, 0.370, and 0.369, for placebo, teriflunomide 7 mg and 14 mg; respective RRR of 31.2% and 31.5%; $P < 0.001$ for both doses vs. placebo).[31] The risk of 12-week confirmed disability progression was also significantly reduced by 29.8% in the teriflunomide 14 mg group ($P = 0.03$ vs. placebo). Both teriflunomide doses were superior to placebo on a range of MRI end-points, including the key MRI evaluation, burden of disease (i.e. total lesion volume); the relative increase in burden of disease was reduced by 39% in the 7 mg group ($P < 0.05$) and 67% in the 14 mg group ($P < 0.001$).[32] Teriflunomide also had dose-dependent effects on other MRI parameters including the number of Gd-enhancing T1 lesions per scan (RRR vs. placebo of 57.2% and 80.4%; $P < 0.001$ for both doses), proportion of patients free from Gd-enhancing T1 lesions ($P < 0.001$ for both doses vs. PBO), and the number of unique active lesions per scan (RRRs vs. placebo of 47.7% and 69.4%; $P < 0.001$ for both doses). The percentage change from baseline in T1 hypointense lesion (black hole) volume was also significantly lower in the 14 mg group ($P = 0.0161$). Notably, teriflunomide was very well tolerated throughout the 108-week study, with similar numbers of TEAEs (87.5%, 89.1%, 90.8%), serious TEAEs (12.8%, 14.1%, 15.9%), and TEAEs leading to treatment discontinuation across the three groups (8.1%, 9.8%, 10.9%). There was no difference between groups in the proportion of patients with ALT increases three times the upper limit of normal (ULN), serious hepatic disorders or serious infections, and no deaths were reported. Together with the other clinical data described previously, TEMSO demonstrates that teriflunomide is an effective new oral monotherapy and a potential first-line treatment option for MS with relapse.[31,32] Full publication of data from TEMSO is anticipated later in 2011.

Teriflunomide adjunctive therapy with conventional DMTs

Teriflunomide has also been investigated as an adjunctive therapy to other DMTs. Two randomized, double-blinded, placebo-controlled, Phase 2 adjunctive therapy studies have evaluated the safety and efficacy of teriflunomide as an adjunct to ongoing IFNβ or GA therapy.[5,6]

In one study, 118 patients already receiving a stable dose of IFNβ-1a for the treatment of MS with relapses were randomized (1:1:1) to additionally receive teriflunomide 7 or 14 mg/day, or placebo, for 24 weeks.[5] Eligible patients were 18–55 years of age, met McDonald's criteria for definite MS diagnosis, and

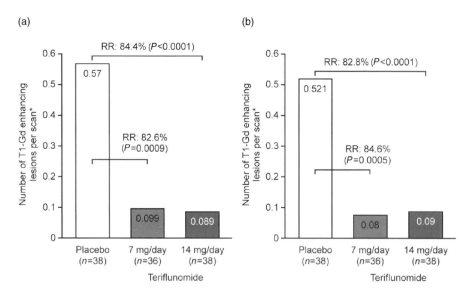

Fig. 35.4. Teriflunomide added to ongoing therapy with interferon-beta: number of Gd-enhancing T1 lesions per scan at (A) 6 months and (B) 1-year.[5,33] RR, relative reduction. *The total number of Gd-enhancing T1-lesion that occurred during the study were divided by the total number of scans during the study. Data were adjusted for the baseline number of Gd-enhancing T1-lesions, region, and IFNβ dose strata using a Poisson model.

were classified as ambulatory (EDSS score ≤5.5). In addition, eligible patients exhibited a relapsing clinical course, with and without progression, had received a stable dose of IFNβ (employing the dosing regimen of the specific IFNβ used) for at least 26 weeks prior to screening, had no relapse in the preceding 60 days and were clinically stable for four weeks prior to randomization. The main objective of the study was to evaluate the safety and tolerability of teriflunomide when administered as an adjunct therapy to IFNβ (reported below). However, related to the efficacy end-points the number of Gd enhancing lesions were reduced in both teriflunomide groups compared with the placebo group (relative reduction: 82.6% and 84.4%, for 7 mg and 14 mg, respectively; both $P < 0.001$ vs. placebo), and a greater proportion of patients remained free from Gd-enhancing lesions with teriflunomide than with placebo (placebo: 57.9%, teriflunomide 7 mg: 69.4%, and teriflunomide 14 mg: 81.6%). Few relapses were reported during the 24-week period (five in the placebo, five in the 7 mg and two in the 14 mg groups). The unadjusted ARR for the study population were 0.279, 0.305, and 0.116 for placebo, teriflunomide 7 mg, and teriflunomide 14 mg, respectively. These results indicate that teriflunomide adjunctive therapy improved disease control beyond that achieved with IFNβ therapy alone over 24 weeks and extension study data over 48 weeks demonstrate that these benefits were maintained over a period of one year of continuing treatment (Fig. 35.4).[33]

In a similar study, teriflunomide was added to therapy with a stable dose of GA.[6] A total of 123 patients with relapsing forms of MS, who were already receiving GA, were randomized to receive either teriflunomide 7 mg or 14 mg once daily, or placebo once daily as adjunctive therapy. As with the teriflunomide/IFNβ adjunctive therapy study, the main objective was to evaluate safety and tolerability; however, for the efficacy end-points it was noted that the addition of teriflunomide to GA significantly improved disease control compared with GA therapy alone, although the effect size did not appear

to be as robust. Compared with placebo, the number of Gd-enhancing lesions were reduced in both the GA+7 mg ($P = 0.011$) and GA+14 mg ($P = 0.1157$) groups, as was the Gd-enhancing lesion volume (GA+7 mg, $P = 0.0886$; GA+14 mg $P = 0.039$). A higher proportion of patients were free from Gd-enhancing lesions in the 14 mg group. However, further interpretation of this study is complicated by differences in baseline disease activity between the different treatment groups.

The results of these two studies indicate that there is also potential for the use of teriflunomide as an adjunctive therapy to other DMTs in some patients, although further Phase 3 investigations are needed to fully establish the clinical benefit of this combination approach to treatment. In this regard, a further Phase 3 trial – TERACLES – has started which will further investigate the efficacy and safety of teriflunomide added to ongoing IFNβ therapy.

Teriflunomide: safety profile

Clinical data indicate that teriflunomide is generally well tolerated with an acceptable safety profile, with no significant safety concerns identified to date.

In the Phase 2 monotherapy study of teriflunomide in MS, TEAEs of nasopharyngitis, mild hair thinning/loss, nausea, increases in alanine aminotransferase (ALT), paraesthesia, back and limb pain, diarrhea, and arthralgia were more frequently reported with teriflunomide than with placebo. An apparent dose-dependent trend in the incidence of mild hair thinning/loss, nausea, paresthesia, back pain, and diarrhea was also reported, and there was a higher frequency of treatment discontinuation due to TEAEs in the 14 mg/day teriflunomide group (14.0%) compared with the placebo (6.6%) and the teriflunomide 7 mg/day (4.9%) groups. However, TEAEs occurring during the double-blind phase of this study were predominantly minor and generally occurred at a similar frequency across all treatment groups. Serious adverse events (SAEs) were evenly distributed throughout the three treatment groups (11.5%, 8.2%, and 12.3%, in the placebo, teriflunomide 7 mg and 14 mg groups, respectively). No deaths were reported. The most frequent SAE was abnormal liver function tests, however, SAEs related to hepatic disorders were equally as frequent or more frequent in patients receiving placebo than in those who received teriflunomide (placebo: 5%; teriflunomide 7 mg: 0%; teriflunomide 14 mg: 5%). Although leukocyte decreases were more frequent in the teriflunomide groups, no patients discontinued study treatment due to leukopenia or neutropenia. It is also notable that there was no evidence of opportunistic infections or impaired immune surveillance in any patient.[8]

Safety data from the open-label extension phase of the study are consistent with the safety profile of teriflunomide observed in the double-blind treatment phase, without the emergence of any new safety concerns.[34] Of the 147 patients entering the long-term extension, 85 (58%) remained permanently on teriflunomide at the most recent published analysis cut-off date, although not all had eight-year teriflunomide exposure. Overall, 28 patients discontinued treatment due to TEAEs, mostly from hepatic disorders ($n = 12$) relating primarily to increases in hepatic enzymes ($n = 11$) (NB threshold for discontinuation was ALT >3x ULN) and one case of abnormal hepatic function. The remaining 34 patients discontinued for non-safety reasons. TEAEs were similar in nature to those reported in the placebo-controlled phase, but exposure-adjusted incidence rates for the most common TEAEs were lower in the long-term extension. The most common TEAEs (per 100 patient–years for teriflunomide 7 mg and 14 mg, respectively; Table 35.1) included nasopharyngitis (12.0 and 17.6), fatigue (12.6 and 13.4), hypoesthesia (11.9 and 13.3), upper respiratory tract infections (8.3 and 12.7), headache (14.7 and 10.1), diarrhoea (6.1 and 11.1), mild hair loss or thinning (4.4 and 6.8), and nausea (5.5 and 6.0). No serious opportunistic infections were reported over the eight-year follow-up. No discontinuations occurred due to leukopenia or neutropenia, and in both groups the incidence of malignancy (0.6 per 100 patient–years across both teriflunomide groups) was within the rates commonly seen in the population at large. Six pregnancies were documented during the course of the study, all occurring in the teriflunomide 7 mg group. Four patients elected to terminate their pregnancy, and two patients permanently discontinued treatment as soon as they were aware of their pregnancy, subsequently giving birth to two healthy babies without structural or functional defects. One death from sudden cardiac disorder (malaise with hypotension and tachycardia) occurred in the teriflunomide 14 mg group, but was considered unlikely to be related to study drug.

Finally, adjunctive therapies show that teriflunomide can be safely combined with other DMTs with no new emerging safety concerns; when teriflunomide was added to ongoing IFNβ or GA therapy over a six-month treatment period, the safety profile of teriflunomide reflected that observed in the Phase 2 monotherapy studies.[5,6]

Table 35.1. *Exposure-adjusted incidence of common treatment-emergent adverse events (per 100 patient–years)*[34]

TEAE	Teriflunomide 7 mg (N = 81)	Teriflunomide 14 mg (N = 66)
Nasopharyngitis	12.0	17.6
Fatigue	12.6	13.4
Hypoaesthesia	11.9	13.3
Upper respiratory tract infection	8.3	12.7
Diarrhea	6.1	11.1
Headache	14.7	10.1
Back pain	7.8	9.6
Influenza	5.7	9.2
Muscular weakness	10.6	9.1
Pain in extremity	11.6	7.8
Paresthesia	6.9	7.5
Pallanesthesia	7.2	6.9
ALT increased	7.0	6.9
Alopecia (mild hair loss/thinning)	4.4	6.8
Sensory disturbance	5.2	6.6
Arthralgia	7.3	6.3
Insomnia	7.8	6.0
Nausea	5.5	6.0
Urinary tract infection	4.8	5.1
Hyperreflexia	4.9	4.8
Dizziness	4.6	4.7

ALT, alanine aminotransferase.
TEAEs presented by MedDRA preferred term and by decreasing order of frequency in the 14 mg dose group (cut-off for inclusion based on ≥10% crude incidence).

Teriflunomide: overview of the clinical program

An extensive clinical development program is ongoing to evaluate the efficacy, safety, and tolerability of teriflunomide in relapsing forms of MS (Fig. 35.5). It is anticipated that over 3000 patients will be enrolled across various clinical trials to evaluate teriflunomide as monotherapy. Clinical studies of teriflunomide have, to date, focused on monotherapy and adjunctive therapy with existing DMTs (IFNβ and GA) in RMS (mostly relapsing–remitting MS). In addition to these studies, the effects of early intervention with teriflunomide in patients with a first event suggestive of demyelination and MRI characteristics suggesting a risk of MS development (CIS) are also being explored in an ongoing pivotal clinical trial (TOPIC). The IFNβ adjunctive therapy program has been expanded into Phase 3 (TERACLES) and a head-to-head study with IFNβ is ongoing (TENERE). Thus, this extensive clinical development program will address a range of issues relevant for the successful treatment of MS.

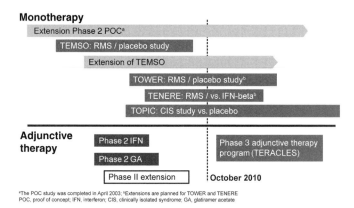

Monotherapy

Extension Phase 2 POCª

TEMSO: RMS / placebo study

Extension of TEMSO

TOWER: RMS / placebo studyᵇ

TENERE: RMS / vs. IFN-betaᵇ

TOPIC: CIS study vs. placebo

Adjunctive therapy

Phase 2 IFN

Phase 2 GA

Phase II extension

Phase 3 adjunctive therapy program (TERACLES)

October 2010

ªThe POC study was completed in April 2003; ᵇExtensions are planned for TOWER and TENERE
POC, proof of concept; IFN, interferon; CIS, clinically isolated syndrome; GA, glatiramer acetate

Fig. 35.5. The teriflunomide clinical development program.
[a]The POC study was completed in April 2003; [b]Extensions are planned for TOWER and TENERE. CIS, clinically isolated syndrome; GA, glatiramer acetate; POC, proof of concept; RMS, relapsing multiple sclerosis; IFN, interferon; RMS, relapsing multiple sclerosis; TEMSO, TEriflunomide Multiple Sclerosis Oral trial; TENERE, TEriflunomide AND REbif; TOPIC, TeriflunOmide in Patients with early multiple sClerosis; TOWER, Teriflunomide Oral in people With relapsing remitting multiplE scleRosis.

Conclusions

Despite advances in MS disease-modifying therapy, existing long-term therapies rely on parenteral administration, with associated issues of convenience, adherence, and tolerability. Oral agents such as teriflunomide therefore represent a major therapeutic advancement for patients. Teriflunomide is one of several oral disease-modifying treatments currently being investigated in clinical trials for the treatment of relapsing forms of MS, and is well advanced in terms of clinical development. Based on currently available data on monotherapy and adjunctive therapy, teriflunomide appears to have a favorable benefit/risk ratio in relapsing MS, and as such, represents a promising new first-line treatment.

References

1. Ruggieri M, Avolio C, Livrea P, Trojano M. Glatiramer acetate in multiple sclerosis: a review. *CNS Drug Rev* 2007; 13:178–91.

2. Wiendl H, Toyka KV, Rieckmann P, Gold R, Hartung HP, Hohlfeld R. Basic and escalating immunomodulatory treatments in multiple sclerosis: current therapeutic recommendations. *J Neurol* 2008;255:1449–63.

3. Gasperini C, Cefaro LA, Borriello G, Tosto G, Prosperini L, Pozzilli C. Emerging oral drugs for multiple sclerosis. *Expert Opin Emerg Drugs* 2008;13:465–77.

4. Gold R, Wolinsky JS. Pathophysiology of multiple sclerosis and the place of teriflunomide. *Acta Neurol Scand* 2011;124:75–84.

5. Freedman MS, Wolinsky JS, Byrnes WJ, *et al.* Oral teriflunomide or placebo added to interferon beta for 6 months in patients with relapsing multiple sclerosis: safety and efficacy results. *Mult Scler* 2009;15:S271–S7. Abs P878.

6. Freedman MS, Wolinsky JS, Frangin GA, *et al.* Oral teriflunomide added to interferon-beta in patients with relapsing multiple sclerosis: 1-year safety and efficacy results. *Mult Scler* 2010;16:996.

7. Limsakun T, Menguy-Vacheron F. Pharmacokinetics of oral teriflunomide, a novel oral disease-modifying agent under investigation for the treatment of multiple sclerosis. *Neurology* 2010;74:9. Abstract P05.032.

8. O'Connor PW, Li D, Freedman MS, *et al.* A Phase II study of the safety and efficacy of teriflunomide in multiple sclerosis with relapses. *Neurology* 2006;66:894–900.

9. Bruneau JM, Yea CM, Spinella-Jaegle S, *et al.* Purification of human dihydro-orotate dehydrogenase and its inhibition by A77 1726, the active metabolite of leflunomide. *Biochem J* 1998;336:299–303.

10. Cherwinski HM, Cohn RG, Cheung P, *et al.* The immunosuppressant leflunomide inhibits lymphocyte proliferation by inhibiting pyrimidine biosynthesis. *J Pharmacol Exp Ther* 1995;275:1043–9.

11. Ruckemann K, Fairbanks LD, Carrey EA, *et al.* Leflunomide inhibits pyrimidine de novo synthesis in mitogen-stimulated T-lymphocytes from healthy humans. *J Biol Chem* 1998;273:21682–91.

12. Siemasko KF, Chong AS, Williams JW, Bremer EG, Finnegan A. Regulation of B cell function by the immunosuppressive agent leflunomide. *Transplantation* 1996;61:635–42.

13. Fox RI, Herrmann ML, Frangou CG, *et al.* Mechanism of action for leflunomide in rheumatoid arthritis. *Clin Immunol* 1999;93:198–208.

14. Dimitrova P, Skapenko A, Herrmann ML, Schleyerbach R, Kalden JR, Schulze-Koops H. Restriction of de novo pyrimidine biosynthesis inhibits Th1 cell activation and promotes Th2 cell differentiation. *J Immunol* 2002; 169:3392–9.

15. Elder RT, Xu X, Williams JW, Gong H, Finnegan A, Chong AS. The immunosuppressive metabolite of leflunomide, A77 1726, affects murine T cells through two biochemical mechanisms. *J Immunol* 1997;159:22–7.

16. Mattar T, Kochhar K, Bartlett R, Bremer EG, Finnegan A. Inhibition of the epidermal growth factor receptor tyrosine kinase activity by leflunomide. *FEBS Lett* 1993;334:161–4.

17. Migita K, Miyashita T, Ishibashi H, Maeda Y, Nakamura M, Yatsuhashi H, *et al.* Suppressive effect of leflunomide metabolite (A77 1726) on metalloproteinase production in IL-1beta stimulated rheumatoid synovial fibroblasts. *Clin Exp Immunol* 2004;137:612–6.

18. Siemasko K, Chong AS, Jack HM, Gong H, Williams JW, Finnegan A. Inhibition of JAK3 and STAT6 tyrosine phosphorylation by the immunosuppressive drug leflunomide leads to a block in IgG1 production. *J Immunol* 1998;160:1581–8.

19. Xu X, Williams JW, Bremer EG, Finnegan A, Chong AS. Inhibition of

protein tyrosine phosphorylation in T cells by a novel immunosuppressive agent, leflunomide. *J Biol Chem* 1995; 270:12398–403.

20. Xu X, Williams JW, Gong H, Finnegan A, Chong AS. Two activities of the immunosuppressive metabolite of leflunomide, A77 1726. Inhibition of pyrimidine nucleotide synthesis and protein tyrosine phosphorylation. *Biochem Pharmacol* 1996;52:527–34.

21. Zeyda M, Poglitsch M, Geyeregger R, et al. Disruption of the interaction of T cells with antigen-presenting cells by the active leflunomide metabolite teriflunomide: involvement of impaired integrin activation and immunologic synapse formation. *Arthritis Rheum* 2005;52:2730–9.

22. Merrill JE. In vitro and in vivo pharmacological models to assess demyelination and remyelination. *Neuropsychopharmacology* 2009;34:55–73.

23. McMonagle-Strucko K, Hanak S, Pu SF, et al. Teriflunomide reduces neurological behaviour and pathology in the Dark Agouti rat model of experimental autoimmune encephalomyelitis. *Mult Scler* 2009;15: S254.

24. Petty M, Lee L, X Y, et al. Teriflunomide treatment reduces infiltration of macrophages, T cells and B cells, and increases survival of oligodendrocytes in the spinal cord of the Dark Agouti rat model of *Exp Allergic Encephalomyelitis*. *Neurology* 2010;74: 9(Suppl 2). Abs P05.033

25. Merrill JE, Hanak S, Pu SF, et al. Teriflunomide reduces behavioral, electrophysiological, and histopathological deficits in the Dark Agouti rat model of experimental autoimmune encephalomyelitis. *J Neurol* 2009;256:89–103.

26. Menguy-Vacheron F, Limsakun T (eds.) Effect of repeated oral doses of teriflunomide on a single oral dose of midazolam in healthy subjects. *Mult Scler* 2010;16:8. Abs P10.

27. Limsakun T, Menguy-Vacheron F (eds.) Effects of cholestyramine on the elimination of teriflunomide in healthy male volunteers. *Mult Scler* 2010;16:8. Abs P11.

28. O'Connor PW, Freedman MS, Bar-Or A, Rice GP, Confavreux C, Traboulsee A. Oral teriflunomide is effective and well tolerated in multiple sclerosis with relapses: results of an open-label 144-week extension study. *Poster presented at 22nd Congress of the European Committee for Treatment and Research in Multiple Sclerosis (ECTRIMS)*. Madrid, Spain, September 27–30, 2006. Abs P379.

29. Li D, O'Connor PW, Confavreux C, et al. Long-term brain MRI and clinical assessments of teriflunomide for the treatment of multiple sclerosis: extension of a Phase II study. *Mult Scler* 2010;16:S142. Abs 431.

30. Bhan V, Grand A, Germe M, Fisk JD. Long-term outcomes in patients who receive teriflunomide for multiple sclerosis: evaluating health-related quality of life and fatigue over 7 years. *Mult Scler* 2010;16:S308; Abs 877.

31. O'Connor PW, Wolinsky JS, Confavreux C, et al. A placebo-controlled phase III trial (TEMSO) of oral teriflunomide in relapsing multiple sclerosis: clinical efficacy and safety outcomes. *Mult Scler* 2010;16:S29. Abs 79.

32. Wolinsky JS, O'Connor PW, Confavreux C, et al. A placebo-controlled phase III trial (TEMSO) of oral teriflunomide in relapsing multiple sclerosis: magnetic resonance imaging (MRI) outcomes. *Mult Scler* 2010;16:S347. Abs 982.

33. Freedman MS, Wolinsky JS, Frangin GA, et al. Oral teriflunomide or placebo added to interferon-beta in relapsing multiple sclerosis patients: 1-year safety and efficacy results. *Mult Scler* 2010;16: 996.

34. Confavreux C, O'Connor PW, Fairbanks LD, Benzedjeb H, Wang S, Bar-Or A. Safety of teriflunomide in the treatment of relapsing multiple sclerosis: results over an 8-year extension. *Mult Scler* 2010;16:S291. Abs 833.

Chapter

36

High-dose methylprednisolone to treat multiple sclerosis

Robert J. Fox and R. Philip Kinkel

Introduction

Treatment of multiple sclerosis (MS) with pulses of high-dose methylprednisolone (HDMP) is currently the treatment of choice for MS relapses in many parts of the world. Evidence suggests that HDMP not only hastens recovery from MS relapses, but may modify the course of relapsing–remitting (RR) MS as well as secondary progressive (SP) MS. In this chapter the evidence supporting the use of HDMP for these indications will be reviewed.

Pharmacology

MP is a synthetic glucocorticoid that differs from hydrocortisone (cortisol) by the addition of a double bond at the 1,2 position and a methyl group at the 6 position.[1] These structural differences increase the relative glucocorticoid effect, decrease the mineralocorticoid effect, and increase the duration of action (Table 36.1). The biologically active sterol is highly insoluble in aqueous solution and must be given as a sodium hemisuccinate ester when administered intravenously (i.v.). Following i.v. administration, 10%–15% of the ester is excreted unchanged in the urine and the rest is converted into MP and eventually into one of several metabolites.[2] The half-life of circulating MP is 1.4 hours, and the half-lives of the active metabolites are about 4 hours.[2] At normal or low concentrations, 80%–90% of glucocorticoids are bound to corticosteroid binding globulin, a protein with high affinity but low capacity for binding corticosteroids. A smaller percentage of glucocorticoids binds to albumin, which displays a higher binding capacity but lower binding affinity. At the high concentrations achieved with HDMP, the protein binding capacity in serum is exceeded and a greater proportion of serum glucocorticoids exist in a free state. An increased proportion of unbound glucocorticoids allows steroids to enter cells and interact with specific receptors, and also allows effective penetration of the central nervous system (CNS), since the blood–brain barrier is relatively impermeable to bound steroids.[3] Accordingly, peak cerebrospinal fluid (CSF) levels are delayed for over 6 hours following a 1500 mg bolus of HDMP, whereas peak plasma levels occur within 2 hours.[4] Thus, high CSF concentrations persist at a time when serum concentrations are much reduced.[5,6] Altered hepatic function will affect both the serum proteins available for binding as well as metabolism.

In addition to i.v. formulations, oral preparations of MP as the parent sterol compound are available up to a maximum strength of 32 mg. While well absorbed, the relatively low strength of the tablet formulation renders oral administration of high doses (500–2000 mg/day) difficult. As an alternative, some studies suggest that the i.v. solution may be taken orally; up to 1000 mg/day are well absorbed and reasonably well tolerated.[5] Concerns regarding a potential increase in gastrointestinal side effects with oral HDMP appear to be unfounded, since oral administration does not increase gastrointestinal permeability or the incidence of endoscopically identified lesions in the gastric mucosa compared with i.v. administration.[7,8] A short-term study of HDMP found no difference in reduction in gadolinium (Gd)-enhancing lesions between the same total dose of i.v. and oral MP.[9] Further studies regarding the tolerability, efficacy, and pharmacokinetics of HDMP pulses administered orally are required before this route is established as an alternative to i.v. administration.

Molecular biology and mechanism of action

Unbound MP freely diffuses across plasma membranes and exerts its effects through interaction with both intracellular and membrane-associated glucocorticoid receptors. The glucocorticoid receptor consists of a DNA-binding domain, a steroid-binding domain, and an immunogenic domain.[10] In the steroid-free state, the intracellular receptor exists as an oligomer complexed to immunophillins and heat-shock protein 90 (HSP), which facilitates its interaction with glucocorticoids.[11] Binding of the sterol to the receptor complex causes dissociation from HSP and immunophillins and allows the steroid-receptor complex to translocate into the nucleus, where it binds in conjunction with other activating proteins to glucocorticoid responsive elements on the 5′-flanking region of various genes.[12–15] This binding leads to an enhancement of transcription in certain instances (i.e. glucose metabolism) or inhibition of transcription in other instances (i.e. many anti-inflammatory effects). Corticosteroids also regulate RNA processing, transport, translation, and final protein secretion.

Multiple Sclerosis Therapeutics, Fourth Edition, ed. Jeffrey A. Cohen and Richard A. Rudick. Published by Cambridge University Press.

Table 36.1. *Relative potency and biological activity of glucocorticosteroids*

Preparation	Glucocorticoid activity	Mineralocorticoid activity	Duration of action	Equivalent strength (mg)
Cortisone	0.8	0.8	Short	25
Cortisol	1	1	Short	20
Prednisone	4	0.8	Intermediate	5
Prednisolone	4	0.8	Intermediate	5
Methylprednisolone	5	0.l5	Intermediate	4
Dexamethasone	25	0	Long	0.75

Corticosteroids also act through a more immediate, non-genomic pathway, involving membrane glucocorticoid receptor interaction with protein kinase C, G proteins, and adenyl cyclase, thereby inducing changes in calcium and potassium currents that lead to alterations in neuronal firing and cell activity.[16] An important non-genomic effect on inflammation is mediated through direct interaction of the steroid-receptor complex with activator protein-1 (AP-1) complex molecules such as c-jun and c-fos.[17,18] The AP-1 complex is activated by proinflammatory stimuli and alters the transcription of many genes involved in the inflammatory response. The steroid–receptor complex modulates expression of target genes through AP-1, which in turn inhibits transcription of proinflammatory growth factors and cytokines.

Corticosteroids have many biological effects of potential therapeutic benefit in MS (Table 36.2). These effects include restoration of the blood–brain barrier function, reduction of tissue edema, suppression of inflammation, and immunomodulation. Animal models of neural tissue injury provide evidence of the efficacy of corticosteroids. Corticosteroids reduce cytokine expression in injured neural tissue in animal models of spinal cord injury.[73] Furthermore, they regulate expression of adhesion molecules at the blood–brain barrier, and in so doing inhibit lymphocyte recruitment into injured tissue and reduce further injury. In a rat model of spinal cord injury, corticosteroids reduced the infiltration of microglia and macrophage cells by 66%–82% over a two-month period following injury.[74] This reduced cellular infiltration was accompanied by a reduction in tissue loss, increased axons near and in the injury site, reduced Wallerian degeneration of axonal fibers, and, perhaps most importantly, increased spouting of neuritic fibers near the lesion. Other potential mechanisms of corticosteroid-induced neural protection include a decrease in after-hyperpolarization, increase synthesis and release of neurotrophic factors and lipocortin feedback regulation of Ca^{2+} currents, and induction of antioxidant enzymes.[21] In very high doses, MP suppresses lipid peroxidation associated with progressive neural degeneration following spinal cord injury.[22] Corticosteroids induce apoptosis in lymphocytes, which may help to curtail the inflammatory response. The mechanism by which apoptosis is induced is unknown, but it may involve interactions with

AP-1, calmodulin, β-galactoside-binding protein, and NKκB and IκBα.[18] Many studies of blood and CSF from MS patients treated with corticosteroids support these potential mechanisms of action.

MP reduces expression of cellular adhesion molecules including very late antigen-4 (VLA-4), which may help restore blood–brain barrier function in areas of inflammation. This effect may also contribute to decreased immune surveillance within the CNS and may have contributed to the development or persistence of the serious viral infectious complication progressive multifocal leukoencephalopathy seen in association with the anti-VLA-4 therapy natalizumab.[77,78]

MP has biologic effects that may be detrimental in MS, too. Apoptosis of immune cells may be helpful in fighting inflammation, but apoptosis of tissue may be harmful. Corticosteroid treatment induces apoptosis of chondrocytes in an experimental arthritis model and airway epithelial cells in an asthma model.[79,80] In the MS animal model experimental autoimmune encephalomyelitis (EAE), severe optic neuritis leads to apoptotic cell death of retinal ganglion cells (RGC). MP treatment significantly increased RGC apoptosis, and this was found to be mediated through suppression of the neuroprotective MAPK phosphorylation pathway.[81,82] The relevance of these animal model findings is unclear, given the clinical and radiologic benefits of HDMP described below, particularly the cessation of brain atrophy progression over five years of treatment with routine pulses of HDMP.

All of these effects are complex, inter-related, and dose dependent in ways that are only partly understood. No particular biological activity of the corticosteroids has been causally linked to the clinical benefits observed in MS patients, in part owing to the pleiotropic effects of corticosteroids on cell function and survival.

Corticosteroids in relapsing MS

The use of corticosteroids as a treatment for MS was first reported in 1951.[83] Several subsequent clinical trials between 1954 and 1979 failed to show a convincing benefit of low to intermediate doses of daily or alternate-day oral corticosteroids, as reviewed by Myers.[84] Although the design of these

Table 36.2. *Glucocorticoids: potential mechanisms of action in MS*

Effects on cellular immune system function and inflammation:
Redistribution of T-cells with transient alterations in T-cell counts[19,20]
Decreased T-cell responses to antigen and mitogen[21]
Decreased synthesis and release of pro-inflammatory cytokines and growth factors (IL-1, IL-2, IL-6, IFNγ, IFNα, IL-8, TNFα, NFκB)[22–26]
Decrease in constitutive HLA-DR expression[19,27,28]
Increase in TGFβ and IL-10 expression[22,24,29–31]
Increased in chemokine receptors CXCR1 and CXCR2[32]
Decreased CXCL10[33]
Increased numbers of monocytes, neutrophils, and T-cells and B-cells[25]
Increased proportion of Fas-expressing CD4+ T-cells and decreased proportion of Fas-expressing CD8+ T-cells[34]
Decreased memory (CD45RO+) CD4+ T-cells and increased CCR5 expression on CD4+ T-cells, the latter lasting over 1 month[35]
Decreased myeloid and plasmacytoid dendritic cells[36]
Increased percentage of CD4+CD25+ and CD4+CD25[hi] T-cells and Foxp3/CD3 ratio[31,36]
Increase leukocyte apoptosis[37]
Inhibition of IFNγ up-regulation of MHC class II expression by macrophages and microglia[38]
Decreased eicosanoid production by monocytes[39]
Decreased Fc receptor expression by macrophages[40]
Decreased immunoglobulin levels 2–4 weeks post-treatment[41]
Increased synthesis of lipocortin 1 and reduced transcription of cyclooxygenase II gene[42,43]
Decreased apoptosis of oligodendrocytes[44]

Effects on endothelial cell function and permeability:
Decreased peripheral blood mononuclear cell adhesion to endothelium[45]
Down-regulation of expression of cell adhesion molecules (VLA-4, VCAM-1, LFA-a, ELAM-1, ICAM-a, ICAM-3) on both circulating cells and after in vitro stimulation[46–49]
Increase in adhesion and trafficking molecules CD11a, CD19, and serum sVCAM[45]
Reduced activity of matrix metalloproteinase (gelatinase B) and increased activity of tissue inhibitors of metalloproteinases in CSF[50]
Decreased serum levels of MMP-9[51]
Decreased transmigration of peripheral mononuclear cells in vitro[52,53]
Decreased mean blood flow velocity[54]

Effects on cerebrospinal fluid immune compartment:
Transient, dose-dependent decrease in CD3, CD4, CD8 T-cell counts[55,56]
Transient, dose-dependent decrease in IgG and IgM synthesis[21,57,55,58–60]
Decreased myelin basic protein and antibodies against myelin basic protein[59,61,62]
Decreased soluble adhesion molecule sICAM[63,64]
Decreased TNFα[65]
Restoration of cortisol levels[66]
Decreased nitric oxide metabolism (nitrite and nitrate)[67–69]
Decrease in the lipid peroxidation marker malondialdehyde[70]
Decreased free radical peroxidation products[71]
Increase in TGF-β1 and soluble TNFα receptor Rp55[59,72]
Decreased chemokine receptor expression: CXCR3 on CD8+ T-cells, and CCR4 on CD4+ T-cells[60]

CSF = cerebrospinal fluid, ELAM = endothelial leukocyte adhesion molecule, HLA = human leukocyte antigen, ICAM = intercellular adhesion molecule, IFN = interferon, IL = interleukin, LFA = leukocyte function antigen, MHC = major histocompatibility complex, MMP = matrix metalloproteinase, NFκB = nuclear factor-kappaB sICAM = soluble ICAM, sVCAM = soluble VCAM, TGF = transforming growth factor, TNF = tumor necrosis factor, VCAM = vascular cell adhesion molecule, VLA = very late antigen.

studies would be considered suboptimal compared with current standards, a consensus developed that chronic corticosteroid administration in low doses does not prevent disease activity. In 1970, an influential clinical trial provided convincing evidence that adrenocorticotrophic hormone (ACTH) improves recovery from MS relapses.[85] Despite the inconvenience of a two-week course of administration and side effects, ACTH was widely adopted as the standard treatment for MS relapses.

During the 1970s, HDMP pulses were reported to be beneficial in acute allograft rejection,[86] and shortly thereafter therapeutic benefits of pulsed HDMP were reported in lupus nephritis,[87] Goodpasture's syndrome,[88] crescentic glomerulonephritis,[89] polyarteritis nodosa,[90] and rheumatoid arthritis.[91] These reports were followed by several uncontrolled, short, open trials of i.v. HDMP for MS relapses. Rapid improvement was reported in the majority of patients with few adverse effects.[21,82–95]

HDMP for MS relapses

After ACTH became the standard of treatment for MS relapses, there followed three randomized trials to assess the relative benefit of i.v. HDMP vs. ACTH (Table 36.3).[96–98] In these trials, a small number of patients were treated with a single course of HDMP or ACTH and followed for a brief period of time. These studies lacked statistical power to detect small but significant differences between treatments, and the trial durations were too short to assess the effects on long-term disease course. The most influential of these trials was a randomized, placebo-controlled, double-blind comparison of i.v. HDMP for three days vs. intramuscular ACTH for 14 days.[98] Both treatment groups improved significantly but there were no significant differences between the groups at 3, 7, 14, 28, and 90 days after treatment. The investigators concluded that i.v. HDMP was

Table 36.3. *Clinical trials of HDMP vs. ACTH for MS relapses*

Study	Treatment regimens	N	Study design	Outcome
Abbruzzese et al.[96]	i.v.MP 20 mg/kg/day for 3 days, 10 mg/kg/day for 4 days, 5 mg/kg/day for 3 days, 1 mg/kg/day for 5 days i.v. ACTH 0.5 twice daily for 15 days	30 30	Open, randomized	No difference at any time point between treatments
Barnes et al.[97]	i.v. MP 1000 mg/day for 7 days IM ACTH 60U/day for 7 days, 40U/day for 7 days, and 20U/day for 7 days	14 11	Single-blind, randomized	MP better at 3, 7, and 28 days but not 3 months after treatment
Thompson et al.[98]	i.v. MP 1000 mg/day for 3 days Intramuscular ACTH 40U twice daily for 7 days, 20U twice daily for 4 days, 20 U/day for 3 days	29 32	Double-blind, randomized	No difference at 3, 7, 14, 28, and 90 days after treatment; MP better tolerated

ACTH = adrenocorticotrophic hormone, i.v. = intravenous, MP = methylprednisolone.

Table 36.4. *Placebo-controlled trials of HDMP for MS relapses and SPMS*

Study	Treatment regimens	N	Study design	Outcome
Durelli et al.[57]	i.v. MP 15 mg/kg/day for 3 days, 10 mg/kg/day for 3 days, 5 mg/kg/day for 3 days, 2.5 mg/kg/day for 3 days, 1 mg/kg/day for 3 days Placebo	12 8	Double-blind, randomized	MP better than placebo at the end of treatment
Milligan et al.[99]	i.v. MP 500 mg/day for 5 days Placebo	13 9	Double-blind, randomized	MP better than placebo at 1 and 4 weeks after treatment
Sellebjerg et al.[100]	Oral MP 500 mg/day for 5 days Placebo	26 25	Double-bind, randomized	More MP treated patients improved 1.0 or more EDSS points at 1, 3, and 8 weeks after treatment
Cazzato et al.[101]	i.v. MP 1000 mg/day for 5 days, prednisone taper for 5 days Placebo	35 35	Double-blind, randomized, cross-over	EDSS improved in MP-treated patients more than placebo

ACTH = adrenocorticotrophic hormone, EDSS = Expanded Disability Status Scale, i.v. =intravenous, MP = methylprednisolone.

an effective alternative to ACTH, required shorter treatment duration, and was better tolerated. This led many clinicians to abandon ACTH treatment for clinical relapses in favor of i.v. HDMP. ACTH is still available for clinical use, although its prohibitive cost and easy availability of oral MP and other corticosteroid preparations made the use of ACTH in MS obsolete.

Ongoing questions about the clinical efficacy of HDMP led to three randomized, double-blind, placebo-controlled trials of i.v. or oral HDMP for relapses in MS (Table 36.4). Although these studies randomized only a small number of patients and were of short duration (2–8 weeks), all three studies found a significant benefit of HDMP compared with placebo. Interestingly, in the studies by Durelli et al.[57] and Milligan et al.[99], patients who entered into the trial up to eight weeks after the onset of their relapse still experienced a significant impact on their clinical recovery when compared with placebo. A meta-analysis and a Cochrane review found convincing evidence to support the use of HDMP to treat acute relapses.[102,103]

Several randomized studies of corticosteroids have focused on the relative benefit of different preparations, dose, and routes of administration (Table 36.5). A randomized trial by Alam et al.[105] compared mean change in Disability Status Scale score (DSS) between the two groups 28 days after the start of treatment with oral vs. i.v. HDMP. There were neither significant

differences in clinical outcome nor increased gastrointestinal side effects in the patients who received oral HDMP. Barnes et al. reported a double-blind, randomized trial comparing i.v. HDMP for three days with low-dose oral MP for three weeks.[107] The authors found no significant difference in the median changes in Expanded Disability Status Scale (EDSS) score 1, 4, 12, and 24 weeks after treatment. In a study by Oliveri et al., low doses (500 mg/day for five days) and high doses (2000 mg/d for five days) of i.v. MP were compared in a double-blind, randomized fashion.[108] All patients showed improved EDSS, but there was no group difference in mean EDSS between the two doses of i.v. MP. These three studies are limited by their reliance on group mean changes in EDSS, thus reducing the power to detect a significant difference in treatments.[109] More importantly, EDSS is an ordinal scale, with unequal differences between each step, rendering mean changes in EDSS statistically inappropriate in measuring differences between groups. The study by Oliveri et al. found significant differences in magnetic resonance imaging (MRI) activity between the two doses of i.v. MP (see below), despite no evidence of clinical difference.[108] These MRI findings highlight the insensitivity of mean EDSS measures in clinical studies.

Lastly, the duration of HDMP therapy required to produce clinical benefits was assessed in a trial comparing a single

Table 36.5. *Clinical trials of different types or doses of glucocorticoids for MS relapses*

Study	Treatment regimens	N	Study design	Outcome
Bindoff et al.[104]	i.v. MP 1000 mg/day for 1 day i.v. MP 1000 mg/day for 5 days	17 15	Unblinded, randomized	Improved EDSS in the 5-day-treated group
Alam et al.[105]	i.v. MP 500 mg/day for 5 days Oral MP 500 mg/day for 5 days	20 15	Double-blind, randomized	No difference at 5 and 28 days after treatment. Side effects minor and equally distributed
La Mantia et al.[106]	i.v. MP 100 mg/day for 3 days, 500 mg/day for 3 days, 250 mg/day for 3 days, 125 mg/day for 3 days, 62.5 mg/day for 2 days i.v. MP 40 mg/day for 7 days, 20 mg/day for 4 days, 10 mg/day for 3 days i.v. dexamethasone 8 mg/day for 7 days, 4 mg/day for 4 days, 2 mg/day for 3 days	10 10 11	Double-blind, randomized	High rate of worsening in low-dose MP group during the month after treatment. Note: groups were of unequal disease duration
Barnes et al.[107]	i.v. MP 1000 mg/day for 3 days Oral MP 48 mg/day for 7 days, 24 mg/day for 7 days, 12 mg/day for 7 days	38 42	Double-blind, randomized	No significant difference in median EDSS change at 1, 4, 12, and 24 weeks after treatment
Oliveri et al.[108]	i.v. MP 2000 mg/day for 5 days i.v. MP 500 mg/day for 5 days	15 14	Double-blind, randomized with MRI	No significant difference in mean EDSS at 7, 15, 30, and 60 days. Lower MRI activity in high-dose group
Marinelli et al.[9]	i.v. MP 1000 mg/d for 5 days Oral MP 1000 mg/d for 5 days	20 20	Neurologist- and radiologist-blinded	No significant difference in reduction in number of gadolinium-enhancing lesions at 7 days

i.v. = intravenous, EDSS = Expanded Disability Status Scale, MP = methylprednisolone.

injection of 1000 mg MP vs. a five-day course of therapy.[104] The superior results of a 5-day course of therapy in this trial suggest that a 3–5-day course of HDMP may be necessary to treat MS relapses effectively.

Impact of HDMP on acute disease course

The benefits of corticosteroid treatment on long-term disease activity have only recently been addressed by clinical trials. The largest and perhaps most influential of these trials was the Optic Neuritis Treatment Trial (ONTT).[110] A total of 457 patients with acute monocular optic neuritis were randomized to acute treatment with oral prednisone (1 mg/kg/day for 14 days), i.v. HDMP (250 mg four times/day for three days followed by oral prednisone 1 mg/kg/day for 11 days), or oral placebo. The two groups receiving oral treatment alone were blinded, but patients receiving i.v. HDMP were not. Compared with placebo, i.v. HDMP resulted in more rapid recovery of vision, most evident during the first two weeks. The extent of improvement in visual field deficits, contrast sensitivity, and color vision were significantly better in the HDMP group at six months, but this difference disappeared by 12 months.[111] Over two years, the rate of recurrent optic neuritis in either eye was 14% in the HDMP group, compared with 16% in the placebo group and 30% in the oral prednisone group. This surprising result suggested that oral prednisone is associated with an increased rate of recurrent optic neuritis, although no other studies in optic neuritis or MS have confirmed this.

In subsequent reports from the ONTT, the rate of conversion to clinically definite MS was evaluated over the following two years in the 389 patients without definite or probable MS at study onset.[111–113] The i.v. HDMP group had a lower rate of conversion to clinically definite MS (7.5%) compared with the placebo (16.7%) and oral prednisone (14.7%) groups. As might be expected, most of this benefit occurred in patients with abnormal MRI scans at study entry, since this group of patients was at highest risk of a recurrent demyelinating event. This benefit on conversion to clinically definite MS was no longer evident 3–5 years after treatment, suggesting that HDMP delays the onset of clinically definite MS, but does not prevent the eventual development of the disease.

Several small prospective studies offer further evidence in support of the prolonged benefits of a single course of HDMP. In the trial by Sellebjerg et al.,[100] one-year follow-up evaluations found that the patients treated with HDMP had a greater median improvement in EDSS and were more likely to maintain an improved EDSS compared with placebo-treated patients. La Mantia et al. reported a randomized double-blind comparison of i.v. dexamethasone and i.v. MP in equivalent low doses vs. i.v. HDMP.[106] i.v. Administration was used to simplify the blinding procedure, but the lower dose preparations could have been administered orally. The authors reported a high rate of symptomatic worsening in the low-dose MP (LDMP) group during the first month after treatment with fewer LDMP patients achieving 1.0 or more step improvement in EDSS. Furthermore, there was a lower relapse rate in the HDMP group than in the

LDMP group during the year after treatment: 66% of HDMP group were relapse free, while only 13% of LDMP group were relapse-free. There was a trend towards a lower relapse rate in the HDMP group compared with the dexamethasone group.

Impact of HDMP on chronic disease course in relapsing MS

There is emerging, though still conflicting, evidence regarding the benefits of HDMP administered in pulses on the course of MS, either alone or in combination with other disease modifying therapy. Zivadinov et al. studied 88 MS patients randomly assigned to receive either regular pulses of i.v. HDMP (1000 mg/day for five days with an oral prednisone taper), or i.v. HDMP in the same fashion, but administered only for clinical relapses.[114] Pulsed HDMP was given every four months for three years, then every six months for another two years. No patients were treated with long-term immunomodulating therapies other than corticosteroids. They found that the onset of sustained EDSS worsening was significantly delayed in the routine-pulsed HDMP group compared with the relapse-only HDMP group. Both patients and examining neurologists were unblinded regarding treatment assignments, so clinical assessment should be interpreted with caution. However, pulsed HDMP was associated with a reduction in the development of brain atrophy and T1-hypointense lesions on MRI (see below), suggesting a potential neuroprotective effect.

The one-year Avonex Combination Trial (ACT) evaluated 313 RRMS patients with persistent MS disease activity despite intramuscular interferon beta-1a (IFNβ-1a).[115] Patients were randomized in a 2×2 factorial design to adjunctive weekly methotrexate 20 mg PO or placebo, with or without bimonthly IVMP 1000 mg/day for three days. Originally planned as a 24-month trial with relapses as the primary outcome for methotrexate and brain atrophy change for i.v. HDMP, the study duration was shortened to 12 months and the primary outcome changed to the number of new and enlarging T2 lesions on brain MRI because of challenges in recruitment. No significant differences were observed in either relapse rate or MS functional composite (MSFC) change between the group that received bimonthly i.v. HDMP and the group that did not receive bimonthly i.v. HDMP. Similarly, no differences were observed in new or enlarging T2 lesions (the primary outcome), Gd-enhancing lesions, and change in brain atrophy. In contrast to the complete cessation in atrophy progression with pulse i.v. HDMP observed by Zivadinov et al.,[61] the ACT study observed a 0.5% progression in atrophy over 1 year of bimonthly pulse HDMP. An explanation for the differing observations between the Zivadinov and ACT studies is not known, although differing trial durations (five years vs. one year) and study populations are two possible explanations.

Two recent trials evaluating the combination of monthly pulses of HDMP with IFNβ-1a shed further light on the potential benefits of this combination treatment. NORMINS was a randomized, placebo-controlled, double-blind trial of HDMP (200 mg oral MP daily for five days, repeated monthly for 96 weeks) or identical placebo in combination with subcutaneous IFNβ-1a 44 μg three times per week.[116] Similar to the ACT study, eligible patients were required to experience disease activity in the 12 months prior to enrollment, despite receiving treatment with subcutaneous IFNβ-1a three times per week. Enrollment for this trial was curtailed for reasons similar to the ACT trial (this was a common problem after the original approval of natalizumab) and only 66 patients were randomized to oral HDMP and 64 patients to placebo. The calculated sample size was 130 per group for 30% reduction in annualized relapse rate. Study participants were typical of well-established relapsing MS patients (age 37.8–39.5, disease duration 6.9–8 years, EDSS 2.5–2.9), though with a shorter disease duration and younger age than ACT study participants. After two years of follow-up, the mean yearly relapse rate was 0.22 for HDMP vs. 0.59 for placebo (62% reduction, 95% confidence interval (CI) 39–77%, $P < 0.0001$). The reduction in annualized relapse rate was identical in years 1 and 2. There was no significant effect on time to EDSS progression, change in MSFC scores, percent change in normalized brain volume, or the number of new or enlarging T2 MRI lesions. The change in T2 lesion volume marginally favored the HDMP group at the end of the study ($P = 0.045$).

There are many potential reasons for differences in relapse rate outcomes between the ACT and NORMINS trials, including differences in study population, length of follow-up, and the administered steroid regimens. One additional explanation is the effect of high titer neutralizing antibodies (NAbs) in the NORMINS trial: 12 of 47 patients (26%) in the HDMP arm and 16 of 46 (35%) patients in the placebo arm were found to have high titer NAbs detected at least once in the study. The amelioration of IFNβ benefit by NAbs may have given HDMP a greater opportunity to exert a beneficial effect. In support of this mechanism, there was a larger relative reduction in relapse rate by HDMP treatment noted in the subgroup of patients positive for NAbs. In contrast, only 5% of subjects in the ACT study had NAbs.

The MECOMBIN study was a multicenter, randomized, double-blind trial of HDMP (500 mg per day orally for three days monthly for 3–4 years) or matching placebo in combination with intramuscular IFNβ-1a in RRMS patients naive to previous disease-modifying therapy.[117] Three hundred and forty one RRMS patients with a recent onset of MS (mean duration of symptoms 1.2 years) were randomized to HDMP (500 mg/day oral MP for three days, repeated every month) or placebo three months after starting intramuscular IFNβ-1a and followed for 3–4 years. There was no difference between groups in the primary outcome, time to six-month, sustained EDSS progression (HR 0.879, 95 % CI 0.566–1.365, $P = 0.57$). The adjusted mean change in MSFC Z-score from baseline to study conclusion favored the HDMP group (estimated difference 0.170, 95 % CI 0.039–0.302, $P = 0.011$). Although not the primary outcome, MSFC may be a more sensitive outcome measure given the low EDSS level of study patients at entry.

This difference in MSFC scores was supported by difference in the patient reported Multiple Sclerosis Impairment Scale ($P = 0.036$). Similar to the NORMINS trial, the HDMP group experienced a significant reduction in annualized relapse rate (0.21 vs. 0.33; relative reduction 38%; $P = 0.04$). This reduction was most notable in the first year (0.24 vs. 1.29; relative reduction 81%, $P < 0.0001$) and became less apparent in years 2 and 3, perhaps as a result of the significant discontinuation rate in the HDMP group during the first year (28%) or a delayed effect of intramuscular IFNβ-1a on relapse rates. The mean number of new or enlarging T2 lesions from baseline to month 39 was reduced in the HDMP group (5.2 vs. 8.0, $P = 0.007$), but there was no difference in the absolute change in brain parenchymal fraction (−0.03 vs. −0.029).

What conclusions can be reached from the results of the aforementioned trials with regard to effect of pulse HDMP on the course of relapsing MS? First, no study has yet to confirm the results of Zivadinov et al. suggesting that long-term pulse HDMP slows disability progression and brain atrophy. Until confirmed by controlled trials, this result must be viewed with caution. Second, multiple studies in both naive patients and patients with breakthrough disease report a significant reduction in relapse rates, particularly in the first year of combined treatment. Even though the ACT study was underpowered to detect an impact on relapses, the clinical and MRI results seemed to favor the HDMP/ intramuscular IFNβ-1a arm (30 % relative reduction in relapse rate). Third, the optimal HDMP regimen is unclear. The most consistent effect on relapse rates was observed with monthly pulses of HDMP orally in doses ranging from 200 mg per day for five days to 500 mg per day for three days, but at a significant cost in terms of side effects and discontinuation rates (52% and 53% withdrawal or discontinuation rates in the HDMP arms of NORMINS and MEDCOMINS trials, respectively). Since the side effects of HDMP are rarely severe and usually manageable, if addressed prior to the onset of therapy, perhaps future studies will attempt to minimize side effects from the beginning of treatment and gradually lengthen the interval between HDMP treatments over time to minimize cumulative adverse effects of treatment. Nonetheless, the current and imminent availability of alternative long-term disease modifying therapies makes it unlikely that HDMP will receive significant future study as an adjuvant treatment to injectable MS therapies.

Impact of HDMP on chronic disease course in secondary progressive MS

A significant proportion of patients with RRMS eventually experience gradual progression of disability occurring between attacks or in the absence of attacks – the SP stage of MS. Two studies evaluated the effect of chronic intermittent corticosteroids in SPMS. (Table 36.6)

A single course of HDMP was evaluated in a double-blind, placebo-controlled trial of 35 patients with a chronic progressive MS.[101] HDMP was found to improve EDSS better than

placebo, with improvements primarily in pyramidal, cerebellar, and sensory systems. The improvement was evident after 10 days, and persisted through to the end of the study, which was 3 months.

Goodkin et al. conducted a double-blind, dose-comparison study of bimonthly i.v. HDMP "pulses" in patients with early SPMS.[118] A total of 109 patients with SPMS were randomized to pulses of i.v. HDMP (500 mg/day for three days followed by oral MP taper starting at 64 mg/day) or i.v. LDMP (10 mg/day for three days followed by oral MP starting at 10 mg/day) every eight weeks for two years. The low-dose regimen was used to improve the success of blinding, since it was anticipated that HDMP pulses would produce side effects that would unmask the patients. The primary outcome measure was the proportion of sustained treatment failures in each treatment arm at the end of the two-year study. Confirmed treatment failure was identified using criteria from a composite outcome involving EDSS, ambulatory index, nine-hole peg test, box and block test, and relapses. Treatment failure was defined as sustained (five months or longer) worsening on any component of the composite outcome measures or three relapses over a 12-month period. Survival analysis using Kaplan–Meier curves to estimate treatment failure rates over the course of the study was a pre-planned secondary analysis. Of the 108 patients who initiated therapy, 29 of 54 (53.7%) patients receiving LDMP and 21 of 54 (38.9%) patients receiving HDMP met the criteria for sustained treatment failure, a 28% reduction in the proportion of treatment failures ($P = 0.18$). The pre-planned secondary analysis, the Kaplan–Meier survival analysis, showed significant differences between groups in estimates of overall sustained treatment failure ($P = 0.04$) Methodological differences account for the slight discrepancy in statistical significance of the primary and secondary outcomes. The primary outcome analysis (the proportion of treatment failures in either arm), utilizes only the entry and exit examination data, while the secondary outcome analysis using survival techniques takes into account the time distribution of treatment failures, as well as available data on patients who dropped out of the study before two years. Therefore, survival curve analysis, which favored the HDMP group, is a more sensitive outcome.

Effects of HDMP on disease activity measured by imaging

Early studies using computed tomography (CT) imaging showed that corticosteroids produce a rapid, dose-dependent reduction in contrast enhancement in MS.[119–121] This effect is evident within eight hours, presumably represents an effect on the blood–brain barrier, and is associated with rapid clinical improvement. Resolution of contrast enhancement raised the possibility that the rapid benefits of corticosteroids therapy could be attributable to abrupt resolution of edema, followed later by reduction of inflammation. Consistent with this interpretation, i.v. mannitol was found to reduce edema rapidly but

Table 36.6. *Controlled trials of pulse HDMP to alter disease course*

Study	Treatment regimens	N	Study design	Outcome
Goodkin et al.[118]	i.v. MP 500 mg/day for 3 days, oral MP taper for 11 days starting at 64 mg/day i.v. MP 10 mg/day for 3 days, oral MP taper for 11 days starting at 10 mg/day	54 54	Double-blind, randomized	No difference in proportion of patients with progression (primary outcome), but high-dose better in time to disease progression (secondary outcome)
Zivadinov et al.[114]	i.v. MP 1000 mg/day for 5 days, repeated every four months for 3 years, then every six months for 2 more years i.v. MP for relapses only	43 45	Unblinded except for image analysis	Lower proportion of patients with EDSS progression, fewer T1 holes, and no atrophy progression in pulse IVMP group
Cohen et al.[115]	IM IFNβ-1a with i.v. MP 1000 mg/d for 3 days, repeated every 2 months with for one year, with or without methotrexate Intramuscular IFNβ-1a without i.v. MP, with or without methotrexate	150 161	Neurologist- and radiologist-blinded	No difference in relapse rate, MS functional composite change, new or enlarging T2 lesions, gadolinium-enhancing lesions, or atrophy progression.
Sorensen, et al.[116]	Subcutaneous IFNβ-1a with 200 mg oral MP daily for 5 days, repeated every month for 2 years Subcutaneous IFNβ-1a with placebo daily for 5 days, repeated every 4 weeks for 2 years	66 64	Double-blind, randomized, with separate treating and evaluating neurologists	Reduction in mean annual relapse rate in MP-treated group, although 22% drop-out rate.
Ravnborg, et al.[117]	Intramuscular IFNβ-1a for 3 months, followed by 500 mg/day oral MP for 3 days, repeated every month for 3–4 years Intramuscular IFNβ-1a for 3 months, followed by oral placebo daily for 3 days, repeated every month for 3–4 years	172 169	Double-blind, randomized, with separate treating and evaluating neurologists Note: all patients were treatment-naive	No difference in time to sustained progression of disability

EDSS = Expanded Disability Status Scale, IFNβ = interferon beta, i.v. = intravenous, MP = methylprednisolone.

improvement in MS symptoms was only transient. In contrast, corticosteroids reduced CT contrast enhancement and clinical symptoms for up to four months.[121,122]

Studies over the past decade found that HDMP produces a rapid reduction in Gd-enhancement on MRI. There is an 84%–96% reduction in Gd-enhancement within 1–4 days after treatment, and this effect correlates with clinical improvement.[123–127] However, some lesions can re-enhance within days of treatment, and new lesions can develop within one month of treatment, despite continued clinical improvement.[124] Although the effects of a course of MP can persist up to 9.7 weeks,[125] some studies have observed that HDMP does not prevent Gd-enhancing lesions from progressing into permanent lesions and does not reduce the overall lesion burden.[128]

The above studies suggested that HDMP has only transient effects on Gd-enhancement and inflammation. However, more recent studies with longer follow-up or using a randomized, placebo-controlled design have found otherwise. A study by Smith et al. followed nine patients with RRMS using monthly Gd-enhanced MRI scans in a natural history study.[129] They found increased total numbers of Gd-enhancing lesions and increased total area of enhancement in the month that preceded clinical worsening. HDMP treatment resulted in a 33% reduction in new lesions over the subsequent six months.

A second study by Oliveri et al. was a double-blind, randomized comparison of two doses of i.v. HDMP (500 mg for five days vs. 2000 mg for five days) using Gd-enhanced MRI obtained at baseline and at 7, 15, 30, and 60 days after the beginning of treatment as the main outcome measure.[108] Both doses of MP resulted in early dramatic reduction in the number of Gd-enhancing lesions followed by a rebound of Gd-enhancing lesions at day 15. However, there was a significant dose-dependent reduction in the total number of Gd-enhancing lesions over the course of the study, and this difference was evident at each time point from day 15 to day 60. These two studies suggest that HDMP has an impact on subsequent MRI disease activity, and that this impact is dose dependent.

A recent study by Martinelli et al. evaluated the effect of oral vs. i.v. HDMP on MRI evidence of active inflammation.[9] Five days of 1000 mg/day i.v. HDMP was compared with five days of 500 mg oral MP given twice a day. All patients were given sucralfate to help with gastrointestinal side effects. No difference was seen in the proportional reduction of Gd-enhancing lesions between the two MP preparations at either week 1 (the primary outcome) or week 4. In addition, there was no difference in the number of new T2 lesions. Both regimens were well tolerated, although dysgeusia was reported more often with oral

MP ($P = 0.05$), and one patient (5%) stopped oral MP because of persistent heartburn and required omerprazole treatment.

The study by Zivadinov *et al.* (see above) suggested that patients receiving intermittent pulses of HDMP had no significant progression of brain atrophy and T1 hypointense lesions over five years, although the short ACT trial did not find a treatment effect on atrophy.[114,115] Neither study observed an impact of intermittent pulse i.v. HDMP on T2 lesions. It is important to recognize that a transient decrease in brain volume can be seen following a course of HDMP, suggesting that brain atrophy measures shortly after HDMP need to be interpreted cautiously.[130–132]

Further support for a possible neuroprotective effect of HDMP therapy comes from studies assessing tissue integrity utilizing magnetization transfer ratio (MTR) analysis. Architectural disruption from inflammation and tissue destruction reduces the transfer of magnetization from tissue structures to free water, which thereby reduces the MTR as measured by MRI. Measurements of MTR are thought to reflect the general tissue integrity, and MTR measurements have been used in MS studies to assess recovery of lesions as well as impact of the disease on normal-appearing white matter. Seventy six Gd-enhancing lesions were studied in a group of MS patients receiving i.v. HDMP (1000 mg/day for five days) and compared with 109 lesions in untreated patients.[133] Recovery of MTR was greater in the HDMP-treated lesions than in the untreated lesions, suggesting that HDMP reduced tissue damage and promoted lesion recovery.

Another study evaluated the effect of corticosteroids on optic nerve cross-sectional area measured by MRI.[134] 66 patients with unilateral optic neuritis were randomized to receive either HDMP (1000 mg/day for three days) or placebo infusion, and clinical and imaging studies were repeated six months later. Optic nerves with neuritis demonstrated progressive atrophy averaging 11% over six months, compared to 2% in unaffected optic nerves. Patients randomized to HDMP demonstrated 14% atrophy progression in optic nerve with neuritis, compared to only 8% in placebo-treated patients, although this difference was not statistically significant. However, there was no association between optic nerve atrophy and clinical measures (visual acuity, visual evoked potentials), which suggests that optic nerve atrophy may not be a valid surrogate measure of permanent optic nerve injury in optic neuritis.

A study of MR spectroscopy after HDMP observed an increased *N*-acetylaspartate (NAA) to creatine (Cr) ratio within both Gd-enhancing and non-enhancing lesions following therapy.[135] This increased NAA/Cr ratio was observed over a three-week period following HDMP treatment and suggests an improved tissue structure over that time period.

The above studies suggest a rationale for pulsed HDMP treatment as a form of disease-modifying therapy in RRMS. However, the negative outcome of the ACT trial and availability of alternative therapies with demonstrated efficacy in RRMS argue against the routine use of pulse HDMP for the treatment of RRMS. Nonetheless, HDMP concurrent with standard long-term MS therapies appears safe and may have some modest synergistic benefits. In a one-year cross-over design utilizing monthly MRI scans as an outcome measure, 68 patients with RRMS were followed for six months before therapy and then for six months after starting IFNβ-1a.[133] Relapses were treated with HDMP (1000 mg/day for six days). When HDMP was administered during the six-month baseline period, there was a brief decline in Gd-enhancing lesions during the first month after HDMP treatment, but then an increase in the second and third months. When HDMP was given during IFNβ-1a treatment, there was a similar decline in Gd-enhancing lesions during the first month after HDMP, but this decline persisted over the next two months.

In summary, several studies provide imaging evidence supporting the use of HDMP as an acute treatment to reduce inflammatory MS disease activity. Additional imaging studies suggest HDMP can improve imaging measure of tissue integrity. However, a large, placebo-controlled trial in RRMS failed to demonstrate a benefit of routine pulses of HDMP in RRMS, suggesting pulse HDMP is not effective in the long-term control of active inflammation in RRMS.

High-dose MP for anti-interferon neutralizing antibodies

NAbs against IFNβ reduce the efficacy of exogenously administered IFNβ.[136–138] The immunomodulatory effect of corticosteroids may alter the prevalence and persistence of anti-IFNβ NAbs. Ravnborg *et al.* treated 13 NAb-positive patients with 500 mg MP i.v. daily for three days, repeated monthly for six months, along with azathioprine 5 mg/kg/day. Anti-IFNβ NAb outcome was measured by in vivo myxovirus resistance protein A (MxA) mRNA response.[139] Comparison was to 14 anti-IFNβ NAb-positive patients who did not receive pulse HDMP treatment. Of the 11 HDMP-treated patients who completed the trial, only two regained MxA-mRNA response, compared to one untreated control.

Hesse *et al.* treated 38 NAb-positive patients who discontinued IFNβ with 500 mg oral MP daily for three days and repeated monthly for six months.[140] The comparison group was 35 NAb-positive patients who discontinued IFNβ but declined HDMP. At six months, eight or 38 treated patients regained in vivo response to IFNβ, as measured by MxA, while only four of 35 untreated patients regained response to IFNβ ($P = 0.35$). Although this was a 50% increase in subjects with regained response to IFNβ, the difference was not significant.

Cohen *et al.* evaluated the effect of HDMP on NAbs in the ACT study using a two-step test: an enzyme-linked immunosorbent assay (ELISA), followed by cytopathic effect assay (see above for trial description).[115] They observed a reduction in anti-IFNβ NAbs in the pulse HDMP-treated patients compared to non-HDMP-treated patients at both six and 12 months of treatment ($P < 0.02$). The ACT study was underpowered to evaluate whether this reduction in anti-IFNβ Nabs was associated with change in MS disease activity. In the NORMINS trial,[116] which evaluated the effect of pulse HDMP in combination with subcutaneous IFNβ-1a 44 μg three times a week (an IFNβ regimen associated with a high incidence of NAbs), NAbs were found in 23% of HDMP-treated patients and 30% of placebo-treated patients. Although this difference was not dramatic, a meaningful improvement in IFN biologic effect was suggested by the absence of a deleterious effect of NAbs in HDMP-treated patients (as measured by relapse rate and new brain lesions), but a significant deleterious effect of NAbs in placebo-treated patients.

A case series reported the effect of HDMP on three patients with anti-IFNβ NAbs.[141] Treatment with 1000 mg/day i.v. MP for five days followed by 1000 mg monthly for one year was associated with a restoration of IFNβ bioactivity. Two additional patients had binding antibodies to IFNβ, which is associated with an 85% risk of developing NAbs. After one year of the same HDMP treatment, binding antibody titers were reduced and neither patient had developed NAbs.

HDMP may have an effect on the development of anti-IFNβ NAbs. In a randomized, controlled trial, monthly pulses of 1000 mg MP decreased the development of NAbs by over 50%.[142] The MECOMBIN study did not report the impact of HDMP on the development of NAbs in previously treatment-naive patients.

Altogether, these studies suggest a possible modest beneficial effect of HDMP on both the development and persistence of NAbs, as well as the deleterious impact of NAbs.

Toxicity of high-dose MP

Side effects of HDMP are listed in Table 36.7. Much of corticosteroid toxicity is probably related to the daily dose, total cumulative dose, and the frequency of administration. In general, corticosteroid toxicity is reduced with short-term "pulsed" administration of HDMP (1000 mg/day for (3–5 days).[143–146] Osteoporosis, aseptic osteonecrosis, Cushingoid features, infections, and suppression of the hypothalamus–pituitary–adrenal (HPA) axis are rare with 3–5 day-pulses of HDMP. The function of the HPA axis was studied in 10 MS patients during and after therapy with HDMP (1000 mg/d for seven days, without subsequent corticosteroid taper). ACTH response was normal, and cortisol response was suppressed only on the first day after ending therapy but recovered two days later.

The impact of many of the common side effects of HDMP can be minimized with proper education. One of the most common side effects is a feeling of well-being or mild euphoria, both of which are often welcomed by the patients and does not require treatment. Moderate to severe anxiety and irritability, especially in newly diagnosed MS patients, is common and should be treated with reassurance and a short-acting anxiolytic medication, if needed. Manic episodes or psychosis are rare and may be avoided in future treatment courses by pre-medication with a phenothiazine antipsychotic or lithium carbonate.[147] Despite the typical activating effects of HDMP, a small study found that compared to daytime treatment,

Table 36.7. *Side effects associated with high-dose methylprednisolone treatment*

Side effects occurring during therapy
Insomnia and mild euphoria
Anxiety
Metallic taste during infusion
Increased appetite and weight gain
Flushing and increased sweating
Headache
Mylagia
Decreased short-term memory
Gastrointestinal upset or pain[b]
Easy bruising[a]
Mania or psychosis[a]
Nausea or vomiting[a]
Pancreatitis[a]
Cardiac arrhythmias[a]
Glaucoma[a]
Intractable hiccups[a]
Hepatitis[a]

Side effects occurring early in patients with underlying risk factors
Peptic ulcer disease
Diabetes mellitus
Hypertension
Acne
Depression

Side effects occurring with repeated use[c]
Osteoporosis
Osteonecrosis, including asymptomatic avascular necrosis
Posterior subcapsular cataracts
Fatty liver
Cushingoid features
Infection diathesis
Impaired healing

[a] rare.
[b] more common with oral administration.
[c] rare compared with chronic daily or alternate day therapy.

nighttime treatment was associated with fewer side effects, greater clinical recovery, and greater preference by patients.[148]

Depression is uncommon, but occurs more frequently than psychosis. Depression can be minimized with judicial co-administration of antidepressants in high-risk patients or patients with a history of depression during corticosteroid therapy. Insomnia is frequent, and many patients benefit from a short-acting sedative-hypnotic. Most other acute side effects require only education, symptomatic treatment if they occur, and dietary modifications for increased appetite. We have found it useful for patients to receive their first dose of HDMP under outpatient medical supervision. This supervision helps with medication educations as well as monitoring and management of side effects. Subsequent doses can be safely administered in the patient's home unless there is a medical contraindication (e.g. cardiac condition, diabetes mellitus). Anaphylactoid reactions are very rare.[149,150] IgE antibodies specific for methylprednisolone succinate were found in one such patient, with skin prick test cross-reactivity with prednisolone succinate.[151] IgE antibodies and positive skin tests confirmed the diagnosis of anaphylactic reaction and suggested succinate as the antigenic culprit. The same patient and one other were treated with prednisolone without ester and i.v. betamethasone without any allergic reactions, further confirming the antigenicity of succinate and providing a treatment alternative for such patients.[151,152] Sensitization protocols are available for those with severe allergic reactions to i.v. HDMP but require admission to an intensive care monitoring unit for each treatment.

Side effects associated with repeated pulses of HDMP were assessed in a study by Goodkin et al.[118] Adverse effects were significantly more frequent in the HDMP than in the LDMP group. Nevertheless, cessation of study drug because of side effects occurred in only one patient. Dose-dependent side effects attributable to HDMP included weight-gain (32% on HDMP, 13% on LDMP), insomnia (35% HDMP, 6% LDMP), depression (26% HDMP, 6% LDMP), infections (39% HDMP, 20% LDMP), and headache (26% HDMP, 13% LDMP). Most of the infections were of the lower urinary tract. Serious adverse effects related to drug were rare and included psychosis, compression fracture, and possibly aseptic meningitis. Only the patient who developed psychosis required treatment cessation.

Two studies have observed a significant impact of HDMP on memory. Thirty patients were studied after receiving HDMP for optic neuritis and MS and were found to have reversible impairment of long-term memory, with relatively spared short-term memory, attention, and alertness.[153] Another study not only confirmed these findings, but also showed that they reversed after two months and were not related to dose of MP (500 mg/day vs. 2000 mg/day, each for five days).[154]

The relative risk of osteoporosis in MS patients treated with repeated pulses of HDMP is highly relevant since bone mineral density (BMD) is decreased and the incidence of fractures is increased in MS patients.[155] Furthermore, HDMP infusions in MS patients are associated with an immediate fall in markers of bone formation and increase in bone resorption.[104,105] Although only one patient experienced a fracture in the study by Goodkin et al., patients were not monitored for osteoporosis.[118] One recent study found no relationship between single or repeated pulses of HDMP and BMD of the lumbar spine or femoral head in MS patients.[158] In fact, BMD of the lumbar spine increased 66 months after a pulse of HDMP, presumably owing to improved mobility with treatment. This finding is consistent with a reported association between low BMD and decreased mobility.[155] It is possible that improved mobility with pulses of HDMP, especially in premenopausal women with MS, may offset declines in BMD related to corticosteroid use. In support of the limited effects of HDMP, markers of bone metabolism normalizes within two weeks of cessation of corticosteroids.[157] This normalization was despite 10 days of HDMP followed by 9 days of oral prednisone. Two relatively large clinical trials of pulse HDMP in combination with IFNβ-1a suggest no effect or minimal effect of monthly HDMP for up to three years on either fracture risk or BMD.[116,117] However, it is important to remember the potential risk of both symptomatic and asymptomatic avascular necrosis (AVN) in MS patients treated with pulse HDMP. One MRI study of steroid-treated MS patients reported that 15.5% of steroid-treated MS patients had

evidence for asymptomatic AVN, while no cases of AVN were found in a non-steroid-treated MS control group.[159]

A study of rheumatoid arthritis patients evaluated the change in BMD and serum biomarkers of osteoporosis in a group of 31 subjects receiving HDMP (1000 mg/day on three alternate days) averaging every 76 days. They found no decline in BMD or serum biomarkers at 6 and 12 months, while control subjects receiving daily corticosteroids demonstrated significant decline in BMD.[160]

Current evidence suggests that pulse HDMP does not significantly reduce BMD in relapsing MS patients but the risk of other osseous complications such as AVN persists. It is still unknown whether certain populations are more vulnerable to BMD loss, particularly those with more disability or older age at onset of therapy. Although additional studies are needed, recommendations for preventing corticosteroid-induced osteoporosis can be made at this time based on guidelines developed by the American College of Rheumatology.[161] Patients starting "pulses" therapy with HDMP should have measurements of BMD in the lumbar spine and femoral heads and should begin vitamin D supplement (50 000 units three times/week) and calcium supplementation to achieve a total daily calcium intake of 1500 mg/day. Patients should be advised to stop smoking and to limit alcohol intake. Regular stretching, strengthening, and aerobic exercise should be instituted to optimize mobility. Additional treatments should be determined by the degree of loss of bone mineral density and directed by a clinician familiar with the treatment of osteoporosis.

Implications for practice

Altogether, numerous clinical and MRI studies suggest that HDMP not only has transient beneficial effects on clinical relapses and established areas of inflammation and demyelination, but may also have a prolonged, dose-dependent benefit involving early events in MS lesion formation, lesion propagation, and lesion recovery. The clinical effectiveness includes acute treatment of relapse in RRMS, chronic treatment of RRMS in combination with IFNβ, and possibly long-term treatment in SPMS. The benefit from a single course of HDMP (i.e. 3–5 days of treatment) lasts for up to six months by MRI measures, and possibly even several years by clinical measures.[108,110] Repeated courses of treatment can be given safely to both RRMS and SPMS patients, although there is a high treatment discontinuation rate due to HDMP side effects, particularly if not managed aggressively from onset of treatment. Further studies on management of HDMP side effects are warranted, given the lack of current consensus and the wide variety of strategies employed by clinicians, all of questionable benefit.

Treatment effects of pulse HDMP in combination with IFNβ include a reduction of relapse rates relative to IFNβ monotherapy in both naive patients and those with breakthrough disease on IFNβ monotherapy. There are modest, inconsistent effects on the development of new T2 lesions, but no effect on the development of sustained disability progression or brain atrophy in RRMS. There are inconsistent data suggesting that pulse HDMP treatment in combination with IFNβ may decrease the risk of developing NAbs and may be associated with a modest reduction in established NAbs against IFNβ.[162] The clinical significance of this effect and the potential to improve IFNβ treatment outcomes by initiating treatment in combination with pulse HDMP, especially when using IFNβ preparations known to be associated with a high rate of NAb formation, requires further study. As more new long-term disease modifying therapies become available, interest in adding HDMP to MS patients with NAbs to IFNβ will likely wane.

Pulse HDMP monotherapy in SPMS requires further study. The study by Goodkin et al. suggests that bimonthly pulses of HDMP (500 mg/day for three days) delays development of disability progression with few significant side effects in secondary progressive patients. In a population of patients who have few treatment options, bimonthly pulses of HDMP appears to be a reasonable treatment option.[118] Further studies are needed to assess the effects of HDMP on the neurodegenerative aspects of progressive MS. HDMP has also been found to be useful in uveitis associated with MS, so the use of HDMP in MS patients may broaden over time.[163]

The optimal dose, route, and frequency of administration for HDMP are unknown. Doses ranging from 500 to 2000 mg/day (i.v. or oral) for 3–5 days have been found to hasten recovery from MS relapses, whereas a single dose of HDMP treatment was found to be minimally effective. One study using 2000 mg/day for five days raised the possibility that doses in excess of 1000 mg/day may be more effective in altering subsequent disease activity. Further studies will hopefully clarify

these issues. In the interim, doses of 500–2000 mg/day (i.v. or oral) for 3–5 days are appropriate for the treatment of MS relapses associated with functional decline. Conventional doses of oral corticosteroids, such as the regimen studied by Barnes et al.,[107] cannot be currently recommended, although further studies of oral corticosteroids use would help clarify the issue. Similarly, there is no evidence that the commonly prescribed single dose of HDMP once monthly is of benefit in either RRMS or SPMS. However, pulse HDMP doses ranging from 200 mg orally for five days monthly to 1000 mg i.v. for three days every two months may be beneficial at reducing relapse rates with concurrent IFNβ therapy.

It is likely that the results of the ONTT[110] can be generalized to other isolated monosymptomatic demyelinating syndromes. The risk of subsequent relapse appears similar between patients with a clinically isolated inflammatory episode of optic neuritis and patients with other monosymptomatic demyelinating syndromes such as transverse myelitis or brainstem syndromes.[164,165] Therefore, such patients are likely to experience the same temporary disease-modifying benefit from HDMP as optic neuritis patients do. More importantly, monosymptomatic patients are not likely to receive significant benefit from LD corticosteroids, which should be avoided in the absence of further controlled clinical trials.

Ongoing studies are evaluating the effect of novel formulations of HD corticosteroids, including polyethylene glycol (PEG)-coated long-circulating liposomes, which may improve pharmacodynamics and increase targeting of drug to the central nervous system, thus decreasing the known side effect profile of corticosteroids.[166]

References

1. Schimmer BP, Parker KL. Adrenocorticotropic hormone, adrenocortical steroids and their synthetic analogs, inhibitors of the synthesis and actions of hormones. In Hardman JG, Limbird LE, eds. *Goodman and Gilman's Pharmacological Basic of Therapeutics.* New York: McGraw-Hill, 1996: 1459–85.

2. Vree TB, Lagerwerf AJ, Verwey-van Wissen CP, Jongen PJ. High-performance liquid chromatography analysis, preliminary pharmacokinetics, metabolism and renal excretion of methylprednisolone with its C6 and C20 hydroxy metabolites in multiple sclerosis patients receiving high-dose pulse therapy. *J Chromatog B, Biomed Sci Appl* 1999;732:337–48.

3. Pardridge WM, Mietus LJ. Transport of steroid hormones through the rat blood-brain barrier. Primary role of albumin-bound hormone. *J Clin Invest* 1979;64:145–54.

4. Defer GL, Barrâe J, Ledudal P, Tillement JP, Degos JD. Methylprednisolone infusion during acute exacerbation of MS: plasma and CSF concentrations. *Eur Neurol* 1995;35:143–8.

5. Hayball PJ, Cosh DG, Ahern MJ, Schultz DW, Roberts-Thomson PJ. High dose oral methylprednisolone in patients with rheumatoid arthritis: pharmacokinetics and clinical response. *Eur J Clin Pharmacol* 1992;42:85–8.

6. Narang PK, Wilder R, Chatterji DC, Yeager RL, Gallelli JF. Systemic bioavailability and pharmacokinetics of methylprednisolone in patients with rheumatoid arthritis following 'high-dose' pulse administration. *Biopharm Drug Dispos* 1983;4:233–48.

7. Chassard D, Banzet O, Lamy F, Gordin J, Viveash D, Thâebault JJ. Tolâerance

gastro-duodâenale de la mâethylprednisolone. Etude de la voie orale versus voie veineuse chez le volontaire sain. *Presse Med* 1994;23:515–17.

8. Metz LM, Sabuda D, Hilsden RJ, Enns R, Meddings JB. Gastric tolerance of high-dose pulse oral prednisone in multiple sclerosis. *Neurology* 1999;53:2093–6.

9. Martinelli V, Rocca MA, Annovazzi P, et al. A short-term randomized MRI study of high-dose oral vs intravenous methylprednisolone in MS. *Neurology* 2009;73:1842–8.

10. Hollenberg SM, Weinberger C, Ong ES, et al. Primary structure and expression of a functional human glucocorticoid receptor cDNA. *Nature* 1985;318:635–41.

11. Smith DF, Toft DO. Steroid receptors and their associated proteins. *Mol Endocrinol* 1993;7:4–11.

12. Boumpas DT, Chrousos GP, Wilder RL, Cupps TR, Balow JE. Glucocorticoid therapy for immune-mediated diseases: Basic and clinical correlates. *Ann Intern Med* 1993;119:1198–208.

13. Diamond MI, Miner JN, Yoshinaga SK, Yamamoto KR. Transcription factor interactions: selectors of positive or negative regulation from a single DNA element. *Science* 1990;249:1266–72.

14. Ing NH, O'Malley BW. The steroid hormone receptor superfamily: molecular mechanisms of action. In Weintraub BD, ed. *Molecular Endocrinology: Basic Concepts and Clinical Correlations*. Raven Press, 1995: 195–215.

15. Rousseau GG. Control of gene expression by glucocorticoid hormones. *Biochem J* 1984;224:1–12.

16. Borski RJ. Nongenomic membrane actions of glucocorticoids in vertebrates. *Trends Endocrinol Metab* 2000;11:427–36.

17. Jonat C, Rahmsdorf HJ, Park KK, *et al.* Antitumor promotion and antiinflammation: down-modulation of AP-1 (Fos/Jun) activity by glucocorticoid hormone. *Cell* 1990;62:1189–204.

18. Planey SL, Litwack G. Glucocorticoid-induced apoptosis in lymphocytes. *Biochem Biophys Res Commun* 2000;279:307–12.

19. Crockard AD, Treacy MT, Droogan AG, McNeill TA, Hawkins SA. Transient immunomodulation by intravenous methylprednisolone treatment of multiple sclerosis. *Mult Scler* 1995;1:20–4.

20. Fauci AS, Dale DC, Balow JE. Glucosorticoid therapy: Mechanisms of action and clinical considerations. *Ann Intern Med* 1976;84:304–15.

21. Trotter JL, Garvey WF. Prolonged effects of large-dose methylprednisolone infusion in multiple sclerosis. *Neurology* 1980;30:702–8.

22. Almawi WY, Beyhum HN, Rahme AA, Rieder MJ. Regulation of cytokine and cytokine receptor expression by glucocorticoids. *J Leukoc Biol* 1996;60:563–72.

23. Joyce DA, Steer JH, Abraham LJ. Glucocorticoid modulation of human monocyte/macrophage function: control of TNF-alpha secretion. *Inflamm Res* 1997;46:447–51.

24. Gayo A, Mozo L, Suâarez A, Tuänon A, Lahoz C, Gutiâerrez C. Glucocorticoids increase IL-10 expression in multiple sclerosis patients with acute relapse. *J Neuroimmunol* 1998;85:122–30.

25. Wandinger KP, Wessel K, Trillenberg P, Heindl N, Kirchner H. Effect of high-dose methylprednisolone administration on immune functions in multiple sclerosis patients. *Acta Neurol Scand* 1998;97:359–65.

26. Eggert M, Goertsches R, Seeck U, Dilk S, Neeck G, Zettl UK. Changes in the activation level of NF-kappa B in lymphocytes of MS patients during glucocorticoid pulse therapy. *J Neurol Sci* 2008;264: 145–50.

27. Crockard AD, Treacy MT, Droogan AG, Hawkins SA. Methylprednisolone attenuates interferon-beta induced expression of HLA-DR on monocytes. *J Neuroimmunol* 1996;70:29–35.

28. Lujâan S, Masjuan J, Roldâan E, Villar LM, Gonzâalez-Porquâe P, Alvarez-Cermeäno JC. The expression of integrins on activated T-cells in multiple sclerosis. Effect of intravenous methylprednisolone treatment. *Mult Scler* 1998;4:239–42.

29. Ossege LM, Sindern E, Voss B, Malin JP. Corticosteroids induce expression of transforming-growth-factor-beta1 mRNA in peripheral blood mononuclear cells of patients with multiple sclerosis. *J Neuroimmunol* 1998;84:1–6.

30. Gelati M, Lamperti E, Dufour A, *et al.* IL-10 production in multiple sclerosis patients, SLE patients and healthy controls: preliminary findings. *Ital J Neurol Sci* 1997;18:191–4.

31. Braitch M, Harikrishnan S, Robins RA, *et al.* Glucocorticoids increase CD4CD25 cell percentage and Foxp3 expression in patients with multiple sclerosis. *Acta Neurol Scand* 2009;119:239–45.

32. Bielecki B, Mazurek A, Wolinski P, Glabinski A. Treatment of multiple sclerosis with methylprednisolone and mitoxantrone modulates the expression of CXC chemokine receptors in PBMC. *J Clin Immunol* 2008;28:122–30.

33. Michalowska-Wender G, Losy J, Szczucinski A, Biernacka-Lukanty J, Wender M. Effect of methylprednisolone treatment on expression of sPECAM-1 and CXCL10

34. Petelin Z, Brinar V, Petravic D, Zurak N, Dubravcic K, Batinic D. CD95/Fas expression on peripheral blood T lymphocytes in patients with multiple sclerosis: effect of high-dose methylprednisolone therapy. *Clin Neurol Neurosurg* 2004;106:259–62.

35. Martâinez-Câaceres EM, Barrau MA, Brieva L, Espejo C, Barberáa N, Montalban X. Treatment with methylprednisolone in relapses of multiple sclerosis patients: immunological evidence of immediate and short-term but not long-lasting effects. *Clin Exp Immunol* 2002;127:165–71.

36. Navarro J, Aristimuno C, Sanchez-Ramon S, *et al.* Circulating dendritic cells subsets and regulatory T-cells at multiple sclerosis relapse: differential short-term changes on corticosteroids therapy. *J Neuroimmunol* 2006;176:153–61.

37. Leussink VI, Jung S, Merschdorf U, Toyka KV, Gold R. High-dose methylprednisolone therapy in multiple sclerosis induces apoptosis in peripheral blood leukocytes. *Arch Neurol* 2001;58:91–7.

38. Loughlin AJ, Woodroofe MN, Cuzner ML. Modulation of interferon-gamma-induced major histocompatibility complex class II and Fc receptor expression on isolated microglia by transforming growth factor-beta 1, interleukin-4, noradrenaline and glucocorticoids. *Immunology* 1993;79:125–30.

39. Kirk PF, Williams JD, Petersen MM, Compston DA. The effect of methylprednisolone on monocyte eicosanoid production in patients with multiple sclerosis. *J Neurol* 1994;241:427–31.

40. Ruiz P, Gomez F, King M, Lopez R, Darby C, Schreiber AD. In vivo glucocorticoid modulation of guinea pig splenic macrophage Fc gamma receptors. *J Clin Invest* 1991;88:149–57.

41. Cupps TR, Gerrard TL, Falkoff RJ, Whalen G, Fauci AS. Effects of in vitro corticosteroids on B cell activation, proliferation, and differentiation. *J Clin Invest* 1985;75:754–61.

42. Gold R, Pepinsky RB, Zettl UK, Toyka KV, Hartung HP. Lipocortin-1 (annexin-1) suppresses activation of

chemokine in serum of MS patients. *Pharmacol Rep* 2006;58:920–3.

autoimmune T cell lines in the Lewis rat. *J Neuroimmunol* 1996;69:157–64.

43. Crofford LJ, Wilder RL, Ristimèaki AP, *et al.* Cyclooxygenase-1 and -2 expression in rheumatoid synovial tissues. Effects of interleukin-1 beta, phorbol ester, and corticosteroids. *J Clin Invest* 1994;93:1095–101.

44. Xu J, Chen S, Chen H, *et al.* STAT5 mediates antiapoptotic effects of methylprednisolone on oligodendrocytes. *J Neurosci* 2009;29:2022–6.

45. Gelati M, Corsini E, Dufour A, *et al.* Reduced adhesion of PBMNCs to endothelium in methylprednisolone-treated MS patients: preliminary results. *Acta Neurol Scand* 1997;96:283–92.

46. Cronstein BN, Kimmel SC, Levin RI, Martiniuk F, Weissmann G. A mechanism for the antiinflammatory effects of corticosteroids: the glucocorticoid receptor regulates leukocyte adhesion to endothelial cells and expression of endothelial-leukocyte adhesion molecule 1 and intercellular adhesion molecule 1. *Proc Natl Acad Sci USA* 1992;89:9991–5.

47. Elovaara I, Lèallèa M, Spêare E, Lehtimèaki T, Dastidar P. Methylprednisolone reduces adhesion molecules in blood and cerebrospinal fluid in patients with MS. *Neurology* 1998;51:1703–8.

48. Gelati M, Corsini E, Dufour A, *et al.* High-dose methylprednisolone reduces cytokine-induced adhesion molecules on human brain endothelium. *Can J Neurol Sci* 2000;27:241–4.

49. Kraus J, Oschmann P, Engelhardt B, *et al.* Soluble and cell surface ICAM-3 in blood and cerebrospinal fluid of patients with multiple sclerosis: influence of methylprednisolone treatment and relevance as markers for disease activity. *Acta Neurol Scand* 2000;101:135–9.

50. Rosenberg GA, Dencoff JE, Correa N, Jr., Reiners M, Ford CC. Effect of steroids on CSF matrix metalloproteinases in multiple sclerosis: relation to blood-brain barrier injury. *Neurology* 1996;46:1626–32.

51. Mirowska D, Wicha W, Czlonkowski A, Czlonkowska A, Weber F. Increase of matrix metalloproteinase-9 in peripheral blood of multiple sclerosis patients treated with high doses of methylprednisolone. *J Neuroimmunol* 2004;146:171–5.

52. Gelati M, Corsini E, De Rossi M, *et al.* Methylprednisolone acts on peripheral blood mononuclear cells and endothelium in inhibiting migration phenomena in patients with multiple sclerosis. *Arch Neurol* 2002;59:774–80.

53. Jalosinski M, Karolczak K, Mazurek A, Glabinski A. The effects of methylprednisolone and mitoxantrone on CCL5-induced migration of lymphocytes in multiple sclerosis. *Acta Neurol Scand* 2008;118:120–5.

54. Ozkan S, Uzuner N, Kutlu C, Ozbabalik D, Ozdemir G. The effect of methylprednisolone treatment on cerebral reactivity in patients with multiple sclerosis. *J Clin Neurosci* 2006;13:214–17.

55. Compston DAS, Milligan NM, Hughes PJ, *et al.* A double-blind controlled trial of high dose methylprednisolone in patients with multiple sclerosis: 2. laboratory results. *J Neurol Neurosurg Psychiatry* 1987;50:517–22.

56. Durelli L, Poccardi G, Cavallo R. CD8+ high CD11b+ low T cells (T suppressor-effectors) in multiple sclerosis cerebrospinal fluid are increased during high dose corticosteroid treatment. *J Neuroimmunol* 1991;31:221–8.

57. Durelli L, Cocito D, Riccio A, Barile C, *et al.* High-dose intravenous methylprednisolone in the treatment of multiple sclerosis: Clinical-immunologic correlations. *Neurology* 1986;36:238–43.

58. Anderson TJ, Donaldson IM, Sheat JM, George PM. Methylprednisolone in multiple sclerosis exacerbation: changes in CSF parameters. *Aust N Z J Med.* 1990;20:794–7.

59. Sellebjerg F, Christiansen M, Jensen J, Frederiksen JL. Immunological effects of oral high-dose methylprednisolone in acute optic neuritis and multiple sclerosis. *Eur J Neurol* 2000;7:281–9.

60. Wang HY, Matsui M, Araya S, Onai N, Matsushima K, Saida T. Immune parameters associated with early treatment effects of high-dose intravenous methylprednisolone in multiple sclerosis. *J Neurol Sci* 2003;216:61–6.

61. Warren KG, Catz I, Jeffrey VM, Carroll DJ. Effect of methylprednisolone on CSF IgG parameters, myelin basic protein and antimyelin basic protein in multiple sclerosis exacerbations. *Can J Neurol Sci* 1986;13:25–30.

62. Barkhof F, Frequin STFM, Hommes OR, *et al.* A correlative triad of gadolinium-DPTA MRI, EDSS, and CSF-MBP in relapsing multiple sclerosis patients treated with high-dose intravenous methylprednisolone. *Neurology* 1992;42:63–7.

63. Franciotta D, Piccolo G, Zardini E, Bergamaschi R, Cosi V. Soluble CD8 and ICAM-1 in serum and CSF of MS patients treated with 6-methylprednisolone. *Acta Neurol Scand* 1997;95:275–9.

64. Trojano M, Avolio C, Simone IL, *et al.* Soluble intercellular adhesion molecule-1 in serum and cerebrospinal fluid of clinically active relapsing-remitting multiple sclerosis: correlation with Gd-DTPA magnetic resonance imaging-enhancement and cerebrospinal fluid findings. *Neurology* 1996;47:1535–41.

65. Spuler S, Yousry T, Scheller A, *et al.* Multiple sclerosis: prospective analysis of TNF-alpha and 55 kDa TNF receptor in CSF and serum in correlation with clinical and MRI activity. *J Neuroimmunol* 1996;66:57–64.

66. Heidbrink C, Hausler SF, Buttmann M, *et al.* Reduced cortisol levels in cerebrospinal fluid and differential distribution of 11beta-hydroxysteroid dehydrogenases in multiple sclerosis: implications for lesion pathogenesis. *Brain Behav Immun* 2010;24:975–84.

67. Yamashita T, Ando Y, Obayashi K, Uchino M, Ando M. Changes in nitrite and nitrate (NO2-/NO3-) levels in cerebrospinal fluid of patients with multiple sclerosis. *J Neurol Sci* 1997;153:32–4.

68. Sait Keles M, Taysi S, Aksoy H, Sen N, Polat F, Akcay F. The effect of corticosteroids on serum and cerebrospinal fluid nitric oxide levels in multiple sclerosis. *Clin Chem Lab Med* 2001;39:827–9.

69. Holzknecht C, Rohl C. Effects of methylprednisolone and glatiramer acetate on nitric oxide formation of cytokine-stimulated cells from the rat oligodendroglial cell line OLN-93. *Neuroimmunomodulation* 2010;17:23–30.

70. Keles MS, Taysi S, Sen N, Aksoy H, Akðcay F. Effect of corticosteroid

therapy on serum and CSF malondialdehyde and antioxidant proteins in multiple sclerosis. *Can J Neurol Sci* 2001;28:141–3.

71. Mitosek-Szewczyk K, Gordon-Krajcer W, Walendzik P, Stelmasiak Z. Free radical peroxidation products in cerebrospinal fluid and serum of patients with multiple sclerosis after glucocorticoid therapy. *Folia Neuropathol* 2010;48:116–22.

72. Franciotta D, Martino G, Zardini E, *et al.* Serum and CSF levels of MCP-1 and IP-10 in multiple sclerosis patients with acute and stable disease and undergoing immunomodulatory therapies. *J Neuroimmunol* 2001;115:192–8.

73. Xu J, Fan G, Chen S, Wu Y, Xu XM, Hsu CY. Methylprednisolone inhibition of TNF-alpha expression and NF-kB activation after spinal cord injury in rats. *Brain Res Mol Brain Res* 1998;59:135–42.

74. Oudega M, Vargas CG, Weber AB, Kleitman N, Bunge MB. Long-term effects of methylprednisolone following transection of adult rat spinal cord. *Eur J Neurosci* 1999;11:2453–64.

75. Abraham IM, Harkany T, Horvath KM, Luiten PGM. Action of glucocorticoids on survivial of nerve cells: promoting neurodegeneration or neuroprotection? *J Neuroendocrinol* 2001;13:749–60.

76. Hall ED. Neuroprotective actions of glucocorticoid and nonglucocorticoid steroids in acute neuronal injury. *Cell Molec Neurobiol* 1993;13:415–32.

77. Langer-Gould A, Atlas SW, Green AJ, Bollen AW, Pelletier D. Progressive multifocal leukoencephalopathy in a patient treated with natalizumab. *New Engl J Med* 2005;353:375–81.

78. Kleinschmidt-DeMasters BK, Tyler KL. Progressive multifocal leukoencephalopathy complicating treatment with natalizumab and interferon beta-1a for multiple sclerosis. *N Engl J Med* 2005;353:369–74.

79. Nakazawa F, Matsuno H, Yudoh K, Watanabe Y, Katayama R, Kimura T. Corticosteroid treatment induces chondrocyte apoptosis in an experimental arthritis model and in chondrocyte cultures. *Clin Exp Rheumatol* 2002;20:773–81.

80. Watters JJ, Campbell JS, Cunningham MJ, Krebs EG, Dorsa DM. Rapid membrane effects of steroids in neuroblastoma cells: effects of estrogen on mitogen activated protein kinase signalling cascade and c-fos immediate early gene transcription. *Endocrinology* 1997;138:4030–3.

81. Meyer R, Weissert R, Diem R, *et al.* Acute neuronal apoptosis in a rat model of multiple sclerosis. *J Neurosci* 2001;21:6214–20.

82. Diem R, Hobom M, Maier K, *et al.* Methylprednisolone increases neuronal apoptosis during autoimmune CNS inflammation by inhibition of an endogenous neuroprotective pathway. *J Neurosci* 2003;23:6993–7000.

83. Glaser GH, Merritt HH. Effects of ACTH and cortisone in multiple sclerosis. *Transact Am Neurol Assoc* 1951;56.

84. Myers LW. Treatment of multiple sclerosis with ACTH and corticosteroids. In Rudick RA, Goodkin DE, eds. *Treatment of Multiple Sclerosis: Trial Design, Results, and Future Perspectives.* London: Springer-Verlag: 1992, 135–56.

85. Rose AS, Kuzma JW, Kurtzke JF, Namerow NS, Sibley WA, Tourtellotte WW. Cooperative study in the evaluation of therapy in multiple sclerosis. ACTH vs. placebo–final report. *Neurology* 1970;20:1–59.

86. Bell PR, Briggs JD, Calman KC, *et al.* Reversal of acute clinical and experimental organ rejection using large doses of intravenous prednisolone. *Lancet* 1971;1:876–80.

87. Cathcart ES, Idelson BA, Scheinberg MA, Couser WG. Beneficial effects of methylprednisolone "pulse" therapy in diffuse proliferative lupus nephritis. *Lancet* 1976;1:163–6.

88. de Torrente A, Popovtzer MM, Guggenheim SJ, Schrier RW. Serious pulmonary hemorrhage, glomerulonephritis, and massive steroid therapy. *Ann Intern Med* 1975;83:218–19.

89. Bolton WK, Couser WG. Intravenous pulse methylprednisolone therapy of acute crescentic rapidly progressive glomerulonephritis. *Am J Med* 1979;66:495–502.

90. Neild GH, Lee HA. Methylprednisolone pulse therapy in the treatment of polyarteritis nodosa. *Postgrad Med J* 1977;53:382–7.

91. Fan PT, Yu DT, Targoff C, Bluestone R. Effect of corticosteroids on the human immune response. Suppression of mitogen-induced lymphocyte proliferation by "pulse" methylprednisolone. *Transplantation* 1978;26:266–7.

92. Dowling PC, Bosch VV, Cook SD. Possible beneficial effect of high-dose intravenous steroid therapy in acute demyelinating disease and transverse myelitis. *Neurology* 1980;30:33–6.

93. Buckley C, Kennard C, Swash M. Treatment of acute exacerbations of multiple sclerosis with intravenous methyl-prednisolone. *J Neurol Neurosurg Psychiatry* 1982;45: 179–80.

94. Newman PK, Saunders M, Tilley PJ. Methylprednisolone therapy in multiple sclerosis. *J Neurol Neurosurg Psychiatry* 1982;45:941–2.

95. Goas JY, Marion JL, Missoum A. High dose intravenous methyl prednisolone in acute exacerbations of multiple sclerosis. *J Neurol Neurosurg Psychiatry* 1983;46:99.

96. Abbruzzese G, Gandolfo C, Loeb C. "Bolus" methylprednisolone versus ACTH in the treatment of multiple sclerosis. *Ital J Neurol Sci* 1983;4:169–72.

97. Barnes MP, Bateman DE, Cleland PG, *et al.* Intravenous methylprednisolone for multiple sclerosis in relapse. *J Neurol Neurosurg Psychiatry* 1985;48: 157–9.

98. Thompson AJ, Kennard C, Swash M, *et al.* Relative efficacy of intravenous methylprednisolone and ACTH in the treatment of acute relapse in MS. *Neurology* 1989;39:969–71.

99. Milligan NM, Newcombe R, Compston DAS. A double-blind controlled trial of high dose methylprednisolone in patients with multiple sclerosis: 1. clinical effects. *J Neurol Neurosurg Psychiatry* 1987;50:511–16.

100. Sellebjerg F, Frederiksen JL, Nielsen PM, Olesen J. Double-blind, randomized, placebo-controlled study of oral, high-dose methylprednisolone in attacks of MS. *Neurology* 1998;51:529–34.

101. Cazzato G, Mesiano T, Antonello R, *et al.* Double-blind, placebo-controlled, randomized, crossover trial of high-dose methylprednisolone in patients with chronic progressive form of multiple sclerosis. *Eur Neurol* 1995;35:193–8.

102. Miller DM, Weinstock-Guttman B, Bâethoux F, et al. A meta-analysis of methylprednisolone in recovery from multiple sclerosis exacerbations. *Mult Scler* 2000;6:267–73.

103. Filippini G, Brusaferri F, Sibley W, Citterio A, Ciucci G, Midgard R. Corticosteroids or ACTH for acute exacerbations in mulitple sclerosis. *Cochrane Database Syst Rev*, 2001.

104. Bindoff L, Lyons PR, Newman PK, Saunders M. Methylprednisolone in multiple sclerosis: a comparative dose study. *J Neurol Neurosurg Psychiatry* 1988;51:1108–9.

105. Alam SM, Kyriakides T, Lawden M, Newman PK. Methylprednisolone in multiple sclerosis: a comparison of oral with intravenous therapy at equivalent high dose. *J Neurol Neurosurg Psychiatry* 1993;56:1219–20.

106. La Mantia L, Eoli M, Milanese C, Salmaggi A, Dufour A, Torri V. Double-blind trial of dexamethasone versus methylprednisolone in multiple sclerosis acute relapses. *Eur Neurol* 1994;34:199–203.

107. Barnes D, Hughes RA, Morris RW, et al. Randomised trial of oral and intravenous methylprednisolone in acute relapses of multiple sclerosis. *Lancet* 1997;349:902–6.

108. Oliveri RL, Valentino P, Russo C, et al. Randomized trial comparing two different doses of methylprednisolone in MS. A clinical and MRI study. *Neurology* 1998;50:1833–6.

109. Barkhof F, Polman C. Oral or intravenous methylprednisolone for acute relapses of MS? *Lancet* 1997;349:893–4.

110. Beck RW, Cleary PA, Anderson MM, et al. A randomized, controlled trial of corticosteroids in the treatment of acute optic neuritis. *N Engl J Med* 1992;326:581–8.

111. Beck RW, Cleary PA. Optic neuritis treatment trial. One-year follow-up results. *Arch Ophthalmol* 1993;111:773–5.

112. Beck RW. The optic neuritis treatment trial: three-year follow-up results. *Arch Ophthalmol* 1995;113:136–7.

113. Cleary PA, Beck RW, Bourque LB, Backlund JC, Miskala PH. Visual symptoms after optic neuritis. Results from the Optic Neuritis Treatment Trial. *J Neuroophthalmol* 1997;17:18–23.

114. Zivadinov R, Rudick RA, De Masi R, et al. Effects of i.v. methylprednisolone on brain atrophy in relapsing-remitting MS. *Neurology* 2001;57:1239–47.

115. Cohen JA, Imrey PB, Calabresi PA, et al. Results of the Avonex Combination Trial (ACT) in relapsing-remitting MS. *Neurology* 2009;72:535–41.

116. Sorensen PS, Mellgren SI, Svenningsson A, et al. NORdic trial of oral Methylprednisolone as add-on therapy to Interferon beta-1a for treatment of relapsing-remitting Multiple Sclerosis (NORMIMS study): a randomised, placebo-controlled trial. *Lancet Neurol* 2009;8:519–29.

117. Ravnborg M, Sorensen PS, Andersson M, et al. Methylprednisolone in combination with interferon beta-1a for relapsing-remitting multiple sclerosis (MECOMBIN study): a multicentre, double-blind, randomised, placebo-controlled, parallel-group trial. *Lancet Neurol* 2010;9:672–80.

118. Goodkin DE, Kinkel RP, Weinstock-Guttman B, et al. A phase II study of i.v. methylprednisolone in secondary-progressive multiple sclerosis. *Neurology* 1998;51:239–45.

119. Sears ES, Tindall RS, Zarnow H. Active multiple sclerosis. Enhanced computerized tomographic imaging of lesions and the effect of corticosteroids. *Arch Neurol* 1978;35:426–34.

120. Troiano R, Hafstein M, Ruderman M, Dowling P, Cook S. Effect of high-dose intravenous steroid administration on contrast-enhancing computed tomographic scan lesions in multiple sclerosis. *Ann Neurol* 1984;15:257–63.

121. Troiano RA, Hafstein MP, Zito G, Ruderman MI, Dowling PC, Cook SD. The effect of oral corticosteroid dosage on CT enhancing multiple sclerosis plaques. *J Neurol Sci* 1985;70:67–72.

122. Stefoski D, Davis FA, Schauf CL. Acute improvement in exacerbating multiple sclerosis produced by intravenous administration of mannitol. *Ann Neurol* 1985;18:443–50.

123. Barkhof F, Hommes OR, Scheltens P, Valk J. Quantitative MRI changes in gadolinium-DPTA enhancement after high-dose intravenous methylprednisolone in multiple sclerosis. *Neurology* 1991;41:1219–22.

124. Miller DH, Thompson AJ, Morrisey SP, et al. High dose steroids in acute relapses of multiple sclerosis: MRI

evidence for a possible mechanism of therapeutic effect. *J Neurol Neurosurg Psychiatry* 1992;55:450–3.

125. Burnham JA, Wright RR, Dreisbach J, Murray RS. The effect of high-dose steroids on MRI gadolinium enhancement in acute demyelinating lesions. *Neurology* 1991;41:1349–54.

126. Barkhof F, Tas MW, Frequin ST, et al. Limited duration of the effect of methylprednisolone on changes on MRI in multiple sclerosis. *Neuroradiology* 1994;36:382–7.

127. Sellebjerg F, Jensen CV, Larsson HB, Frederiksen JL. Gadolinium-enhanced magnetic resonance imaging predicts response to methylprednisolone in multiple sclerosis. *Mult Scler* 2003;9:102–7.

128. Kesselring J, Miller DH, MacManus DG, et al. Quantitative magnetic resonance imaging in multiple sclerosis: the effect of high dose intravenous methylprednisolone. *J Neurol Neurosurg Psychiatry* 1989;52:14–7.

129. Smith ME, Stone LA, Albert PS, et al. Clinical worsening in multiple sclerosis is associated with increased frequency and area of gadopentetate dimeglumine-enhancing magnetic resonance imaging lesions. *Ann Neurol* 1993;33:480–9.

130. Fox RJ, Fisher E, Tkach J, Lee JC, Cohen JA, Rudick RA. Brain atrophy and magnetization transfer ratio following methylprednisolone in multiple sclerosis: short-term changes and long-term implications. *Mult Scler* 2005;11:140–5.

131. Rao AB, Richert N, Howard T, et al. Methylprednisolone effect on brain volume and enhancing lesions in MS before and during IFNbeta-1b. *Neurology* 2002;59:688–94.

132. Hoogervorst EL, Polman CH, Barkhof F. Cerebral volume changes in multiple sclerosis patients treated with high-dose intravenous methylprednisolone. *Mult Scler* 2002;8:415–19.

133. Gasperini C, Pozzilli C, Bastianello S, et al. Effects of steroids on Gd-enhancing lesions before and during recombinant beta interferon 1a treatment in relapsing remitting multiple sclerosis. *Neurology* 1998;50:403–6.

134. Hickman SJ, Kapoor R, Jones SJ, Altmann DR, Plant GT, Miller DH. Corticosteroids do not prevent optic

nerve atrophy following optic neuritis. *J Neurol Neurosurg Psychiatry* 2003;74:1139–41.

135. Schocke MF, Berger T, Felber SR, *et al.* Serial contrast-enhanced magnetic resonance imaging and spectroscopic imaging of acute multiple sclerosis lesions under high-dose methylprednisolone therapy. *Neuroimage* 2003;20:1253–63.

136. Francis GS, Rice GP, Alsop JC. Interferon beta-1a in MS: results following development of neutralizing antibodies in PRISMS. *Neurology* 2005;65:48–55.

137. Kappos L, Clanet M, Sandberg-Wollheim M, *et al.* Neutralizing antibodies and efficacy of interferon beta-1a: a 4-year controlled study. *Neurology* 2005;65:40–7.

138. Pachner AR, Cadavid D, Wolansky L, Skurnick J. Effect of anti-IFNb antibodies on MRI lesions of MS patients in the BECOME study. *Neurology* 2009;73:1485–92.

139. Ravnborg M, Bendtzen K, Christensen O, *et al.* Treatment with azathioprine and cyclic methylprednisolone has little or no effect on bioactivity in anti-interferon beta antibody-positive patients with multiple sclerosis. *Mult Scler* 2009;15:323–8.

140. Hesse D, Frederiksen J, Koch-Henriksen N, *et al.* Methylprednisolone does not restore biological response in multiple sclerosis patients with neutralizing antibodies against interferon-beta. *Eur J Neurol* 2009;16:43–7.

141. Pachner AR, Brady J, Steiner I, Narayan K. Management of neutralizing antibodies against beta-IFN in beta-IFN-treated multiple sclerosis patients. *J Neurol* 2008;255:1815–7.

142. Pozzilli C, Antonini G, Bagnato F, *et al.* Monthly corticosteroids decrease neutralizing antibodies to IFNbeta1 b: a randomized trial in multiple sclerosis. *J Neurol* 2002;249:50–6.

143. Lyons PR, Newman PK, Saunders M. Methylprednisolone therapy in multiple sclerosis: a profile of adverse effects. *J Neurol Neurosurg Psychiatry* 1988;51:285–7.

144. Smith MD, Ahern MJ, Roberts-Thomson PJ. Pulse methylprednisolone therapy in rheumatoid arthritis: unproved therapy, unjustified therapy, or effective adjunctive treatment? *Ann Rheum Dis* 1990;49:265–7.

145. Leviâc Z, Miciâc D, Nikoliâc J, *et al.* Short-term high dose steroid therapy does not affect the hypothalamic-pituitary-adrenal axis in relapsing multiple sclerosis patients. Clinical assessment by the insulin tolerance test. *J Endocrinol Invest* 1996;19:30–4.

146. Mirâo J, Amado JA, Pesquera C, Lâopez-Cordovilla JJ, Berciano J. Assessment of the hypothalamic-pituitary-adrenal axis function after corticosteroid therapy for MS relapses. *Acta Neurol Scand* 1990;81:524–8.

147. Falk WE, Mahnke MW, Poskanzer DC. Lithium prophylaxis of corticotropin-induced psychosis. *J Am Med Assoc* 1979;241:1011–12.

148. Glass-Marmor L, Paperna T, Ben-Yosef Y, Miller A. Chronotherapy using corticosteroids for multiple sclerosis relapses. *J Neurol Neurosurg Psychiatry* 2007;78:886–8.

149. Pryse-Phillips WEM, Chandra RK, Rose B. Anaphylactoid reaction to methylprednisolone pulsed therapy for multiple sclerosis. *Neurology* 1984;34:1119–21.

150. van den Berg JS, van Eikema Hommes OR, Wuis EW, Stapel S, van der Valk PG. Anaphylactoid reaction to intravenous methylprednisolone in a patient with multiple sclerosis. *J Neurol Neurosurg Psychiatry* 1997;63:813–14.

151. Burgdorff T, Venemalm L, Vogt T, Landthaler M, Stolz W. IgE-mediated anaphylactic reaction induced by succinate ester of methylprednisolone. *Ann Allergy Asthma Immunol* 2002;89:425–8.

152. Kuga A, Futamura N, Funakawa I, Jinnai K. Allergic skin rashes by methylprednisolone in a case with multiple sclerosis. *Clinical Neurol* 2004;44:691–4.

153. Brunner R, Schaefer D, Hess K, Parzer P, Resch F, Schwab S. Effect of corticosteroids on short-term and long-term memory. *Neurology* 2005;64:335–7.

154. Uttner I, Mèuller S, Zinser C, *et al.* Reversible impaired memory induced by pulsed methylprednisolone in patients with MS. *Neurology* 2005;64:1971–3.

155. Cosman F, Nieves J, Komar L, *et al.* Fracture history and bone loss in patients with MS. *Neurology* 1998;51:1161–5.

156. Dovio A, Perazzolo L, Osella G, *et al.* Immediate fall of bone formation and transient increase of bone resorption in the course of high-dose, short-term glucocorticoid therapy in young patients with multiple sclerosis. *J Clin Endocrinol Metab* 2004;89:4923–8.

157. Ardissone P, Rota E, Durelli L, Limone P, Isaia GC. Effects of high doses of corticosteroids on bone metabolism. *J Endocrinol Invest* 2002;25:129–33.

158. Schwid SR, Goodman AD, Puzas JE, McDermott MP, Mattson DH. Sporadic corticosteroid pulses and osteoporosis in multiple sclerosis. *Arch Neurol* 1996;53:753–7.

159. Ce P, Gedizlioglu M, Gelal F, Coban P, Ozbek G. Avascular necrosis of the bones: an overlooked complication of pulse steroid treatment of multiple sclerosis. *Eur J Neul* 2006;13:857–61.

160. Frediani B, Falsetti P, Bisogno S, *et al.* Effects of high dose methylprednisolone pulse therapy on bone mass and biochemical markers of bone metabolism in patients with active rheumatoid arthritis: a 12-month randomized prospective controlled study. *J Rheum* 2004;31:1083–7.

161. Recommendations for the prevention and treatment of glucocoerticoid-induced osteoporosis. American College of Rheumatology Task Force on Osteoporosis Guidelines. *Arthritis Rheumatism* 1996;39:1791–801.

162. Zarkou S, Carter JL, Wellik KE, Demaerschalk BM, Wingerchuk DM. Are corticosteroids efficacious for preventing or treating neutralizing antibodies in multiple sclerosis patients treated with beta-interferons? A critically appraised topic. *Neurologist* 2010;16:212–14.

163. Wakefield D, Jennings A, McCluskey PJ. Intravenous pulse methylprednisolone in the treatment of uveitis associated with multiple sclerosis. *Clin Exp Ophthalmol* 2000;28:103–6.

164. Kinkel RP, Simon JH, Baron B. Bimonthly cranial MRI activity following an isolated monosymptomatic demyelinating

syndrome: potential outcome measures for future multiple sclerosis 'prevention' trials. *Mult Scler* 1999;5:307–12.

165. Jacobs LD, Beck RW, Simon JH, *et al.* The effect of initiating Interfereon beta-1a therapy during a first demyelinating event on the development of clinically definite multiple sclerosis. *N Eng J Med* 2000;343:898–904.

166. Schmidt J, Metselaar JM, Gold R. Intravenous liposomal prednisolone downregulates in situ TNF-alpha production by T-cells in experimental autoimmune encephalomyelitis. *J Histochem Cytochem* 2003;51:1241–4.

Chapter 37

Use of immunosuppressants to treat multiple sclerosis

James M. Stankiewicz and Howard L. Weiner

Introduction

Multiple sclerosis (MS) is an inflammatory cell-mediated autoimmune disease that affects the central nervous system. It follows logically, then, that suppression of the immune system can attenuate or truncate disease activity. Drugs with an immunosuppressive effect have been successfully employed in other autoimmune diseases, so it is not surprising that they have been tried in MS as well. Generally, therapies considered immunosuppressive have direct effects on DNA synthesis or immune cell activation, with primary targeting of the bone marrow or other lymphoid tissue. Cyclophosphamide interferes with DNA and RNA synthesis to have its effects, while the other immunosuppressives discussed in this chapter inhibit purine synthesis pathways, inhibiting DNA replication in B-cells and T-cells, subsequently decreasing the production and effectiveness of these cells.

Cyclophosphamide

Cyclophosphamide (Cytoxan) is a synthetic compound related to nitrogen mustards that becomes an alkylating agent after being metabolized in the liver. Because it interferes with DNA synthesis within organs with rapidly dividing cells, it disproportionately affects the bone marrow, bladder, and gastrointestinal epithelium. This helps account for both its beneficial effects on autoimmune disease and potential toxicities. It is standard therapy in lupus nephritis, and also employed in autoimmune neuropathies, and vasculidities such as Wegener's granulomatosis and polyarteritis nodosa.

Cyclophosphamide and the immune system

Cyclophosphamide affects the immune system by a dual mechanism: depletion of CD4+ T-cells and promotion of a shift from a Th1 immune profile to a less deleterious Th2 response. Cyclophosphamide has been shown to either reduce or prevent development of disease in a well-accepted experimental autoimmune encephalitis animal model.[1] Multiple studies have shown a pronounced suppression of CD4+ T-cells.[2-5] Cytokines typically present with activation of a Th2 response are found at increased levels in patients treated with cyclophos-

phamide. Specifically, increased interleukin-4 (IL-4), IL-5, IL-10, transforming growth factor beta, and eosinophils are observed.[6,7] Interferon-gamma (IFNγ) is reduced, also consistent with increased Th2 activity. A reduction in Th1 response also probably occurs, as IL-12, a cytokine typically up-regulated with Th1 response, is reduced in cyclophosphamide-treated patients.[6] CCR5+ and CXCR3+ CD8+ IFNγ-producing T-cells are less frequent with cyclophosphamide treatment.[8] Myelin autoantigen responses in cyclophosphamide-treated patients also deviate toward a more benign Th2/Th3 response. Work by Takashima found that cyclophosphamide treatment causes myelin reactive T-cells to secrete IL-4.[9] Our group reported that an increased frequency of IL-4-secreting myelin basic protein- and proteolipid protein reactive-cells are found in cyclophosphamide-treated MS patients when compared to MS patients treated with i.v. methylprednisolone. IFNγ production by CD8+ T-cells is reduced in cyclophosphamide treated secondary progressive MS patients.[8] Taken together, these results suggest that not only does cyclophosphamide deplete immune cells, but also encourages a benign deviation of the immune system that is helpful for reducing disease activity.

Cyclophosphamide trials

Cyclophosphamide was initially successfully employed in a case of progressive MS.[10] This led to an open-label study by Girard et al. in 30 patients treated with i.v. cyclophosphamide 200 mg/d for 4–6 weeks. At two years, 50% of patients were improved or stable.[11] Hommers et al.[12] reported that 39 progressive patients receiving 400 mg/day of cyclophosphamide and 100 mg/day of prednisone for 20 days resulted in stabilization of 69% of treated patients for an average of two years. A third of patients did not experience progression during the study follow-up. Further analysis showed that patients with an earlier disease onset (<28 years), shorter disease duration (six years), faster disease progression, or lower initial disability were likely to respond better to treatment. The first randomized trial was reported in 1983. Hauser et al.[13] randomized 58 patients to either adrenocorticotropic hormone (ACTH) alone, ACTH combined with plasma exchange and oral cyclophosphamide, or ACTH and i.v. cyclophosphamide to achieve leukopenia with white blood cell

---

Multiple Sclerosis Therapeutics, Fourth Edition, ed. Jeffrey A. Cohen and Richard A. Rudick. Published by Cambridge University Press.
© Cambridge University Press 2011.

(WBC) count of 2000/mm^3. Investigators were not blinded to treatment type. Patients receiving i.v. cyclophosphamide and ACTH did best with 80% of patients improved or stable at one year, in contrast to only 20% in the ACTH treated group. Additional analysis suggested that the effect of a cyclophosphamide induction lasted an average of 18 months, with some patients experiencing return of clinical activity at six months. A study by Carter et al.[14] using the same protocol as the Hauser study found that patients stabilized with treatment but then progressed within 30 months of treatment.

Because it was clear that disease activity did eventually return after cyclophosphamide induction a single-blind multicenter trial, the Northeast Cooperative Treatment Group, was undertaken to explore whether maintenance pulse therapy might help lengthen treatment response.[15] Two hundred and sixty one progressive patients were randomized to four treatments. All patients received induction treatment, with groups 1 and 2 receiving the induction regimen used by Hauser et al.,[13] groups 3–4 a dose of i.v. cyclophosphamide 600 mg/m^2 with a modified ACTH regimen essentially every-other-day for eight days. The regimen previously published consisted of 125 mg i.v. cyclophosphamide four times per day over 8 to 18 days until the WBC count decreased below 4000/mm^3 plus i.v. ACTH. Patient groups 2 and 4 received every other month i.v. cyclophosphamide boosters (700 mg/m^2) for two years, while groups 1 and 3 did not receive further treatment. There was no placebo group. No difference was seen between the published versus the modified induction regimen either by stabilization at 12 and 24 months or subsequent progression by the time-to-failure analysis. Booster therapy, however, modestly delayed progression at 24 and 30 months ($P = 0.04$). Patients were more likely to respond to booster therapy if they were younger or had a more recent disease onset.

Two controlled single-blinded trials using protocols different from previously published studies yielded negative results. The Kaiser study[16] randomized 43 progressive patients to receive folic acid or i.v. cyclophosphamide induction of 400 to 500 mg/d for five days per week until the WBC count fell below 4000/mm^3. It found no difference in the primary outcome measure, Expanded Disability Status Scale (EDSS) change at one year, with the cyclophosphamide treated group having a mean increase 0.5, the folic acid group 0.53. Interestingly, at two years, EDSS increase in the cyclophosphamide group was 0.58 vs. 0.97 in the folic acid group, though the result still might be attributed to chance, given the small number of patients enrolled. The Canadian Cooperative MS Study group[17] randomized 55 progressive patients to one of three groups. Group 1 received 1 gram i.v. cyclophosphamide every-other-day to either a WBC of 4500/mm^3 or 9000 mg total (whichever occurred first) in addition to prednisone 40 mg/d for 10 days with subsequent taper, group 2 received plasmapheresis combined with cyclophosphamide by mouth for 22 weeks with alternate day oral prednisone (20 mg every other day tapered over 22 weeks), and group 3 was a placebo control. No difference was seen in the primary outcome measure,

a comparison over time of the cumulative treatment failure rates.

A retrospective open-label study found that 30 progressive patients treated for one year with 700 mg/m^2 of pulse monthly i.v. cyclophosphamide showed improvements in cognitive measures including global intelligence, verbal and visuospatial memory, and executive function.[18]

Cyclophosphamide MRI effects

A number of open-label studies with both clinical and MRI outcomes have been conducted. In the first study with MRI metrics, Gobbini et al. gave monthly i.v. cyclophosphamide 1 g/m^2 to patients who on average had failed three other MS treatments. Three of five patients showed a decreased T2 lesion load after 5 months of treatment, and all showed a reduction in gadolinium (Gd) enhancement compared to interferon-beta (IFNβ) alone pre-trial.[19] Other small open-label studies adding cyclophosphamide treatment to patients failing IFNβ showed similar results.[20,21] A larger retrospective open-label study of 490 progressive MS patients treated with monthly pulse i.v. cyclophosphamide (700 mg/m^2) in combination with 1 g i.v. methylprednisolone found that 78.6% of secondary progressive patients and 73.5% of primary progressive patients had a stable EDSS at one year.[22] Patients were more likely to respond to therapy if they had lower disease duration (5.1 years in responders vs. 7.1 years in non-responders). If patients showed a response at six months, they were also likely to have a better outcome at one year.

A single-blind multicenter study randomized 59 relapsing–remitting (RR) MS patients with continued disease activity on IFNβ to either IFNβ and 1 g monthly i.v. methylprednisolone or a combination of IFNβ, monthly i.v. cyclophosphamide, and 1 g i.v. methylprednisolone. Patients were treated for six months, and then given IFNβ in follow-up. At six months there was a reduction in Gd-enhancing lesions in the group that received cyclophosphamide and steroids in addition to IFNβ ($P = 0.04$). Time to treatment failure was also significantly delayed ($P = 0.02$).[23]

Cyclophosphamide in clinical practice

Though there is still debate in the literature, we consider the question of cyclophosphamide's effectiveness for MS settled. We believe that, given careful patient selection, the literature supports cyclophosphamide's use. Though two placebo-controlled trials failed to reveal a benefit with cyclophosphamide therapy, the patient populations were older, the cyclophosphamide administered differently, and the degree of progression in the placebo arm lower. Multiple open-label studies, single-blinded studies, and studies employing MRI support the notion that patients with evidence of inflammation on MRI, patients with relapses, younger patients, and patients with early progressive disease may benefit from cyclophosphamide (Table 37.1).

Table 37.1. *Immunosuppressive drug dosages and side effects*

Drug	Dosage	Common side effects	Recommended monitoring
Azathioprine	1–3 mg/kg orally daily	Infection, macrocytosis, rash, anemia, leukopenia, thrombocytopenia, pancytopenia, hepatotoxicity	CBC, LFTs weekly during the first month, twice monthly for second and third months, then monthly
Cyclophosphamide	Variable*	Nausea, alopecia, menstrual disorders, infertility, leukopenia, infection, bladder toxicity, cancer	WBC count at mid-month and yearly during treatment, cystoscopy if abnormal cytology and yearly after third year of treatment. Lifetime maximum dose = 80–100 g.
Methotrexate	7.5–20 mg orally once weekly	Nausea, vomiting, diarrhea, infection	CBC, LFTs, BMP at weeks 1, 2, 4 then monthly
Mycophenolate mofetil	1 g orally twice daily, titrated over one month	Nausea, diarrhea, leukopenia, infection	CBC, LFTs weekly during the first month, twice monthly for second and third months, then monthly

Specific recommendation at www.partnersmscenter.org.
BMP = basic metabolic panel, CBC = complete blood count, LFTs = liver function tests.

Based on the results of the Northeast cooperative trial our center generally defers induction treatment and gives cyclophosphamide pulses most typically in conjunction with 1 g of i.v. methylprednisolone. In the first year the combination is given monthly, the second year every other month, and in the third year every two months. Treatment is generally administered for three years, though this is an individualized decision between patient and physician. Cyclophosphamide dose is adjusted per protocol to keep WBC count nadir between 1500–2000/mm^3 up to a maximum dose of 1600 mg/m^2. Nadir most typically occurs 1 to 2 weeks after treatment. More specific details of our protocol may be found at www. partnersmscenter.org. In line with previously published results, a retrospective study conducted by our group[24] found that patients earlier in progressive disease do better and that primary progressive patients do not respond well, two factors we consider before selecting a particular patient for treatment.

Newer uses of cyclophosphamide

A small open-label trial of high dose (50 mg/kg/d for four days) i.v. cyclophosphamide in patients with active disease showed a reduction in EDSS and T2 lesions.[25] Some open-label trials of patients undergoing immunoablation with cyclophosphamide with subsequent autologous stem cell transplantation have reported impressive efficacy,[26] though concerns about possible neurotoxicity from these aggressive treatments urge caution against over-application.[27] Open-label reports of cyclophosphamide's efficacy in an active pediatric MS population also exist.[28]

Cyclophosphamide tolerability and safety

Our experience has been that monthly pulses of cyclophosphamide are generally well tolerated (Table 37.2). At our center it is given in conjunction with i.v. methylprednisolone, antiemetics, and aggressive i.v. fluid hydration (3 liters) on the day of treatment and the day after. There is some evidence to suggest that methylprednisolone may augment cyclophosphamide's effects and lessen renal toxicity.[29] Alopecia is

Table 37.2. *Factors associated with a positive response to cyclophosphamide*

Rapidly progressive course
Gadolinium-enhancing MRI lesions
Relapses in the prior year
Less than 2 years in the progressive phase
Younger age
Lower initial disability score

common with induction therapy, though less so with monthly pulses. In a study of lupus patients, premature menopause was found to be more likely in cyclophosphamide treated patients over the age of 25 or receiving >300 mg/kg.[30] Malignancies have been reported in patients receiving cyclophosphamide in the oncology and rheumatology literature, with risk thought to increase after a cumulative dose of 100 g.[31] Because bladder cancers have been reported we perform a yearly urine cytology, and cytoscopy after three years. Opportunistic infections have been reported, including progressive multifocal leukoencephalopathy, though other factors such as disease-related immunosuppression or combination with other medications make it difficult to determine how much cyclophosphamide actually contributed.[32,33] Despite these concerns, a single follow-up study of MS patients undergoing pulse cyclophosphamide treatment found that it was well tolerated, with amenorrhea (33.3%), hypogammaglobulinemia (5.4%), and hemorrhagic cystitis (4.5%) being the most commonly reported side effects. Malignancies were diagnosed in four (3.6%) subjects, three of whom were previously treated with azathioprine. Interestingly, 81.8% of the patients judged the treatment regimen as very or relatively acceptable and tolerable.[34]

Mycophenolate mofetil

Mycophenolate mofetil (Cellcept) is a potent immunosuppressant which selectively inhibits inosine 5′-monophosphate dehydrogenase type II, the enzyme responsible for the de novo synthesis of the purine nucleotide guanine within activated T-cells and B-cells, and macrophages. It has been used increasingly in post-transplant patients because it is considered less toxic than azathioprine and cyclophosphamide. Though no placebo-controlled trials have been completed in MS, open-label trial reports are available. A trial of mycophenolate in seven progressive patients[35] found that mycophenolate was well tolerated and either offered improvement or halted progression in five patients. MRI was available for only two patients, but was improved. One patient reduced dose because of frequent non-serious infections. Nausea was common. A retrospective review of 79 patients on mycophenolate, 15 with monotherapy, 44 on IFNβ, and 20 on glatiramer acetate found that mycophenolate was well tolerated, with 70% of patients continuing therapy.[36] Again, gastrointestinal side effects such as nausea and diarrhea were common. A case of cytomegalovirus diarrhea occurred, though no other serious infections were reported. Seven patients had disease progression, and clinical impressions were that the rest remained stable on therapy, though no formal evaluations were performed. An open-label study in 30 active RR patients treated with a combination of IFNβ-1a and mycophenolate reported a reduction in relapse rate (2 to 0.57), improvement in mean EDSS (2.9 to 2.6), and absence of Gd-enhancing lesions on MRI follow-up.[37] Six patients reported diarrhea, with one discontinuation. Eight patients reported transient abdominal pains and five reported transient nausea. During the six month study, relapses occurred more commonly in the first two months, suggesting some latency of drug effect. It should also be noted that a retrospective review also suggests that mycophenolate might have efficacy in neuromyelitis optica.[38]

At our center, we tend to employ mycophenolate in MS patients with insidious progression despite treatment with IFNβ or glatiramer acetate. We have also had successful results in patients with neuromyelitis optica. We use the same dosing that was used in the open-label studies: 250 mg twice daily for one week, then 500 mg twice daily for week 2; 750 mg twice daily for week 3; and then 1 g twice daily thereafter. Laboratory studies are performed weekly during the first month, twice monthly during the second and third month, then monthly and consist of liver function testing, a complete blood count, and basic metabolic panel. Though in trials mycophenolate was well tolerated, immunosuppressive complications are known to occur and can include progressive multifocal leukoencephalopathy (http://www.fda.gov/downloads/Safety/MedWatch/Safety Information/SafetyAlertsforHumanMedicalProducts/ ucm093666.pdf). Confirmed cases have been seen in solid organ transplant patients and patient with lupus, all of which were on concomitant immunosuppression.

Methotrexate

Methotrexate is a general immunosuppressant that acts primarily by inhibition of dihydrofolate reductase.[39] Goodkin et al.[40] randomized 31 progressive patients to 7.5 mg of methotrexate and 29 to placebo for 36 months. RRMS patients were excluded, with 30% of patients enrolled with primary progressive MS and 70% with secondary progressive MS. Neither sustained EDSS progression nor time to first relapse differed between the

groups. MRI metrics were reported separately later,[41] but also were unimpressive, with no change in new T2 or Gd-enhancing lesions demonstrated between groups. Though it is fair to say that these results do not favor the use of methotrexate, some caveats should be offered. The first is that the trial did show a favorable effect of methotrexate on its primary outcome measure, a combination of EDSS, ambulation index, box and block test, and 9-hole peg test. This effect was driven primarily by a more pronounced effect on the 9-hole peg test. A second caveat is that T2 lesion area was significantly reduced compared to placebo when accounting for study week and baseline T2 lesion area.

Calabresi et al.[42] added 20 mg of methotrexate to intramuscular IFNβ-1a for 6 months in 15 relapsing patients and found a 44% reduction in number of Gd-enhancing lesions when compared with baseline scans of patients on IFNβ-1a alone. These results led to the Avonex Combination Trial (ACT) in RR patients. ACT randomized patients with breakthrough disease on intramuscular IFNβ-1a to combination treatment with either oral methotrexate 20 mg weekly, i.v. methylprednisolone 1 g bimonthly, or both.[43] Patients receiving IM IFNβ-1a combined with methotrexate had no additional benefit compared to those receiving IM IFNβ-1a and steroids on a number of metrics including new or enlarged T2 lesions, Gd-enhancing lesions, multiple sclerosis functional composite, or brain parenchymal fraction. A recent open-label study found that 89% of unresponsive progressive patients receiving methotrexate intrathecally every 8–11 weeks for eight cycles were improved compared to their baseline.[44]

Methotrexate appears safe for use in an MS patient population. In the Goodkin trial, side effects were reported no more frequently in the methotrexate-treated group than in the placebo arm. In ACT, no serious adverse events occurred and again treatment was well tolerated. It is our impression that, unless better support in the form of randomized controlled trials emerges, methotrexate should be employed sparingly.

Azathioprine

Azathioprine (Imuran) is a purine analog that is metabolized to 6-mercaptopurine and thioinosine acid, which compete with DNA nucleotides, causing immunosuppression.[39] It has found use in autoimmune disorders such as myasthenia gravis, and to prevent post-transplant organ rejection. The largest trial of azathioprine in MS[45] randomized 354 patients to either azathioprine 2.5 mg/kg daily or placebo with 3-year followup. Little change in EDSS (azathioprine 0.62 vs. placebo 0.80) or relapse rate (azathioprine 2.2 vs. placebo 2.5) was observed between the two groups, though ambulation index (azathioprine 0.84 vs. placebo 1.25, 95% confidence interval 0.03–0.80) was significantly improved. About a third of patients were classified as having progressive disease, but a subgroup analysis revealed that neither disease course responded particularly to azathioprine. Mild side effects were seen especially in the first year of azathioprine treatment, but no serious adverse

Table 37.3. *Selected randomized trials of immunosuppressive drugs in multiple sclerosis*

Author	Blinding	Length	N	Patient profile	Treatments	Outcome
Azathioprine						
British Dutch[45]	Double	3 years	354	67% RRMS, 18% SPMS, 15% PPMS	AZA vs. PLC	EDSS change (P = NS), mean relapse number (P = NS)
Ellison[46]	Double	3 years	65	Progressive	AZA + MP vs. AZA vs. PLC	Mean DSS change (P = NS)
Goodkin[47]	Double	2 years	59	RRMS	AZA vs. PLC	AZA ARR 0.3 vs. placebo 0.79 (P < 0.05), EDSS change (P = NS)
Milanese[48]	Double	3 years	40	47.5% RRMS, 25% SPMS, 27.5% PPMS	AZA vs. PLC	Mean relapse frequency (P = NS)
Etemadifar[50]	Single	1 year	94	RRMS	IFNβ vs. AZA	AZA ↓ ARR 0.28 vs. IFNβ 0.64 (P < 0.05), AZA EDSS ↓ 1.34 vs. IFNβ 0.96 (P < 0.01)
Havrdova[51]	Double	2 years	181	RRMS	IM IFNβ-1a vs. IFNβ-1a + AZA vs. IFNβ-1a + AZA + prednisone	ARR (P = NS)
Cyclophosphamide						
Hauser[13]	Single	1 year	58	Progressive	i.v. CTX+ ACTH vs. PO CTX + ACTH + PLEX vs. ACTH	Disease progression CTX + ACTH vs. ACTH (P < 0.01), CTX + ACTH vs. PLEX (P = 0.087)
Weiner[15]	Single	3 years	256	Progressive	Fixed i.v. CTX no booster + ACTH vs. variable i.v. CTX no booster + ACTH vs. fixed i.v. CTX + ACTH with booster vs. variable i.v. CTX + ACTH with booster	Slower progression in booster group at 2 years (P = 0.04), variable vs. fixed induction differences (P = NS)
Likosky[16]	Single	2 years	42	Progressive	i.v. CTX vs. folic acid	EDSS change (P = NS)
CCMSG[17]	Double	1 year	168	Progressive	i.v. CTX + prednisone vs. PO CTX + prednispone + PLEX vs. PLC	Rate of treatment failure (P = NS)
Smith[23]	Single	2 years	59	RRMS	CTX + MP + IM IFNβ-1a vs. MP + IFNβ-1a	Mean change Gd-enhancing lesions from baseline lower in CTX + MP group (P = 0.02)
Methotrexate						
Goodkin[40]	Double	2 years	56	Progressive	MTX vs. PLC	Sustained progression MTX 51.6% vs. PLC 82.8% (P = 0.01)
Cohen[43]	Double	1 year	313	RRMS	IM IFNβ-1a + MTX vs. IFNβ-1a + PLC vs. IFNβ-1a + MTX + MP vs. IFNβ-1a + PLC + MP	New or enlarging T2 lesions (P = NS)

ACTH = adrenocorticotrophic hormone, ARR = annualized relapse rate, AZA = azathioprine, CCMSG = Canadian Cooperative MS Study Group, CTX = cyclophosphamdie, DSS = Disability Status Scale, EDSS = Expanded Disability Status Scale, MP = methylprednisolone, Gd = gadolinium, IFNβ = interferon-beta, MS = multiple sclerosis, MTX = methotrexate, NS = not significant, PLC = placebo, PLEX = plasma exchange, PP = primary progressive, RR = relapsing–remitting, SP = secondary progressive,

events that could be linked to azathioprine treatment were observed. Leukopenia was seen in 26% of patients at the end of year 1, though this was seen in only 8% of patients by year 3. Ellison *et al.*[46] randomized 98 chronic progressive MS patients for 3 years to one of three groups: azathioprine and steroids, azathioprine and placebo, or placebo. Azathioprine dose was adjusted to bring the WBC count between 3000–4000/mm³. Using an intention-to-treat analysis, EDSS change did not differ between groups. It should be noted that little progression on EDSS was seen in any of the groups (0.10 in placebo, 0.05 in azathioprine group). Effects on relapse rate were seen (annualized relapse rate = 0.24 azathioprine group vs. 0.48 placebo, P = 0.04). Again, leukopenia, macrocytic anemia, and liver function abnormalities were observed. Three patients in the azathioprine group withdrew due to drug fevers, eight

in the azathioprine and steroid group withdrew. A study by Goodkin *et al.*[47] randomized 59 ambulatory RR patients to receive either 3 mg/kg daily of azathioprine or placebo. The trial found that azathioprine-treated patients benefited from a reduced mean relapse rate (azathioprine 0.30 vs. placebo 0.79, P = 0.05). Mean change in EDSS and ambulatory index did not differ at 2 years between the two groups, though the proportion of patients worsening was statistically better in the azathioprine treated group compared to placebo for EDSS (P = 0.04) and ambulatory index (P = 0.03). The treatment again was well tolerated, with leukopenia and liver function abnormalities seen in a small proportion of the azathioprine group. Milenese *et al.*[48] conducted a three year double-blind placebo-controlled trial in patients with either RR or secondary progressive MS. Azathioprine was given at a dose of 2 mg/kg/day. Treatment with azathioprine did not lead to a statistically significant benefit in EDSS change, the primary outcome measure. Mean relapse frequency also was not improved in the azathioprine treated group. Other outcome measures were explored with results approaching statistical significance, but these analyses were not predetermined. A case of pancytopenia, two cases of intractable vomiting, and a case of herpes zoster were observed. Mild leukopenia and macrocytosis were reported, but again no malignancies were observed. The authors concluded that these results favored the use of azathioprine in MS.

A meta-analysis looking at 698 patients included in placebo-controlled double-blind randomized trials of azathioprine in MS was recently conducted.[49] The authors concluded that at two years, relapse rate did decline when compared to placebo (relative risk reduction 23%, 95% confidence interval 12%–33%). Only 87 patients could be included to examine whether azathioprine treatment reduced risk of progression by EDSS. At three years there was a statistically significant reduction in risk of progression (relative risk reduction = 42%, 95% confidence interval 7%–64%).

A one-year single-blind study comparing IFNβ-1b or IM or subcutaneous IFNβ-1a with 3 mg/kg a day of azathioprine found that 57% of patients on IFNβ remained relapse free compared with 77% of patients on azathioprine ($P < 0.05$).[50] Mean EDSS in IFNβ-treated patients at one year was 1.34, azathioprine-treated patients 0.96 ($P < 0.01$), at study entry EDSS was 1.6 in the IFNβ group, 1.4 in the azathioprine group, a non-statistically significant difference The neurologist assessing outcome was blinded to treatment, though patients were aware of their treatment allocation.

A study randomizing 181 RRMS patient to either IM IFNβ-1a vs. IFNβ-1a and 50 mg daily azathioprine vs. IFNβ-1a, 50 mg oral daily azathioprine, and 10 mg oral prednisone every other day found no difference on annualized relapse rate at two years.[51] Cumulative probably of sustained disability progression also did not differ. An MRI metric did show a significant benefit to adding azathioprine to IFNβ-1a, with percent T2 lesion volume change significantly lower for the combination (14.5% vs. IFNβ-1a alone (30.3%, $P < 0.05$).

Hematologic malignancies are probably increased with long-term azathioprine use. Lhermitte et al.[52] identified 131 patients treated with azathioprine treated for a mean duration of 73 months (range 12–184) and a mean follow-up from treatment onset of 121 months (range 30–187) treated with an average daily dose of 100 mg. Ten cancers were seen in this group, with a frequency of almost 10% for patients having at least five years of follow-up. An age- and sex-matched control group developed only four cancers. Reported cancers were solid tumors rather than hematologic. A case control study undertaken using the Lyon MS database found that 14 patients from a database of 1191 patients had both developed cancer and been exposed to azathioprine at least one month. Risk of developing cancer with 5–10 years of azathioprine treatment was double that in patients not treated with azathioprine, and over four-fold higher when treated for more than 10 years. When examining cumulative dose rather than duration of treatment similar effects were found, with five years of treatment being equivalent to a cumulative dose of 300 g. Solid tumors were most common, though a few hematologic malignancies were seen. Another study found that MS patient on azathioprine were less likely to develop cancer when compared to untreated patients.[53]

Conclusion

Table 37.3 lists randomized trials of immunosuppressives in MS. In the right patient, cyclophosphamide has been demonstrated effective, while work with methotrexate and mycophenolate mofetil has been less conclusive. Azathioprine also is likely to have a favorable effect on MS, and is relatively safe. Recent novel uses of immunosuppressives in active patients, or new disease populations have broadened the possible uses of these drugs. Further work seeking to better clarify proper use of these medications needs to be done.

References

1. Paterson PY, Drobish DG. Cyclophosphamide: effect on experimental allergic encephalomyelitis in Lewis rats. *Science* 1969;165:191–2.

2. Moody DJ, Fahey JL, Grable E, Ellison GW, Myers LW. Administration of monthly pulses of cyclophosphamide in multiple sclerosis patients. Delayed recovery of several immune parameters following discontinuation of long-term cyclophosphamide treatment. *J Neuroimmunol* 1987;14:175–82.

3. Moody DJ, Kagan J, Liao D, Ellison GW, Myers LW. Administration of monthly-pulse cyclophosphamide in multiple sclerosis patients. Effects of long-term treatment on immunologic parameters. *J Neuroimmunol* 1987;14:161–73.

4. Hafler DA, Orav J, Gertz R, Stazzone L, Weiner HL. Immunologic effects of cyclophosphamide/ACTH in patients with chronic progressive multiple sclerosis. *J Neuroimmunol* 1991;32:149–58.

5. Mickey MR, Ellison GW, Fahey JL, Moody DJ, Myers LW. Correlation of clinical and immunologic states in multiple sclerosis. *Arch Neurol* 1987;44:371–5.

6. Comabella M, Balashov K, Issazadeh S, Smith D, Weiner HL, Khoury SJ. Elevated interleukin-12 in progressive multiple sclerosis correlates with disease activity and is normalized by pulse cyclophosphamide therapy. *J Clin Invest* 1998;102:671–8.

7. Smith DR, Balashov KE, Hafler DA, Khoury SJ, Weiner HL. Immune deviation following pulse cyclophosphamide/methylprednisolone treatment of multiple sclerosis: increased interleukin-4 production and associated eosinophilia. *Ann Neurol* 1997;42:313–18.

8. Karni A, Balashov K, Hancock WW, *et al.* Cyclophosphamide modulates CD4+ T cells into a T helper type 2 phenotype and reverses increased IFN-gamma production of CD8+ T cells in secondary progressive multiple

sclerosis. *J Neuroimmunol* 2004;146: 189–98.

9. Takashima H, Smith DR, Fukaura H, Khoury SJ, Hafler DA, Weiner HL. Pulse cyclophosphamide plus methylprednisolone induces myelin-antigen-specific IL-4-secreting T cells in multiple sclerosis patients. *Clin Immunol Immunopathol* 1998;88: 28–34.

10. Aimard G, Girard PF, Raveau J. [Multiple sclerosis and the autoimmunization process. Treatment by antimitotics]. *Lyon Med* 1966;215: 345–52.

11. Girard PF, Aimard G, Pellet H. [Immunodepressive therapy in neurology]. *Presse Med* 1967;75:967–8.

12. Hommes OR, Lamers KJ, Reekers P. Effect of intensive immunosuppression on the course of chronic progressive multiple sclerosis. *J Neurol* 1980;223: 177–90.

13. Hauser SL, Dawson DM, Lehrich JR, *et al.* Intensive immunosuppression in progressive multiple sclerosis. A randomized, three-arm study of high-dose intravenous cyclophosphamide, plasma exchange, and ACTH. *N Engl J Med* 1983;308: 173–80.

14. Carter JL, Hafler DA, Dawson DM, Orav J, Weiner HL. Immunosuppression with high-dose i.v. cyclophosphamide and ACTH in progressive multiple sclerosis: cumulative 6-year experience in 164 patients. *Neurology* 1988;38(Suppl 2): 9–14.

15. Weiner HL, Mackin GA, Orav EJ, *et al.* Intermittent cyclophosphamide pulse therapy in progressive multiple sclerosis: final report of the Northeast Cooperative Multiple Sclerosis Treatment Group. *Neurology* 1993; 43:910–18.

16. Likosky WH, Fireman B, Elmore R, *et al.* Intense immunosuppression in chronic progressive multiple sclerosis: the Kaiser study. *J Neurol Neurosurg Psychiatry* 1991;54:1055–60.

17. The Canadian cooperative trial of cyclophosphamide and plasma exchange in progressive multiple sclerosis. The Canadian Cooperative Multiple Sclerosis Study Group. *Lancet* 1991;337:441–6.

18. Zephir H, de Seze J, Dujardin K, *et al.* One-year cyclophosphamide treatment combined with methylprednisolone improves cognitive dysfunction in progressive forms of multiple sclerosis. *Mult Scler* 2005;11:360–3.

19. Gobbini MI, Smith ME, Richert ND, Frank JA, McFarland HF. Effect of open label pulse cyclophosphamide therapy on MRI measures of disease activity in five patients with refractory relapsing-remitting multiple sclerosis. *J Neuroimmunol* 1999;99:142–9.

20. Patti F, Cataldi ML, Nicoletti F, Reggio E, Nicoletti A, Reggio A. Combination of cyclophosphamide and interferon-beta halts progression in patients with rapidly transitional multiple sclerosis. *J Neurol Neurosurg Psychiatry* 2001;71:404–7.

21. Perini P, Gallo P. Cyclophosphamide is effective in stabilizing rapidly deteriorating secondary progressive multiple sclerosis. *J Neurol* 2003;250: 834–8.

22. Zephir H, de Seze J, Duhamel A, *et al.* Treatment of progressive forms of multiple sclerosis by cyclophosphamide: a cohort study of 490 patients. *J Neurol Sci* 2004;218: 73–7.

23. Smith DR, Weinstock-Guttman B, Cohen JA, *et al.* A randomized blinded trial of combination therapy with cyclophosphamide in patients-with active multiple sclerosis on interferon beta. *Mult Scler* 2005;11:573–82.

24. Hohol MJ, Olek MJ, Orav EJ, *et al.* Treatment of progressive multiple sclerosis with pulse cyclophos-phamide/methylprednisolone: response to therapy is linked to the duration of progressive disease. *Mult Scler* 1999;5: 403–9.

25. Krishnan C, Kaplin AI, Brodsky RA, *et al.* Reduction of disease activity and disability with high-dose cyclophosphamide in patients with aggressive multiple sclerosis. *Arch Neurol* 2008;65:1044–51.

26. Martino G, Franklin RJ, Van Evercooren AB, Kerr DA. Stem cell transplantation in multiple sclerosis: current status and future prospects. *Nat Rev Neurol* 2010;6:247–55.

27. Chen JT, Collins DL, Atkins HL, Freedman MS, Galal A, Arnold DL. Brain atrophy after immunoablation and stem cell transplantation in multiple sclerosis. *Neurology* 2006; 66:1935–7.

28. Makhani N, Gorman MP, Branson HM, Stazzone L, Banwell BL, Chitnis T. Cyclophosphamide therapy in pediatric multiple sclerosis. *Neurology* 2009;72: 2076–82.

29. Illei GG, Austin HA, Crane M, *et al.* Combination therapy with pulse cyclophosphamide plus pulse methylprednisolone improves long-term renal outcome without adding toxicity in patients with lupus nephritis. *Ann Intern Med* 2001;135: 248–57.

30. Boumpas DT, Austin HA, 3rd, Vaughan EM, Yarboro CH, Klippel JH, Balow JE. Risk for sustained amenorrhea in patients with systemic lupus erythematosus receiving intermittent pulse cyclophosphamide therapy. *Ann Intern Med* 1993;119:366–9.

31. Talar-Williams C, Hijazi YM, Walther MM, *et al.* Cyclophosphamide-induced cystitis and bladder cancer in patients with Wegener granulomatosis. *Ann Intern Med* 1996;124:477–84.

32. Morgenstern LB, Pardo CA. Progressive multifocal leukoencephalopathy complicating treatment for Wegener's granulomatosis. *J Rheumatol* 1995; 22:1593–5.

33. Yokoyama H, Watanabe T, Maruyama D, Kim SW, Kobayashi Y, Tobinai K. Progressive multifocal leukoencephalopathy in a patient with B-cell lymphoma during rituximab-containing chemotherapy: case report and review of the literature. *Int J Hematol* 2008;88:443–7.

34. Portaccio E, Zipoli V, Siracusa G, Piacentini S, Sorbi S, Amato MP. Safety and tolerability of cyclophosphamide 'pulses' in multiple sclerosis: a prospective study in a clinical cohort. *Mult Scler* 2003;9:446–50.

35. Ahrens N, Salama A, Haas J. Mycophenolate-mofetil in the treatment of refractory multiple sclerosis. *J Neurol* 2001;248:713–14.

36. Frohman EM, Brannon K, Racke MK, Hawker K. Mycophenolate mofetil in multiple sclerosis. *Clin Neuropharmacol* 2004;27:80–3.

37. Vermersch P, Waucquier N, Michelin E, *et al.* Combination of IFN beta-1a (Avonex) and mycophenolate mofetil (Cellcept) in multiple sclerosis. *Eur J Neurol* 2007;14:85–9.

38. Jacob A, Matiello M, Weinshenker BG, *et al.* Treatment of neuromyelitis optica

with mycophenolate mofetil: retrospective analysis of 24 patients. *Arch Neurol* 2009;66:1128–33.

39. Neuhaus O, Kieseier BC, Hartung HP. Immunosuppressive agents in multiple sclerosis. *Neurotherapeutics* 2007;4: 654–60.

40. Goodkin DE, Rudick RA, VanderBrug Medendorp S, *et al.* Low-dose (7.5 mg) oral methotrexate reduces the rate of progression in chronic progressive multiple sclerosis. *Ann Neurol* 1995;37: 30–40.

41. Goodkin DE, Rudick RA, VanderBrug Medendorp S, Daughtry MM, Van Dyke C. Low-dose oral methotrexate in chronic progressive multiple sclerosis: analyses of serial MRIs. *Neurology* 1996;47:1153–7.

42. Calabresi PA, Wilterdink JL, Rogg JM, Mills P, Webb A, Whartenby KA. An open-label trial of combination therapy with interferon beta-1a and oral methotrexate in MS. *Neurology* 2002; 58:314–17.

43. Cohen JA, Imrey PB, Calabresi PA, *et al.* Results of the Avonex Combination Trial (ACT) in relapsing-remitting MS. *Neurology* 2009;72:535–41.

44. Sadiq SA, Simon EV, Puccio LM. Intrathecal methotrexate treatment in multiple sclerosis. *J Neurol* 2010;257: 1806–11.

45. British and Dutch Multiple Sclerosis Azathioprine Trial Group. Double-masked trial of azathioprine in multiple sclerosis. *Lancet* 1988;2: 179–83.

46. Ellison GW, Myers LW, Mickey MR, *et al.* A placebo-controlled, randomized, double-masked, variable dosage, clinical trial of azathioprine with and without methylprednisolone in multiple sclerosis. *Neurology* 1989; 39:1018–26.

47. Goodkin DE, Bailly RC, Teetzen ML, Hertsgaard D, Beatty WW. The efficacy of azathioprine in relapsing-remitting multiple sclerosis. *Neurology* 1991; 41:20–5.

48. Milanese C, La Mantia L, Salmaggi A, Eoli M. A double blind study on azathioprine efficacy in multiple sclerosis: final report. *J Neurol* 1993; 240:295–8.

49. Casetta I, Iuliano G, Filippini G. Azathioprine for multiple sclerosis. *Cochrane Database Syst Rev* 2007(4): CD003982.

50. Etemadifar M, Janghorbani M, Shaygannejad V. Comparison of interferon beta products and azathioprine in the treatment of relapsing-remitting multiple sclerosis. *J Neurol* 2007;254:1723–8.

51. Havrdova E, Zivadinov R, Krasensky J, *et al.* Randomized study of interferon beta-1a, low-dose azathioprine, and low-dose corticosteroids in multiple sclerosis. *Mult Scler* 2009;15:965–76.

52. Lhermitte F, Marteau R, Roullet E. Not so benign long-term immunosuppression in multiple sclerosis? *Lancet* 1984;1:276–7.

53. Amato MP, Pracucci G, Ponziani G, Siracusa G, Fratiglioni L, Amaducci L. Long-term safety of azathioprine therapy in multiple sclerosis. *Neurology* 1993;43:831–3.

Chapter

38

Intravenous immunoglobulin to treat multiple sclerosis

Franz Fazekas, Siegrid Fuchs, Per Soelberg Sørensen, and Ralf Gold

Introduction

Intravenous immunoglobulin (IVIG) is an important treatment option for various autoimmune neurologic diseases like the Guillain–Barré syndrome, chronic inflammatory demyelinating polyneuropathy, or multifocal motor neuropathy.[1-3] This is a consequence of the broad range of immunologic activities of IVIG, although its exact mechanism(s) of action are still elusive for the majority of the disorders.[4] These beneficial effects have prompted similar expectation in multiple sclerosis (MS) as the most frequent autoimmune disorder of the central nervous system.

IVIG affects with the immune system at several levels possibly relevant to MS (Table 38.1).[5] Immunomodulatory mechanisms are composed of the regulation of antibody production and elimination, and of effects on T-cells, macrophages, cytokine production, and the complement system. IVIG was also reported to inhibit the differentiation of dendritic cells[6] and most recent data suggest an inhibition of the differentiation, amplification, and function of Th17 T-cells as a further mechanism of action of IVIG for achieving a therapeutic effect in autoimmune and allergic diseases.[7] Furthermore, experiments have drawn attention to the possibility of improving remyelination with IVIG, although the respective studies have been equivocal in their outcomes, and such capacity could be contributed to specific monoclonal IgM antibodies rather than to the effects of polyclonal immunoglobulin.[8] Nevertheless, the possibility of diverse effects of IVIG and its overall good tolerability has led to the exploration of IVIG treatment in various conditions and stages of MS, unfortunately, with quite divergent results.

IVIG treatment of acute relapses

The currently recommended practice for treating acute disabling MS relapses is a pulse of high-dose intravenous methylprednisolone (IVMP). This treatment has been shown to hasten recovery, but often cannot produce complete remission. The first historic uncontrolled study reported that 68% of patients treated with IVIG during a relapse improved within 24 hours.[9] Several studies attempted to confirm such benefit (Table 38.2).

The Treatment of Acute Relapse in MS (TARIMS) study was the largest of these trials and included patients with clinically

Table 38.1. *Suggested mechanisms of IVIG in the treatment of MS*

Target	Regulatory effects
T-cells	Regulation of cytokine production
	Neutralization of T-cell superantigens
B-cells	Inhibition of B-cell differentiation
	Selective regulation of antibody production
Fc Receptors	Blocking the effector cells by FcR saturation and FcR down-regulation
	Inhibition of antibody-dependent cellular cytotoxicity
	Elimination of autoantibodies by increased catabolism
Antibodies	Inhibition of pathogenic antibodies by anti-idiotypic network
Cytokines	Modulation of mononuclear cell cytokine production
	Induction of anti-inflammatory cytokines
Complement	Binding of complement components
	Attenuation of complement activation

IVIG = intravenous immunoglobulin, MS = multiple sclerosis.
Adopted from Humle-Jorgensen & Soelberg-Sorensen.[5]

or laboratory-supported definite MS and magnetic resonance imaging (MRI) changes consistent with a diagnosis of MS with a relapsing–remitting (RR) or relapsing–progressive (defined here as secondary progressive [SP] with relapses) course.[10] The patients had to be between 18 and 55 years old, with an Expanded Disability Status Scale (EDSS) score ≤6.0 prior to relapse, and ≥2.0 at the time of inclusion. Patients were randomized to receive either IVIG (10% IVIG-C, Bayer Vital GmbH, Leverkusen, Germany) at a dose of 1 g/kg body weight (maximum 80 g) or placebo (0.1% human albumin and 10% maltose) between 24 hours and 14 days after the onset of symptoms of an acute relapse. The study drug infusion was given 24 hours before starting steroid treatment, which consisted of 1 g IVMP for three days. Relapses had to involve visual acuity, upper limb motor function, or gait with a deterioration of at least one step in the relevant Functional System Scale or ≥1 point on the EDSS. This served to identify a so-called target deficit, which was assessed by measures of visual acuity, the nine-hole peg test (9-HPT), or timed walking on days 3, 4, 12,

Multiple Sclerosis Therapeutics, Fourth Edition, ed. Jeffrey A. Cohen and Richard A. Rudick. Published by Cambridge University Press.
© Cambridge University Press 2011.

Table 38.2. *IVIG for the treatment of acute relapses*

Reference	Patients	Study design	IVIG administration	Primary outcome	Results
Sorensen et al.[10]	76 MS patients with acute relapse 24 hours to 14 days after onset	Randomized, double-blind	1 × 1 g/kg IVIG vs. placebo (0.1% human albumin and 10% maltose)	Change in z-score of target deficit after 6 months	Negative. No difference in relapse-free patients or change in global scores (MSIS, EDSS).
Visser et al.[11]	19 MS patients with acute relapse within 22 days of onset	Randomized, double-blind	500 mg IVMP + 0.4 g/kg IVIG or placebo (2% human albumin) on 5 consecutive days	Change in EDSS score from baseline to week 4	Negative.
Roed et al.[12]	68 patients with optic neuritis (23 MS, 45 CIS) within 30 days of onset	Randomized, double-blind	0.4 g/kg IVIG vs. placebo at days 0, 1, 2, 30, and 60	Recovery of contrast sensitivity at 6 months	Negative. No difference in contrast-enhancing lesions on MRI follow-up or in relapses.
Tselis et al.[13]	23 MS patients with optic neuritis refractory to IVMP 60 to 90 days after onset of visual loss	Open-label, non-randomized	0.4 g/kg IVIG on 5 consecutive days and then monthly for 5 months vs. no IVIG treatment	Improvement of visual acuity 1 year after onset of optic neuritis	18/23 (78%) of IVIG-treated patients reached near normal to normal visual acuity vs. 3/24 (12.5%) of those without treatment ($P < 0.0001$).

CIS = clinically isolated syndrome, EDSS = Expanded Disability Status Scale, IVIG = intravenous immunoglobulin, IVMP = intravenous methylprednisolone, MRI = magnetic resonance imaging, MS = multiple sclerosis, MSIS = Multiple Sclerosis Impairment Scale.

and 26 weeks after infusion of study medication. Because of slow recruitment and expiration of study medication, the trial was terminated after inclusion of 76 patients, which was less than half of the calculated sample size of 172 patients. The 36 patients treated with IVIG and the 40 allocated to placebo all improved in the z-score of the target deficit from baseline to 12 weeks after infusion, which had been defined as the primary outcome of the trial, and the mean change was not significantly different between both groups (IVIG: 0.72 ± 1.0 vs. placebo: 0.64 ± 1.0; $P = 0.89$). There was a somewhat better recovery as measured by the Multiple Sclerosis Impairment Scale and the EDSS in the IVIG group, but the differences relative to the placebo group did not reach statistical significance. There was also no significant difference in the proportion of patients who had not experienced a further relapse at the end of the six-month follow-up; IVIG: 24 (67%) vs. placebo: 22 (55%); $P = 0.3$.

Another study assessed a different treatment regimen, 0.4 g/kg IVIG plus IVMP over five consecutive days vs. IVMP only, but was mainly exploratory and intended to generate data for the planning of a larger trial rather than to provide conclusive results.[11] Nineteen patients (IVIG: 10; placebo: 9) were included and the EDSS was used as the primary outcome variable. No meaningful signal of a treatment response was noted, and this approach was, therefore, not carried further.

To circumvent the problem of how to measure recovery within the broad spectrum of deficits that can be caused by an MS relapse, two further trials focused specifically on optic neuritis (ON). The larger of the two studies[12] included 68 patients aged between 18 and 59 years with a symptom duration of less than 4 weeks. Thirty-four patients received 0.4 g/kg body weight IVIG (Immunoglobulin SSI liquid; Statens Serum Institute, Copenhagen, Denmark) over there days, and on days 30 and 60, and 34 patients were randomized to placebo. The recovery in contrast sensitivity after six months as defined by Arden

gratings (worst score 150) was similar in both groups (IVIG: median score 93; placebo: median score 89; $P = 0.16$). There was also no significant difference in the secondary outcome measures such as recovery of visual acuity, color vision, or regarding visual evoked potential results between treatment groups. During the six-month follow-up, seven patients in each treatment group had one or more relapses (IVIG: nine relapses, placebo: 10 relapses). The number of gadolinium (Gd)-enhancing lesions on MRI was comparable between IVIG and placebo treatment at day 30 and day 180.

The other trial investigated the effect of IVIG treatment on corticosteroid refractory ON in MS in an open-label prospective design and in a post-acute setting.[13] The study considered all patients with clinically definite RRMS who had experienced unilateral ON and did not sufficiently recover following IVMP 1 g per day for five days, i.e. still had a visual acuity ≤20/400 on the Snellen chart 60–90 days after onset of visual loss. A total of 23 patients then received IVIG at a dose of 0.4 g/kg body-weight per day for five days followed by once monthly infusion (0.4 g/kg) for five months. Comparison was made against a so-called untreated or control group of 24 RRMS patients with similar persistence of visual loss that could either not be screened for treatment with IVIG within the pre-specified 90-day time frame, could not be treated with IVIG, or refused such therapy. There was significant improvement in the IVIG group with 18 of 23 (78%) subjects reaching near-normal vision (20/30 or better) while only three of 24 (12.5%) recovered to a similar extent in the control group ($P < 0.0001$). The afferent pupillary defect resolved one year after the onset of ON in 19 of 23 (82%) patients treated with IVIG but in only 4 of 24 (16.6%) patients in the control group ($P = 0.0001$). These results suggest that IVIG may be an alternative to a further IVMP pulse or to plasmapheresis in cases of insufficient recovery of ON, but such a conclusion will have to be confirmed by a randomized trial.

Table 38.3. *Randomized double-blind placebo-controlled trials of IVIG for long-term treatment of MS*

Reference	Patients	IVIG administration	Primary outcome	Results
CIS:				
Achiron *et al.*[14]	91 patients with a first symptom suggestive of MS	0.4 g/kg for 5 consecutive days and once every 6 weeks for 1 year vs. placebo (0.9% saline)	Number of patients experiencing a second attack within 1 year	26% of IVIG patients converted to clinically definite MS vs. 50% on placebo, $P = 0.03$); significant positive effect on change in volume and number of T2-weighted lesions.
RRMS:				
Fazekas *et al.*[15]	150 patients with RRMS and EDSS 1.0–6.0 and 2 relapses in prior 2 years	0.15–0.2 g/kg every month for 2 years vs. placebo (0.9% saline)	Absolute change of EDSS and proportion of patients who improved, remained stable or worsened in disability	EDSS change over 2 years: IVIG -0.23 vs. 0.12, $P = 0.008$; IVIG: 91% improved and 16% deteriorated vs. 14% and 23%; IVIG: significantly greater reduction in annual relapse rate and higher proportion of relapse-free patients.
Achiron *et al.*[16]	40 patients with MRI-confirmed RRMS	0.4 g/kg for 5 consecutive days and then once every 2 months for 2 years vs. placebo (0.9% saline)	Change in annual relapse rate and proportion of relapse-free patients	Significantly lower annual relapse rate over 2 years (IVIG 0.59 vs. placebo 1.61; $P = 0.0006$); larger number of relapse-free patients (6 vs. 0; $P = 0.001$); beneficial shift on disability improvement/worsening.
Sørensen *et al.*[17]	26 patients with RRMS or SPMS with relapses	1 g/kg on 2 consecutive days at monthly intervals vs. albumin 2% over 6 months in crossover design	Total number of Gd-enhancing lesions and the number of new Gd-enhancing lesions on monthly MRI	Significant reduction of mean number of new and total Gd-enhancing lesions (IVIG: 1.3 ± 2.3 vs. 2.9 ± 5.4; $P = 0.003$); significantly greater number of relapse-free patients when receiving IVIG
Lewanska *et al.*[18]	49 patients with RRMS	0.2 g/kg vs. 0.4g/kg vs. 0.9% saline monthly over 1 year	Annual relapse rate	Annual relapse rate lower in both IVIG groups (0.88 vs. 0.87 vs. 1.24) but difference not significant; significant reduction of Gd-enhancing lesions over trial period in both IVIG arms compared with placebo with corresponding effects on lesion number and volume
Fazekas *et al.*[21]	127 patients with MS according to McDonald criteria	0.2 g/kg vs. 0.4 g/kg vs. placebo 0.1% albumin every 4 months for 48 weeks	Proportion of relapse-free patients	No difference in proportion of relapse-free patients (57% vs. 60% vs. 68%); no difference regarding the cumulative number of newly active MRI lesions.
PMS:				
Hommes *et al.*[22]	318 patients with SPMS and clinically active disease	1g/kg vs. placebo (0.1% albumin) every month for 27 months	Confirmed worsening of disability	No difference in confirmed EDSS progression (48.4% vs. 44%); similar annual relapse rate in both treatment groups and no difference in other clinical outcome measures or in the change of T2 lesion load
Pohlau *et al.*[23]	231 patients with SPMS ($n = 197$) and PPMS ($n = 34$)	0.4 g/kg vs. placebo (0.1% albumin) every month for 24 months	Time to sustained progression of disease and improvement of neurologic functions defined by a patient's best EDSS score	Longer time to sustained progression in IVIG than placebo group (74 vs. 62 weeks; $P = 0.04$) with effect mainly in PPMS but not SPMS. No effect on improvement of neurologic functions.

CIS = clinically isolated syndrome, EDSS = Expanded Disability Status Scale, Gd = gadolinium, IVIG = intravenous immunoglobulin, MS = multiple sclerosis, PMS = progressive MS, PP = primary progressive, RR = relapsing–remitting, SP = secondary progressive.

IVIG as a long-term treatment

Repeated administration of IVIG to improve the course of MS has now been tested in almost all stages of the disease, although to a variable extent and with various study designs (Table 38.3).

Clinically isolated syndrome

In a single-center trial, Achiron *et al.* enrolled 91 patients within six weeks of a clinically isolated syndrome (CIS) suggestive of MS to test the potential of IVIG to delay conversion to

clinically definite MS.[14] Patients were randomly assigned to receive either a loading dose of IVIG (0.4 g/kg bodyweight for five consecutive days; Omr-IgG-am, Omrix Biopharmaceuticals Ltd., Ramat-Gann, Israel) followed by 0.4 g/kg body weight per day of IVIG once every six weeks for a period of one year or placebo (0.9% saline) in an identical setting and regime. Examinations occurred every three months and the determination of a relapse was based on a neurological examination by two evaluating neurologists both unaware of treatment assignment. At one year, the cumulative probability of fulfilling the clinical criteria for the diagnosis of MS, i.e. of having had a second attack, was 26% in the IVIG treatment group and 50% in the placebo group ($P = 0.03$). Thus, IVIG treatment reduced the relative probability of reaching a clinically definite diagnosis, which had been the primary end-point of this study, by 48%. Regarding secondary outcome measures, IVIG also resulted in a significant reduction in the volume and number of T2-weighted MRI lesions compared with the placebo group after adjustment for baseline volume and number of lesions. Similarly, at 12 months, the volume of Gd-enhancing lesions was lower in the patients treated with IVIG compared with placebo, but the mean number of Gd-enhancing lesions did not differ significantly between treatment groups.

Relapsing–remitting MS

The findings of this study were in line with four earlier controlled clinical trials in RRMS, which suggested a long-term benefit of IVIG with regard to several aspects (Table 38.3).[15–19] The largest of these trials was the Austrian Immunoglobulin in MS (AIMS) trial that randomized 150 patients to receive IVIG treatment in a dosage of 0.15–0.2 g/kg body weight (Sero Merieux, Austria) or physiologic saline every month over a period of two years. Inclusion criteria were a diagnosis of clinically definite RRMS, baseline EDSS score 1.0–6.0, and a history of at least two clearly identified and documented relapses during the previous two years. A centralized, computer-generated randomization schedule stratified patients by centre, age, sex, and progression rate, i.e. the actual EDSS score divided by the duration of the disease in years. Patients were seen and cared for monthly in their centre by the treating physician. Study assessments were performed at scheduled intervals (baseline and every six months) or in the event of a possible relapse by a neurologist who was unaware of treatment allocation and different from the treating physician. The study met both primary outcome measures which were the between-group differences in the absolute change of the mean EDSS score and the proportion of patients who improved, remained stable, or worsened in disability, defined as an increase or a decrease of at least 1.0 grade of the EDSS score by the end of the study. The intention-to-treat analysis showed a slight but significant decrease of the EDSS score in IVIG-treated patients compared to an increase in the placebo group (-0.23 vs. 0.12; $P = 0.008$). Accordingly, the proportions of patients improving or deteriorating on the EDSS favored IVIG (31% improved and 16% deteriorated in the IVIG group vs. 14% improved and 23% deteriorated with placebo; $P = 0.041$). In the IVIG group there was also a significantly higher proportion of relapse-free patients (53% vs. 26%; $P = 0.03$) and a 59% reduction of the annual relapse rate compared with placebo (0.52 vs. 1.26; $P = 0.0037$). Unfortunately, regular MRI evaluations to confirm the reduction of disease activity radiographically were not part of the study protocol.

A significant reduction in the annual relapse rate was also reported in a further study by Achiron et al. in 40 patients with clinically definite and MRI-confirmed RRMS. Twenty of these individuals received IVIG at the dose of 0.4 g/kg body weight per day for five consecutive days and subsequently once every two months. In this trial the annual relapse rate of IVIG-treated patients dropped from 1.85 ± 0.26 in the pre-study period to 0.75 ± 0.16 in the first year and 0.42 ± 0.14 in the second year ($P < 0.05$ compared with baseline): this was significantly lower than the relapse rate in the placebo group that remained at 1.42 ± 0.23 in the second year of the trial. The number of relapse-free patients was also significantly higher with IVIG treatment during both study years and there was a trend towards reduced neurologic disability in the IVIG group (baseline EDSS: 2.9 ± 0.43; study completion EDSS: 2.6 ± 2.2). The distribution of patients who improved or worsened by at least one point in the EDSS score was again in favor of IVIG treatment (23.5% and 13.7% vs. 10.8% and 17.1%; $P = 0.03$). Parallel MRI examinations at 0.5T showed no significant between-group differences. However, imaging studies were performed in only 30 patients at the end of the study, and images were analyzed in a semi-quantitative manner by scoring the number and diameter of demyelinating plaques.

More solid MRI data were generated by Sørensen et al. who examined the effect of IVIG using frequent Gd-enhanced MRI in a cross-over study of 26 patients with RRMS or SPMS with relapses.[17] IVIG treatment consisted of infusions of 1 g/kg body weight per day for two consecutive days at monthly intervals. Human albumin (2%) administered with an identical regimen served as placebo. MRI was performed using 1.5 T scanners and a conventional double spin-echo sequence with a slice thickness of 4 mm and no inter-slice gap. Post-contrast T1-weighted scans were obtained 10 minutes after injection of Gd at a dosage of 0.1 mmol/kg bodyweight. All scans were evaluated blindly by two independent radiologists for the presence of Gd-enhancing lesions. IVIG treatment reduced the mean number of new and total Gd-enhancing lesions significantly by approximately 60% compared with placebo, both in the per-protocol population (total number – baseline: 3.8 ± 8.3; IVIG: 1.2 ± 2.2; placebo 3.2 ± 5.9; $P = 0.03$) and according to intention-to-treat analysis (total number – baseline: 3.6 ± 7.7; IVIG: 1.3 ± 2.3; placebo 2.9 ± 5.4; $P = 0.003$). Disease activity on MRI decreased after one month of treatment with IVIG and then remained stable, whereas no changes in activity were observed during treatment with placebo. The average percentage of per-protocol patients with active scans on six-monthly serial MRIs was 37% during IVIG treatment compared with 68% when receiving placebo ($P < 0.01$). No significant between-group differences were found in regard to the total T2 lesion load.

Clinically, a significantly greater number of patients were relapse free when receiving IVIG than placebo medication (71% vs. 33%; $P = 0.02$); but although a greater number of patients improved on IVIG than on placebo, no significant differences were found with regard to changes of the EDSS score between the two treatment groups. The study also experienced a very high number of acute and chronic adverse events consisting of headaches, nausea, and urticarial rashes. A reduction in the infusion rate of IVIG significantly decreased the occurrence of post-infusion headache and nausea, and urticarial rashes could be abolished or diminished by administration of an antihistamine drug before the infusion. The most common major chronic side effect was severe eczema observed in 11 patients during treatment with IVIG. It was speculated that both the high dosage of IVIG and differences in the concentration of cytokines between the commercially available preparations of IVIG might have contributed to this unusual adverse event profile. In addition, one patient developed hepatitis C and one experienced deep venous thrombosis with a fatal pulmonary embolism.

A fourth, randomized, double-blind, placebo-controlled study of IVIG in RRMS compared the efficacy of two different doses of IVIG against placebo based on clinical and MRI outcome measures.[18] Patient inclusion criteria were duration of MS for more than two years, a baseline EDSS score between 0.0 and 6.5, and a history of at least two clearly documented relapses during the previous two years. A total of 49 patients were randomly allocated to three treatment groups with either 0.2 g/kg or 0.4 g/kg of IVIG or saline as placebo given at monthly intervals for one year. The annual relapse rate, the primary clinical outcome, was lower in both IVIG groups than in the placebo group (IVIG 0.2 g/kg: 0.88 ± 1.26; IVIG 0.4 g/kg: 0.87 ± 0.99; placebo: 1.24 ± 0.75), but these differences did not reach statistical significance. Also, the proportion of relapse-free patients during the study was higher in both IVIG groups (IVIG 0.2 g/kg: 47%; IVIG 0.4 g/kg: 50%) than in patients receiving placebo (12%) but this difference was also not statistically significant. A Kaplan–Meier analysis of EDSS progression assessed at every three months suggested significant beneficial effects on MS progression in both IVIG-treated groups.

The MRI results of this study were in parallel with the clinical findings. The cumulative number of Gd-enhancing lesions between baseline and study conclusion was significantly reduced in both IVIG groups compared with the placebo group, and was not different between the 0.2 and 0.4 g/kg groups. Similarly, the cumulative number of new lesions on T2-weighted images during the study was markedly higher in the placebo group compared with both IVIG groups. Accordingly, there was an increase in the total T2 lesion volume of the placebo group by 13.6% while lesion volume decreased by –3.95% in the 0.4 g/kg and increased by 3.6% in the 0.2 g/kg IVIG group.

The results of these four trials were summarized in a meta-analysis, which provided information on 265 patients with relapsing MS.[19] The combined data showed a significant reduction in the yearly relapse rate during IVIG treatment with an effect size of -0.5 (95% confidence interval [CI] -0.73 to -0.27, $P = 0.00003$; effect size calculated as the difference in mean results for IVIG and placebo/common standard deviation of study population). Similarly, there was also a highly significant effect on the proportion of relapse-free patients in favor of IVIG (0.29, 95% CI 0.18–0.39; $P = 2.1 \times 10^{-8}$). All studies showed a trend towards a greater reduction of the EDSS following treatment with IVIG, and the difference between treatment groups

with an effect size of -0.25 (95% CI -0.46 to -0.01) just reached statistical significance ($P = 0.0429$). Accordingly, the proportion of patients who deteriorated was significantly smaller in the IVIG than placebo group ($P = 0.03$). MRI data could not be incorporated in this analysis because they had been obtained in only two studies with different methodology.

The results of these four trials and their meta-analysis are supported by a retrospective multicentre observational study from Germany.[20] It was conducted by an independent research organization that aimed to document the clinical course of MS patients who were treated with IVIG for a period of at least two years in routine clinical practice. A total of 1122 patients in 22 centers in Germany and Austria were screened for their eligibility. This led to the identification of 300 patients, 80.8% of whom gave their consent for source data verification. In these individuals treatment with IVIG had resulted in a 69% reduction of the mean annual relapse rate from 1.74 ± 1.15 before to 0.53 ± 0.61 during IVIG treatment. Also, the mean EDSS values of the identified patients remained stable throughout the observational period. About 61% of the patients had not received any previous immunomodulatory or immunosuppressive treatment. Contraindications for other therapies such as the desire to have children, lactation period, psychiatric disturbances, or social reasons were the most important reasons for using IVIG as a first-choice therapy. In those 39% of patients that had been switched from other immunomodulatory or immunosuppressive treatment to IVIG, side effects and/or continued disease activity under the previous immunoprophylactic treatment were the main reasons for switching to IVIG. Treatment schemes of IVIG varied between patients with a mean dose of 0.24 ± 0.15 g/kg body weight per month, and no dose-dependent effects could be observed. While the results of this observational study are thus in line with those of the randomized, placebo-controlled trials, it has to be noted that the analysis did not account for patients who had prematurely terminated IVIG treatment ($n = 138$) or had entered a SP course ($n = 149$).

In view of the different dosages and dosing schemes of IVIG applied in the above studies and other limitations such as their relatively small patient groups, a partly single-centre study design, and the lack of more comprehensive documentation of MRI effects, the Prevention of Relapse with IVIG (PRIVIG) trial was initiated.[21] It attempted to assess the safety and efficacy of two different doses of a new formulation of IVIG (IVIG-C 10%: Talecris Biotherapeutics, formerly Bayer Healthcare AG) with regard to both clinical and MRI markers of MS disease activity. The study comprised two treatment arms of IVIG, 0.2 g/kg ($n = 44$) or 0.4 g/kg ($n = 42$), which was given every four weeks for 48 weeks and a placebo arm ($n = 41$), which received an equal volume of 0.1% of albumin. The primary end-point was the proportion of relapse-free patients. The main secondary end-point was lesion activity assessed by six-weekly MRI. Patient randomization to treatment groups was performed with stratification for the presence or absence of one or more Gd-enhancing lesions on the first of two MRI run-in examinations obtained at an interval of six weeks, i.e. before the initiation of treatment. The MRI protocol included a dual echo T2-weighted sequence and a T1-weighted sequence before and after administration of Gd-DTPA in a dosage of 0.1 mmol/kg body weight. Slice thickness was 3 mm and the MR image analysis was performed centrally and fully blinded to all clinical information. At study termination there was no significant between-group difference regarding the proportion of relapse-free subjects based on all reported relapses. In fact, the placebo group performed better with 68.3% of patients remaining relapse free during the study period compared with 58.1% of patients in the combined IVIG group ($P = 0.29$). There was also no difference between the combined IVIG and placebo groups regarding the cumulative number of unique newly active lesions: the median number of unique newly active lesions in IVIG-treated patients was 5.0 (range 0.0–538.0) compared with 7.2 (range 0.0–218.0) in the placebo group ($P = 0.46$) or between the two dose-groups of IVIG. All other exploratory efficacy variables, like the change in burden of disease volume, were also negative except for a smaller reduction in the brain fractional ratio of IVIG-treated patients at 48 weeks.

Progressive MS

To date, two clinical trials have tested the effects of IVIG on progressive forms of MS. The European Study on IVIG-Treatment in Secondary Progressive MS (ESIMS)[22] was a European-Canadian multicentre, double-blind, placebo-controlled, randomized Phase 3 trial of two parallel treatment groups. Eligible patients were age 18–55, had an EDSS score of 3.0–6.5, and had to have evidence for active SPMS, defined as a documented deterioration over the preceding 12 months with or without interposed relapses following an initial RR course. Pre-study disease activity was defined as a documented deterioration of 1.0 EDSS point for a baseline EDSS score $\leq$ 5.5 or of 0.5 EDSS points for a baseline EDSS score $\geq$ 6.0, or two relapses and a documented deterioration of at least 0.5 EDSS points in the two years preceding the trial. Patients were treated with monthly infusions of IVIG 10% in a dosage of 1 g/kg body weight up to a maximum of 80 g. Placebo medication consisted of the same volume of 0.1 % albumin. All infusions were administered at the study site. Regular visits for neurological evaluation occurred every three months for a total of 30 months and MRI was performed at baseline, year 1, and year 2. No difference between the treatment groups was found in the primary outcome measure, i.e. the time to the start of a confirmed treatment failure defined as deterioration of 1.0 EDSS point if the initial EDSS score was $\leq$5.5 or of 0.5 EDSS points if the initial EDSS score was $\geq$6.0. Treatment failure was observed in 77 patients in the IVIG group and in 70 patients of the placebo group. Accordingly, the mean EDSS score increased to a similar extent in both treatment arms (IVIG: 5.3 $\pm$ 1.1 to 5.8 $\pm$ 1.4; placebo: 5.2 $\pm$ 1.1 to 5.7 $\pm$ 1.4). There were also no significant differences in other secondary outcome measures like the patients' performance on the 9-HPT and the annual relapse rate, which was

identical in both groups (0.46). Lesion volume on T2-weighted MRI did not change significantly in both groups over the two years of the study and there were also no significant differences between the treatment groups in other MRI variables except that the brain volume decreased significantly less in the IVIG group than in the placebo group (brain parenchymal fraction: -0.62 ± 0.88 vs. $-0.88 \pm 0.91\%$; $P = 0.009$).

The second trial investigated IVIG in both primary progressive (PP) ($n = 34$) and SP ($n = 197$) MS patients who were randomly assigned to a monthly treatment with IVIG 0.4 g/kg body weight (Sandoglobulin, 3% solution in saline, Novartis) or placebo (0.1% albumin).[23] For inclusion into the trial, patients had to have an EDSS score between 3.0 and 7.0 with documentation of active disease as indicated by a deterioration of $\geq$0.5 points on the EDSS during the preceding 12 months. The study had two primary end-points defined as (1) progression of disease and (2) improvement of neurological functions defined by a patient's best EDSS score. Progression was identified as a worsening of the EDSS score by $\geq$1.0 point if the EDSS score was $\leq$5.0 at baseline or by $\geq$0.5 points if the EDSS score was >5.0 at baseline and sustained for three months. In the combined intention-to-treat population, the mean time to sustained progression was 74 weeks in the IVIG and 62 weeks in the placebo group which was significantly different and in favor of IVIG ($P = 0.04$). This difference, however, was driven primarily by the small PPMS subgroup, although time to sustained progression was not significantly different to placebo in within-subgroup analysis. There was no IVIG-mediated improvement in neurological functions. In the per-protocol analysis, PPMS patients showed a slightly favorable IVIG effect on the best EDSS score, which was not seen in the patients with SPMS. There were also fewer patients with sustained progression in the IVIG than in the placebo group (48% vs. 63%; $P = 0.0284$) and this difference was also significant in the PPMS subgroup (29% vs. 71%; $P = 0.0164$). However, this comparison was based on only 17 of 34 patients who reached sustained progression. Other secondary end-points such as the relapse rate and patients' performance on several functional tests and a questionnaire on quality of life did not show treatment-related differences. It was concluded from these results that monthly IVIG infusion could delay progression of disease in patients with PPMS and that there was a trend in favor of IVIG treatment in patients with SPMS.

Post-partum use of IVIG

Approved disease-modifying treatments of MS cannot be given during pregnancy or in the post-partum period during breastfeeding. While the rate of relapses appears to naturally decline during pregnancy, especially in the third trimester, the Pregnancy in MS (PRIMS) study indicated a marked resurgence of relapses within the first three months after delivery.[24] Consequently, possibilities for prophylactic treatment, i.e. protection during the high-risk post-partum period, would be desirable. In this context first observational studies suggested a significant reduction of relapses compared to historical controls following immediate application of IVIG after delivery.[25,26]

In a further investigation, Achiron *et al.* retrospectively evaluated the data of 108 pregnant patients with RRMS who were followed at their center.[27] Three groups were compared: the first that was not treated during the pregnancy or post-partum period; the second that received IVIG (0.4 g/kg body weight per day for five consecutive days within the first week after delivery with an additional booster dose of 0.4 g/kg body weight per day at six and 12 weeks post-partum) and the third group that was treated continuously with IVIG during gestation and post-partum (0.4 g/kg body weight per day for five consecutive days within 6 to 8 weeks of gestation with an additional booster dose of 0.4 g/kg body weight per day once every six weeks until 12 weeks post-partum). The decision to treat patients with IVIG was based on the willingness of the health-insurance provider to supply the treatment. Relapse rates were lowest in women who were treated with IVIG for the whole pregnancy and post-partum period with 78% of patients remaining relapse free. Patients treated with IVIG only during the post-partum period also showed a decrease in relapse rate compared with untreated patients (0.58 vs. 1.33; $P = 0.012$); 51% of them and only 31% of untreated patients had been relapse free for the pregnancy and post-partum period. No severe adverse events were associated with IVIG treatment, either during the pregnancy or post-partum period in both patients and newborns, and all women delivered live births with only one neonatal ventricular septal defect.

In a prospective, multicentre, randomized, open-label, parallel study design, the GAmmaglobulins Post Pregnancy (GAMPP) trial assessed the effects of two different dosages of IVIG on the relapse rate during the post-partum period.[28] A formal comparison against placebo, however, was not performed. In total, 173 pregnant patients with RRMS and at least one relapse in the two years before pregnancy were enrolled and randomized to receive either 0.15 g/kg IVIG on day 1 with placebo infusions on days 2 and 3 or a loading dose of IVIG 0.4 g/kg, 0.3 g/kg, and 0.15 g/kg on days 1, 2, and 3, respectively. Both groups then received 0.15 g/kg of IVIG five times at four-weekly intervals. The mean annual relapse rate before the actual pregnancy, calculated from the number of relapses over the preceding 24 months was 1.0 in both groups. During pregnancy, 78% women remained relapse free (low dose: 65%; high dose: 63%; with annual relapse rates of 0.3 ± 0.6 and 0.4 ± 0.7, respectively). In the first 3 months post-partum, the annualized relapse rate increased to 1.1 ± 2.0 for the low dose and 0.7 ± 1.7 for the high dose (combined 0.9), and 76% in the low-dose group and 82% of patients in the high-dose group remained relapse free. In the period from 4–6 months after delivery, the annualized relapse rate increased to 1.3 ± 2.2 in the low-dose and 0.8 ± 1.8 in the high-dose group. Thus, the mean annualized relapse rate after pregnancy did not show a markedly higher risk for relapse, but returned to pre-pregnancy levels independently of IVIG dosage. The ratio of patients remaining relapse free during the first three months post-partum also did not significantly differ between both groups (75.6% vs. 81.5%).

Trials of IVIG to reverse fixed deficits

Following earlier observations in small case series[29,30], two randomized, double-blind, placebo-controlled trials attempted to confirm the capacity of IVIG to reverse fixed deficits from demyelinating lesions in larger patient cohorts. One trial in 67 patients with MS was performed to ameliorate an apparently irreversible motor deficit.[31] To be defined as the targeted neurologic deficit in the trial, the weakness had to have been present and stable for between four and 18 months and to involve at least one limb with >25% loss of power. The primary end-point was the change from baseline to six months in the mean percentage of normal strength of muscles chosen as the targeted neurologic deficit. Secondary outcome measures included various disability scales and measures of neurologic functions. MRI studies were also performed in five patients of each treatment group. Treatment consisted of 0.4 g/kg IVIG in a 10% solution or placebo (0.1% human serum albumin in 10% maltose) given intravenously for five days and every two weeks thereafter for three months for a total of 11 infusions.

At six months, muscle strength had worsened mildly in both treatment groups and IVIG failed to improve isometric strength of the muscles representing the targeted neurologic deficit as well as that in other muscle groups. The deterioration in mean percentage of normal muscle strength of targeted neurologic deficit muscle groups from baseline to six months was even somewhat more pronounced in the IVIG group (-2.5 ± 12.5% vs. -0.3 ± 14.2%). This difference was, however, not statistically significant. Analysis of secondary outcome variables, including the EDSS, the 9-HPT and the ambulation index, also showed no evidence of a beneficial effect of IVIG.

The same group of investigators also examined the potential of IVIG to repair functional deficits in the visual system in another cohort of 55 MS patients.[32] Inclusion criteria of this study included one or more episodes of demyelinating ON, which had occurred in the setting of clinically definite or laboratory-supported definite MS or in the presence of cranial MRI changes consistent with MS. Visual acuity had to be worse than 20/40 (logMAR value worse than 0.3) for a period of at least six months with no change on at least two standardized examinations separated by at least one month. Optical disk pallor and an abnormal visual field were further prerequisites. The primary outcome measure was the change in visual acuity from baseline to six months. Secondary outcome measures included other tests for visual function, neurologic impairment, and clinical measures of disease activity. Patients received 0.4 g/kg IVIG in a 10% solution or placebo (0.1% human serum albumin in 10% maltose) intravenously for five days, and thereafter at four-weekly intervals for a total of eight infusions. At the end of the study, no significant differences between treatment groups were noted to suggest that IVIG had reversed pre-existing visual or neurologic dysfunction. Visual acuity was essentially unchanged for both groups at six months and a slight positive trend in favor of IVIG at 12 months was non-significant.

Current recommendations on the use of IVIG in MS[2,33,34]

As outlined before, the efficacy of IVIG has been explored in several stages and settings of MS ranging from attempts to ameliorate the acute attack via investigations on the effects of long-term immunomodulation to attempts of restoration of fixed deficits. Limitations of many studies are the investigation of only a small number of patients often in one center and the quite variable dosage used. It also needs to be considered that the various studies used different preparations of IVIG. Although there is no evidence from the use of IVIG in other autoimmune disorders of obvious differences in efficacy between preparations, it cannot be excluded that differences in study results might have also come from yet unidentified components which have been contained in one or the other brand but might have been eliminated in newer formulations because of increased safety standards. It has also been argued that the use of albumin as a placebo might have impacted on trial results.[35] In fact, five of the seven randomized, placebo-controlled, double-blind studies using saline or dextrose as placebo led the authors to conclude on positive effects of IVIG while no differences were seen in the eight studies which used albumin as placebo. It has been speculated that albumin itself is active in suppressing inflammation and might have led to an obscuration of the effects of IVIG. On the other hand, it could be argued that the use of albumin as placebo allows for a more effective blinding of patients and medical personnel administering study medication than saline and even dextrose. Unfortunately, most of the trials that used saline or dextrose as placebo did not include MRI evaluations to substantiate the possible effects of IVIG in an unbiased way by complementary morphologic data. Thus, a final verdict on the role of IVIG in MS is not yet possible although many aspects argue for a very restrictive attitude. Table 38.4 summarizes current recommendations based on a consensus of German-speaking MS experts.[34]

At present, there is clearly no indication for adding IVIG to the acute treatment of an MS relapse, and there is no evidence that IVIG might be able to reverse fixed neurologic deficits. Based on the trial of Tselis et al.,[13] it may be discussed if IVIG should be explored further in patients with severe relapses who do not respond to a high-dose steroid pulse.

Regarding IVIG as a long-term treatment for ameliorating the course of MS, data from the PRIVIG study[21] certainly created doubt of a beneficial effect of IVIG treatment in RRMS, despite the positive results of the meta-analysis of four earlier, randomized, placebo-controlled trials.[19] The report of positive treatment effects from the retrospective observational study by Haas et al.[20] cannot compensate for the lack of efficacy seen in the PRIVIG trial and it has to be considered that there was also no evidence for an impact on relapse activity in the

Table 38.4. *Current recommendations on the use of IVIG in MS*

Indication	Evidence[a]	Recommendation
Relapse treatment		
Acute relapse	Class I	Not recommended
Severe relapse refractory to steroids	Class II	Controversial
Disease modifying		
Relapsing–remitting MS	Class I/II	Second-line treatment in some countries
Secondary progressive MS	Class I	Not recommended
Primary progressive MS	Insufficient data	Not recommended
Reduction of post-partum relapses	Class III	Possibly efficacious, may be used on an individual basis
Induction of regeneration		
Repair of fixed deficits	Class I	Not recommended

[a] Evidence classes: I, randomized, placebo-controlled trial available.
II, randomized study with small patient numbers or non-randomized, controlled study.
III, non-controlled studies available.
Modified from Stangel & Gold.[34]

ESIMS trial, though in patients with SPMS. At the same time, in view of the above-noted uncertainties and the conflicting trial results, it appears premature to take a fully negative position, and this is the reason why IVIG is still considered a second- or third-line treatment option in some countries. Clearly, a large clinical and MRI-controlled trial in RRMS would be needed for a definitive statement on the utility of IVIG. In this regard, it should also be considered that IVIG might be specifically attractive for those subtypes of MS in which antibody-mediated mechanisms may play a more important role. Such strategies could also be tested in conditions like acute demyelinating encephalomyelitis where several case reports and small case series have suggested the efficacy of IVIG,[36,37] but unfortunately this has not yet been explored in any controlled clinical trial.

Current evidence argues against the use of IVIG in progressive forms of MS. The ESIMS trial with more than 300 patients was clearly negative,[22] and the study by Pohlau et al.[23] also did not show any promising effects in SPMS. The small benefit seen in the time to progression of disability was primarily due to a few patients with PPMS. Thus, in the absence of other supporting evidence, these data are insufficient to recommend the use of IVIG in progressive MS.

Because of the good tolerability of IVIG, it has been recommended as a possible means to lessen disease activity that may be seen after delivery in some MS patients. The GAMPP study suggested a positive effect of IVIG, as a significant increase of the relapse rate after delivery was not seen with IVIG, but this effect was not tested against placebo and such treatment was also unable to preserve the low relapse rate observed during pregnancy.[28] Therefore, the effect of IVIG can be considered modest at most.

Concerning the safety and tolerability of IVIG treatment, no further concerns have been raised by the newly added trials. The side effects observed at lower dosages of IVIG have been uniformly minor and consisted primarily of headaches, malaise, or a transient rash.[38] An increased risk of thrombosis or prolonged skin reactions appears to be conferred primarily by doses of ≥ 1 g/kg body weight of IVIG,[17,22] which are currently not recommended in MS – as there is no evidence for a better efficacy over low-dose treatment – and anaphylaxis

is rare. Other severe complications such as acute renal failure, stroke, and myocardial infarction have been observed in elderly patients with multiple cardiovascular risk factors and in those with pre-existing renal failure, but these risks usually do not apply for patients with MS.[39] Thus, the good tolerability of IVIG, has even led to considerations of a preferred use in children with MS. However, proof of efficacy must be present before safety and convenience can be discussed. In this regard, further positive studies would be needed to justify the use of IVIG on a regular basis in this specific patient group.[40,41]

References

1. Dalakas M. Intravenous immunoglobulin in autoimmune neuromuscular diseases. *J Am Med Assoc* 2004;291:2367–75.

2. Elovaara I, Apostolski S, van Doorn P, *et al.* EFNS guidelines for the use of intravenous immunoglobulin in treatment of neurological diseases: EFNS task force on the use of intravenous immunoglobulin in treatment of neurological diseases. *Eur J Neurol* 2008;15:893–908.

3. Hughes RA, Dalakas MC, Cornblath DR, *et al.* Clinical applications of intravenous immunoglobulins in neurology. *Clin Exp Immunol* 2009;1589(Suppl 1):34–42.

4. Kazatchkine M, Kaveri S. Immunomodulation of autoimmune and inflammatory diseases with intravenous immune globulin. *N Engl J Med* 2001;345:747–55.

5. Humle-Jorgensen S, Soelberg-Sorensen P. Intravenous immunoglobulin treatment of multiple sclerosis and its animal model, experimental autoimmune encephalomyelitis. *J Neurol Sci* 2005;233:61–5.

6. Misra N, Bayary J, Dasgupta S, *et al.* Intravenous immunoglobulin and dendritic cells. *Clin Rev Allergy Immunol* 2005;29:201–5.

7. Maddur MS, Janakiraman V, Hegde P, *et al.* Inhibition of differentiation, amplification, and function of human T(h)17 cells by intravenous immunoglobulin. *J Allergy Clin Immunol* 2011;127:823–30.

8. Rodriguez M, Miller D, Lennon V. Immunoglobulins reactive with myelin basic protein promote CNS remyelination. *Neurology* 1996;46:538–45.

9. Soukop W, Tschabitscher H. Gamma globulin therapy in multiple sclerosis. Theoretical considerations and initial clinical experience with 7s immunoglobulins in MS therapy. *Wien Med Wochenschr* 1986;136:477–80.

10. Sorensen PS, Haas J, Sellebjerg F, Olsson T, Ravnborg M. IV immunoglobulins as add-on treatment to methylprednisolone for acute relapses in MS. *Neurology* 2004;63:2028–33.

11. Visser L, Beekman R, Tijssen C, *et al.* A randomized, double-blind, placebo-controlled pilot study of i.v. Immune globulins in combination with i.v. methylprednisolone in the treatment of relapses in patients with MS. *Mult Scler* 2004;10:89–91.

12. Roed H, Langkilde A, Sellebjerg F, *et al.* A double-blind, randomized trial of iv immunoglobulin treatment in acute optic neuritis. *Neurology* 2005;64:804–10.

13. Tselis A, Perumal J, Caon C, *et al.* Treatment of corticosteroid refractory optic neuritis in multiple sclerosis patients with intravenous immunoglobulin. *Eur J Neurol* 2008;15:1163–7.

14. Achiron A, Kishner I, Sarova-Pinhas I, *et al.* Intravenous immunoglobulin treatment following the first demyelinating event suggestive of multiple sclerosis: a randomized, double-blind, placebo-controlled trial. *Arch Neurol* 2004;61:1515–20.

15. Fazekas F, Deisenhammer F, Strasser-Fuchs S, Nahler G, Mamoli B, for the Austrian Immunoglobulin in Multiple Sclerosis Study Group. Randomised placebo-controlled trial of monthly intravenous immunoglobulin

therapy in relapsing–remitting multiple sclerosis. *Lancet* 1997;349:589–93.

16. Achiron A, Gabbay U, Gilad R, *et al.* Intravenous immunoglobulin treatment in multiple sclerosis: effect on relapses. *Neurology* 1998;50:398–402.

17. Sørensen P, Wanscher B, Jensen C, *et al.* Intravenous immunoglobulin g reduces MRI activity in relapsing multiple sclerosis. *Neurology* 1998;50:1273–81.

18. Lewanska M, Siger-Zajdel M, Selmaj K. No difference in efficacy of two different doses of intravenous immunoglobulins in MS: clinical and MRI assessment. *Eur J Neurol* 2002;9:565–72.

19. Sørensen P, Fazekas F, Lee M. Intravenous immunoglobulin G for the treatment of relapsing-remitting multiple sclerosis: a meta-analysis. *Eur J Neurol* 2002;2002:557–63.

20. Haas J, Maas-Enriquez M, Hartung HP. Intravenous immunoglobulins in the treatment of relapsing remitting multiple sclerosis – results of a retrospective multicenter observational study over five years. *Mult Scler* 2005;11:562–7.

21. Fazekas F, Lublin FD, Li D, *et al.* Intravenous immunoglobulin in relapsing–remitting multiple sclerosis: a dose-finding trial. *Neurology* 2008;71:265–71.

22. Hommes O, Soerensen P, Fazekas F, *et al.* Intravenous immunoglobulin in secondary progressive multiple sclerosis: randomised, placebo-controlled trial. *Lancet* 2004;364:1149–56.

23. Pohlau D, Przuntek H, Sailer M, *et al.* Intravenous immunoglobulin in primary and secondary chronic progressive multiple sclerosis: a randomized placebo controlled

multicentre study. *Mult Scler*
2007;13:1107–17.

24. Confavreux C, Hutchinson M, Hours M, *et al.* Rate of pregnancy-related relapse in multiple sclerosis. *N Engl J Med* 1998;339:285–91.

25. Achiron A, Rotstein Z, Noy S, *et al.* Intravenous immunoglobulin treatment in the prevention of childbirth-associated acute exacerbations in multiple sclerosis: a pilot study. *J Neurol* 1996;243:25–8.

26. Haas J. High dose IVIG in the post partum period for prevention of exacerbations in ms. *Mult Scler* 2000;6(Suppl 2):S18–20.

27. Achiron A, Kishner I, Dolev M, *et al.* Effect of intravenous immunoglobulin treatment on pregnancy and postpartum-related relapses in multiple sclerosis. *J Neurol* 2004;251:1133–7.

28. Haas J, Hommes OR. A dose comparison study of IVIG in postpartum relapsing-remitting multiple sclerosis. *Mult Scler* 2007;13:900–8.

29. Van Engelen B, Hommes O, Pinckers A, Cruysberg J, Barkhof F, Rodriguez M. Improved vision after intravenous immunoglobulin in stable

demyelinating optic neuritis. *Ann Neurol* 1992;32:834–5.

30. Stangel M, Boegner F, Klatt C, Hofmeister C, Seyfert S. Placebo controlled pilot trial to study the remyelinating potential of intravenous immunoglobulins in multiple sclerosis. *J Neurol Neurosurg Psychiatry* 2000;68:89–92.

31. Noseworthy J, O'Brien P, Weinshenker B, *et al.* IV immunolobulin does not reverse established weakness in MS. *Neurology* 2000;55:1135–43.

32. Noseworthy J, O`Brien P, Petterson T, *et al.* A randomized trial of intravenous immunoglobulin in inflammatory demyelinating optic neuritis. *Neurology* 2001;56:1514–22.

33. Multiple Sclerosis Therapy Consensus Group (MSTCG), Wiendl H, Toyka K, *et al.* Basic and escalating immunomodulatory treatments in multiple sclerosis: current therapeutic recommendations. *J Neurol* 2008;255:1449–63.

34. Stangel M, Gold R. [administration of intravenous immunoglobulins in neurology: an evidence-based consensus: Update 2010.]. Nervenarzt.

35. Hommes OR, Haas J, Soelberg-Sorenson P, Friedrichs M. IVIG trials

in MS. Is albumin a placebo? *J Neurol* 2009;256:268–70.

36. Marchioni E, Ravaglia S, Piccolo G, *et al.* Postinfectious inflammatory disorders: Subgroups based on prospective follow-up. *Neurology* 2005;65:1057–65.

37. Ravaglia S, Piccolo G, Ceroni M, *et al.* Severe steroid-resistant post-infectious encephalomyelitis: General features and effects of IVIG. *J Neurol* 2007;254:1518–23.

38. Stangel M, Kiefer R, Pette M, *et al.* Side effects of immunoglobulins in neurological autoimmune disorders – a prospective study. *J Neurol* 2003;250:818–21.

39. Caress JB, Kennedy BL, Eickman KD. Safety of intravenous immunoglobulin treatment. *Expert Opin Drug Safety*; 9:971–9.

40. Tenembaum SN. Therapy of multiple sclerosis in children and adolescents. *Clin Neurol Neurosurg*; 112:633–40.

41. Kuntz NL, Chabas D, Weinstock-Guttman B, *et al.* Treatment of multiple sclerosis in children and adolescents. *Expert Opin Pharmacother*; 11:505–20.

Chapter

39

Plasma exchange treatment for CNS inflammatory demyelinating disease

Brian G. Weinshenker, B. Mark Keegan, Jeffrey L. Winters, Ichiro Nakashima, and Kazuo Fujihara

Introduction

Research into therapeutic applications of apheresis is limited by the rarity of many of the diseases for which plasma exchange (PLEX) is indicated and by the uncommon and often dire circumstances in which apheresis is considered for common diseases (e.g. myasthenic crisis and acute severe demyelinating disease attacks unresponsive to standard treatment). It is often difficult to perform randomized or appropriately powered studies for these reasons. As a result, case reports, case series, and underpowered trials dominate the literature with respect to clinical application of apheresis. To address this weakness, the American Society for Apheresis (ASFA) Apheresis Categories Subcommittee reviews the medical literature concerning the use of apheresis to treat disease every three years and publishes evidence-based guidelines in a special edition of the *Journal of Clinical Apheresis.*[1] The guidelines include an apheresis category and a recommendation grade for each evaluated disease. The categories define the role of apheresis in disease treatment: Category I – first-line therapy, Category II – second-line therapy, Category III – role of apheresis not established so decisions should be individualized, and Category IV – apheresis is ineffective or harmful. The recommendation grade defines strength of recommendation, either strong (grade 1) or weak (grade 2), and provides an assessment of the literature quality: A – high, B – moderate, or C – low or very low quality evidence.[1] In the recently published special edition, multiple sclerosis (MS), neuromyelitis optica (NMO), acute disseminated encephalomyelitis (ADEM), and progressive multifocal leukoencephalopathy (PML) associated with natalizumab were assigned categories and recommendation grades (see Table 39.1). Strong recommendations were given for its use for acute severe attacks of central nervous system (CNS) demyelination and for NMO. Over the past decade, apheresis has been applied frequently for these indications. This chapter will review the history and current use of these techniques for CNS demyelinating diseases, as well as apheresis techniques and their complications.

Apheresis methods

Patients with inflammatory demyelinating disease have been treated with a variety of apheresis techniques including PLEX,[2-8] double filtration plasmapheresis (DFPP),[9] and immunoadsorption. The immunoadsorption techniques include anti-human polyclonal immunoglobulin columns,[10] staphylococcal protein A agarose columns,[11] and tryptophan or phenylalanine polyvinyl alcohol gel columns.[12-15] Characteristics of these techniques are summarized and compared in Table 39.2.

In PLEX, a device separates whole blood into the cellular components and plasma. The plasma is discarded and replaced with a colloid replacement fluid that is returned with the cellular elements.[1] The replacement fluid is most commonly 5% human serum albumin, fresh frozen plasma, or a combination. PLEX differs from plasmapheresis as plasmapheresis involves the removal of plasma without replacement of the discarded volume.[1]

Two separation techniques, centrifugation or filtration, are used for PLEX. With filtration-based devices, a filter separates plasma from the cellular elements. In centrifugal-based devices, whole blood is pumped into a centrifuge where the components are separated based upon density. With both techniques, as well as the other techniques described later, an anticoagulant, either citrate, heparin, or a mixture of both, is added to the whole blood at the site of removal to prevent clotting of the extracorporeal circuit; in Japan, nafamostat mesylate is used as an anticoagulant.

DFPP (also known as differential filtration plasmapheresis, cascade filtration plasmapheresis) is widely available in Europe and Asia but not in the United States, where the Food and Drug Administration (FDA) has not approved a device. With this technique, plasma is separated from whole blood using a filter and then filtered through a plasma fractionator, which determines the size of molecules to be discarded. For example, a filter with a pore size that would remove immunoglobulin (Ig) G would retain molecules the size of IgG and larger while returning smaller molecules, such as albumin. Plasma fractionators do not have strict size cutoffs, so some small molecules are discarded while some of the larger molecules will pass through the filter. The loss of plasma proteins may require albumin replacement fluid but in volumes smaller than needed with PLEX.

In immunoadsorption, plasma is treated with a device that removes Ig or other humoral factors.[1] A number of devices

---

Multiple Sclerosis Therapeutics, Fourth Edition, ed. Jeffrey A. Cohen and Richard A. Rudick. Published by Cambridge University Press.
© Cambridge University Press 2011.

Table 39.1. *American Society for Apheresis categorization and recommendation grades for central nervous system demyelinating diseases[1]*

Disease	Apheresis procedure	ASFA category	Recommendation grade
Acute central nervous system demyelination unresponsive to steroids	Plasma exchange	II – Accepted second-line therapy	1B – Strong recommendation with moderate quality evidence. Can be applied to most patients in most circumstances without reservation.
Acute disseminated encephalomyelitis	Plasma exchange	II – Accepted second-line therapy	2C – Very weak recommendation. Other alternatives may be equally reasonable.
Chronic progressive multiple sclerosis	Plasma exchange	III – Optimal role uncertain	2B – Weak recommendation with moderate quality evidence. Best action may differ depending upon circumstances.
Neuromyelitis optica	Plasma exchange	II – Accepted second-line therapy	1C – Strong recommendation with weak quality evidence. Recommendation may change with higher-quality evidence.
Progressive multifocal leukoencephalopathy due to natalizumab	Plasma exchange	III – Optimal role uncertain	2C – Very weak recommendation. Other alternatives may be equally reasonable.

Table 39.2. *Characteristics of apheresis technologies*

Technique	Basis of selectivity	Replace-ment fluid required	Plasma volumes effectively treated by device	Availability in USA	Complexity	Relative cost	Other considerations
Plasma exchange (centrifugation or filtration)	None	Yes	1.0–1.5	Yes	Low	Low	Removes desirable substances
Double filtration plasmapheresis	Molecular size	Usually no	1.0–1.5	No	Intermediate	Intermediate	Removes some desirable substances
Anti-human Ig column	Ig	No	Theoretically unlimited; practically 3.0	No	High	High	Exposure to animal protein
Staphylococcal protein A column	Ig	No	Theoretically unlimited; practically 3.0	No	High	High	Limited removal of IgM and IgG3
Tryptophan or phenylalanine polyvinyl alcohol gel column	Ig	No	2.0 before column saturation	No	Intermediate	High	Removes Ig and complement

Ig = immunoglobulin.

are available that can perform this function, but none has been licensed by the FDA and, therefore, none is available in the United States. The devices used for immunoadsorption include staphylococcal A protein columns, anti-human polyclonal immunoglobulin columns, dextran sulfate columns, tryptophan polyvinyl alcohol gel columns, and phenylalanine polyvinyl alcohol gel columns. Only a few of these devices have been reported as being used to treat MS and NMO. As each device uses a different immunosorbent, they may differ in efficacy. All of these devices use filtration or centrifugation to separate plasma from whole blood. An Ig binding column is then perfused with the plasma and the "cleansed" plasma and cellular components are returned to the patient.

Ig-Therasorb (Plasmaselect, Teterow Germany) contains two columns packed with polyclonal sheep anti-human Ig bound to sepharose beads. One column is perfused with plasma until it becomes saturated. Flow is then switched to the second column while the first column is regenerated with a buffer solution that removes the bound Ig. The first column is then available to treat additional plasma. The Immunosorba column (Fresenius Kabi AG, Bad Homburg, Germany) is part of a system consisting of two columns and an elution monitor. Each

column contains staphylococcal protein A linked to sepharose beads. Plasma collected by a separate apheresis device is pumped into the elution monitor that directs plasma through one column. The staphylococcal protein A in the column binds the Fc portion of Ig removing it. After a column is saturated, plasma is directed to the other column and the first column is regenerated. The Immusorba PH and TR columns (Ashai Kasei Kuraray Medical, Tokyo Japan) contain phenylalanine or tryptophan, respectively, bound to polyvinyl alcohol gel. Ig binds to the column through hydrophobic and ionic interactions with the amino acid. This column cannot be regenerated, so once it has become saturated, the treatment is complete and the column is discarded. The column is available in different sizes (250 and 350 ml) to allow for treatment of different plasma volumes.

Use of PLEX in CNS demyelinating disease
Acute attacks of MS and other CNS demyelinating disease

PLEX has now become a widely used treatment in select patients with acute relapses of inflammatory demyelinating disease in

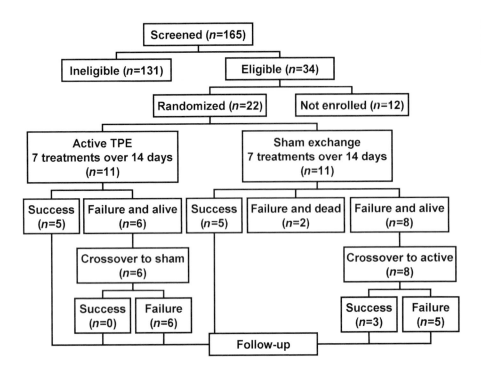

Fig. 39.1. Patient flow in the Mayo Clinic randomized double-masked sham-controlled study of therapeutic plasma exchange in acute, severe, steroid-refractory demyelinating disease.

a variety of contexts (MS, ADEM, idiopathic transverse myelitis, idiopathic optic neuritis, and NMO) when such patients have a severe episode sufficient to justify the complexity and costs of this treatment and when they have been refractory to corticosteroids, the standard treatment for acute attacks. As reviewed in the previous edition of this textbook, a variety of anecdotal case reports were the basis of two controlled studies of PLEX.[16] One, a multicenter study ($n = 116$) provided weak support for this treatment as an adjunct to corticosteroids and cyclophosphamide.[17] A second much smaller study ($n = 22$) focused on patients with more severe attacks than the Harvard multicenter study who did not respond to a course of high-dose intravenous methylprednisolone (HIMP) and showed a robust treatment effect.[18]

The Harvard study reported by Weiner *et al.* was a randomized, controlled, parallel-design trial of 11 courses of true vs. sham exchange over eight weeks as a supplement to oral cyclophosphamide and ACTH in 116 relapsing–remitting or progressive MS patients with acute exacerbations.[17] The primary end-point was improvement by one disability status scale (DSS) point. The overall difference between the patients and controls was not significant, but there was a trend in favor of treatment at one month that was most evident in patients with relapsing-remitting forms of MS with the most severe attacks. The limitations of this study included: (1) patients with attacks of varying degrees of severity were included, including patients with mild attacks. (2) Patients with progressive MS were also included. (3) All patients received ACTH and cyclophosphamide in addition to being randomized to receive true or sham plasma exchange. (4) The end-point was the DSS rather than the deficit targeted to the patient's specific attack-related neurological deficit. The

DSS is insensitive to major improvements of cognitive or upper-extremity function, which limits its responsiveness in instances where these were the neurological deficits caused by the attack.

The Mayo Clinic study[18] included 22 patients between the ages of 18 and 60 who had a recent (between three weeks and three months from onset) severe neurological deficit caused by an attack of MS ($n = 12$) or other inflammatory demyelinating disease ($n = 10$) including transverse myelitis, ADEM, NMO, recurrent myelitis and localized cerebral inflammatory demyelination. All patients had been refractory to treatment with high-dose intravenous corticosteroids (typically HIMP). Patients were randomly assigned to receive either true or sham PLEX, seven exchanges (54 ml/kg or 1.1 plasma volumes per exchange) every other day for 14 days. At the conclusion of two weeks, two neurologists, who were masked to the treatment assignment, decided if moderate to marked improvement occurred. Patients who experienced less than moderate improvement crossed over to the opposite treatment. The results of the study are summarized in the patient flowchart (Fig. 39.1). Nine patients experienced moderate to marked (had a significant impact on function) improvement during treatment. Eight of nine had been receiving the active treatment at the time of improvement. Of 19 courses of true PLEX that were administered, eight resulted in moderate to marked improvement (42% of courses of active treatment). In comparison, one of 17 (5.9%) courses of sham treatment resulted in moderate to marked improvement. The predefined end-point that compared the distribution of patients according to the three possible outcomes (improved in first phase, did not crossover; failed in first phase, crossed over and improved in second phase; failed in both treatment phases) and the result was positive ($P = 0.01$).

Table 39.3. *Retrospective analysis of PLEX treatment of acute, severe attacks of CNS demyelinating disease*

Author	N	Exchanges median (range)	Diagnosis	Syndrome	Response	EDSS median (range) Baseline	Improvement
Bennetto (UK)[21]	6	5 (3–5)	MS 4; TM1; NMO 1	quadriplegia 2; paraplegia 3; cerebellar 1	6 of 6	7.5 (6.5–9.5)	1.5 (0.5–4.5)
Meca-Lallana (Spain)[19]	11	6	MS 9; ADEM 1; TM 1	paraplegia 8; ataxia 4; dysphagia 3	7 of 11 improved in first month	6 (5–8)	1.5 (0–8)
Ruprecht (Germany)[20]	10	5 (3–5)	RRMS 4; CIS 6	ON 10	7 of 10	VA: logmar 0.0 (0.0–0.4)	logmar 0.2; 2 lines of VA
Llufriu (Spain)[7]	41	6 (5–15)	RRMS 18; SPMS3; CIS 2; ADEM 7; NMO 4 Marburg 2; TM 1; ON 4	ON 4; others varied	15 (37%) at 12 days [non ON]; 1 (25%) at 12 days [ON]	7.0 [except ON]; Visual FS 5–6 [ON]	1.5 (1–3.5) [non ON]; logmar 0.2; 2 lines of VA

ADEM = acute disseminated encephalomyelitis; CIS = clinically isolated demyelinating syndrome; EDSS = expanded disability status scale (Kurtzke); FS = functional score; MS = multiple sclerosis; NMO = neuromyelitis optica; ON = optic neuritis; RR = relapsing–remitting; SP = secondary progressive; TM = idiopathic transverse myelitis; VA = visual acuity.

Favorable responses occurred early in the course of treatment and benefits were sustained after treatments stopped. Of the eight patients who improved on active treatment, four of eight had further attacks during the six-month follow-up. In some cases, the subsequent attacks were severe. Some patients did not experience subsequent attacks at three years of follow-up.

Several groups have since reported patient experience that was designed to recapitulate the design of the Mayo Clinic trial using a systematic prospective, though unblinded, study design.[19–21] Specifically, patients with severe attacks of CNS demyelinating disease with varied deficits who had failed courses of intravenous corticosteroids were treated with PLEX and assessed for clinically important improvement. These studies have uniformly confirmed the benefits of PLEX and are summarized in Table 39.3. As found in the Mayo Clinic study, the benefit occurred in patients in a variety of clinical syndromes and for a broad range of neurological deficits, including ataxia, paralysis, and optic neuritis.

To identify predictive factors of benefit, two groups have analyzed treatment responses. Keegan *et al.* analyzed all patients with acute, severe attacks of CNS demyelinating diseases treated with PLEX at Mayo Clinic from 1984–2000 using the same criteria for success as used in the prospective clinical trial.[22] Fifty-nine patients were treated, most of whom had severe attacks of relapsing remitting MS ($N = 22$), NMO ($N = 10$), and ADEM ($N = 10$). Moderate or marked improvement occurred in 44.1% of treated patients. Improvement occurred in most disease subtypes, but was somewhat more common in NMO and Marburg variant MS. Male gender, preserved reflexes, and early initiation of treatment (within 20 days of onset) predicted treatment success.

A retrospective analysis of 41 patients treated in Spain between 1995 and 2007 with a similar distribution of underlying demyelinating disease contexts to the Mayo Clinic study with a median Expanded Disability Status Scale (EDSS) score 7.0 (range 3.0–9.5) documented a similar rate of improvement (39% at hospital discharge, 63% at 6-month follow-up).[7]

The major predictor of improvement was early initiation of treatment (odds ratio 6.29; 95% CI 1.18–52.96) and improvement at hospital discharge (odds ratio 7.32; 95% CI 1.21–44.38).

Removal of natalizumab

Therapy with natalizumab is associated with the opportunistic JC virus infection of the CNS, progressive multifocal leukoencephalopathy (PML). Natalizumab inhibits CNS lymphocyte trafficking by blocking α4-integrin and its serological clearance is enhanced by PLEX. Khatri and colleagues reported that serum natalizumab concentrations were reduced by a mean of 92% following three PLEX procedures of 1.5 plasma volumes.[23] However, saturation of α 4-integrin receptors (and therefore therapeutic effect) by natalizumab remained until serum concentrations were extremely low (<1 μg/ml). For this reason, the authors recommended five PLEX sessions, each of 1.5 plasma volumes, two days apart to reduce natalizumab serum concentrations to this very low level aiming to reduce α4-integrin saturation levels to less than 50%.[23] While the benefit of PLEX in natalizumab-associated PML remains uncertain, rare patients have been reported to respond favorably with PLEX in addition to other potential anti-JC virus therapy.[24] Some patients may worsen clinically despite successful treatment due to immune reconstitution inflammatory syndrome.

Progressive MS

Vamvakas *et al.*[25] reported a meta-analysis of six prospective studies[26–31] that included patients with clinically definite, progressive MS and had a concurrent comparison group. The design and results of the individual studies were summarized in the paper. Of the six studies, four were randomized[26–29] and two were double-blinded with respect to the use of PLEX.[26,29] One study was multicenter.[27] The treatment regimens were variable (4–20 treatments) as was the duration over which they were administered (two weeks to one year), making comparison between the studies difficult. The homogeneity of the

Table 39.4. *Meta-analysis of effect of plasma exchange in progressive multiple sclerosis*

	Follow-up			
	6 months		12 months	
	All	**Controlled**	**All**	**Controlled**
Change in Disability Status Scale score	−0.171	−0.177 (−0.149)[a]	−0.212	0.204 (−0.167)[a]
Relative odds of worsening	0.746	0.879	0.436[b]	0.441[b]
Relative odds of improvement	1.981[b]	2.321[b]	2.129[b]	2.258[b]

- Based on review of six studies, four of which were controlled, by Vamvakas *et al.*[25]
- Values shown reflect difference in change in mean Disability Status Scale score or relative odds of worsening/improvement by 1 point in treatment vs. control group.

[a] after exclusion of four outliers.
[b] $P < 0.05$.

behavior of patients in these studies, assessed using the Q statistic,[32] allowed for meta-analysis. However, for analysis of mean change in DSS, some patients in one study[26] were excluded because the conditions for homogeneity could not otherwise be met as these patients were "outliers." The results of the meta-analysis are given in Table 39.4. There was evidence for significant, though modest efficacy in reducing odds of worsening at 12 months, and in enhancing the odds of improving at 6 and 12 months after PLEX. Follow-up at 24–36 months revealed significant results only for the relative odds of worsening at 24 months.

The conclusions from this meta-analysis must remain tentative because:

1. The "control groups" were not strictly comparable (e.g. in the Canadian Cooperative Study, the "control group" for the purposes of this meta-analysis had received high-dose intravenous cyclophosphamide rather than oral cyclophosphamide as did the PLEX group because the trial was designed to evaluate several therapeutic claims for different regimens, particularly ones including cyclophosphamide, and not to expressly evaluate the efficacy of PLEX.).
2. The effects of PLEX and the other immunosuppressive treatments administered in these studies are difficult to disentangle.
3. The PLEX regimes differed considerably in terms of the intensity of the exchanges and the durations over which they were applied.

Further investigation of PLEX for progressive MS is limited because: (1) existing studies did not adequately differentiate between patients with secondary and primary progressive MS and did not identify a subgroup likely to respond and (2) PLEX is an expensive, cumbersome treatment not well suited for chronic management, particularly if benefit is transient and requires maintenance therapy.

Neuromyelitis optica

NMO is an uncommon inflammatory neurologic disease characterized by severe optic neuritis and transverse myelitis.

Aquaporin-4 (AQP4) autoantibody, otherwise known as NMO-IgG, is an NMO-specific, pathogenic autoantibody. More than half of patients with NMO are seropositive for AQP4 antibody.[33] AQP4 is the dominant water channel in the CNS, and is highly expressed in astrocytes. Other features that distinguish NMO from MS include dramatic female preponderance (80%–90% of cases), severe functional disability, optic chiasmal lesions, longitudinally extensive myelitis (T2 lesions over longer than three vertebral segments on MRI), negative test for oligoclonal IgG bands in cerebrospinal fluid, and high frequency of coexisting autoimmune disorders.[34,35] More than half of patients with NMO have brain lesions, and the spectrum of NMO defined by AQP4 autoantibody is wider than just opticomyelitis. Perivascular deposition of Ig and complement and severe astrocytic damage are cardinal pathological feature of NMO, suggesting the importance of humoral immunity in the unique astrocytopathy of NMO.[36–39] These findings indicate that NMO is clinically, pathologically, and therapeutically distinct from MS.

As in MS, HIMP is the first-line therapy for acute attacks of NMO. However, since NMO attacks fail to respond adequately to HIMP much more frequently than MS, PLEX is frequently used as a rescue therapy in those cases. AQP4 antibody titers decline steadily in every session of PLEX if patients receive sufficient doses of oral prednisolone. Case reports and retrospective studies support the efficacy of PLEX for acute attacks of NMO. Keegan *et al.*[22] analyzed 10 NMO patients and 49 with other inflammatory CNS demyelinating diseases who received PLEX. Functionally significant improvement was seen in six NMO patients following PLEX. Analysis of all 59 cases revealed that male gender, preserved reflexes and early initiation of PLEX were associated with better prognosis. Watanabe *et al.*[40] reported the therapeutic outcome of PLEX in six NMO-IgG-seropositive patients who did not respond to HIMP. Three of them had functionally important improvement, one showed a mild improvement, and two had no improvement following PLEX. The clinical improvement was noted after just one or two PLEX procedures. These results also support a pivotal pathogenetic role of humoral immunity in NMO. Llufriu *et al.*[7] reviewed 41 patients with inflammatory CNS demyelination including four NMO cases that were treated with PLEX after inadequately effective HIMP. In three of the four, the EDSS scores were lower six months after PLEX. Although early initiation of PLEX was associated with a favorable response, some patients responded well even if they were treated after 60 days of relapse. Bonnan et al.[41] reported a retrospective analysis of 29 severe spinal attacks in 18 NMO patients who received PLEX from two days after the initiation of HIMP (3–10 g of methylprednisolone). They performed PLEX daily for five days and exchanged one volume of plasma with 5% albumin solution in each session. Residual EDSS, EDSS lowering (EDSS difference between basal EDSS and acute EDSS), and mean Δ EDSS (difference between residual EDSS and basal EDSS) were significantly lower in the PLEX-treated group than in the steroid-only group. Interestingly, favorable results in PLEX-treated patients were observed in both NMO-IgG-seropositive and -seronegative patients, suggesting PLEX should be initiated regardless of NMO-IgG serological status.

In addition to PLEX, immunoadsorption has been widely used in Japan with tryptophan immobilized on a polyvinyl alcohol gel carrier as the absorbent. The amino acids adsorb pathogenic substances by hydrophobic and electrostatic interactions. Ohashi et al.[42] reported the efficacy of immunoadsorption in four patients with severe acute exacerbations of NMO unresponsive to HIMP. Alternate-day immunoadsorption was performed three to seven times. Immunoadsorption was well tolerated and a significant reduction of EDSS was observed during the treatment period in all patients.

PLEX may be useful to prevent recurrence as well as to treat acute exacerbations in NMO. Recently, the therapeutic effect of intermittent plasmapheresis (four to six times a year) in combination with immunosuppressants to prevent long-term recurrence in two patients with NMO that were poorly controlled with oral immunosuppressive drugs alone was reported.[43] PLEX, immunoadsorption and DFPP were similarly effective in this report.

Acute disseminated encephalomyelitis

ADEM is an acute, monophasic encephalomyelitis with multifocal white matter lesions in the brain and spinal cord. ADEM may be post-infectious, post-vaccinal, or idiopathic. Although ADEM affects all age groups, the disease is more commonly seen in children and adolescents than in adults. ADEM is often difficult to distinguish from a severe inaugural event of MS; 30% or more individuals given this diagnosis are ultimately diagnosed with MS. An ADEM syndrome may occur as an attack, even rarely an inaugural attack, of NMO.

HIMP is usually applied as the first-line treatment and most of the patients respond well. However, some patients with ADEM are refractory to the HIMP and require additional immunosuppressive therapies such as PLEX and intravenous immunoglobulin (IVIG). There is no large-scale randomized trial of PLEX for ADEM, but there have been some case reports suggesting the therapeutic benefits of PLEX in ADEM.[44–47] In the analysis done by Keegan et al.,[22] four out of ten patients with ADEM showed moderate to marked improvement following PLEX while no improvement was seen in five. Khurana et al.[47] reported six pediatric patients with severe ADEM who received PLEX after they failed to respond to HIMP or IVIG. They had a prolonged intensive care; all but one eventually improved with varying degrees of residual neurologic deficits. Further investigations are needed to establish the therapeutic role of PLEX versus HIMP and IVIG in ADEM.

Mechanism of action
General considerations

Circulating pathologic antibodies directed against myelin oligodendrocyte glycoprotein and myelin basic protein have been implicated in subsets of MS patients.[48] In NMO, IgG autoantibodies to AQP4 (NMO-IgG) have been implicated in the pathogenesis of the disease.[49] Removal of these antibodies as well as circulating cytokines, chemokines, complement, and other humoral factors could influence the course of these diseases.

Removal of 1.5 plasma volumes by PLEX, a non-selective method, results in a 70% reduction of all substances present in the plasma. Treatment of each additional 1.5 plasma volume results in removal of 70% of remaining substances such that treating additional plasma volumes fails to produce significant additional reduction but does increase risks. PLEX cannot reduce a pathologic substance to zero and, as a result, the standard of care is to limit the treated volume to 1.5 plasma volumes.[1] The reduction of a given substance by DFPP is determined by the properties of the plasma fractionator; therefore, general statements about efficacy in substance removal cannot be made. Immunoadsorption techniques remove primarily Ig, with minimal effect on other plasma components. Treatment of 1.5 to 2.0 plasma volumes with the anti-human polyclonal immunoglobulin column removes 70% of IgG1, IgG2, IgG3, IgG4, IgM, and IgA. The staphylococcal protein A column removes 97% of IgG1, 98% of IgG2, 77% of IgG4, 56% of IgM, and 55% of IgA but only 40% of IgG3. The limited IgG3 removal has been found to influence response to treatment in disorders where an IgG3 is the dominant pathologic antibody. The pathogenic NMO-IgG autoantibodies seem to be exclusively IgG1. Finally, the tryptophan polyvinyl alcohol column removes 45% of IgG, though greater removal has been reported with some specific autoantibodies.

It is assumed that the effects of these apheresis treatments result from the removal of pathologic immunoglobulins and, in the case of the less selective techniques, other circulating substances. However, the mechanisms may be more complex; alterations in immune function have been reported with the staphylococcal A protein columns including clonal deletion of some B-cells and generation of biologically active complement fragments.

MS-specific considerations

The mechanism of action underlying the functional improvements resulting from therapeutic PLEX in MS patients is incompletely understood. Suspected mechanisms include the removal of circulating autoantibodies, complement components or other inflammatory mediators. Historically, MS was assumed to be a primarily, if not exclusively, a T-cell-mediated disease process, which would argue against an effect on antibodies as being responsible for the robust response to PLEX. Nonetheless, the effects of PLEX may also modulate cellular immunity and may shift the balance from T-helper 1 to T-helper 2 effects.[50] The substantial contribution of B-cell and humorally mediated pathology to the pathogenesis of MS is now increasingly accepted.[51] The role of B-cells in MS pathogenesis is further supported by the efficacy of medications that target B-cells, such as rituximab (anti-CD20) for relapsing–remitting MS.[52] However, rituximab may act, at least in part, through effects on T-cell proliferation.[53]

Further evidence regarding the role of humoral immunity comes from pathological examination of acute lesions by biopsy or autopsy in MS patients who have suffered acute severe attacks of demyelination treated with PLEX. Functional improvement is seen exclusively in those who had pattern II pathology in acute demyelinating plaques obtained approximately at the time of PLEX, and this may be a critical determinant of positive treatment response of acute, severe, corticosteroid-unresponsive MS attacks.[54] Pattern II pathology is defined based on the presence of Ig and terminal activated complement (C9neo antigen) in the plaque. Furthermore, some patients with acute attacks or progressive disease course that have shown improvement with PLEX had similar pathology suggesting an important role of Ig and complement.[55]

Neuromyelitis optica – specific considerations

In neuropathological studies of autopsied cases of NMO, the immunoreactivity of AQP4 and glial fibrillary acidic protein, two astrocytic proteins, was extensively lost in the perivascular areas and accompanied by deposition of immunoglobulins and activated complement.[37–39] The concentration of glial fibrillary acidic protein in the cerebrospinal fluid is remarkably elevated during acute exacerbations of NMO.[56] Recent experimental studies demonstrated that purified IgG derived from AQP4 antibody-seropositive NMO patients is pathogenic in vitro and in vivo.[57–61] AQP4 antibodies, predominantly IgG1 subclass, bind to AQP4 expressed on cultured astrocytes or AQP4-transfected HEK293 cells, activate complement at the cell surface, and eventually destroy the cells in vitro.[57,58] In vivo studies revealed that T-cell-mediated brain inflammation in the context of experimental autoimmune encephalomyelitis is a necessary pathological substrate for induction of NMO-like lesions by passive transfer of immunoglobulin; such lesions are characterized by AQP4 and astrocyte loss, granulocytic infiltrates, T-cells and activated macrophages/microglia cells,

and an extensive deposition of Ig and complement on astrocytic processes of the perivascular and superficial glia limitans.[58,60,61]

Based on these findings, the removal of pathogenic AQP4 antibodies and complement by PLEX is highly likely to be associated with the therapeutic efficacy of this treatment in NMO. In addition, interleukins 6 and 17, and other proinflammatory cytokines and chemokines are up-regulated during acute exacerbations of NMO[62,63] and they probably play a crucial role in enhancing the pathogenic immunological reactions of NMO. Thus, immunomodulation resulting from lowering the levels of those humoral immune factors by PLEX might also be linked to clinical improvement following PLEX.

Adverse effects
Frequency of complications

Complications occur in 4.75% to 36% of PLEX procedures.[64–66] The majority are mild, easily treated, and self-limited and include paresthesias and muscle cramping due to hypocalcemia from citrate anticoagulant, bleeding and hematoma formation from vascular access, urticaria/pruritus and fever from blood products, hypotension, pallor, nausea, and vomiting. Severe reactions that are potentially life threatening are rare and occur in 0.12% of procedures in the series reported by Basic-Jukic et al.[64] They include anaphylaxis, arrhythmia, air embolism, tetany from citrate anticoagulant, transfusion related acute lung injury from blood products, and pneumothorax/hemothorax from central line placement. Couriel and Weinstein observed a higher severe reaction rate of 6.15% in their series with all severe reactions resulting from central line placement. In their series, only 23% of the patients underwent apheresis using peripheral venous access[65] while in the series of Basic-Jukic et al., 72% of the procedures used peripheral venous access.[64] Therefore, the frequency of reactions directly attributable to PLEX when performed using peripheral access is less than the frequency of complications related to central line placement.[65]

Reactions to DFPP occur in 4.7 to 26% of procedures.[67,68] In 2502 procedures, the most common reactions attributed to DFPP were hemolysis (20%) and hypotension (3.3%).[68] Hemolysis resulted from red cell damage during plasma separation and was clinically insignificant with an average decline in hemoglobin of 0.2 g/dl.[68] In a report examining 2021 procedures, the most common reactions were hypotension (2.1%), hematoma/bleeding (0.8%), and dizziness (0.6%). Hemolysis was uncommon in this series and only 1.2% of reactions required intervention.[67]

Moldenhauer et al. performed 164 procedures using anti-human polyclonal Ig column in patients with MS and reported "occasional bruising" as the major side effect.[69] Jansen et al. performed 89 treatments in patients with coagulation factor inhibitors and reported reactions in 5.6% of treatments, the most common of which were nausea, vomiting, and vascular access issues.[70] Hauser et al. performed 842 treatments in patients with MS and reported "no serious side effects."[3]

Studies of 134 European patients and 54 US patients undergoing 891 and 300 staphylococcal protein A agarose column procedures reported adverse reactions in 26% and 30% of procedures. Pain was the most frequent side effect in Europe (9.5%), while nausea and vomiting (8.5%) and hypotension (8.5%) were most common in the USA.[71] A unique problem reported with this system has been the occurrence of mercury poisoning as these columns were originally stored in Thimerosal, a mercury-containing preservative. Replacement of the original preservative with a mercury-free preservative by the manufacturer has eliminated this problem.

The most frequently reported side effect using the phenylalanine polyvinyl alcohol column to treat Guillain–Barré syndrome was transient hypotension that occurred in 6% of patients. Another study of 16 patients with MS treated with this column reported that there were no side effects.[14]

Specific complications

Angiotensin-converting enzyme (ACE) inhibitors

Angiotensin-converting enzyme (ACE) inhibitors are associated with severe reactions consisting of flushing, hypotension, bradycardia, and dyspnea in patients undergoing immunoadsorption. As plasma contacts the negatively charged surfaces of the columns, the kinin system is activated, generating bradykinin. Normally, bradykinin is rapidly metabolized but the necessary enzymes are inactivated by ACE inhibitors resulting high bradykinin levels. These reactions can be avoided by withholding ACE inhibitors for 24–48 hours prior to treatment. The manufacturers of the immunoadsorption columns described recommend withholding or discontinuing ACE inhibitors prior to treatment.

Vascular access

Complications of central line placement are more common than reactions due to PLEX procedures themselves. In the study by Couriel and Weinstein, severe reactions were exclusively associated with central line placement.[65] While it is frequently assumed that all patients undergoing apheresis require central line placement, studies have demonstrated that the majority of patients (72 to 96%) can satisfactorily undergo PLEX using peripheral vascular access.[65,72]

Infectious complications

While severe infections due to removal of Ig are a potential risk, the incidence of infection appears to be small and is primarily related to central line placement. Note that the use of central venous catheters is not mandatory and this risk can be minimized. Bambauer et al. examined complications in 332 central venous catheters placed for apheresis. The infection rates varied according to the portal for venous access: 28.5% for femoral, 19.1% for subclavian, and 5.2% for internal jugular catheters.[73] Early studies using PLEX and immunosuppressive agents such as cyclophosphamide to treat systemic lupus erythematosus, polyarteritis nodosa,

and glomerulonephritis reported increased incidence of severe infections.[74–76] More recent series examining PLEX, DFPP, and immunoadsorption fail to report a significant incidence of infection.[2,5,6,10,13]

Patients with CNS demyelinating disease

Plasma exchange is well tolerated by patients treated for severe attacks of CNS demyelinating disease as evidenced by the adverse events documented in the largest case series. In a case series of 59 consecutive patients, ten patients (16.9%) experienced symptomatic hypotension. Significant anemia (hemoglobin ≤ 8.0 g/dl) occurred in three patients (5.1%). Two patients (3.4%) developed heparin-induced thrombocytopenia.[22] Central venous catheter placement was necessary in 26 patients (44.1%). Two patients had catheter thrombosis, two required multiple line insertions (maximum three insertions) and one patient developed a pneumothorax during line placement. No patients developed catheter-related sepsis. Citrate-related paresthesias occurred in nine patients (15.3%). Five patients (8.5%) developed urticaria and two patients had reactivation of latent viral infections (herpes simplex virus, $n = 1$; and varicella zoster virus, $n = 1$). A separate large case series reported no serious major events in 41 patients treated.[7] Ten patients (24%) had symptomatic hypotension, two (5%) had central line-associated bacteremia, one with venous line thrombosis, and one corticosteroid-responsive skin rash. The most serious potential complications of treatment seem to be those related to central line placement, including risk of sepsis, and these complications are dependent upon technical factors relating to central access and management of central catheters.

Conclusions

PLEX is now an accepted treatment for acute attacks of CNS demyelinating disease, including MS and NMO, and is thought to suppress inflammatory reactions by removing plasma containing putative pathogenic humoral immune factors such as antibodies, complement components, cytokines and chemokines by centrifugation or membrane filtration. DFPP and immunoabsorption are alternative techniques to accomplish antibody depletion that are currently only available outside the USA. PLEX is a well-tolerated procedure in most patients. Adverse reactions, mainly hemodynamic and hematological, are occasionally encountered but are manageable; the major risk is related to the frequent, but not universal, need for central venous access.

Based on available evidence, PLEX appears to be effective as a rescue therapy in patients with severe attacks of MS and other inflammatory CNS demyelinating disorders who fail to respond to HIMP, the first-line therapy for the diseases, in severe attacks, although randomized, double-blind placebo-controlled clinical trials are few.

In MS, therapeutic efficacy has been retrospectively associated strongly in a small series with the presence of Ig accompanied by activated terminal components of complement using immunopathological stains in biopsied lesions. Evidence of therapeutic efficacy of PLEX in progressive MS is sparse, but high-quality long-term studies with PLEX in this situation are difficult to conduct. Some argue that CNS compartmentalization in the face of restored blood–brain barrier integrity in the progressive phase of MS might limit the ability of PLEX to alter humoral mediators trafficking into the CNS; furthermore, neurodegeneration that characterizes this type of MS may not respond to PLEX.

One unique use of PLEX in MS is to remove natalizumab (an anti-α4 integrin monoclonal antibody) from the blood in patients who developed PML during natalizumab treatment. PLEX restores leukocyte function by reducing α4-integrin saturation in those patients, and the resulting immune-reconstitution can lead to suppression of PML.

PLEX seems highly effective in patients with NMO, a condition associated with a pathogenic autoantibody. By comparison with MS, much higher percentage of relapses in NMO is refractory to HIMP, but clinical improvement is seen in more than half of the patients treated with PLEX. Since experimental studies showed the pathogenicity of AQP4 antibody and the need of T-cell-mediated brain inflammation in the development of NMO-like pathology, the therapeutic efficacy of PLEX is probably related with the removal of AQP4 antibody and other humoral factors modulating cellular and humoral immunity. PLEX could theoretically be effective as a maintenance treatment to prevent relapse in NMO, but this has not been adequately studied to provide recommendations about its use in this regard. PLEX may also be effective in some patients with ADEM that is unresponsive to HIMP and IVIG, but further investigations are needed to prove the efficacy.

In acute exacerbations of any inflammatory CNS demyelinating disease, the earlier PLEX is started, the more efficacious the therapy is expected to be; however, benefit seems to occur even beyond three months from onset of the demyelinating syndrome in some patients. Elucidating the clinical significance and pathogenic roles of plasma immune factors in MS and related diseases and developing devices and methods to remove them selectively merits further research.

References

1. Szczepiorkowski ZM, Winters JL, Bandarenko N, et al. Guidelines on the use of therapeutic apheresis in clinical practice–evidence-based approach from the Apheresis Applications Committee of the American Society for Apheresis. *J Clin Apher* 2010;25:83–177.

2. Tindall RS, Walker JE, Ehle AL, et al. Plasmapheresis in multiple sclerosis: prospective trial of pheresis and immunosuppression versus immunosuppression alone. *Neurology* 1982;32:739–43.

3. Hauser SL, Dawson DM, Lehrich JR, et al. Intensive immunosuppression in progressive multiple sclerosis. A randomized, three-arm study of high-dose intravenous cyclophosphamide, plasma exchange, and ACTH. *N Engl J Med* 1983;308:173–80.

4. Khatri BO, McQuillen MP, Harrington GJ, et al. Chronic progressive multiple sclerosis: double-blind controlled study of plasmapheresis in patients taking immunosuppressive drugs. *Neurology* 1985;35:312–19.

5. Weiner HL, Dau PC, Khatri BO, et al. Double-blind study of true vs. sham plasma exchange in patients treated with immunosuppression for acute attacks of multiple sclerosis. *Neurology* 1989;39:1143–9.

6. Weinshenker BG, O'Brien PC, Petterson TM, et al. A randomized trial of plasma exchange in acute central nervous system inflammatory demyelinating disease. *Ann Neurol* 1999;46:878–86.

7. Llufriu S, Castillo J, Blanco Y, et al. Plasma exchange for acute attacks of CNS demyelination: Predictors of improvement at 6 months. *Neurology* 2009;73:949–53.

8. The Canadian cooperative trial of cyclophosphamide and plasma exchange in progressive multiple sclerosis. The Canadian Cooperative Multiple Sclerosis Study Group. *Lancet* 1991;337:441–6.

9. Ramunni A, De Robertis F, Brescia P, et al. A case report of double filtration plasmapheresis in an acute episode of multiple sclerosis. *Ther Apher Dial* 2008;12:250–4.

10. Moldenhauer A, Haas J, Wascher C, et al. Immunoadsorption patients with multiple sclerosis: an open-label pilot study. *Eur J Clin Invest* 2005;35:523–30.

11. Schneidewind JM, Winkler R, Ramlow W, et al. Immunoadsorption–a new therapeutic possibility for multiple sclerosis? *Transfusion Science* 1998;19 Suppl:59–63.

12. Schmitt E, von Appen K, Behm E. Immunoadsorption with phenylalanine-immobilized polyvinyl alcohol versus plasma exchange – a controlled pilot study in multiple sclerosis. *Therapeutic Plasmapheresis* 1993;12:239–42.

13. Schmitt E, Behm E, Buddenhagen F, et al. Immunoadsorption (IA) versus plasma exchange (PE) in multiple sclerosis–first results of a double blind controlled trial. *Prog Clin Biol Res* 1990;337:289–92.

14. Hosokawa S, Oyamaguchi A, Yoshida O. Successful immunoadsorption with membrane plasmapheresis for multiple sclerosis. *ASAIO Trans* 1989;35:576–7.

15. Palm M, Behm E, Schmitt E, et al. Immunoadsorption and plasma exchange in multiple sclerosis: complement and plasma protein behaviour. *Biomat Artif Cells Immobilization Biotechnol* 1991;19:283–96.

16. Weinshenker B. Therapeutic plasma exchange for multiple sclerosis. In Rudick R, Goodkin D, eds. *Multiple Sclerosis: Experimental and Applied Therapeutics*. London: Martin Dunitz, 1999:323–33.

17. Weiner HL, Dau PC, Khatri BO, et al. Double-blind study of true vs. sham plasma exchange in patients treated with immunosuppression for acute attacks of multiple sclerosis. *Neurology* 1989;39:1143–9.

18. Weinshenker B, O'Brien P, Petterson T, et al. A randomized trial of plasma exchange in acute CNS inflammatory

demyelinating disease. *Ann Neurol* 1999;46:878–86.

19. Meca-Lallana JE, Rodríguez-Hilario H, Martínez-Vidal S, *et al.* Plasmapheresis: Its use in multiple sclerosis and other demyelinating processes of the central nervous system. An observation study. *Revista Neurologia* 2003;37:917–26.

20. Ruprecht K, Klinker E, Dintelmann T, *et al.* Plasma exchange for severe optic neuritis – treatment of 10 patients. *Neurology* 2004;63:1081–3.

21. Bennetto L, Totham A, Healy P, *et al.* Plasma exchange in episodes of severe inflammatory demyelination of the central nervous system – A report of six cases. *J Neurol* 2004;251:1515–21.

22. Keegan M, Pineda AA, McClelland RL, *et al.* Plasma exchange for severe attacks of CNS demyelination: predictors of response. *Neurology* 2002;58:143–6.

23. Khatri BO, Man S, Giovannoni G, *et al.* Effect of plasma exchange in accelerating natalizumab clearance and restoring leukocyte function. *Neurology* 2009;72:402–9.

24. Wenning W, Haghikia A, Laubenberger J, *et al.* Treatment of progressive multifocal leukoencephalopathy associated with natalizumab. *N Engl J Med* 2009;361:1075–80.

25. Vamvakas EC, Pineda AA, Weinshenker BG. Meta-analysis of clinical studies of the efficacy of plasma exchange in the treatment of chronic progressive multiple sclerosis. *J Clin Apher* 1995;10:163–70.

26. Khatri BO, McQuillen MP, Harrington GJ, *et al.* Chronic progressive multiple sclerosis: double-blind controlled study of plasmapheresis in patients taking immunosuppressive drugs. *Neurology* 1985;35:312–19.

27. Noseworthy JH, Vandervoort MK, Penman M, *et al.* Cyclophosphamide and plasma exchange in multiple sclerosis. *Lancet* 1991;337:1540–1.

28. Hauser SL, Dawson DM, Lehrich JR, *et al.* Intensive immunosuppression in progressive multiple sclerosis. A randomized, three-arm study of high-dose intravenous cyclophosphamide, plasma exchange, and ACTH. *N Engl J Med* 1983;308: 173–80.

29. Gordon PA, Carroll DJ, Etches WS, *et al.* A double-blind controlled pilot study of plasma exchange versus sham apheresis in chronic progressive

multiple sclerosis. *Can J Neurol Sci* 1985;12:39–44.

30. Tindall RS, Walker JE, Ehle AL, *et al.* Plasmapheresis in multiple sclerosis: prospective trial of pheresis and immunosuppression versus immunosuppression alone. *Neurology* 1982;32:739–43.

31. Trouillas P, Neuschwander P, Nighoghossian N, *et al.* [Intensive immunosuppression in progressive multiple sclerosis. An open study comparing 3 groups: cyclophosphamide, cyclophosphamide-plasmapheresis and control subjects. Results after 3 years] Immunosuppression intensive dans la sclerose en plaques progressive. Etude ouverte comparant trois groupes: cyclophosphamide, cyclophosphamide-plasmaphereses et temoins. Resultats a trois ans. *Rev Neurol* 1989;145:369–77.

32. Yusuf S, Peto R, Lewis J, *et al.* Beta blockade during and after myocardial infarction: an overview of the randomized trials. *Prog Cardiovasc Dis* 1985;27:335–71.

33. Lennon VA, Wingerchuk DM, Kryzer TJ, *et al.* A serum autoantibody marker of neuromyelitis optica: Distinction from multiple sclerosis. *Lancet* 2004;364:2106–12.

34. Takahashi T, Fujihara K, Nakashima I, *et al.* Anti-aquaporin-4 antibody is involved in the pathogenesis of NMO: a study on antibody titre. *Brain* 2007;130:1235–43.

35. Wingerchuk DM, Lennon VA, Lucchinetti CF, *et al.* The spectrum of neuromyelitis optica. *Lancet Neurol* 2007;6:805–15.

36. Lucchinetti CF, Mandler RN, McGavern D, *et al.* A role for humoral mechanisms in the pathogenesis of Devic's neuromyelitis optica. *Brain* 2002;125:1450–61.

37. Misu T, Fujihara K, Nakamura M, *et al.* Loss of aquaporin-4 in active perivascular lesions in neuromyelitis optica: a case report. *Tohoku J Exp Med* 2006;209:269–75.

38. Roemer SF, Parisi JE, Lennon VA, *et al.* Pattern-specific loss of aquaporin-4 immunoreactivity distinguishes neuromyelitis optica from multiple sclerosis. *Brain* 2007;130:1194–205.

39. Misu T, Fujihara K, Kakita A, *et al.* Loss of aquaporin 4 in lesions of

neuromyelitis optica: distinction from multiple sclerosis. *Brain* 2007;130: 1224–34.

40. Watanabe S, Nakashima I, Misu T, *et al.* Therapeutic efficacy of plasma exchange in NMO-IgG-positive patients with neuromyelitis optica. *Mult Scler* 2007;13:128–32.

41. Bonnan M, Valentino R, Olindo S, *et al.* Plasma exchange in severe spinal attacks associated with neuromyelitis optica spectrum disorder. *Mult Scler* 2009;15:487–92.

42. Ohashi T, Ota K, Shimizu Y, *et al.* Immunoadsorption plasma pheresis for the treatment of neuromyelitis optica spectrum disorder. *Mult Scler* 2008;14: S170-S170.

43. Miyamoto K, Kusunoki S. Intermittent plasmapheresis prevents recurrence in neuromyelitis optica. *Ther Apher Dial* 2009;13:505–8.

44. Kanter DS, Horensky D, Sperling RA, *et al.* Plasmapheresis in fulminant acute disseminated encephalomyelitis. *Neurology* 1995;45:824–7.

45. Lin CH, Jeng JS, Yip PK. Plasmapheresis in acute disseminated encephalomyelitis. *J Clin Apher* 2004;19:154–9.

46. Stricker RB, Miller R, Kiprov DD. Role of plasmapheresis in acute disseminated (postinfectious) encephalomyelitis. *J Clin Apher* 1992;7:173–9.

47. Khurana DS, Melvin JJ, Kothare SV, *et al.* Acute disseminated encephalomyelitis in children: discordant neurologic and neuroimaging abnormalities and response to plasmapheresis. *Pediatrics* 2005;116:431–6.

48. Berger T, Reindl M. Biomarkers in multiple sclerosis: role of antibodies. *Disease Markers* 2006;22: 207–12.

49. Weinshenker BG, Wingerchuk DM, Pittock SJ, *et al.* NMO-IgG: a specific biomarker for neuromyelitis optica. *Dis Markers* 2006;22:197–206.

50. Goto H, Matsuo H, Nakane S, *et al.* Plasmapheresis affects T helper type-1/T helper type-2 balance of circulating peripheral lymphocytes. *Ther Apher* 2001;5:494–6.

51. Racke MK. The role of B cells in multiple sclerosis: rationale for B-cell-targeted therapies. *Curr Opin Neurol* 2008;21 Suppl 1:S9–18.

463

52. Hauser SL, Waubant E, Arnold DL, *et al*. B-cell depletion with rituximab in relapsing-remitting multiple sclerosis. *N Engl J Med* 2008;358:676–88.

53. Bar-Or A, Fawaz L, Fan B, *et al*. Abnormal B-cell cytokine responses a trigger of T-cell-mediated disease in MS? *Ann Neurol* 2010;67:452–61.

54. Keegan M, Konig F, McClelland R, *et al*. Relation between humoral pathological changes in multiple sclerosis and response to therapeutic plasma exchange. *Lancet* 2005;366:579–82.

55. Zettl UK, Hartung HP, Pahnke A, *et al*. Lesion pathology predicts response to plasma exchange in secondary progressive MS. *Neurology* 2006;67: 1515–16.

56. Takano R, Misu T, Takahashi T, *et al*. Astrocytic damage is far more severe than demyelination in NMO: a clinical CSF biomarker study. *Neurology* 2010;75:208–16.

57. Hinson SR, Pittock SJ, Lucchinetti CF, *et al*. Pathogenic potential of IgG binding to water channel extracellular domain in neuromyelitis optica. *Neurology* 2007;69:1–11.

58. Kinoshita M, Nakatsuji Y, Kimura T, *et al*. Neuromyelitis optica: passive transfer to rats by human immunoglobulin. *Biochem Biophys Res Commun* 2009;386:623–7.

59. Kinoshita M, Nakatsuji Y, Moriya M, *et al*. Astrocytic necrosis is induced by anti-aquaporin-4 antibody-positive serum. *Neuroreport* 2009;20:508–12.

60. Bennett JL, Lam C, Kalluri SR, *et al*. Intrathecal pathogenic anti-aquaporin-4 antibodies in early neuromyelitis optica. *Ann Neurol* 2009;66:617–29.

61. Bradl M, Misu T, Takahashi T, *et al*. Neuromyelitis optica: pathogenicity of patient immunoglobulin in vivo. *Ann Neurol* 2009;66:630–43.

62. Ishizu T, Osoegawa M, Mei FJ, *et al*. Intrathecal activation of the IL-17/IL-8 axis in opticospinal multiple sclerosis. *Brain* 2005;128:988–1002.

63. Yanagawa K, Kawachi I, Toyoshima Y, *et al*. Pathologic and immunologic profiles of a limited form of neuromyelitis optica with myelitis. *Neurology* 2009;73:1628–37.

64. Basic-Jukic N, Kes P, Glavas-Boras S, *et al*. Complications of therapeutic plasma exchange: experience with 4857 treatments. *Ther Apher Dial* 2005; 9:391–5.

65. Couriel D, Weinstein R. Complications of therapeutic plasma exchange: a recent assessment. *J Clin Apher* 1994; 9:1–5.

66. Shemin D, Briggs D, Greenan M. Complications of therapeutic plasma exchange: a prospective study of 1,727 procedures. *J Clin Apher* 2007;22:270–6.

67. Klingel R, Fassbender C, Fassbender T, *et al*. Rheopheresis: rheologic, functional, and structural aspects. *Ther Apher* 2000;4:348–57.

68. Yeh J-H, Chen W-H, Chiu H-C. Complications of double-filtration plasmapheresis. *Transfusion* 2004; 44:1621–5.

69. Moldenhauer A, Haas J, Wascher C, *et al*. Immunoadsorption patients with multiple sclerosis: an open-label pilot study. *Eur J Clin Invest* 2005;35:523–30.

70. Jansen M, Schmaldienst S, Banyai S, *et al*. Treatment of coagulation inhibitors with extracorporeal immunoadsorption (Ig-Therasorb). *Br J Haematol* 2001;112:91–7.

71. Huestis DW, Morrison FS. Adverse clinical effects of immune sorption with staphylococcal protein A columns. *Transfus Med Rev* 1996;10:62–70.

72. Noseworthy JH, Shumak KH, Vandervoort MK. Long-term use of antecubital veins for plasma exchange. The Canadian Cooperative Multiple Sclerosis Study Group. *Transfusion* 1989;29:610–13.

73. Bambauer R, Schneidewind-Muller J-M, Schiel R, *et al*. Side-effects and complications in large-bore catheters for apheresis. *Ther Apher Dial* 2003; 7:221–4.

74. Lhote F, Guillevin L, Leon A, *et al*. Complications of plasma exchange in the treatment of polyarteritis nodosa and Churg–Strauss angiitis and the contribution of adjuvant immunosuppressive therapy: a randomized trial in 72 patients. *Artificial Organs* 1988;12:27–33.

75. Aringer M, Smolen JS, Graninger WB. Severe infections in plasmapheresis-treated systemic lupus erythematosus. *Arthritis Rheum* 1998;41:414–20.

76. Wing EJ, Bruns FJ, Fraley DS, *et al*. Infectious complications with plasmapheresis in rapidly progressive glomerulonephritis. *J Am Med Assoc* 1980;244:2423–6.

Chapter

40

Statins in multiple sclerosis

Martin S. Weber, Emmanuelle Waubant, and Scott S. Zamvil

Introduction

Statins are orally administered inhibitors of the enzyme 3-hydroxy-3-methylglutaryl coenzyme A (HMG-CoA) reductase, which catalyzes the conversion of HMG-CoA to L-mevalonate, a key intermediate for cholesterol biosynthesis[1] (Fig. 40.1(a)). Since 1987, when lovastatin was the first statin to be approved in the United States for treatment of hypercholesterolemia, statins have established themselves as safe and well-tolerated drugs. A number of statins have been approved for treatment of dyslipidemia: simvastatin (Zocor®, Lipex®), mevastatin (Compactin®), lovastatin (Mevacor®, Altocor®) and pravastatin (Pravachol®) are natural fungal derivatives, whereas fluvastatin (Lescol®), cerivastatin (Baycol®), atorvastatin (Lipitor®) and rosuvastatin (Crestor®) are synthetic statins. All statins resemble HMG-CoA in its chemical structure and thereby competitively bind and inhibit the HMG-CoA reductase (Fig. 40.1(b)). Although synthetic statins are considered the more potent agents, there is no significant difference in the recommended total daily dose between natural and synthetic statins.

Recent studies in animal models showed that statins have immunomodulatory properties that might be of benefit in the treatment of neuroinflammatory disorders, such as multiple sclerosis (MS). Statins are especially attractive candidates for the treatment of MS, because until recently all approved immunomodulatory agents, namely interferon-beta (IFNβ) and glatiramer acetate (GA), were administered parenterally and only partially effective.

Current concept of immunomodulation by statins

The immunomodulatory potential of statins surfaced in 1995, when it was discovered that cardiac transplant patients treated with pravastatin had a reduced incidence of hemodynamically significant rejection episodes, and showed decreased mortality that did not correlate with cholesterol reduction.[2] This landmark observation was followed by a number of studies that established the immunoregulatory and anti-inflammatory properties of statins.[3]

The molecular mechanisms responsible for statin-mediated immune modulation can be generally divided into HMG-CoA reductase-dependent- and HMG-CoA reductase-independent mechanisms. Statins directly bind the cellular adhesion molecule leukocyte function antigen 1 (LFA1), thereby inhibiting activation and migration of pro-inflammatory leukocytes.[4] Most of the currently known statin-mediated immunomodulatory effects seem to be related to the inhibition of HMG-CoA reductase though, as they can be reversed by addition of its downstream product mevalonate. Mevalonate is a key substrate not only for the synthesis of cholesterol, but also for the synthesis of isoprenoid intermediates, including farnesylpyrophosphate (FPP) and geranylgeranylpyrophosphate (GGPP). These two molecules participate in the post-translational modification of GTP-binding proteins, such as Ras and Rho, which have important roles in cellular differentiation and proliferation. Isoprenylation of these proteins is necessary for their intracellular trafficking and localization at the cytoplasmic surface of the plasma membrane, where they function. Therefore, prevention of isoprenylation of Ras and Rho by statins can lead to accumulation of inactive molecules in the cytosol and inhibition of cellular functions that are vital for the activation of various cell types, including immune cells. (Fig. 41.2)[5]

Statins in treatment of experimental CNS autoimmunity

Our current understanding regarding the therapeutic potential of statins in central nervous system (CNS) autoimmune diseases evolved from studies in mice with experimental autoimmune encephalomyelitis (EAE).[6] In EAE, activated pro-inflammatory CD4+ T-cells, which recognize one of the candidate CNS myelin antigens, cause demyelination of axons, resulting in chronic or relapsing paralysis. Oral treatment with statins at the onset of EAE prevented the development of chronic or relapsing paralysis, and clinical symptoms were reversed when statin treatment was initiated after EAE onset.[7–9] When treatment was discontinued, only a few animals developed EAE, suggesting a sustained treatment effect.

Multiple Sclerosis Therapeutics, Fourth Edition, ed. Jeffrey A. Cohen and Richard A. Rudick. Published by Cambridge University Press.
© Cambridge University Press 2011.

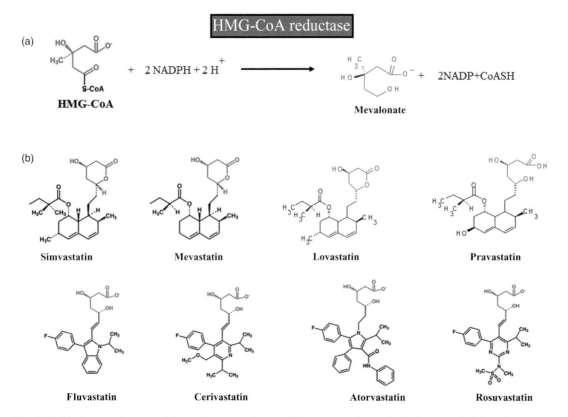

Fig. 40.1. Mechanism of action and chemical structure of statins. (a) Statins are inhibitors of 3-hydroxy-3-methylglutaryl coenzyme A (HMG-CoA) reductase, which catalyzes the conversion of HMG-CoA to L-mevalonate, a key intermediate for cholesterol biosynthesis. (b) Due to chemical similarities with HMG-CoA statins are competitively binding and inhibiting HMG-CoA reductase. Simvastatin, mevastatin, lovastatin, and pravastatin are natural fungal derivatives, whereas fluvastatin, cerivastatin, atorvastatin, and rosuvastatin are synthetic statins.

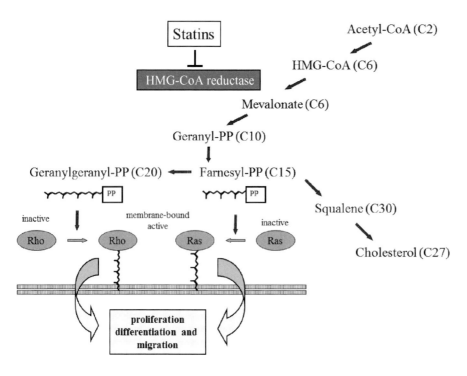

Fig. 40.2. Cholesterol biosynthesis and isoprenylation of Ras and Rho. Farnesylpyrophosphate (farnesyl-PP) and its derivative geranylgeranyl-PP are lipid attachments for the posttranslational modification of immunologically important proteins, such as Ras and Rho. This 'isoprenylation' permits subsequent activation and membrane translocation of these proteins, which is crucial for various cellular functions, such as migration, differentiation, and proliferation. Inhibition of the 3-hydroxy-3-methylglutaryl coenzyme A (HMG CoA) reductase by statins leads to prevention of isoprenylation and accumulation of inactive Ras and Rho molecules in the cytosol.

Table 40.1. Summary of potentially beneficial effects of statins in treatment of CNS autoimmunity

Immunological effect
Inhibit secretion of pro-inflammatory cytokines[5,7,8,10,11,12]
Promote secretion of anti-inflammatory cytokines[7,10,11,12]
Reduce T-cell activation and proliferation[5,7,8,13,14,15]
Suppress upregulation of MHC II and costimulatory molecules on APC[7,14,16]
Reduce expression of adhesion molecules on leukocytes[4]
Inhibit lymphocyte migration into and within the CNS[13,17,18]

Statins might have beneficial effects at several steps in the pathogenesis of CNS autoimmune disease. They might inhibit the presentation of myelin antigen, which is required for T-cell activation, differentiation of T-cells into pro-inflammatory T-cells and T-cell entry into the CNS. In addition, they might suppress the secretion of numerous inflammatory mediators. These different possibilities are summarized in Table 40.1 and discussed in the following sections.

Expression of molecules required for antigen presentation and T-cell activation

The activation of CD4$^+$ T-cells requires recognition of linear peptide antigen bound in the context of the major histocompatibility complex (MHC) class II molecules, termed human leukocyte antigens (HLA) in humans. MHC class II is constitutively expressed in mature professional antigen-presenting cells (APC), and is inducible by interferon-gamma (IFNγ) in non-professional antigen presenting cells (APC).[19] The MHC class II transactivator (CIITA) directs both IFNγ-inducible and constitutive expression of MHC class in APC.[19] One report demonstrated that statins inhibit IFNγ-inducible MHC class II expression on different non-professional APC.[16] It was also shown that atorvastatin inhibits IFNγ-inducible MHC class II expression on microglia, a residential APC population that is thought to have a key role in antigen presentation in the CNS.[7]

In addition to binding of the T-cell receptor to antigen presented in the context of the MHC class II molecule, a second signal is necessary for T-cell activation.[20] Antigen-activated T-cells express the CD40 ligand, which recognizes the co-stimulatory molecule CD40 on the surface of APC. Cross-linking of CD40 and CD40 ligand enhances expression of other co-stimulatory molecules on APC, such as B7–1 (CD80) and B7–2 (CD86), which are required for CD28-mediated T-cell co-stimulation. Atorvastatin treatment inhibits IFNγ-inducible expression of co-stimulatory molecules CD40, CD80 (B7–1) and CD86 (B7–2) on APC.[7] Decreased expression of the molecules that are involved in antigen presentation was found to be associated with reduced secretion of APC-derived cytokines that are involved in the differentiation of T-cells into pro-inflammatory Th1 cells.

Differentiation of pro-inflammatory T lymphocytes

CD4$^+$ T-cells can be categorized into pro- and anti-inflammatory T-cell subsets, mainly based on the profile of cytokines that they secrete.[21] CD4$^+$ Th1 cells, which have a key role in initiating and sustaining EAE disease activity, secrete pro-inflammatory cytokines, including IFNγ, interleukin (IL)-2 and IL-12, and tumor necrosis factor (TNF). IFNγ is thought to have an important role in MS pathogenesis,[22] and Th1-cell-derived cytokines are also strongly associated with clinical disease in EAE.[23,24] More recently, IL-17 producing Th17 cells have been described as a probably equally important pro-inflammatory T-cell subset in development and progression of CNS autoimmune disease. In contrast, Th2 cytokines, such as IL-4, IL-5, IL-10, and IL-13, have down-regulatory properties on the inflammatory cascade in EAE, and are thought to have a beneficial role in MS pathogenesis. Besides Th2 cells, FoxP3$^+$ regulatory T-cells which primarily control development of pro-inflammatory Th1 and Th17 cells are another T-cell subset with anti-inflammatory properties.

The effects of statins on T-cell activation and differentiation perhaps provide one of the most compelling arguments for their use in the treatment of MS and other autoimmune diseases. Several independent studies indicate that statin treatment inhibits antigen-specific stimulation of myelin-specific CD4$^+$ T-cells, which is accompanied by a reduced secretion of pro-inflammatory Th1 cytokines. At least in the case of simvastatin, a similar inhibitory effect has been reported recently for Th17 cell differentiation.[25] Many, but not all studies have further demonstrated that statin treatment may enhance secretion of (protective) Th2 cytokines.[7,8,10,11]

A more mechanistic study confirmed that these immunomodulatory effects on T-cell activation and differentiation are indeed related to the assumed mechanism of statins inhibiting prenylation of regulatory proteins. It was shown that atorvastatin treatment inhibited production of farnesyl-PP and geranylgeranyl-PP in T-cells.[5] The lowered abundance of these isoprenoid intermediates decreased the membrane association of Ras and Rho and compromised the downstream activation of ERK and DNA binding of the c-fos transcription factor. As c-fos transactivates the IFNγ promoter and represses the IL-4 promoter,[26] these results could explain how atorvastatin can bias T-cells to produce higher amounts of IL-4 in the early period of antigen signaling, and subsequently trigger GATA-3 expression and the Th2 program of differentiation.

Migration of immune cells into the CNS

Migration of leukocytes from the blood into the CNS involves multiple steps, including chemoattraction, cell adhesion, extravasation, and proteolytic degradation of biological membranes. Lymphocyte function-associated antigen 1 (LFA-1), and its ligand intracellular adhesion molecule 1 (ICAM-1), have an important role in leukocyte adhesion to brain endothelium. Both molecules have been identified on the surface of inflammatory cells and endothelial cells in perivascular MS lesions.[27] Independent of its effect on HMG CoA reductase, lovastatin binds LFA-1 and directly inhibits LFA-1- and ICAM-1-mediated cell adhesion.[4]

Recent studies showed that ICAM-1 on brain endothelium not only functions as a leukocyte adhesion molecule, but, on engagement, results in intracellular signaling responses, leading to facilitation of lymphocyte transendothelial migration.[28–31] The efficient transduction of ICAM-1-mediated signaling responses in brain endothelium cells, and consequently transendothelial migration of T-cells, is critically dependent on functional Rho GTPase.[28,32] It was shown that in vitro treatment of brain endothelium cells with lovastatin inhibited transendothelial T-cell migration, owing to the absence of activated membrane-bound Rho.[13] Following their passage across the endothelial barriers, leukocytes still have to traverse the basement membrane (basal lamina) of brain venules to access CNS parenchyma. Matrix metalloproteinases (MMPs) are proteolytic enzymes that are considered to be the physiologic mediators of cell migration through biological membranes and extracellular matrix.[33] Two independent reports demonstrated that statins reduce the secretion of MMP-9 by monocytes.[13,18] Therefore, statins interfere with multiple steps of leukocyte recruitment and migration into the CNS.

Statins in treatment of multiple sclerosis

Statin-mediated immunomodulation observed in mice may translate to humans.[34] In vitro, statins inhibit the expression of ICAM-1 and various chemokine receptors on activated peripheral mononuclear cells from both patients with MS and controls.[14] Expression of HLA-DR was found to be reduced when peripheral blood APC were cultured in the presence of statins, which correlated with decreased antigen presentation and T-cell activation. Antigen-independent proliferation of T-cells was also inhibited in a dose-dependent manner.[14]

As some MS patients are treated with statins for the indication of hypercholesterolemia, one might ask whether there is already epidemiological evidence supporting their use in MS. This question is difficult to address for at least three reasons. First, the various statins in use differ in their efficacy for treatment of hypercholesterolemia and, likewise, may differ in their capability to induce immune modulation. Second, lower approved doses of statins are used for the majority of patients treated for hypercholesterolemia. Data from animal studies suggest that the immunomodulatory effects of statins may be evident only at the higher approved doses. Third, data suggest that statins may be beneficial in the earlier, "inflammatory phase" of MS. The mean age of onset of MS is about 32 and the mean age of an individual on a statin for treatment of hypercholesterolemia is 62,[35] a time when many patients are experiencing more advanced (secondary progressive) MS. Thus, at this time the evidence supporting use of statins in MS is insufficient and it is advised that physicians and patients should wait for the results

of controlled clinical trials before using these drugs in MS clinical practice.

Thus, clinical trials evaluating statins in MS are needed. In a single open-label study, 30 MS patients with at least one gadolinium (Gd)-enhancing lesion in the three-month pretreatment period were treated with the highest FDA-approved dose of 80 mg simvastatin daily over six months. Simvastatin once daily was found to decrease the number of new T2-hyperintense lesions on brain MRI scans compared to pretherapy.[36]

To evaluate whether statins may have a clinical and/or MRI effect in a more controlled manner, we recently conducted a placebo-controlled trial with patients who have experienced their first demyelinating attack or "clinically isolated syndrome."[37] The primary end-point (PEP) of the study was development of ≥ 3 new T2 lesions, or one clinical relapse within 12 months. Subjects meeting the PEP were offered additional weekly IFNβ-1a. Due to slow recruitment, enrollment was stopped after 81 subjects were randomized. Based on this number of patients the study failed to show a significant difference between atorvastatin and placebo in regard to the PEP. However, patients receiving atorvastatin showed a significantly reduced number of new brain MRI T2 lesions, a finding which may still warrant conduct of a larger trial evaluating the clinical effect of atorvastatin alone in treatment of MS.

Statins as candidates for combination therapy

Current trials might determine that statins are only partially effective as monotherapy in treatment of MS. However, because they are well tolerated and orally administered, statins might be useful in combination with existing disease-modifying medications.[38] Ideally, medications chosen for combination therapy should have a different mode of action without overlapping toxicities, and should provide an additive or synergistic effect when given in combination. In this regard, an in vitro study revealed that IFNβ and statins had an additive effect, inhibiting activation of T-cells.[14] In a smaller single-center study ($n = 26$), the addition of atorvastatin 40 or 80 mg once daily to subcutaneous IFNβ-1a resulted in a lesser decrease of MS activity compared to subjects receiving IFNβ-1a alone.[39] One theoretical possibility for such potential antagonism may relate to the opposing activity of type I interferon on STAT1 phosphorylation, in which statins inhibit STAT1 phosphorylation,[40] whereas activation of the type I IFN receptor activates STAT1 phosphorylation.[41] However, no other clinical trials or observational studies have confirmed antagonism of IFNβ therapy by statins.[42–46] In our CIS trial mentioned above,[35] we did not observe that the addition of intramuscular IFNβ-1a to atorvastatin in the rescue phase of this trial decreased IFNβ-1a treatment effect on new T2 and Gd-enhancing lesions.

GA is a polypeptide-based therapy for MS that seems to preferentially cause a Th2 deviation of T-cells that are specific for CNS autoantigens.[47,48] Recent data indicate that GA also has immunomodulatory activity on APC, promoting the secretion of anti-inflammatory cytokines and inhibiting the secretion of pro-inflammatory cytokines.[40–51] One can envisage that an agent that augments the immunomodulatory activity induced by GA treatment on myelin-reactive lymphocytes or APC could enhance the efficacy of GA in MS therapy. In this regard, it was recently observed that the combination of GA and atorvastatin synergistically ameliorated CNS autoimmunity in EAE.[52] Combination of both agents at individually suboptimal doses was found to facilitate differentiation of T-cells into anti-inflammatory Th2 cells. In vitro studies revealed that atorvastatin and GA also altered the cytokine profile of activated monocytes in an additive manner. Primarily on the basis of these findings, a trial testing atorvastatin in combination with GA is currently being conducted and its results are anticipated with high expectations.

Potential toxicities

Although statins are considered safe and well-tolerated drugs, they have side effects that should be considered, particularly when they are administered in combination with other agents. Stains are metabolized by the cytochrome P450 pathway, thereby occasionally causing hepatotoxicity (<3% of patients), predominantly with a reversible elevation of transaminases.

Another side effect for which the mechanisms remain obscure is myopathy, which occurs in less than 0.2% of statin-treated patients.[53–55] In severe cases (<0.05%), skeletal muscle injury leads to rhabdomyolysis with myoglobinuria, which can result in kidney failure.[56] In 2001, cerivastatin (Lipobay®) was voluntarily removed from the US market after the rate of fatal rhabdomyolysis associated with cerivastatin therapy was found to be 16–80 times higher than the rates for any other statin.[57] Most notably, rhabdomyolysis is more likely to occur when statins are used with other lipid-lowering drugs, including fibrates, and compounds that are also metabolized by the cytochrome-P450 pathway.

Another occasional side effect is polyneuropathy. However, in a study on the relative risk of polyneuropathy under statin treatment, the incidence was found to be only slightly higher in users of statins (0.73 per 10 000 person–years) than in the hyperlipidemia non-treated cohort and the general population cohort (0.40 vs. 0.46 per 10 000 person–years).[58,59]

Conclusions

Statins have pleiotropic immunomodulatory effects that may have applications in various inflammatory conditions. They have been shown to target key elements of the immunological cascade associated with glial and neural tissue damage in MS. Encouraging results have been obtained from small open-label studies testing statins alone or in combination with established disease-modifying treatments. In a recent placebo-controlled trial in patients with early MS, statin treatment reduced development of newly occurring CNS inflammatory lesions, a finding which supports usefulness of statins in future MS treatment regimens.

References

1. Ginsberg HN. Effects of statins on triglyceride metabolism. *Am J Cardiol* 1998;81(4A):32B–5B.

2. Kobashigawa JA, Katznelson S, Laks H, et al. Effect of pravastatin on outcomes after cardiac transplantation. *N Engl J Med* 1995;333:621–7.

3. Steinman L. Immune therapy for autoimmune diseases. *Science* 2004;305:212–16.

4. Weitz-Schmidt G, Welzenbach K, Brinkmann V, et al. Statins selectively inhibit leukocyte function antigen-1 by binding to a novel regulatory integrin site. *Nat Med* 2001;7:687–92.

5. Dunn SE, Youssef S, Goldstein MJ, et al. Isoprenoids determine Th1/Th2 fate in pathogenic T cells, providing a mechanism of modulation of autoimmunity by atorvastatin. *J Exp Med* 2006;203:401–12.

6. Weber MS, Youssef S, Dunn SE, et al. Statins in the treatment of central nervous system autoimmune disease. *J Neuroimmunol* 2006;178:140–8.

7. Youssef S, Stuve O, Patarroyo JC, et al. The HMG-CoA reductase inhibitor, atorvastatin, promotes a Th2 bias and reverses paralysis in central nervous system autoimmune disease. *Nature* 2002;420:78–84.

8. Aktas O, Waiczies S, Smorodchenko A, et al. Treatment of relapsing paralysis in experimental encephalomyelitis by targeting Th1 cells through atorvastatin. *J Exp Med* 2003;197:725–33.

9. Stanislaus R, Gilg AG, Singh AK, Singh I. Immunomodulation of experimental autoimmune encephalomyelitis in the Lewis rats by Lovastatin. *Neurosci Lett* 2002;333:167–70.

10. Nath N, Giri S, Prasad R, Singh AK, Singh I. Potential targets of 3-hydroxy-3-methylglutaryl coenzyme a reductase inhibitor for multiple sclerosis therapy. *J Immunol* 2004;172:1273–86.

11. Hakamada-Taguchi R, Uehara Y, Kuribayashi K, et al. Inhibition of hydroxymethylglutaryl-coenzyme a reductase reduces Th1 development and promotes Th2 development. *Circ Res* 2003;93:948–56.

12. Pahan K, Sheikh FG, Namboodiri AM, Singh I. Lovastatin and phenylacetate inhibit the induction of nitric oxide synthase and cytokines in rat primary astrocytes, microglia, and macrophages. *J Clin Invest* 1997;100: 2671–9.

13. Greenwood J, Walters CE, Pryce G, et al. Lovastatin inhibits brain endothelial cell Rho-mediated lymphocyte migration and attenuates experimental autoimmune encephalomyelitis. *FASEB J* 2003;17:905–7.

14. Neuhaus O, Strasser-Fuchs S, Fazekas F, et al. Statins as immunomodulators: comparison with interferon-beta 1b in MS. *Neurology* 2002;59:990–7.

15. Waiczies S, Prozorovski T, Infante-Duarte C, et al. Atorvastatin induces T cell anergy via phosphorylation of ERK1. *J Immunol* 2005;174:5630–5.

16. Kwak B, Mulhaupt F, Myit S, Mach F. Statins as a newly recognized type of immunomodulator. *Nat Med* 2000;6:1399–402.

17. Ganne F, Vasse M, Beaudeux JL, *et al.* Cerivastatin, an inhibitor of HMG-CoA reductase, inhibits urokinase/urokinase-receptor expression and MMP-9 secretion by peripheral blood monocytes–a possible protective mechanism against atherothrombosis. *Thromb Haemost* 2000;84:680–8.

18. Bellosta S, Via D, Canavesi M, *et al.* HMG-CoA reductase inhibitors reduce MMP-9 secretion by macrophages. *Arterioscler Thromb Vasc Biol* 1998;18:1671–8.

19. Chang CH, Flavell RA. Class II transactivator regulates the expression of multiple genes involved in antigen presentation. *J Exp Med* 1995;181:765–7.

20. Dustin ML, Shaw AS. Costimulation: building an immunological synapse. *Science* 1999;283:649–50.

21. Abbas AK, Murphy KM, Sher A. Functional diversity of helper T lymphocytes. *Nature* 1996;383:787–93.

22. Panitch HS, Hirsch RL, Haley AS, Johnson KP. Exacerbations of multiple sclerosis in patients treated with gamma interferon. *Lancet* 1987;1:893–5.

23. Khoury SJ, Hancock WW, Weiner HL. Oral tolerance to myelin basic protein and natural recovery from experimental autoimmune encephalomyelitis are associated with downregulation of inflammatory cytokines and differential upregulation of transforming growth factor beta, interleukin 4, and prostaglandin E expression in the brain. *J Exp Med* 1992;176:1355–64.

24. Begolka WS, Vanderlugt CL, Rahbe SM, Miller SD. Differential expression of inflammatory cytokines parallels progression of central nervous system pathology in two clinically distinct models of multiple sclerosis. *J Immunol* 1998;161:4437–46.

25. Zhang X, Jin J, Peng X, Ramgolam VS, Markovic-Plese S. Simvastatin inhibits IL-17 secretion by targeting multiple IL-17-regulatory cytokines and by inhibiting the expression of IL-17 transcription factor RORC in CD4+ lymphocytes. *J Immunol* 2008;180:6988–96.

26. Jorritsma PJ, Brogdon JL, Bottomly K. Role of TCR-induced extracellular signal-regulated kinase activation in the regulation of early IL-4 expression in naive CD4+ T cells. *J Immunol* 2003;170:2427–34.

27. Cannella B, Raine CS. The adhesion molecule and cytokine profile of multiple sclerosis lesions. *Ann Neurol* 1995;37:424–35.

28. Etienne S, Adamson P, Greenwood J, Strosberg AD, Cazaubon S, Couraud PO. ICAM-1 signaling pathways associated with Rho activation in microvascular brain endothelial cells. *J Immunol* 1998;161:5755–61.

29. Adamson P, Etienne S, Couraud PO, Calder V, Greenwood J. Lymphocyte migration through brain endothelial cell monolayers involves signaling through endothelial ICAM-1 via a rho-dependent pathway. *J Immunol* 1999;162:2964–73.

30. Etienne-Manneville S, Manneville JB, Adamson P, Wilbourn B, Greenwood J, Couraud PO. ICAM-1-coupled cytoskeletal rearrangements and transendothelial lymphocyte migration involve intracellular calcium signaling in brain endothelial cell lines. *J Immunol* 2000;165:3375–83.

31. Adamson P, Wilbourn B, Etienne-Manneville S, *et al.* Lymphocyte trafficking through the blood-brain barrier is dependent on endothelial cell heterotrimeric G-protein signaling. *FASEB J* 2002;16:1185–94.

32. Walters CE, Pryce G, Hankey DJ, *et al.* Inhibition of Rho GTPases with protein prenyltransferase inhibitors prevents leukocyte recruitment to the central nervous system and attenuates clinical signs of disease in an animal model of multiple sclerosis. *J Immunol* 2002;168:4087–94.

33. Yong VW, Chabot S, Stuve O, Williams G. Interferon beta in the treatment of multiple sclerosis: mechanisms of action. *Neurology* 1998;51:682–9.

34. Weber MS, Prod'homme T, Steinman L, Zamvil SS. Drug Insight: using statins to treat neuroinflammatory disease. *Nat Clin Pract Neurol* 2005;1:106–12.

35. Bonet S, Garcia Villena I, Tomas Santos P, Tapia Mayor I, Gussinye Canabal P, Mundet Tuduri X. [When and how do we treat our hypercholesterolemic patients?]. *Aten Primaria* 1999;24:397–403.

36. Vollmer T, Durkalsi V, Tyor W, *et al.* An open-label, single arm study of simvastatin as a therapy for multiple sclerosis (MS). *Neurology* 2003;60:A84 (abstract).

37. Waubant P, Mass JA, Cohen, *et al.* ITN020AI Study Management Team, Spencer and Zamvil. A randomized double-blind controlled study of atorvastatin in patients with clinically isolated syndrome: the STAyCIS study. submitted.

38. Costello F, Stuve O, Weber MS, Zamvil SS, Frohman E. Combination therapies for multiple sclerosis: scientific rationale, clinical trials, and clinical practice. *Curr Opin Neurol* 2007;20: 281–5.

39. Birnbaum G, Cree B, Altafullah I, Zinser M, Reder AT. Combining beta interferon and atorvastatin may increase disease activity in multiple sclerosis. *Neurology* 2008;71:1390–5.

40. Lee SJ, Qin H, Benveniste EN. Simvastatin inhibits IFN-gamma-induced CD40 gene expression by suppressing STAT-1alpha. *J Leukoc Biol* 2007;82:436–47.

41. Darnell JE, Jr., Kerr IM, Stark GR. Jak-STAT pathways and transcriptional activation in response to IFNs and other extracellular signaling proteins. *Science* 1994;264:1415–21.

42. Rudick RA, Pace A, Rani MR, *et al.* Effect of statins on clinical and molecular responses to intramuscular interferon beta-1a. *Neurology* 2009;72:1989–93.

43. Paul F, Waiczies S, Wuerfel J, *et al.* Oral high-dose atorvastatin treatment in relapsing-remitting multiple sclerosis. *PLoS ONE* 2008;3:e1928.

44. Lanzillo R, Orefice G, Quarantelli M, *et al.* Atorvastatin combined to interferon to verify the efficacy (ACTIVE) in relapsing-remitting active multiple sclerosis patients: a longitudinal controlled trial of combination therapy. *Mult Scler* 2010;16:450–4.

45. Togha M, Karvigh SA, Nabavi M, *et al.* Simvastatin treatment in patients with relapsing-remitting multiple sclerosis receiving interferon beta 1a: a double-blind randomized controlled trial. *Mult Scler* 2010;16:848–54.

46. Sellner J, Weber MS, Vollmar P, Mattle HP, Hemmer B, Stuve O. The combination of interferon-beta and

HMG-CoA reductase inhibition in multiple sclerosis: enthusiasm lost too soon? *CNS Neurosci Ther* 2010;16:362–73.

47. Neuhaus O, Farina C, Wekerle H, Hohlfeld R. Mechanisms of action of glatiramer acetate in multiple sclerosis. *Neurology* 2001;56:702–8.

48. Duda PW, Schmied MC, Cook SL, Krieger JI, Hafler DA. Glatiramer acetate (Copaxone) induces degenerate, Th2-polarized immune responses in patients with multiple sclerosis. *J Clin Invest* 2000;105:967–76.

49. Weber MS, Starck M, Wagenpfeil S, Meinl E, Hohlfeld R, Farina C. Multiple sclerosis: glatiramer acetate inhibits monocyte reactivity in vitro and in vivo. *Brain* 2004;127:1370–8.

50. Kim HJ, Ifergan I, Antel JP, *et al.* Type 2 monocyte and microglia differentiation mediated by glatiramer acetate therapy in patients with multiple sclerosis. *J Immunol* 2004;172:7144–53.

51. Weber MS, Prod'homme T, Youssef S, *et al.* Type II monocytes modulate T cell-mediated central nervous system autoimmune disease. *Nat Med* 2007;13:935–43.

52. Stuve O, Youssef S, Weber MS, *et al.* Immunomodulatory synergy by combination of atorvastatin and glatiramer acetate in treatment of CNS autoimmunity. *J Clin Invest* 2006;116:1037–44.

53. Randomised trial of cholesterol lowering in 4444 patients with coronary heart disease: the Scandinavian Simvastatin Survival Study (4S). *Lancet* 1994;344:1383–9.

54. Jukema JW, Bruschke AV, van Boven AJ, *et al.* Effects of lipid lowering by pravastatin on progression and regression of coronary artery disease in symptomatic men with normal to moderately elevated serum cholesterol levels. The Regression Growth Evaluation Statin Study (REGRESS). *Circulation* 1995;91:2528–40.

55. Prevention of cardiovascular events and death with pravastatin in patients with coronary heart disease and a broad range of initial cholesterol levels. The Long-Term Intervention with Pravastatin in Ischaemic Disease (LIPID) Study Group. *N Engl J Med* 1998;339:1349–57.

56. Graham DJ, Staffa JA, Shatin D, *et al.* Incidence of hospitalized rhabdomyolysis in patients treated with lipid-lowering drugs. *J Am Med Assoc* 2004;292:2585–90.

57. Staffa JA, Chang J, Green L. Cerivastatin and reports of fatal rhabdomyolysis. *N Engl J Med* 2002;346:539–40.

58. Gaist D, Jeppesen U, Andersen M, Garcia Rodriguez LA, Hallas J, Sindrup SH. Statins and risk of polyneuropathy: a case-control study. *Neurology* 2002;58:1333–7.

59. Gaist D, Garcia Rodriguez LA, Huerta C, Hallas J, Sindrup SH. Are users of lipid-lowering drugs at increased risk of peripheral neuropathy? *Eur J Clin Pharmacol* 2001;56:931–3.

Chapter

41

T-cell-based therapies for multiple sclerosis

Tanuja Chitnis and Samia J. Khoury

Role of T-cells in multiple sclerosis

T-cells play a central role in the pathogenesis of multiple sclerosis (MS).[1] Both CD4+ and CD8+ T-cells have been demonstrated in MS lesions, with CD4+ T-cells predominating in acute lesions, and CD8+ T-cells being observed more frequently in chronic lesions.[2] Additionally, T-cells are found in all four of the recently described histopathological subtypes of MS.[3] Activated myelin-reactive CD4+ T-cells are present in the blood and cerebrospinal fluid (CSF) of MS patients; in contrast, only non-activated myelin-reactive T-cells are present in the blood of controls.[4] The success of several T-cell-targeted therapies in MS reinforces the important role of the T-cell in MS pathogenesis. Here, we summarize potential molecular therapeutic targets in T-cell activation and function, and the current state of T-cell based therapies in MS.

Targeting stages of the T-cell response

T-cells originate and differentiate in the thymus. Every T-cell that leaves the thymus is conferred with a unique specificity for recognizing antigens through its T-cell receptor (TCR). The TCR consists of two glycosylated polypeptide chains, the alpha (α) and beta (ß) chain, which are linked by disulfide bonds. Each chain consists of variable (V), joining (J), and constant (C) regions closely resembling immunoglobulin chains. T-cells that recognize self-antigens with high affinity are either deleted or rendered tolerant within the thymus, through a process called central tolerance.

T-cells may be divided into two groups on the basis of their expression of either the CD4+ or CD8+ surface molecules. Functionally, CD4+ T-cells are involved in delayed-type hypersensitivity (DTH) responses and also provide help for B-cell differentiation, and, hence, are termed helper T-cells. In contrast, CD8+ T-cells are involved in class I restricted lysis of antigen-specific targets, and, hence, are termed cytotoxic T-cells. The CD4 molecule binds to a non-polymorphic site on the major histocompatability complex (MHC) class II beta chain that is expressed by antigen-presenting cells (APCs). In contrast CD8 binds to the alpha-3 domain of the MHC class I molecule expressed by most T-cell types. The MHC molecule serves to present antigen to the T-cell via the TCR.

Signaling through surface molecules by second messengers deliver signals for cell division to the nucleus. The CD3 molecule is part of the TCR complex, and although the TCR interacts with the MHC-peptide complex on APCs, the signals for the subsequent enactment of T-cell activation and proliferation are delivered by the CD3 antigen. The cytoplasmic tail of the CD3 protein contains one copy of a sequence motif important for signaling functions, called the immunoreceptor tyrosine-based activation motif (ITAM). Phosphorylation of the ITAM initiates intracellular signaling events. The interaction of MHC peptide complex with T-cells, while necessary, is insufficient for T-cell activation. Additional classes of molecules are involved in T-cell antigen recognition, activation, intracellular signaling, adhesion, and trafficking of T-cells to their target organs.

Two signals are required for T-cell activation. According to this "two-signal" model,[5] "signal 1" consists of the interaction of the TCR with antigen, presented by the major MHC on the surface of antigen-presenting cells (APC). "Signal 2" consists of the engagement of co-stimulatory receptors on the T-cell, by ligands present on the surface of APCs.[6,7] After contact with specific antigen-MHC complex and adequate costimulatory signals, T-cells proliferate, differentiate, and deliver a series of signals enabling effector functions of other cells such as B-cells and natural killer cells. T-cells can thereby orchestrate the immune response.

Costimulatory molecules may deliver either a stimulatory (positive) or inhibitory (negative) signal for T-cell activation.[8] Examples of molecules delivering a positive costimulatory signal for T-cell activation include the B7-CD28, CD40-CD154 pathways. Examples of molecular pathways delivering a negative signal for T-cell activation include B7-CTLA4 and PD1-PD ligand. The delicate balance between positive and negative regulatory signals can determine the outcome of a specific immune response. Importantly, in the absence of adequate costimulatory signals, T-cells can die or become anergic in vitro, and, thus, fail to initiate an effective immune response in vivo. Therefore, manipulation of costimulatory signals represents an important mechanism to inhibit immune-activation.

Molecules primarily involved in cell migration into tissues, include chemokines, integrins, selectins, and matrix

Multiple Sclerosis Therapeutics, Fourth Edition, ed. Jeffrey A. Cohen and Richard A. Rudick. Published by Cambridge University Press.
© Cambridge University Press 2011.

metalloproteinases (MMPs). Chemokines constitute a large family of chemoattractant peptides that regulate the vast spectrum of leukocyte migration events. The chemokine family and their receptors are described in detail elsewhere in this book. The integrin family includes vascular cell adhesion molecule 1 (VCAM-1), intercellular adhesion molecule (ICAM-1), leukocyte function antigen 3 (LFA-3), CD45, and CD2. The integrin family also mediates T-cell adhesion, facilitates interaction with the APCs, as well as mediating adhesion to non-hematopoietic cells such as endothelial cells and guiding cell traffic. L-selectins facilitate the rolling of leucocytes along the surface of endothelial cells and function as a homing receptor to target peripheral lymphoid organs. The MMPs are a family of proteinases, secreted by inflammatory cells, which digest specific components of the extracellular matrix, thereby facilitating lymphocyte entry through basement membranes, including the blood-brain barrier. Inhibition of molecular pathways involved in T-cell migration has been effective in reducing MS relapses;[9] however, recent clinical trials with an α4-integrin antibody (natalizumab) led to several cases of progressive multifocal leukoencephalopathy, resulting in the re-evaluation of the role of such drugs in MS therapeutics.[10-12] This topic is discussed in more detail in other chapters of this book.

The helper T-cells play a critical role in the orchestration of the immune response, in part, through the production of cytokines that provide secondary signals to other cells in the immune cascade. Two major types of helper T-cell responses have been described. Th1 cells produce interleukin-2 (IL-2), tumor necrosis factor alpha (TNFα) and interferon gamma (IFNγ), while Th2 cells produce IL-4, IL-5, IL-10 and IL-13. A Th3 cell that primarily secretes transforming growth factor beta (TGFβ) has been described in the context of oral tolerance to myelin antigens[13,14] and in other immune-mediated settings.[15] Th1 cytokines are generally found in the brains of MS patients, while levels of Th2 cytokines, in particular TGFβ and IL-10, are low.[16-18] Moreover, several studies have demonstrated enhanced production of Th1 cytokines from peripheral blood mononuclear cells (PBMCs) restimulated ex vivo in MS patients compared to controls.[19,20] Thus, in the context of MS, Th1 cytokines are thought to mediate disease, while Th2 cytokines are believed to play a protective role. However, as our understanding of the disease evolves, it is clear that this paradigm is an over-simplification.

More recently, a subset of T-cells that predominantly produce IL-17 have been described.[21] These cells are believed to represent a distinct subset from IFNγ-producing Th1 cells, evidenced by the dependence of Th17 cells on IL-6 and TGFβ for differentiation[22-24] and IL-23 for expansion,[25,26] as opposed to Th1 cells which are dependent on IL-12 and IL-2, respectively, for differentiation and expansion. Both Th1 and Th2 cytokines have been shown to suppress the development of Th17 cells.[27,28] Th17 cells facilitate the recruitment of neutrophils and participate in the response to Gram-negative organisms. These cells

may also play a role in the initiation of autoimmune disease. Studies in the experimental autoimmune encephalomyelitis (EAE) model demonstrated that transfer of Th17 cells induces a more acute and fulminant disease compared to that induced by Th1 cells. Interestingly, in a study of MS patients, IFNγ and IL-17 were found to co-localize in cultured T-cells.[29] Moreover, pathological studies in MS patients and in the EAE model demonstrated cells expressing both cytokines efficiently cross the blood–brain barrier and accumulate within the central nervous system (CNS).[29]

The most prevalent theory of the etiology of MS is "molecular mimicry" whereby CD4+ T-cells are activated by a foreign antigen that cross-reacts with myelin antigens. These activated T-cells then migrate to the CNS where they undergo reactivation in response to nascent myelin antigens. The reactivation of T-cells heralds an inflammatory response within the CNS, resulting in more tissue damage and release of secondary antigens. Subsequent T-cell reactivity to secondary antigens is termed "epitope spreading" (Fig. 41.1). Evidence of epitope spreading has been demonstrated in animal models of MS,[30,31] and may play an important role in the pathogenesis of the human disease.

Upon exposure to an antigen, antigen-specific T-cells proliferate and differentiate into effector T-cells.[32] The vast majority of effector T-cells, undergo apoptosis as the immune response progresses, but the few lymphocytes that survive become long-lived memory T-cells.[33] Memory T-cells are specific to the antigen encountered during the primary immune response and react rapidly and vigorously when they re-encounter with the same antigen. Functionally, in terms of activation requirements, memory T-cells can be activated by lower concentrations of anti-CD3,[34] require less costimulation by anti-CD28,[35] and readily secrete more effector cytokines[36-38] than naive T-cell counterparts, indicating a state of hyper-responsiveness. In MS patients, T-cells that can be activated in the absence of CD28 have been detected.[39] This suggests that memory T-cells play a role in MS pathogenesis, and are an important consideration when designing immunomodulatory therapies.

Several populations of regulatory or suppressor T-cells have been described in humans. These include CD4+CD25+Foxp3+ regulatory T-cells,[40-43] CD8+CD28- T-cells,[44] IL-10-producing Th2 cells,[45] and TGFβ-producing Th3 cells.[46,47] Regulatory T-cells exert their effects through a variety of mechanisms, including the production of immunosuppressive cytokines or through T–T-cell interactions. Several studies demonstrated that these cells play an important role in the control of the immune response in MS, and that the function of regulatory T-cells may be enhanced by immunomodulatory therapies.[13,14,48-50]

Many of the molecular pathways described above involved in T-cell activation and function have been utilized as therapeutic targets in the treatment of MS. Others remain to be explored. Below, is a summary of the current knowledge of T-cell-based therapies in MS.

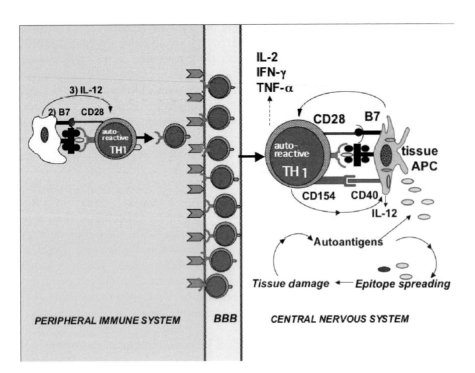

Fig. 41.1. Role of T-cells in the initiation and propagation of autoimmune disease in MS. In the peripheral immune system, a foreign antigen is presented to T-cells via the T-cell receptor interaction with the major histocompatibility complex molecule present on antigen presenting cells (APCs). The presence of costimulatory signals facilitates T-cell activation, while interleukin-12 (IL-12) cytokine facilitates Th1 differentiation. These activated T-cells traverse the blood–brain barrier (BBB) and reach the central nervous system (CNS) compartment. Within the CNS, T-cells are re-activated by presentation of cross-reactive myelin antigens by local APCs. The inflammatory environment can induce upregulation of additional costimulatory molecules, and can facilitate presentation of antigens to T-cells by CNS APCs. Re-activation of T-cells induces production of cytokines, in particular tumor necrosis factor alpha as well as recruitment of macrophages into the CNS, which facilitates tissue damage. This results in a release of additional tissue antigens, which can be taken up by potential APCs in the CNS, such as macrophages/microglia, and astrocytes and presented to T-cells (epitope spreading), thus, inciting further T-cell activation and tissue damage.

Specific therapies classified by mechanism of action

Therapies targeting specific T-cells

Altered peptide ligands

An altered peptide ligand (APL) may be defined as "any peptide that serves as a receptor ligand, in which substitutions of a single or multiple amino acids lead to changes in the functional outcome of receptor signaling".[51] APLs have most commonly been used as TCR ligands, to alter T-cell responses to presumed immunogenic or target antigens. APLs are purported to work via two major mechanisms: the first is to produce partial agonism or TCR antagonism to the target antigen resulting in immune suppression or immune deviation; and the second is to induce a regulatory T-cell population reactive to the APL itself, which then serves to down-regulate the inflammatory disease process through bystander suppression. Because of the interest in myelin basic protein (MBP) as a potential autoantigen in MS,[52–54] and the ability of the MS disease associated MHC class II allele, DRB1*1501 to present this antigen,[55,56] considerable interest has developed in the modulation of T-cell responses to MBP using APLs. Glatiramer acetate (GA; Copaxone) may be classified as an APL, and its purported mechanism of action is through bystander suppression of the immune response. Additional APLs have been tested in MS, with less successful results.

An altered peptide ligand of MBP$_{87-99}$ peptide was shown to be effective in ameliorating disease in the EAE model.[57] Similar APLs have been tested in MS, that differ from the native MBP$_{83-99}$ peptide by three to four amino acids related to MHC class II and TCR binding sites. An initial Phase 1 clinical trial tested four doses (1, 5, 20, and 50 mg) of an APL to MBP$_{83-99}$

administered subcutaneously for four weeks and demonstrated no safety concerns.[51] However, ex vivo studies demonstrated expansion of APL-reactive T-cell populations. Two Phase 2 trials using MBP$_{83-99}$ APLs were initiated: a small NIH-based trial tested the highest dose of APL CGP77116 (50 mg) administered weekly for nine months. Three out of eight patients developed atypical MS relapses, characterized by a numerous gadolinium-enhancing lesions, tumefactive-type lesion, or a flaccid paralysis with inflammatory involvement of the peripheral nervous system.[58] Two out of three relapses correlated with enhanced reactivity to MBP.[58] A second, larger multicenter study testing three doses of APL NBI-5788 (5, 20 or 50 mg) vs. placebo in 144 patients was terminated because of the occurrence of APL-induced systemic hypersensitivity reactions in 9% of enrolled patients.[59] In both studies, enhanced ex vivo T-cell responses to APL were observed following treatment. In patients who developed hypersensitivity reactions, enhanced Th2 responses to the APL were demonstrated.[59] Although, in the lower dose arm of the multicenter study, modest improvements in the volume of contrast-enhancing lesions were demonstrated, the potential adverse effects of this form of APL therapy have limited this therapeutic approach. Any additional studies in this area must address issues related to the structure of the APL and cross-reactivity to nascent antigens, optimal dose of antigen, as well as the question of tailoring individual patients' APL therapies to their existing T-cell repertoire and MHC class II phenotype.

Glatiramer acetate

GA, an approved therapy for the treatment of relapsing–remitting (RR) MS, is an APL originally developed to mimic

MBP. It is a random sequence of the amino acids glutamic acid, lysine alanine and tyrosine present in a specific molar ratio (0.14:0.34:0.43:0.09). GA is administered by daily subcutaneous injection, and in a Phase 3 clinical trial was found to reduce relapse frequency by 29%, as well as decrease the incidence of new gadolinium-enhancing lesions on MRI.[60-62] Despite its crude resemblance to MBP, evidence from several studies showing GA stimulates several non-myelin antigen T-cell lines, suggests that GA acts as a "universal" or degenerate T-cell antigen.[63] GA displays a high affinity for the MHC class II groove, and may bind the MHC molecule directly,[64] or may be processed by the cell, and then displayed on the cell surface by MHC molecules resulting in antigen-presentation. GA has been shown to inhibit responses to MBP-specific T-cell lines in vitro,[65] and in vivo treatment with GA induces a hypo-responsiveness to this antigen.[66] Interestingly, GA-reactive T-cells lines isolated from both treated patients as well as untreated controls were found to cross-react with a variety of peptides, suggesting degenerate antigenicity.[63] In vivo treatment with GA enhanced Th2 cytokine production in GA-reactive human T-cell lines.[63] In the EAE model, Th2-cytokine-producing GA-reactive T-cells were shown to accumulate in the CNS and attenuate disease.[67] Recent EAE studies have shown that GA induces anti-inflammatory type II monocytes, which preferentially produce IL-10 and TGFβ, with decreased production of IL-12 and TNFα associated with reduced STAT-1 signaling.[68] These type II monocytes subsequently were found to direct differentiation of Th2 cells and CD4+CD25+FoxP3+ regulatory T-cells, independent of antigen specificity. A study in humans found that MS patients had reduced numbers of GA-reactive CD8+T-cells, which corrected after GA treatment.[69] Thus, the principal mechanism of action of GA may be through monocyte-induction of Th2 and populations of regulatory T-cells, which exert bystander suppression of inflammation within the CNS.

Oral tolerance

Immunological tolerance to antigens may be achieved through the deletion or induction of anergy of T-cell clones.[70] One practical mechanism of inducing tolerance to a specific antigen is through the continuous exposure of the antigen to the gut mucosa, termed "oral tolerance" or "mucosal tolerance." This process induces tolerance to the antigen through the induction of TGFβ-producing Th3 cells, Th2 cells, and CD4+CD25+ regulatory T-cells, as well as deletion of antigen-reactive T-cell clones.[71] This process can be exploited in disease states. Due to the interest in MBP as a target antigen in MS, pilot clinical trials tested administering oral myelin to MS patients and were encouraging.[72] However, a subsequent larger randomized controlled double-blinded trial failed to reproduce these results.[73] Oral GA was effective in the EAE model,[74] and showed some effects on immunomodulation in a Phase 1 trial in MS.[75] However, further clinical trials failed to show a benefit in MS. The lack of efficacy in both oral myelin and oral GA trials may be due to dose of antigen used or to other factors related to antigen administration.

T-cell vaccination

T-cell vaccination strategies attempt to eliminate pathogenic T-cells through the enhancement of regulatory immune responses to autoreactive T-cells. This approach requires the isolation of autoreactive T-cell clones from the individual patient's blood or CSF, and subcutaneous re-injection in the form of an immunizing vaccine. Pilot trials of T-cell vaccination with autologous MBP-specific T-cells from peripheral blood, in 28 RRMS and 26 secondary progressive (SP) MS patients, demonstrated a modest reduction in post-treatment relapse rate.[76,77] In this study, the frequency of gadolinium-enhancing lesions was largely unchanged post-treatment. A second pilot trial using autologous MBP and myelin oligodendrocyte glycoprotein (MOG)-reactive T-cell vaccines in 20 RRMS non-responders demonstrated a significant reduction in relapse rate ($P = 0.026$) as well as gadolinium-enhancing and T2 lesion load.[78] In both studies, no serious adverse events were noted. In a small study utilizing myelin-reactive CD4+ T-cells derived from autologous CSF, no adverse effects were observed in any of the five treated patients.[79] The precise mechanism of action of T-cell vaccination in MS is unclear; however, ex vivo immunological studies have demonstrated enhanced T-cell responses to the T-cell vaccine, consisting of varying combinations of CD4+, CD8+, CD4-CD8- and γδ-T-cells.[80] MHC class I-restricted CD8+ T-cell cytolytic responses as well as CD4+ T-cell responses are believed to be the major mediators of vaccine-induced tolerance.[76,81-83] Further larger Phase 2 trials using T-cell vaccination are planned.

T-cell receptor vaccination

TCR vaccination strategies target TCR sequences believed to be critical in the immunopathogenesis of MS. Certain variable-region (V-region) genes of TCR have been shown to be over-expressed in peripheral T-cells and CNS plaques from MS patients.[84] Vβ5.2/5.3+ has been identified as a dominant TCR variable region sequence involved in MBP T-cell reactivity.[85-87] TCR vaccines are thought to exert their effects by enhancing the function of regulatory T-cell populations and Th2 cells recognizing TCR determinants.[88,89] TCR peptides derived from the Vβ5.2 region of the TCR has been used as a vaccine in MS patients. In a double-blind pilot study, 23 patients were treated with weekly to monthly injections of the peptide. No major adverse events were observed in treated patients. All patients carried the HLADRB1*1501 allele. Enhanced Th2 cell responses to the immunizing peptide correlated with clinical improvement.[88,90] Th1 cell responses to MBP trended downwards in responders. A follow-up study demonstrated increased frequencies of CD4+CD25+Foxp3 and IL-10-producing T-cells in immunized patients, which persisted until the end of the study at 12 months.[91]

ATM-027 is an antibody specifically targeting the Vβ5.2/5.3 sequence of TCR. Results from a multicenter Phase 2 study in 47 MS patients treated with a run-in regimen of ATM-027 monthly for six months, showed no significant reduction in new gadolinium MRI lesions post-treatment despite a significant reduction in Vβ5.2/5.3+ T-cells.[92,93] MS relapses occurred in three treated patients, but no other adverse events directly related to drug were observed. These negative results suggest that there is considerable variability in Vβ profiling in individual MS patients. An alternative explanation is that, by the time the disease presents clinically, epitope spreading has occurred, negating the use of a single Vβ-depleting agent.

Therapies targeting T-cells non-specifically

Lymphocytapheresis

Lymphocytapheresis can induce prolonged lymphocyte depletion. Initial small studies using lymphocytapheresis showed varying results, with modest effects on relapse rate and progression.[94–98] A Phase 2 study combining lymphocytapheresis and azathioprine treatment was recently initiated.

Total lymphoid irradiation

Total lymphoid irradiation is another strategy used to induce prolonged lymphocyte depletion. A small randomized controlled double-blind study in progressive MS patients showed modest effects on slowing progression;[99–101] however, these findings require validation in randomized control trials. Improvement of MRI measures grossly correlated with prolonged suppression of CD3+ and CD4+ T-cell counts.[102]

Anti-CD4 antibody

CD4 is a cell surface marker of helper T-cells. In a randomized Phase 2 double-blind trial, anti-CD4 antibody (cM-T412) was administered intravenously to 35 RR and SPMS patients.[103] Administration of the antibody resulted in a rapid and sustained reduction in circulating CD4+ T-cells. Infusion related side effects including nausea, fever, and tachycardia were limited to 24 hours post-infusion. After nine months, treated patients demonstrated an approximately 40% reduction in relapse rate compared to placebo controls; however, there was no significant change in the number of gadolinium enhancing lesions on MRI. Lack of efficacy on the primary MRI measures led to questions regarding the effectiveness of anti-CD4 therapy in MS.

Anti-CD3 antibody

Intravenous anti-CD3 antibody treatment is a well-established therapy for acute allograft rejection. Recent studies testing anti-CD3 in type I diabetes[104] suggested utility in the treatment of autoimmune diseases. There is renewed interest in the use of anti-CD3 therapy in MS. Studies in EAE demonstrated that oral administration of anti-CD3 induces CD4+ CD25- LAP+ regulatory T-cells that contain latency-associated peptide (LAP) on their surface and that function in vitro and in vivo through a TGFβ-dependent mechanism.[105] Studies of human T-cells stimulated in vitro with plate-bound anti-CD3 showed induction of a population of regulatory CD4+ T-cells that markedly suppressed the proliferation and cytokine production of autologous PBMCs in a non-MHC dependent manner and produced lower levels of IFNγ, TNFα and IL-2, and higher levels of TGFβ than controls.[106] Phase 1 studies of oral anti-CD3 therapy in MS are under way.

CTLA4Ig

Blockade of the CD28-B7 pathway results in increased T-cell death, anergy induction, and blockade of cell differentiation. CTLA4Ig has been shown to be an effective treatment in EAE through blockade of the CD28-B7 pathway.[107] CTLA4Ig also has another potentially immunosuppressive effect by interacting with B7 on dendritic cells inducing indole 2,3-dioxygenase, a derivative of trytophan, which indirectly blocks naive T-cell activation.[108] Abatacept is an intravenously administered form of CTLA4Ig. Based on results of Phase 3 studies, monthly intravenous Abatacept (Orencia, Bristol-Myers Squibb) is approved as monotherapy or combination therapy for adult[109–111] and juvenile rheumathoid arthritis.[112] Safety results in the arthritis studies were excellent, with nasopharyngitis reported as the most frequent side effect. Phase 2 studies in RRMS using Abatacept are currently ongoing. Use of CTLA4Ig is being explored in other autoimmune disorders. Studies in patients with the T-cell-mediated skin disease, psoriasis vulgaris, demonstrated that treatment with CTLA4Ig caused a marked reduction in skin-infiltrating T-cells, associated with excellent clinical results with no significant adverse events.[113]

Anti-CD154 antibody

In MS, the CD40-CD154 (CD40L) pathway is believed to play an important role in T-cell costimulation and the production of the proinflammatory cytokines IL-12 and IL-18.[19,114] Both CD40 and CD154 are over-expressed in CNS lesions from MS brains compared with controls.[115] CD40 is expressed on macrophages and microglia, while CD154 co-localized with the CD4 T-cell marker. In addition, expression of CD154 was found to be higher in peripheral blood monocytes isolated from SPMS compared with RRMS or healthy controls,[116,117] and was reduced by IFNβ treatment.[118] Clinical trials with an intravenously administered anti-CD154 antibody (Biogen-idec) in autoimmune diseases such as immune thrombocytopenia purpura and lupus were terminated because of the occurrence of thromboembolic events. A Phase 1 clinical trial in MS patients was performed with good safety data, although concerns about thromboembolic complications observed in other trials has made further development of this product unlikely.

Cytokine modulation

Interleukin-12

IL-12 is a cytokine that is critical for the differentiation of Th1 cells. IL-12 is a disulfide-linked heterodimer p70 complex, composed of one p40 and one p35 subunit. The p35 component is synthesized by most T-cell sub-types, while the p40 component is synthesized only by mononuclear phagocytes and dendritic cells. In humans, IL-12 was found to be up-regulated in patients with MS; IL12p40 expression is increased in acute MS plaques.[119] IL-12 p40 mRNA levels in unstimulated PBMCs were increased in SP and RR patients compared with controls, and correlated with the development of active lesions on MRI. In contrast, IL-12 p35 levels were decreased in both groups compared with controls.[120] Serum levels of IL-12p70 were reported to be increased in progressive patients[121] and production of IL-12 p70 by stimulated PBMCs was higher in progressive patients than controls or patients with acute MS.[122]

Importantly, therapies such as cyclophosphamide normalize the high levels of IL-12 expressed by monocytes in progressive MS.[20] Furthermore, IFNβ, an approved MS therapy, inhibits IL-12[123] and induces reciprocal changes in IL-10.[124] Salbutamol (Albuterol) administered in vivo was found to down-regulate the expression of IL-12 by monocytes in MS patients.[125] A clinical trial of Albuterol in combination with GA showed improvement in the MS Functional Composite in the GA+albuterol group at the six-month and 12-month time points.[126] Clinical trials with anti-IL-12 antibodies (ABT-874; CNTO-1275) have been initiated for treatment of MS.

Tumor necrosis factor alpha

Expression of TNFα in the CNS is up-regulated in MS lesions, predominantly in macrophages, microglia, and astrocytes.[16,127–129] Several studies found a positive correlation between TNFα levels and MS relapses.[128,130–134] TNFα levels in serum and CSF correlated with MRI disease activity.[135] However, a clinical trial using a TNF antagonist (soluble TNF receptor-IgG p55, Lenercept) had the unexpected outcome of increased enhancing lesions on MRI.[136] In addition, treatment with an anti-TNFα antibody (Infliximab) led to worsened disease.[137] Possible explanations for these confounding results may be a prolongation of TNFα half-life in the serum induced by antagonist binding. Alternatively in certain situations, TNF may play a protective role differentially mediated by the TNF receptors 1 and 2. At present, TNFα blockade does not appear to have utility in MS treatment.

Interferon gamma

IFNγ is a proinflammatory Th1 cytokine. Increased expression of IFNγ after anti-CD3 stimulation of PBMCs was reported in patients with SPMS compared to RRMS or controls.[138] MS patients experiencing a relapse have significantly increased PBMC IFNγ production after mitogen stimulation compared with patients in remission, but this production was reduced after treatment with IFNβ.[139] Similar results were found in patients with primary progressive MS.[140] Clinical attacks correlate with increased IFNγ production in vitro[134] and administration of IFNγ to MS patients precipitated clinical relapses.[141,142]

Transforming growth factor beta

Because of its association with disease remissions, TGFβ is an attractive candidate for immunotherapy in MS. In a Phase 1 safety trial 12 chronic progressive MS patients were treated with TGFβ2 three times a week for four weeks. Results showed no change in Expanded Disability Status Scale scores or MRI but a significant decline in renal glomerular filtration rate was observed.[143] Glomerular nephrotoxicity had been previously observed in a TGFβ1 transgenic murine model and is associated with an accumulation of glomerular extracellular matrix protein.[144] Thus, high doses of TGFβ are considered to be unsuitable treatment choices for MS.

Drugs with secondary effects on T-cell measures

Although the T-cell is not the primary target of several drugs that are currently approved or are under investigation for the treatment of MS, many of these therapies have secondary effects on T-cell measures. Examples of such therapies include the IFNβ, minocycline, rituximab, and the statin family of drugs. Therapies that affect T-cell migration including fingolimod (Gilenya) and natalizumab (Tysabri) are covered elsewhere in this textbook.

Conclusions

The T-cell plays a critical role in the pathogenesis of MS, and is an important target in MS therapeutics. The success of several drugs that specifically target the T-cell and T-cell responses reinforces this point. Further success of T-cell directed therapies depends on the appropriate targeting of phases of T-cell activation and function, as well as the accurate identification of antigens driving T-cell responses at various phases of disease. Phase 2 and 3 clinical trials are required to validate initial efficacy observations in many of the newer specific immunotherapies, as well as to assess long-term safety.

References

1. Zhang J, Weiner HL, Hafler DA. Autoreactive T-cells in multiple sclerosis. *Int Rev Immunol* 1992;9:183–201.

2. Raine CS. The Dale E. McFarlin Memorial Lecture: the immunology of the multiple sclerosis lesion. *Ann Neurol* 1994;36 Suppl:S61–72.

3. Lucchinetti C, Bruck W, Parisi J, Scheithauer B, Rodriguez M, Lassmann H. Heterogeneity of multiple sclerosis lesions: implications for the pathogenesis of demyelination. *Ann Neurol* 2000;47:707–17.

4. Zhang J, Markovic-Plese S, Lacet B, Raus J, Weiner HL, Hafler DA. Increased frequency of interleukin 2-responsive T-cells specific for myelin basic protein and proteolipid protein in peripheral blood and cerebrospinal fluid of patients with multiple sclerosis. *J Exp Med* 1994;179:973–84.

5. Bretscher P, Cohn M. A theory of self-nonself discrimination. *Science* 1970;169:1042–9.

6. Bretscher PA. A two-step, two-signal model for the primary activation of precursor helper T-cells. *Proc Natl Acad Sci USA* 1999;96:185–90.

7. Alegre ML, Frauwirth KA, Thompson CB. T-cell regulation by CD28 and CTLA-4. *Nat Rev Immunol* 2001;1:220–8.

8. Brunet JF, Denizot F, Luciani MF, *et al.* A new member of the immunoglobulin superfamily–CTLA-4. *Nature* 1987;328:267–70.

9. Miller DH, Khan OA, Sheremata WA, *et al.* A controlled trial of natalizumab for relapsing multiple sclerosis. *N Engl J Med* 2003;348:15–23.

10. Van Assche G, Van Ranst M, Sciot R, *et al.* Progressive multifocal leukoencephalopathy after natalizumab therapy for Crohn's disease. *N Engl J Med* 2005;353:362–68.

11. Langer-Gould A, Atlas SW, Bollen AW, Pelletier D. Progressive Multifocal leukoencephalopathy in a patient treated with natalizumab. *N Engl J Med* 2005.

12. Kleinschmidt-Demasters BK, Tyler KL. Progressive multifocal leukoencephalopathy complicating treatment with natalizumab and interferon beta-1a for multiple sclerosis. *N Engl J Med* 2005.

13. Hafler DA, Kent SC, Pietrusewicz MJ, Khoury SJ, Weiner HL, Fukaura H. Oral administration of myelin induces antigen-specific TGF-beta 1 secreting T-cells in patients with multiple sclerosis. *Ann N Y Acad Sci* 1997;835:120–31.

14. Fukaura H, Kent SC, Pietrusewicz MJ, Khoury SJ, Weiner HL, Hafler DA. Induction of circulating myelin basic protein and proteolipid protein-specific transforming growth factor-beta1-secreting Th3 T-cells by oral administration of myelin in multiple sclerosis patients. *J Clin Invest* 1996;98:70–7.

15. Minguela A, Torio A, Marin L, *et al.* Implication of Th1, Th2, and Th3 cytokines in liver graft acceptance. *Transplant Proc* 1999;31:519–20.

16. Cannella B, Raine CS. The adhesion molecule and cytokine profile of multiple sclerosis lesions [see comments]. *Ann Neurol* 1995;37:424–35.

17. Hofman FM, von Hanwehr RI, Dinarello CA, Mizel SB, Hinton D, Merrill JE. Immunoregulatory molecules and IL 2 receptors identified in multiple sclerosis brain. *J Immunol* 1986;136:3239–45.

18. Woodroofe MN, Cuzner ML. Cytokine mRNA expression in inflammatory multiple sclerosis lesions: detection by non-radioactive in situ hybridization. *Cytokine* 1993;5:583–8.

19. Balashov KE, Smith DR, Khoury SJ, Hafler DA, Weiner HL. Increased interleukin 12 production in progressive multiple sclerosis: induction by activated CD4 +T-cells via CD40 ligand. *Proc Natl Acad Sci USA* 1997;94:599–603.

20. Comabella M, Balashov K, Issazadeh S, Smith D, Weiner HL, Khoury SJ. Elevated interleukin-12 in progressive multiple sclerosis correlates with disease activity and is normalized by pulse cyclophosphamide therapy. *J Clin Invest* 1998;102:671–8.

21. Yao Z, Painter SL, Fanslow WC, *et al.* Human IL-17: a novel cytokine derived from T-cells. *J Immunol* 1995;155:5483–6.

22. Veldhoen M, Hocking RJ, Atkins CJ, Locksley RM, Stockinger B. TGFbeta in the context of an inflammatory cytokine milieu supports de novo differentiation of IL-17-producing T-cells. *Immunity* 2006;24:179–89.

23. Bettelli E, Carrier Y, Gao W, *et al.* Reciprocal developmental pathways for the generation of pathogenic effector TH17 and regulatory T-cells. *Nature* 2006;441:235–8.

24. Mangan PR, Harrington LE, O'Quinn DB, *et al.* Transforming growth factor-beta induces development of the T(H)17 lineage. *Nature* 2006;441:231–4.

25. Aggarwal S, Ghilardi N, Xie MH, de Sauvage FJ, Gurney AL. Interleukin-23 promotes a distinct CD4 T-cell activation state characterized by the production of interleukin-17. *J Biol Chem* 2003;278:1910–14.

26. Langrish CL, Chen Y, Blumenschein WM, *et al.* IL-23 drives a pathogenic T-cell population that induces autoimmune inflammation. *J Exp Med* 2005;201:233–40.

27. Park H, Li Z, Yang XO, *et al.* A distinct lineage of CD4 T-cells regulates tissue inflammation by producing interleukin 17. *Nat Immunol* 2005;6:1133–41.

28. Harrington LE, Hatton RD, Mangan PR, *et al.* Interleukin 17-producing CD4 +effector T-cells develop via a lineage distinct from the T helper type 1 and 2 lineages. *Nat Immunol* 2005;6:1123–32.

29. Kebir H, Ifergan I, Alvarez JI, *et al.* Preferential recruitment of interferon-gamma-expressing TH17 cells in multiple sclerosis. *Ann Neurol* 2009;66:390–402.

30. McMahon EJ, Bailey SL, Castenada CV, Waldner H, Miller SD. Epitope spreading initiates in the CNS in two mouse models of multiple sclerosis. *Nat Med* 2005;11:335–9.

31. Vanderlugt CL, Begolka WS, Neville KL, *et al.* The functional significance of epitope spreading and its regulation by co-stimulatory molecules. *Immunol Rev* 1998;164:63–72.

32. Sprent J, Surh CD. T-cell memory. *Annu Rev Immunol* 2002;20:551–79.

33. Dutton RW, Bradley LM, Swain SL. T-cell memory. *Annu Rev Immunol* 1998;16:201–23.

34. Byrne JA, Butler JL, Cooper MD. Differential activation requirements for virgin and memory T-cells. *J Immunol* 1988;141:3249–57.

35. Kuiper H, Brouwer M, de Boer M, Parren P, van Lier RA. Differences in responsiveness to CD3 stimulation between naive and memory CD4+ T-cells cannot be overcome by CD28 costimulation. *Eur J Immunol* 1994;24:1956–60.

36. Lee WT, Yin XM, Vitetta ES. Functional and ontogenetic analysis of murine CD45Rhi and CD45Rlo CD4+ T-cells. *J Immunol* 1990;144:3288–95.

37. Ehlers S, Smith KA. Differentiation of T-cell lymphokine gene expression: the in vitro acquisition of T-cell memory. *J Exp Med* 1991;173:25–36.

38. Bird JJ, Brown DR, Mullen AC, *et al.* Helper T-cell differentiation is controlled by the cell cycle. *Immunity* 1998;9:229–37.

39. Markovic-Plese S, Cortese I, Wandinger KP, McFarland HF, Martin R. CD4+CD28-costimulation-independent T-cells in multiple sclerosis. *J Clin Invest* 2001;108:1185–94.

40. Stephens LA, Mottet C, Mason D, Powrie F. Human CD4(+)CD25(+) thymocytes and peripheral T-cells have

immune suppressive activity in vitro. *Eur J Immunol* 2001;31:1247–54.

41. Dieckmann D, Plottner H, Berchtold S, Berger T, Schuler G. Ex vivo isolation and characterization of CD4(+)CD25(+) T-cells with regulatory properties from human blood. *J Exp Med* 2001;193:1303–10.

42. Baecher-Allan C, Brown JA, Freeman GJ, Hafler DA. CD4+CD25high regulatory cells in human peripheral blood. *J Immunol* 2001;167:1245–53.

43. Levings MK, Sangregorio R, Roncarolo MG. Human cd25(+)cd4(+) t regulatory cells suppress naive and memory T-cell proliferation and can be expanded in vitro without loss of function. *J Exp Med* 2001;193:1295–302.

44. Koide J, Engleman EG. Differences in surface phenotype and mechanism of action between alloantigen-specific CD8+ cytotoxic and suppressor T-cell clones. *J Immunol* 1990;144:32–40.

45. Bacchetta R, Bigler M, Touraine JL, *et al.* High levels of interleukin 10 production in vivo are associated with tolerance in SCID patients transplanted with HLA mismatched hematopoietic stem cells. *J Exp Med* 1994;179:493–502.

46. Kitani A, Chua K, Nakamura K, Strober W. Activated self-MHC-reactive T-cells have the cytokine phenotype of Th3/T regulatory cell 1 T-cells. *J Immunol* 2000;165:691–702.

47. Roncarolo MG, Levings MK. The role of different subsets of T regulatory cells in controlling autoimmunity. *Curr Opin Immunol* 2000;12:676–83.

48. Viglietta V, Baecher-Allan C, Weiner HL, Hafler DA. Loss of functional suppression by CD4+CD25+ regulatory T-cells in patients with multiple sclerosis. *J Exp Med* 2004;199:971–9.

49. Karaszewski JW, Reder AT, Anlar B, Kim WC, Arnason BG. Increased lymphocyte beta-adrenergic receptor density in progressive multiple sclerosis is specific for the CD8+, CD28-suppressor cell. *Ann Neurol* 1991;30:42–7.

50. Crucian B, Dunne P, Friedman H, Ragsdale R, Pross S, Widen R. Alterations in levels of CD28-/CD8 +suppressor cell precursor and CD45RO+/CD4+ memory T lymphocytes in the peripheral blood of multiple sclerosis patients. *Clin Diagn Lab Immunol* 1995;2:249–52.

51. Bielekova B, Martin R. Antigen-specific immunomodulation via altered peptide ligands. *J Mol Med* 2001;79:552–65.

52. Zhang J, Markovic-Plese S, Lacet B, Raus J, Weiner HL, Hafler DA. Increased frequency of interleukin 2-responsive T-cells specific for myelin basic protein and proteolipid protein in peripheral blood and cerebrospinal fluid of patients with multiple sclerosis. *J Exp Med* 1994;179:973–84.

53. Allegretta M, Nicklas JA, Sriram S, Albertini RJ. T-cells responsive to myelin basic protein in patients with multiple sclerosis. *Science* 1990;247:718–21.

54. Chou YK, Bourdette DN, Offner H, *et al.* Frequency of T-cells specific for myelin basic protein and myelin proteolipid protein in blood and cerebrospinal fluid in multiple sclerosis. *J Neuroimmunol* 1992;38:105–13.

55. Wucherpfennig KW, Catz I, Hausmann S, Strominger JL, Steinman L, Warren KG. Recognition of the immunodominant myelin basic protein peptide by autoantibodies and HLA-DR2-restricted T-cell clones from multiple sclerosis patients. Identity of key contact residues in the B-cell and T-cell epitopes. *J Clin Invest* 1997;100:1114–22.

56. Wucherpfennig KW, Hafler DA, Strominger JL. Structure of human T-cell receptors specific for an immunodominant myelin basic protein peptide: positioning of T-cell receptors on HLA-DR2/peptide complexes. *Proc Natl Acad Sci USA* 1995;92:8896–900.

57. Karin N, Mitchell DJ, Brocke S, Ling N, Steinman L. Reversal of experimental autoimmune encephalomyelitis by a soluble peptide variant of a myelin basic protein epitope: T-cell receptor antagonism and reduction of interferon gamma and tumor necrosis factor alpha production. *J Exp Med* 1994;180:2227–37.

58. Bielekova B, Goodwin B, Richert N, *et al.* Encephalitogenic potential of the myelin basic protein peptide (amino acids 83–99) in multiple sclerosis: results of a phase II clinical trial with an altered peptide ligand. *Nat Med* 2000;6:1167–75.

59. Kappos L, Comi G, Panitch H, *et al.* Induction of a non-encephalitogenic type 2 T helper-cell autoimmune response in multiple sclerosis after administration of an altered peptide ligand in a placebo-controlled, randomized phase II trial. The Altered Peptide Ligand in Relapsing MS Study Group. *Nat Med* 2000;6:1176–82.

60. Johnson KP, Brooks BR, Cohen JA, *et al.* Copolymer 1 reduces relapse rate and improves disability in relapsing-remitting multiple sclerosis: results of a phase III multicenter, double-blind placebo-controlled trial. The Copolymer 1 Multiple Sclerosis Study Group. *Neurology* 1995;45:1268–76.

61. Ge Y, Grossman RI, Udupa JK, *et al.* Glatiramer acetate (Copaxone) treatment in relapsing-remitting MS: quantitative MR assessment. *Neurology* 2000;54:813–17.

62. Johnson KP, Brooks BR, Cohen JA, *et al.* Copolymer 1 reduces relapse rate and improves disability in relapsing-remitting multiple sclerosis: results of a phase III multicenter, double-blind, placebo-controlled trial. 1995. *Neurology* 2001;57:S16–24.

63. Duda PW, Schmied MC, Cook SL, Krieger JI, Hafler DA. Glatiramer acetate (Copaxone) induces degenerate, Th2-polarized immune responses in patients with multiple sclerosis. *J Clin Invest* 2000;105:967–76.

64. Fridkis-Hareli M, Teitelbaum D, Arnon R, Sela M. Synthetic copolymer 1 and myelin basic protein do not require processing prior to binding to class II major histocompatibility complex molecules on living antigen-presenting cells. *Cell Immunol* 1995;163:229–36.

65. Racke MK, Martin R, McFarland H, Fritz RB. Copolymer-1-induced inhibition of antigen-specific T-cell activation: interference with antigen presentation. *J Neuroimmunol* 1992;37:75–84.

66. Schmied M, Duda PW, Krieger JI, Trollmo C, Hafler DA. In vitro evidence that subcutaneous administration of glatiramer acetate induces hyporesponsive T-cells in patients with multiple sclerosis. *Clin Immunol* 2003;106:163–74.

67. Aharoni R, Teitelbaum D, Leitner O, Meshorer A, Sela M, Arnon R. Specific Th2 cells accumulate in the central nervous system of mice protected against experimental autoimmune

encephalomyelitis by copolymer 1. *Proc Natl Acad Sci USA* 2000;97:11472–7.

68. Weber MS, Prod'homme T, Youssef S, *et al.* Type II monocytes modulate T-cell-mediated central nervous system autoimmune disease. *Nat Med* 2007;13:935–43.

69. Karandikar NJ, Crawford MP, Yan X, *et al.* Glatiramer acetate (Copaxone) therapy induces CD8(+) T-cell responses in patients with multiple sclerosis. *J Clin Invest* 2002;109:641–9.

70. Burnet M. The clonal selection theory of acquired immunity. In: Vanderbilt University Press; 1959; Nashville, Tennessee, USA, 1959.

71. Faria AM, Weiner HL. Oral tolerance. *Immunol Rev* 2005;206:232–59.

72. Weiner HL, Mackin GA, Matsui M, *et al.* Double-blind pilot trial of oral tolerization with myelin antigens in multiple sclerosis. *Science* 1993;259:1321–4.

73. Faria AM, Weiner HL. Oral tolerance: mechanisms and therapeutic applications. *Adv Immunol* 1999;73:153–264.

74. Teitelbaum D, Arnon R, Sela M. Immunomodulation of experimental autoimmune encephalomyelitis by oral administration of copolymer 1. *Proc Natl Acad Sci USA* 1999;96:3842–7.

75. de Seze J, Edan G, Labalette M, Dessaint JP, Vermersch P. Effect of glatiramer acetate (Copaxone) given orally in human patients: interleukin-10 production during a phase 1 trial. *Ann Neurol* 2000;47: 686.

76. Medaer R, Stinissen P, Truyen L, Raus J, Zhang J. Depletion of myelin-basic-protein autoreactive T-cells by T-cell vaccination: pilot trial in multiple sclerosis. *Lancet* 1995;346:807–8.

77. Zhang JZ, Rivera VM, Tejada-Simon MV, *et al.* T-cell vaccination in multiple sclerosis: results of a preliminary study. *J Neurol* 2002;249:212–18.

78. Achiron A, Lavie G, Kishner I, *et al.* T-cell vaccination in multiple sclerosis relapsing-remitting nonresponders patients. *Clin Immunol* 2004;113:155–60.

79. Van Der Aa A, Hellings N, Medaer R, *et al.* T-cell vaccination in multiple sclerosis patients with autologous CSF-derived activated T-cells: results

from a pilot study. *Clin Exp Immunol* 2003;131:155–68.

80. Hermans G, Medaer R, Raus J, Stinissen P. Myelin reactive T-cells after T-cell vaccination in multiple sclerosis: cytokine profile and depletion by additional immunizations. *J Neuroimmunol* 2000;102:79–84.

81. Zhang J, Medaer R, Stinissen P, Hafler D, Raus J. MHC-restricted depletion of human myelin basic protein-reactive T-cells by T-cell vaccination. *Science* 1993;261:1451–4.

82. Zhang J, Vandevyver C, Stinissen P, Raus J. In vivo clonotypic regulation of human myelin basic protein-reactive T-cells by T-cell vaccination. *J Immunol* 1995;155:5868–77.

83. Hermans G, Denzer U, Lohse A, Raus J, Stinissen P. Cellular and humoral immune responses against autoreactive T-cells in multiple sclerosis patients after T-cell vaccination. *J Autoimmun* 1999;13:233–46.

84. Offner H, Vandenbark AA. T-cell receptor V genes in multiple sclerosis: increased use of TCRAV8 and TCRBV5 in MBP-specific clones. *Int Rev Immunol* 1999;18:9–36.

85. Kotzin BL, Karuturi S, Chou YK, *et al.* Preferential T-cell receptor beta-chain variable gene use in myelin basic protein-reactive T-cell clones from patients with multiple sclerosis. *Proc Natl Acad Sci USA* 1991;88:9161–5.

86. Oksenberg JR, Panzara MA, Begovich AB, *et al.* Selection for T-cell receptor V beta-D beta-J beta gene rearrangements with specificity for a myelin basic protein peptide in brain lesions of multiple sclerosis. *Nature* 1993;362:68–70.

87. Lozeron P, Chabas D, Duprey B, Lyon-Caen O, Liblau R. T-cell receptor V beta 5 and V beta 17 clonal diversity in cerebrospinal fluid and peripheral blood lymphocytes of multiple sclerosis patients. *Mult Scler* 1998;4:154–61.

88. Vandenbark AA, Chou YK, Whitham R, *et al.* Treatment of multiple sclerosis with T-cell receptor peptides: results of a double-blind pilot trial. *Nat Med* 1996;2:1109–15.

89. Vandenbark AA. TCR peptide vaccination in multiple sclerosis: boosting a deficient natural regulatory network that may involve TCR-specific CD4+CD25 +Treg cells. *Curr Drug Targets Inflamm Allergy* 2005;4:217–29.

90. Bourdette DN, Whitham RH, Chou YK, *et al.* Immunity to TCR peptides in multiple sclerosis. I. Successful immunization of patients with synthetic V beta 5.2 and V beta 6.1 CDR2 peptides. *J Immunol* 1994;152:2510–19.

91. Vandenbark AA, Culbertson NE, Bartholomew RM, *et al.* Therapeutic vaccination with a trivalent T-cell receptor (TCR) peptide vaccine restores deficient FoxP3 expression and TCR recognition in subjects with multiple sclerosis. *Immunology* 2008; 123:66–78.

92. Killestein J, Olsson T, Wallstrom E, *et al.* Antibody-mediated suppression of Vbeta5.2/5.3(+) T-cells in multiple sclerosis: results from an MRI-monitored phase II clinical trial. *Ann Neurol* 2002;51:467–74.

93. Olsson T, Edenius C, Ferm M, *et al.* Depletion of Vbeta5.2/5.3 T-cells with a humanized antibody in patients with multiple sclerosis. *Eur J Neurol* 2002;9:153–64.

94. Rose J, Klein H, Greenstein J, McFarlin D, Gerber L, McFarland H. Lymphocytapheresis in chronic progressive multiple sclerosis: results of a preliminary trial. *Ann Neurol* 1983;14:593–4.

95. Hauser SL, Fosburg M, Kevy SV, Weiner HL. Lymphocytapheresis in chronic progressive multiple sclerosis: immunologic and clinical effects. *Neurology* 1984;34:922–6.

96. Medaer R, Eeckhout C, Gautama K, Vermijlen C. Lymphocytapheresis therapy in multiple sclerosis, a preliminary study. *Acta Neurol Scand* 1984;70:111–15.

97. Ghezzi A, Zaffaroni GA, Caputo D, *et al.* Lymphocytoplasmapheresis in multiple sclerosis: one-year results in 6 patients. *Ital J Neurol Sci* 1986;7: 119–23.

98. Maida E, Hocker P, Mann E. Long-term lymphocytapheresis therapy in multiple sclerosis. Preliminary observations. *Eur Neurol* 1986;25:225–32.

99. Cook SD, Devereux C, Troiano R, *et al.* Effect of total lymphoid irradiation in chronic progressive multiple sclerosis. *Lancet* 1986;1:1405–9.

100. Cook SD, Devereux C, Troiano R, *et al.* Total lymphoid irradiation in multiple sclerosis: blood lymphocytes and clinical course. *Ann Neurol* 1987;22:634–8.

101. Troiano R, Devereux C, Oleske J, *et al.* T-cell subsets and disease progression after total lymphoid irradiation in chronic progressive multiple sclerosis. *J Neurol Neurosurg Psychiatry* 1988;51:980–3.

102. Rohowsky-Kochan C, Molinaro D, Devereux C, *et al.* The effect of total lymphoid irradiation and low-dose steroids on T lymphocyte populations in multiple sclerosis: correlation with clinical and MRI status. *J Neurol Sci* 1997;152:182–92.

103. van Oosten BW, Lai M, Hodgkinson S, *et al.* Treatment of multiple sclerosis with the monoclonal anti-CD4 antibody cM-T412: results of a randomized, double-blind, placebo-controlled, MR-monitored phase II trial. *Neurology* 1997;49:351–7.

104. Herold KC, Hagopian W, Auger JA, *et al.* Anti-CD3 monoclonal antibody in new-onset type 1 diabetes mellitus. *N Engl J Med* 2002;346:1692–8.

105. Ochi H, Abraham M, Ishikawa H, *et al.* Oral CD3-specific antibody suppresses autoimmune encephalomyelitis by inducing CD4+ CD25- LAP+ T-cells. *Nat Med* 2006;12:627–35.

106. Abraham M, Karni A, Dembinsky A, *et al.* In vitro induction of regulatory T-cells by anti-CD3 antibody in humans. *J Autoimmun* 2008;30:21–8.

107. Khoury SJ, Akalin E, Chandraker A, et al. CD28-B7 costimulatory blockade by CTLA4Ig prevents actively induced experimental autoimmune encephalomyelitis and inhibits Th1 but spares Th2 cytokines in the central nervous system. *J Immunol* 1995;155:4521–4.

108. Bluestone JA, St Clair EW, Turka LA. CTLA4Ig: bridging the basic immunology with clinical application. *Immunity* 2006;24:233–8.

109. Schiff M, Keiserman M, Codding C, *et al.* Efficacy and safety of abatacept or infliximab vs placebo in ATTEST: a phase III, multi-centre, randomised, double-blind, placebo-controlled study in patients with rheumatoid arthritis and an inadequate response to methotrexate. *Ann Rheum Dis* 2008;67:1096–103.

110. Genovese MC, Becker JC, Schiff M, *et al.* Abatacept for rheumatoid arthritis refractory to tumor necrosis factor alpha inhibition. *N Engl J Med* 2005;353:1114–23.

111. Kremer JM, Genant HK, Moreland LW, *et al.* Effects of abatacept in patients with methotrexate-resistant active rheumatoid arthritis: a randomized trial. *Ann Intern Med* 2006;144:865–76.

112. Ruperto N, Lovell DJ, Quartier P, *et al.* Abatacept in children with juvenile idiopathic arthritis: a randomised, double-blind, placebo-controlled withdrawal trial. *Lancet* 2008;372:383–91.

113. Abrams JR, Kelley SL, Hayes E, *et al.* Blockade of T lymphocyte costimulation with cytotoxic T lymphocyte-associated antigen 4-immunoglobulin (CTLA4Ig) reverses the cellular pathology of psoriatic plaques, including the activation of keratinocytes, dendritic cells, and endothelial cells. *J Exp Med* 2000;192:681–94.

114. Karni A, Koldzic DN, Bharanidharan P, Khoury SJ, Weiner HL. IL-18 is linked to raised IFN-gamma in multiple sclerosis and is induced by activated CD4(+) T-cells via CD40-CD40 ligand interactions. *J Neuroimmunol* 2002;125:134–40.

115. Gerritse K, Laman JD, Noelle RJ, *et al.* CD40-CD40 ligand interactions in experimental allergic encephalomyelitis and multiple sclerosis. *Proc Natl Acad Sci USA* 1996;93:2499–504.

116. Filion LG, Matusevicius D, Graziani-Bowering GM, Kumar A, Freedman MS. Monocyte-derived IL12, CD86 (B7–2) and CD40L expression in relapsing and progressive multiple sclerosis. *Clin Immunol* 2003;106:127–38.

117. Jensen J, Krakauer M, Sellebjerg F. Increased T-cell expression of CD154 (CD40-ligand) in multiple sclerosis. *Eur J Neurol* 2001;8:321–8.

118. Teleshova N, Bao W, Kivisakk P, Ozenci V, Mustafa M, Link H. Elevated CD40 ligand expressing blood T-cell levels in multiple sclerosis are reversed by interferon-beta treatment. *Scand J Immunol* 2000;51:312–20.

119. Windhagen A, Newcombe J, Dangond F, *et al.* Expression of costimulatory molecules B7–1 (CD80), B7–2 (CD86), and interleukin 12 cytokine in multiple sclerosis lesions. *J Exp Med* 1995;182:1985–96.

120. van Boxel-Dezaire AH, Hoff SC, van Oosten BW, *et al.* Decreased interleukin-10 and increased interleukin-12p40 mRNA are associated with disease activity and characterize different disease stages in multiple sclerosis [see comments]. *Ann Neurol* 1999;45:695–703.

121. Nicoletti F, Patti F, Cocuzza C, *et al.* Elevated serum levels of interleukin-12 in chronic progressive multiple sclerosis. *J Neuroimmunol* 1996;70:87–90.

122. Ferrante P, Fusi ML, Saresella M, *et al.* Cytokine production and surface marker expression in acute and stable multiple sclerosis: altered IL-12 production and augmented signaling lymphocytic activation molecule (SLAM)-expressing lymphocytes in acute multiple sclerosis. *J Immunol* 1998;160:1514–21.

123. Wang X, Chen M, Wandinger KP, Williams G, Dhib-Jalbut S. IFN-beta-1b inhibits IL-12 production in peripheral blood mononuclear cells in an IL-10-dependent mechanism: relevance to IFN-beta-1b therapeutic effects in multiple sclerosis. *J Immunol* 2000;165:548–57.

124. Byrnes AA, McArthur JC, Karp CL. Interferon-beta therapy for multiple sclerosis induces reciprocal changes in interleukin-12 and interleukin-10 production. *Ann Neurol* 2002;51:165–74.

125. Makhlouf K, Comabella M, Imitola J, Weiner HL, Khoury SJ. Oral salbutamol decreases IL-12 in patients with secondary progressive multiple sclerosis. *J Neuroimmunol* 2001;117:156–65.

126. Khoury SJ, Healy BC, Kivisakk P, *et al.* A randomized controlled double-masked trial of albuterol add-on therapy in patients with multiple sclerosis. *Arch Neurol*; 67:1055–61.

127. Cannella B, Raine CS. The adhesion molecule and cytokine profile of multiple sclerosis lesions. *Ann Neurol* 1995;37:424–35.

128. Selmaj K, Raine CS, Cannella B, Brosnan CF. Identification of lymphotoxin and tumor necrosis factor in multiple sclerosis lesions. *J Clin Invest* 1991;87:949–54.

129. Hofman FM, Hinton DR, Johnson K, Merrill JE. Tumor necrosis factor identified in multiple sclerosis brain. *J Exp Med* 1989;170:607–12.

130. Andrews T, Zhang P, Bhat NR. TNFalpha potentiates

IFNgamma-induced cell death in oligodendrocyte progenitors. *J Neurosci Res* 1998;54:574–83.

131. Huberman M, Shalit F, Roth-Deri I, Gutman B, Kott E, Sredni B. Decreased IL-3 production by peripheral blood mononuclear cells in patients with multiple sclerosis. *J Neurol Sci* 1993;118:79–82.

132. van Oosten BW, Barkhof F, Scholten PE, von Blomberg BM, Ader HJ, Polman CH. Increased production of tumor necrosis factor alpha, and not of interferon gamma, preceding disease activity in patients with multiple sclerosis. *Arch Neurol* 1998;55:793–8.

133. Zipp F, Weber F, Huber S, *et al.* Genetic control of multiple sclerosis: increased production of lymphotoxin and tumor necrosis factor-alpha by HLA-DR2 +T-cells. *Ann Neurol* 1995;38:723–30.

134. Beck J, Rondot P, Catinot L, Falcoff E, Kirchner H, Wietzerbin J. Increased production of interferon gamma and tumor necrosis factor precedes clinical manifestation in multiple sclerosis: do cytokines trigger off exacerbations? *Acta Neurol Scand* 1988;78:318–23.

135. Spuler S, Yousry T, Scheller A, *et al.* Multiple sclerosis: prospective analysis of TNF-alpha and 55 kDa TNF receptor in CSF and serum in correlation with clinical and MRI activity. *J Neuroimmunol* 1996;66:57–64.

136. TNF neutralization in MS: results of a randomized, placebo-controlled multicenter study. The Lenercept Multiple Sclerosis Study Group and The University of British Columbia MS/MRI Analysis Group. *Neurology* 1999;53:457–65.

137. van Oosten BW, Barkhof F, Truyen L, *et al.* Increased MRI activity and immune activation in two multiple sclerosis patients treated with the monoclonal anti-tumor necrosis factor antibody cA2. *Neurology* 1996;47:1531–4.

138. Balashov KE, Comabella M, Ohashi T, Khoury SJ, Weiner HL. Defective regulation of IFNgamma and IL-12 by endogenous IL-10 in progressive MS. *Neurology* 2000;55:192–8.

139. Becher B, Giacomini PS, Pelletier D, McCrea E, Prat A, Antel JP. Interferon-gamma secretion by peripheral blood T-cell subsets in multiple sclerosis: correlation with disease phase and interferon-beta therapy. *Ann Neurol* 1999;45:247–50.

140. Noronha A, Toscas A, Jensen MA. Interferon beta decreases T-cell activation and interferon gamma production in multiple sclerosis. *J Neuroimmunol* 1993;46:145–53.

141. Panitch HS, Hirsch RL, Haley AS, Johnson KP. Exacerbations of multiple sclerosis in patients treated with gamma interferon. *Lancet* 1987;1:893–5.

142. Panitch HS, Hirsch RL, Schindler J, Johnson KP. Treatment of multiple sclerosis with gamma interferon: exacerbations associated with activation of the immune system. *Neurology* 1987;37:1097–102.

143. Calabresi PA, Fields NS, Maloni HW, *et al.* Phase 1 trial of transforming growth factor beta 2 in chronic progressive MS. *Neurology* 1998;51:289–92.

144. Kopp JB, Factor VM, Mozes M, *et al.* Transgenic mice with increased plasma levels of TGF-beta 1 develop progressive renal disease. *Lab Invest* 1996;74:991–1003.

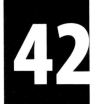

Chapter

B-cell-based therapies for multiple sclerosis

Emmanuelle Waubant and Amit Bar-Or

Introduction

The predominant view of pathogenic mechanisms in multiple sclerosis (MS), in large part driven by insights from studies of animal models, has traditionally held that inflammation is principally mediated by CD4$^+$ and CD8$^+$ T-cells. In keeping with this, studies of therapeutic mechanisms of action of approved immune therapies have tended to focus on T-cells as the primary therapeutic target. While these therapies are proven to decrease clinical and MRI focal inflammatory activity, they are partially effective, have a limited impact on accumulation of disability, and are associated with variable tolerability and/or safety limitations. There is also a growing appreciation that immune responses that are relevant to MS, and as a corollary to MS therapeutics, involve multiple interacting immune cell subsets, and a range of adaptive, innate, and humoral responses. Indeed, the cellular and molecular mechanisms underlying the spectrum of immune-mediated injury in MS, as well as those underlying the more smoldering CNS injury contributing to progressive axonal degeneration and progressive disability, remain to be fully elucidated and adequately targeted.

The abnormal presence of immunoglobulins (Ig) in the central nervous system (CNS) of many MS patients, often exhibiting an oligoclonal band (OCB) pattern, the demonstration of anti-myelin antibodies within MS plaques, as well as the identification of intraclonally expanded B-cells and plasmacytes in the cerebrospinal fluid (CSF) and CNS plaques of MS patients have long been recognized. However, how and to what extent these B-cell-related mediators contribute to the disease process throughout its different phases and anatomical compartments has not been resolved. Recent observations that selective targeting of B-cells can substantially diminish new focal inflammatory CNS lesions and clinical relapses in patients with MS confirms an important role for B-cells and the question is no longer "whether" but rather "how" B-cells contribute to the MS disease process. Advances in the basic fields of immunology, together with accumulating results from clinical studies of B-cell targeting in MS and other autoimmune diseases, have engendered a renewed interest in the potential roles of both antibody-dependent, as well as antibody-independent B-cell mechanisms and their roles in MS and its animal models.

These insights have also prompted re-evaluation of the potential impact of existing as well as emerging interventions for MS on the range of potentially disease-relevant B-cell responses. This includes revisiting the impact and underlying mechanisms of action of plasma exchange (PLEX) and intravenous Ig (IVIg); the approved MS immune therapies, interferon beta (IFNβ) formulations, glatiramer acetate (GA, Copaxone), natalizumab (Tysabri), mitoxantrone (Novantrone), and fingolimod (Gilenya); as well as the growing range of emerging therapies. Understanding the relevant biological impact of selective B-cell interventions such as rituximab (Rituxan), ocrelizumab, and ofatumumab in MS becomes of particular interest.

Here, we aim to provide an overview of treatments targeting B-cells and humoral responses in MS, with particular focus on results of the recent clinical trials of B-cell depletion. While a complete review of the data implicating Ig and B-cell responses in MS and its animal models is beyond the scope of this chapter (please refer to Chapter 3), we will present some of the relevant published and emerging studies that provide the rationale for discussion of B-cell based therapies in MS.

Treatments that non-selectively target B-cells and the humoral response

Impacting B-cell and humoral responses in MS and related disease can be considered in three contexts: (i) therapies traditionally viewed as targeting humoral responses such as IVIg and PLEX, (ii) therapies developed with a view of targeting T-cells, or more broadly targeting immune responses, that may also have important effects on disease relevant aspects of B-cell biology, and (iii) therapies specifically designed to target B-cells and, as a consequence, their contribution to both antibody-related and non-antibody related aspects of the disease (Table 42.1).

IVIg and PLEX

Detailed discussion of IVIg and PLEX and their evaluation in MS and related diseases can be found elsewhere in this book. Early reports of successful treatment of active MS relapses or

Multiple Sclerosis Therapeutics, Fourth Edition, ed. Jeffrey A. Cohen and Richard A. Rudick. Published by Cambridge University Press.
© Cambridge University Press 2011.

Table 42.1. *Approved, off-label, and promising MS therapies targeting potentially relevant B-cell and humoral responses*

	Therapies	Among reported mechanisms of action	Predicted impact on B-cell and humoral responses
Therapies traditionally viewed as targeting humoral responses	IVIg	• Anti-idiotypic antibodies • Fc-receptor blockade • Stimulation of inhibitory Fc-γ receptor type 2B • Change in cytokine profile • Binding of complement through constant domain • Changes in CD4+ helper and CD8+ suppressor-cytotoxic T-cells • ? Promotion of remyelination	• Decreases availability of humoral (B-cell products) such as antibodies in peripheral blood
	Plasma exchange	• Depletion of Ig of all classes, immune complexes, cryoglobulins, cholesterol-containing lipoproteins • ? Depletion of IFNγ, TNFα, and complement • ? Alters T suppressors • ? Removes conduction blocking substances	• Decreases availability of humoral (B-cell products) such as antibodies in peripheral blood
Therapies traditionally viewed as targeting T-cell responses	IFNβ	Modulation of MHC class II and co-stimulatory molecules (decreased lymphocyte activation) Decreased up-regulation of adhesion molecules and MMPs (decreased cell trafficking)	Decreases B-cell migration to CNS ? Decreased B-cell activation
	Natalizumab	Blocks alpha-4-beta1 (VLA-4) integrin (decreased trafficking)	Decreases B-cell migration to CNS
	GA	Immune deviation in CD4+ T-cells from a Th1 to a Th2 phenotype Induction of anergy, regulatory T-cells population Modulation of antigen presentation and APC responses activation of B-cells with development if anti-GA antibodies	• ? Modulation of B-cell activation • ? Modulation of B-cell populations
	Glucocorticosteroids	• Restoration of blood–brain barrier • Decreased transcription of AP-1 and NFkB • Decreased MMP secretion • Induction of T-cell apoptosis • Suppression of Ig levels	• ? Likely pleotropic
	Cyclophosphamide	Crosslinks DNA Kills rapidly dividing cells including lymphocytes	• Moderate B-cell depletion in peripheral blood
	Mitoxantrone	Abrogates B-cell and T-cell proliferation, Diminishes antibody production Deactivates macrophages	• Moderate B-cell depletion in peripheral blood • ? Modulation of B-cell response profile
	Azathioprine, mycophenolate mofetil	• Partial inhibition of purine, DNA, RNA and membrane glycoprotein synthesis. • Viewed as largely impacting T-cell function	Mild decrease in peripheral blood B-cells
	Alemtuzumab (CAMPATH)	• Depleting humanized antibody that recognizes CD52 present on all lymphocytes	• Profound depletion of B-cells in peripheral blood

(cont.)

Table 42.1. *(cont.)*

	Therapies	Among reported mechanisms of action	Predicted impact on B-cell and humoral responses
	Methotrexate	• Potent folate analog • Binds to and inhibits dihydrofolate reductase, an enzyme that is essential for the production of reduced cofactors necessary for the synthesis of both DNA and RNA	? Likely to impact B-cell proliferation
	Fingolimod	Sphingosine 1-phosphate receptor modulator Induces aberrant internalization of this receptor in lymphocytes Deprives lymphocytes of a signal necessary to egress from secondary lymphoid tissues	• ? Likely to impact B-cell mobilization to CNS
Therapies specifically targeting B-cells	Rituximab Ocrelizumab Ofatumumab	• Profoundly depletes B-cell in peripheral blood • Lesser depletion of CSF B-cells	• ? Alters APC compartment, thereby decrease T-cell activation, • ? Modulates immune regulatory function of B-cells • ? Impacts role of B-cells in formation and maintenance of new lymphoid foci • ? Limits precursor pool for plasma cells and hence production of pathogenic anti-CNS antibody production • ? Decreases EBV pool and hence reduces chronically activated B-cells

APC = antigen presenting cell, CNS = central nervous system, CSF = cerebrospinal fluid, EBV = Epstein–Barr virus, IFN = interferon, Ig = immunoglobulin, i.v. = intravenous, GA = glatiramer acetate, MHC = major histocompatability complex, MMP = matrix metalloproteinase, TNF= tumor necrosis factor.

prevention of relapses with IVIg or PLEX implicated humoral mechanisms in the disease process,[1–4] though subsequent studies have not demonstrated a consistent effect on disability progression.[5] The assumption that any benefit from these therapies implicates anti-CNS antibodies in the disease process may be an over-simplification, as the mechanisms of action of these interventions may be pleotropic. Various immunoregulatory properties have been suggested as contributors to an IVIg effect: anti-idiotypic antibodies binding Fab fragments (that may neutralize autoantibodies and down-regulate antibody production); Fc-receptor blockade; stimulation of inhibitory Fcγ receptor type 2B; change in cytokine profile; binding of complement through constant domain; changes in CD4+ helper and CD8+ suppressor-cytotoxic T-cells; and finally possible promotion of remyelination.[6] PLEX has been used with some success to treat severe acute relapses that do not initially respond to steroids,[4] but there is no evidence that such intervention alters ongoing disease course including prevention of subsequent relapses or accrual of disability. PLEX removes many plasma proteins (Ig of all classes, immune complexes, cryoglobulins, cholesterol-containing lipoproteins, and possibly proinflammatory factors such as IFNγ, tumor necrosis factor-alpha (TNFα), and complement). It is unknown, whether PLEX removes conduction blocking substances. Substances smaller than 15 kDa are more efficiently removed. Ninety percent of the removal occurs within five exchanges over 7–10 days.

Immune modulators and suppressors developed to target T-cells

Essentially, all US Food and Drug Administration (FDA)-approved therapies as well as off-label drugs used in MS have potential impact on B-cell biology. In view of the increasing implication of B-cell responses in MS disease pathophysiology, it becomes important to consider how any immune therapy introduced to patients may impact on B-cells and their products. For example, while the approved IFNβ therapies have largely been viewed as T-cell directed therapies, human B-cells use similar (though not identical) molecular machinery as T-cells to traffic across the blood–brain barrier.[7] These include particular adhesion molecules and matrix proteases that are known targets for IFNβ therapies. For example, B-cells express the adhesion molecule VLA-4 at higher levels than T-cells, and are likely also to be targeted by natalizumab (anti-VLA-4 antibody therapy). GA also has generally been viewed as mediating its effects through modulation of T-cell as well as monocyte/dendritic cell responses.[8–11] Therapy with GA has also been shown to modulate the proliferation, population dynamics, and response profiles of B-cells in experimental autoimmune encephalomyelitis (EAE)[12,13] and in patients with MS.[14,15] Mitoxantrone, FDA-approved for therapy in patients with active and progressive MS, has also been shown to have a range of effects on B-cell biology[16,17] in addition to impacting T-cells. Steroids, and non-selective

Table 42.2. *Expression of CD19 and CD20 on the B-cell lineages*

	Surface expression of Ig	CD19	CD20
Stem cell	0	0	0
Pro-B-cell	0	+	0
Pre-B-cell	+	+	+
Immature B-cell	+	+	+
Mature B-cell	++	+	+
Activated B-cell	++	+	+
Memory B-cell	++	+	+
Plasma cell	0	0	0

immune suppressants used occasionally off label in MS (e.g. methotrexate, azathioprine, mycophenolate mofetil, cyclophosphamide), as well as experimental agents that non-selectively target or deplete T-cells and B-cells (e.g. alemtuzumab, αCD52, CAMPATH-1) all impact B-cell biology in ways that may be relevant to their efficacy and toxicity in MS (Table 42.1).

Rituximab

Rituximab (MabThera®/Rituxan®) is a glycosylated IgG1 κ chimeric mouse/human antibody that binds to the CD20 antigen present on the majority of circulating B-cells.[18] CD20 expression is restricted to the B-cell lineage, ranging from the pre–B-cell stage through to plasmablasts, but is generally not expressed on stem cells or fully differentiated plasma cells (Table 42.2).[18] CD20 is an attractive target, as its turn-over is slow with no internalization and no soluble forms of the protein are released into serum.[19] Treatment with rituximab induces a pronounced, rapid (within hours), and prolonged (over three months) near-depletion of circulating B-cells in humans. In vitro, rituximab has been demonstrated to mediate complement-dependent cytotoxicity (CDC) and antibody-dependent cellular cytotoxicity (ADCC) of B-cells, as well as induce B-cell apoptosis.[20,21] The relative extent to which these individual mechanisms account for the observed depletion of B-cells in vivo is unknown, but is likely influenced by the tissue where depletion is occurring. Several investigator-driven and industry (Genentech and Biogen IDEC) sponsored studies of rituximab were performed in MS, based on insights from other autoimmune disease states.

Rituximab in lymphoma and autoimmune disease

Rituximab was approved in the USA in 1997 for the treatment of different forms of non-Hodgkin's (B-cell) lymphoma. Useful insights into administration, safety, and tolerability profiles have been gained through more than 1 000 000 lymphoma patient exposures to rituximab, either as monotherapy, in combination with immunosuppressant drugs, or as maintenance therapy for up to two years.[22,23] More recently, rituximab has been evaluated for its potential to treat autoimmune states in which B-cells and autoantibodies have been

thought to contribute to disease pathophysiology.[24] To date, rituximab has been reported to have potential benefits on signs and symptoms of rheumatoid arthritis (RA),[25,26] systemic lupus erythematosus,[27,28] immune thrombocytopenia,[29] autoimmune anemia,[30] autoimmune neuropathy,[31] and paraneoplastic opsoclonus–myoclonus syndrome.[32] Based on the data in RA, rituximab gained FDA-approval in 2006 for the treatment of patients with moderate to severe RA who had an inadequate response to TNF antagonists. The rapid onset of clinical effect of rituximab in RA and lupus argues for a therapeutic mechanism of action that is not merely related to removal of pathogenic antibodies, since these would not be expected to deplete as rapidly. Rituximab was initially approved in lymphoma at a dose of 375 mg/m² weekly for four doses. Subsequently, the regimen was changed to a fixed dose of 2 g (two infusions of 1 gram, two weeks apart) based on safety, pharmacokinetic, pharmacodynamic and efficacy data in lymphoma, RA, and autoimmune polyneuropathy.[26]

Open-label add-on study of rituximab in breakthrough relapsing–remitting MS

In an investigator-initiated open-label trial of rituximab as add-on therapy in patients with relapsing–remitting (RR) MS exhibiting suboptimal response despite standard treatment with either IFNβ or GA (annualized baseline relapse rate 1.27), including at least one gadolinium (Gd)-enhancing lesion at baseline, 30 participants (median disease duration 7.5 years, median Expanded Disability Status Scale (EDSS) 4.0) completed the regimen of four weekly infusions of 375 mg/m² each.[33,34] The primary end-point was change in number of Gd-enhancing lesions on three post-treatment vs. three pre-treatment brain MRI scans. Treatment with rituximab was associated with an 88% reduction in the mean number of Gd-enhancing lesions at weeks 12, 16, and 20 after treatment compared to pre-treatment (P < 0.0001).[34] Twenty-five of 30 participants had a reduction of 50% or more in the number of Gd-enhancing lesions. Annualized relapse rate during the 52-week study was 0.23. MS Functional Composite (MSFC) scores improved over baseline after 32 weeks.

Phase 1 re-treatment trial of rituximab in relapsing MS

Twenty-six participants with RRMS were enrolled in this 72-week open-label, multi-center, Phase 1 re-treatment trial with rituximab.[35] Subjects received two courses of rituximab six months apart. Each course consisted of two doses of 1000 mg, administered two weeks apart, such that infusions were given on weeks 0 and 2, and weeks 24 and 26. All patients participated through the week 24 visit and 22 (84.6%) participants completed the week 72 visit. At baseline, mean age was 40.4 ± 8.7 years, females 73.1%, mean EDSS 2.3, mean disease duration 7.2 years and mean of 1.27 relapses during the prior year prior. Over 75% of enrolled participants had received one or more disease-modifying therapies (mostly IFNβ or GA).

Over the 72 weeks, 21 (80.8%) participants remained relapse free; four participants (15.4%) reported one relapse, and one participant (3.8%) reported two relapses. The unadjusted annualized relapse rate was 0.25 from baseline to week 24, and 0.18 from baseline to week 72. The mean relapse rate was 0.25 from baseline to week 24 and 0.22 from baseline to week 72. After the first course of rituximab (week 0 and 2 infusions), the mean number of Gd-enhancing lesions decreased from 1.31 at baseline to 0.73 at week 4. After the second course (weeks 24 and 26), the mean number of Gd-enhancing lesions decreased to 0.05 (week 48) and 0 (week 72). The mean number of new T2-hyperintense lesions decreased from 0.92 at week 4 to 0 at week 72.

Phase 2 placebo-controlled trial of rituximab in RRMS

A 48-week, randomized, placebo-controlled, multicenter trial of rituximab in RRMS enrolled 104 participants.[36] Patients received rituximab 1000 mg twice two weeks apart ($n = 69$), or placebo ($n = 35$) at week 0 and week 2. Baseline demographics, clinical characteristics, and use of prior disease-modifying therapies were essentially the same as for the patients who participated in the open-label re-treatment trial described above, and were generally well balanced between treatment groups. However, at baseline, the proportion of participants without Gd-enhancing lesions was greater in the placebo than the rituximab group (85.7% vs. 63.8%, respectively). Of 104 participants, 96 (92.3%) completed 24 weeks, and 79 (76%) completed 48 weeks, including 84.1% in the rituximab group and 60% in the placebo group. Twelve of the 25 participants who discontinued the study treatment early completed the safety follow-up through the end of the study, including 10.1% of participants in the rituximab group and 14.3% of participants in the placebo group.[36]

Primary-end-point

Rituximab-treated participants demonstrated a substantial reduction in total Gd-enhancing lesion counts at weeks 12, 16, 20, and 24 compared with placebo recipients (intent-to-treat analysis, $P < 0.001$). During the first 24 weeks, those receiving rituximab had a mean total Gd-enhancing lesion count of 0.5, compared with 5.5 in those receiving placebo, a relative reduction of 91%. Beginning at week 12, rituximab significantly reduced the number of Gd-enhancing lesions at each subsequent study visit compared with placebo ($P = 0.003$ to < 0.001).

Key secondary end-points

The proportion of participants with clinical relapses was significantly reduced in the rituximab group compared with placebo at week 24 (14.5% vs. 34.3%, $P = 0.02$) and week 48 (20.3% vs. 40.0%, $P = 0.04$). At week 24, placebo recipients were at more than double the risk (relative risk = 2.31) of relapse compared with rituximab-treated participants; at week 48, the relative risk

of relapse was 1.90. Rituximab-treated participants had a lower annualized relapse rate compared with placebo-treated patients at 24 weeks (0.37 vs. 0.84, $P = 0.04$), and at 48 weeks (0.37 vs. 0.72, $P = 0.09$). Rituximab significantly reduced *new* Gd-enhancing lesions at weeks 12, 16, 20, and 24 compared with placebo ($P < 0.001$). Beginning at week 12, rituximab also significantly reduced the number of *new* Gd-enhancing lesions at each study week ($P = 0.002$ to < 0.001). This effect was seen until week 48.

Phase 2/3 trial of rituximab in primary progressive MS

A two-year Phase 2/3 multicenter randomized trial (OLYMPUS) tested the effect of rituximab vs. placebo in participants with primary progressive (PP) MS.[37] Using 2:1 randomization, 439 participants received either two 1000 mg rituximab infusions or two placebo infusions (separated by two weeks) intravenously, every 24 weeks for a total of four treatment courses through 96 weeks. Sixty-five percent of the participants had not received any prior MS disease-modifying therapy. Mean baseline EDSS was 4.8 (more than 50% of the participants had an EDSS of 4.0 or more). Half of the participants were males. Median age at baseline was 51 years; 84.4% and 82.5% of the participants completed 96 weeks, respectively, in the placebo and the rituximab groups.

Primary end-point

The primary efficacy end-point in this study was the time to confirmed disease progression (CDP), defined by a pre-specified increase in EDSS sustained for 12 weeks (increased by at least 1.0 point from baseline if EDSS between 2.0 and 5.5 inclusive; increased by at least 0.5 point if EDSS > 5.5). The difference in time to CDP between treatment arms was not statistically significant ($P = 0.14$, stratified log-rank test). Kaplan–Meier estimates for the proportion of participants with CDP at 96 weeks were 38.5% for placebo and 30.2% for rituximab (i.e. a 24% reduction in the risk of progression in rituximab recipients). Stratified hazard ratio was 0.77.

Secondary imaging end-points

Rituximab recipients had significantly less T2 lesion volume increase than placebo recipients: median increase 302.95 mm^3 for rituximab-treated participants vs. 809.50 mm^3 for placebo recipients ($P < 0.001$). Brain volume change was similar in both groups ($P = 0.62$).

Exploratory end-points

Compared with placebo, rituximab-treated participants had less worsening in the timed 25-foot walk at weeks 48 ($P = 0.04$), 96 ($P = 0.076$), and 122 ($P = 0.015$). Other MSFC items (nine-hole-peg test and paced auditory serial addition test) showed no difference between groups. Pre-planned sub-group analysis showed that rituximab-treated participants under 51 years of age (hazard ratio = 0.52, P = 0.01) or participants who had Gd-enhancing lesions at baseline (hazard ratio = 0.41, P = 0.007) were less likely to experience CDP compared with placebo.

Clinical safety and tolerability of rituximab

The overall rituximab experience

The most common side effects of rituximab are infusion reactions including fever, chills, rigors, hypotension, and general flu-like symptoms. These generally occur during the first infusion when the majority are classified as mild or moderate, and dissipate in both frequency and intensity with subsequent infusions. To mitigate these common infusion reactions, slow administration over several hours with prophylactic use of acetaminophen or an equivalent antipyretic agent and anti-histamine such as diphenhydramine HCl an hour prior to the start of rituximab use is recommended. Infusions are often started at 50 mg/hour, and the rate is increased by 50 mg/hour every half hour if tolerability is good. Rarely, severe and even fatal infusion-related reactions have occurred in lymphoma patients. Risk factors for serious infusion reactions in lymphoma patients include high tumor burden, high circulating lymphocyte counts, and concurrent cardiovascular or pulmonary disease. Rituximab does not appear to increase the rate of serious infections in most studies to date.[22,23,38] However, cases of progressive multifocal leukoencephalopathy (PML) have been reported in patients receiving rituximab and concurrent or prior therapy with other immunosuppressive therapies for lymphoma, RA, or lupus. No PML case has been reported to date in patients with MS, or in patients with other conditions receiving rituximab as a monotherapy who had not been exposed to prior immunosuppression.

Safety and tolerability of rituximab in MS clinical trials

All three industry-sponsored trials rituximab monotherapy in RRMS and PPMS confirmed a side effect profile similar to that previously reported in RA and other autoimmune disorders.[35–37] The most common (≥10%) drug-related adverse events (AEs) in MS patients receiving rituximab were infusion-associated. Most infusion-related AEs occurring with the first infusion were mild or moderate (>90%), while 7% were grade 3 and none were grade 4. Rates of infusion-related AEs were comparable to placebo upon successive infusions. In the Phase 2 trial in RRMS,[36] grade 4 events were reported in three rituximab recipients: ischemic coronary artery disorder (n =1), malignant thyroid neoplasm (n =1), and acute and progressive MS symptoms (n =1). Serious AEs (SAEs) were reported in 14.3% of placebo recipients and 13% of rituximab recipients. A total of 5.7% placebo participants and 4.3% of rituximab participants withdrew from the study due to AEs. One death (homicide) occurred in the rituximab group. The incidence of any infections was similar in the placebo (71.4%) and rituximab (69.6%) groups. The most common (≥10%)

infections in rituximab recipients were nasopharyngitis, upper respiratory tract infections, urinary tract infections and sinusitis. Urinary tract infections (14.5% rituximab vs. 8.6% placebo) and sinusitis (13.0% vs. 8.6%) were more common in rituximab recipients. No opportunistic infections were reported. Infectious SAEs were reported by 5.7% of placebo and 2.9% of rituximab recipients. Of the two infection-related SAEs in the rituximab group (gastroenteritis, bronchitis), both resolved without sequelae; the last recorded values for Ig levels prior to these infections were above the lower limit of normal in both participants.

In the PPMS Phase 2/3 trial, infection-related SAEs were higher in the rituximab group than the placebo group (4.5% vs. <1.0%). Three participants died, one from each group with pneumonia, and one from the placebo group due to cardiopulmonary failure.[37] There was no evidence for increased incidence of infection or other AE in participants with Ig levels below the lower limit of normal, although this group is likely too small to be conclusive.

Pharmacodynamics and immunogenicity of rituximab in MS trials

The aforementioned trials in MS provided a wealth of details on the pharmacodynamics and immunogenicity of rituximab.[35–37] In these trials, rituximab induced near-complete depletion (>95% reduction from baseline) of peripheral B-cells (measured by CD19 expression since residual circulating rituximab may mask CD20 on any residual B-cells) by week 2. In the Phase 2 trial, after one course of rituximab at weeks 0 and 2, depletion was sustained through 24 weeks, while by week 48, CD19-positive cells had returned to 30.7% of baseline values.[36,39] CD3+ T-cells in the blood were not appreciably altered by rituximab. Similarly, in the Phase 1 study (two courses of 1000 mg rituximab at weeks 0 and 2, and at weeks 24 and 26), B-cell depletion was essentially complete up to week 48, with reconstitution to mean 34.5% of baseline by week 72.[35] The majority of reconstituting cells were CD19+ CD27− naive B-cells (mean 51% of baseline) rather than CD19+ CD27+ memory B-cells (mean 14% of baseline) indicating that naive B-cells recover faster than memory B-cells.[39] This kinetic of reconstitution is similar to what has been seen with rituximab use in other indications, as circulating B-cells are replenished from bone marrow pro-B-cells within four to 12 months after depletion, sometimes longer.

Median levels of serum IgM, IgG, and IgA in the Phase 1 re-treatment study and in the Phase 2 monotherapy study of rituximab in RRMS, remained above the lower limit of normal in both treatment groups throughout the trial. In the Phase 2 study,[36] at any time through week 48, IgG levels were below lower limit of normal in 7.9% of rituximab recipients and 3.0% of placebo recipients, while IgM levels were below the lower limit of normal in 22.4% of rituximab participants and 8.6% of placebo participants. No participant had IgA levels below the normal limit during the study. In the OLYMPUS Phase 3 study in PPMS, IgG, and IgA levels were below lower limit of normal range in less than 5% of participants in either active or placebo-treated groups. IgM were below lower limit of normal at some time during the study in 31.7% of rituximab, and 5.9% of placebo, recipients.[37] With respect to pathogen-specific immunity assessed in the Phase 1 study, serum IgG titers for tetanus generally remained unchanged over the 72 weeks and no participant who was seropositive for mumps or rubella at baseline became seronegative during the study.[39]

In the Phase 2 RRMS trial, human anti-chimeric antibodies (HACA) to rituximab were measured at week 48 in 14 (23.1%) of the 58 participants who completed the treatment period; no placebo participant tested positive at any time. There was no apparent association between HACA positivity and the type or severity of AEs or efficacy response at weeks 24, 36, or 48 but this trial did not evaluate rituximab re-administration.[36] In the Phase 1 re-treatment trial in RRMS, at week 72, all six participants positive for HACA as well as 15 of 20 HACA-negative participants were relapse free.[35] In the open-label add-on trial, 13% of participants developed HACA by 24 weeks after therapy.[34] Surprisingly, in the PPMS trial,[37] 7% of rituximab recipients and 6.3% of placebo recipients were positive for HACA. The reason for the presence of HACA in placebo recipients in this study is not clear.

Ocrelizumab

Ocrelizumab is a humanized anti-CD20 monoclonal antibody (IgG1) that recognizes an epitope that overlaps with that recognized by rituximab. In vitro, ocrelizumab mediates efficient lysis of CD20+ cells by ADCC, CDC, and apoptosis while, in vivo, apoptosis seems to play a limited role. The increased ADCC activity seen in vitro with ocrelizumab correlates with increased binding affinity for human FcγRIII. As a humanized antibody, ocrelizumab is expected to have lower immunogenicity and possibly impart lesser infusion-related reactions. Ocrelizumab was first evaluated in RA in the Phase 1/2 ACTION trial comparing methotrexate plus ocrelizumab vs. methotrexate plus placebo.[40] Dual doses of 200 mg of ocrelizumab and higher showed better clinical responses. Human anti-human antibodies (HAHA) were detected in 19% and 10% of patients receiving 10 mg or 50 mg doses of ocrelizumab, respectively, compared with 0%–5% of those receiving 200, 500, and 1000 mg doses. Infusion-related reactions were experienced by 45% to 65% of patients receiving their first infusions of ocrelizumab depending on the dose regimen.[40]

A Phase 2, multicenter, randomized, placebo-controlled study of ocrelizumab in RRMS is ongoing. In an interim report,[41] 220 patients with at least two MS relapses in the three years prior to enrolment (at least one of which had to occur during the year prior to screening), were randomized to two doses of either ocrelizumab 300 mg ($n = 55$) or 1000 mg ($n = 55$), 2 weeks apart, vs. placebo ($n = 54$), or to open-label IFNβ-1a ($n = 54$) for the first 24 weeks. At week 24, all patients

received ocrelizumab. The primary end-point of this study was the total number of Gd-enhancing on brain MRI scans obtained at week 12, 16, 20, and 24. Both ocrelizumab-treated groups experienced significantly fewer new Gd-enhancing lesions than placebo ($P < 0.001$) and IFNβ-1a ($P < 0.001$) recipients. Relative to placebo, reductions in the total number of Gd-enhancing foci at weeks 12, 16, 20, and 24 were 89% in the ocrelizumab 300 mg × 2 group and 96% in the 1000 mg × 2 group. Relative to IFNβ-1a, reductions in the total number of Gd-enhancing foci at weeks 12, 16, 20, and 24 were 91% in the ocrelizumab 300 mg × 2 group and 97% in the 1000 mg × 2 group. Secondary endpoints included annualized relapse rate, which was significantly lower in both ocrelizumab arms (unadjusted annualized relapse rate reduction: 80% in the 300 mg × 2, and 73% in the 1000 mg × 2, compared to placebo, and 66% in the 300 mg × 2 and 54% in the 1000 mg × 2, compared to IFNβ-1a). No opportunistic infection was reported. One death was reported in the ocrelizumab 1000 mg × 2 arm attributable to an acute disseminated intravascular coagulation. Two infectious SAEs were reported (one in the 1000 mg × 2 and one in the placebo group).

In RA, the development of ocrelizumab has been discontinued due to the perceived lack of improved risk/benefit ratio compared to rituximab. This decision was based, in part, on several opportunistic infections that were reported in ocrelizumab recipients who were also receiving oral methotrexate. No such AE has been reported in the MS trial with ocrelizumab as a monotherapy and, given the promising efficacy results, Phase 3 trials in RRMS and PPMS have been launched.

Ofatumumab

Several other humanized anti-CD20 molecules are being developed and include both monoclonal antibodies and small molecules. Ofatumumab (Arzerra, HuMax-CD20) is a humanized monoclonal antibody. It was FDA-approved in 2009 for the treatment of chronic lymphocytic leukemia refractory to other treatments. Ofatumumab targets an epitope different from rituximab and most other anti-CD20 antibodies. Several trials are ongoing in RA, as well as a Phase 1/2 dose-finding study in RRMS. In a multicenter randomized double-blind, placebo-controlled trial of ofatumumab in RRMS,[42] patients with at least two MS relapses during the prior 24 months or one MS relapse during the prior 12 months or one MS relapse between 12–24 months and one Gd-enhancing lesions in the prior 12 months, were successively randomized 2 : 1 to increasing doses of ofatumumab (100 ($n = 8$), 300 ($n = 11$) or 700 ($n = 7$) mg i.v. at weeks 0 and 2) or placebo ($n = 12$). All doses of ofatumumab depleted circulating B-cells. MRI scans were obtained four weeks prior to enrollment, at baseline, and at weeks 4, 8, 12, 16, 20, and 24. The mean cumulative number of Gd-enhancing lesions from week 8 to 24 after treatment was 0.04 (0.20) in the combined ofatumumab group and 9.69 (24.86) in the placebo group. The estimated relative reduction in the number of Gd-enhancing lesion was 99.8% (90% confidence interval 94.7–100.0, $P < 0.001$). At week 24, a dose-dependent B-cell depletion was seen with a mean CD19+ B-cell count reduced by 78%, 95%, and 98% in the 100, 300, and 700 mg groups.

What have we learned from B-cell depletion trials in humans?

The initial pursuit of clinical trials with rituximab in MS was based on the consideration that such an approach would serve to decrease precursors to plasma cells, thereby reducing synthesis of potentially pathogenic CNS-directed antibodies.[24,43] The four completed trials of rituximab and the ongoing trial of ocrelizumab that have been reported in RRMS and PPMS have all shown a benefit in terms diminishing the accrual of focal brain MRI T2 and Gd-enhancing lesions. When early follow-up MRIs were available, the effect on Gd-enhancing lesion reduction appeared to be very prompt in onset (i.e. beginning within a few weeks after initial infusion). This rapid impact of rituximab and ocrelizumab argues for a main effect related to antibody-independent B-cell functions. While the effect of rituximab and ocrelizumab on focal inflammatory lesions and relapses appears evident, the effect on insidious disability progression such as occurs in PPMS is unclear.

While anti-CD20 treatment efficiently depleted the great majority of circulating B-cells, there have been inconsistent reports regarding treatment effects on other circulating immune cells subsets in part due to the nature of the observation reported (within-patient differences vs. inter-patient differences). A 12% within-patient reduction in circulating T-cells was reported in one of the open-label studies of rituximab as an add-on therapy in RRMS which may reflect decreases in specific CD4+ and CD8+ T-cell subsets.[44] We have made a similar observation that within-patient CD3+ T-cell counts decrease after treatment with rituximab by approximately 20% (E.W. personal observation). In our cohort, a 20% decrease in CD4+ and 23% in CD8+ T-cell counts were seen after rituximab therapy compared to pre-treatment. No significant differences in circulating CD4 or CD8 T-cell subsets, or of T-cells with Treg phenotype, were seen in the Phase 1 (re-treatment) or Phase 2 studies of rituximab in RRMS,[39] though larger multicenter studies are more susceptible to pre-analytical variables. We have not seen an effect of rituximab treatment on CD56+ cells (E.W. personal observation). In lupus, treatment with rituximab did reportedly increase the frequency of Tregs which has been considered a potential therapeutic mode of action of B-cell depletion. Other circulating T-cell subsets did not appear impacted in rituximab add-on studies in lupus and RA, though assessment in these diseases may be confounded by the other concurrent immune therapies.

As expected, CD20-mediated B-cell depletion in a variety of human diseases has generally been found to have little if any effects on circulating IgG levels (many of which are thought to be generated by long-lived plasma cells that would not be susceptible to B-cell depletion), and modest to moderate effects on IgM levels. Whether these changes are relevant to disease modification in MS is unknown. Modest reductions in serum

antibodies to the myelin antigens, myelin-oligodendrocyte glycoprotein (MOG) and myelin basic protein (MBP), were seen in some participants 24 weeks following rituximab therapy.[33] A surprising insight, however, reported by several groups was that, in spite of the substantial peripheral B-cell depletion achieved, treatment with rituximab was not associated with changes in CSF IgG concentrations, IgG index, or OCB number or pattern.[33,44–46] These results strongly support the premise that the ability of anti-CD20 therapy to limit new relapsing disease activity in patients with MS reflects non-antibody dependent mechanisms rather than antibody-dependent mechanisms of injury. While circulating B-cells were consistently depleted with rituximab treatment, studies in RRMS and PPMS,[33,44,45,47] as well as in opsoclonus–myoclonus syndrome,[32] indicated that the number of CSF B-cells was only partially reduced in some, but not all, participants. It is unclear whether the decreased B-cell numbers (up to 90% decrease) observed in the CSF of patients following rituximab treatment (typically assessed in follow-up CSF obtained 3–6 months after depletion), reflects B-cell targeting within the CNS, vs. peripheral depletion of a trafficking pool of B-cells. Of interest is whether rituximab affects centroblasts (germinal center-like cells) reported to be present in the CNS of patients, and whether this is required for rituximab to have clinical benefit. Peripherally infused rituximab may access the CNS at variable levels achieving concentrations that are probably 100-fold less than those reached in peripheral blood (potentially related to the degree of blood–brain barrier disruption).[38] It is also not clear whether the mechanisms underlying peripheral depletion (for example, ADCC) can be fully recapitulated in the CNS. An ongoing study involving intrathecal administration of rituximab in patients SPMS (RIVITaLISe) should provide important insights in this regard.

Interestingly, rituximab treatment also resulted in decreased numbers of T-cells in the CSF of treated MS patients, in the range 50%.[33,44] Such decreases in CSF T-cells following targeted B-cell therapy could conceivably reflect diminished T-cell activation in the periphery due to peripheral B-cell depletion (resulting in decreased T-cell trafficking into the CNS), as well as decreased activation and/or chemoattraction of T-cells by B-cells within the CNS. Recent work has demonstrated that B-cell depletion in MS patients, both ex vivo and in vivo, results in diminished pro-inflammatory Th1 and Th17 responses of both CD+ and CD8+ T-cells.[39] Intriguingly, soluble products from activated B-cells of untreated MS participants were able to reconstitute the diminished T-cell responses observed following in vivo B-cell depletion in the same participants. This effect appeared to be largely mediated by B-cell derived lymphotoxin (LT) and TNFα. Decreased peripheral T-cell activation and proliferation in the absence of B-cells would be expected to result in lesser T-cell trafficking into the CSF compartment, and likely reflects an important antibody-independent mechanism (see further below) by which B-cells contribute to new MS disease activity. With respect to the possibility that B-cell depletion within the CNS, even if partial, can result in lesser chemoattraction to T-cells, CSF levels of CXCL13 and CCL19, two chemokines involved in the organization of lymphoid follicles, were found to be selectively decreased after rituximab administration, and CXCL13 decreases correlated modestly with CSF T-cell reduction.[44]

B-cell reconstitution in patients with MS following rituximab treatment generally follows similar kinetics as reported in other populations.[17,39] Naive (CD27-) B-cells re-emerge earlier and more rapidly than memory (CD27+) B-cells. The B-cells that reconstitute following rituximab treatment in MS patients have been shown to produce lower levels of the pro-inflammatory cytokine LT, and higher levels of the anti-inflammatory cytokine interleukin (IL)-10, as compared with pre-treatment B-cells isolated from the same patients.[17] This indicates that the biological response profile of B-cells re-emerging after anti-CD20 therapy are distinct from the pre-existing B-cells, which may be an important consideration with respect to re-treatment decisions as well as our evolving understanding of the different roles of functionally distinct B-cell subsets.

Overall, the studies of B-cell depletion in MS have been very instructive in highlighting an important contribution of B-cells to the MS disease process. The implication of antibody-independent roles of B-cells does not preclude pathophysiologic roles of antibodies in MS, but does highlight the emerging appreciation of the multiple functions whereby distinct B-cell subsets can participate in both normal and pathologic immune responses, as discussed in more detail below.

Putative mechanisms of B-cell and antibody contributions to CNS inflammation in MS

Accumulating evidence suggests that the contribution of B lineage cells and their secreted products to CNS inflammatory disease may relate to the abilities of B-cells to: (1) differentiate into plasmacytes that produce antibodies; (2) function as antigen-presenting cells (APC), contributing to T-cell activation; (3) produce effector cytokines that may modulate the local immune environment; (4) function at the innate-adaptive interface, for example, by harboring the Epstein–Barr virus (EBV) in a chronically activated state; and (5) play a role in formation and maintenance of new lymphoid foci, including within the CNS.

Early studies into the roles of B-cells and antibodies in EAE yielded, at times, conflicting results. In Lewis rats, intact B-cell activity was described as essential for complete expression of EAE[48] and presence of Ig was implicated in EAE development.[49] In contrast, other groups did not identify B-cells as critical for EAE onset. Subsequent work noted that B-cell-deficient mice were susceptible to clinical EAE when immunized with an encephalitogenic myelin peptide (MOG$_{35-55}$), but not with the whole MOG protein,[50] and was thought to implicate non-antibody roles of B-cells in EAE onset. In other EAE studies, transfer of MOG-specific autoantibodies was shown to lead to demyelination and clinical disease.[51,52] It was also suggested that CNS-directed autoantibodies in EAE may contribute to ongoing disease.[53]

Roles of antibodies in MS

Antibodies directed against CNS epitopes could theoretically participate in CNS damage through both antigen-specific and indirect mechanisms.[51,52,54–57] Binding to their CNS targets, autoantibodies could promote Fc-mediated complement activation, resulting in local damage and further recruitment of inflammatory cells.[58] Bound antibodies could also promote macrophage/microglia and possibly dendritic cell activation via Fc–Fc-receptor interaction. This could contribute to target-specific injury through phagocytosis of the antibody and its target antigen, but also promote the local pro-inflammatory response and subsequent injury in a non-antigen specific way. Pathogenic antibodies may also mediate end-organ damage through the formation of immune complexes. It is also worth noting that some CNS-directed antibodies may have a beneficial effect, possibly through support of remyelination[59] or by blocking "myelin-associated inhibitory molecules" that might otherwise limit axonal regeneration.[60,61] The extent to which these CNS auto-antibody-related mechanisms contribute to MS injury or repair has been an area of active study.

The presence of CSF OCBs and increased intrathecal IgG synthesis compared with serum IgG synthesis in MS have long been recognized and suggest plasmocyte activation to particular antigens within the CNS compartment.[62–64] The latter notion is further supported by molecular analyses of Ig gene somatic mutation of B-cells in CSF and MS lesions, demonstrating intraclonal expansion patterns that invoke local antigen driven B-cell differentiation and expansion.[65–68] The oligoclonal pattern of Ig and B-cells may remain stable in a given patient over time.[69–71] The presence of OCBs, increased free light chains, and increased intrathecal IgM synthesis in MS CSF have been reported to correlate with MS activity and subsequent outcome in some, but not all studies.[72–75]

The identity of OCBs in MS patients has been studied extensively with the hope that this will provide clues to the disease-causing antigen(s). However, studies have not confirmed the consistent presence of autoantibodies against recognizable myelin components.[76,77] In contrast, OCBs detected in several CNS infectious processes, including subacute sclerosing panencephalitis (a complication of live measles infection), human T-lymphotropic virus, mumps, meningitis, neurosyphilis, PML, and cryptococcal meningitis, have been confirmed to represent antibodies directed against the disease-specific causative agent.

Pathologic studies identified prominent deposition of Ig and complement (in addition to T-cell and macrophage infiltration) was a commonly observed pattern of MS demyelinating injury.[78,79] A study of brain tissues in early MS noted the prominent presence of Ig and immune complexes in association with non-degraded myelin, and the authors suggested a possible role for Ig and complement in the earliest stages of lesion development.[80] Autoantibodies directed against MOG have been detected within acute EAE and MS lesions[55] where they were seen to specifically bind disintegrating myelin around axons, and antibodies recognizing MOG have been extracted directly from inflamed MS lesions.[81] Together, these findings suggest that anti-myelin autoantibodies can participate in damage in both animal and human inflammatory CNS diseases.

Ongoing efforts have been made to measure, characterize and define the significance of anti-CNS antibodies in patients with MS. Anti-myelin antibodies, such as those directed against MOG, MBP, and protein lipid protein, have been variably reported in the serum[82–85] as well as CSF[44,63,84,85] of patients with MS. Their significance remains unclear, as similar serum observations can be made in healthy as well as inflammatory-disease controls. In a selected population of patients with clinically isolated demyelinating events (clinically isolated syndromes, CIS) and high risk MRI and CSF profiles, measures of serum anti-MOG and anti-MBP antibodies were initially described as markers of early conversion to the diagnosis of clinically definite MS.[86] These findings were not replicated in a broader population of CIS patients with both high- and low-risk profiles for development of MS.[87] Together, the suggestion is that serum measures of anti-CNS antibodies may be less useful in discriminating MS from non-MS, but may provide a marker of disease activity and thus predict earlier transition from a high-risk CIS event to definite RRMS.[57,86] More recently, a study of anti-myelin antibodies in pediatric-onset MS, indicated that, while such antibodies may be present in the serum of children as part of the normal humoral repertoire, their presence in children who were also developing CNS inflammation as part of MS, was associated with a more severe clinical phenotype.[88] This suggest that presence of anti-myelin antibodies may not be abnormal in and of itself but, when present, may modulate the expression of CNS inflammatory disease, a concept that is in keeping with results of adoptive transfer EAE studies where passive administration of anti-CNS antibodies alone was insufficient to induce disease, but its presence modulated the expression of disease induced by peripheral immune activation.

Additional types of antibodies, such as those directed against ganglioside, galactocerebroside, neurofilament, and the myelin-associated inhibitory molecule Nogo, have been observed in patients with MS and may eventually be validated as useful biomarkers.[60,89–91] Recent studies have emphasized methodological challenges in CNS auto-antibody measurements, and underscore the relevance of antigen conformation and the affinity and avidity of antibody-antigen interaction in detecting disease-relevant autoantibodies.[81,92–100] For example, anti-myelin antibodies in MS patient CSF and serum appear to be of relatively low affinity, in contrast to anti-pancreatic antibodies in serum of Type-I diabetes patients, which are of high affinity and are also of considerable prognostic value.[92] Newer approaches are being developed and employed to measure relevant anti-CNS antibodies in adult as well as pediatric MS cohorts, and ultimately elucidate their antigen-specific roles in pathogenesis and repair, or presence as non-specific markers of inflammation.

B-cells as antigen-presenting cells

Over the years antibody-independent functions of B-cells such as antigen presentation, have been implicated in animal models of several autoimmune diseases including lupus,[101,102] diabetes,[103] and EAE.[50,104] Early on, a role for B-cells as APC was suggested in MS based on observations that B-cells can regulate expression of T-cell costimulatory molecules and may be enriched in certain MS patient populations.[105,106] Indeed, activated antigen-specific B-cells are viewed as very potent APC that can endocytose, process and present antigen at east 10 000-fold more efficiently than other professional APC,[107] largely because B-cells can selectively internalize antigen through the B-cell receptor, and efficiently costimulatory molecules such as CD80 (B7.1) and CD86 (B7.2). Further evidence for antigen-specific B-cell : T-cell interaction in MS comes from studies identifying shared B-cell and T-cell myelin epitopes.[108] Recent studies of B-cell depletion in MS, point to an important capacity of human B-cells to support CD4+ and CD8+ T-cell activation,[39] also supported by observations in animal models that further highlight the distinct pro-inflammatory and anti-inflammatory roles that B-cells may play in context of CNS inflammation.[109,110] The identification of chronically activated B-cells in the meninges of patients with MS further points to the potential for B lineage cells chronically residing in the CNS to act as APC to T-cells and contribute to propagation of local disease-relevant immune responses.[111–113] Such a process may take place relatively independently of ongoing waves of activated immune cells infiltrating from the periphery, which would be consistent with the paucity of clinical relapses and new Gd-enhancing lesions in patients who nonetheless accrue relentless disability in the progressive forms of the disease.

B-cells as immune regulators

In addition to presenting antigen, B-cells may also influence the immune response through expression of distinct profiles of accessory molecules and/or production an array of effector cytokines, including immune regulatory cytokines like IL-10 and transforming growth factor-beta, polarizing cytokines such as IL-4, and lymphoid tissue-organizing cytokines such as TNFα and LT.[17,114,115] B-cell production of certain cytokines, such as IL-6 and IL-10, may have important autocrine B-cell growth and differentiation functions, but may also influence other cells in the local environment, including dendritic cells, macrophages and T-cells. In earlier EAE studies, animals depleted of B-cells failed to remit,[116] an effect that was attributed to the role of IL-10 from B-cells in regulating the expression of the autoimmune disease.[117] The emerging appreciation of regulatory B-cell subsets (Bregs) described in both animal and human systems, underscores the importance of functionally distinct B-cell subsets that could either induce or inhibit local immune responses, and provides an explanation for the variable effects targeting B-cells may have in vivo.[109,110] Several abnormalities in B-cell cytokine regulation in patients with MS have been described, including deficient capacity to produce the down-regulatory cytokine IL-10,[17,118] as well as an over-propensity to produce the pro-inflammatory cytokines TNFα and LT.[39] The latter has been suggested to contribute to abnormal "bystander" T-cell activation in patients with MS, providing a plausible therapeutic mechanism of action to explain why B-cell depletion, with consequent decreases in T-cell activation (effects that may be relevant both in the periphery and in the CNS), results in diminished new relapsing disease activity as seen in patients with MS.[39]

B-cells and neolymphogenesis

An important function of B-cells has emerged as their contribution to the formation and maintenance of new lymphoid foci. B-cells and ectopic neolymphogenesis may be important in several autoimmune diseases, including Sjogren's, RA, and MS.[111,113,119–121] There may be distinct molecular mechanisms underlying the capacity of certain B-cell populations to migrate into the particular compartments such as the CNS.[122,123] The follicle-like structures that have been described in the meningeal compartment in MS may harbor chronically activated B-cells that could act as APC, as regulators of local immune responses and as potential precursors of Ig-secreting plasma cells within the CNS compartment. If true, such B-cell lineage cells may contribute to smoldering CNS injury, relatively independent of newly invading waves of peripherally activated immune cells. As indicated above, the potential to more effectively target CNS compartmentalized B-cells is of considerable interest and studying the effects of intrathecal rituximab treatment should provide important insights.

B-cells harbor Epstein–Barr virus

There is growing evidence for a role of EBV infection in MS pathogenesis.[124–128] In addition to observations in epidemiological studies of adults with MS,[124] a robust association between EBV infection and pediatric onset MS has been reported.[124,126] It is noteworthy that, after the initial infection, EBV remains dormant in the body mostly in B-cells that can become chronically activated. It is also interesting to speculate on the potential relevance of the reported "molecular mimicry" between EBV epitopes and epitopes of putative CNS targets such as MBP.[108,125] Treatments that target B-cells could decrease significantly the EBV reservoir. Whether EBV is involved in the above noted chronically activated B-cells identified in the CNS of MS patients has been controversial.[129]

Future developments and challenges

As emerging therapies targeting MS relapses are setting the bar higher, the safety profiles of these therapies become key in defining favorable risk–benefit balance, in keeping with threshold of acceptable toxicity over time. B-cell depletion studies in MS have looked quite promising, though there remains the possibility that sustained depletion with repeat cycles of treatment may present result in limiting safety issues. Non-depleting therapeutic strategies that target B-cells are of interest in this regard. One instructive example is ataciccep, a fusion protein bound to the TACI receptor of Blyss (B-cell lymphocyte stimulating factor) and APRIL, two molecules that play important roles in B-cell differentiation, survival, and class switching. The Phase 2 study of atacicept in MS was discontinued early when patients receiving active drug were found to experience more relapses than the placebo treated group. While challenges remain, given our still limited understanding of the different ways in which B-cell subsets and their humoral products actually contribute to the pathophysiology of MS in its different compartments, the success of B-cell depletion in MS has opened the door to a therapeutic strategy and a growing range of related molecules to be pursued with interest in the upcoming years.

References

1. Fazekas F, Deisenhammer F, Strasser-Fuchs S, et al. Randomised placebo-controlled trial of monthly intravenous immunoglobulin therapy in relapsing-remitting multiple sclerosis. Lancet 1997;349:589–93.

2. Achiron A, Gabbay U, Gilad R, et al. Intravenous immunoglobulin treatment in multiple sclerosis. Effect on relapses. Neurology 1998;50:398–402.

3. Sorensen PS, Wanscher B, Jensen CV, et al. Intravenous immunoglobulin G reduces MRI activity in relapsing remitting multiple sclerosis. Neurology 1998;50:1273–81.

4. Weinshenker BG, O'Brien PC, Petterson PM, et al. A randomized trial of plasma exchange in acute central nervous system inflammatory demyelinating disease. Ann Neurol 1999;46:878–86.

5. Hommes OR, Sorensen PS, Fazekas F, et al. Intravenous immunoglobulin in secondary progressive multiple sclerosis: randomised placebo-controlled trial. Lancet 2004;364:1149–56.

6. Yu Z, Lennon VA. Mechanism of intravenous immune globulin therapy in antibody-mediated autoimmune diseases. N Engl J Med 1999;340:227–8.

7. Alter A, Duddy M, Hebert S, et al. Determinants of human B cell migration across brain endothelial cells. J Immunol 2003;170:4497–505.

8. Yong VW. Differential mechanisms of action of interferon-beta and glatiramer acetate in MS. Neurology 2002;59:802–8.

9. Kim HJ, Ifergan I, Antel JP, et al. Type 2 monocyte and microglia differentiation mediated by glatiramer acetate therapy in patients with multiple sclerosis. J Immunol 2004;172:7144–53.

10. Weber MS, Starck M, Wagenpfeil S, et al. Multiple sclerosis: glatiramer acetate inhibits monocyte reactivity in vitro and in vivo. Brain 2004;127:1370–8.

11. Weber MS, Prod'homme T, Youssef S, et al. Type II monocytes modulate T cell-mediated central nervous system

autoimmune disease. *Nat Med* 2007;13:935–43.

12. Begum-Haque S, Christy M, Ochoa-Reparaz J, *et al.* Augmentation of regulatory B cell activity in experimental allergic encephalomyelitis by glatiramer acetate. *J Neuroimmunol* 2011;232:136–44.

13. Kala M, Rhodes SN, Piao WH, *et al.* B cells from glatiramer acetate-treated mice suppress experimental autoimmune encephalomyelitis. *Exp Neurol* 2010;221:136–45.

14. Farina C, Weber MS, Meinl E, Wekerle H, Hohlfeld R. Glatiramer acetate in multiple sclerosis: update on potential mechanisms of action. *Lancet Neurol* 2005;4:567–75.

15. Bar-Or A, Oger J, Gibbs E, *et al.* Serial combination therapy: is immune modulation in multiple sclerosis enhanced by initial immune suppression? *Mult Scler* 2009;15:959–64.

16. Martin F, Chan AC. B cell immunobiology in disease – evolving concepts from the clinic. *Annual Rev Immunol* 2006;24:467–496.

17. Duddy, M, Niino M, Adatia F, *et al.* Distinct effector cytokine profiles of memory and naive human B cell subsets and implication in multiple sclerosis. *J Immunol* 2007;178: 6092–9.

18. Stashenko, P, Nadler LM, Hardy R, Schlossman SF. Characterization of a human B lymphocyte–specific antigen. *J Immunol* 1980;125:1678–85.

19. Cragg MS, Walshe CA, Ivanov A, Glennie MJ. The biology of CD20 and its potential as a target for mAb therapy. *In Curr Dir Autoimmun vol* 8:140–174, Karger: Basel, 2005.

20. Maloney DG, Smith B, Appelbaum FR. The anti-tumor effect of monoclonal anti CD20 antibody (mAb) therapy includes direct anti-proliferative activity and induction of apoptosis in CD20 positive non-Hodgkin's lymphoma cell lines. *Blood* 1996;88(Suppl 1):637a.

21. Manches O, Lui G, Chaperot L, *et al.* In vitro mechanisms of action of rituximab on primary non-Hodgkin lymphomas. *Blood* 2003;101:949–54.

22. Hainsworth JD, Litchy S, Barton JH, *et al.* Single-agent rituximab as first-line and maintenance treatment for patients with chronic lymphocytic leukemia or small lymphocytic lymphoma: a Phase II trial of the Minnie Pearl Cancer Research Network. *J Clin Oncol* 2003;21:1746–51.

23. Hainsworth JD, Litchy S, Burris HA III, *et al.* Rituximab as first-line and maintenance therapy for patients with indolent non-Hodgkin's lymphoma. *J Clin Oncol* 2002;20:1–67.

24. Edwards JC, Leandro MJ, Cambridge G. B-lymphocyte depletion therapy in rheumatoid arthritis and other autoimmune disorders. *Biochem Soc Trans* 2002;30:824–8.

25. Leandro MJ, Edwards JC, Cambridge G. Clinical outcome in 22 patients with rheumatoid arthritis treated with B-cell depletion. *Ann Rheum Dis* 2002;61:883–8.

26. Edwards JC, Szczepanski L, Szechinski J, *et al.* Efficacy of B-cell-targeted therapy with rituximab in patients with rheumatoid arthritis. *N Engl J Med* 2004;350:2572–81.

27. Leandro MJ, Edwards JC, Cambridge G, *et al.* An open study of B lymphocyte depletion in systemic lupus erythematosus. *Arthritis Rheum* 2002;46:2673–77.

28. Eisenberg R. SLE-rituximab in lupus. *Arthritis Res Ther* 2003;5:157–9.

29. D'Arena G, Luigiavigliotti M, Coccaro M, *et al.* Late and long-lasting response in an adult chronic idiopathic thrombocytopenic purpura after extended course of rituximab. *Leuk Lymphoma* 2003;44:561–2.

30. Zaja F, Iacona I, Masolini P, *et al.* B-cell depletion with rituximab as treatment for immune hemolytic anemia and chronic thrombocytopenia. *Haematologica* 2002;87:189–95.

31. Pestronk A, Florence J, Miller T, *et al.* Treatment of IgM antibody associated polyneuropathies using rituximab. *J Neurol Neurosurg Psychiatry* 2003;74:485–9.

32. Pranzatelli MR, Tate ED, Travestead AL, Verhultst SJ. CSF B cell over-expansion in paraneoplastic opsoclonus-myoclonus syndrome: effect of rituximab, an anti–B-cell monoclonal antibody. *Neurology* 2003 60(Suppl 1):A395.

33. Cross AH, Stark JL, Lauber J, *et al.* Rituximab reduces B cells and T cells in cerebrospinal fluid of multiple sclerosis patients. *J Neuroimmunol* 2006;180:63–70.

34. Naismith RT, Piccio L, Lyons JA, *et al.* Rituximab add-on therapy for breakthrough relapsing multiple sclerosis: a 52-week phase II trial. *Neurology* 2010;74:1860–7.

35. Bar-Or A, Calabresi PA, Arnold D, *et al.* Rituximab in relapsing-remitting multiple sclerosis: a 72-week, open-label, phase I trial. *Ann Neurol* 2008;63:395–400.

36. Hauser SL, Waubant E, Arnold DL, *et al.* B-cell depletion with rituximab in relapsing-remitting multiple sclerosis. *N Engl J Med* 2008;358:676–88.

37. Hawker K, O'Connor P, Freedman MS, *et al.* Rituximab in patients with primary progressive multiple sclerosis: results of a randomized double-blind placebo-controlled multicenter trial. *Ann Neurol* 2009;66:460–71.

38. Ruhstaller TW, Ambler U, Cerny T. Rituximab: active treatment of central nervous system involvement by non-Hodgkin lymphoma? *Ann Oncol* 2000;11:374–5.

39. Bar-Or A, Fawaz L, Fan B, *et al.* Abnormal B cell cytokine responses: a trigger of T-cell-mediated disease in MS? *Ann Neurol* 2010;67: 452–61.

40. Genovese MC, Kaine JL, Lowenstein MB, *et al.* Ocrelizumab, a humanized anti-CD20 monoclonal antibody, in the treatment of patients with rheumatoid arthritis: a phase I/II randomized, blinded, placebo-controlled, dose-ranging study. *Arthritis Rheum* 2008;58:2652–61.

41. Kappos L, Calabresi P, O'Connor P, *et al.* Efficacy and safety of ocrelizumab in patients with relapsing-remitting multiple sclerosis: results of a phase II randomized placebo-controlled multicenter trial. *Mult Scler* 2010;16:S114.

42. Soelberg Sorensen P, Drulovic J, Havrdova E, *et al.* Magnetic resonance imaging efficacy of ofatumumab in relapsing-remitting multiple sclerosis – 24-week results of a phase II study. *Mult Scler* 2010;16:S136.

43. Cambridge G, Leandro MJ, Edwards JC, *et al.* Serologic changes following B lymphocyte depletion therapy for rheumatoid arthritis. *Arthritis Rheum* 2003;48:2146–54.

44. Piccio L, Naismith RT, Trinkaus K, *et al.* Changes in B and T lymphocytes and chemokines with rituximab

treatment in multiple sclerosis. *Arch Neurol* 2010;67:707–14.

45. Monson N, Cravens P, Frohman E, *et al.* Effect of rituximab on the peripheral blood and cerebrospinal fluid B cells in patients with primary progressive multiple sclerosis. *Arch Neurol* 2005;62:258–64.

46. Petereit HF, Moeller-Hartmann W, Reske D, Rubbert A. Rituximab in a patient with multiple sclerosis–effect on B cells, plasma cells and intrathecal IgG synthesis. *Acta Neurol Scand* 2008;117:399–403.

47. Stuve O, Cepok S, Elias B, *et al.* Clinical stabilization and effective B-lymphocyte depletion in the cerebrospinal fluid and peripheral blood of a patient with fulminant relapsing-remitting multiple sclerosis. *Arch Neurol* 2005;62:1620–3.

48. Gausas J, Paterson PY, Day ED, Dal Canto MS. Intact B-cell activity is essential for complete expression of experimental allergic encephalomyelitis in Lewis rats. *Cell Immunol* 1982;72:360–6.

49. Willenborg DO, Sjollema P, Danta G. Immunoglobulin deficient rats as donors and recipients of effector cells of allergic encephalomyelitis. *J Neuroimmunol* 1986;11:93–103.

50. Lyons JA, San M, Happ MP, Cross AH. B-cells are critical to induction of experimental allergic encephalomyelitis by protein but not by a short encephalitogenic peptide. *Eur J Immunol* 1999;29:3432–9.

51. Genain CP, Nguyen MH, Letvin NL, *et al.* Antibody facilitation of multiple sclerosis-like lesions in nonhuman primate. *J Clin Invest* 1995;96:2966–74.

52. Schluesener HJ, Sobel RA, Linington C, Weiner HL. A monoclonal antibody against myelin oligodendroctye glycoprotein induces relapses and demyelination in central nervous system autoimmune disease. *J Immunol* 1987;139:4016–20.

53. Robinson WH, Fontoura P, Lee BJ, *et al.* Protein microarrays guide tolerizing DNA vaccine treatment of autoimmune encephalomyelitis. *Nat Biotechnol* 2003;21:1033–9.

54. Esiri MM. Immunoglobulin-containing cells in multiple sclerosis plaques. *Lancet* 1977;ii:478–80.

55. Genain CP, Cannella B, Hauser SL, Raine CS. Identification of autoantibodies associated with myelin damage in multiple sclerosis. *Nat Med* 1999;5:170–5.

56. Lyons JA, Ramsbottom MJ, Cross AH. Critical role of antigen-specific antibody in EAE induced by recombinant MOG. *Eur J Immunol* 2002;32:1905–13.

57. Antel JP, Bar-Or A. Do myelin antibodies predict the diagnosis of multiple sclerosis? *N Engl J Med* 2003;349:107–9.

58. Lou YH, Park KK, Agersborg S, *et al.* Retargeting T Cell-mediated inflammation: a new perspective on autoantibody action. *J Immunol* 2000;164:5251–7.

59. Rodriguez M, Miller D, Lennon V. Immunoglobulins reactive with myelin basic protein promote CNS remyelination. *Neurology* 1996;46:538–45.

60. Reindl M, Khantane S, Ehling R, *et al.* Serum and cerebrospinal fluid antibodies to Nogo-A in patients with multiple sclerosis and acute neurological disorders. *J Neuroimmunol* 2003;145:139–47.

61. Fontoura P, Ho PP, DeVoss J, *et al.* Immunity to the extracellular domain of Nogo-A modulates experimental autoimmune encephalomyelitis. *J Immunol* 2004;173:6981–92.

62. Siden A. Isoelectric focusing and crossed immunoelectrofocusing of CSF immunoglobulins in MS. *J Neurol* 1979;221:39–51.

63. Andersson M, Yu M, Soderstrom M, *et al.* Multiple MAG peptides are recognized by circulating T and B lymphocytes in polyneuropathy and multiple sclerosis. *Eur J Neurol* 2002;9:243–51.

64. O'Connor KC, Bar-Or A, Hafler DA. The neuroimmunology of multiple sclerosis: possible roles of T and B lymphocytes in immunopathogenesis. *J Clin Immunol* 2001;21:81–92.

65. Qin Y, Duquette P, Zhang Y, *et al.* Clonal expansion and somatic hypermutation of V(H) genes of B cells from cerebrospinal fluid in multiple sclerosis. *J Clin Invest* 1998;102:1045–50.

66. Owens GP, Kraus H, Burgoon MP, *et al.* Restricted use of VH4 germline segments in an acute multiple sclerosis brain. *Ann Neurol* 1998;43: 236–43.

67. Baranzini SE, Jeong MC, Butunoi C, *et al.* B cell repertoire diversity and clonal expansion in multiple sclerosis brain lesions. *J Immunol* 1999;163:5133–44.

68. Colombo M, Dono M, Gazzola P, *et al.* Accumulation of clonally related B lymphocytes in the cerebrospinal fluid of multiple sclerosis patients. *J Immunol* 2000;164:2782–9.

69. Cepok S, Rosche B, Grummel V *et al.* Short lived plasma blasts are the main B cell effector subset during the course of MS. *Brain* 2005;128:1667–76.

70. Walsh MJ, Tourtelotte WW. Temporal invariance and clonal uniformity of brain and cerebrospinal IgG, IgA and IgM in multiple sclerosis. *J Exp Med* 1986;163:41–53.

71. Hemmer B, Cepok S, Nessler S, Sommer N. Pathogenesis of multiple sclerosis: an update on immunology. *Curr Opin Neurol* 2002;15:227–31.

72. Rudick MA, Medendorp SV, Namey M, *et al.* Multiple sclerosis progression in a natural history study: predictive value of cerebrospinal fluid free kappa light chains. *Mult Scler* 1995;1:150–5.

73. Zeman D, Adam P, Kalistova H, *et al.* Cerebrospinal fluid cytologic findings in multiple sclerosis. A comparison between patient subgroups. *Acta Cytol* 2001;45:51–9.

74. Izquierdo G, Angulo S, Garcia-Moreno JM, *et al.* Intrathecal IgG synthesis: marker of progression in multiple sclerosis patients. *Acta Neurol Scand* 2002;105:158–63.

75. Villar LM, Masjuan J, Gonzalez-Porque P, *et al.* Intrathecal IgM synthesis is a prognostic factor in multiple sclerosis. *Ann Neurol* 2003;53:222–6.

76. Trotter JL, Rust RL. Human cerebrospinal Fluid immunology. In: Brumbach R, Herndon R, eds. *Cerebrospinal Fluid, Martinus* Nyhoff: Amsterdam, 1989;179–226.

77. Cross AH, Trotter JL, Lyons JA. B cells and antibodies in CNS demyelinating disease. *J Neuroimmunol* 2001;122:1–14.

78. Lucchinetti CF, Bruck W, Parisi J, *et al.* Heterogeneity of multiple sclerosis lesions: implications for the pathogenesis of demyelination. *Ann Neurol* 2000;47:707–17.

79. Storch MK, Piddlesden S, Haltia M, *et al.* Multiple sclerosis: in situ evidence

for antibody- and complement-mediated demyelination. *Ann Neurol* 1998;43:465–71.

80. Gay FW, Drye TJ, Dick GW, Esiri MM. The application of multifactorial cluster analysis in the staging of plaques in early MS. Identification and characterization of the primary demyelinating lesions. *Brain* 1997;120:1461–83.

81. O'Connor KC, Appel H, Bregoli L, *et al.* Antibodies from inflamed central nervous system tissue recognize myelin oligodendrocyte glycoprotein. *J Immunol* 2005;175:1974–82.

82. Cruz M, Olsson T, Ernerudh J, *et al.* Immunoblot detection of oligoclonal anti-myelin basic protein IgG antibodies in cerebrospinal fluid in multiple sclerosis. *Neurology* 1987;37:1515–19.

83. Olsson T, Baig S, Hojeberg B, Link H. Antimyelin basic protein and antimyelin antibody-producing cells in multiple sclerosis. *Ann Neurol* 1990;27:132–6.

84. Reindl M, Linington C, Brehm U, *et al.* Antibodies against the myelin oligodendrocyte glycoprotein and the myelin basic protein in multiple sclerosis and other neurological diseases: a comparative study. *Brain* 1999;122:2047–56.

85. Egg R, Reindl M, Deisenhammer F, *et al.* Anti-MOG and anti-MBP antibody subclasses in multiple sclerosis. *Mult Scler* 2001;7:285–9.

86. Berger T, Rubner P, Schautzer F, *et al.* Antimyelin antibodies as a predictor of clinically definite multiple sclerosis after a first demyelinating event. *N Engl J Med* 2003;349:139–45.

87. Lim ET, Berger T, Reindl M, *et al.* Anti-myelin antibodies do not allow earlier diagnosis of multiple sclerosis. *Mult Scler* 2005;11:492–4.

88. O'Connor KC, Lopez-Amaya C, Gagne D, *et al.* Anti-myelin antibodies modulate clinical expression of childhood multiple sclerosis. *J Neuroimmunol.* 2010;223:92–9.

89. Sadatipour BT, Greer JM, Pender MP. Increased circulating antiganglioside antibodies in primary and secondary progressive multiple sclerosis. *Ann Neurol* 1998;44:980–3.

90. Mata S, Lolli F, Soderstrom M, *et al.* Multiple sclerosis is associated with enhanced B cell responses to the ganglioside GD1a. *Mult Scler* 1999;5:379–88.

91. Menge T, Lalive PH, von Budingen HC, *et al.* Antibody responses against galactocerebroside are potential stage-specific biomarkers in multiple sclerosis. *J Allergy Clin Immunol* 2005;116:453–9.

92. O'Connor KC, Chitnis T, Griffin DE, *et al.* Myelin basic protein-reactive autoantibodies in the serum and cerebrospinal fluid of multiple sclerosis patients are characterized by low-affinity interactions. *J Neuroimmunol* 2003;136:140–8.

93. Lily O, Palace J, Vincent A. Serum autoantibodies to cell surface determinants in multiple sclerosis: a flow cytometric study. *Brain* 2004;127:269–79.

94. Menge T, Lalive PH, von Budingen HC, *et al.* Antibody responses against galactocerebroside are potential stage-specific biomarkers in multiple sclerosis. *J Allergy Clin Immunol* 2005;116:453–9.

95. Zhou D, Srivastava R, Nessler S, *et al.* Identification of a pathogenic antibody response to native myelin oligodendrocyte glycoprotein in multiple sclerosis. *Proc Natl Acad Sci USA* 2006;103:19057–62.

96. Lalive PH, Menge T, Delarasse C, *et al.* Antibodies to native myelin oligodendrocyte glycoprotein are serologic markers of early inflammation in multiple sclerosis. *Proc Natl Acad Sci USA* 2006;103:2280–5.

97. O'Connor KC, McLaughlin KA, De Jager PL, *et al.* Self-antigen tetramers discriminate between myelin autoantibodies to native or denatured protein. *Nat Med* 2007;13:211–17.

98. McLaughlin KA, Chitnis T, Newcombe J, *et al.* Age-dependent B cell autoimmunity to a myelin surface antigen in pediatric multiple sclerosis. *J Immunol* 2009;183:4067–76.

99. Brilot F, Dale RC, Selter RC, *et al.* Antibodies to native myelin oligodendrocyte glycoprotein in children with inflammatory demyelinating central nervous system disease. *Ann Neurol* 2009;66:833–42.

100. Chan A, Decard BF, Franke C, *et al.* Serum antibodies to conformational and linear epitopes of myelin oligodendrocyte glycoprotein are not elevated in the preclinical phase of multiple sclerosis. *Mult Scler* 2010;16:1189–92.

101. Shlomchik MJ, Madaio MP, Ni D, *et al.* The role of B cells in lpr/lpr-induced autoimmunity. *J Exp Med* 1994;180:1295–306.

102. Chan O T, Hannum LG, Haberman AM, *et al.* A novel mouse with B cells but lacking serum antibody reveals an antibody-independent role for B cells in murine lupus. *J Exp Med* 1999;189:1639–48.

103. Falcone M, Lee J, Patstone G, *et al.* B lymphocytes are crucial antigen-presenting cells in the pathogenic autoimmune response to GAD65 antigen in nonobese diabetic mice. *J Immunol* 1998;161:1163–8.

104. Constant SL. B lymphocytes as antigen-presenting cells for CD4+ T cell priming in vivo. *J Immunol* 1999;162:5695–703.

105. Genc K, Dona DL, Reder AT. Increased CD80(+) B cells in active multiple sclerosis and reversal by interferon beta-1b therapy. *J Clin Invest* 1997;99:2664–71.

106. Bar-Or A, Oliveira EML, Anderson DE, *et al.* Immunological memory: contribution of memory B cells expressing costimulatory molecules in the resting state. *J Immunol* 2001;167:5669–77.

107. Lanzavecchia A. Receptor-mediated antigen uptake and its effect on antigen presentation to class II restricted T lymphocytes. *Annu Rev Immunol* 1990;8:773–93.

108. Wucherpfennig KW, Strominger JL. Molecular mimicry in T cell-mediated autoimmunity: viral peptides activate human T cell clones specific for myelin basic protein. *Cell* 1995;80:695–705.

109. Matsushita T, Yanaba K, Bouaziz JD, Fujimoto M, Tedder TF. Regulatory B cells inhibit EAE initiation in mice while other B cells promote disease progression. *J Clin Invest* 2008;118:3420–30.

110. Weber MS, Prod'homme T, Patarroyo JC, *et al.* B-cell activation influences T-cell polarization and outcome of anti-CD20 B-cell depletion in central nervous system autoimmunity. *Ann Neurol* 2010;68:369–83.

111. Corcione A, Casazza S, Ferretti E, *et al.* Recapitulation of B cell differentiation in the central nervous system of

patients with multiple sclerosis. *Proc Natl Acad Sci USA* 2004;101:11064–9.

112. Uccelli A, Aloisi F, Pistoia V. Unveiling the enigma of the CNS as a B-cell fostering environment. *Trends Immunol* 2005;26:254–9.

113. Magliozzi R, Howell O, Vora A, *et al.* Meningeal B-cell follicles in secondary progressive multiple sclerosis associate with early onset of disease and severe cortical pathology. *Brain* 2007;130:1089–104.

114. Lund FE, Garvy BA, Randall TD, Harris DP. Regulatory roles for cytokine-producing B cells in infection and autoimmune disease. *Curr Dir Autoimmun* 2005;8:25–54.

115. Duddy ME, Alter A, Bar-Or A. Distinct profiles of human B cell effector cytokines: A role in immune regulation? *J Immunol* 2004;172:3422–7.

116. Wolf SD, Dittel BN, Hardardottir F, Janeway CA, Jr. Experimental autoimmune encephalomyelitis induction in genetically B cell-deficient mice. *J Exp Med* 1996;184:2271–8.

117. Fillatreau S, Sweenie CH, McGeachy MJ, *et al.* B cells regulate autoimmunity by provision of IL-10. *Nat Immunol* 2002;3:944–50.

118. Correale J, Farez M, Razzitte G. Helminth infections associated with multiple sclerosis induce regulatory B cells. *Ann Neurol* 2008;64:187–99.

119. Serafini B, Rosicarelli B, Magliozzi R, *et al.* Detection of ectopic B-cell follicles with germinal centers in the meninges of patients with secondary progressive multiple sclerosis. *Brain Pathol* 2004;14:164–74.

120. Barone F, Bombardieri M, Manzo A, *et al.* Association of CXCL13 and CCL21 expression with the progressive organization of lymphoid-like structures in Sjogren's syndrome. *Arthritis Rheum* 2005;52:1773–84.

121. Weyand CM, Kurtin PJ, Goronzy JJ. Ectopic lymphoid organogenesis: a fast track for autoimmunity. *Am J Pathol* 2001;159:787–93.

122. Alter A, Duddy M, Hebert S, *et al.* Determinants of human B cell migration across brain endothelial cells. *J Immunol* 2003;170:4497–505.

123. Bar-Or A, Nuttall RK, Duddy M, *et al.* Analyses of all matrix metalloproteinase members in leuckocytes: monocytes as major inflammatory mediators in multiple sclerosis. *Brain* 2003;126: 2738–49.

124. Ascherio A, Munger KL, Lennette ET, *et al.* Epstein–Barr virus antibodies and risk of multiple sclerosis: a prospective study. *J Am Med Assoc* 2001;286:3083–8.

125. Lang HL, Jacobsen H, Ikemizu S, *et al.* A functional and structural basis for TCR cross-reactivity in multiple sclerosis. *Nat Immunol* 2002;3: 940–3.

126. Alotaibi S, Kennedy J, Tellier R, Stephens D, Banwell B. Epstein-Barr virus in pediatric multiple sclerosis. *J Am Med Assoc* 2004;291:1875–9.

127. Pender MP. Infection of autoreactive B lymphocytes with EBV, causing chronic autoimmune diseases. *Trends Immunol* 2003;24:584–8.

128. Banwell B, Krupp L, Tellier R, *et al.* Clinical features and viral serologies in children with multiple sclerosis: results of a multinational cohort study. *Lancet Neurology* 2007;6:773–81.

129. Ascherio A, Bar-Or A. EBV and brain matter(s)? *Neurology* 2010;74:1092–5.

Chapter

43

Sex hormones and other pregnancy-related factors with therapeutic potential in multiple sclerosis

Rhonda R. Voskuhl

Introduction

It has been appreciated for decades that symptoms of patients with autoimmune diseases are affected by pregnancy and the post-partum period. The most well-characterized observations include those in multiple sclerosis (MS), rheumatoid arthritis, and psoriasis. These patients experience clinical improvement during pregnancy with a temporary "rebound" exacerbation post-partum.[1-7] This chapter will focus on possible mechanisms which may underlie the disease protection during pregnancy in MS. This phenomenon of an improvement in disease during pregnancy is a unique opportunity to gain insight into MS disease pathogenesis and to capitalize on a naturally occurring situation in which the disease is down-regulated. Understanding disease-modifying mechanisms during pregnancy may lead to the identification of factors with therapeutic potential for MS. Further, the therapeutic potential of an identified factor might be beneficial not only in MS, but also in other autoimmune diseases characterized by significant improvement during pregnancy.

The effect of pregnancy on MS

During decades of observations that MS improved with late pregnancy, the early studies did not separate the MS patients into relapsing–remitting and secondary progressive groups.[1,2,8] However, what was generally described was that there was a period of relative "safety" with regard to relapses during pregnancy followed by a period of increased relapses post-partum. These clinical observations were supported by a small study of two patients who underwent serial cerebral MRIs during pregnancy and post-partum. In both women there was a decrease in MR disease activity (T2 lesion number) during the second half of pregnancy and a return of MR disease activity to pre-pregnancy levels in the first months post-partum.[9] Other studies found that in addition to having a decrease in disease

activity in patients with established MS, the risk of developing the first episode of MS was decreased during pregnancy as compared with non-pregnant states.[6] The most definitive study of the effect of pregnancy on MS came in 1998 by the Pregnancy in Multiple Sclerosis (PRIMS) Group.[3] Relapse rates were significantly reduced from 0.7 per woman–year in the year before pregnancy to 0.2 during the third trimester. Rates then increased to 1.2 during the first 3 months post-partum before returning to pre-pregnancy rates.

In a two-year follow-up report by the PRIMS group, clinical factors that predicted post-partum relapses were examined. Neither breast feeding nor epidural anesthesia affected likelihood to relapse post-partum. The best predictor of which subjects would relapse post-partum was their pre-pregnancy relapse rates. Those with the most active disease before pregnancy were the most likely to relapse post-partum.[10]

Since latter pregnancy is associated with a reduction in relapses and the post-partum period with a transient increase in relapses, what is the net effect of pregnancy on the accumulation of disability? Short-term follow-up after pregnancy showed no effect on permanent disability,[10] and some long-term follow-up studies also showed no effect.[11] However, other long-term studies addressing time to reach a given disability suggested a protective effect of pregnancy on disability with some, but not all, studies having groups matched initially for deficit, disease duration, and age.[5,6,12,13] An effect of multiple pregnancies on permanent disability would be unexpected since it is known that three to five, years of continuous dosing with immunomodulatory treatments have only a modest impact on disability. Thus, a temporary anti-inflammatory effect of the third trimester of pregnancy would not be expected to impact long-term disability. This could perhaps be reconciled if a pregnancy associated neuroprotective factor were discovered.

There are no conclusive data supporting a long-term effect of pregnancy in healthy individuals and their subsequent risk

Disclosures

The University of Los Angeles, California (UCLA) holds a use patent for estriol treatment of MS for which Dr. Voskuhl is an inventor. Dr. Voskuhl provides consulting advice about MS treatments to Adeona Pharmaceuticals with compensation capped at a maximum of $10 000 per year.

Multiple Sclerosis Therapeutics, Fourth Edition, ed. Jeffrey A. Cohen and Richard A. Rudick. Published by Cambridge University Press.
© Cambridge University Press 2011.

to develop MS. One study reported that women of parity 0–2 developed MS twice as often as women of parity 3 or more, thereby implying a protective effect of multiple pregnancies, but the difference did not reach statistical significance.[14] Another found no association between parity and the subsequent risk of developing MS.[15] Together, these data indicate that pregnancy in healthy women has no long-lasting effects with regard to reducing their risk of developing MS in the future and hence pregnancy does not have a permanent effect on the immunopathogenesis of MS. However, if women with MS get pregnant, it will indeed be associated with a temporary reduction in relapses during late pregnancy. The effect of pregnancy appears to be similar to what is observed when patients take the approved anti-inflammatory therapies for MS: relapses are reduced temporarily when patients are on the treatments but when they are discontinued, relapses return.

The immunology of pregnancy

Since mechanisms of action of the approved therapies for MS involve anti-inflammatory effects, and since these treatments result primarily in a reduction in relapse rates, it is logical to hypothesize that mechanisms of action of the protective effect of pregnancy on MS relapses involve anti-inflammatory effects.

MS is a demyelinating disease of the central nervous system (CNS) which is thought to be mediated by myelin protein-specific CD4+ T-cells of the T helper 1 (Th1) and Th17 type.[16] T-cells and macrophages infiltrate the CNS and set off a cascade of events ultimately leading to demyelination of axons. This acute demyelination leads to conduction block of neurons and a clinical relapse results: a deficit in the function served by the affected neuronal pathway.[17] In contrast to the deleterious Th1 and Th17 responses described above, Th2 responses are thought to be beneficial in MS. In murine systems, Th1 and Th2 immune responses are counter-regulatory and, in states of health, the two responses exist in a delicate balance.[18] While there are clearly differences in human and murine systems, therapies for MS have nevertheless aimed to either reduce Th1 responses or increase Th2 responses.[19,20]

So how do these immune abnormalities of MS relate to the immune changes during pregnancy? From the mother's standpoint, the fetus is an allograft since it harbors antigens inherited by the father. Thus, it is evolutionarily advantageous for the mother to transiently suppress cell-mediated, Th1 type immune responses involved in fetal rejection during pregnancy. However, not all immune responses should be suppressed since humoral, Th2 type immunity is needed for passive transfer of antibodies to the fetus. Thus, a shift in immune responses with a down-regulation of Th1 and an up-regulation of Th2 is thought to be necessary for fetal survival.[18,21] This shift in immune responses from Th1 to Th2 occurs both locally at the maternal–fetal interface[18,22,23] as well as systemically.[24,25] A shift from Th1 to Th2 was shown at both the mRNA and protein level in peripheral blood immune responses in MS patients followed

longitudinally during pregnancy and post-partum.[26–28] However, another study failed to detect such a shift.[29] While it is plausible that a Th2 shift in the immune response could underlie the decrease in relapses in cell-mediated autoimmune diseases during late pregnancy, other immune changes involving natural killer cells have also been described and could contribute.[30,31]

Candidate pregnancy factors with therapeutic potential

Sex hormones (estrogens and progesterone) in animal models of MS

It had been previously shown that experimental autoimmune encephalomyelitis (EAE) in guinea pigs, rats, rabbits, and mice improved during pregnancy.[1,32,33] While no preclinical model is a perfect MS model, and caution must always be used in translating animal to human data, EAE is the MS model most widely used. Therefore, this model was used in an attempt to ascertain mechanisms underlying pregnancy-related disease protection. Two estrogens (estradiol and estriol) and progesterone each increase progressively during pregnancy. While estradiol and progesterone are present at much lower fluctuating levels during the menstrual cycle in non-pregnant women and female mice, estriol is made by the fetal placental unit and is not otherwise present in nonpregnant states. It has been shown that estrogen treatment (both estriol and estradiol) can ameliorate both active and adoptive EAE in several strains of mice (SJL, C57BL/6, B10.PL, B10.RIII).[34–42] Estriol treatment has also been shown to be effective in reducing clinical signs in EAE when administered after disease onset.[41] Finally, both estradiol and estriol have been shown to be efficacious in both female and male mice with EAE.[43] In contrast, treatment with progesterone had minimal effect on EAE when used alone,[41,44] but appeared to be additive with estrogen in offering protection when given in combination.[45] On the other hand, another study showed that progesterone treatment was deleterious in EAE in Lewis rats.[46]

In translational research, careful attention must be given to dose. A clinical amelioration of EAE occurred when estriol was used at doses to induce serum levels which were physiologic with pregnancy.[40,41] On the other hand, estradiol had to be used at doses several-fold higher than pregnancy levels in order to induce the same degree of disease protection.[40] Since ovariectomy removes physiologic levels of estradiol, as well as progesterone, data on the effect of ovariectomy on EAE are somewhat informative. Some reports have found that ovariectomy of female mice makes EAE worse,[37] while others have found that ovariectomy does not have a significant effect on the disease.[33]

Estrogen treatment in an MS animal model: mechanisms

Protective mechanisms of estrogen treatment (both estriol and estradiol) in EAE clearly involve anti-inflammatory processes,

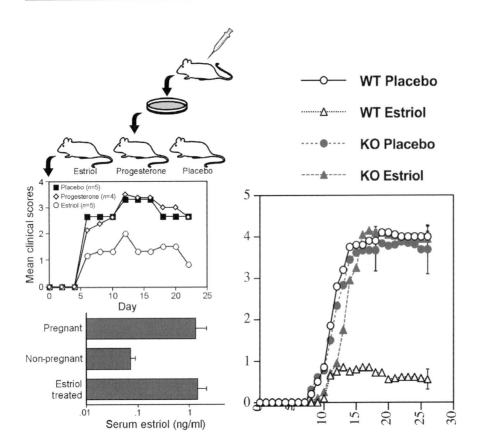

Fig. 43.1. Estriol treatment decreases EAE disease severity. SJL mice which received myelin basic protein-lymph node cells through adoptive transfer were treated 10–14 days previously with 90-day release pellets of estriol, progesterone, or placebo. Upper left: Estriol-treated mice had a significantly less severe course of EAE as compared to placebo, while progesterone-treated mice had a disease course indistinguishable from placebo. n = the number of mice in each treatment group. Lower left: Estriol levels were assessed by ELISA in sera from mice treated with estriol, from pregnant untreated mice, and non-pregnant untreated mice. An estriol dose that was effective in decreasing EAE severity gave a serum level which approximated that found in untreated pregnant mice during day 18 of the 19 day gestation period. Right: Estriol treatment at this same dose was also used in myelin-oligodendrocyte glycoprotein peptide fragment 35–55-induced active EAE in C57BL/6 mice. A reduction in mean clinical EAE scores occurred in estriol treated WT, but not ERα KO, mice. There were a total of 40 mice, with 10 mice in each of four groups: WT treated with placebo (WT Placebo), WT treated with estriol (WT Estriol), homozygous ERα KO treated with placebo (KO Placebo), and homozygous ERα KO treated with estriol (KO Estriol). Error bars represent variation in scores between mice within each group.[41,42] EAE = experimental autoimmune encephalomyelitis, ELISA = enzyme-linked immunosorbent assay, ER = estrogen receptor, KO = knockout, WT = wild type.

with estrogen-treated mice having fewer inflammatory lesions in the CNS.[41] In adoptive EAE in SJL mice, an increase in interleukin-10 (IL-10), with no change in interferon-gamma (IFNγ), was observed in ex vivo stimulated myelin basic protein (MBP) specific responses.[41] In active EAE in C57BL/6 mice, a decrease in tumor necrosis factor-alpha, IFNγ, and IL-6 has been observed, with an increase in IL-5.[34,35,42,43] Estrogen treatment has also been shown to down-regulate chemokines in the CNS of mice with EAE and may affect expression of matrix matalloprotease-9, each leading to impaired recruitment of cells to the CNS.[37,39,47] In addition, estrogen treatment has been shown to impair the ability of dendritic cells to present antigen.[36,48,49] Finally, estrogen treatment has recently been shown to induce CD4+CD25+ regulatory T-cells in EAE.[50] Relevant to the dose issue, estradiol at pregnancy levels, but not below, reduced IL-17 and increased programmed death 1 (PD-1) in regulatory T-cells.[51] Thus, estrogen treatment has been shown to be anti-inflammatory through a variety of mechanisms.

An anti-inflammatory effect of estrogen treatment in EAE does not preclude an additional more direct neuroprotective effect. Estrogens are lipophilic, readily traversing the blood–brain barrier, with the potential to be directly neuroprotective,[52] and numerous reviews have described estrogen's neuroprotective effects, both in vitro and in vivo in other model systems.[52,53] Thus, it was next determined whether estrogen treatment might be neuroprotective in EAE. Estradiol treatment not only reduced clinical disease severity and was anti-inflammatory with respect to cytokine production in peripheral immune cells, it also decreased CNS white matter inflammation and demyelination, while preserving axonal counts in spinal cords of mice with EAE.[54]

Selective estrogen receptor modifiers, which aim to maximize efficacy and minimize toxicity, could be employed if the receptor was identified through which anti-inflammatory and neuroprotective effects occurred. The actions of estrogen are mediated primarily by nuclear estrogen receptors, ERα and ERβ,[55] although non-genomic membrane effects have also been described.[56] Global estrogen receptor knockout mice showed that the protective effect of estrogen treatment (estradiol and estriol) in EAE was dependent upon the presence of ERα, not ERβ[38,42] (Fig. 43.1). A highly selective ERα ligand, propyl pyrazole triol (PPT) was then used to show that stimulation of ERα in developmentally normal mice was sufficient for protection in EAE.[54,57] Subsequently, bone marrow chimeras were used by Garidou et al. to show that the disease-ameliorating effects of estradiol treatment in EAE were not dependent upon ERα signaling in blood-derived inflammatory cells.[58] This observation suggested that the functionally significant target for estrogen's actions in vivo during EAE are cells within the CNS.

Since treatment with an ERα ligand is highly anti-inflammatory in the peripheral immune system of EAE mice, it is difficult to discern whether the effect of ERα ligand treatment is solely anti-inflammatory (and only indirectly neuroprotective) vs. whether it is both anti-inflammatory and directly neuroprotective. In this context, direct neuroprotection refers to protection of CNS cells which is not merely due to reducing the immune attack. However, differential neuroprotective and anti-inflammatory effects of ERα and ERβ ligand treatment revealed insights into whether estrogen treatment might be directly neuroprotective in EAE.[59] ERβ ligand (diarylpropionitrile, DPN) treatment did not affect peripheral immune responses (Fig. 43.2), but was nevertheless able to reduce demyelination and preserve axon numbers (Fig. 43.3)[60,61] while inducing functional remyelination.[62] Thus, neuroprotective effects of estrogen treatment were not necessarily dependent upon anti-inflammatory properties. It remains unknown whether neuroprotective effects of estrogen treatments in EAE are directly mediated by binding estrogen receptors on neurons, versus indirectly mediated by binding estrogen receptors on glial cells (oligodendrocytes, astrocytes and microglia) since these also express estrogen receptors.[63]

Estrogen treatment in MS

Levels of estrogens that are in oral contraceptives or hormone replacement therapy may not be high enough to be protective in MS. While some studies have attempted to simulate a situation of treatment with oral contraceptives in EAE mice and have shown an effect on disease,[34,39] doses used in mice are not readily translatable to humans. In fact, the data in humans thus far have suggested that treatment with oral contraceptives is not likely to suppress MS incidence.[64] Together, these reports suggest that it is likely that a sustained level of a sufficient dose of an estrogen will be necessary to ameliorate disease activity in MS. Previous retrospective studies on oral contraceptives and hormone replacement in MS are problematic, as they have grouped together patients who were on low-dose estrogens, high-dose estrogens, and even progestin only treatments. Prospective studies which maintain a given dose, of a given hormone, over all days of the month are needed.

Since estriol is the major estrogen of pregnancy and since an estriol dose which yielded a pregnancy level in mice was protective in disease,[41] estriol was administered in a prospective pilot clinical trial to women with MS, in an attempt to recapitulate the protective effect of pregnancy on disease.[65] A crossover study was used whereby patients were followed for six months pretreatment to establish baseline disease activity which included cerebral MRI every month and neurologic examination every three months. The patients were then treated with oral estriol (8 mg/day) for six months, then observed for six more months in the post-treatment period. There were six RR patients and four SP patients who finished the 18-month study period. The RRMS subjects were then retreated with oral estriol and progesterone in a four month extension phase. Estriol treatment resulted in serum estriol levels which approximated levels observed in untreated healthy control women who were six months pregnant. Interestingly, a significant decrease in a prototypic in vivo Th1 response, the delayed type hypersensitivity response to the recall antigen tetanus, was observed at the end of

the six-month treatment period as compared with the pretreatment period. When PBMCs were stimulated ex vivo, a favorable shift in cytokine profile (decreased TNFα, increased IL-10 and IL-5) was observed during treatment as compared with baseline.[66] Estriol treatment also decreased expression of matrix matalloprotease-9.[47] On serial MRIs, RR patients demonstrated an 80% reduction in gadolinium enhancing lesions within three months of treatment, as compared with pretreatment,[65] and this improvement in enhancing lesions correlated with the favorable shift in cytokine profiles.[66] Importantly, gadolinium-enhancing disease activity gradually returned to baseline in the posttreatment period, and the favorable cytokine shift also returned to baseline. Further, in the four-month extension phase of the study, both the decrease in brain enhancing lesions and the favorable immune shift, returned upon retreatment with estriol in combination with progesterone in the RRMS group. These latter data have important translational implications since progesterone treatment is needed in combination with estrogen treatment to prevent uterine endometrial hyperplasia when estrogens are administered for a year or more in duration. These results indicate that treatment with progesterone in combination with estriol did not neutralize the beneficial effect of estriol treatment on these biomarkers of disease. A multicenter, double-blind, placebo-controlled trial of estriol treatment in RRMS is now ongoing in the United States.

Other candidate pregnancy factors with therapeutic potential
General considerations

Numerous factors other than sex hormones have been identified in sera during pregnancy and have been shown to be immunosuppressive either in cultures of immune cells in vitro or in EAE models. Hence numerous factors have been proposed as possibly contributing to disease protection during pregnancy. The two key issues which should be considered when one weighs the possibility of whether a candidate factor is or is not likely to be responsible for the decrease in disease relapse in MS include: (1) is the factor increased early or late during pregnancy? and (2) are doses of the factors used in the in vitro and in vivo models to demonstrate an immunosuppressive effect associated with levels of the factor which are similar to what occurs during natural pregnancy? Regarding the first issue, if a factor is increased only transiently very early during pregnancy, then it seems unlikely that it would be responsible for disease activity reduction in the third trimester followed by post-partum relapse. On the other hand, if a factor gradually increases in concentration to peak in the last trimester followed by a precipitous drop post-partum, then it seems more likely that this factor might be responsible for alterations in the disease course. Regarding the second issue, if the factor is immunosuppressive only at a dose which is much higher than that which occurs during pregnancy, it would be unlikely that

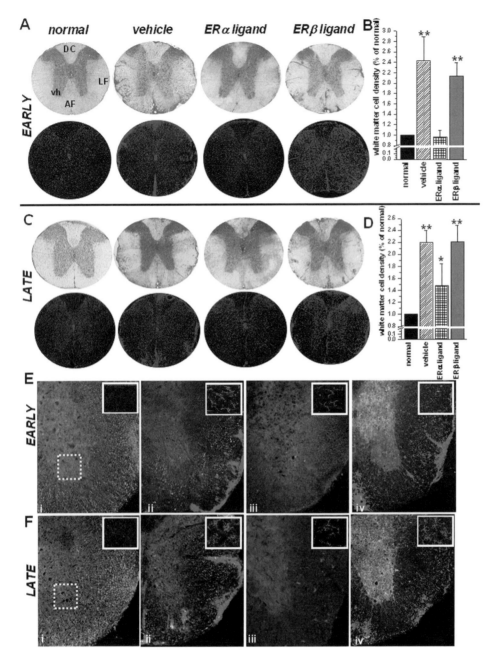

Fig. 43.2. Treatment with an ERα ligand, not an ERβ ligand, reduced inflammation in spinal cords of mice with EAE. (a) Representative H&E-stained and DAPI-stained thoracic spinal cord sections (4X magnification) from normal (healthy control), as well as vehicle-, ERα ligand PPT-treated, and ERβ ligand (DPN)-treated EAE mice all sacrificed at day 19 (early) post-disease induction. Compared to normal controls and PPT-treated spinal cords, vehicle-treated EAE spinal cord shows multifocal to coalescing areas of inflammation in the leptomeninges and white matter, around blood vessels, and in the parenchyma of the white matter. (b) The increase in total number of infiltrating cells after induction of EAE was quantified by counting DAPI+ cells in the entire delineated white matter (including dorsal, lateral, and ventral funiculi) and presented as percent of normal. Vehicle-treated and DPN-treated EAE mice had a significant increase in white matter cell density compared to healthy normal control, while the ERα ligand PPT-treated groups did not. (c) At day 40 (late) after disease induction, representative H&E-stained and DAPI-stained vehicle, DPN-treated, and PPT-treated EAE thoracic spinal cord sections showed significantly increased inflammation compared to controls. (d) Total number of infiltrating cells after induction of EAE quantified by counting DAPI+ cells as in (B). Number of mice = 3 per treatment group, number of T1–T5 sections per mouse = 6, total number of sections per treatment group = 18. Statistically significant compared with normals (*P < 0.05; **P < 0.001), 1 x 4 ANOVAs. Consecutive thoracic spinal cord sections were also co-immunostained with NF200 (green) and CD45 (red) at 10X magnification. Shown are partial images (lateral funniculus, a portion of anterior funniculus and gray matter) from normal control, vehicle-treated EAE, PPT-treated EAE, and DPN-treated EAE mice at day 19 (e) and day 40 (f) after disease induction. Vehicle-treated EAE cords had large areas of CD45+ cells associated with reduced NF200 axonal staining in white matter as compared to the normal control, while PPT-treated EAE mice had only occasional CD45 positivity, with intact NF200 axonal staining. ERβ ligand DPN-treated EAE mice had large areas of CD45+ cells with normal NF200 axonal staining. Consecutive sections from the same mice were also scanned at 40X magnification (within the section of the ventral horn designated by the dotted line square area in normal panel confocal microscopy) to show the morphology of CD45+ cells in the gray matter.[61] AF = anterior funnicilus, ANOVA = analysis of variance, DAPI-4',6-diamidino-2-phenylindole, DC = dorsal column, DPN = diarylpropionitrile, EAE = experimental autoimmune encephalomyelitis, ER = estrogen receptor, H&E = hematoxylin and eosin, LF = lateral funiculus, PPT = propyl pyrazole triol, vh = ventral horn (see also color plate section).

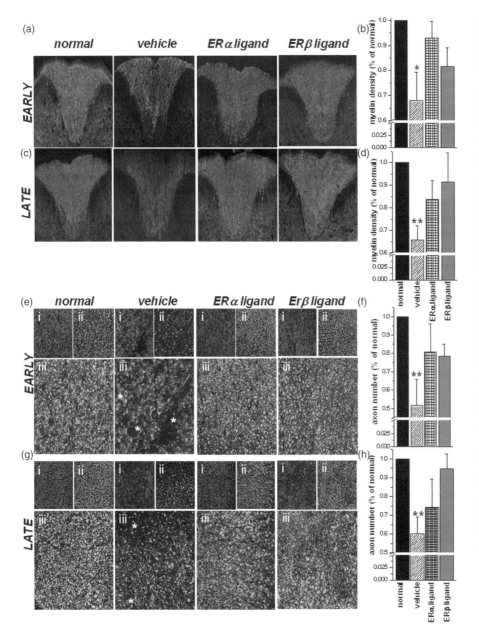

Fig. 43.3. Treatment with an ERα ligand and an ERβ ligand each preserved MBP immunoreactivity and spared axonal pathology in white matter of spinal cords of mice with EAE. Dorsal columns of thoracic spinal cord sections were imaged at 10X magnification from mice in Fig. 43.2 that were immunostained with anti-MBP (red). At day 19 (a) and day 40 (c) after disease induction, vehicle-treated mice had reduced MBP immunoreactivity as compared to normal controls, while PPT-treated EAE and DPN-treated EAE mice showed relatively preserved MBP staining. Upon quantification (b, d), MBP immunoreactivity in dorsal column was significantly lower in vehicle-treated EAE mice as compared to normal mice, while PPT-treated and DPN-treated EAE mice demonstrated no significant decreases. Myelin density is presented as percent of normal. Statistically significant compared with normal (*$P < 0.01$; **$P < 0.005$), 1 x 4 ANOVAs. Part of the anterior funiculus of thoracic spinal cord sections was imaged at 40X magnification from mice in Fig. 43.2 that were co-immunostained with anti-NF200 (green, i) and anti-MBP (red, ii). Merged images of smaller (i) and (ii) panels are shown in (iii). Distinct green axonal centers surrounded by red myelin sheaths can be seen in normal controls, PPT-treated, and DPN-treated EAE mice from 19 day (e) and 40 day (g) after disease induction. Vehicle-treated mice show reduced axonal numbers and myelin, along with focal demyelination (white stars) and loss of axons. Upon quantification (f, h), neurofilament-stained axon numbers in white matter were significantly lower in vehicle-treated EAE mice as compared to normal mice, while PPT-treated and DPN-treated EAE mice demonstrated no significant reduction in axon numbers. Axon number is presented as percent of normal. Statistically significant compared with normal (*$P < 0.01$; **$P < 0.005$), 1 x 4 ANOVAs.[61] ANOVA = analysis of variance, DPN = diarylpropionitrile, EAE = experimental autoimmune encephalomyelitis, ER = estrogen receptor, MBP = myelin basic protein, PPT = propyl pyrazole triol (see also color plate section).

the factor is responsible for disease amelioration during pregnancy. On the other hand, if the factor is immunosuppressive at doses that are similar to those that occur during pregnancy, then it is plausible that the factor may be responsible, at least in part, for the immunosuppression and disease activity alteration during pregnancy. Unfortunately, for many of the proposed factors (e.g. alpha-fetoprotein, early pregnancy factor, human chorionic gonadotropin, pregnancy-specific glycoproteins), these two key issues have not been addressed and, therefore, it becomes difficult to ascertain what the contribution of each factor might be to the improvement in disease activity in MS during late pregnancy. Another candidate, IFNτ, is clearly not responsible for the decrease in disease activity in the last trimester of *human* pregnancy, since its expression is restricted to the embryonic trophectoderm of ruminants

during early pregnancy.[67] Two candidates with a high level of potential for contributing at least in part for some of the disease protection during late pregnancy include cortisol and vitamin D.

Cortisol

The full protective effect of pregnancy on putative Th1-mediated diseases such as MS and rheumatoid arthritis may result from a synergistic effect of numerous factors that occur during pregnancy. One factor in addition to sex hormones that may contribute to disease protection is cortisol. During late pregnancy it is known that serum cortisol levels are persistently in the high normal range. Cortisol is known to be immunosuppressive in both EAE and MS, and the third trimester of pregnancy is characterized by a mildly hyperactive hypothalamic-pituitary-adrenal (HPA) axis, driven by elevated circulating levels of corticotrophin releasing hormone of placental origin.[68,69] Given the profound immunosuppressive effect of cortisol on MS and EAE, it would seem likely that even mild elevations of serum cortisol which occur during late pregnancy might contribute, at least in part, to the state of disease protection during this time.

Vitamin D

Vitamin D has been proposed as a factor that is increased during pregnancy, which might contribute to disease protection during this time. In one study, 23 women with normal pregnancies were studied in the second and third trimesters and post-partum. 1,25-dihydroxyvitamin D levels in the second and third trimesters were two-fold higher than post-partum values. The increase in serum 1,25-dihydroxyvitamin D values during pregnancy is thought to be important in providing for the increase in maternal calcium requirements during pregnancy.[70] Interestingly, higher vitamin D levels have been associated with a lower incidence of MS in women but not in men.[71] In EAE, diets high in vitamin D reduced disease severity in female but not in male mice, suggesting a role for estrogen in vitamin D mediated inhibition of EAE.[72] When MS patients were supplemented with vitamin D treatment for six months, increases in the protective cytokine transforming growth factor beta-1 were detected in serum,[73] but no effects on clinical disease or MRI were reported. Thus, whether a synergistic effect exists between estrogen and vitamin D during late pregnancy remains unknown.

Post-partum hormones

Evidence in animal models suggests not only that high levels of estrogens are protective in Th1-mediated autoimmune diseases during pregnancy, but that the precipitous drop in estrogens post partum may lead to disease exacerbation. In type II collagen-induced arthritis in DBA/1 mice, a characteristic feature is the remission during gestation and the exacerbation of the disease during the post-partum period. Two possibilities were pursued with regard to hormonal changes underlying the post partum flare: (1) the precipitous fall in estrogens post-partum and (2) the surge of prolactin after delivery. It was shown that treatment with high dose estrogens during a short period immediately after parturition protected mice from post-partum flares, while treatment with bromocriptine, a drug known to inhibit the endogenous prolactin release, has a less marked effect. Further, studies of lactating (i.e. animals with physiological stimulation of endogenous prolactin release) and non-lactating arthritic mice revealed no clear-cut differences in flares, indicating that prolactin was of minor importance in the induction of post-partum flares.[74] These data in arthritis in mice are consistent with data in MS in women. The PRIMS group found that whether women were or were not breast feeding had no effect on the increase in relapse rates post-partum.[10] Together, these data suggest that the precipitous drop in estrogens or progesterone after delivery may be responsible, at least in part, for post-partum exacerbations. Notably, there is an ongoing placebo-controlled clinical trial in Europe in which high dose progesterone and low dose estradiol are given for three months, beginning within 24 hours of delivery in an effort to reduce post-partum relapses.[75]

The post-partum period is complex, involving more than a pro-inflammatory state. On the one hand, prolactin has pro-inflammatory properties and treatment with bromocriptine to block prolactin ameliorated EAE.[76] In addition, small studies suggested that hyperprolactinemia may be associated with MS relapses.[77,78] However, on the other hand, pregnant mice were shown to have an enhanced ability to remyelinate non-inflammatory white matter lesions, and prolactin was shown to regulate oligodendrocyte precursor proliferation and mimic this regenerative effect of pregnancy.[79] Thus, when considering any pregnancy factor, its effects on both the CNS and the immune system must be considered. So what is the net effect of the post-partum period? A large study showed no difference between those who did or did not breast feed with respect to the post-partum relapse rate in MS.[10] Rather, the best predictor of post-partum relapse was pre-pregnancy relapse rate.[3,10] One small study suggested that exclusive breast feeding (with elevated prolactin) might be associated with a decreased relapse rate as compared to no or partial breast feeding, but this was confounded by the fact that it appeared that those with less active disease were more likely to exclusively breast feed.[80] The latter is a critical confound, since it is known that those with the most active disease before pregnancy are the most likely to relapse post-partum.[10]

Conclusions

Pregnancy is a state that is clearly protective with regard to relapses, while the effect on long-term disability remains unclear. Two important changes occur during pregnancy. First, there is a down-regulation of cellular immune responses. This likely occurs to prevent fetal rejection. Second, pregnancy is characterized by the presence of potentially neuroprotective hormones. It would seem evolutionarily advantageous to have such neuroprotective factors present, as neuronal and oligodendrocyte lineage cells in the fetus progress through critical developmental windows.[81] Together, the combined anti-inflammatory and neuroprotective state of pregnancy, perhaps aimed at protecting the fetus, may be precisely what is needed to protect the CNS of a mother with MS.

Acknowledgments

This work was supported by grants RO1 NS051591, R21 NS071210 and K24 NS062117 from the NIH (RRV), grants RG3915, RG4033 and RG4363 from the National Multiple Sclerosis Society (RRV) as well as the Skirball Foundation, the Hilton Foundation and the Sherak Family Foundation.

References

1. Abramsky O. Pregnancy and multiple sclerosis. *Ann Neurol.* 1994;36 Suppl(1):S38–41.

2. Birk K, Ford C, Smeltzer S, Ryan D, Miller R, Rudick RA. The clinical course of multiple sclerosis during pregnancy and the puerperium. *Arch Neurol* 1990;47(7):738–42.

3. Confavreux C, Hutchinson M, Hours MM, Cortinovis-Tourniaire P, Moreau T. Rate of pregnancy-related relapse in multiple sclerosis. Pregnancy in Multiple Sclerosis Group [see comments]. *N Engl J Med.* 1998;339(5):285–91.

4. Da Silva JA, Spector TD. The role of pregnancy in the course and aetiology of rheumatoid arthritis. *Clin Rheumatol.* 1992;11(2):189–94.

5. Damek DM, Shuster EA. Pregnancy and multiple sclerosis. *Mayo Clin Proc.* 1997;72(10):977–89.

6. Runmarker B, Andersen O. Pregnancy is associated with a lower risk of onset and a better prognosis in multiple sclerosis [see comments]. *Brain* 1995;118(1)(10):253–61.

7. Whitacre CC, Reingold SC, O'Looney PA. A gender gap in autoimmunity. *Science* 1999;283(5406):1277–8.

8. Birk K, Smeltzer SC, Rudick R. Pregnancy and multiple sclerosis. *Semin Neurol* 1988;8(3):205–13.

9. van Walderveen MA, Tas MW, Barkhof F, *et al.* Magnetic resonance evaluation of disease activity during pregnancy in multiple sclerosis. *Neurology* 1994;44(2):327–9.

10. Vukusic S, Hutchinson M, Hours M, *et al.* Pregnancy and multiple sclerosis (the PRIMS study): clinical predictors of post-partum relapse. *Brain* 2004;127(6):1353–60.

11. Roullet E, Verdier-Taillefer MH, Amarenco P, Gharbi G, Alperovitch A, Marteau R. Pregnancy and multiple sclerosis: a longitudinal study of 125 remittent patients. *J Neurol Neurosurg Psychiatry* 1993;56(10): 1062–5.

12. Verdru P, Theys P, D'Hooghe MB, Carton H. Pregnancy and multiple sclerosis: the influence on long term disability. *Clin Neurol Neurosurg* 1994;96(1):38–41.

13. D'Hooghe M B, Nagels G, Uitdehaag BM. Long-term effects of childbirth in MS. *J Neurol Neurosurg Psychiatry* 2010;81(1):38–41.

14. Villard-Mackintosh L, Vessey MP. Oral contraceptives and reproductive factors in multiple sclerosis incidence. *Contraception* 1993;47(2):161–8.

15. Hernan MA, Hohol MJ, Olek MJ, Spiegelman D, Ascherio A. Oral contraceptives and the incidence of multiple sclerosis. *Neurology* 2000;55(6):848–54.

16. Martin R, McFarland HF, McFarlin DE. Immunological aspects of demyelinating diseases. *Ann Rev Immunol* 1992;10(5):153–87.

17. Waxman SG. Demyelinating diseases – new pathological insights, new therapeutic targets [editorial; comment]. *N Engl J Med* 1998;338(5):323–5.

18. Wegmann TG, Lin H, Guilbert L, Mosmann TR. Bidirectional cytokine interactions in the maternal-fetal relationship: is successful pregnancy a TH2 phenomenon? [see comments]. *Immunol Today* 1993;14(7):353–6.

19. Duda PW, Schmied MC, Cook SL, Krieger JI, Hafler DA. Glatiramer acetate (Copaxone) induces degenerate, Th2-polarized immune responses in patients with multiple sclerosis. *J Clin Invest* 2000;105(7):967–76.

20. Kozovska ME, Hong J, Zang YC, *et al.* Interferon beta induces T-helper 2 immune deviation in MS. *Neurology* 1999;53(8):1692–7.

21. Raghupathy R. Th1-type immunity is incompatible with successful pregnancy [see comments]. *Immunol Today* 1997;18(10):478–82.

22. Lin H, Mosmann TR, Guilbert L, Tuntipopipat S, Wegmann TG. Synthesis of T helper 2-type cytokines at the maternal-fetal interface. *J Immunol* 1993;151(9):4562–73.

23. Sacks GP, Clover LM, Bainbridge DR, Redman CW, Sargent IL. Flow cytometric measurement of intracellular Th1 and Th2 cytokine production by human villous and extravillous cytotrophoblast. *Placenta* 2001;22(6):550–9.

24. Hill JA, Polgar K, Anderson DJ. T-helper 1-type immunity to trophoblast in women with recurrent spontaneous abortion [see comments]. *J Am Med Assoc* 1995;273(24):1933–6.

25. Marzi M, Vigano A, Trabattoni D, *et al.* Characterization of type 1 and type 2 cytokine production profile in physiologic and pathologic human pregnancy. *Clin Exp Immunol* 1996;106(1):127–33.

26. Al-Shammri S, Rawoot P, Azizieh F, *et al.* Th1/Th2 cytokine patterns and clinical profiles during and after pregnancy in women with multiple sclerosis. *J Neurol Sci* 2004 ; 222(1–2):21–7.

27. Gilmore W, Arias M, Stroud N, Stek A, McCarthy KA, Correale J. Preliminary studies of cytokine secretion patterns associated with pregnancy in MS patients. *J Neurol Sci* 2004;224(1–2):69–76.

28. Lopez C, Comabella M, Tintore M, Sastre-Garriga J, Montalban X. Variations in chemokine receptor and cytokine expression during pregnancy in multiple sclerosis patients. *Mult Scler* 2006;12(4):421–7.

29. Langer-Gould A, Gupta R, Huang S, *et al.* Interferon-gamma-producing T cells, pregnancy, and postpartum relapses of multiple sclerosis. *Arch Neurol* 2010;67(1):51–7.

30. Airas L, Saraste M, Rinta S, Elovaara I, Huang YH, Wiendl H. Immunoregulatory factors in multiple sclerosis patients during and after pregnancy: relevance of natural killer cells. *Clin Exp Immunol* 2008;151 (2): 235–43.

31. Saraste M, Vaisanen S, Alanen A, Airas L. Clinical and immunologic evaluation of women with multiple sclerosis during and after pregnancy. *Gend Med* 2007;4(1):45–55.

32. Langer-Gould A, Garren H, Slansky A, Ruiz PJ, Steinman L. Late pregnancy suppresses relapses in experimental autoimmune encephalomyelitis: evidence for a suppressive pregnancy-related serum factor. *J Immunol* 2002;169(2):1084–91.

33. Voskuhl RR, Palaszynski K. Sex hormones and experimental autoimmune encephalomyelitis: Implications for multiple sclerosis. *Neuroscientist* 2001;7(3):258–70.

34. Bebo BF, Jr., Fyfe-Johnson A, Adlard K, Beam AG, Vandenbark AA, Offner H. Low-dose estrogen therapy ameliorates experimental autoimmune encephalomyelitis in two different

inbred mouse strains. *J Immunol* 2001;166:2080–9.

35. Ito A, Bebo BF, Jr., Matejuk A, Zamora A, *et al.* Estrogen treatment down-regulates TNF-alpha production and reduces the severity of experimental autoimmune encephalomyelitis in cytokine knockout mice. *J Immunol* 2001;167(1):542–52.

36. Liu HY, Buenafe AC, Matejuk A, *et al.* Estrogen inhibition of EAE involves effects on dendritic cell function. *J Neurosci Res* 2002;70(2):238–48.

37. Matejuk A, Adlard K, Zamora A, Silverman M, Vandenbark AA, Offner H. 17beta-estradiol inhibits cytokine, chemokine, and chemokine receptor mRNA expression in the central nervous system of female mice with experimental autoimmune encephalomyelitis. *J Neurosci Res* 2001;65(6):529–42.

38. Polanczyk M, Zamora A, Subramanian S, *et al.* The protective effect of 17beta-estradiol on experimental autoimmune encephalomyelitis is mediated through estrogen receptor-alpha. *Am J Pathol* 2003;163(4):1599–605.

39. Subramanian S, Matejuk A, Zamora A, Vandenbark AA, Offner H. Oral feeding with ethinyl estradiol suppresses and treats experimental autoimmune encephalomyelitis in SJL mice and inhibits the recruitment of inflammatory cells into the central nervous system. *J Immunol* 2003; 170(3):1548–55.

40. Jansson L, Olsson T, Holmdahl R. Estrogen induces a potent suppression of experimental autoimmune encephalomyelitis and collagen-induced arthritis in mice. *J Neuroimmunol* 1994;53(2):203–7.

41. Kim S, Liva SM, Dalal MA, Verity MA, Voskuhl RR. Estriol ameliorates autoimmune demyelinating disease: implications for multiple sclerosis. *Neurology* 1999;52(6):1230–8.

42. Liu HB, Loo KK, Palaszynski K, Ashouri J, Lubahn DB, Voskuhl RR. Estrogen receptor alpha mediates estrogen's immune protection in autoimmune disease. *J Immunol* 2003;171(12):6936–40.

43. Palaszynski KM, Liu H, Loo KK, Voskuhl RR. Estriol treatment ameliorates disease in males with experimental autoimmune

encephalomyelitis: implications for multiple sclerosis. *J Neuroimmunol* 2004;149(1–2): 84–9.

44. Voskuhl RR, Palaszynski KM. Female sex hormones at supraphysiologic, but not physiologic, levels decrease EAE severity in female SJL mice. *FASEB J* 2001;15(4):A372.

45. Garay L, Gonzalez Deniselle MC, Gierman L, *et al.* Steroid protection in the experimental autoimmune encephalomyelitis model of multiple sclerosis. *Neuroimmunomodulation* 2008;15(1):76–83.

46. Hoffman GE, Le WW, Murphy AZ, Koski CL. Divergent effects of ovarian steroids on neuronal survival during experimental allergic encephalitis in Lewis rats. *Exp Neurol* 2001;171(2):272–84.

47. Gold SM, Sasidhar MV, Morales LB, *et al.* Estrogen treatment decreases matrix metalloproteinase (MMP)-9 in autoimmune demyelinating disease through estrogen receptor alpha (ERalpha). *Lab Invest* 2009;89(10):1076–83.

48. Du S, Sandoval F, Trinh P, Umeda E, Voskuhl R. Estrogen receptor-beta ligand treatment modulates dendritic cells in the target organ during autoimmune demyelinating disease. *Eur J Immunol* 2011;41(1):140–50.

49. Zhang QH, Hu YZ, Cao J, Zhong YQ, Zhao YF, Mei QB. Estrogen influences the differentiation, maturation and function of dendritic cells in rats with experimental autoimmune encephalomyelitis. *Acta Pharmacol Sin* 2004;25(4):508–13.

50. Polanczyk MJ, Carson BD, Subramanian S, *et al.* Cutting edge: estrogen drives expansion of the CD4+CD25+ regulatory T cell compartment. *J Immunol* 2004;173(4):2227–30.

51. Wang C, Dehghani B, Li Y, Kaler LJ, Vandenbark AA, Offner H. Oestrogen modulates experimental autoimmune encephalomyelitis and interleukin-17 production via programmed death 1. *Immunology* 2009;126(3):329–35.

52. Wise PM, Dubal DB, Wilson ME, Rau SW, Bottner M. Minireview: neuroprotective effects of estrogen-new insights into mechanisms of action. *Endocrinology* 2001;142(3):969–73.

53. Garcia-Segura LM, Azcoitia I, DonCarlos LL. Neuroprotection by

estradiol. *Prog Neurobiol* 2001;63(1):29–60.

54. Morales LB, Loo KK, Liu HB, Peterson C, Tiwari-Woodruff S, Voskuhl RR. Treatment with an estrogen receptor alpha ligand is neuroprotective in experimental autoimmune encephalomyelitis. *J Neurosci* 2006;26(25):6823–33.

55. Enmark E, Gustafsson JA. Oestrogen receptors – an overview. *J Intern Med* 1999;246(2):133–8.

56. Weiss DJ, Gurpide E. Non-genomic effects of estrogens and antiestrogens. *J Steroid Biochem* 1988;31(4B):671–6.

57. Elloso MM, Phiel K, Henderson RA, Harris HA, Adelman SJ. Suppression of experimental autoimmune encephalomyelitis using estrogen receptor-selective ligands. *J Endocrinol* 2005;185(2):243–52.

58. Garidou L, Laffont S, Douin-Echinard V, *et al.* Estrogen receptor alpha signaling in inflammatory leukocytes is dispensable for 17beta-estradiol-mediated inhibition of experimental autoimmune encephalomyelitis. *J Immunol* 2004;173(4):2435–42.

59. Tiwari-Woodruff S, Morales LB, Lee R, Voskuhl RR. Differential neuroprotective and antiinflammatory effects of estrogen receptor (ER){alpha} and ERbeta ligand treatment. *Proc Natl Acad Sci USA* 2007;104(37):14813–8.

60. Du S, Sandoval F, Trinh P, Voskuhl RR. Additive effects of combination treatment with anti-inflammatory and neuroprotective agents in experimental autoimmune encephalomyelitis. *J Neuroimmunol* 2010;219 (1–2):64–74.

61. Tiwari-Woodruff S, Voskuhl RR. Neuroprotective and anti-inflammatory effects of estrogen receptor ligand treatment in mice. *J Neurol Sci* 2009;286(1–2):81–5.

62. Crawford DK, Mangiardi M, Song B, *et al.* Oestrogen receptor beta ligand: a novel treatment to enhance endogenous functional remyelination. *Brain* 2010;133(10):2999–3016.

63. Platania P, Laureanti F, Bellomo M, *et al.* Differential expression of estrogen receptors alpha and beta in the spinal cord during postnatal development: localization in glial cells. *Neuroendocrinology* 2003;77(5): 334–40.

64. Thorogood M, Hannaford PC. The influence of oral contraceptives on the risk of multiple sclerosis. *Br J Obstet Gynaecol* 1998;105(12):1296–9.

65. Sicotte NL, Liva SM, Klutch R, *et al.* Treatment of multiple sclerosis with the pregnancy hormone estriol. *Ann Neurol* 2002;52(4):421–8.

66. Soldan SS, Retuerto AI, Sicotte NL, Voskuhl RR. Immune modulation in multiple sclerosis patients treated with the pregnancy hormone estriol. *J Immunol* 2003;171(11):6267–74.

67. Senda T, Saitoh SI, Mitsui Y, Li J, Roberts RM. A three-dimensional model of interferon-tau. *J Interferon Cytokine Res* 1995;15(12):1053–60.

68. Magiakou MA, Mastorakos G, Rabin D, *et al.* The maternal hypothalamic-pituitary-adrenal axis in the third trimester of human pregnancy. *Clin Endocrinol* 1996;44(4):419–28.

69. Magiakou MA, Mastorakos G, Webster E, Chrousos GP. The hypothalamic-pituitary-adrenal axis and the female reproductive system. *Ann N Y Acad Sci* 1997;816:42–56.

70. Seely EW, Brown EM, DeMaggio DM, Weldon DK, Graves SW. A prospective study of calciotropic hormones in pregnancy and post partum: reciprocal changes in serum intact parathyroid hormone and 1,25- dihydroxyvitamin D. *Am J Obstet Gynecol* 1997;176(1, 1):214–7.

71. Kragt J, van Amerongen B Killestein J, *et al.* Higher levels of 25-hydroxyvitamin D are associated with a lower incidence of multiple sclerosis only in women. *Mult Scler* 2009;15(1):9–15.

72. Spach KM, Hayes CE. Vitamin D3 confers protection from autoimmune encephalomyelitis only in female mice. *J Immunol* 2005;175(6):4119–26.

73. Mahon BD, Gordon SA, Cruz J, Cosman F, Cantorna MT. Cytokine profile in patients with multiple sclerosis following vitamin D supplementation. *J Neuroimmunol* 2003;134(1–2):128–32.

74. Mattsson R, Mattsson A, Holmdahl R, Whyte A, Rook GA. Maintained pregnancy levels of oestrogen afford complete protection from post-partum exacerbation of collagen-induced arthritis. *Clin Exp Immunol* 1991;85(1):41–17.

75. Vukusic S, Ionescu I, El-Etr M, *et al.* The Prevention of Post-Partum Relapses with Progestin and Estradiol in Multiple Sclerosis (POPART'MUS) trial: rationale, objectives and state of advancement. *J Neurol Sci* 2009;286(1–2):114–18.

76. Riskind PN, Massacesi L, Doolittle TH, Hauser SL. The role of prolactin in autoimmune demyelination: suppression of experimental allergic encephalomyelitis by bromocriptine. *Ann Neurol* 1991;29(5):542–7.

77. Nociti V, Frisullo G, Tartaglione T, Patanella AK, Iorio R, Tonali PA, *et al.* Multiple sclerosis attacks triggered by hyperprolactinemia. *J Neurooncol* 2010;98(3):407–9.

78. Yamasaki K, Horiuchi I, Minohara M, *et al.* Hyperprolactinemia in optico-spinal multiple sclerosis. *Intern Med* 2000;39(4):296–9.

79. Gregg C, Shikar V, Larsen P, *et al.* White matter plasticity and enhanced remyelination in the maternal CNS. *J Neurosci* 2007;27(8):1812–23.

80. Langer-Gould A, Huang SM, Gupta R, *et al.* Exclusive breastfeeding and the risk of postpartum relapses in women with multiple sclerosis. *Arch Neurol.* 2009;66:958.

81. Craig A, Ling Luo N, Beardsley DJ, *et al.* Quantitative analysis of perinatal rodent oligodendrocyte lineage progression and its correlation with human. *Exp Neurol* 2003;181(2): 231–40.

Chapter

Hematopoietic stem cell transplantation to treat multiple sclerosis

Richard K. Burt and Francesca Milanetti

Types of stem cells

Stem cells are capable of both self-renewal and differentiation into more specialized cells and tissue, and are broadly categorized as either embryonic stem cells (ESCs) or adult stem cells (Fig. 44.1). Fertilization of the oocyte results in the generation of totipotent cells that can form both the placenta and all tissues within the developing fetus. The initial differentiation of post-fertilized totipotent cells leads to the delineation of an outer layer of trophoblast that develops into the placenta, and an inner cell mass (ICM) of pluripotent ESCs that can differentiate into all three germ layers: mesoderm, endoderm, and ectoderm. An ESC line may be obtained by culturing the ICM over a feeder layer of fibroblasts.[1–3] A major disadvantage of ESCs is a tendency to form teratomas when injected in vivo.[4,5] This complication may be overcome by ex vivo-directed differentiation of ESCs into adult stem cells prior to in vivo application.[5] Another disadvantage of using ESCs in clinical studies is that current culture requirements for a feeder layer and/or xenogenic-derived products for maintenance culture must meet Food and Drug Administration (FDA) requirements for human application. While ESCs may be differentiated into neuronal stem cells, neurons, or oligodendrocyte progenitor cells,[6–8] clinical trials in the US depended on developing ex vivo culture and expansion techniques that satisfy FDA requirements for human trials. Recently, the first human trial using ESC-derived cells was approved by the FDA for acute spinal cord injury (http://www.geron.com/).

For the rest of this chapter, we focus on adult hematopoietic stem cell sources in current clinical transplant trials for multiple sclerosis (MS). Adult stem cells are obtained from differentiated tissue compartments during or after birth, and are lineage-restricted (multipotent) to differentiate into and replenish a particular tissue or organ system. Most adult stem cells are difficult to collect safely in clinically relevant numbers. For example, neuronal stem cells are located in the periventricular area of the brain while liver stem cells (ovalocytes) are located in the periductal area of the liver parenchyma, making harvest in a living patient impractical. In contrast, hematopoietic stem cells (HSCs) may be easily and safely collected in clinically significant number from the bone marrow, blood, or placenta

(umbilical cord blood, UCB). For UCB, safe and rapid engraftment, following myeloablative (marrow ablative) therapy, depends on infusion of more than 2.5×10^7 mononuclear cells/kg of recipient weight (Cord Blood Registry Guidelines), which limits the use of UCB to children, although some centers infuse multiple UCB units from different deliveries to achieve sufficient HSCs for adult recipients. In adults, HSCs are generally collected from the blood, and termed peripheral blood stem cells (PBSCs).

Since negligible HSCs are detectable in the peripheral blood during steady state, either a hematopoietic growth factor such as granulocyte colony-stimulating factor (G-CSF) or chemotherapy (usually cyclophosphamide) with or without G-CSF is necessary to mobilize HSCs and subsequently collect them from the blood. Hematopoietic growth factors used to mobilize stem cells also have immune-modulating effects and, depending on the growth factors, may exacerbate autoimmune disease. G-CSF may precipitate clinical flares of MS, sometimes with significant and irreversible neurological deterioration.[9–11] G-CSF-induced MS flare may be prevented by either administration of corticosteroids or mobilization with combined cyclophosphamide and G-CSF.

HSCs mobilized into the peripheral blood are collected by apheresis, which is an outpatient procedure performed through a double lumen catheter inserted into either the antecubital or internal jugular vein. Blood is drawn from one lumen of the catheter, and mononuclear cells are separated by an external centrifuge (Baxter Fenwall or COBE Spectra) and returned to the patient through the second catheter lumen. Approximately 10–15 liters of blood are processed as an out-patient procedure that requires several hours. The PBSCs are cryopreserved or further processed by immunoselection for a HSC phenotype and then cryopreserved. Purification or enrichment ex vivo for HSCs may be performed using antibodies to select for CD34 or CD133, or by negative selection using antibodies to remove lymphocytes. In practice, the most common method of purging lymphocytes is via CD34-positive selection using either the Baxter Isolex (Deerfield, IL) cell separator device, which is no longer commercially available or the Miltenyi CliniMACS (Bergish Gladbach, Germany). In general, a minimum number of

Multiple Sclerosis Therapeutics, Fourth Edition, ed. Jeffrey A. Cohen and Richard A. Rudick. Published by Cambridge University Press.
© Cambridge University Press 2011.

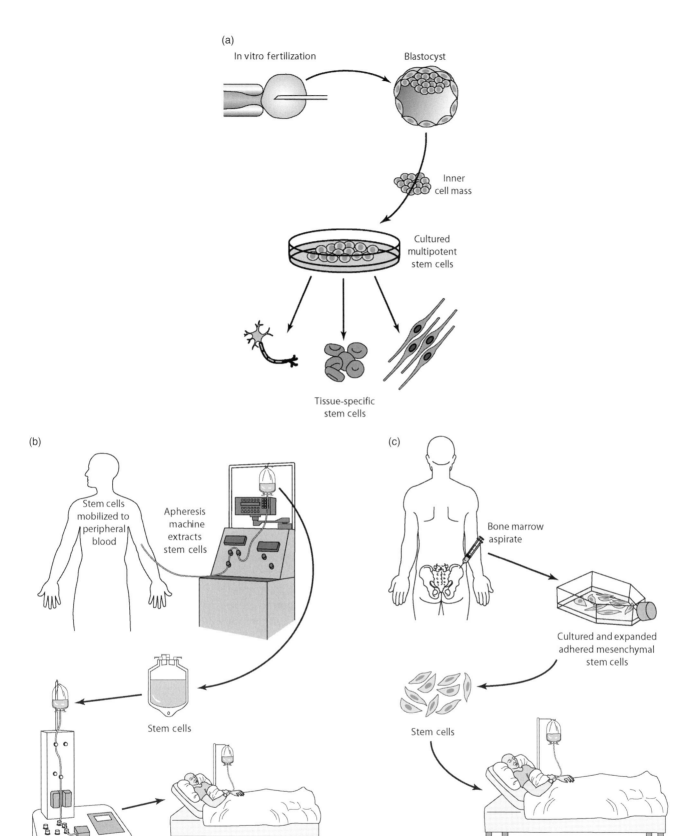

Fig. 44.1. Different types of stem cells. (a) Pluripotent embryonic stem cells (ESCs) can differentiate into cells of all three germ layers: mesoderm, ectoderm, entoderm origin. (b) Hematopoietic stem cells (HSCs) are collected from peripheral blood. (c) Mesenchymal stem cells (MSCs) are obtained from bone marrow as cells that adhere to and expand on the culture dish surface.

2×10^6 CD34+ cells/kg of recipient weight will ensure engraftment.

HSCs can be either allogeneic (from another person) or autologous (from the recipient). HSCs differentiate and replenish all types of blood cells, including red blood cells, platelets, vascular endothelial cells, and immune cells such as neutrophils, dendritic cells, monocytes, and T-cells, and B-cells. Some studies have suggested that HSCs may, under certain conditions, transdifferentiate into non-hematopoietic tissues such as liver, muscle, brain, etc.[12–15] However, most of these experiments have been performed ex vivo, with little evidence of significant in vivo transdifferentiation, and have relied on tissue-specific antigen presentation without evidence of tissue-specific function. Transdifferentiation remains an ex vivo laboratory culture-related phenomenon and is not clinically relevant. While of interest, the in vivo transdifferentiation of HSCs to replace damaged oligodendrocytes or neurons is, at best, theoretical, and, therefore, will not be discussed further.

Rationale for autologous hematopoietic stem cell transplantation

Traditional therapies for MS (interferon-beta and glatiramer acetate) have achieved modest therapeutic benefits for patients with less aggressive MS, offering the ability to slow or delay the accumulation of disabilities but rarely reducing or reversing preexisting disabilities. Now, more potent agents that interfere with immune function (mitoxantrone, natalizumab, cladribine, fingolimod, and alemtuzumab) have shown better activity at suppressing MS relapses but do not significantly reverse disability. Autologous hematopoietic stem cell transplantation (HSCT) was first suggested by Burt et al. as a form of intense immune-suppressive therapy.[16] The transplant conditioning regimen ablates the aberrant disease-causing immune cells resulting in an immediate immune cease fire. The HSCs then regenerate, within a non-inflammatory environment, a new immune system. The manner in which antigen is presented helps determine the immune response. That is, presentation of antigen without co-stimulation (without inflammation) biases the immune system towards anergy.[17]

The mechanism of autologous transplant-induced remission of MS may be either transient immune suppression-related lymphopenia and/or a more durable "immune reset" due to the regeneration of an antigen-naive immune system from the HSCs. By analyzing T-cell receptor (TCR) repertoires with flow cytometry, polymerase chain reaction (PCR) spectratyping, and sequenced-based clonotyping, as well as recent thymic emigrant output by T-cell receptor excision circle (TREC), Muraro et al. demonstrated in M patients undergoing HSCT that a new and antigen-naive T-cell repertoire arises from the stem cell compartment via thymic regeneration.[18] This suggests that intense immune suppression via HSCT results in long-term immune reset independent of transient immune-suppression-mediated lymphopenia. However, the observed persistence post-therapy of some pre-existing T-cell clones suggested the potential for disease recurrence. Dubinsky et al. investigated whether TCRs that reappear after a myeloablative conditioning regimen and HSCT were reintroduced with the autologous, CD34-selected, HSC graft. In-frame TCR sequences were detectable in only one of four patient grafts and no TCR sequences were found to be shared between the graft and pre- or post-HSCT samples. These findings suggest that T-cells in selected autologous grafts are unlikely to be a major source of carryover of T-cell expansions potentially involved in MS.[19]

Animal results

HSCT was proposed as a treatment for MS in 1995 by Burt et al. based on favorable results in experimental autoimmune encephalomyelitis (EAE), an animal model of MS[16] (Fig. 44.2). EAE is an autoimmune demyelinating disease of the central nervous system (CNS) induced either by in vivo immunization with myelin peptides or by adoptive transfer of ex vivo primed CD4+ T-cells. HSCs are acquired from an euthanized animal of a different strain (allogeneic HSCT), of the same highly inbred strain (syngeneic HSCT), or from a syngeneic animal with the same stage of disease (pseudoautologous HSCT). Any of three donor HSC sources (allogeneic, syngeneic, or pseudoautologous) is capable of improving neurological disability when performed during the acute phase of disease.[20–25] In contrast, HSCT does not improve neurological impairment when performed during the chronic progressive phase of EAE (Fig. 44.2).[20]

In contrast to the initial relapsing–remitting course of EAE, Theiler's murine encephalomyelitis virus (TMEV) induces a CNS demyelinating disease manifesting at onset as progressive neurological deterioration. TMEV is a small RNA virus (picornavirus) acquired in the wild by oral inoculation. Disease-resistant strains of mice clear the virus within two weeks of infection, while disease susceptible strains have a persistent CNS infection. Both virus- and myelin-specific T-cell responses occur in TMEV-induced demyelinating disease.[26] Unlike the beneficial effect of HSCT seen in relapsing EAE, syngeneic HSCT of TMEV-infected mice results in exacerbation of neurological disability and high mortality due to CNS viral hyperinfection following immune ablation.[27] Therefore, a functional immune system appears important to prevent lethal neuropathic effects from a persistent viral-induced CNS demyelinating disease. Since several hundred patients with MS have undergone HSCT world-wide without experiencing viral encephalomyelitis, it is unlikely that patients with MS harbor a persistent neuropathic viral infection. However, this caveat needs to be kept in mind if HSCT is considered for a patient with acute disseminated viral encephalomyelitis.

In summary, animal models such as EAE and TMEV-induced demyelinating disease suggest that: (1) most cases of MS are, at onset, an autoimmune-initiated disease similar to EAE, and not a persistent viral-related demyelinating disease

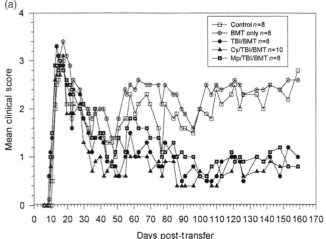

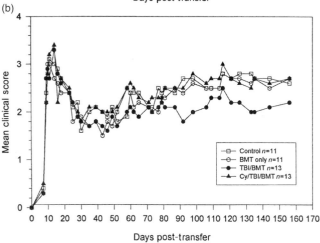

Fig. 44.2. Bone marrow transplantation of experimental autoimmune encephalomyelitis (EAE). (a) Bone marrow (BMT) transplant during acute (relapsing) stage of EAE, in which transplant causes disease to remit. (b) Bone marrow transplant (BMT) during chronic (progressive) stage of EAE, in which transplant has no effect on neurological disability. TBI, total body irradiation; Cy, cyclophosphamide; Mp, methylprednisolone. This research was originally published in *Blood*. Burt RK, Padilla J, Begolka WS, Canto MC, Miller SD. Effect of disease stage on clinical outcome after syngeneic bone marrow transplantation for relapsing experimental autoimmune encephalomyelitis.1998;91(7):2609–16[20] © the American Society of Hematology.

akin to TMEV; (2) to be effective, HSCT should be performed in the relapsing phase of MS while it is still an immune-mediated inflammatory process, rather than in its chronic progressive phase when axonal degeneration predominates. This emphasizes that HSCT is a method of HSC-derived immune regeneration and not a method for transdifferentiation of HSC and neuronal or oligodendrocyte regeneration.

Conditioning regimen

The toxicity and efficacy of an autologous HSCT is entirely a consequence of the conditioning regimen. Before receiving a transplant, patients with MS receive "conditioning" chemotherapy or radiation that destroys lymphocytes, inducing

an immediate immune ceasefire. Subsequently, HSCs are infused to regenerate a new self-tolerant immune system. Some centers advocate conditioning regimens based on myeloablative cancer drugs and or total body irradiation (TBI). These extreme regimens cause irreversible bone marrow failure, thus requiring mandatory HSC reinfusion to recover. In contrast, we advocate less extreme non-myeloablative regimens based on standard immune suppressive medications, which can halt inflammation without altering the bone marrow's ability to recover. For non-myeloablative regimens, HSC reinfusion is not mandatory for recovery but infused to shorten duration of hospitalization and post-conditioning regimen related cytopenias. In addition to patient safety benefits from lower toxicity, non-myeloablative regimens are less expensive and less likely to be associated with late complications such as infertility or secondary leukemias.[28,29]

The conditioning regimen must also avoid further damage to already injured axons and oligodendrocytes. By definition, myeloablative agents are lethal to HSCs, and apart from their myeloablative effect on bone marrow may be similarly cidal to tissue-specific stem cells such as oligodendrocyte progenitor cells or neural stem cells. In animal models, cranial radiation impairs CNS repair by causing neural stem cell apoptosis, an alteration in cell cycle progression, and/or destruction of the neural stem cell niche or milieu through invasion of macrophages and microglia.[30] This raises concerns about using a TBI-based or otherwise stem cell-ablative regimen in the treatment of MS. Non-myeloablative regimens that are immune suppressive without myeloablative adverse effects may be designed by using agents or combinations of agents such as cyclophosphamide (CY) and/or antilymphocyte antibodies such as anti-thymocyte globulin (ATG) or rituximab. Due to the high risk of alemtuzumab-associated late immune cytopenias (immune thrombocytopenic purpura, autoimmune haemolytic anemia, etc.) when included in the conditioning regimen,[31] we do not currently recommend the use of alemtuzumab in autologous transplant conditioning regimens for MS. Fever-related deterioration of neural function in MS, termed pseudoexacerbations, due to conduction blocks in marginally functioning demyelinated axons should be avoided during transplant by minimizing fever from pyrogenic agents such as ATG in the conditioning regimen with prophylactic corticosteroids. Similarly, the risk of infection-related fever should be minimized during transplant by the use of prophylactic antibiotics.

In summary, for MS, the rationale behind the transplant conditioning regimen should be to: (1) dose-escalate conventional immune-suppressive agents for MS, (2) maximize immune suppression without using cancer regimen-based myeloablative drugs or radiation, (3) avoid conditioning regimen agents that may cause injury to already disease-affected and damaged CNS tissue, (4) avoid injury to tissue-specific stem cell compartments that may be important for CNS repair, (5) minimize risk of fever. The above principles are essential in designing regimens where the potential toxicity is justified for the morbidity and mortality of the disease being treated.

Results of first-generation myeloablative hematopoietic stem cell transplantation protocols for secondary progressive multiple sclerosis

Initial HSCT protocols generally did not follow the above concepts that argue for non-myeloablative regimens used during the inflammatory stage of MS, but rather employed aggressive malignancy-specific myeloablative regimens in patients with progressive MS (Table 44.1). As a consequence, treatment was complicated by relatively high mortality and failure to reverse neurologic deficits. However, these studies confirmed that autologous HSCT is an effective therapy to halt inflammation on magnetic resonance imaging (MRI). In fact, there is no other therapy that may provide such a striking and long-term effect on suppressing MRI gadolinium enhancement and new T2-weighted lesions.

In 1995, Fassas *et al.* (Thessaloniki, Greece) performed the first HSCT for MS by using a low intensity myeloablative lymphoma regimen (BEAM / ATG) to treat patients with progressive MS.[50] This regimen was adopted in a study by an Italian cooperative group led by Mancardi (Genoa) that demonstrated HSCT to be highly effective at eliminating active inflammation in the brain.[36] Fassas' approach was also adopted by the multicenter European MS randomized trial (ASTIMS) comparing HSCT to mitoxantrone treatment that was recently stopped after inclusion of 30 patients due to slow accrual.[51]

On the American side of the Atlantic, initial protocols by Chicago and Seattle utilized a high groups in intensity myeloablative leukemia conditioning regimen, containing TBI, for patients with late secondary progressive MS. While patient selection and treatment were similar in these two non-randomized Phase 1/2 trials, the interpretation of treatment outcome reported in the same issue of *Blood* by both centers was divergent. The Seattle (Sullivan/Nash) consortium interpreted the outcome as clinically "promising" because transplant may have slowed the rate of progressive disability compared with historical controls and coined the term high-dose immune suppressive therapy (HDIT) for treatment of autoimmune diseases with intense myeloablative conditioning regimens.[38] The concept behind HDIT is that maximal ablation of pathologic disease causing immune cells will translate into longer and more durable disease remission. However, subsequently, Seattle selected MS patients with more inflammatory disease and less disability and TBI was abandoned in favor of the European (Fassas) low-intensity myeloablative regimen in a non-randomized Phase 2 trial (the HALT-MS study).[52]

In contrast, because disability did not improve and over time progressed, Chicago (Burt *et al.*) interpreted and reported their results using an intense myeloablative TBI regimen as "failure of treatment."[37] Importantly, lymphocytes from the Chicago trial were harvested before and after HSCT and analyzed by Muraro and colleagues at the NIH intramural program. As mentioned earlier, this immune analysis confirmed an immune regeneration following HSCT.[18] To the Chicago group, immune regeneration without clinical improvement in neurologic disability indicated that: (1) late progressive MS is an axonal degenerative disorder for which no immune based therapy including HSCT would be effective; (2) optimal benefit from HSCT would occur by offering HSCT to patients with frequent relapses earlier in disease course, i.e. relapsing remitting (RR) MS. Results by Saiz *et al.* (Spain)[34] supported Chicago's interpretations of an early therapeutic treatment window and prompted the pertinent question for treating late-stage MS: "Too much too late, or too late for much".[53] In terms of risk–benefit, treatment earlier in disease course, that is treatment of RRMS, must be performed with safer and less intense regimens. Thus, Chicago abandoned cancer-based myeloablative regimens and introduced the term autologous non-myeloablative HSCT for autoimmune diseases in general and MS in specific.[29]

Numerous Phase 1/2 studies have subsequently been reported in the literature but these trials are often a mixture of different types of MS: RR, secondary progressive (SP), primary progressive (PP), or relapsing progressive (RP) and in some cases a mixture of diverse conditioning regimens making interpretation of results difficult. Some of these trials also report improvement as a decline in the Extended Disability Status Scale (EDSS) by 0.5 points. However, an EDSS change of less than 1.0 point is within the range of intra- and inter-neurologist examination error upon repeat scoring. We, therefore, prefer the more conservative decline of 1.0 or more points in EDSS to define improvement (Table 44.1). Finally, the natural history of progressive MS is to remain stable for an extended period of time at some EDSS steps. This makes short-term follow-up of EDSS stabilization difficult to separate from the natural history of the disease.

In a European retrospective analysis, involving 143 patients with different types of MS and treated with diverse conditioning regimens, stabilization or improvement occurred in 90 and worsening in 53, with younger patients, transplanted within five years from diagnosis, having a significantly better progression-free survival (PFS) (89%). The PFS was not related to the intensity of the conditioning regimen[40,41].

The importance of selecting patients with inflammatory disease was demonstrated in three of the registry patients with "malignant" MS, i.e. striking gadolinium-enhancing lesions, and severe deficits (non-ambulatory with EDSS scores of 7.5, 8.0, and 9.0) after a short clinical duration of disease (one and three years), who were able to ambulate again, without aid, by six months after HSCT. The effect was long lasting, as demonstrated by a sustained efficacy over a two-year period in two subjects and 12 months in the third case. In addition, a striking effect on inflammation-related MRI findings was obtained.[54]

Lack of general benefit in terms of reversing neurologic disability was reported from two European single center studies treating SPMS. In a Rotterdam, the Netherlands trial using a TBI-based myeloablative regimen in 14 patients with SPMS, only one improved by an EDSS of 1.0, three remained stable, and nine had continued post-transplant progression of

Table 44.1. *Autologous hematopoietic stem cell transplant trials for multiple sclerosis*

Authors	Predominate type MS/predominate regimen	Regimen	# of Patients (# died)	(# patients) Cause of death/time after transplant	Progression free survival	Number of patients (%) in whom EDSS significantly improved, i.e. declined ≥ 1.0 point
Fassas et al.[32]	SPMS Myeloablative	BEAM / ATG	24 (1)	(1) aspergillosis at day +65	100%, 92%, and 39% at 4 years in RRMS, SPMS, and PPMS respectively	9 (37%)
Kozak et al.[33]	SPMS Myeloablative	BEAM / ATG	10 (0)	None	80 % and 64,3% at 5 years in the group with purged or not purged graft respectively	1 (10%)
Saiz et al.[34,35]	SPMS Myeloablative	BCNU / Cy / ATG	14 (0)	None	86% and 62.5% at 3 and 6 years	N/A
Mancardi et al.[36]	SPMS Myeloablative	BEAM	10 (0)	None	NA	0%
Burt et al.[37]	SPMS Myeloablative	Cy / TBI	21 (2)	(2) DP at 13 and 18 mo	NA	1 (5%)
Nash et al.[38]	SPMS Myeloablative	TBI / Cy / ATG	26 (2)	(1) EBV PTLD at day +53 (1) DP at 23 mo	76% at 40 mo	0
Openshaw et al.[39]	SPMS Myeloablative	Bu / Cy / ATG	5 (2)	(1) influenza A pneumonia at day +22, (1) pneumonia sepsis at 19 mo	NA	0
Atkins (verbal communication)	SPMS Myeloablative	Bu / Cy / ATG	11 (1)	(1) VOD of liver	NA	N/A
EBMT[40,41]	SPMS Myeloablative	Multiple regimens	143 (9)	(6) toxicity infection at day +7 to 19 months, (2) DP at 3 months, (1) acquired Factor VIII inhibitor	63%	N/A – EDSS decreased or remained stable in 63%
Fassas and Passweg[40] Saccardi et al.[41]						
Xu et al.[42,43]	SPMS Myeloablative	BEAM	22 (0)	None	77% at 59 mo	13 (59%)
Ni et al.[44]	SPMS Myeloablative	TBI / Cy (1) BEAM (20)	21 (2)	(1) pneumonia at 4.5 mo, (1) VZV hepatitis, at 15 mo	75% at 42 mo	N/A –
Samijn et al.[45]	SPMS Myeloablative	Cy / TBI / ATG	14 (1)	(1) DP (5 years)	36% at 3 years	N/A – 2 (14%) improved but EDSS not given
Shevchenko et al.[46]	SPMS Myeloablative	BEAM	45 (1)	(1) leukemia	72% at 6 years	17 (38%)
Fagius et al.[47]	RRMS Myeloablative and non-myeloablative	Cy / ATG (1) BEAM / ATG (8)	9 (0)	None	100%	9 (100%)
Burt[48]	RRMS Non-myeloablative	CY / CAMPATH CY / rATG	21 (0)	None	100% at 3 years	17 (81%)
Hamerschlak et al.[49]	SPMS Myeloablative vs. non-myeloablative	BEAM / hATG Versus CY / rATG	21 (3) versus 20 (0)	Myeloablative –(1) pneumonitis, (1) CMV pneumonia (1) alveolar hemorrhage Non-myeloablative- (0)	Myeloablative – 47% at 3 years Non-myeloablative- 70% at 3 years	Myeloablative – 1 (5%) Non-myeloablative- 1 (5%)

ATG, antithymocyte globulin; BEAM, carmustine (BCNU), etoposide, ara-c (cytosine arabinoside), melphalan; Bu, busulfan; CAMPATH, alemtuzumab; Cy, cyclophosphamide; DP, disease progression; EBV, Epstein–Barr virus; EDSS, Expanded Disability Status Scale; Flu, fludarabine; hATG, horse ATG; MDS, myelodysplastic syndrome; mo, month; PPMS, primary progressive multiple sclerosis; PTLD, post-transplant lymphoproliferative disorder; rATG, rabbit ATG; RRMS, relapsing–remitting multiple sclerosis; SPMS, secondary progressive multiple sclerosis; TBI, total body irradiation; VOD, veno-occlusive disease.

disability.[45] In a Prague, Czech Republic trial treated with a low intensity myeloblative regimen of BEAM, only one of 11 patients improved by at least 1 point.[33]

Compared with experiences in America and Europe, the Chinese and Russians have reported more favorable outcomes in terms of neurologic improvement after myeloablative HSCT for predominately SPMS. In Beijing, China, Xu reported 22 patients with SPMS treated with BEAM. Thirteen patients improved by 1.0 EDSS point, four remained stable, and five progressed.[43] In Nanjing, China, Ni reported 21 patients with progressive MS treated with conditioning regimen of either cyclophosphamide and TBI or BEAM: three patients worsened, eight were stable and eight were reported to improve but the actual change in EDSS was not reported.[44] In a Russian (Moscow) study of 45 patients that included RRMS, SPMS, PPMS, and PRMS treated with myeloablative BEAM, EDSS improved in 28, stabilized in 17, or worsened in 4.[46] Compared with American and European results, it is unclear why the Chinese and Russians report significant reversal of neurologic disability in progressive MS following HSCT. One possible explanation is that American and European trials generally enrolled late progressive MS while Asian studies may be enrolling patients with MS that are transitioning into progressive disease but still inflammatory. Of interest, unlike most European and American trials, the Russian and Chinese trials did not utilize ATG in the conditioning regimen and avoided use of a potentially significant pyrogenic agent which would otherwise cause fever unless thoughtful prophylaxis with corticosteroids is prescribed during transplant hospitalization.

Mortality from myeloablative regimens

The initial myeloablative regimens have been associated with treatment-related deaths and serious toxicities (Table 44.1). A Phase 1 study performed at the City of Hope (Duarte, CA) utilizing a maximum-dose myeloablative cancer-specific regimen of busulfan and cyclophosphamide, also known as "Big BuCy", along with ATG and CD34+ selection, resulted in the treatment-related death of two of five patients.[39] A similar "Big BuCy" regimen performed in Ottawa, Canada, resulted in a treatment-related death due to hepatic venoocclusive disease in one of 11 patients (MS Freedman, personal communication). A slightly less-intense regimen using a leukemia-specific protocol of myeloablative TBI, cyclophosphamide, ATG and CD34+ selection performed at the Fred Hutchinson Cancer Center resulted in one reported transplant-related death out of 26 patients.[38] A similar TBI-based regimen performed in Rotterdam, the Netherlands, that enrolled 14 patients ended with one patient developing radiation-related pre-leukemic myelodysplasia and another developing Epstein–Barr virus-associated lymphoproliferative disease.[45]

In a retrospective European analysis of 85 patients treated with a lymphoma-specific regimens, mostly BEAM: carmustine (BCNU), etoposide, cytosine arabinoside (ara-c),

melphalan, five treatment-related deaths were reported.[40] A later analysis from the EBMT showed a decreased treatment-related mortality with no deaths recorded after 2001, probably because of better patient selection and due to the experience accumulating at transplantation centers. The study also confirmed that a more aggressive conditioning regimen, including busulfan, is associated with higher risk of mortality. Although there was a trend for an increased risk of mortality in more disabled patients, this item was not statistically significant.[41]

An Italian trial of the BEAM regimen in MS showed better safety, with no deaths in 19 patients.[55] In the Ni et al. study (Nanjing, China), two patients (9.5%) died of severe pneumonia and varicella-zoster viral hepatitis at 4.5 and 15 months after transplant.[44] The Shevchenko et al. (Russian) study reported a single fatality at long-term follow-up after transplantation. The patient developed acute promyelocytic leukemia at 43 months after transplantation and died of cerebral hemorrhage.[46]

Second-generation non-myeloablative autologous stem cell transplant protocols for relapsing–remitting multiple sclerosis

As mentioned above, the Chicago group (Burt et al.) based on experience in the animal model EAE[27] and initial clinical trial in late SPMS, first reported the fallacy of myeloablative regimens and the futility of treating late progressive MS with therapy directed towards regenerating the immune system.[37] Therefore, rather than selecting for rapidly progressive disease, that is, an increase in EDSS score of one or more points in the preceding 12 months, as performed in prior myeloablative studies, in second-generation non-myeloablative protocols, transplant candidates are selected for frequent relapses with less accumulated disability (EDSS score of 2.0–6.0) and active inflammation on MRI. Criteria include RR or RP MS with, in the preceding 12 months, more than two acute relapses treated with corticosteroids despite interferon-beta treatment, or one relapse and at a time separate from the relapse gadolinium-enhancing lesions on MRI. Patients with higher EDSS scores could be considered if they have "malignant" MS manifested by rapid clinical deterioration and striking gadolinium enhancement on MRI. Based on these entry criteria, the Chicago group recently reported the outcome using a non-myeloablative regimen on 21 RRMS patients who had frequent relapses despite treatment with interferon-beta. The patients experienced little acute toxicity following treatment with a low-intensity conditioning regimen, CY 200 mg/kg followed by a single dose of 20 mg of alemtuzumab and in the last four cases, after it was shown that alemtuzumab can cause immune thrombocytopenic purpura, CY 200 mg/kg and rabbit ATG 6 mg/kg. With a median follow-up of three years, 17 of the 21 patients had a 1-point or greater improvement (decline) in their EDSS score compared to baseline (seven improved by 1.0 to 1.5 points, six improved by 2.0 to 2.5 points, and four improved by 3 or more points) (Table 44.1).[48]

Utilizing either a low-intensity myeloablative regimen of BEAM and ATG or a non-myeloablative regimen of cyclophosphamide and ATG, Fagius *et al.* in Sweden performed HSCT in nine young patients with "malignant" RRMS of recent onset and documented similar reversal of neurologic disability. Median EDSS at HSCT was 7.0 and median EDSS improvement was 3.5 at a median follow-up of 29 months, clearly surpassing previous reports. Eight of nine patients remained stable, median EDSS being 2.0. Before HSCT, 61 relapses occurred in 82 patient–months; during follow-up, one relapse in 289 patient–months.[47] Safety of the non-myeloablative approach compared with a low-intensity myeloablative regimen was reported by a Brazilian study that retrospectively compared sequential cohorts of patients who underwent transplantation for MS in Brazil and found that patients receiving a low intensity myeloablative BEAM and horse ATG regimen had a higher regimen-related morbidity and mortality (3 deaths out of 20 patients) than patients who received the non-myeloablative regimen of CY and rabbit ATG with no reported mortality (0 of 20).[49] Importantly, none of the HSCT studies for RRMS (Chicago, Sweden, Brazil) using non-myeloablative regimens have reported deaths, while both studies (Chicago and Sweden) that treated relapsing MS reported marked reversal (81% and 100%, respectively) of neurologic disability.

On-going controlled trials of autologous HSCT for patients with multiple sclerosis

Several non-randomized autologous HSCT trials utilizing myeloablative regimens have recently been closed. The European ASTIMS (Autologous Stem Cell Transplantation International Multiple Sclerosis) Trial[51] (www.astims.org), which employed a low-intensity myeloablative lymphoma specific regimen (BEAM) was recently closed due to poor accrual. In the last report from ASTIMS, 75% of patients remained stable while 25% progressed.[41] The HALT-MS (High-Dose Immunosuppression and Autologous Stem Cell Transplantation for Poor Prognosis Multiple Sclerosis) Trial[52] (www.halt-ms.org), which also utilized a BEAM-based regimen, was closed to new accrual with results pending. The Canadian trial of autologous stem cell transplantation for poor prognosis Multiple Sclerosis[56] (www.clinicaltrials.gov NCT01099930) that employs an intense myeloablative regimen based on busulfan and cyclophosphamide is no longer accruing and as mentioned earlier had one treatment-related death.

The Chicago based trial using a non-myeloablative regimen in RRMS,[48] reported above, is the only trial that has been expanded into a randomized controlled Phase 3 trial of non-myeloablative HSCT (cyclophosphamide and rATG regimen) vs. FDA approved drugs that are standard of care for patients failing interferon-beta (currently natalizumab or mitoxantrone). Patient eligibility requires two or more corticosteroid-treated relapses in the prior 12 months despite interferon-beta. Upon FDA approval, the option for newly approved standard of care drugs such as fingolimod will be incorporated in the control arm. While it is impossible to blind the patient to treatment arm, both the evaluating neurologist and MRI reading center are blinded to patient treatment. The study can be accessed at www.clinicaltrials.gov (NCT00273364), is accruing patients in Chicago (USA), Calgary (Canada), and Ribeirao Preto (Brasil), and will soon be opened in Uppsala (Sweden). Currently, this trial, termed MIST (Multiple Sclerosis International Stem cell Transplant Trial), is the only randomized autologous stem cell transplant trial for MS world-wide (see Table 44.2).[57]

Rationale for allogeneic hematopoietic stem cell transplantation for multiple sclerosis

Unlike autologous HSCT, the immune compartment arising from an allogeneic stem cells will have a different and presumably more disease-resistant genetic predisposition towards disease recurrence. Compared with autologous HSCT, allogeneic HSCT is, therefore, thought to be more likely to cure or prevent the recurrence of immune-mediated diseases such as MS. However, the traditional complications arising from allogeneic HSCT are more serious than after an autologous transplant due predominantly to graft vs. host disease (GVHD), a disease mediated by donor immune cells that recognize host tissue as foreign, and which in severe cases is lethal.

GVHD may be eliminated by infusing a graft enriched for donor HSCs through aggressive purging of donor lymphocytes. In patients with malignancies, depleting donor lymphocytes to prevent GVHD results in leukemia relapse rates similar to patients receiving autologous HSC transplants. Donor lymphocytes convey both a beneficial graft vs. leukemia (GVL) or graft vs. tumor (GVT) effect and a detrimental GVHD. In terms of risk–benefit for malignant disease, GVHD is often, depending upon the cancer considered, an acceptable risk. For autoimmune diseases, the risk of trading one immune-initiated disease (MS) for another even more lethal immune-mediated disease (GVHD) would not be acceptable. Further GVHD associated fever and cytokine storm may accelerate axonal injury and, although in normal patients GVHD is not thought to target the CNS, in patients with MS undergoing HSCT for malignant diagnosis, histologic study of post-mortem brain tissue showed high numbers of CD3+ and CD8+ T-cells and CD68+ microglia/macrophages in demyelinated CNS plaques.[58] Clinical neurological worsening and increased MRI brain lesion load occurred in an allogeneic HSCT recipient with chronic myelogenous leukemia and coincident MS with 100% donor chimerism who developed GVHD.[59] Thus, for MS, allogeneic HSCT must be performed without risk of GVHD, i.e. by using a HSC-enriched and/or lymphocyte-depleted allogeneic graft.

Unlike the relationship between GVL and GVHD, both of which result from donor lymphocytes, in animal models, a graft vs. autoimmune effect appears to be separable from GVHD. NOD (non-obese diabetic) mice develop spontaneous diabetes due to an autoimmune-mediated insulitis. ESCs may be differentiated ex vivo into HSC without differentiation into, or

Table 44.2. *Summary of ongoing Phase 2 and Phase 3 autologous HSCT trials for the treatment of MS*

Study	MIST [57]	ASTIMS [51]	HALT-MS [52]	Canadian MS-BMT [56]
Center	Chicago, Northwestern, Calgary, Canada Ribeirao Preto, Brasil Uppsulla, Sweden	European multicenter	Seattle, FHCRC	Ottawa
MS subtype	RRMS failing IFNβ or Copaxone	Aggressive RR or SPMS	RR or SPMS with relapses failing standard therapy	Active RR or SPMS
Entry EDSS	2.0–6.0	3.5–6.5	3.0–5.5	3.0–6.0
Trial design	Randomized Phase 3	Randomized Phase 2	Phase 2	Phase 2
Control arm	Current FDA approved treatments	Mitoxantrone	None	None
Mobilization regimen	CY+G-CSF	CY+G-CSF	G-CSF	CY+G-CSF
CD34 graft selection	None	None	Baxter isolex	CliniMACS
Conditioning regimen	CY + rATG	BEAM+ rATG	BEAM	BuCY+ rATG
Trial status	Active	Recently closed	Closed to accrual	Closed to accrual

ASTIMS, trial Autologous Stem Cell Transplantation International Multiple Sclerosis sponsored by European Group for Blood and Marrow Transplantation; CY, cyclophosphamide; EDSS, expanded disability status scale; FHCRC, Fred Hutchinson Cancer Research Center; G-CSF = granulocyte colony stimulating factor; HALT-MS, trial of High-Dose Immunosuppression and Autologous Stem Cell Transplantation for Poor Prognosis Multiple Sclerosis sponsored by the Immune Tolerance Network and the National Institutes of Health; IFNβ-interferon beta; MIST, Multiple Sclerosis International Stem Cell Transplant trial; MS multiple sclerosis; rATG, rabbit antithymocyte globulin; RRMS, relapsing remitting MS; SPMS, secondary progressive MS with or without relapses.

contamination with, lymphocytes.[5] In NOD mice, ESC-derived HSC conveyed a GVA effect and reintroduced islet cell tolerance without adverse events such as GVHD. ESC-derived HSC engraftment as low as 5% exerted a profound antidiabetic effect as confirmed by glucose levels, survival, histology, and antigen-specific non-responsiveness to GAD65, a diabetic-specific islet cell antigen.[60] Since the prevention of diabetes did not require the complete replacement of host hematopoietic and immune systems, it appears that the reintroduction of even small numbers of non-diabetic-prone hematopoietic stem cells is capable of favorably modulating impaired mechanisms of tolerance in autoimmune diseases.[60] Future clinical trials would be needed to determine if lymphocyte-depleted allogeneic hematopoietic stem cell transplantation can achieve a favorable graft vs. autoimmune effect without GVHD in MS.

Hematopoietic stem cell transplantation using a composite graft of hematopoietic stem cells and mesenchymal stem cells

Both autologous and allogeneic HSCT require a chemotherapy conditioning regimen to suppress or "ablate" the immune system. However, mesenchymal stem cells (MSCs) have unique regenerative and immune-modulating effects independent of chemotherapy.[61,62] MSCs are defined by their adherence capabilities. When bone marrow is placed in culture, hematopoietic cells float within the medium and are removed with each passage, while MSCs remain adhered to the flask. These adherent MSCs are morphologically heterogeneous and may be spindle-like, polygonal, or cuboidal in shape. MSCs are negative for hematopoietic markers such as CD34 and CD45, positive for

adhesion molecules (CD44, CD62), and generally positive for stem cell antigen-1 (Sca-1), stromal-derived factor-1 (STRO-1) and D105/endoglin.[61–64]

For autoimmune diseases, unlike either autologous HSCT in which immune suppression is a consequence of chemotherapy or allogeneic HSCT in which engraftment with subsequent alteration of genetic susceptibility to disease requires the administration of chemotherapy, MSCs appear to have a direct immunomodulatory effect which occurs independent of any chemotherapeutic drug or cytotoxic agent. Although the exact mechanism(s) is unclear, MSC-mediated immune suppression occurs through both direct cell contact and cytokine secretion.[64] It has been reported that intravenous injection of MSCs can ameliorate EAE, without the use of any chemotherapy or immune-suppressive medications.[62,65,66] In fact, MSCs have already been tested as an immune-modulating agent for the treatment of severe GVHD, successfully salvaging patients with steroid-refractory GVHD with little toxicity.[67] Preliminary human applications using intrathecal and/or intravenous MSC have begun with promising results.[68,69]

Nevertheless, many questions and concerns about MSCs remain unanswered. (1) What are the late complications of MSC infusions? For example, will they lodge in tissue such as the pulmonary vascular bed resulting in local proliferation and differentiation into fibroblasts with late fibrosis? (2) MSC cultured ex vivo develop cytogenetic abnormalities.[70] Can cultured MSCs proliferate in vivo to form tumors when placed outside their normal bone marrow niche? (3) What are the exact mechanisms of MSC-mediated immune suppression? Do MSCs normally suppress immune reactions in vivo or is an immune-suppressive phenotype the consequence of extended passage in tissue culture? (4) Since MSCs are a heterogeneous population of cells, is there a unique identifiable MSC marker? (5) What is the best method to isolate, purify and assay MSCs? (6) Are MSCs true stem cells that can be transplanted, isolated and re-transplanted in serial generations of recipients? (7) Is their immune suppressive effect durable, or will repeated infusions be required? Will immunological sensitization or rejection occur with repeated exposure? (8) Will non-specific MSC-mediated immune suppression lead to increased opportunistic infections? These questions notwithstanding, the application of MSCs for immune modulation may allow MS-directed stem cell therapy that results in favorable immune modulation without exposure to chemotherapy, or the use of combined allogeneic HSC and MSC transplantation for engraftment without GVHD.

Conclusions

The leading indication for autologous HSCT of autoimmune diseases is MS and over 500 patients with MS have undergone this procedure. Clinical studies showed a decrease of disease progression in almost 70% of cases, at least in the first three years of follow-up, and a dramatic reduction of relapses. The MRI studies demonstrated that autologous HSCT has the capacity of a profound and long-lasting suppression of gadolinium-enhancing lesions. New active lesions were rarely detected. Furthermore, the MRI studies showed that the volume of brain atrophy decreased significantly with time after 2–3 years following autologous HSCT.[71,72]

Initial autologous HSCT protocols employed malignancy-specific myeloablative regimens, enrolled predominately late secondary progressive MS, were complicated by some treatment-related deaths, and generally failed to stop continued decline in neurological disability, (increase in EDSS), despite the effective suppression of CNS inflammation. These results helped to clarify the pathogenesis of late progressive MS as predominantly an axonal degenerative disease, and raised questions about the use of any immune-suppressive medication to treat late progressive MS. The current goal of autologous HSCT studies in MS is to intervene earlier in the disease course with safer MS-specific non-myeloablative regimens not only to prevent or delay the onset of progressive neurological disability but also to reverse neurologic deficits. In patients with inflammatory MS defined by frequent active relapses and gadolinium-enhancing lesions on MRI, non-myeloablative HSCT is the only therapy to consistently demonstrate improvement in neurological disability (i.e. lower EDSS score by ≥ 1.0 point) in the majority of patients. The duration of autologous non-myeloablative HSCT-induced MS remission is unknown. The risk of mortality, which is still the main problem of this powerful therapy has significantly dropped with experience and the advent of non-myeloablative regimens.[28,29]

References

1. Wobus AM, Holzhausen H, Jakel P, Schoneich J. Characterization of a pluripotent stem cell line derived from a mouse embryo. *Exp Cell Res* 1984; 152:212–19.

2. Carpenter MK, Rosler E, Rao MS. Characterization and differentiation of human embryonic stem cells. *Cloning Stem Cells* 2003; 5:79–88.

3. Edwards RG. Stem cells today: A. Origin and potential of embryo stem cells. *Reprod Biomed Online* 2004; 8:275–306.

4. Edwards RG. In vitro fertilization: past and future. *Ann Biol Clin* 1987; 45:321–9.

5. Burt RK, Verda L, Kim DA, *et al.* Embryonic stem cells as an alternate marrow donor source: engraftment without graft-versus-host disease. *J Exp Med* 2004; 199:895–904.

6. Zhang S-C, Wernig M, Duncan ID, *et al.* In vitro differentiation of transplantable neural precursors from human embryonic stem cells. *Nat Biotechnol* 2001; 19:1129–33.

7. Reubinoff BE, Itsykson P, Turetsky T, *et al.* Neuralprogenitors from human embryonic stem cells. *Nat Biotechnol* 2001; 19:1134–40.

8. Xian HQ, McNichols E, St Clair A, Gottlieb DI. A subset of ES-cell-derived neural cells marked by gene targeting. *Stem Cells* 2003; 21:41–9.

9. Burt RK, Fassas A, Snowden J, *et al.* Collection of hematopoietic stem cells from patients with autoimmune diseases. *Bone Marrow Transpl* 2001; 28:1–12.

10. Openshaw H, Stuve O, Antel JP, *et al.* Multiple sclerosis flares associated with recombinant granulocyte colonystimulating factor. *Neurology* 2000; 54:2147–50.

11. Verda L, Luo K, Kim DA, *et al.* Effect of hematopoietic growth factors on severity of experimental autoimmune encephalomyelitis. *Bone Marrow Transpl* 2006; 38(6):453–60.

12. Petersen BE, Bowen WC, Patrene KD, *et al.* Bone marrow as a potential source of hepatic oval cells. *Science* 1999; 284:1168–70.

13. Krause DS, Theise ND, Collector MI, *et al.* Multiorgan, multi-lineage engraftment by a single bone marrow-derived stem cell. *Cell* 2001; 105:369–77.

14. Orlic D, Kajstura J, Chimenti S, *et al.* Bone marrow cells regenerate infarcted myocardium. *Nature* 2001; 410: 701–5.

15. Eglitis MA, Mezey E. Hematopoietic cells differentiate into both microglia and macroglia in the brains of adult mice. *Proc Natl Acad Sci USA* 1997; 94:4080–5.

16. Burt RK, Burns W, Hess A. Bone marrow transplantation for multiple sclerosis. *Bone Marrow Transpl* 1995; 16:1–6.

17. Schwartz RH. T cell anergy. *Annu Rev Immunol* 2003; 21:305–34.

18. Muraro PA, Douek DC, Packer A, *et al.* Thymic output generates a new and diverse TCR repertoire after autologous stem cell transplantation in multiple sclerosis patients. *J Exp Med* 2005; 201:805–16.

19. Dubinsky AN, Burt RK, Martin R, Muraro PA. T-cell clones persisting in the circulation after autologous hematopoietic SCT are undetectable in the peripheral CD34+ selected graft.

Bone Marrow Transpl 2010 Feb; 45(2):325–31.

20. Burt RK, Padilla J, Begolka WS, *et al.* Effect of disease stage on clinical outcome after syngeneic bone marrow transplantation for relapsing experimental autoimmune encephalomyelitis. *Blood* 1998; 91:2609–16.

21. Karussis DM, Slavin S, Lehmann D, *et al.* Prevention of experimental autoimmune encephalomyelitis and induction of tolerance with acute immunosuppression followed by syngeneic bone marrow transplantation. *J Immunol* 1992; 148:1693–8.

22. van Gelder M, van Bekkum DW. Effective treatment of relapsing experimental autoimmune encephalomyelitis with pseudoautologous bone marrow transplantation. *Bone Marrow Transpl* 1996; 18:1029–34.

23. van GelderM, Mulder AH, van Bekkum DW. Treatment of relapsing experimental autoimmune encephalomyelitis with largely MHC-mismatched allogeneic bone marrow transplantation. *Transplantation* 1996; 62:810–18.

24. Karussis DM, Vourka-Karussis U, Lehmann D, *et al.* Prevention and reversal of adoptively transferred, chronic relapsing experimental autoimmune encephalomyelitis with a single high-dose cytoreductive treatment followed by syngeneic bone marrow transplantation. *J Clin Invest* 1993; 92:765–72.

25. van Gelder M, Kinwel-Bohré EP, van Bekkum DW. Treatment of experimental allergic encephalomyelitis in rats with total body irradiation and syngeneic BMT. *Bone Marrow Transpl* 1993; 11:233–41.

26. Miller SD, Vanderlugt CL, Begolka WS, *et al.* Persistent infection with Theiler's virus leads to CNS autoimmunity via epitope spreading. *Nat Med* 1997; 3:1133–6.

27. Burt RK, Padilla J, Dal Canto MC, Miller SD. Viral hyperinfection of the central nervous system and high mortality after hematopoietic stem cell transplantation for treatment of Theiler's murine encephalomyelitis virus-induced demyelinating disease. *Blood* 1999; 94:2915–22.

28. Burt RK, Abinun M, Farge-Bancel D, *et al.* Risks of immune system treatments. *Science* 2010; 328(5980):825–6.

29. Burt RK, Loh Y, Pearce W, Clinical applications of blood-derived and marrow-derived stem cells for nonmalignant diseases. *J Am Med Assoc* 2008 Feb 27; 299(8):925–36.

30. Monje ML, Mizumatsu S, Fike JR, *et al.* Irradiation induces neural precursor-cell dysfunction. *Nat Med* 2002; 8:955–62.

31. Loh Y, Oyama Y, Statkute L, *et al.* Development of a secondary autoimmune disorder after hematopoietic stem cell transplantation for autoimmune diseases: role of conditioning regimen used. *Blood* 2007 Mar 15; 109(6):2643–8.

32. Fassas A, Anagnostopoulos A, Kazis A, *et al.* Autologous stem cell transplantation in progressive multiple sclerosis – an interim analysis of efficacy. *J Clin Immunol* 2000; 20:24–30.

33. Kozak T, Havrdova E, Pit'ha J, *et al.* Immunoablative therapy with autologous stem cell transplantation in the treatment of poor risk multiple sclerosis. *Transplant Proc* 2001; 33:2179–81.

34. Saiz A, Blanco Y, Carreras E, *et al.* Clinical and MRI outcome after autologous hematopoietic stem cell transplantation in MS. *Neurology* 2004; 62:282–4.

35. Saiz A, Blanco Y, Berenguer J, *et al.* Clinical outcome 6 years after autologous hematopoietic stem cell transplantation in multiple sclerosis. *Neurologia* 2008 Sep; 23(7):405–7.

36. Mancardi GL, Saccardi R, Filippi M, *et al.* Autologous hematopoietic stem cell transplantation suppresses Gd enhanced MRI activity in MS. *Neurology* 2001; 57:62–8.

37. Burt RK, Cohen BA, Russell E, *et al.* Hematopoietic stem cell transplantation for progressive multiple sclerosis: failure of a total body irradiation-based conditioning regimen to prevent disease progression in patients with high disability scores. *Blood* 2003; 102:2373–8.

38. Nash RA, Bowen JD, McSweeney PA, *et al.* High-dose immunosuppressive therapy and autologous peripheral blood stem cell transplantation for severe multiple sclerosis. *Blood* 2003; 102:2364–72.

39. Openshaw H, Lund BT, Kashyap A, *et al.* Peripheral blood stem cell transplantation in multiple sclerosis with busulfan and cyclophosphamide conditioning: report of toxicity and immunological monitoring. *Biol Blood Marrow Transpl* 2000; 6:563–75.

40. Fassas A, Passweg JR, Anagnostopoulos A, *et al.* Hematopoietic stem cell transplantation for multiple sclerosis. A retrospective multi-center study. *J Neurol* 2002; 249:1088–97.

41. Saccardi R, Kozak T, Bocelli-Tyndall C, *et al.* Autoimmune Diseases Working Party of EBMT. Autologous stem cell transplantation for progressive multiple sclerosis: update of the European Group for Blood and Marrow Transplantation autoimmune diseases working party database. *Mult Scler* 2006; 12(6):814–23.

42. Su L, Xu J, Ji BX, *et al.* Autologous peripheral blood stem cell transplantation for severe multiple sclerosis. *Int J Hematol* 2006; 84(3):276–81.

43. Xu J, Ji BX, Su L, *et al.* Clinical outcomes after autologous haematopoietic stem cell transplantation in patients with progressive multiple sclerosis. *Chin Med J (Engl)* 2006; 119(22):1851–5.

44. Ni XS, Ouyang J, Zhu WH, Wang C, Chen B. Autologous hematopoietic stem celltransplantation for progressive multiple sclerosis: report of efficacy and safety at three yr of follow up in 21 patients. *Clin Transpl* 2006; 20(4):485–9.

45. Samijn JPA, te Boekhurst PAW, Mondria T, *et al.* Intense T cell depletion followed by autologous bone marrow transplantation for severe multiple sclerosis. *J Neurol Neurosurg Psychiatry* 2006; 77:46–50.

46. Shevchenko YL, Novik AA, Kuznetsov AN, *et al* High-dose immunosuppressive therapy with autologous hematopoietic stem cell transplantation as a treatment option in multiple sclerosis. *Exp Hematol* 2008; 36(8):922–8.

47. Fagius J, Lundgren J, Oberg G. Early highly aggressive MS successfully treated by hematopoietic stem cell transplantation. *Mult Scler* 2009; 15(2):229–37.

48. Burt RK, Loh Y, Cohen B, *et al.*
Autologous non-myeloablative
haemopoietic stem cell transplantation
in relapsing-remitting multiple
sclerosis: a phase I/II study. *Lancet
Neurol.* 2009; 8(3):244–53. Epub 2009
Jan 29. Erratum in: *Lancet Neurol.*
2009;8(4):309.

49. Hamerschlak N, Rodrigues M, Moraes
DA, *et al.* Brazilian experience with two
conditioning regimens in patients with
multiple sclerosis: BEAM/horse ATG
and CY/rabbit ATG. *Bone Marrow
Transpl* 2010; 45(2):239–48.

50. Fassas A, Anagnostopoulos A, Kazis A,
et al. Peripheral blood stem cell
transplantation in the treatment of
progressive multiple sclerosis: first
results of a pilot study. *Bone Marrow
Transpl* 1997; 20(8):631–8.

51. ASTI MS (Autologous Stem cell
Transplantation International Multiple
Sclerosis). Available from: http://www.
astims.org.

52. HALT-MS (High Dose
Immunosuppression and Autologous
Stem Cell Transplantation for Poor
Prognosis Multiple Sclerosis). Available
from: http://www.halt-ms.org and
www.clinicaltrials.gov/ct21/show/
record/NCT00288626.

53. Freedman MS, Atkins HL. Suppressing
immunity in advancing MS: too much
too late, or too late for much? *Neurology*
2004; 62(2):168–9.

54. Mancardi GL, Murialdo A, Rossi P,
et al. Autologous stem cell
transplantation as rescue therapy in
malignant forms of multiple sclerosis.
Mult Scler 2005; 11(3):367–71.

55. Saccardi R, Mancardi GL, Solari A,
et al. Autologous HSCT for severe
progressive multiple sclerosis in a
multicenter trial: impact on disease
activity and quality of life. *Blood* 2005;
105:2601–7.

56. Autologous Stem Cell Transplant for
Multiple Sclerosis (MS/BMT). Available
from: http://www.halt-ms.org and
www.clinicaltrials.gov/ct21/show/
record/ NCT01099930.

57. Multiple Sclerosis International Stem
Cell Transplant trial (MIST). Available
from: http://www.clinicaltrials.gov
(NCT00273364).

58. Lu JQ, Joseph JT, Nash RA *et al.*
Neuroinflammation and demyelination
in multiple sclerosis after allogeneic
hematopoietic stem cell
transplantation. *Arch Neurol* 2010;
67(6):716–22.

59. Lu JQ, Storek J, Metz L, *et al.*
Continued disease activity in a patient
with multiple sclerosis after allogeneic
hematopoietic cell transplantation.
Arch Neurol. 2009; 66(1):116–20.

60. Verda L, Kim DA, Ikehara S, *et al.*
Hematopoietic mixed chimerism
derived from allogeneic embryonic
stem cells prevents autoimmune
diabetes mellitus in NOD mice. *Stem
Cells* 2008; 26(2):381–6.

61. Di Nicola M, Carlo-Stella C, Magni M,
et al. Human bone marrow stromal
cells suppress T-lymphocyte
proliferation induced by cellular or
nonspecific mitogenic stimuli. *Blood*
2002; 99:3838–43.

62. Zappia E, Casazza S, Pedemonte E,
et al. Mesenchymal stem cells
ameliorate experimental autoimmune
encephalomyelitis inducing T-cell
anergy. *Blood* 2005; 106:1755–61.

63. Aggarwal S, Pittenger MF. Human
mesenchymal stem cells modulate
allogeneic immune cell responses.
Blood 2005; 105:1815–22.

64. Zhao RC, Liao L, Han Q. Mechanisms
of and perspectives on the
mesenchymal stem cells in
immunotherapy. *J Lab Clin Med* 2003;
143:284–91.

65. Bai L, Lennon DP, Eaton V, *et al.*
Human bone marrow-derived
mesenchymal stem cells induce
Th2-polarized immune response and
promote endogenous repair in animal
models of multiple sclerosis. *Glia* 2009;
57:1192–203.

66. Rafei M, Birman E, Forner K, Galipeau
J. Allogeneic mesenchymal stem cells
for treatment of experimental
autoimmune encephalomyelitis. *Mol
Ther* 2009; 17:1799–803.

67. Le Blanc K, Frassoni F, Ball L, *et al.*
Mesenchymal stem cells for treatment
of steroidresistant, severe, acute
graft-versus-host disease: a phase II
study. *Lancet* 2008; 371:1579–86.

68. Liang J, Zhang H, Hua B, *et al.*
Allogeneic mesenchymal stem cells
transplantation in treatment of multiple
sclerosis. *Mult Scler* 2009; 15:644–6.

69. Mohyeddin Bonab M, Yazdanbakhsh S,
et al. Does mesenchymal stem cell
therapy help multiple sclerosis patients?
Report of a pilot study. *Iran J Immunol*
2007; 4:50–7.

70. Josse C, Schoemans R, Niessen NA,
et al. Systematic chromosomal
aberrations found in murine bone
marrow-derived mesenchymal stem
cells. *Stem Cells Dev* 2010;
19(8):1167–73.

71. Chen JT, Collins DL, Atkins HL, *et al*;
Canadian MS BMT Study Group. Brain
atrophy after immunoablation and stem
cell transplantation in multiple
sclerosis. *Neurology* 2006;66(12):
1935–7.

72. Roccatagliata L, Rocca M, Valsasina P
et al. Italian GITMO-NEURO
Intergroup on Autologous Stem Cell
Transplantation. The long-term effect of
AHSCT on MRI measures of MS
evolution: a five-year follow-up study.
Mult Scler 2007; 13(8):1068–70.

Chapter

45

Mesenchymal stem cell transplantation to treat multiple sclerosis

Don Mahad, Sarah M. Planchon, and Jeffrey A. Cohen

Introduction

As outlined in Chapters 1–5, multiple sclerosis (MS) pathogenesis is multifactorial, resulting in multifocal central nervous system (CNS) lesions with varying perivenular inflammation, demyelination, axonal transection, neuronal degeneration, and gliosis in both white and gray matter. Inflammatory mechanisms predominate in early disease, reflected most directly in relapses and magnetic resonance imaging (MRI) focal lesion activity, but gradual worsening in primary progressive and late secondary progressive MS may be due to neurodegeneration. Also, although intrinsic repair processes exist in MS, they do not sufficiently compensate for ongoing damage in most patients. Currently approved MS treatments primarily reduce CNS inflammation. Treatment strategies to prevent tissue damage and/or augment both remyelination and axonal regeneration are greatly needed.

Transplantation of several types of stem cells has been considered as a way to augment repair. As outlined in Table 45.1, each cell type has potential advantages and disadvantages. Embryonic stem cells, neural stem cells, and induced pluripotent stem cells are not appropriate for extensive human testing as yet. In contrast, the immunomodulatory, tissue protective, and repair-promoting properties of mesenchymal stem cells (MSCs) make them an attractive candidate therapy to test now to address the multifactorial pathologic processes in MS.

Overview of mesenchymal stem cells

Stromal cells in the bone marrow (BM) connective tissue provide scaffolding and cytokines/growth factors essential for normal hematopoiesis.[1] Besides hematopoietic stem cells (HSCs), the BM microenvironment contains pluripotent non-hematopoietic precursor cells that generate stromal cells. These precursor cells can be isolated and culture expanded to purity from BM aspirates from animals and humans and induced to differentiate in vitro and in vivo into mesodermal derivatives, including osteoblasts, chondrocytes, adipocytes, and myocytes.[2,3] Therefore, these cells are referred as multipotent stromal cells or mesenchymal stem cells (MSCs). MSCs with similar properties exist in a variety of other tissues, including adipose tissue, peripheral and umbilical cord blood, placenta,

Table 45.1. *Potential cell sources for neural repair*

Embryonic stem cells
Source: inner cell mass of blastocyst-stage embryos
Advantages: indefinite self-renewal capacity, pluripotency (ability to generate all tissues)
Disadvantages: practical and ethical issues, lack of protocols to direct in vivo differentiation and avoid teratocarcinoma formation
Neural stem/precursor cells
Source: embryonic, fetal, neonatal, or adult CNS
Advantages: culture conditions can be manipulated to promote proliferation or differentiation, multipotent (potentially able to differentiate into neurons, astrocytes, or oligodendrocytes)
Disadvantages: practical and ethical issues, limited proliferation capacity, protocols to direct/maintain differentiation in vivo are lacking
Induced pluripotent stem cells (iPSCs)
Source: genetic reprogramming to dedifferentiate then redifferentiate adult somatic cells
Advantages, adult autologous cells, pluripotent
Disadvantages: highly manipulated, clinical protocols do not yet exist
Mesenchymal stem cells
Source: stromal cells that can be isolated from many adult tissues
Advantages: can be isolated from adult tissues and cultured to purity in high numbers; immunomodulatory, tissue-protective, and repair-promoting properties, immuno-privileged, can be administered peripherally (i.v.) and seek areas of damage and/or inflammation, significant clinical experience exists
Disadvantages: finite proliferative capacity, significant neural transdifferentiation is unlikely

amniotic fluid, fetal tissues, synovial membrane, and deciduous teeth, but BM MSCs are the best characterized. It recently was postulated that the normal MSC niche is the perivascular space, that MSC correspond to pericytes, and their normal function is to maintain vascular and immunologic homeostasis and facilitate tissue repair.[4]

No single marker or combination specifically defines MSCs. Minimal criteria listed in Table 45.2 were proposed by the Mesenchymal and Tissue Stem Cell Committee of the International Society for Cellular Therapy.[5] A number of studies have phenotypically characterized MSCs.[2,8–15] A partial list of the large

---

Multiple Sclerosis Therapeutics, Fourth Edition, ed. Jeffrey A. Cohen and Richard A. Rudick. Published by Cambridge University Press.
© Cambridge University Press 2011.

Table 45.2. *Minimal criteria for MSC proposed by the Mesenchymal and Tissue Stem Cell Committee of the International Society for Cellular Therapy*[5]

- Plastic adherent under standard culture conditions.
- Positive for CD105 (SH2, endoglin)[6] and CD73 (SH3 and SH4, ecto-5'-nucleotidase).[7]
- Negative for hematopoietic surface markers CD34 (primitive hematopoietic progenitors and endothelial cells), CD45 (leukocyte common antigen, pan-leukocyte), CD14 (lipopolysaccharide receptor) or CD11b (Mac-1, monocytes and macrophages), CD79α or CD19 (B-cells), and MHC class II (except after IFNγ stimulation).
- Multipotent differentiation potential in vitro: osteoblasts (demonstrated by Alizarin Red or von Kossa staining), adipocytes (demonstrated by Oil Red O staining), and chondroblasts (demonstrated by Alcian Blue staining or immunohistochemistry for collagen type II).
- Extensively passaged cells should be karyotyped.

IFN = interferon, MHC = major histocompatibility.

Table 45.3. *Phenotypic characterization MSCs. A partial list of markers reported to be expressed by MSCs includes*[2,6,8–16]

- Surface markers
  - Positive: CD105 (SH2, endoglin), CD73 (SH3 and SH4, ecto-5'-nucleotidase).
  - Negative for hematopoietic markers: CD34 (primitive hematopoietic progenitors and endothelial cells), CD45 (leukocyte common antigen, pan-leukocyte), CD14 (lipopolysaccharide receptor) or CD11b (Mac-1) (monocytes and macrophages), CD79α or CD19 (B-cells), and MHC class II (except after IFNγ stimulation).
- Adhesion molecules
  - Positive: CD166 (ALCAM), CD54 (ICAM-1), CD102 (ICAM-2), CD50 (ICAM-3), CD62L (L-selectin), CD58 (LFA-3), CD56 (NCAM), CD44 (HCAM), CD106 (VCAM), CD44 (hyaluronate receptor, Hermes antigen).
  - Negative: CD62E (E-selectin), CD62P (P-selectin), CD144 (cadherin), CD31 (PECAM-1).
- Integrins
  - Positive: CD49a (VLA-α1), CD49b (VLA-α2), CD49c (VLA-α3), CD49e (VLA-α5), CD49f (VLA-α6), CD29 (VLA-β), CD104 (β4 integrin), CD61 (vitronectin R β chain).
  - Negative: CD49d (VLA-α4), CD11a (LFA-1 α chain), CD18 (LFA-1 β chain), CD 51 (vitronectin R α chain), CD11c (CR4 α chain).
- Growth factor and cytokine receptors
  - Positive: CD121 (IL-1R), CD123 (IL-3R), CD124 (IL-4R), CD126 (IL-6R), CD127 (IL-7R), CDw119 (IFNγ R), CD120a (TNFα-1R), CD120b (TNFα-2R), FGFR, CD140a (PDGFR), CD71 (transferrinR).
  - Negative: CD25 (IL-2R), CD40 (nerve growth factor receptor),
- Growth factors and cytokines
  - Expressed in culture without induction: IL-6, IL-7, IL-8, IL-11, IL-12, IL-14, IL-15, LIF, M-CSF, Flt-3 ligand, SCF, PGE2, VEGF.
  - Induced by IL-1: IL-1, IL-1β, IL-6, IL-8, IL-11, G-CSF, GM-CSF, LIF.
  - Induced by ischemic rat brain extract: BDNF, NGF, VEGF, HGF.
  - Not expressed: IL-2, IL-3, IL-4, IL-10, IL-13.
- Miscellaneous
  - MHC class I expressed
  - MHC class II induced by IFNγ in some experiments
  - Negative: CD1a (T6), CD3, CD4, CD8, CD15 (LewisX), CD80 (B7–1), CD83 (HB-15), CD86 (B7–2), CD133.

ALCAM = activated leukocyte cell adhesion molecule, BDNF = brain-derived neurotrophic factor, FGFR = fibroblast growth factor receptor, G-CSF = granulocyte colony stimulating factor, HCAM = homing cell adhesion molecule, HGF = hepatocyte growth factor), ICAM = intercellular cell-adhesion molecule, IFN = interferon, IL = interleukin, IL-2R = IL-2 receptor, LFA = lymphocyte function-associated antigen, LIF = leukocyte inhibitory factor, M-CSF = macrophage colony stimulating factor, MHC = major histocompatibility complex, NCAM = neural cell adhesion molecule, NGF = nerve growth factor, PDGFR = platelet derived growth factor receptor, PECAM = platelet endothelial cell adhesion molecule, PGE = prostaglandin E, SCF = stem cell factor, TNF = tumor necrosis factor, VCAM = vascular cell adhesion molecule, VEGF = vascular endothelial growth factor, VLA = very late antigen.

number of markers expressed by MSCs and factors produced by them are summarized in Table 45.3.

In vitro immune effects of MSCs

The potent immunomodulatory properties of MSCs are particularly relevant for MS.[12,17,18] They inhibit both innate and adaptive immunity, including a variety of potent immunosuppressive effects on T-cells, natural killer (NK) cells, B-cells, and antigen-presenting cells. Whether MSCs play a role in normal immune regulation is unknown. A wide variety of in vitro immune effects have been described.

Effects on T-cells

MSCs inhibit T-cell proliferation stimulated by polyclonal activators (e.g. concanavalin A, phytohemagglutinin, Protein A, interleukin-2 (IL-2), anti-CD3, and anti-CD28),[11,19–26] cognate antigen,[25,27,28] and allogeneic mixed lymphocyte reaction.[19–23,29,30] Both primary and secondary T-cell responses are affected. There is some selectivity as cellular responses to alloantigens but not recall antigens are targeted. MSCs inhibit proliferation of both CD4+ and CD8+ T-cells.[20,24,28]

The precise mechanism of MSC inhibition of T-cell activation is unclear, but MSC-derived soluble factors,[20,23–25,27] cell-contact,[27] and indirect effects through other cells including CD8+ regulatory cells[23] or antigen-presenting cells[31] have been implicated. Proposed MSC-derived soluble factors include inoleamine-2,3-dioxygenase, transforming growth factor-β, hepatic growth factor, nitric oxide, and soluble HLA-G.[20–25,27,32–34] The inhibition of proliferation has features of anergy in some studies[25] but not others,[28] and is not due to T-cell apoptosis.[20] In addition to reduced proliferation, T-cell production of interferon-gamma (IFNγ) and tumor necrosis factor-alpha (TNFα) are inhibited, and production of IL-4 is stimulated.[11,28,35] Recent studies confirmed in vitro inhibition by MSC supernatants of Th1 T-cell proliferation and production of the Th1 cytokine IFNγ but, surprisingly, showed stimulation of Th17 proliferation and production of IL-17A.[26] Thus,

in vivo, MSC transplantation could have both pro- and anti-inflammatory effects in MS.

Effects on B-cells

MSCs inhibit B-cell proliferation in culture[28,36] via soluble factors,[36] accompanied by inhibition of B-cell differentiation and production of IgM, IgG, and IgA.[36] MSCs inhibit B-cell expression in culture of CXCR4, CXCR5, and CCR7 and chemotaxis to CXCL12 (CXCR4 ligand) and CCL13 (CXCR5 ligand).[36] However, in one study,[37] MSCs from normal donors co-cultured with purified B-cells from healthy donors or patients with pediatric systemic lupus erythematosis stimulated proliferation and differentiation into immunoglobulin-secreting cells, and strongly enhanced differentiation of memory B-cells into plasma cells. This finding suggests caution using MSC to treat autoimmune disorders involving B-cells in pathogenesis, such as MS.

Effects on natural killer cells

MSCs inhibit IL-2-induced proliferation[38] and IFNγ production[11] by resting natural killer (NK) cells. Activated NK cells are affected to a lesser extent.[38] MSCs do not inhibit NK cell lysis of K562 tumor cells.[32]

Effects on antigen-presenting cells

Some of the inhibitory effects of MSCs on T-cell responses are mediated by contact-dependent induction of IL-10 production by antigen-presenting cells.[11,31] In addition, MSCs reversibly inhibit the differentiation and function of monocyte-derived dendritic cells, including morphologic change, expression of CD83, major histocompatibility complex (MHC) class I and class II expression, expression of co-stimulatory molecules (CD80 and CD86), and secretion of IL-12 and TNFα.[11,39,40] The overall net effect is to impair ability to present antigen.

In vivo immunomodulatory effects of MSCs

MSCs prolong survival of transplanted allogeneic/xenogeneic tumor cells in mice[23] and skin grafts in baboons.[19] In MRL/lpr mice with a spontaneous autoimmune disease resembling systemic lupus erythematosis, transplantation of BM cells and bone (as a source of stromal cells) prevented development of lymphadenopathy, nephritis, arthritis, circulating immune complexes, and abnormal T-cells.[41] Of particular relevance to MS, in acute[25] and chronic[35,42–44] experimental autoimmune encephalomyelitis (EAE) mice, intravenous (i.v.) MSC administration ameliorated clinical manifestations, central nervous system (CNS) inflammatory infiltrates, demyelination, and axonal damage. In some studies, donor cells were identified in recipient CNS, particularly in inflammatory demyelinated areas.[42–44] Increased brain-derived neurotrophic factor (BDNF) production by CNS cells was demonstrated in transplanted animals, suggesting the possibility of a neuroprotective/reparative effect. In other studies, very few donor MSCs were detected in recipient CNS.[25,35] The majority of transplanted MSCs trafficked to lymph nodes and spleen, and the clinical and pathological benefit appeared to be mediated by inhibition of peripheral encephalitogenic T-cells, as also was proposed for neurospheres in EAE.[45]

MSCs are immunopriviledged

MSCs are minimally immunogenic. In vitro, they do not stimulate proliferation or IFNγ production by allogeneic T-cells.[21,22,27,29,31,46] They are not lysed and do not induce production of IFNγ or TNFα by allogeneic cytotoxic T-cells.[32,47] In vivo, allogeneic and xenogeneic MSCs are not rejected in mice.[23] Numerous studies demonstrate that allogeneic MSCs are not rejected in humans (see Table 45.4). This property allows for use of universal donor allogeneic culture-expanded MSCs, the approach taken by several companies developing MSCs as therapy. Use of MSCs as an "off-the-shelf" reagent is expected to improve convenience and allow purified MSCs to be use to treat acute conditions, e.g. acute myocardial infarction or MS relapse. In addition, this approach could address the theoretical concern that, due to an underlying disease or its treatment, autologous MSCs could have "defective" immunomodulatory, tissue protective, or reparative properties.

Neural repair potential of MSCs

The other property of MSCs relevant to MS is their potential ability to lessen damage and augment repair in numerous tissue injury models. Experimental rodent stroke is the most-studied animal model of the neural repair potential of MSCs. Several general points can be concluded from these studies.[102–108] MSCs were effective when administered by various routes, including direct tissue, intraventricular, intra-arterial, and i.v. injection. Importantly, MSCs were capable of entering the CNS from the blood, survived in host tissue, migrated along fiber tracts, and preferentially accumulated in the area of damage or inflammation. Although some transplanted cells transdifferentiated into neuron- and glial-like cells, the number was very small and the cells maintained primitive morphology. Thus, transdifferentiation, neurogenesis, and integration probably were not the major mechanisms of improved functional recovery. Rather, the rapidity of the observed improvement, small number of transplanted MSCs in the CNS, and very small percentage with neuronal or glial features suggest that the benefit was due to neuroprotection, trophic effects, enhanced endogenous repair mechanisms, and/or angiogenesis mediated by elaboration of cytokines and growth factors, which would serve to magnify the benefit of the small number of cells getting into damaged tissue. For example, in culture MSCs promote neuronal or oligodendrocytic differentiation of neural stem cells via soluble factors.[109,110]

Benefit of MSC transplantation also was shown in other animal models of neural injury, including focal spinal cord demyelination produced by X-irradiation then ethidium bromide injection,[111] sciatic nerve transection,[112] SOD-G93A mouse model of amyotrophic lateral sclerosis,[113,114] MPTP-induced parkinsonism,[115] Huntington's disease model induced by striatal injection of quinolinic acid,[116] cerebral contusion,[117,118] and spinal cord contusion.[119–121] Many other animal tissue injury models also have been studied showing benefit, including acute and chronic myocardial infarction,[122–129] bleomycin- or endotoxin-induced acute lung injury,[130–132] ischemia/reperfusion- and cisplatin-induced acute renal injury,[133–136] acute and chronic hepatic failure,[137,138] articular cartilage injury,[139] ovariectomy-induced osteoporosis,[140] chemical corneal wound,[141] streptozocin- or alloxan-induced diabetes,[142] chemotherapy-induced ovarian

Table 45.4. *Published studies of MSC transplantation in conditions other than MS. Unless otherwise noted, MSCs were isolated from bone marrow and administered i.v.*

Reference	Indication	Patients	MSC Source
48	Hematologic malignancy	23	Autologous cultured MSCs
49	Breast cancer	32	Autologous cultured MSCs and PBSCs
50	Acute myelogenous leukemia	1	Allogeneic cultured MSCs and PBSCs
51	Acute leukemia	15	Haploidentical parental cultured MSCs and unrelated donor umbilical cord blood
52	Leukemia in remission	27	Allogeneic cultured MSCs and haploidentical HSCs
53	GVHD	31	Allogeneic cultured MSCs and HSCs
54	GVHD	1	Allogeneic cultured MSCs
55	GVHD	8	Allogeneic cultured MSCs
56	GVHD	10	Allogeneic cultured MSCs
57	GVHD	1	Allogeneic cultured MSCs
58	GVHD	55	Allogeneic cultured MSCs
59	GVHD	32	Universal donor allogeneic cultured MSCs
60	GVHD	12	Universal donor allogeneic cultured MSCs
61	GVHD	4	Allogeneic cultured MSCs administered intra-BM
62	GVHD	3	Allogeneic cultured MSCs administered by regional intra-arterial injection
63	Aplastic anemia	1	Allogeneic cultured MSCs
64	Acute myocardial infarction	20	Autologous BM or blood progenitor cells
65	Acute myocardial infarction	10	Autologous BM aspirate
66	Acute myocardial infarction	6	Autologous cultured MSCs
67	Acute myocardial infarction	35	Autologous percoll gradient purified MSCs
68	Acute myocardial infarction	11	Autologous ficoll gradient/plastic adherence purified MSCs
69	Acute myocardial infarction	39	Universal donor allogeneic cultured MSCs
70	Refractory angina pectoris	8	Autologous BM aspirate
71	Refractory angina pectoris	10	Autologous cultured MSCs and fresh gradient-purified BM MNCs
72	Peripheral arterial disease with limb ischemia	22	Autologous BM aspirate
73	Peripheral arterial disease with limb ischemia	10	Autologous cultured MSCs and fresh gradient-purified BM MNCs
74	Systemic sclerosis with limb ischemia	1	Autologous cultured MSCs
75	Thromboangiitis obliterans	8	Fresh autologous BM cells
76	Non-healing skin ulcer	3	Autologous BM aspirate and cultured adherent cells
77	Non-healing skin ulcer	12	Autologous cultured MSCs
78	Non-healing bone fracture	3	Autologous cultured MSCs
79	Cartilage defects in osteoarthritis	24	Autologous cultured MSCs in collagen gel
80	Infantile hypophosphatemia	1	Allogeneic HSCs and bone fragments
81	Infantile hypophosphatemia	1	HSCs and BM stromal cells
82,83,84	Osteogenesis imperfecta	9	Allogeneic cultured MSCs
85	Lysosomal or peroxisomal disorders	11	Allogeneic cultured MSCs
80	Hunter syndrome	1	Allogeneic HSC and bone fragments
86	End-stage hepatic cirrhosis	8	Autologous cultured MSCs administered into peripheral or portal vein
87	Crohn's disease	10	Autologous cultured MSCs
80	Childhood systemic vasculitis	1	Allogeneic HSCs and bone fragments
88	Systemic lupus erythematosus	16	Allogeneic cultured umbilical cord derived MSCs
89	Systemic lupus erythematosus	15	Allogeneic cultured MSCs

(cont.)

Table 45.4. (cont.)

Reference	Indication	Patients	MSC Source
90	Acute stroke	5	Autologous cultured MSCs
91	Acute stroke	16	Autologous cultured MSCs
92	Traumatic spinal cord injury	2	Autologous MSCs and autologous myelin autoreactive T-cells
43,93	Traumatic spinal cord injury	3	Autologous cultured MSCs administered i.v. and i.t.
94	Traumatic spinal cord injury	30	Autologous cultured MSCs administered i.t.
95	Traumatic spinal cord injury	44	Autologous cultured MSCs administered i.t. monthly X6
96	Traumatic cerebral injury	7	Autologous cultured MSCs administered i.v. and i.t.
97,98	Amyotrophic lateral sclerosis	9	Autologous cultured MSCs
99	Amyotrophic lateral sclerosis	10	Autologous cultured MSCs administered into the spinal cord
100	Amyotrophic lateral sclerosis	19	Autologous cultured MSCs i.v. and i.t.
43,93	Multisystem atrophy	1	Autologous cultured MSCs administered i.v. and i.t.
101	Parkinson's disease	7	Autologous cultured MSCs administered by stereotaxic surgery into the sublateral ventricular zone

BM = bone marrow, GVHD = graft vs. host disease, HSC = hematopoietic stem cell, i.t. = intrathecal, i.v. = intravenous, MNC = mononuclear cell, MSC = mesenchymal stem cell, PBSC = peripheral blood stem cell.

failure,[143] radiation sickness,[144] and a transgenic mouse model of osteogenesis imperfecta.[145] The wide range of tissue injury models in which MSCs are effective further supports the hypothesis that they promote intrinsic repair mechanisms rather than differentiating into and directly replacing cellular elements.

Trafficking of MSCs after i.v. administration

After i.v. administration in rodents and primates, MSCs have been shown by a variety of tracking techniques to distribute widely to normal tissues, predominantly lung but also liver, kidney, bone, skeletal muscle, heart, spleen, lymph node, thymus, and BM.[117,118,145–153] MSCs have prominent ability to home from the blood to sites of tissue injury and inflammation, including in chronic cardiac rejection,[151] localized prostatic inflammation,[154] stroke,[148] traumatic brain injury,[117,118] demyelinated spinal cord lesions,[155] intracranial glioma xenografts,[156] and multiple tissues affected by acute radiation sickness.[144] In chronic murine EAE, labeled MSCs were detected in CNS in proportion to the degree of inflammation.[42,43] However, in other studies of murine EAE, labeled MSCs were detected in lymph node and spleen after i.v. administration but not brain parenchyma,[25,35] suggesting the beneficial effects of MSCs occurred via peripheral immune mechanisms. The factors that attract MSCs to areas of tissue injury or inflammation and the mechanisms by which they enter these tissues are poorly understood.

Donor MSCs are difficult to detect in human recipient tissues after transplantation, and long-term engraftment was not demonstrated in most studies. BM-derived MSCs remained host-derived in 13 patients 1–14 yrs after allogeneic hematopoietic stem cell (HSC) transplantation for lysosomal or peroxisomal disease despite complete donor hematopoietic engraftment.[157] In three children with osteogenesis imperfecta transplanted with unmanipulated allogeneic BM cells, donor osteoblasts subsequently were demonstrated.[82] Six children with osteogenesis imperfecta were transplanted with allogeneic MSCs transfected with the neomycin phosphotransferase gene (NeoR).[83] Five of six patients subsequently showed engraftment in one or more sites, including bone, skin, and marrow stroma. In nine patients with graft vs. host disease (GVHD) treated with allogeneic MSCs, donor DNA was detected in one patient in colon and lymph node.[55] Donor DNA was not detected in multiple organs in two patients. In general, the extent and duration of survival of donor MSCs after transplantation in humans is unknown.

Factors affecting the characteristics of isolated MSCs

It is unclear whether MSCs isolated from patients with disease are normal, as studies have yielded conflicting results. MSCs from patients with aplastic anemia,[158] advanced osteoarthritis,[159] and connective tissue diseases[160,161] had altered proliferation and/or function. In contrast, in two studies, MSCs from patients with systemic lupus erythematosis, rheumatoid arthritis, systemic sclerosis, Sjogren's syndrome, polymyalgia rheumatic, or diabetes had similar surface phenotype, plaque-forming ability, differentiation capacity, ability to support hematopoiesis, and immunomodulatory properties as control MSCs, with no apparent effect of disease activity or immunosuppressant therapy.[162,163] BM stromal cells from 15 MS patients supported hematopoiesis normally, with no effect of recent interferon-beta treatment.[164] MSCs from five MS patients had similar proliferation, differentiation potential, and cell surface antigen expression as five healthy

Table 45.5. *Published studies of mesenchymal stem cell transplantation in multiple sclerosis. Unless otherwise noted, MSCs were isolated from bone marrow and administered i.v.*

Reference	Indication	Patients	MSC source
171	Chronic MS	6	Fresh BM cells enriched for MSCs
172	Treatment-refractory MS	3	Autologous non-expanded adipose MSCs
173	PP MS	1	Allogeneic umbilical cord MSCs administered i.v. and i.t. after cyclophosphamide
174	MS	24	Autologous cultured MSCs
175	Treatment-refractory MS	10	Autologous cultured MSCs administered i.t.
176	Advanced MS	7	Autologous cultured MSCs administered i.t.
100	RR, SP, PP MS	15	Autologous cultured MSCs administered i.v. and i.t.

BM = bone marrow, i.t. = intrathecal, i.v. = intravenous, MS = multiple sclerosis, MSC = mesenchymal stem cell, PP = primary progressive, RR = relapsing–remitting, SP = secondary progressive.

donors.[165] MSCs isolated from 10 MS patients had similar proliferation, differentiation capacity, toll-like receptor expression, immunomodulatory actions, ability to inhibit dendritic cell differentiation and activation, but significantly greater lipopolysaccharide stimulated IP10 production compared to six healthy controls.[166] It remains uncertain whether MSCs from MS patients have altered immunomodulatory and/or repair capacity. Studies of the phenotype and function of MSCs isolated as part of planned trials will address this issue.

In contrast, aspects of cell harvest and culture may have dramatic effects.[167] Key factors include freshness of the starting material, starting cell number, culture medium, serum lot, the specific plasticware used, culture density, timing of passages, etc. Experience in our facility and others, confirms that it is possible to cryopreserve and thaw cells and maintain viability, proliferation, differentiation, and surface marker expression.[49,168,169] Several factors at the time of administration also are important. For example, prolonged storage in the syringe and rapid injection through a small-bore needle decrease cell viability.[170] Attention to these procedural issues will be important in planned trials.

Therapeutic transplantation of MSCs in humans

MSCs have been tested in a variety of conditions, sometimes with dramatic responses. Published human MSC transplantation experience is limited, only ~800 recipients as of this writing in January 2011 (see Table 45.4). The largest studies were in hematologic malignancy, breast cancer, GVHD, and coronary artery disease and myocardial infarction. There have been individual patients or small series with a large number of other conditions, including neurologic disorders such as acute stroke, spinal cord injury, cerebral trauma, Parkinson's disease, multisystem atrophy, and amyotrophic lateral sclerosis.

There are several individual case reports and case series of MSC transplantation in MS (Table 45.5). Scolding et al. performed a small pilot study of freshly isolated BM cells enriched for MSCs in six participants with chronic MS.[171]

Detailed results have not been published. Riordan et al. reported administration of non-expanded autologous adipose stromal fraction-derived MSCs in three treatment-refractory MS patients.[172] There were no adverse events (AEs) but also no definite benefit. Liang et al. reported intravenous (i.v.) and intrathecal (i.t.) transplantation of allogeneic umbilical-cord-derived MSCs following cyclophosphamide induction in one patient with primary progressive MS.[173] No acute GVHD or other toxicity was observed, and neurologic status appeared to stabilize. There is an ongoing Phase 1/2 study of autologous MSC administered i.v. in MS at Cambridge University by Chandran et al.[174] No results have been presented.

An Iranian group reported i.t. administration of autologous culture-expanded MSCs in ten treatment-unresponsive MS patients.[175] There were no acute or chronic AEs. Improvement was seen in one recipient, no change in four, and continued progression in five.

Yamout et al.[176] reported i.t. injection of autologous culture-expanded MSCs in seven patients with severe MS. In three additional patients, culture did not yield sufficient cells. Assessment at 3–6 months demonstrated Expanded Disability Status Scale (EDSS) improvement in five, stabilization in one, and worsening in one. MRI at three months showed new or enlarged T2 lesions in five and gadolinium (Gd)-enhancing lesions in three. There were no serious AEs.

The largest experience to date is that of Karussis et al.[100] In 15 patients with MS treated with autologous culture-expanded MSCs administered both i.v. and i.t. and 6–25 months of follow-up, no serious AEs were noted. The most common AE was headache related to lumbar puncture and i.t. injection, with one case of documented aseptic meningitis. Mean EDSS score improved from 6.7 to 5.9 over the first six months. MRI after injection of ferumoxides-labeled MSCs showed signal in the meninges, subarachnoid space, and spinal cord. Studies of peripheral blood mononuclear cells 24 hours after transplantation showed an increase in the proportion of CD4+ CD25+ regulatory T-cells; decreased lymphocyte proliferative response; and decreased expression of CD40, CD83, CD86, and MHC class II on myeloid dendritic cells.

Potential safety issues with MSC transplantation

In general, MSC transplantation in humans, including with allogeneic MSCs, has been very well tolerated. Up to 10 × 10⁶ cells per kg can be infused safely.[85] Neither acute nor long-term clinically significant AEs attributable to MSCs have been reported. Nevertheless, several potential AEs will require close attention in planned trials.

Infusion-related toxicity

Most studies have reported no infusion-related AEs. One patient developed encephalopathy, stroke, and myocardial infarction related to dimethyl sulfoxide in the freezing medium.[177] Anti-fetal bovine serum antibodies are common but usually not clinically significant.[178] One study reported a participant with an urticarial rash following a second allogeneic MSC infusion[83] and associated 150-fold increase in anti-fetal bovine serum antibodies. Because MSCs are relatively large cells (20–60 μm)[179] and cell clumping is possible, pulmonary embolism is a potential concern. No study has reported pulmonary symptoms, change in O_2-saturation, or change in chest X-ray. Adherence to established procedures for thawing and infusing cells should minimize the potential for these AEs.

Infection

MSCs might become contaminated during harvest, manipulation, or infusion. One series reported a patient with GVHD who developed central line infection and cellulitis,[180] a not uncommon experience in critically ill patients. Aseptic technique during BM aspiration and infusion, strict culture protocols, and stringent microbiologic screening are needed to minimize the risk of infusion-related infection.

Also, due to immunologic actions of MSCs, recipients potentially are at increased risk for infection. MSCs inhibit lymphocyte proliferative responses to herpes viruses, candida, and *Staphlococcus aureus* Protein A.[181] MSC effects on virus-specific T-cell responses appear to be less than on other immune responses, e.g. to alloantigens.[182] Infections have occurred relatively frequently in some series. However, all of the reported cases involved already immunocompromised patients with cancer or GVHD following HSC transplantation.[55,58,183] There have been no reports of opportunistic infection attributable to MSC transplantation.

Cancer

The potential for malignant transformation would not be unexpected, given some of the biologic similarities between stem cells and cancer cells. MSCs in adults may become tumorigenic[184,185] and have been implicated in several human or experimental tumors, including childhood leukemia,[186] gastric epithelial cancers,[187] and osteogenic sarcoma.[188] In the study of Tolar et al.,[188] the high frequency of osteogenic sarcoma in lung after MSC transplantation in mice appeared to be related to the propensity of mouse cells to develop frequent karyotypic abnormalities even with short-term culture. Karyotypic abnormalities were not seen in some studies of human MSCs[180] but were reported in others,[127,190,191] predominantly with prolonged culture. An important factor appears to be continuing cultures following senescent crisis.[192,193]

A number of studies demonstrated homing of MSCs to primary and metastatic cancers where they may form tumor stroma.[194] In addition, trophic or immunosuppressive effects of MSCs could create a permissive environment for cancer development. For example, MSC-derived adipocytes reduced apoptosis of acute promyelocytic leukemia cells in culture.[195] Human MSCs mixed with human breast cancer cells injected as a subcutaneous xenograft in mice led to marked increase in metastatic potential.[196] MSCs prolonged B16 melanoma tumor cell survival when coinjected subcutaneously in mice.[23] In a randomized trial in hematologic malignancy of MHC-identical sibling matched HSCs +/− MSCs, there was decreased GVHD in MSC recipients (11.1% vs. 53.3%) but increased leukemia relapse: 6/10 (60.0%) vs. 3/15 (20.0%).[183] Despite these theoretical concerns, there are no reports of de novo tumor formation complicating MSC transplantation in humans, either derived directly from transplanted MSCs or from other cells due to a permissive effect of MSCs. Nevertheless, in planned trials, MSCs should be passaged the minimum times needed to obtain sufficient cell yield to lessen potential for cytogenetic abnormalities. Also, initial trials should exclude participants with a cancer history.

Ectopic tissue formation

MSCs can differentiate into a number of mesodermal tissues and, possibly, cells derived from other germ layers. Ectopic calcification and/or ossification was observed with direct MSC injection into infarcted mouse heart.[127] Ectopic tissue formation has not been reported in human studies. It was not seen when specifically looked for in seven patients with MSC-HSC co-transplantation with 3+ years follow-up and autopsy in one participant.[180]

Rejection

MSCs are non-immunogenic in general, allowing allogeneic and xenogeneic transplantation (see Table 45.4). Rejection should not be an issue with planned studies of transplantation of autologous cells.

Graft vs. host disease

GVHD should not be an issue with removal of lymphocytes during culture expansion and, particularly when autologous cells are transplanted.

Autoimmunity

There have been no reports of autoimmune phenomena with MSC transplantation. However, experience in immune-mediated disorders such as MS is extremely limited. Other treatments in MS have produced unanticipated autoimmune phenomena, e.g. alemtuzumab[147] or increased MS disease activity, e.g. TNF blockers.[148] Because MSCs have both anti- and pro-inflammatory immune effects discussed above, monitoring for systemic autoimmune phenomena and paradoxical disease activation should be a focus of preliminary studies of MSC transplantation in MS.

Planned studies of MSC transplantation in MS

Several groups have initiated formal studies of MSC transplantation in MS. Our group recently received funding from the US Department of Defense and National Institutes of Health to carry out a Phase 1 trial and mechanistic immunologic studies. Briefly, we will enroll 24 men and women ages 18–55, with active relapsing forms of MS, EDSS 3.0–6.5, documented involvement of the anterior afferent visual system, and brain MRI demonstrating T2-hyperintense lesions satisfying diagnostic criteria for MS.[199,200] Participants will be followed for two months pre-treatment and six months after i.v. infusion of autologous, culture-expanded MSCs ($1–2 \times 10^6$ per kg), meeting strict release criteria for sterility, viability, and purity. In addition to intensive general safety monitoring, clinical immunology safety assessments will include serologic studies (thyroid stimulating hormone, anti-thyroglobulin antibodies, anti-microsomal antibodies, sedimentation rate, C-reactive protein, anti-nuclear antibodies, SSA antibodies, SSB antibodies, rheumatoid factor), quantitative immunoglobulin levels, and lymphocyte subsets measured by flow cytofluorometry. Efficacy assessments will include participant global impression, relapse rate, neurologic and visual impairment (EDSS, MS Functional Composite, visual acuity, Sloan low-contrast letter acuity), brain MRI (T2-hyperintense, T1-hypointense, and Gd-enhancing lesions, whole brain and gray matter atrophy, and whole brain magnetization transfer imaging and diffusion tensor imaging), visual evoked potentials (P100 latency), and optical coherence tomography (overall mean and quadrantic peripapillary retinal nerve fiber layer thickness, foveal thickness, macular volume).

Ancillary mechanistic immunologic studies will examine the in vivo effects of autologous MSC transplantation on MS relevant T-cell and B-cell immune responses at several timepoints before and after MSC transplantation. The immunologic effects of MSC transplantation will be correlated with clinical and imaging measures of MS disease activity/severity, and potential AEs. Finally, exploratory in vitro studies will evaluate molecular mechanisms of MSC-induced

Table 45.6. *Potential issues with stem cell transplantation in multiple sclerosis (MS)*

- Anti-inflammatory, neuroprotective, and repair strategies need to be combined.
- The route of administration needs to account for the multifocality of lesions.
- MS is a chronic disease. Repeated transplantation may be necessary.
- The MS disease process evolves over time. The appropriate time window for transplantation needs to be identified.
- Functional restoration requires appropriate terminal differentiation and functional integration of neural cells.
- The MS immune system, central nervous system, or therapies may create an inhospitable environment for stem cells.
- Stem cells from MS patients may be "defective."
- MS patients may be at increased risk for allergic phenomena
- Stem cell transplantation may lead to paradoxical disease activation as has been observed with some other therapies.

immunomodulation and predict the in vivo effects of MSC transplantation.

Recommendations of the MSC consensus conference

A meeting of investigators with expertise in MSCs, MS immunology, and MS clinical trials was held in Paris in March 2009[201] to review the biology of MSCs, clinical experience with MSC transplantation, the rationale in MS, and the preliminary experience in MS and to develop a consensus protocol for future Phase 2 clinical trials of MSC transplantation in MS. The hope was that as groups develop formal studies to evaluate MSCs in MS, that the core elements of the protocols will be sufficiently consistent to allow "pooling" of data.

Conclusions

There are a number of theoretical issues that will need to be addressed for stem cell therapy to be successful in MS (Table 45.6). There is significant overall experience with immunoablation and hematopoietic reconstitution, so-called "rebooting the immune system." The efficacy-safety balance in MS remains uncertain. Embryonic, neural, and inducible pluripotent stem cell transplantation are promising based on in vitro and animal studies but largely untested. MSCs have potential immunomodulatory, tissue protective, and repair-promoting properties. There is rapidly accumulating experience with both autologous and allogeneic MSC transplantation in a number of conditions. The modest experience in MS so far is encouraging. Several groups are initiating formal studies, the results of which should be of great interest.

References

1. Wilson A, Trumpp A. Bone-marrow haematopoietic-stem-cell niches. *Nature Rev Immunol* 2006;6:93–106.

2. Prockop DJ. Marrow stromal cells as stem cells for nonhematopoietic tissues. *Science* 1997;276:71–4.

3. Pittenger MF, Mackay AM, Beck SC, *et al.* Multilineage potential of adult human mesenchymal stem cells. *Science* 1999;284:143–7.

4. Da Silva Meirelles L, Caplan AI, Nardi NB. In search of the in vivo identity of

mesenchymal stem cells. *Stem Cells* 2008;26:2287–99.

5. Dominici M, Le Blanc K, Mueller I, *et al.* Minimal criteria for defining multipotent mesenchymal stromal cells. The International Society fo Cellular

Therapy position statement. *Cytotherapy.* 2006;8:315–17.

6. Barry FP, Boynton RE, Haynesworth S, Murphy JM, Zaia J. The monoclonal antibody SH-2, raised against human mesenchymal stem cells, recognizes an epitope on endoglin (CD 105). *Biochem Biophys Res Commun* 1999;265:134–9.

7. Barry F, Boynton R, Murshy M, Zaia J. The SH-3 and SH-4 antibodies recognize distinct epitopes on CD73 from human mesenchymal stem cells. *Biochem Biophys Res Commun* 2001;289:519–24.

8. Majumdar MK, Thiede MA, Mosca JD, Moorman M, Gerson SL. Phenotypic and functional comparison of cultures of marrow-derived mesenchymal stem cells (MSCs) and stromal cells. *J Cell Physiol* 1998;176:57–66.

9. Deans RJ, Moseley AB. Mesenchymal stem cells: Biology and potential clinical uses. *Exp Hematol* 2000;28:875–84.

10. Roufosse CA, Direkze NC, Otto WR, Wright NA. Circulating mesenchymal stem cells. *Int J Biochem Cell Biol* 2004;36:585–97.

11. Aggarwal S, Pittenger MF. Human mesenchymal stem cells modulate allogeneic immune cell responses. *Blood* 2005;105:1815–22.

12. Le Blanc K, Ringden O. Immunobiology of human mesenchymal stem cells and future use in hematopoietic stem cell transplantation. *Biol Blood Marrow Transplant* 2005;11:321–34.

13. Stagg J. Immune regulation by mesenchymal stem cells: two sides to the coin. *Tissue Antigens* 2006;69:1–9.

14. Noel D, Djouad F, Bouffi C, Mrugala D, Jorgensen C. Multipotent mesenchymal stromal cells and immune tolerance. *Leuk Lymphoma* 2007;48:1283–9.

15. Pelagiadis I, Dimitriou H, Kalmanti M. Biologic characteristics of mesenchymal stromal cells and their clinical applications in pediatric patients. *J Pediatr Hematol Oncol* 2008;30:301–9.

16. Chen X, Li Y, Wang L, *et al.* Ischemic rat brain extracts induce human bone marrow stromal cell growth factor production. *Neuropathology* 2002;22:275–9.

17. Uccelli A, Moretta L, Pistoia V. Immunoregulatory function of mesenchymal stem cells. *Eur J Immunol.* 2006;36:2566–73.

18. Newman RE, Yoo D, LeRoux MA, Danilkovitch-Miagkova A. Treatment of inflammatory diseases with mesenchymal stem cells. *Inflammation Allergy–Drug Targets* 2009;8:110–23.

19. Bartholomew A, Sturgeon C, Siatskas M, *et al.* Mesenchymal stem cells suppress lymphocyte proliferation in vitro and prolong skin graft survival in vivo. *Exp Hematol* 2002;30:42–8.

20. Di Nicola M, Carlo-Stella C, Magni M, *et al.* Human bone marrow stromal cells suppress T-lymphocyte proliferation induced by cellular or nonspecific mitogenic stimuli. *Blood* 2002;99:3838–43.

21. Le Blanc K, Tammik L, Sundberg B, Haynesworth SE, Ringden O. Mesenchymal stem cells inhibit and stimulate mixed lymphocyte cultures and mitogenic responses independently of the major histocompatability complex. *Scand J Immunol* 2003;57:11–20.

22. Tse WT, Pendleton JD, Beyer WM, Egalka MC, Guinan EC. Suppression of allogeneic T-cell proliferation by human marrow stromal cells: implications in transplantation. *Transplantation.* 2003;75:389–97.

23. Djouad F, Pience P, Bony C, *et al.* Immunosuppressive effect of mesenchymal stem cells favors tumor growth in allogeneic animals. *Blood* 2003;102:3837–44.

24. Le Blanc K, Rasmusson I, Gotherstrom C, *et al.* Mesenchymal stem cells inhibit the expression of CD25 (interleukin-2 receptor) and CD38 on phytohaemagglutinin-activated lymphocytes. *Scand J Immunol* 2004;60:307–15.

25. Zappia E, Casazza S, Pedemonte E, *et al.* Mesenchymal stem cells ameliorate experimental autoimmune encephalomyelitis inducing T-cell anergy. *Blood* 2005;106:1755–61.

26. Darlington PJ, Boivin M-N, Renoux C, *et al.* Reciprocal Th1 and Th17 regulation by mesenchymal stem cells: implications for MS. *Ann Neurol* 2010;68:540–5.

27. Krampera M, Glennie S, Dyson J, *et al.* Bone marrow mesenchymal stem cells inhibit the response of naive and memory antigen-specific T cells to their cognate peptide. *Blood* 2003;101:3722–9.

28. Glennie S, Soeiro I, Dyson PJ, Lam EW-F, Dazzi F. Bone marrow mesenchymal stem cells induce division arrest anergy of activated T cells. *Blood* 2005;105:2821–7.

29. Potian JA, Aviv H, Ponzio NM, Harrison JS, Rameshwar P. Veto-like activity of mesenchymal stem cells: functional discrimination between cellular responses to alloantigens and recall antigens. *J Immunol* 2003;171:3426–34.

30. Meisel R, Zibert A, Laryea M, *et al.* Human bone marrow stromal cells inhibit allogeneic T-cell responses by indoleamine 2,3-dioxygenase-mediated tryptophan degradation. *Blood* 2004;103:4619–21.

31. Beyth S, Borovsky Z, Mevorach D, *et al.* Human mesenchymal stem cells alter antigen-presenting cell maturation and induce T-cell unresponsiveness. *Blood.* 2005;105:2214–19.

32. Rasmusson I, Ringden O, Sundberg B, Le Blanc K. Mesenchymal stem cells inhibit the formation of cytotoxic T lymphocytes, but not activated cytotoxic T lymphocytes or natural killer cells. *Transplantation* 2003;76:1208–13.

33. Chabannes D, Hill M, Merieau E, *et al.* A role for heme oxygenase-1 in the immunosuppressive effect of adult rat and human mesenchymal stem cells. *Blood* 2007;110:3691–4.

34. Nasef A, Mathieu N, Chapel A, *et al.* Immunosuppressive effects of mesenchymal stem cells: involvement of HLA-G. *Transplantation* 2007;84:231–7.

35. Gerdoni E, Gallo B, Casazza S, *et al.* Mesenchymal stem cells effectively modulate pathogenic immune response in experimental autoimmune encephalomyelitis. *Ann Neurol* 2007;61:219–27.

36. Corcione A, Benvenuto F, Ferretti E, *et al.* Human mesenchymal stem cells modulate B-cell functions. *Blood* 2006;107:367–72.

37. Traggiai E, Volpi S, Schena FP, *et al.* Bone marrow-derived mesenchymal stem cells induce both polyclonal expansion and differentiation of B cells isolated from healthy donors and

systemic lupus erythematosus patients. *Stem Cells* 2008;26:562–9.

38. Spaggiari GM, Capobianco A, Becchetti S, Mingari MC, Moretta L. Mesenchymal stem cell-natural killer cell interactions: evidence that activated NK cells are capable of killing MSCs, whereas MSCs can inhibit IL-2-induced NK-cell proliferation. *Blood* 2006;107:1484–90.

39. Jiang X-X, Zhang Y, Liu B, *et al.* Human mesenchymal stem cells inhibit differentiation and function of monocyte-derived dendritic cells. *Blood* 2005;105:4120–6.

40. Ramasamy R, Fazekasova H, Lam EW-F, *et al.* Mesenchymal stem cells inhibit dendritic cell differentiation and function by preventing entry into the cell cycle. *Transplantation* 2007;83:71–6.

41. Ishida T, Inaba M, Hisha H, *et al.* Requirement of donor-derived stromal cells in the bone marrow for successful allogeneic bone marrow transplantation. Complete prevention of recurrence of autoimmune diseases in MRL/MP-lpr/lpr mice by transplantation of bone marrow plus bones (stromal cells) from the same donor. *J Immunol* 1994;152:3119–27.

42. Karussis DM, Grigoriadis N, Ben-Hur T, *et al.* Mesenchymal bone marrow stem cells migrate in CNS lesions in experimental autoimmune encephalomyelitis, differentiate into neuronal and glial line and downregulate EAE (abstract). *Neurology* 2005;64(Suppl 1):A407.

43. Karussis D, Kassis I. Use of stem cells for the treatment of multiple sclerosis. *Expert Rev Neurotherap.* 2007;7:1189–201.

44. Zhang J, Li Y, Chen J, *et al.* Human bone marrow stromal cell treatment improves neurological functional recovery in EAE mice. *Exp Neurol* 2005;195:16–26.

45. Einstein O, Fainstein N, Vaknin I, *et al.* Neural precursors attenuate autoimmune encephalomyelitis by peripheral immunosuppression. *Ann Neurol* 2007;61:209–18.

46. Klyushnenkova E, Mosca JD, Zernetkina V, *et al.* T cell responses to allogeneic human mesenchymal stem cells: immunogenicity, tolerance, and

suppression. *J Biomed Sci* 2005;12:47–57.

47. Rasmusson I, Uhlin M, Le Blanc K, Levitsky V. Mesenchymal stem cells fail to trigger effector functions of cytotoxic T lymphocytes. *J Leukoc Biol* 2007;82:887–93.

48. Lazarus HM, Haynesworth SE, Gerson SL, Rosenthal NS, Caplan AI. Ex vivo expansion and subsequent infusion of human bone marrow-derived stromal progenitor cells (mesenchymal progenitor cells): implications for therapeutic use. *Bone Marrow Transplant* 1995;16:557–64.

49. Koc ON, Gerson SL, Cooper BW, *et al.* Rapid hematopoietic recovery after coinfusion of autologous-blood stem cells and culture-expanded marrow mesenchymal stem cells in advanced breast cancer patients receiving high-dose chemotherapy. *J Clin Oncol* 2000;18:307–16.

50. Lee ST, Jang JH, Cheong J-W, Kim JS, Maemg H-Y. Treatment of high-risk acute myelogenous leukaemia by myeloablative chemoradiotherapy followed by co-infusion of T cell depleted haematopoietic stem cells and culture-expanded marrow mesenchymal cells from a related donor with one fully mismatched human leucocyte antigen haplotype. *Br J Haematol* 2002;118:1128–31.

51. MacMillan ML, Blazar BR, DeFor TE, Wagner JE. Transplantation of ex-vivo culture-expanded parental haploidentical mesenchymal stem cells to promote engraftment in pediatric recipients of unrelated donor umbilical cord blood: results of a phase I–II clinical trial. *Bone Marrow Transplant* 2009;43:447–54.

52. Liu K, chen Y, Xu L, *et al.* A randomized controlled clinical study: co-infusion of mesenchymal stromal cells facilitates platelet recovery without increasing leukemia recurrence in haploidentical hematopoietic stem cell transplantation. *Stem Cells Dev* 2011;in press.

53. Frassoni F, Labopin M, Bacigalupo A, *et al.* Expanded mesenchymal stem cells (MSC), co-infused with HLA identical hematopoietic stem cell transplants, reduce acute and chronic graft versus host disease: a matched pair analysis (abstract). *Bone Marrow Transplant* 2002;29(Suppl 2):S2.

54. Le Blanc K, Rasmusson I, Sundberg B, *et al.* Treatment of severe acute graft-versus-host disease with third party haploidentical mesenchymal stem cells. *Lancet* 2004;363:1439–41.

55. Ringden O, Uzunel M, Rasmusson I, *et al.* Mesenchymal stem cells for treatment of therapy-resistant graft-versus-host disease. *Transplantation* 2006;81:1390–7.

56. Ringden O, Uzunel M, Sundberg B, *et al.* Tissue repair using allogeneic mesenchymal stem cells for hemorrhagic cystitis, pneumomediastinum and perforated colon. *Leukemia* 2007;21:2271–6.

57. Ball L, Bredius R, Klankester A, *et al.* Third party mesenchymal stromal cell infusions fail to induce tissue repair despite successful control of severe grade i.v. acute graft-versus-host disease in a child with juvenile myelo-monocytic leukemia. *Leukemia,* 2008;22:1256–7.

58. Le Blanc K, Frassoni F, Ball L, *et al.* Mesenchymal stem cells for treatment of steroid-resistant, severe, acute graft-versus-host disease: a phase II study. *Lancet* 2008;371:1579–86.

59. Kebriaei P, Isola L, Bahceci E, *et al.* Adult human mesenchymal stem cells added to corticosteroid therapy for the treatment of acute graft-versus-host disease. *Biol Blood Marrow Transplant* 2009;15:804–11.

60. Prasad VK, Lucas KG, Kleiner GI, *et al.* Efficacy and safety of ex-vivo cultured adult mesenchymal stem cells (Prochymal) in pediatric patients with severe refractory acute graft-versus-host disease in a compassionate use study. *Biol Blood Marrow Transpl* 2011;17:534–41.

61. Zhou H, Guo M, Bian C, *et al.* Efficacy of bone marrow-derived mesenchymal stem cells in the treatment of sclerodermatous chronic graft-versus-host disease: clinical report. *Biol Blood Marrow Transplant* 2010;16:404–12.

62. Arima N, Nakamura F, Fukunaga A, *et al.* Single intra-arterial injection of mesenchymal stromal cells for treatment of steroid-refractory acute graft-versus-host disease: a pilot study. *Cytotherapy* 2010;12:265–8.

63. Fouillard L, Bensidhoum M, Bories D, *et al.* Engraftment of allogeneic mesenchymal stem cells in the bone

marrow of a patient with severe idiopathic aplastic anemia improves stroma. *Leukemia* 2003;17:474–6.

64. Assmus B, Schachinger V, Teupe C, *et al*. Transplantation of progenitor cells and regeneration enhancement in acute myocardial infarction (TOPCARE-AMI). *Circulation* 2002;106:3009–17.

65. Strauer BE, Brehm M, Zeus T, *et al*. Repair of infarcted myocardium by autologous intracoronary mononuclear bone marrow cell transplantation in humans. *Circulation* 2002;106:1913–8.

66. Stamm C, Westphal B, Kleine H-P, *et al*. Autologous bone-marrow stem-cell transplantation for myocardial regeneration. *Lancet* 2003;361:45–6.

67. Chen S-l, Fang W-w, Ye F, *et al*. Effect on left ventricular function of intracoronary transplantation of autologous bone marrow mesenchymal stem cell in patients with acute myocardial infarction. *Am J Cardiol* 2004;94:92–5.

68. Katritsis DG, Sotiropoulou PA, Karvouni E, *et al*. Transcoronary transplantation of autologous mesenchymal stem cells and endothelial progenitors into infarcted human myocardium. *Catheter Cardiovasc Interv* 2005;65:321–9.

69. Hare JM, Traverse JH, Henry TD, *et al*. A randomized, double-blind, placebo-controlled, dose-escalation study of entravenous adult human mesenchymal stem cells (Prohymal) after acute myocardial infarction. *J Am Coll Cardiol* 2009;54:2277–86.

70. Tse H-F, Kwong Y-L, Chan JKF, *et al*. Angiogenesis in ischaemic myocardium by intramyocardial autologous bone marrow mononuclear cell implantation. *Lancet* 2003;361:47–9.

71. Lasala GP, Silva JA, Kusnick BA, Minguell JJ. Combination stem cell therapy for the treatment of medically refractory coronary ischemia: a Phase I study. *Cardiovasc Revasc Med* 2011;12:29–34.

72. Tateishi-Yuyama E, Matsubara H, Murohara T, *et al*. Therapeutic angiogenesis for patients with limb ischaemia by autologous transplantation of bone-marrow cells: a pilot study and a randomised controlled trial. *Lancet* 2002;360:427–35.

73. Lasala GP, Silva JA, Gardner PA, Minguell JJ. Combination stem cell therapy for the treatment of severe limb ischemia: safety and efficacy analysis. *Angiology* 2010;61:551–6.

74. Guiducci S, Porta F, Saccardi R, *et al*. Autologous mesenchymal stem cells foster revascularization of ischemic limbs in systemic sclerosis. A case report. *Ann Intern Med* 2010;153:650–4.

75. Miyamoto K, Nishigami K, Nagaya N, *et al*. Unblinded pilot study of autologous transplantation of bone marrow mononuclear cells in patients with thromboangiitis obliterans. *Circulation* 2006;114:2679–84.

76. Badiavas EV, Falanga V. Treatment of chronic wounds with bone marrow-derived cells. *Arch Dermatol* 2003;139:510–6.

77. Dash NR, Dash SN, Routray P, Mohapatra S, Mohapatra PC. Targeting nonhealing ulcers of lower extremity in human through autologous bone marrow-derived mesenchymal stem cells. *Rejuvenation Res* 2009;12:359–66.

78. Quarto R, Mastrogiacomo M, Cancedda R, *et al*. Repair of large bone defects with the use of autologous bone marrow stromal cells (letter). *N Engl J Med* 2001;344:385–6.

79. Wakitani S, Imoto K, Yamamoto T, *et al*. Human autologous culture expanded bone marrow mesenchymal cell transplantation for repair of cartilage defects in osteoarthritic knees. *Osteoarthritis Cartilage* 2002;10:199–206.

80. Cahill RA, Jones OY, Klemperer M, *et al*. Replacement of recipient stromal/mesenchymal cells after bone marrow transplantation using bone fragments and cultured osteoblast-like cells. *Biol Blood Marrow Transplant* 2004;10:709–17.

81. Whyte MP, Kurtzberg J, McAlister WH, *et al*. Marrow transplantation for infantile hypophosphatemia. *J Bone Miner Res* 2003;18:624–36.

82. Horwitz EM, Prockop DJ, Fitzpatrick LA, *et al*. Transplantability and therapeutic effects of bone marrow-derived mesenchymal cells in children with osteogenesis imperfecta. *Nat Med* 1999;5:309–13.

83. Horwitz EM, Gordon PL, Koo WKK, *et al*. Isolated allogeneic bone marrow-derived mesenchymal cells engraft and stimulate growth in children with osteogenesis imperfecta: Implications for cell therapy of bone. *Proc Natl Acad Sci USA* 2002;99:8932–7.

84. Horwitz EM, Prockop DJ, Gordon PL, *et al*. Clinical responses to bone marrow transplantation in children with severe osteogenesis perfecta. *Blood* 2001;97:1227–31.

85. Koc ON, Day J, Nieder M, *et al*. Mesenchymal stem cells. Allogeneic mesenchymal stem cell infusion for treatment of metachromatic leukodystrophy (MLD) and Hurler syndrome (MPS-IH). *Bone Marrow Transplant* 2002;30:215–22.

86. Kharaziha P, Hellstrom PM, Noorinayer B, *et al*. Improvement of liver function in live cirrhosis patients after autologous mesenchymal stem cell injection: a phase I-II clinical trial. *Eur J Gastroenterol Hepatol* 2009;21:1199–205.

87. Duijvestein M, Vos ACW, Roelofs H, *et al*. Autologous bone marrow-derived mesenchymal stromal cell treatment for refractory luminal Chrohn's disease: results of a phase I study. *Gut* 2010;59:1662–9.

88. Sun L, Wang D, Liang J, *et al*. Umbilical cord mesenchymal stem cell transplantation in severe and refractroy systemic lupus erythematosus. *Arthritis Rheum* 2010;62:2467–75.

89. Liang J, Zhang H, Hua B, *et al*. Allogenic mesenchymal stem cell transplantation in refractory systemic lupus erythematosus: a pilot clinical study. *Ann Rheum Dis* 2010;69:1423–9.

90. Bang OY, Lee JS, Lee PH, Lee G. Autologous mesenchymal stem cell transplantation in stroke patients. *Ann Neurol* 2005;57:874–82.

91. Lee JS, Hong JM, Moon GJ, *et al*. A long-term follow-up study of intravenous autologous mesenchymal stem cell transplantation in patients with ischemic stroke. *Stem Cells* 2010;28:1099–106.

92. Moviglia GA, Fernandez Vina R, Brizuela JA, *et al*. Combined protocol of cell therapy for chronic spinal cord injury. Report on the electrical and functional recovery of two patients. *Cytotherapy* 2006;8:202–9.

93. Karussis D, Kassis I, Kurkalli BGS, Slavin S. Immunomodulation and neuroprotection with mesenchymal

bone marrow stem cells (MSCs): a proposed treatment for multiple sclerosis and other neuroimmunological/neurodegenerative diseases. *J Neurol Sci* 2008;265:131–5.

94. Pal R, Venkataramana NK, Jan M, *et al.* Ex vivo-expanded autologous bone marrow-derived mesenchymal stromal cells in human spinal cord injury/paraplegia: a pilot study. *Cytotherapy* 2009;11:897–911.

95. Kishk NA, Gabr H, Hamdy S, *et al.* Case control series of intrathecal autologous bone marrow mesenchymal stem cell therapy for chronic spinal cord injury. *Neurorehabil Neural Repair* 2010;24:702–8.

96. Zhang Z-X, Guan L-X, Zhang K, Zhang Q, Dai L-J. A combined procedure to deliver autologous mesenchymal stromal cells to patients with traumatic brain injury. *Cytotherapy* 2008;10: 134–9.

97. Mazzini L, Fagioli F, Boccaletti R, *et al.* Stem cell therapy in amyotrophic lateral sclerosis: a methodological approach in humans. ALS and other motor neuron disorders. *Amyotroph Lateral Scler Other Motor Neuron Diserd* 2003; 4:158–61.

98. Mazzini L, Mareschi K, Ferrero I, *et al.* Autologous mesenchymal stem cells: clinical applications in amyotrophic lateral sclerosis. *Neurol Res* 2006; 28:523–6.

99. Mazzini L, Ferrero I, Luparello V, *et al.* Mesenchymal stem cell transplantation in amyotrophic lateral sclerosis: a Phase I clinical trial. *Exp Neurol* 2010;223: 229–37.

100. Karussis D, Karageorgiou C, Vaknin-Dembinsky A, *et al.* Safety and immunologic effects of mesenchymal stem cell transplantation in patients with multiple sclerosis and amyotrophic lateral sclerosis. *Arch Neurol* 2010;67:1187–94.

101. Venkataramana NK, Kumar SKV, Balaraju S, *et al.* Open-labeled study of unilateral autologous bone-marrow-derived mesenchymal stem cell transplantation in Parkinson's disease. *Translational Res* 2010;155: 62–70.

102. Brass LM. Bone marrow for the brain? *Exp Neurol.* 2006;199:16–19.

103. Bliss T, Guzman R, Daadi M, Steinberg GK. Cell transplantation therapy for stroke. *Stroke* 2007;38:817–26.

104. Phinney DG, Isakova I. Plasticity and therapeutic potential of mesenchymal stem cells in the nervous system. *Curr Pharm Des* 2005;11:1255–65.

105. English D, Klasko SK, Sanberg PR. Elusive mechanisms of "stem-cell"-mediated repair of cerebral damage. *Exp Neurol* 2006;199:10–15.

106. Phinney DG, Prockop DJ. Mesenchymal stem/multipotent stromal cells: the state of transdifferentiation and modes of tissue repair – current views. *Stem Cells* 2007;25:2896–902.

107. Chopp M, Li Y, Zhang J. Plasticity and remodeling of brain. *J Neurol Sci* 2008;265:97–101.

108. Dharmasaroja P. Bone marrow-derived mesenchymal stem cells for the treatment of ischemic stroke. *J Clin Neurosci.* 2009;16:12–20.

109. Munoz JR, Stoutenger BR, Robinson AP, Spees JL, Prockop DJ. Human stem/progenitor cells from bone marrow promote neurogenesis of endogenous neural stem cells in the hippocampus of mice. *Proc Natl Acad Sci USA* 2005;102:18171–6.

110. Rivera F, Couillard-Despres S, Pedre X, *et al.* Mesenchymal stem cells instruct oligodrogenic fate decision on adult neural stem cells. *Stem Cells* 2006;24: 2209–19.

111. Akiyama Y, Radtke C, Honmou O, Kocsis JD. Remyelination of the spinal cord following intravenous delivery of bone marrow cells. *Glia* 2002;39: 229–36.

112. Dezawa M, Takahashi I, Esaki M, Takano M, Sawada H. Sciatic nerve regeneration in rats induced by transplantation of in vitro differentiated bone-marrow stromal cells. *Eur J Neurosci* 2001;14: 1771–6.

113. Zhao C-P, Zhang C, Zhou S-N, *et al.* Human mesenchymal stromal cells ameliorate the phenotype of SOD1-G93A ALS mice. *Cytotherapy* 2007;9:414–26.

114. Zhang C, Zhou C, Teng J-J, Zhao R-L, Song Y-Q. Multiple administrations of human marrow stromal cells through cerebrospinal fluid prolong survival in a transgenic mouse model of amyotrophic lateral sclerosis. *Cytotherapy* 2009;11:299–306.

115. Li Y, Chen J, Wang L, *et al.* Intracerebral transplantation of bone

marrow stromal cells in a 1-methyl-4-phenyl-1,2,3,6-tetrahydropyridine mouse model of Parkinson's disease. *Neurosci Lett* 2001;315:67–70.

116. Sadan O, Shemesh N, Barzilay R, *et al.* Migration of neurotrophic factor-secreting mesenchymal stem cells toward a quinolinic acid lesion as viewed by magnetic resonance imaging. *Stem Cells* 2008;26:2542–51.

117. Mahmood A, Lu D, Wang L, *et al.* Treatment of traumatic brain injury in female rats with intravenous administration of bone marrow stromal cells. *Neurosurgery* 2001;49:1196–204.

118. Lu P, Tuszynski MH. Can bone marrow-derived stem cells differentiate into functional neurons? *Exp Neurol* 2005;193:273–8.

119. Chopp M, Zhang XH, Li Y, *et al.* Spinal cord injury in rat: treatment with bone marrow stromal cell transplantation. *Neuroreport* 2000;11:3001–5.

120. Hofstetter CP, Schwarz EJ, Hess D, *et al.* Marrow stromal cells form guiding strands in the injured spinal cord and promote recovery. *Proc Natl Acad Sci USA* 2002;99:2199–204.

121. Wu S, Suzuki Y, Ejiri Y, *et al.* Bone marrow stromal cells enhance differentiation of cocultured neurosphere cells and promote regeneration of injured spinal cord. *J Neurosci Res* 2003;72:343–51.

122. Orlic D, Kajstura J, Chimenti S, *et al.* Mobilized bone marrow cells repair the infarcted heart, improving function and survival. *Proc Natl Acad Sci USA* 2001; 98:10344–9.

123. Wang J-S, Shum-Tim D, Chedrawy E, Chiu RC-J. The coronary delivery of marrow stromal cells for myocardial regeneration: Pathophysiologic and therapeutic implications. *J Thorac Cardiovasc Surg* 2001;122(699–705).

124. Martin B, Caparelli D, Kuang J-Q, *et al.* Implantation of allogeneic mesenchymal stem cells results in improved cardiac performance in a swine model of myocardial infarction (abstract). *Bone Marrow Transplant* 2002;29(Suppl 2):S2.

125. Tomita S, Mickle DAG, Weisel RD, *et al.* Improved heart function with myogenesis and angiogenesis after autologus porcine bone marrow stromal cell transplantation. *J Thorac Cardiovasc Surg* 2002;123: 1132–40.

126. Kawada H, Fujita J, Kinjo K, *et al.* Nonhematopoietic mesenchymal stem cells can be mobilized and differentiate into cardiomyocytes after myocardial infarction. *Blood* 2004;104:3581–7.

127. Breitbach M, Bostani T, Roell W, *et al.* Potential risks of bone marrow cell transplantation into infarcted hearts. *Blood* 2007;110:1362–9.

128. Van't Hof W, Mal N, Huang Y, *et al.* Direct delivery of syngeneic and allogeneic large-scale expanded multipotent adult progenitor cells improves cardiac function after myocardial infarct. *Cytotherapy* 2007;9:477–87.

129. Mirotsou M, Zhang Z, Deb A, *et al.* Secreted frizzled related protein 2 (sfrp2) is the key Akt-mesenchymal stem cell-released paracrine factor mediating myocardial survival and repair. *Proc Nat Acad Sci USA* 2007;104:1643–8.

130. Ortiz LA, Gambelli F, McBride C, *et al.* Mesenchymal stem cell engraftment in lung is enhanced in response to bleomycin exposure and ameliorates its fibrotic effects. *Proc Natl Acad Sci USA* 2003;100:8407–11.

131. Ortiz LA, DuTreil M, Fattman C, *et al.* Interleukin 1 receptor antagonist mediates the antiinflammatory and antifibrotic effect of mesenchymal stem cells during lung injury. *Proc Nat Acad Sci USA* 2007;104:11002–7.

132. Gupta N, Su X, Popov B, *et al.* Intrapulmonary delivery of bone marrow-derived mesenchymal stem cells improves survival and attenuates endotoxin-induced acute lung injury in mice. *J Immunol* 2007;179:1855–63.

133. Togel F, Hu Z, Weiss K, *et al.* Administered mesenchymal stem cells protect against ischemic acute renal failure through differentiation-independent mechanisms. *Am J Physiol Renal Physiol* 2005;289:F31–F42.

134. Kunter U, Rong S, Djuric Z, *et al.* Transplanted mesenchymal stem cells accelerate glomerular healing in experimental glomerulonephritis. *J Am Soc Nephrol* 2006;17:2202–12.

135. Morigi M, Introna M, Imberti B, *et al.* Human bone marrow mesenchymal stem cells accelerate recovery of acute renal injury and prolong survival in mice. *Stem Cells* 2008;26:2075–82.

136. Imberti B, Morigi M, Tomasoni S, *et al.* Insulin-like growth factor-1 sustains stem cell-mediated renal repair. *J Am Soc Nephrol* 2007;18:2921–8.

137. Parekkadan B, van Poll D, Suganuma K, *et al.* Mesenchymal stem-derived molecules reverse fulminant hepatic failure. *PLoS ONE* 2007;2:e941.

138. Carvalho AB, Quintanilha LF, Dias JV, *et al.* Bone marrow multipotent mesenchymal stromal cells do not reduce fibrosis or improve function in a rat model of severe chronic liver injury. *Stem Cells* 2008;26:1307–14.

139. Wakitani S, Yamamoto T. Response of the donor and recipient cells in mesenchymal cell transplantation to cartilage defect. *Microsc Res Tech* 2002;58:14–18.

140. Uejima S, Okada K, Kagami H, Taguchi A, Ueda M. Bone marrow stromal cell therapy improves femoral bone mineral density and mechanical strength in ovariectomized rats. *Cytotherapy* 2008;10:479–89.

141. Oh JY, Kim MK, Shin MS, *et al.* The anti-inflammatory and anti-angiogenic role of mesenchymal stem cells in corneal wound healing following chemical injury. *Stem Cells* 2008; 26:1047–55.

142. Chang C, Niu D, Zhou H, *et al.* Mesenchymal stroma cells improve hyperglycemia and insulin deficiency in the diabetic porcine pancreatic microenvironment. *Cytotherapy* 2008;10:796–805.

143. Fu X, He Y, Kie C, Liu W. Bone marrow mesenchymal stem cell transplantation improves ovarian function and structure in rats with chemotherapy-induced ovarian failure. *Cytotherapy* 2008;10:353–63.

144. Chapel A, Bertho JM, Bensidhoum M, *et al.* Mesenchymal stem cells home to injured tissues when co-infused with hematopoietic cells to treat a radiation-induced multi-organ failure syndrome. *J Gene Med* 2003;5: 1028–38.

145. Pereira RF, O'Hara MD, Laptev AV, *et al.* Marrow stromal cells as a source of progenitor cells for nonhematopoietic tissues in transgenic mice with a phenotype of osteogenesis imperfecta. *Proc Natl Acad Sci USA* 1998;95:1142–7.

146. Pereira RF, Halford KW, O'Hara MD, *et al.* Cultured adherent cells from marrow can serve as long-lasting precursor cells for bone, cartilage, and lung in irradiated mice. *Proc Natl Acad Sci USA* 1995;92:4857–61.

147. Li Y, Hisha H, Inaba M. Evidence for migration of donor bone marrow stromal cells into recipient thymus after bone marrow transplantation plus bone grafts: A role of stromal cells in positive selection. *Exp Hematol* 2000;28: 950–60.

148. Chen J, Li Y, Wang L, *et al.* Therapeutic benefit of intravenous administration of bone marrow stromal cells after cerebral ischemia in rats. *Stroke* 2001;32:1005–11.

149. Devine SM, Bartholomew AM, Mahmud N, *et al.* Mesenchymal stem cells are capable of homing to the bone marrow of non-human primates following systemic infusion. *Exp Hematol* 2001;29:244–55.

150. Gao J, Dennis JE, Muzic RF, Lundberg M, Caplan AI. The dynamic in vivo distribution of bone marrow-derived mesenchymal stem cells after infusion. *Cells Tissues Organs* 2001;169: 12–20.

151. Wu GD, Nolta JA, Jin Y-S, *et al.* Migration of mesenchymal stem cells to heart allografts during chronic rejection. *Transplantation* 2003; 75:679–85.

152. Allers C, Sierralta WD, Neubauer S, *et al.* Dynamic of distribution of human bone marrow-derived mesenchymal stem cells after transplantation into adult unconditioned mice. *Transplantation.* 2004;78:503–8.

153. Niemeyer P, Vohrer J, Schmal H, *et al.* Survival of human mesenchymal stromal cells from bone marrow and adipose tissue after xenogenic transplantation in immunocompetent mice. *Cytotherapy* 2008;10:784–95.

154. Sokolova IB, Zin'kova NN, Shvedova EV, Kruglyakov PV, Polyntsev DG. Distribution of mesenchymal stem cells in the area of tissue inflammation after transplantation of the cell material via different routes. *Bull Exp Biol Med* 2007;143:143–6.

155. Inoue M, Honmou O, Oka S, *et al.* Comparative analysis of remyelinating potential of focal and intravenous administration of autologous bone marrow cells into the rat demyelinated spinal cord. *Glia* 2003;44:111–8.

156. Nakamizo A, Marini F, Amano T, *et al.* Human bone marrow-derived mesenchymal stem cells in the

treatment of gliomas. *Cancer Res* 2005;65:3307–18.

157. Koc ON, Peters C, Auborg P, *et al.* Bone marrow-derived mesenchymal stem cells remain host-derived despite successful hematopoietic engraftment after allogeneic transplantation in patients with lysosomal and peroxisomal storage diseases. *Exp Hematol* 1999;27:1675–81.

158. Bacigalupo A, Valle M, Podesta M, *et al.* T-cell suppression mediated by mesenchymal stem cells is deficient in patients with severe aplastic anemia. *Exp Hematol* 2005;33:819–27.

159. Murphy JM, Dixon K, Beck S, *et al.* Reduced chondrogenic and adipogenic activity of mesenchymal stem cells from patients with advanced osteoarthritis. *Arthritis Rheum* 2002;46:704–13.

160. Del Papa N, Quirici N, Soligo D, *et al.* Bone marrow endothelial progenitors are defective in systemic sclerosis. *Arthritis Rheum* 2006;54:2605–15.

161. Kastrinaki M-C, Sidiropoulos P, Roche S, *et al.* Functional, molecular and proteomic characterisation of bone marrow mesenchymal stem cells in rheumatoid arthritis. *Ann Rheum Dis* 2008;67:741–9.

162. Bocelli-Tyndall C, Bracci L, Spagnoli G, *et al.* Bone marrow mesenchymal stromal cells (BM-MSCs) from healthy donors and auto-immune disease patients reduce the proliferation of autologous- and allogeneic-stimulated lymphocytes in vitro. *Rheumatology (Oxf)* 2007;46:403–8.

163. Larghero J, Farge D, Braccini A, *et al.* Phenotypical and functional characteristics of in vitro expanded bone marrow mesenchymal stem cells from patients with systemic sclerosis. *Ann Rheum Dis* 2008;67:443–9.

164. Papadaki HA, Tsagournisakis M, Mastorodemos V, *et al.* Normal bone marrow hematopoietic stem cell reserves and normal stromal cell function support the use of autologous stem cell transplantation in patients with multiple sclerosis. *Bone Marrow Transplant* 2005;36:1053–63.

165. Mallam E, Kemp K, Wilkins A, Rice C, Scolding N. Characterization of in vitro expanded bone marrow-derived mesenchymal stem cells from patients with multiple sclerosis. *Mult Scler* 2010;16:909–18.

166. Mazzanti B, Aldinucci A, Biagioli T, *et al.* Differences in mesenchymal stem cell cytokine profiles between MS patients and healthy donors: Implications for assessment of disease activity and treatment. *J Neuroimmunol* 2008;199:142–50.

167. Ho AD, Wagner W, Franke W. Heterogeneity of mesenchymal stromal cell preparations. *Cytotherapy* 2008;10:320–30.

168. Haack-Sorensen M, Bindslev L, Mortensen S, Friis T, Kastrup J. The influence of freezing and storage on the characteristics and functions of human mesenchymal stromal cells isolated for clinical use. *Cytotherapy* 2007;9:328–37.

169. Samuelsson H, Ringden O, Lonnies H, Le Blanc K. Optimizing in vitro conditions for immunomodulation and expansion of mesenchymal stromal cells. *Cytotherapy* 2009;11:129–36.

170. Agashi K, Chau DYS, Shakesheff KM. The effect of delivery via narrow-bore needles on mesenchymal cells. *Regenerat Med* 2009;4:49–64.

171. Scolding N, Marks D, Rice C. Autologous mesenchymal bone marrow stem cells: practical considerations. *J Neurol Sci* 2008;265:111–5.

172. Riordan NH, Ichim TE, Min W-P, *et al.* Non-expanded adipose stromal vascular fraction cell therapy for multiple sclerosis. *J Translat Med* 2009;7:29.

173. Liang J, Zhang H, JHua B, *et al.* Allogeneic mesenchymal stem cells transplantation in treatment of multiple sclerosis. *Mult Scler* 2009;15:644–6.

174. Chandran S, Hunt D, Joannides A. Myelin repair: the role of stem and precursor cells in multiple sclerosis. *Phil Trans R Soc Lond B Biol Sci* 2008;363:171–83.

175. Moyeddin Bonab M, Yazdanbakhsh S, Loft J, *et al.* Does mesenchymal stem cell therapy help multiple sclerosis patients? *Iran J Immunol* 2007;4:50–7.

176. Yamout B, Hourani R, Salti H, *et al.* bone marrow mesenchymal stem cell transplantation in patients with multiple sclerosis: A pilot study. *J Neuroimmunol* 2010;227:185–9.

177. Chen-Plotkin AS, Vossel KA, Samuels MA, Chen MH. Encephalopathy, stroke and myocardial infarction with DMSO use in stem cell transplantation. *Neurology* 2007;68:859–61.

178. Sundin M, Ringden O, Sundberg B, *et al.* No alloantibodies against mesenchymal stromal cells, but presence of anti-fetal calf serum antibodies, after transplantation in allogeneic hematopoietic stem cell recipients. *Haematologia (Budap)* 2007;92:1208–15.

179. Brooke G, Cook M, Blair C, *et al.* Therapeutic applications of mesenchymal stromal cells. *Semin Cell Dev Biol* 2007;18:846–58.

180. Le Blanc K, Samuelsson H, Gustafsson B, *et al.* Transplantation of mesenchymal stem cells to enhance engraftment of hematopoietic stem cells. *Leukemia* 2007;21:1733–8.

181. Sundin M, Orvell C, Rasmusson I, *et al.* Mesenchymal stem cells are susceptible to human herpesviruses, but viral DNA cannot be detected in the healthy seropositive individual. *Bone Marrow Transplant* 2006;37:1051–9.

182. Karlsson H, Samarasinghe S, Ball LM, *et al.* Mesenchymal stem cells exert differential effects on alloantigen and virus-specific T-cell responses. *Blood* 2008;112:532–41.

183. Ning H, Yang F, Jiang M, *et al.* The correlation between cotransplantation of mesenchymal stem cells and higher recurrence rate in hematologic malignancy patients: outcome of a pilot clinical study. *Leukemia* 2008;22:593–9.

184. Prindull G, Zipori D. Environmental guidance of normal and tumor cell plasticity: epithelial mesenchymal transitions as a paradigm. *Blood* 2004;103:2892–9.

185. Serakinci N, Guldberg P, Burns JS, *et al.* Adult human mesenchymal stem cell as a target for neoplastic transformation. *Oncogene* 2004;23:5095–8.

186. Greaves M. Molecular genetics, natural history and the demise of childhood leukaemia. *Eur J Cancer* 1999;35:1941–53.

187. Houghton JM, Stoicov C, Nomura S, *et al.* Gastric cancer originating from bone marrow-derived cells. *Science* 2004;306:1568–1571.

188. Tolar J, Nauta AJ, Osborn MJ, *et al.* Sarcoma derived from cultured mesenchymal stem cells. *Stem Cells* 2007;25:371–9.

189. Bernardo ME, Zaffaroni N, Novara F, *et al.* Human bone marrow-derived mesenchymal stem cells do not undergo

transformation after long-term in vitro culture and do not exhibit telomere maintenance mechanisms. *Cancer Res* 2007;67:9142–9.

190. Wang Y, Huso DL, Harrington J, *et al.* Outgrowth of a transformed cell population derived from normal human BM mesenchymal stem cell culture. *Cytotherapy* 2005;7:509–19.

191. Rubio D, Garcia-Castro J, Martin MC, *et al.* Spontaneous human adult stem cell transformation. *Cancer Res* 2005;65:3035–9.

192. Kim J, Kang JW, Park JH, *et al.* Biological characterization of long-term cultured human mesenchymal stem cells. *Arch Pharm Res* 2008;32:117–26.

193. Rosland GV, Svendsen A, Torsvik A, *et al.* Long-term cultures of bone marrow-derived human mesenchymal stem cells frequently undergo spontaneous malignant transformation. *Cancer Res.* 2009;69:5331–9.

194. Kidd S, Spaeth E, Klopp A, *et al.* The (in)auspicious role of mesenchymal stromal cells in cancer: be it friend or foe. *Cytotherapy* 2008;10:657–67.

195. Tabe Y, Konopleva M, Munsell MF, *et al.* PML-RARα is associated with leptin-receptor induction: the role of mesenchymal stem cell-derived adipocytes in APL survival. *Blood* 2004;103:1815–22.

196. Karnoub AE, Dash AB, Vo AP, *et al.* Mesenchymal stem cells within tumour stroma promote breast cancer metastasis. *Nature* 2007;449: 557–65.

197. Coles AJ, The CAMMS223 Study Group. Efficacy of alemtuzumab in treatment-naive relapsing-remitting multiple sclerosis: analysis after two years of study CAMMS223 (S12.004). *Neurology* 2007;68(Suppl 1):A100.

198. The Lenercept Multiple Sclerosis Study Group, The University of British Columbia MS/MRI Analysis Group. TNF neutralization in MS. Results of a randomized, placebo-controlled multicenter study. *Neurology* 1999; 53:457–65.

199. Barkhof F, Rocca M, Francis G, *et al.* Validation of diagnostic magnetic resonance imaging criteria for multiple sclerosis and response to interferon β1a. *Ann Neurol* 2003;53: 718–24.

200. Tintore M, Rovira M, Rio J, *et al.* New diagnostic criteria for multiple sclerosis. Application in first demyelinating episode. *Neurology* 2003;60:27–30.

201. Freedman MS, Bar-Or A, Atkins HL, *et al.* The therapeutic potential of mesenchymal stem cell transplantation as a treatment for multiple sclerosis: consensus report of the International MSCT Study Group. *Mult Scler* 2010;16:503–10.

Chapter

46

Neuroprotection in multiple sclerosis

Avindra Nath and Peter A. Calabresi

Introduction

The pathological substrate of permanent disability in multiple sclerosis (MS) is neuronal injury and axonal loss. While axonal loss is initiated early in the disease process, the mechanisms for axonal damage likely vary at different stages of the disease. In this chapter, we review the mechanisms for both inflammatory and non-inflammatory mediated neural degeneration in MS and discuss potential therapeutic targets for neuroprotection. While this is a convenient manner in which to divide these topics, it should be recognized that there is likely a continuum of inflammatory and non-inflammatory neurodegenerative mechanisms occurring simultaneously in most patients. Therefore, treatment strategies need to address both aspects of the disease.

Effect of immunomodulatory drugs on cerebral atrophy and black holes

The interferon-beta (IFNβ) trials revealed that the most potent effect of this class of drugs is at the blood–brain barrier as evidenced by reductions in new T2 weighted lesions and gadolinium (Gd)-enhancing lesions. Further, IFNβ may offer some neuroprotective effect by reducing inflammation and thereby preventing the formation of new black holes. IFNβ-1a was shown to reduce the rate of brain atrophy significantly between the first and second year of the trial but not between baseline and year 1 suggesting that the reduction of inflammation in year 1 might result in fewer damaging plaques that evolve into black holes in year 2.[1] Importantly, another MRI-based trial found that IFNβ had no effect on the likelihood of T1 hole formation after a Gd-enhancing lesion has already occurred providing further evidence that IFNβs act systemically and are probably not neuroprotective within the central nervous system (CNS).[2] Alternatively, glatiramer acetate (GA) has a more modest effect on reducing Gd-enhancing lesions than IFNβ drugs but seems to have equal efficacy in reducing relapse rate. An MRI-based study of GA suggested that fewer of the Gd-enhancing lesions that occurred on GA became permanent T1 black holes, which raises the possibility that GA may have neuroprotective effects within the CNS.[3] This

supports data from experimental autoimmune encephalomyelitis (EAE) studies and in vitro where GA-reactive T-cells can be found within the CNS and secrete brain-derived neurotrophic factor (BDNF).[4] Natalizumab reduced the rate of brain atrophy in year 2 of the Phase 3 trials.[5,6] Interestingly, fingolimod was also shown to reduce the rate of brain atrophy, but unlike other drugs, its effect was seen in the first six-month epoch of treatment.[7] Whether the earlier reduction in the rate of atrophy reflects the known CNS penetration of this lipophilic drug or possibly bioactivity on neural and or glial cells, which express sphingosine 1-phosphate receptors, is unknown.

Several lines of evidence suggest that inflammatory infiltrates may be key factors in mediating cerebral atrophy and black holes or axonal transaction in patients with MS. For example, neuroimaging studies suggest that ring Gd-enhancing patterns on MRI contribute to severe brain atrophy over a three-month period in patients with relapsing–remitting (RR) MS.[8] Patients exhibit significant brain atrophy in the earliest stages of MS and CNS atrophy and axonal loss may develop at a faster rate in the first few years of disease onset. Other reports have suggested that the rate of progression of CNS atrophy, especially gray matter atrophy, may be greater in more advanced RR phases of disease.[9] Because none of these anti-inflammatory treatments is completely effective, it remains important to identify the downstream mechanism(s) by which the infiltrating cells lead to neuronal and myelin injury to develop complementary neuroprotective strategies.

Limitations of anti-inflammatory therapies

Although axonal damage has been described pathologically dating back to Charcot, only recently was there more definitive and quantitative pathological evidence associating the number of axonal transections with the extent of inflammation in both the gray and white matter of MS brain tissue, suggesting that inflammation is an important mechanism in mediating damage to the axon.[10] Unfortunately, presently available drugs have minimal efficacy in purely progressive forms of MS.[11] Clinical trials testing the efficacy of immunomodulatory drugs in primary progressive MS have been uniformly negative, except in subsets of younger patients with active Gd-enhancing lesions

Multiple Sclerosis Therapeutics, Fourth Edition, ed. Jeffrey A. Cohen and Richard A. Rudick. Published by Cambridge University Press.
© Cambridge University Press 2011.

535

on MRI. In secondary progressive (SP) MS, IFNβ drugs only seem to have benefit in cohorts that are still having relapses and MRI activity or only provide benefit in slowing less affected parts of the neuraxis such as the upper extremities.[12] However, early institution of immunomodulating drugs in RR disease or at the time of a clinically isolated demyelinating syndrome does appear to have some benefit in delaying progression of disability in a more robust and reliable fashion. This suggests suppression of inflammation early in the course of the illness is needed for any meaningful reduction or slowing of later disability.

Assessing neuronal injury in MS

Role of MRI

MRI offers the potential to probe MS-affected tissues serially in patients and occasionally make correlations with pathology in cases of tissue biopsy, resection, or post-mortem analysis. T1-weighted low signal lesions that persist for months after Gd-enhancement has resolved represent areas in which there has been significant axonal loss. Indeed, the darkness of these so-called black holes correlates with the extent of axonal loss seen pathologically. Another useful MRI measure that may reflect loss of myelin and axons is whole-brain atrophy. Both of these measures have been found to be useful outcomes in clinical trials to quantify protection of brain tissues.[13] Brain tissues imaged by MRI can now be accurately segmented and reveal that not only does the gray matter atrophy contribute significantly to total brain tissue loss in MS, but that gray matter atrophy accelerates in later stages of the disease.[9] While both cortical and deep gray matter structures are atrophic in MS, the underlying tissue component leading to loss of volume remains unclear and, thus, gray matter atrophy may represent a composite of myelin, neuronal, and axonal loss. The hippocampus has been shown to be atrophic in MS, but when inspected pathologically it appears that hippocampal neurons are relatively preserved in CA1 despite extensive demyelination in some cases.[14]

Diffusion tensor imaging (DTI) utilizes information obtained from measuring directional diffusion of water in different planes. Free water, as in cerebrospinal fluid (CSF), will diffuse in an isotropic or spherical fashion; whereas, water constrained by anatomical boundaries, such as white matter fiber tracts will diffuse preferentially along the long axis plane of the axons in an anisotropic fashion. The fractional anisotropy (FA) can then be measured to provide information about integrity of that tract. As axons degenerate, the FA decreases. In addition to examining the FA, one can individually measure the principal Eigen vector called lamda1 in the parallel (axial) plane and the two orthogonal vectors, lamda2 and 3, in the radial planes perpendicular to the axon. While lamda1 (parallel diffusion) decreases acutely in axonal injury models, it increases in states of chronic injury.[15] Increased perpendicular diffusion has been suggested to be a marker of demyelination, but also appears to occur in acute axonal injury.

A study of DTI change over time in the brain suggested DTI indices can be reproducibly measured and change over a

two-year timeframe.[16] Whether these novel DTI indices will be useful in clinical trials remains untested.

Magnetic resonance proton spectroscopy studies have examined peaks of the neuronal marker N-acetylaspartate (NAA) in MS brain tissue and found lower NAA in areas of active inflammation as well as in normal appearing white and gray matter providing further support for the notion of an early axonal damage even in the absence of overt inflammation.[17] In purely progressive MS cases, the major disabling pathology is often in the spinal cord where the resolution is less good and it is more difficult to quantify inflammation and degeneration. Indeed, axonal injury has been documented pathologically in the absence of T2 plaques.[18] Despite these obstacles, spinal cord atrophy and more recently decreases in the magnetic transfer ratios (MTR) in cervical spinal cord have been positively correlated with disease severity, again suggesting that tissue loss is linked with disability and is in some cases separate from inflammation.[19–23]

Role of optical coherence tomography

Optical coherence tomography (OCT) allows quantitative measurement of retinal structures by examining the backscatter of infrared light shined through the pupil. Several groups have shown that OCT scanner measurements of the retinal nerve fiber layer (RNFL), which are the axons that coalesce to become optic nerve, reveal RNFL thinning not only after an episode of acute optic neuritis (AON), but also in MS patients with no clinical history of AON.[24] RNFL thinning is significantly correlated with loss of visual acuity, especially on low contrast (Sloan) charts, Expanded Disability Status Scale (EDSS), and brain volume on MRI.[25] Longitudinal changes in OCT can be detected in MS patients in the absence of AON suggesting that subclinical axonal damage occurs in MS perhaps related to microscopic inflammation in the optic nerve or the consequences of prior demyelination.[26] While primary retinal neuronal injury was postulated many years ago based on electroretinogram abnormalities, there is now pathological and OCT evidence of neuronal injury in the inner nuclear layer (amacrine and bipolar cells) and outer nuclear layer (rods and cones) by OCT retinal segmentation. The mechanism underlying retinal neuronal injuries are unclear, but may be informative as to how neurons are injured in other parts of the brain in MS.

The latest generation OCT scanners, which utilize spectral domain technology (SD-OCT) allow resolution of 3–4 microns and have been shown to be a reliable and reproducible method that can be used across clinical centers to quantify RNFL and macular thicknesses. OCT can potentially be used in a six-month clinical trial of patients with AON to quantify the neuroprotective effects of a study drug. Sample size estimates suggest that 120 patients would be required in a two-arm study to see a 50% effect size assuming a mean loss of RNFL of 10 microns. The utility of OCT in large Phase 3 trials in which patients are not having AON events frequently is less clear, but at this time appears to be similar to EDSS in that approximately 20% of patients will have detectable changes over the course of a two-year trial. This proportion of patients who change in a focal (quadrantic change) manner is likely to be higher and may be better assessed using SD-OCT.

Mechanisms of neurodegeneration in MS

Inflammatory

T-cell activation

The classical pathological description of the MS lesion has focused on the perivenular inflammatory infiltrate characterized predominantly by lymphocytes and monocytes. The development of monoclonal antibodies has allowed further definition of these cells allowing us to subtype them. Reports differ as to the prevalence of CD4+ and CD8+ T-cells, but clearly both are present with CD4+ being more common in the perivenular location and more CD8+ extravasating into the tissue parenchyma.[27] The T-cells are widely held to be the cell type responsible for initiating the pathological process in MS because of their ability to respond specifically to autoantigens and foreign proteins and release proinflammatory cytokines. T-cells are directly pathogenic to neurons and may also facilitate activation of secondary effector cells such as monocytes and glial cells by secreting cytokines such as IFNγ, interleukin (IL)-17 and IL-6. Key among T-cell-derived inflammatory molecules that may stimulate neuronal damage are proteinases. Such enzymes include cathepsins and granzymes that may be released from cytotoxic granules, and matrix metalloproteinases (MMPs), which are typically secreted as proforms and activated extracellularly. Examples of toxicity by such proteinases include neuronal apoptosis that results from microglial cell-derived cathepsin B. Granzyme B has been shown to cause neurotoxicity and impairment of proliferation and differentiation of neural progenitor cells via interactions with a G-protein-coupled receptor. Further, CSF levels of granzyme B are elevated in patients with MS.[28] MMPs, which have been shown to target myelin proteins and to influence oligodendroglial cell process outgrowth, may also be neurotoxic. A study using intravital dual photon microscopy in EAE documented the formation of synapse-like contacts between T-cells and neurons that resulted in intraneuronal calcium fluxes, and in some cases neuronal apoptosis. However, it is also clear that there is significant lesion heterogeneity and that while some MS lesions are predominantly characterized by T-cell inflammation, a humoral component including evidence for B-cells, immunoglobulin deposition, and complement activation is present in many MS lesions.[29] As was described for T-cells a direct pathogenic effect of Ig deposition on both myelin and axons has been described.[30]

Macrophage and microglial activation

Despite the therapeutic emphasis on targeting the upstream lymphocytic arm of the immune system, it has not escaped attention that the MS parenchymal infiltrate is predominantly composed of CD68+ macrophages and microglia, and in some cases microglial activation may precede the lymphocytic infiltrate. Whether any of the present immunomodulating therapies target these cells is also unclear, although a recent report did suggest that in GA-treated EAE mice there is less microglial activation perhaps as a result of the Th2 phenotype of the GA-reactive T-cells.[31] The microglia are likely an important effector cell in the MS plaque as it has been well documented that macrophages and microglia can mediate several pathogenic processes, including phagocytosis of myelin, antigen presentation, and release of molecules that may cause axonal and neuronal death.[32] Active stripping of myelin off axons has been shown in by electron microscopy, but whether this is truly causative or reactive to already damaged myelin is unclear. Alternatively, it has been recently suggested that the phagocytic properties of macrophages and microglia may be beneficial in order to clear myelin debris, which inhibits neuroregeneration.[33] Indeed, the triggering receptor expressed on myeloid cells (TREM) 2 has been linked with phagocytic function, and blocking it worsens EAE, whereas other effector functions of macrophages and microglia may still be detrimental. The capacity to present antigen within the CNS is thought to be one mechanism by which microglia propagate compartmentalized inflammation, and it has been hypothesized that the CNS may then become a tertiary lymphoid tissue. Certainly, it is clear that activated T-cells have access to the CNS continuously, but if they are not presented their cognate antigen or provided chemotactic gradients by which to extravasate into tissues they egress through cervical lymphatics without causing damage. Macrophages and microglia also release IL-1b, tumor necrosis factor (TNF)α, IL-12, and IL-23, which have important functions in both activating other immune cells and mediating downstream damage.[34] Indeed, the release of high levels of TNFα can mediate direct damage to oligodendrocytes, although low levels of TNF may have neuroprotective properties. Production of nitric oxide (NO), which is converted to peroxynitrite in the presence of superoxides is likely a mechanism by which the macrophages and microglia cause nerve tissue damage.[35] Inflammation-induced nitric oxide synthetase (iNOS) or neuronal NOS both lead to increased NO, which in conjunction with influx of calcium into neurons, activates damaging calpains.[36] In addition, NO was recently shown to initiate a non-caspase-dependent cell death pathway mediated by polyadenylated ADP-ribose polymerase (PARP), which facilitates transfer of apoptosis inducing factor from the mitochondrion to the nucleus.[37] In most neurodegenerative diseases there has been substantial interest to determine if oxidative stress or mitochondrial injury plays a role in neuronal injury in part because there are a large number of antioxidants available for human use. Several pathological studies from MS patients also suggest that significant amount of oxidative stress occurs in chronic active plaques[38] and plays a role in neurodegeneration. However, most of the antioxidants agents do not readily cross the blood–brain barrier. The neurophilin ligands are of special interest, since they have substantial anti-oxidative properties and favorable pharmacokinetic profiles that include good CNS penetration. The pathogenic role of microglia in MS has been difficult to quantify because of the CNS localization and inability to track these cells in vivo. Several recent EAE studies have confirmed a pathogenic role for microglia in autoimmune demyelination, whereas in virally mediated CNS disease microglia may play a critical role in mounting a protective immune response.[39] The role of microglia in non-inflammatory injuries and in reparative settings is just beginning to be elucidated. Perhaps newer imaging approaches that allow quantification of activated microglia will provide more information regarding their role in MS as discussed later in the section on outcome measures.

Astrocyte activation

Although there is known to be a marked astroglial reaction in MS plaques, the contribution of astroglial cells to tissue damage is less clear. While not part of the peripheral immune system, astrocytes likely play a critical role in mediating immune responses in the brain. Astrocytes may have some role in presenting antigens; however, a major function is the production of soluble mediators of inflammation including cytokines and chemokines.[40] Astroglia are a major source of IL-6 and chemokines. As producers of IL-6, it is possible that astrocytes could play both a neuroprotective role by releasing low levels of IL-6 or a neurotoxic role by releasing high levels of IL-6 as was recently documented in transverse myelitis.[41] In this study IL-6 levels in the CSF were correlated with NO and predicted the likelihood of future disability. Another potentially important role of glial cells is in the regulation of glutamate levels in the synapse. It has been well described in amyotrophic lateral sclerosis that sustained elevated levels of glutamate in the synapse are neurotoxic by allowing excessive influx of calcium through α-amino-3-hydroxyl-5-methyl-4-isoxazole-proprionate (AMPA) receptors. Since glial cells are known to express glutamate transport receptors that function to take up glutamate and thereby regulate glutamate levels, it has been hypothesized in amyotrophic lateral sclerosis and more recently MS that there may be a defect in this mechanism.[42] Interestingly, beta lactam antibiotics were recently shown to block accumulation of glutamate and may be neuroprotective. Further, studies of the AMPA receptor blocker NBQX in EAE suggested a protective role for this approach in inflammatory mediated nerve damage.[43]

Non-inflammatory

Sodium channel redistribution

In normal myelinated axons, sodium channels are clustered at the nodes of Ranvier, allowing rapid saltatory conduction along the axon. Sodium channels in the axon membrane beneath myelin (internodal and paranodal axolemma) are present at too low a density to support effective conduction. Following demyelination, conduction failure occurs because current dissipates through the sodium channel-poor portions of the axon membrane, resulting in clinical deficit. This conduction can

be restored by expression of sodium channels along demyelinated (previously sodium channel-poor) axon regions – this phenomenon may be largely responsible for spontaneous clinical remission following relapse in RRMS.[44] Sodium channels may, however, also have a deleterious effect in MS. Studies over the past decade have shown that sustained sodium influx through voltage-gated sodium channels on CNS axons triggers reverse sodium-calcium exchange, importing damaging levels of calcium into axons and inducing axonal degeneration.[45] Consistent with a possible role for sodium channels in MS-associated axonal injury, pharmacological blockade of sodium channels prevents axonal degeneration induced by NO, which is present at increased levels in MS lesions. In addition, it has been demonstrated that the sodium channel blockers, phenytoin, lamotrigene, and flecainide have a protective effect in EAE, preventing CNS axonal degeneration and improving clinical outcome.[46,47] There exist several voltage-gated sodium channel isoforms (Nav1.1–Nav1.9), all sharing a common motif but with different sequences and kinetics. Recent work suggested that specific sodium channel isoforms are associated with the restoration of conduction and with axonal degeneration in MS. It was proposed that Nav1.2 channel expression along demyelinated axons support conduction, but expression of Nav1.6 channels may predispose axons to injury.[44] Hence, according to this hypothesis, strategies that induce expression of Nav1.2 may promote restoration of conduction in MS, and subtype-specific blockade of Nav1.6 may prevent axonal degeneration in MS.

Kv channel expression

Activated effector memory lymphocytes express a subtype of the voltage gated potassium channels, called Kv1.3 on their cell surface. Blocking this channel prevents lymphocyte activation. Increased expression of this channel has also been found in the inflammatory infiltrates in the brains of patients with MS.[48] Similarly, neurons when exposed to activated lymphocytes also express increased amounts of Kv1.3 channel on the cell membrane, possibly as part of the apoptotic cascade, and blocking of this channel prevents neurotoxicity (Nath and Calabresi unpublished observations). This suggests that blockers of Kv1.3 may be excellent targets of neuroprotection in inflammatory diseases, since they have a dual effect with the ability to protect neurons and also prevent T-cell activation. Dalfampridine (4-amino-pyridine), a K^+ channel blocker that improves gait in a subset of MS patients, is thought to act by blockade of Kv1.4 channels on axons. However, it remains unknown if it has any long-term neuroprotective properties.[49]

Loss of trophic support by myelin

There is a wealth of evidence that in the absence of inflammation, chronically demyelinated axons undergo Wallerian degeneration in the context of impaired trophic support and myelin signaling.[50] A classic example is Charcot–Marie–Tooth disease, the most common inherited peripheral neuropathy. In the demyelinating forms of Charcot–Marie–Tooth disease, abnormal myelination can be detected in early childhood, but the clinical manifestations often occur only years later, and are due to progressive axonal loss in the peripheral nerves.[51] In addition, secondary axonal damage has been demonstrated in animal models of demyelination, including PMP22 transgenic rats, and mice with P0 and connexin 32 mutations. Bjartmar and colleagues found a progressive loss of nerve fiber numbers in the lumbar corticospinal tract of MS patients with longer duration of disease,[52] a finding consistent with ongoing low-level axonal degeneration even at disease stages when inflammation is infrequent. They suggested that "demyelinated axons may degenerate from lack of myelin-derived trophic support."

Our group has recently shown the relevance of myelin-associated glycoprotein (MAG), a myelin protein located in the adaxonal oligodendrocyte plasmalemma, in axonal stability.[53] We observed that mice genetically engineered to lack MAG have progressive spontaneous distal axonal degeneration in the CNS and peripheral nervous system (PNS). Furthermore, axons in these animals have phenotypic changes similar to those produced by demyelination in terms of reduced neurofilament phosphorylation, neurofilament spacing, and axonal caliber.[54] Of note, MAG is not necessary for myelination, and myelin sheaths from MAG-/- mice are largely normal.[54] Hence, MAG-induced signaling likely plays an important role in axonal maintenance, and may be a necessary means by which oligodendrocytes normally signal to axons.

Strategies for neuroprotection in MS

Progressive axonal loss occurs in the CNS of patients with MS, and the extent of this axonal loss correlates with the degree of permanent neurological deficit. As discussed above, there are several possible causes for axonal degeneration in MS. These causes include direct axonal damage by inflammatory mediators, and the effects of demyelination on the underlying axon, namely loss of trophic signaling by myelin, and calcium-mediated injury via sodium channel redistribution. In addition, demyelination may render the underlying, naked axon more vulnerable to damage by inflammatory mediators.

Strategies to prevent axonal degeneration can be considered direct and indirect (Table 46.1). **"Direct" neuroprotective strategies** are those that directly target the axon, increasing intrinsic axonal stability and resistance to degeneration. Examples of these strategies include the use of recombinant human erythropoietin (EPO), the non-immunosuppressive neuroimmunophilin ligands and sodium channel blockers. These will be discussed later as candidate agents for clinical trials in MS. It should be pointed out that it does not necessarily follow that an agent that prevents neuronal death will prevent axonal degeneration, as it is now well recognized that the two processes may exploit different signaling pathways.[55] This was beautifully illustrated by a study in a mouse model of motor neuron disease, which pointed to the overriding importance of axonal degeneration rather than motor neuronal death in this neurodegenerative disease.[56] The ability to prevent axonal

Table 46.1. *Neuroprotective strategies in MS*

Candidate drugs
DIRECT (increase intrinsic axonal resistance to degeneration)
- Growth factors/neurotrophins
- Non-immunosuppressive neuroimmunophilin ligands
- Sodium channel blockers
- AMPA antagonists
- SSRIs
- Intense exercise
- Kv1.3 channel blockers
- BG12 (fumarate)
- Antioxidants

INDIRECT
- Strategies to promote remyelination
  - Prevention of oligodendrocyte death (e.g., PARP inhibitors)
  - Differentiation of OPCs to myelin-producing oligodendrocytes (e.g., anti-LINGO)
- Strategies modulating autoimmune response that injures axons/neurons, myelin/oligodendrocytes and neural progenitor cells

Drugs that have failed
- Lamotrigine (brain atrophy outcome)
- Glatiramer (PPMS)
- Rituximab (PPMS)
- Interferon-beta (PPMS)
- Cyclophospamide (PMS)
- Cyclosporine A
- IVIg (recovery from attack)
- Sulfasalazine
- Pentoxyphylline

AMPA = α-amino-3-hydroxyl-5-methyl-4-isoxazole-proprionate, IVIg = intravenous immunoglobulin, PARP = polyadenylated ADP-ribose polymerase, POCs = oligodendrocyte progenitor cells, PMS = progressive MS, PPMS = primary progressive MS, SSRIs = selective serotonin reuptake inhibitors.

degeneration should thus be specifically assessed when considering the efficacy of a neuroprotective agent, as axonal dysfunction rather than neuronal loss is often the dominant pathology in human neurodegenerative diseases (and MS), particularly early on in the disease when therapeutic intervention is still possible.

"Indirect" neuroprotective strategies prevent axonal degeneration by mechanisms that do not directly increase intrinsic axonal stability. They include several strategies, including modulation of the autoimmune process that damages axon, myelin, and oligodendrocytes, and promotion of remyelination via inhibitors of oligodendrocyte death and growth factors that promote the differentiation of oligodendrocyte precursor cells (OPCs) into myelin-producing oligodendrocytes.

Clinical trials of neuroprotective drugs in MS

To translate neuroprotective candidate drugs into proven therapies, an efficient system of testing these agents will have to be established. One of the reasons that immunomodulatory drugs have been easier to test and get Food and Drug Administration (FDA) approval is that RR disease is easier to quantify than progressive MS and agents have been approved solely based on a reduction of relapse rate. Further, the measurement of Gd-enhancing lesions on MRI has gained acceptance as a secondary outcome measure in pivotal Phase 3 trials and has served as a useful screening tool in early Phase 1 or 2 trials.

It is important to consider the mechanism of action of the drug being tested before designing a clinical trial and considering outcome measures. In neuroprotective trials, it is likely that any benefit on sustained disability may not occur or be detectable for a substantial period of time, possibly 3–5 years. As discussed above, even when targeting upstream inflammation the effect on preserving brain tissue as measured by brain parenchymal fraction was not seen until the second year of the trial except in the case of fingolimod, which enters the CNS well and may target glial or neuronal sphingosine 1-phosphate receptors. As such, brain atrophy is now the only imaging tool for which we have sufficient data to power clinical trials for neuroprotective agents. Unfortunately, the slow and small rate of change of this measure requires that hundreds of patients be enrolled to see an effect. Some studies are now assessing the conversion rate of new lesions to permanent T1 black holes, and suggest this might be a useful short-term measure as in the Ibudilast study,[57] but the ultimate collapse of tissue in these areas makes it difficult to use this measure to confirm sustained loss of tissue. This same phenomenon has limited the use of spectroscopy since voxels of tissue with reduced NAA often are filled in by normal tissue giving one the paradoxical result of increased NAA at late time points. For these reasons some investigators have preferred whole-brain measures of global tissue damage such as MTR histograms, and this approach has shown some promise as MT changes appear to be fairly robust and may not only reflect focal inflammation but are more sensitive to structural changes in adjacent tissues including demyelination and even axonal loss.[14] Recent progress has also been made in detecting focal areas of remyelination using voxel-based analysis of MT signal changes.[58]

Candidate drugs

Careful consideration to the pathophysiology of MS is necessary to identify candidate drugs for therapeutic trials. Just because a drug has been used safely in another neurological condition does not necessarily mean that it could be used safely in MS as well. For example, phenytoin that has been used safely for treatment of seizures for several decades has been shown to cause a rebound effect in EAE with increased mortality. Similarly, memantine that is used as a neuroprotective agent in Alzheimer's disease can cause worsening of MS.[59] Similarly, statins have been shown to have neuroprotective properties in a variety of in vitro and in vivo models but have shown mixed results in MS. They may inhibit remyelination and can also cause increased disease activity in MS.[60] Inosine a precursor of uric acid failed to show any neuroprotective effect in MS, even though uric acid has been shown to boost the endogenous neuroprotection in EAE.[61] GA has neuroprotective properties in EAE and other animal models of neuronal injury but failed to be of any benefit in primary progressive MS. Several other immunomodulatory drugs have failed to show neuroprotection in MS in clinical trials. These include rituximab, cyclosporine A, sulfasalizine, intravenous immunoglobulin, and pentoxyphylline.[62]

Growth factors

Recombinant human erythropoietin

EPO is an FDA-approved agent that has been used for several years to treat anemia. EPO and its receptor, EPOR, are also present in the CNS and PNS, and EPO is a potent neuroprotective agent. EPO-treated EAE animals had reduced axonal damage, inflammatory cell infiltration, and demyelination.[63] Once considered a leading candidate for clinical trials in MS or transverse myelitis, EPO has been abandoned due to the risk for polycythemia and an attendant prothrombotic risk in non-anemic patients.

Leukemia inhibitory factor

Leukemia inhibitory factor (LIF) may play a crucial role in neuroprotection and axonal regeneration as well as the prevention of demyelination. LIF is also an important survival factor for stem cells and neuronal precursors. Therefore, it is a potential therapeutic candidate for MS. However, some caution in its use may be necessary because under certain circumstances it may have pro-inflammatory properties.[64] Ligands to the beta subtype of the estrogen receptor promote remyelination and axonal protection in EAE and are being developed for treatment of MS.[65]

Alemtuzumab

Peripheral blood mononuclear cells derived from patients treated with the CD52+ lymphocyte-depleting humanized monoclonal antibody, alemtuzamab, produced increased concentrations of BDNF, platelet-derived growth factor, and ciliary neurotrophic factor, but only when stimulated with MBP.[66] The conditioned media from these cultures promoted survival of rat neurons and increased axonal length in vitro.

Recombinant human insulin-like growth factor-I and insulin-like growth factor *binding protein-3*

These recombinant proteins are currently in clinical trials for a number of diseases including myotonic dystrophy. Experimental studies show that these factors are important for growth and migration of oligodendrocytes and in neuroprotection and regeneration. Hence they may have potential for treatment of MS, but also may have proinflammatory properties.[67]

Exercise

Intense exercise has been shown to induce BDNF production leading to proliferation of endogenous stem cells. In a pilot study we found that patients with SPMS showed increases in BDNF levels in the CSF upon using a modified exercise bicycle that provides forced exercise (unpublished observations).

Neuroimmunophilin ligands

The neuroimmunophilins are a highly conserved group of chaperone proteins that are enriched in neurons of both the CNS and PNS. Neuroimmunophilin ligands include the immunosuppressants, FK506 and cyclosporin A, which are FDA-approved drugs primarily used to prevent organ transplant rejection. These ligands have also been demonstrated to have neuroprotective properties, preventing neuronal death in in vitro excitotoxicity paradigms and in in vivo stroke models. Cyclosporin A, however, failed to provide any clinically meaningful benefit in patients with SPMS even though the effects were statistically significant. Of note, non-immunosuppressive analogs of FK506, such as GPI-1046, exist and have been shown to exhibit similar neuroprotective properties.[68] Consistent with this, FK506's neuroprotective effect is not dependent upon its immunosuppressive properties, as FK506 is still neuroprotective in the absence of FKBP-12, the immunophilin mediating calcineurin inhibition and FK506-mediated immunosuppression. It has been hypothesized that neuroprotection is instead mediated by binding to FKBP-52, which results in activation of the extracellular signal-regulated kinase pathway.[69] FK506 at a low, non-immunosuppressive dose and a non-immunosuppressant derivative (FK1706) both significantly reduced axonal injury in chronic relapsing EAE.[70] The above evidence suggests that neuroimmunophilin ligands may be effective neuroprotective agents in MS, and are certainly worthy of investigation by clinical trial.

Minocycline

Minocycline is a tetracycline antibiotic widely used for the treatment of acne. It has known anti-inflammatory properties, including inhibition of MMPs and reduction of microglial activation. Minocycline administration has been shown to reduce CNS inflammation and clinical severity of EAE.[71] Of pertinence to this discussion, minocycline appears to have neuroprotective properties in addition to its anti-inflammatory effect. In a pilot study, minocycline reduced the appearance of new Gd-enhancing lesions in patients with MS,[72] and appeared to be well tolerated. A larger trial of minocycline in MS is presently being conducted. However, it should be noted that potential detrimental effects of minocyline on remyelination have been described in a non-inflammatory animal model of ethidium bromide induced oligodendrocyte damage.[73] In a clinical trial in patients with amyotrophic lateral sclerosis, the drug made the patients worse.[74]

Sodium channel blockers

As discussed above, it has been demonstrated that the sodium channel blockers phenytoin, lamotrigine, and flecainide ameliorate axonal degeneration and improve clinical outcome in EAE. Of note, a protective effect was observed even when administration of phenytoin and flecainide was delayed until 7–10 days after disease induction in EAE. These data provide rationale to begin clinical studies that aim to test the neuroprotective efficacy of sodium channel blockers in MS. A potential concern is that these agents may cause decompensation of demyelinated axons, as sodium channel redistribution along the demyelinated axon may be responsible for clinical remission due to restoration of axonal conduction ability. More subtype specific blockade of Nav1.6 channels may obviate this concern, as preliminary evidence suggests that these channels are closely linked to axonal injury, in contrast to Nav1.2 channels whose expression in demyelinated axons promotes impulse conduction. A clinical trial with lamotrigine in patients with SPMS, however, failed to show any benefit in reducing the rate of brain atrophy.[75]

Glutamate antagonists

Glutamate excitotoxicity has been postulated to play a role in MS pathogenesis. In EAE and MS, brain microglia and macrophages release excessive amounts of glutamate, which potentially can damage axons and oligodendrocytes via AMPA-mediated excitotoxicity.[76] AMPA/kainate antagonists have been shown to ameliorate EAE-induced axonal injury.[43] Riluzole, a glutamate antagonist that is FDA-approved for the treatment of ALS, attenuated the clinical severity of myelin oligodendrocyte glycoprotein-induced EAE, reducing CNS demyelination and axonal damage. An open-label clinical trial of riluzole in primary progressive MS revealed preliminary evidence of a benefit in slowing cervical cord atrophy.[77] Other agents that act through this mechanism and have the potential for neuroprotection include talampanel and beta-lactam antibiotics.

Other novel neuroprotective strategies

Additional strategies include compounds, such as heat-shock protein co-inducers, which upregulate cell stress responses, and agents promoting autophagy and mitochondriogenesis, such as lithium and rapamycin. Cannabinoids exert anti-glutamatergic and anti-inflammatory actions through activation of the CB(1) and CB(2) receptors, respectively. Activation of CB(1) receptors may therefore inhibit glutamate release from presynaptic nerve terminals and reduce the postsynaptic calcium influx in response to glutamate receptor stimulation. Meanwhile, CB(2) receptors may influence inflammation, whereby receptor activation reduces microglial activation, resulting in a decrease in microglial secretion of neurotoxic mediators. Finally, cannabinoid agents may also exert anti-oxidant actions by a receptor-independent mechanism. Therefore, the ability of cannabinoids to target multiple neurotoxic pathways in different cell populations may increase their therapeutic potential in MS.[78] In a pilot study low dose *naltrexone* was shown to improve several quality of life measures.[79] It is proposed that the μ-opioid receptor antagonist, naltrexone, acts by reducing apoptosis of oligodendrocytes. It does this by reducing inducible NO synthase activity. This results in a decrease in the formation of peroxynitrites, which in turn prevent the inhibition of the glutamate transporters. *Resveratrol* and its derivatives,

SRT501 and SRT1720, have a neuroprotective effect in EAE without affecting the inflammatory response. They act via activation of SIRT1, an NAD-dependent deacetylase that promotes mitochondrial function.[80] *Ibudilast*, a phosphodiesterase inhibitor, has in vitro neuroprotectant properties by modulating inflammatory mediators such as TNF-α, leukotrienes, and NO, with some effects in animal models of CNS damage. In a trial of RRMS patients there was less atrophy in the treatment group, and inflammatory plaques were less likely to evolve into black holes.[57] *BG00012* (BG-12) is a fumaric acid ester. Its active agent, dimethyl fumarate has been used for treatment of psoriasis. It has both anti-inflammatory and neuroprotective properties and is administered orally. It is currently in clinical trials for MS.[81] NRF2 is a transcription factor that regulates a number of anti-oxidant pathways. Hence, compounds such as *bromocriptine* and *beta-naphthoflavone* that activate NRF2 have potential as neuroprotective.[82] It is also possible that a single agent may not be sufficient in providing neuroprotection, but rather a combination of agents acting on different pathways may be needed.

Neuroregenerative strategies in MS

Stem cells are immature cells that have the ability to self-renew and differentiate into multiple mature cell types. Several sources of stem cells exist, including pre-implantation embryos, and fetal and adult tissues. Stem cells exist within the adult CNS of higher mammals, and recently, several groups have successfully isolated and expanded human stem cells from specific regions of the brain and spinal cord. There are several potential ways by which stem cells could be therapeutically used. The conceptually simplest is to utilize endogenous or transplanted stem cells to replace cells damaged by age or disease. In MS, for example, transplanted OPCs may remyelinate host axons, serving both to augment axonal function and to protect the axon from degeneration. However, although conceptually simple, the "insertion" and functional integration of new cells or tissues into a mature organ is exceptionally complex and in many systems the ability of stem cells to achieve this is largely or completely unproven. As a simpler task, stem cells may serve to enhance the function of host tissues, to provide missing chemicals or enzymes or to halt a degenerative or neoplastic process. In MS, such a scenario may be manifest as stem cells which are transplanted in order to secrete trophic factors which support axonal function.

Stimulating endogenous stem cell function in the CNS

Stem cells exist within the adult, mammalian nervous system and neurogenesis, the formation of mature neural cells from precursor cells, occurs in discrete germinal centers throughout the life of all mammals including humans. Most of these studies suggest that new neurons are only generated in the subventricular zone and the hippocampal dentate gyrus. External factors such as enriched environment, physical activity and stress, or application of neurotrophins differentially modulate the generation of new neurons and oligodendrocytes from neural stem cells in the mammalian brain. Antidepressants, particularly the selective serotonin reuptake inhibitors, can induce proliferation and differentiation of neural stem cells.

Endogenous progenitor cells can be recruited to non-neurogenic areas following injury, and contribute to repair of the injured area.[83] However, it may be that new neurons and oligodendrocytes generated within these regions rapidly die and do not contribute to structural or functional recovery. Endogenous stem cells also exist within another non-neurogenic region of the nervous system, the spinal cord, although these cells do not contribute to the generation of new neural cells under normal conditions or following injury.[84] When transplanted into neurogenic regions of the nervous system, endogenous stem cells from non-neurogenic region do differentiate into neurons,[85] confirming that these stem cells are not inherently different from those found in neurogenic regions of the CNS. In part, the failure of stem cells present in non-neurogenic regions to differentiate into neurons may be due to the host environment which favors an astrocytic differentiation pathway[84] rather than one which favors the generation of oligodendrocytes or neurons. Modification of the signaling pathways or immune cell activation[86] within the spinal cord may alter the differentiation of stem cells in non-neurogenic regions such that occasional neurons are developed, though it is not clear that those neurons are capable of integrating into neural circuits or restoring function.

Applications of stem cells to demyelinating disease

Demyelination of axons is seen in many CNS disorders including spinal cord injury, MS, and stroke and likely contributes to the observed clinical dysfunction in all of these disorders. Schwann cells and neural precursor cells derived from adult human brain (subventricular zone) and from bone marrow have been studied anatomically and physiologically after transplantation into the demyelinated rat spinal cord.[87] Schwann cells and olfactory ensheathing cells (OECs) facilitated axonal regeneration and restoration of conduction across the lesioned area.[88] Myelinating OECs resemble myelinating Schwann cells in forming peripheral myelin sheaths around CNS axons and in the transcriptional pattern of myelin proteins.[89] Schwann cells and neural precursor cells derived from adult human brain and from bone marrow remyelinate axons after transplantation into the demyelinated rat spinal cord.[90] Highly purified OPCs can be expanded and purified from human embryonic stem cells and that, when transplanted into inflammatory demyelinating models, results in thin myelin lamella around host axons.[91]

Other researchers are investigating strategies that enhance the remyelinative potential of endogenous stem cells. Many studies have suggested that remyelination is minimal in the human CNS because endogenous OPCs fail to fully differentiate and assume a myelinating phenotype.[92] In rodents, there are abundant NG2+/PDGFRa+ OPCs.[93] These cells can be induced to differentiate by a variety of strategies including; thyroid hormones, retinoids (RXR agonists), and blockade of inhibitory pathways such as LINGO. LINGO is a molecule that is expressed on OPCs and naturally inhibits differentiation.[94] Blockade of LINGO results in rapid differentiation of OPCs into myelinating cells in vitro and in vivo in a variety of animal models.[95,96] This approach is now in Phase 1 trials in MS.

The paradigm has changed over time from the original prediction that mesenchymal stem cells (MSCs) would enhance tissue repair through their transdifferentiation into somatic cells to the current paradigm that they can produce therapeutic benefits without engraftment into the injured tissues. In particular, MSCs have the remarkable ability to modulate the immune response mainly by inhibiting proliferation of T-cells and to protect injured tissues through paracrine mechanisms. In an open label clinical trial autologous MSCs were injected intrathecally and/or intravenously.[97] The MSCs were well tolerated and could be localized to the occipital horn of the lateral ventricle. The mean (standard deviation) EDSS score improved from 6.7 (1.0) to 5.9 (1.6). This was accompanied with an increase in regulatory T-cells, a decrease in the proliferative responses of lymphocytes, and the expression of CD40, CD83, CD86, and HLA-DR on myeloid dendritic cells at 24 hours after MSC transplantation. Larger trials are now needed to confirm these observations.

Immunologic considerations

It is likely that, in some circumstances, transplanted cellular grafts may be recognized as foreign and rejected by the host immune system. Therefore, strategies must be employed that avoid rejection and in some cases, patients may need long-term immunosuppression. Alternatively, strategies may be employed to inhibit the rejection of transplanted cells by genetic or immunologic approaches. Genetic modification of major histocompatibility gene expression in transplanted cells may be achieved so that the transplant more closely resembles the host and is ignored by the host immune system. The introduction of immunosuppressive molecules such as Fas-ligand into cells prior to transplantation or knockdown of antigen presentation molecules such as B7 or CD40 could reduce immune rejection

of transplanted cells.[98] Somatic cell nuclear transplantation is another strategy which would eliminate the potential immune rejection by the host. In this approach, the nucleus from a normal somatic cell of the recipient is extracted and injected into an enucleated oocyte. The cytoplasm of this oocyte has the required potential to reprogram the differentiated nucleus injected and re-establishes an embryonic gene expression pattern in the chromatin of the somatic cell nucleus. The blastocyst formed from this oocyte would be the source for the derivation of new embryonic stem cell lines which would be genetically matched for each recipient.[99] In this case, whole major histocompatibility complex regions and other relevant proteins in immune rejection will be identical to that of the patient with the exception of minor molecules derived from mitochondrial genes.

Conclusions

It is now widely appreciated that substantial axonal loss occurs in the brains of patients with multiple sclerosis, and the degree of this axonal loss correlates with the severity of permanent neurological disability in patients. As the currently available immunomodulatory treatments for MS have only a modest impact on progressive axonal loss and disability particularly in advanced stages of the disease, there exists a pressing need to develop strategies to prevent this axonal loss. It is likely that axonal loss occurs in MS secondary to inflammation as well as due to demyelination and subsequent loss of trophic signaling to the axon from myelin. Hence, if one could discover the signaling mechanisms underpinning myelin-induced axonal protection, therapeutic strategies could be devised that exploit this protective signaling. In addition, there are a number of promising neuroprotective and remyelinating strategies but challenges remain in determining the appropriate trial design and outcome measures.

Acknowledgments

The authors have received grant support from the National MS Society (TR 3760-A-3, RO1 NS 41435 (PAC), and the Nancy Davis Center Without Walls.

References

1. Rudick RA, Lee JC, Simon J, Ransohoff RM, Fisher E. Defining interferon beta response status in multiple sclerosis patients. *Ann Neurol* 2004;56:548–55.

2. Brex PA, Molyneux PD, Smiddy P, *et al.* The effect of IFNbeta-1b on the evolution of enhancing lesions in secondary progressive MS. *Neurology* 2001;57:2185–90.

3. Filippi M, Rovaris M, Rocca MA, *et al.* Glatiramer acetate reduces the proportion of new MS lesions evolving into "black holes". *Neurology* 2001;57: 731–3.

4. Chen M, Valenzuela RM, Dhib-Jalbut S. Glatiramer acetate-reactive T cells produce brain-derived neurotrophic factor. *J Neurol Sci* 2003;215:37–44.

5. Miller DH, Soon D, Fernando KT, *et al.* MRI outcomes in a placebo-controlled trial of natalizumab in relapsing MS. *Neurology* 2007;68:1390–401.

6. Radue EW, Stuart WH, Calabresi PA, *et al.* Natalizumab plus interferon

beta-1a reduces lesion formation in relapsing multiple sclerosis. *J Neurol Sci* 2010;292:28–35.

7. Kappos L, Freedman MS, Polman CH, *et al.* Long-term effect of early treatment with interferon beta-1b after a first clinical event suggestive of multiple sclerosis: 5-year active treatment extension of the phase 3 BENEFIT trial. *Lancet Neurol* 2009;8:987–97.

8. Zivadinov R LL, Cookfair D, Srinivasaraghavan B, *et al.* Interferon

beta-1a slows progression of brain atrophy in relapsing-remitting multiple sclerosis predominantly by reducing gray matter atrophy. *Mult Scler* 2007; 13:490–501.

9. Fisher E, Lee JC, Nakamura K, Rudick RA. Gray matter atrophy in multiple sclerosis: a longitudinal study. *Ann Neurol* 2008;64:255–65.

10. Peterson JW, Bo L, Mork S, Chang A, Trapp BD. Transected neurites, apoptotic neurons, and reduced inflammation in cortical multiple sclerosis lesions. *Ann Neurol* 2001; 50:389–400.

11. Leary SM, Thompson AJ. Primary progressive multiple sclerosis : current and future treatment options. *CNS Drugs* 2005;19:369–76.

12. Kappos L. Effect of drugs in secondary disease progression in patients with multiple sclerosis. *Mult Scler* 2004; 10(Suppl 1):S46–54; discussion S-5.

13. Filippi M, Grossman RI. MRI techniques to monitor MS evolution: the present and the future. *Neurology* 2002;58:1147–53.

14. Sicotte NL, Kern KC, Giesser BS, *et al.* Regional hippocampal atrophy in multiple sclerosis. *Brain* 2008;131: 1134–41.

15. Naismith RT, Xu J, Tutlam NT, *et al.* Increased diffusivity in acute multiple sclerosis lesions predicts risk of black hole. *Neurology* 2010;74: 1694–701.

16. Harrison DM, Caffo BS, Shiee N, *et al.* Longitudinal changes in diffusion tensor-based quantitative MRI in multiple sclerosis. *Neurology* 2011; 76:179–86.

17. Filippi M, Bozzali M, Rovaris M, *et al.* Evidence for widespread axonal damage at the earliest clinical stage of multiple sclerosis. *Brain* 2003;126:433–7.

18. Bergers E, Bot JC, De Groot CJ, *et al.* Axonal damage in the spinal cord of MS patients occurs largely independent of T2 MRI lesions. *Neurology* 2002; 59(11):1766–71.

19. Waesberghe V. Axonal loss in multiple sclerosis lesions: magnetic resonance imaging insights into substrates of disability. *Ann Neurol* 1999;46: 747–54.

20. Lycklama G TA, Filippi M, Miller D, *et al.* Spinal-cord MRI in multiple sclerosis. *Lancet Neurol* 2003;2:555–62.

21. Smith SA, Golay X, Fatemi A, *et al.* Magnetization transfer weighted imaging in the upper cervical spinal cord using cerebrospinal fluid as intersubject normalization reference (MTCSF imaging). *Magn Reson Med* 2005;54:201–6.

22. Losseff NA, Wang L, Miller DH, Thompson AJ. T1 hypointensity of the spinal cord in multiple sclerosis. *J Neurol* 2001;248:517–21.

23. Losseff NA, Webb SL, O'Riordan JI, *et al.* Spinal cord atrophy and disability in multiple sclerosis. A new reproducible and sensitive MRI method with potential to monitor disease progression. *Brain* 1996;119:701–8.

24. Frohman E, Costello F, Zivadinov R, *et al.* Optical coherence tomography in multiple sclerosis. *Lancet Neurol* 2006;5:853–63.

25. Gordon-Lipkin E, Chodkowski B, Reich DS, *et al.* Retinal nerve fiber layer is associated with brain atrophy in multiple sclerosis. *Neurology* 2007; 69:1603–9.

26. Talman LS, Bisker ER, Sackel DJ, *et al.* Longitudinal study of vision and retinal nerve fiber layer thickness in multiple sclerosis. *Ann Neurol* 2010;6:749–60.

27. Lassmann H, Raine CS, Antel J, Prineas JW. Immunopathology of multiple sclerosis: report on an international meeting held at the Institute of Neurology of the University of Vienna. *J Neuroimmunol* 1998;86:213–7.

28. Wang T, Lee MH, Johnson T, *et al.* Activated T-cells inhibit neurogenesis by releasing granzyme B: rescue by Kv1.3 blockers. *J Neurosci* 2010;30: 5020–7.

29. Lucchinetti C, Bruck W, Parisi J, *et al.* Heterogeneity of multiple sclerosis lesions: implications for the pathogenesis of demyelination. *Ann Neurol* 2000;47:707–17.

30. Raine CS, Cannella B, Hauser SL, Genain CP. Demyelination in primate autoimmune encephalomyelitis and acute multiple sclerosis lesions: a case for antigen-specific antibody mediation. *Ann Neurol* 1999;46:144–60.

31. Aharoni R, Arnon R, Eilam R. Neurogenesis and neuroprotection induced by peripheral immunomodulatory treatment of experimental autoimmune encephalomyelitis. *J Neurosci* 2005;25:8217–28.

32. Sriram S, Rodriguez M. Indictment of the microglia as the villain in multiple sclerosis. *Neurology* 1997;48:464–70.

33. Piccio L, Buonsanti C, Cella M, *et al.* Identification of soluble TREM-2 in the cerebrospinal fluid and its association with multiple sclerosis and CNS inflammation. *Brain* 2008;131:3081–91.

34. Becher B, Durell BG, Noelle RJ. IL-23 produced by CNS-resident cells controls T cell encephalitogenicity during the effector phase of experimental autoimmune encephalomyelitis. *J Clin Invest* 2003; 112:1186–91.

35. De Groot CJ RS, Theeuwes JW, Dijkstra CD, Van Der Valk P. Immunocytochemical characterization of the expression of inducible and constitutive isoforms of nitric oxide synthase in demyelinating multiple sclerosis lesions. *J Neuropathol Exp Neurol* 1997;56:10–20.

36. Araujo IM, Carvalho CM. Role of nitric oxide and calpain activation in neuronal death and survival. *Curr Drug Targets CNS Neurol Disord* 2005;4: 319–24.

37. Koh DW, Dawson TM, Dawson VL. Mediation of cell death by poly(ADP-ribose) polymerase-1. *Pharmacol Res* 2005;52:5–14.

38. Lu F, Selak M, O'Connor J, *et al.* Oxidative damage to mitochondrial DNA and activity of mitochondrial enzymes in chronic active lesions of multiple sclerosis. *J Neurol Sci* 2000; 177:95–103.

39. Heppner FL, Greter M, Marino D, *et al.* Experimental autoimmune encephalomyelitis repressed by microglial paralysis. *Nat Med* 2005;11: 146–52.

40. Constantinescu CS TM, Ransohoff RM, Wysocka M, *et al.* Astrocytes as antigen-presenting cells: expression of IL-12/IL-23. *J Neurochem* 2005;95:331–40.

41. Kaplin AI, Deshpande DM, Scott E, *et al.* IL-6 induces regionally selective spinal cord injury in patients with the neuroinflammatory disorder transverse myelitis. *J Clin Invest* 2005;115: 2731–41.

42. Pitt D, Nagelmeier IE, Wilson HC, Raine CS. Glutamate uptake by oligodendrocytes: Implications for excitotoxicity in multiple sclerosis. *Neurology* 2003;61:1113–20.

43. Pitt D, Werner P, Raine CS. Glutamate excitotoxicity in a model of multiple sclerosis. *Nat Med* 2000;6:67–70.

44. Waxman SG, Craner MJ, Black JA. Na$^+$ channel expression along axons in multiple sclerosis and its models. *Trends Pharmacol Sci* 2004;25:584–91.

45. Stys PK. General mechanisms of axonal damage and its prevention. *J Neurol Sci* 2005;233:3–13.

46. Bechtold DA KR, Smith KJ. Axonal protection using flecainide in experimental autoimmune encephalomyelitis. *Ann Neurol* 2004;55:607–16.

47. Lo AC, Saab CY, Black JA, Waxman SG. Phenytoin protects spinal cord axons and preserves axonal conduction and neurological function in a model of neuroinflammation in vivo. *J Neurophysiol* 2003;90:3566–71.

48. Rus H, Pardo CA, Hu L, et al. The voltage-gated potassium channel Kv1.3 is highly expressed on inflammatory infiltrates in multiple sclerosis brain. *Proc Natl Acad Sci USA* 2005;102:11094–9.

49. Goodman AD, Brown TR, Krupp LB, et al. Sustained-release oral fampridine in multiple sclerosis: a randomised, double-blind, controlled trial. *Lancet* 2009;373:732–8.

50. Simon JH, Kinkel RP, Jacobs L, Bub L, Simonian N. A Wallerian degeneration pattern in patients at risk for MS. *Neurology* 2000;54:1155–60.

51. Krajewski KM, Lewis RA, Fuerst DR, et al. Neurological dysfunction and axonal degeneration in Charcot–Marie–Tooth disease type 1A. *Brain* 2000;123:1516–27.

52. Bjartmar C, Wujek JR, Trapp BD. Axonal loss in the pathology of MS: consequences for understanding the progressive phase of the disease. *J Neurol Sci* 2003;206:165–71.

53. Nguyen T, Mehta NR, Conant K, et al. Axonal protective effects of the myelin-associated glycoprotein. *J Neurosci* 2009;29:630–7.

54. Yin X, Crawford TO, Griffin JW, et al. Myelin-associated glycoprotein is a myelin signal that modulates the caliber of myelinated axons. *J Neurosci* 1998;18:1953–62.

55. Raff MC, Whitmore AV, Finn JT. Axonal self-destruction and neurodegeneration. *Science* 2002;296:868–71.

56. Sagot Y, Dubois-Dauphin M, Tan SA, et al. Bcl-2 overexpression prevents motoneuron cell body loss but not axonal degeneration in a mouse model of a neurodegenerative disease. *J Neurosci* 1995;15:7727–33.

57. Barkhof F, Hulst HE, Drulovic J, et al. Ibudilast in relapsing-remitting multiple sclerosis: a neuroprotectant? *Neurology* 2010;74:1033–40.

58. Chen JT, Kuhlmann T, Jansen GH, et al. Voxel-based analysis of the evolution of magnetization transfer ratio to quantify remyelination and demyelination with histopathological validation in a multiple sclerosis lesion. *Neuroimage* 2007;36:1152–8.

59. Villoslada P, Arrondo G, Sepulcre J, Alegre M, Artieda J. Memantine induces reversible neurologic impairment in patients with MS. *Neurology* 2009;72:1630–3.

60. Birnbaum G, Cree B, Altafullah I, Zinser M, Reder AT. Combining beta interferon and atorvastatin may increase disease activity in multiple sclerosis. *Neurology* 2008;71:1390–5.

61. Gonsette RE, Sindic C, D'Hooghe M B, et al. Boosting endogenous neuroprotection in multiple sclerosis: the ASsociation of Inosine and Interferon beta in relapsing–remitting Multiple Sclerosis (ASIIMS) trial. *Mult Scler* 2010;16:455–62.

62. Prieto JM, Dapena D, Lema M, et al. [Pentoxifylline: is it useful in multiple sclerosis?]. *Rev Neurol* 2001;32:529–31.

63. Agnello D, Bigini P, Villa P, et al. Erythropoietin exerts an anti-inflammatory effect on the CNS in a model of experimental autoimmune encephalomyelitis. *Brain Res* 2002;952:128–34.

64. Slaets H, Hendriks JJ, Stinissen P, Kilpatrick TJ, Hellings N. Therapeutic potential of LIF in multiple sclerosis. *Trends Mol Med* 2010;16:493–500.

65. Crawford DK, Mangiardi M, Song B, et al. Oestrogen receptor beta ligand: a novel treatment to enhance endogenous functional remyelination. *Brain* 2010;133:2999–3016.

66. Jones JL, Anderson JM, Phuah CL, et al. Improvement in disability after alemtuzumab treatment of multiple sclerosis is associated with neuroprotective autoimmunity. *Brain* 2010;133:2232–47.

67. Chesik D, De Keyser J, Bron R, Fuhler GM. Insulin-like growth factor binding protein-1 activates integrin-mediated intracellular signaling and migration in oligodendrocytes. *J Neurochem* 2010;113:1319–30.

68. Steiner JP, Hamilton GS, Ross DT, et al. Neurotrophic immunophilin ligands stimulate structural and functional recovery in neurodegenerative animal models. *Proc Natl Acad Sci USA* 1997;94:2019–24.

69. Gold BG, Zhong YP. FK506 requires stimulation of the extracellular signal-regulated kinase 1/2 and the steroid receptor chaperone protein p23 for neurite elongation. *Neurosignals* 2004;13:122–9.

70. Gold BG, Voda J, Yu X, McKeon G, Bourdette DN. FK506 and a nonimmunosuppressant derivative reduce axonal and myelin damage in experimental autoimmune encephalomyelitis: neuroimmunophilin ligand-mediated neuroprotection in a model of multiple sclerosis. *J Neurosci Res* 2004;77:367–77.

71. Popovic N, Schubart A, Goetz BD, et al. Inhibition of autoimmune encephalomyelitis by a tetracycline. *Ann Neurol* 2002;51:215–23.

72. Metz LM, Zhang Y, Yeung M, et al. Minocycline reduces gadolinium-enhancing magnetic resonance imaging lesions in multiple sclerosis. *Ann Neurol* 2004;55:756.

73. Li WW, Setzu A, Zhao C, Franklin RJ. Minocycline-mediated inhibition of microglia activation impairs oligodendrocyte progenitor cell responses and remyelination in a non-immune model of demyelination. *J Neuroimmunol* 2005;158:58–66.

74. Gordon PH, Moore DH, Miller RG, et al. Efficacy of minocycline in patients with amyotrophic lateral sclerosis: a phase III randomised trial. *Lancet Neurol* 2007;6:1045–53.

75. Kapoor R, Furby J, Hayton T, et al. Lamotrigine for neuroprotection in secondary progressive multiple sclerosis: a randomised, double-blind, placebo-controlled, parallel-group trial. *Lancet Neurol* 2010;9:681–8.

76. McDonald JW, Althomsons SP, Hyrc KL, Choi DW, Goldberg MP. Oligodendrocytes from forebrain are

highly vulnerable to AMPA/kainate receptor-mediated excitotoxicity. *Nat Med* 1998;4:291–7.

77. Killestein J, Kalkers NF, Polman CH. Glutamate inhibition in MS: the neuroprotective properties of riluzole. *J Neurol Sci* 2005;233:113–5.

78. Bisogno T, Di Marzo V. Cannabinoid receptors and endocannabinoids: role in neuroinflammatory and neurodegenerative disorders. *CNS Neurol Disord Drug Targets* 2010;9:564–73.

79. Cree BA, Kornyeyeva E, Goodin DS. Pilot trial of low-dose naltrexone and quality of life in multiple sclerosis. *Ann Neurol* 2010;68:145–50.

80. Shindler KS, Ventura E, Dutt M, *et al.* Oral resveratrol reduces neuronal damage in a model of multiple sclerosis. *J Neuroophthalmol* 2010;30:328–39.

81. Papadopoulou A, D'Souza M, Kappos L, Yaldizli O. Dimethyl fumarate for multiple sclerosis. *Expert Opin Investig Drugs* 2010;19:1603–12.

82. Nannelli A, Rossignolo F, Tolando R, *et al.* Effect of beta-naphthoflavone on AhR-regulated genes (CYP1A1, 1A2, 1B1, 2S1, Nrf2, and GST) and antioxidant enzymes in various brain regions of pig. *Toxicology* 2009;265:69–79.

83. Magavi SS, Leavitt BR, Macklis JD. Induction of neurogenesis in the neocortex of adult mice. *Nature* 2000;405:951–5.

84. Yamamoto S, Yamamoto N, Kitamura T, Nakamura K, Nakafuku M. Proliferation of parenchymal neural progenitors in response to injury in the adult rat spinal cord. *Exp Neurol* 2001;172:115–27.

85. Shihabuddin LS, Horner PJ, Ray J, Gage FH. Adult spinal cord stem cells generate neurons after transplantation in the adult dentate gyrus. *J Neurosci* 2000;20:8727–35.

86. Mikami Y, Okano H, Sakaguchi M, *et al.* Implantation of dendritic cells in injured adult spinal cord results in activation of endogenous neural stem/progenitor cells leading to de novo neurogenesis and functional recovery. *J Neurosci Res* 2004;76:453–65.

87. Akiyama Y, Radtke C, Kocsis JD. Remyelination of the rat spinal cord by transplantation of identified bone marrow stromal cells. *J Neurosci* 2002;22:6623–30.

88. Fouad K, Schnell L, Bunge MB, *et al.* Combining Schwann cell bridges and olfactory-ensheathing glia grafts with chondroitinase promotes locomotor recovery after complete transection of the spinal cord. *J Neurosci* 2005;25:1169–78.

89. Franklin RJ, Gilson JM, Franceschini IA, Barnett SC. Schwann cell-like myelination following transplantation of an olfactory bulb-ensheathing cell line into areas of demyelination in the adult CNS. *Glia* 1996;17:217–24.

90. Kocsis JD, Akiyama Y, Radtke C. Neural precursors as a cell source to repair the demyelinated spinal cord. *J Neurotrauma* 2004;21:441–9.

91. Groves AK, Barnett SC, Franklin RJ, *et al.* Repair of demyelinated lesions by transplantation of purified O-2A progenitor cells. *Nature* 1993;362:453–5.

92. Zhao C, Fancy SP, Kotter MR, Li WW, Franklin RJ. Mechanisms of CNS remyelination – the key to therapeutic advances. *J Neurol Sci* 2005;233:87–91.

93. Kang SH, Fukaya M, Yang JK, Rothstein JD, Bergles DE. NG2+ CNS glial progenitors remain committed to the oligodendrocyte lineage in postnatal life and following neurodegeneration. *Neuron* 2010;68:668–81.

94. Mi S, Miller RH, Lee X, *et al.* LINGO-1 negatively regulates myelination by oligodendrocytes. *Nat Neurosci* 2005;8:745–51.

95. Mi S, Hu B, Hahm K, *et al.* LINGO-1 antagonist promotes spinal cord remyelination and axonal integrity in MOG-induced experimental autoimmune encephalomyelitis. *Nat Med* 2007;13:1228–33.

96. Mi S, Miller RH, Tang W, *et al.* Promotion of central nervous system remyelination by induced differentiation of oligodendrocyte precursor cells. *Ann Neurol* 2009;65:304–15.

97. Karussis D, Karageorgiou C, Vaknin-Dembinsky A, *et al.* Safety and immunological effects of mesenchymal stem cell transplantation in patients with multiple sclerosis and amyotrophic lateral sclerosis. *Arch Neurol* 2010;67:1187–94.

98. Harlan DM, Kirk AD. The future of organ and tissue transplantation: can T-cell costimulatory pathway modifiers revolutionize the prevention of graft rejection? *JAMA* 1999;282:1076–82.

99. Hochedlinger K, Rideout WM, Kyba M, *et al.* Nuclear transplantation, embryonic stem cells and the potential for cell therapy. *Hematol J* 2004;5 (Suppl 3):S114–17.

Chapter

47

Combination therapy in multiple sclerosis

Michelle Fabian and Fred D. Lublin

Introduction

Since 1993, the field of multiple sclerosis (MS) therapeutics has changed dramatically with the approval by North American and European regulatory agencies of interferon beta-1b (IFNβ-1b, Betaseron), IFNβ-1a by intramuscular injection, (IFNβ-1a (IM), Avonex), IFNβ-1a by subcutaneous injection (IFNβ-1a (SC), Rebif), glatiramer acetate (GA, Copaxone), natalizumab (Tysabri), and most recently in the United States, fingolimod (Gilenya), for the treatment of relapsing–remitting MS (RRMS). In Europe, IFNβ-1b has also been approved for use in secondary progressive MS (SPMS), and in the US Mitoxantrone (mitox, Novantrone) has this indication. Although these agents are clearly beneficial, efficacy is only partial. In the pivotal trials that led to approval, all produced only an approximately 30%–68% reduction in relapse rate and approximately 10% absolute reduction of the proportion of patients with sustained worsening of disability.[1-8] Experience in clinical practice corroborates this observation: a sizable proportion of patients have continued relapses or worsening disability despite these therapies. A variety of factors probably contribute to this incomplete response:

- Pharmacogenomic and pathogenic heterogeneity leading to responders and non-responders.
- Non-compliance because of route of administration and/or side effects.
- Emergence of biological resistance.
- Development of neutralizing antibodies (NAbs) vs. IFNβ or natalizumab.

Thus, there is a clear need for more effective and better tolerated therapies. Several approaches have been considered for future experimental therapeutics in MS:

1. *Trials to define the optimal use of currently available agents* For example, multiple prospective therapeutic trials using either IFNβ or GA have now shown that the initiation of a disease-modifying agent at the time of a clinically isolated syndrome (CIS) results in a delay of the occurrence of the second neurological episode.[9-11] There is a suggestion that starting therapy at an early stage of the disease improves efficacy of the drug as well. Another example of this approach would be trials that utilize an increased understanding of disease pathogenesis and biomarkers. These trials would hopefully provide evidence that will allow the physician to choose from established therapies on an individualized basis, according to a patient's unique disease characteristics.

2. *Trials of monotherapies with novel agents* As the pathophysiology of the MS is further elucidated, it is likely that drugs will be developed that will be superior to currently available agents in terms of efficacy, safety, or tolerability.

3. *Trials based on new approaches to treatment* An example of this approach is trials of new therapies based on the known beneficial effects of pregnancy on MS.[12-14] Better understanding of the biological mechanisms by which the differences in the immunogenicity of the fetus are tolerated during pregnancy may lead to new and different approaches in therapy. Another interesting approach would involve employment of neuroprotective or repair strategies.[15]

4. *Trials of combination therapies* The use of combinations of disease-modifying agents may lead to additive or even synergistic effects. This approach is the subject of this chapter.

Rationale for combination therapy

Combination therapy has been used successfully for a number of years in a variety of conditions including cancer, hypertension, diabetes, infectious diseases, and immune-mediated diseases. In fact, the standard of care for the majority of serious, chronic diseases dictates the use of combination therapies in order to achieve optimal disease control.

As an example, in infectious disease, the combination of various antibiotics is necessary to effectively treat multi-drug resistant tuberculosis.[16] In a similar manner, the introduction of highly active anti-retroviral therapy regimens in the management human immunodeficiency virus infection dramatically changed the clinical course and prognosis for these patients.[17] In cancer treatment, the use of combinations of chemotherapeutic agents is commonplace. Additionally,

Multiple Sclerosis Therapeutics, Fourth Edition, ed. Jeffrey A. Cohen and Richard A. Rudick. Published by Cambridge University Press.
© Cambridge University Press 2011.

combination therapy is often essential for management of hypertension.

More closely analogous to the use of combination therapies in MS is the use of combination therapies in autoimmune diseases such as rheumatoid arthritis (RA). In RA, multiple studies of combination therapies have proven its use to be extremely efficacious, affording much better disease control with acceptable toxicity profiles.[18] For example, in a combination trial with rituximab and methotrexate (MTX), the combination of medications led to greater than 50% of the patients in the combination therapy group achieving at least a 20% improvement in clinical disease activity compared to 24% of the MTX monotherapy group achieving the same disease control.[19] In support of combination therapies in RA, a systematic review of multiple randomized, active comparator trials found that clinical disease remission was 74% more likely and radiographic disease stability was 30% more likely with the use of a biologic plus MTX when compared to MTX alone.[20] Of note, not all combination regimens that have been studied in RA have shown additive or synergistic effects. For example, the addition of gold[21] or azathioprine (AZA)[22] to MTX was no more effective than monotherapy. The addition of hydroxychloroquine to gold was marginally more effective, but also more toxic than gold alone.[23]

Several lines of evidence suggest that combination therapy could be an effective approach in the treatment of MS (Table 47.1). It appears that multiple environmental and genetic factors play a role in the disease.[24] Viruses may trigger the disease, although this has not been definitively demonstrated.[25] Chronic immune dysregulation ultimately targeting central nervous system myelin is postulated to result in tissue injury. Due in part to epitope spreading, there are likely multiple myelin antigens involved in MS pathogenesis.[26] An important mechanism is thought to be cell-mediated autoimmunity, possibly due to defective T-cell regulatory function, and by altered immunological balance with a shift away from anti-inflammatory response towards pro-inflammatory responses.[27] There is also increasing evidence of a role for B-cell mechanisms and innate immunity in the disease process.[28-29] For these and other reasons there are presumably multiple different subtypes of MS.[30] This immunopathogenic heterogeneity may explain why patients respond to each of the available agents to variable degrees and supports the hypothesis that a combination of synergistic agents would be more likely to achieve optimal disease control when compared to a monotherapy approach.

Considerations for designing trials of combination therapies

The first and most important question is which therapies to include in the combination. To improve the chances of additive or, even better, synergistic beneficial effects, candidate drugs for combination therapy should have demonstrated stand alone efficacy and distinct mechanisms of action. In the case of MS, drugs could be directed at different therapeutic domains such

Table 47.1. *Rationale for combination therapy in multiple sclerosis (MS)*

Factors supporting the use of combination therapy in MS
- The pathogenesis of MS is complex with numerous contributory mechanisms.
- The pathogenesis of MS may be heterogeneous across patients and in individual patients over time.
- Agents with partial efficacy individually may have additive or synergistic efficacy in combination.
- Use of agents in combination may allow for lower doses with decreased side effects.
- Combination therapy has proven useful in other disorders.

Caveats in the testing of combination therapy in MS
- Overlapping mechanisms of action of agents can lead to no additional efficacy when used in combination.
- Interfering mechanisms of action may lead to decreased efficacy incombination.
- There may be additive, synergistic, or unanticipated toxicities.
- The number of potential combinations is large.
- Dose-finding for each component is necessary.
- Incomplete understanding of MS pathogenesis, incomplete understanding of mechanisms of action of potential therapies, and lack of reliable animal model makes selection of combinations largely empirical.
- The logistics of securing funding for trials of combination therapy can be difficult.
  - Definitive trials require large numbers of patients and, thus, are expensive.
  - The agents to be tested in combination may be marketed by different companies.
  - The agents to be tested may be off-patent and, as such, it may be difficult to secure funding from industry sponsors.

as tissue destruction and tissue repair. But the concept also holds within a given therapeutic domain. For example, currently available therapies act through modulating the immune system, but at different levels. Theoretically, in vitro or animal data could direct the choice among several candidate therapies. Unfortunately, results from such experiments do not necessarily predict successful results when tested in humans.

The safety and tolerability of the candidate treatments must also be taken into account. Each therapy in the combination must have an acceptable safety profile. Ideally, toxicity might be lessened with the combination by decreasing the dosage of each individual agent. This potential advantage has been one of the rationales for combining AZA and steroids in the treatment of myasthenia gravis.[31-32] In practice, in a disease such as MS which afflicts young patients and does not reduce life expectancy significantly, drugs with a good long-term safety and tolerability profile should be selected preferentially.

The second question is how to test combination therapy in MS patients. A Phase 1 study should serve as a preliminary evaluation of safety and tolerability of the combination. The rationale for this is three-fold: (1) checking via monitoring clinical and biological parameters at regular intervals that the combination is acceptably safe and well tolerated – this includes close monitoring for toxicities as well as for opportunistic infections; (2) assessing by means of appropriate pharmacological assessments the impact of the combination on the pharmacokinetics and pharmacodynamics of each individual drug in the

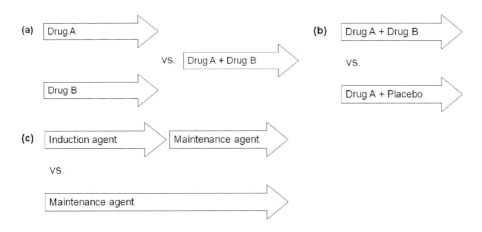

Fig. 47.1. Possible designs for Phase 2 combination trials: (a) combination therapy compared retrospectively to monotherapy, (b) combination therapy compared to contemporaneous monotherapy, (c) induction/maintenance compared to maintenance therapy alone.

combination (3) searching for trends towards efficacy or conversely, adverse interactions by using relatively sensitive markers such as MRI activity measured as new or enlarging T2-hyperintense lesions or gadolinium (Gd)-enhancing lesions. These early assessments should also exclude a detrimental effect of the combination on MS. Dose-finding for the agents used in combination must also be done at this stage.

The design of Phase 2 studies is straightforward when the combination consists of two drugs, A and B. Potential designs include either testing two agents alone in a run-in period followed by the combination as illustrated in Fig. 47.1(a), or testing one agent vs. the combination and placebo as illustrated in Fig. 47.1(b). It becomes more complex when the goal is to test combinations of more than two agents. For combination strategies of the sequential type, e.g. an induction phase followed by a maintenance phase, or escalation strategies, a conventional parallel design is appropriate, such as the design in Fig. 47.1(c).

Such Phase 2 studies should take place before a large Phase 3 efficacy study, but this strategy may prove time-consuming and may delay a Phase 3 study. This is a major problem in MS, where definitive Phase 3 trials require years with currently available outcome criteria. In order to save time and resources, an alternative would be to combine Phase 2 and 3 studies, with rigorous monitoring of safety and tolerability of the drug combination during the initial stages of the trial. Expansion to a sample size and duration of treatment required for a pivotal trial could be contingent on the results of interim analysis of the initial part of the trial.

The third question is how to best design the Phase 3 pivotal efficacy trial. Although there are many possible designs, ideally a full factorial 2 × 2 design is preferable. The 2 × 2 design results in four groups: Active A/Active B, Active A/Placebo B, Placebo A/Active B, and Placebo A/Placebo B. The advantage of the 2x2 factorial design is that, in addition to testing the combination of agents against placebo, this design also allows for both monotherapies to be tested against the combination and against each other in a head-to-head fashion. In practice, such a design becomes unrealistic when the goal is to assess all possible combinations of three or more agents. Also, at the present time,

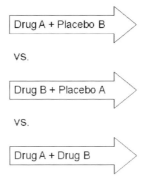

Fig. 47.2. Design for a Phase 3 combination trial. This trial design allows for the combination of agents to be tested against each monotherapy. Additionally, the two monotherapies are compared to one another in a head-to-head fashion.

a double placebo arm is difficult to justify on ethical grounds for most trials in RRMS and thus a three-arm design, such as the depicted in Fig. 47.2, will be more likely to be employed in future Phase 3 combination trials.

Selected trials of combination therapies

A sizable number of trials of combination therapy are planned, are in progress, or have been completed (see Table 47.2). Selected trials are discussed below.

CombiRx

A pilot trial of 33 participants with RRMS demonstrated that combined therapy with IFNβ-1a (IM) and GA was safe as measured by clinical, laboratory and MRI assessments over six months.[33] A large-scale, National Institutes of Health-funded trial (CombiRx) is currently fully enrolled (1008 participants) and will be completed in January 2012.[34] Key eligibility criteria include a diagnosis of RRMS, Expanded Disability Status Scale (EDSS) score 0–5.5, at least two relapses in the prior three years, and no prior treatment with IFNβ or GA. Participants are randomized to IFNβ-1a (IM) and placebo, GA and placebo, or both active drugs in combination. The primary outcome measure is annualized relapse rate (ARR) over three years of follow-up. There is a focus on obtaining key biomarker information during this time as well. This study will provide definitive evidence as to whether combination therapy with IFNβ-1a (IM) and GA is

Table 47.2. *Selected from notable, ongoing, and recently completed trials of combination disease therapy in multiple sclerosis (MS)*

Agents	Type of MS	Subjects	Investigator/Reference	Status
IFNβ-1a (IM) + GA	RR	1008	CombiRx[34]	Ongoing
Natalizumab + IFNβ-1a (IM)	RR	1171	SENTINEL[35]	Completed
Natalizumab + GA	RR	110	GLANCE[36]	Completed
Cladribine + IFNβ-1a (SC)	RR, SP with relapse	200	ONWARD[37]	Ongoing
Mitox induction + GA	RR, PR	30	Vollmer et al.[38]	Completed
Daclizumab + IFNβ	RR	230	CHOICE[39]	Completed
Teriflunomide + IFNβ	RR	120	Freedman et al.[40]	Completed
Teriflunomide + GA	RR	116	Freedman et al.[41]	Completed
Mycophenalate mofetil + IFNβ-1a (IM)	RR	24	Frohman et al.[42]	Completed
PO MP + IFNβ-1a (IM)	RR	341	MECOMBIN[43]	Completed
PO MP + IFNβ1-a (SC)	RR	130	NORMIMS[44]	Completed
MTX + i.v. MP + IFNβ-1a (IM)	RR	313	ACT[45]	Completed
AZA + prednisone + IFNβ-1a (IM)	RR	182	ASA[46]	Completed
Estriol + GA	RR, women	130	Voksuhl et al.[47]	Ongoing
Etinilestradiol + desogestrel + IFNβ-1a (SC)	RR, women	180	Pozzilli et al.[48]	Ongoing
Albuterol + GA	RR	44	Khoury et al.[49]	Completed
Simvastatin + IFNβ-1a (IM)	RR	380	SIMCOMBIN[50]	Completed
Minocycline + IFNβ-1a (SC)	RR	380	RECYCLINE[51]	Ongoing
Minocycline + GA	RR	50	Godin et al.[52]	Completed
Doxycycline + IFNβ-1a (IM)	RR	15	Minagar et al.[53]	Completed
Sunphenon + GA	RR	100	Bellmann-Strobl et al.[54]	Ongoing
Lamotrigine + IFNβ-1a (IM)	RR	88	Putzki et al.[55]	Ongoing
Riluzole + IFNβ-1a (IM)	CIS, RR	40	Waubant et al.[56]	Ongoing

Adapted from *Clinical Trials in Multiple Sclerosis: 2010*, available on the website of the National MS Society. (http://www.nationalmssociety.org/research/clinical-trials/participate-in-clinical-trials/index.aspx)

AZA = azathioprine, CIS = clinically isolated yndrome, GA = glatiramer acetate, IFNβ = interferon beta, IM = intramuscular, i.v. = intravenous, mitox = mitoxantrone, MP = methylprednisolone, MTX = methotrexate, RR = relapsing–remitting, SP = secondary progressive.

more efficacious than either therapy alone. In addition, there is a head-to-head component that will allow comparison of IFNβ-1a (IM) to GA. As some participants will be on study in excess of 7 years, the study will allow for a better assessment of the factors that lead to irreversible worsening than previously possible. The biomarker study will provide data on genomic, RNA expression, and proteomic expression in MS and potentially provide profiles for responders and non-responders to the study agents as well as prognostic information.

Combination trials with natalizumab

Currently, natalizumab is approved only as a monotherapy. This is due to concern over combined toxicity because of the two cases of progressive multifocal leukoencephalopathy (PML) that occurred in patients enrolled in the combination arm of the SENTINEL trial as discussed below. However, natalizumab combination trials remain important examples of combination therapy trials in MS.

Sentinel

The largest completed trial of combination therapy in MS to date has been SENTINEL (Safety and Efficacy of Natalizumab in Combination with Interferon β-1a in Patient with Relapsing-Remitting MS), a randomized, double-blind, placebo-controlled multicenter Phase 3 trial that assessed the efficacy, tolerability and safety of natalizumab combined with IFNβ-1a (IM).[35] This trial is discussed in detail elsewhere in the book. Briefly, a total of 1171 participants with RRMS at 124 centers in the USA and Europe, with one or more relapses in the 12 months prior to randomization despite IFNβ-1a (IM) therapy, were randomized to receive either natalizumab 300 mg or placebo intravenously every four weeks as add-on therapy to IFNβ-1a (IM). Primary end-points were the relapse rate at one year and disability progression at two years.

In general, the combination was well tolerated. There were no apparent increases in overall rates of standard infections or malignancy. As discussed in detail elsewhere in this book, the trial was stopped approximately one month early due to two reports of PML in patients in the combination arm. Natalizumab added to IFNβ-1a (IM) reduced the ARR by 55% (0.34 vs. 0.75, $P < 0.001$) and disability (EDSS) progression by 24% (hazard ratio 0.76, $P = 0.02$) compared with IFNβ-1a plus placebo. The number of new and enlarging T2-hyperintense MRI lesions was reduced by 83% ($P < 0.001$), and the number of Gd-enhancing lesions by 89% ($P < 0.001$).

This trial illustrates several important points. First, a large sample size is necessary to definitively demonstrate an efficacy advantage of combination therapy over monotherapy. This trial confirmed superior efficacy of natalizumab /IFNβ-1a (IM) combination over IFNβ-1a (IM) alone. However, the second point is that the design precluded confirmation that the combination was superior to natalizumab alone. This is a problem that is unavoidable if a trial does not include an arm testing the new agent as monotherapy in addition to testing the combination. Finally, SENTINEL illustrates the potential for unanticipated toxicity to arise when agents are used in combination, as the two patients who developed PML were in the combination arm. However, subsequent experience with natalizumab has shown that PML can occur with use of natalizumab as monotherapy.

GLANCE

GLANCE (Glatiramer Acetate and Natalizumab Combination Evaluation) was a Phase 2 trial that enrolled 110 participants between June, 2003 and March, 2004. Eligibility requirements included a diagnosis of RRMS and therapy with GA for ≥ 12 months with one or more relapses during that time. This randomized, double-blind placebo-controlled 24-week trial compared the combination of natalizumab and GA against GA alone by utilizing a novel primary end-point of rate of new lesion formation.[36] Secondary end-points included additional MRI parameters, annualized relapse rate, incidence of adverse events (AEs), and prevalence of serum anti-natalizumab antibodies in the combination group.

This trial was conducted in large part as a safety trial to address the concern that the combination of natalizumab and GA might not provide additive efficacy, as natalizumab's inhibition of leukocyte egress across the blood–brain barrier might prevent GA from its theorized beneficial actions in the central nervous system. The results of GLANCE did not support the concerns about potential negative effects of natalizumab and GA in combination. The rate of new lesion formation over 24 weeks was decreased in the combination group vs. the GA alone group (0.11 vs. 0.03, $P = 0.03$). Additionally, there was a nonsignificant trend towards a decrease in ARR with combination therapy vs. GA alone (0.4 vs. 0.67, $P = 0.24$). The combination was well tolerated with no evidence of increase of serious AEs in the combination group. Of note, there was a 13% incidence of natalizumab neutralizing antibody formation in GLANCE compared with 6% of patients in Phase 3 trials of natalizumab. The authors hypothesized that the addition of GA allowed for an immune shift that promoted the production of more antibodies, including those against natalizumab. In the patients that were persistently positive for NAbs, there was a trend towards

increased ARR and infusion-related AEs compared to the transiently positive and never positive participants.

Combination trials with steroids

Perhaps the most frequently used combination therapy approach utilized in clinical practice for patients with RRMS and continued disease activity while on platform therapy is the ad hoc addition of periodic courses of corticosteroids, most often intravenous methylprednisolone (i.v. MP). There have now been multiple trials assessing whether there is a role for corticosteroids in the management of MS outside of treatment for relapses, although none has answered this question conclusively.

Mecombin

Mecombin (methylprednisolone in combination with interferon beta-1a for relapsing–remitting MS) was a 39-month randomized double-blind, placebo-controlled trial comparing patients on IFNβ-1a (IM) combined with monthly, three-day pulses of 500 mg of oral methylprednisolone (PO MP) starting three months after initiation of IFNβ therapy vs. those on IFNβ-1a (IM) alone.[43] Inclusion criteria included EDSS <4 and relapse in the past year. The primary outcome was time to sustained disability progression. A sample size of 192 participants per group would have been powered to detect a 35% relative difference in disability progression between the groups, assuming a 15% dropout rate. Secondary end-points included mean change in the MS Functional Composite (MSFC), ARR, and absolute change in brain parenchyma fraction on MRI.

The study initially enrolled 341 participants, well under the target number. Furthermore, because of high dropout rates (66/169 participants in the placebo arm and 90/172 participants in the active arm withdrew before the study end) it is difficult to make any firm conclusions based on its findings. Nonetheless, there was no significant difference in time to sustained progression between the two groups. However, there was a 38% relative decrease ($P = 0.002$) in ARR in the PO MP group compared to the placebo group as well as a 35% relative reduction in number of new or enlarging T2 lesions ($P = 0.007$). The authors were unable to determine what the cause of the high dropout rate was because of incomplete discontinuation information, but they postulated that it was AEs secondary to steroid in the combination group and lack of treatment effect or AEs related to IFNβ-1a (IM) in the IFNβ only group. In summary, this trial suggested that there was a benefit to treatment with PO MP but was unable to provide convincing evidence, in part because of suboptimal enrollment coupled with a large attrition rate.

NORMIMS

NORMIMS (NORdic trial of oral Methylprednisolone as add-on therapy to Interferon beta-1a for treatment of relapsing–remitting Multiple Sclerosis) was a randomized, double-blind, placebo-controlled, add-on trial comparing IFNβ-1a (SC) alone vs. IFNβ-1a (SC) in combination with monthly, five day oral pulses of 200 mg daily MP.[44] Participants were eligible for inclusion in the trial if they were on treatment with IFNβ-1a (SC) for at least the previous 12 months, on a stable dose of 44 μg three times weekly for at least three months, and had at least one relapse during the previous 12 months. The primary end-point was defined as mean yearly relapse rate at 48 and 96 weeks. Secondary end-points included time to worsening of sustained disability, changes in MSFC score, number of active lesions (new or enlarging lesions) on T2-weighted MRI, and the presence of NAbs at any point up to week 96.

This study was also hampered by slow enrollment and high dropout rates. Although initially planned for 130 participants in each arm, the study eventually enrolled 66 participants in the IFNβ-1a (SC)/PO MP arm and 64 participants in the IFNβ-1a (SC)/placebo arm. 35/66 participants withdrew from treatment early in the active arm (18 because of AEs) and 20/64 withdrew early from the placebo arm (nine due to lack of efficacy). Using intention-to-treat analysis there was a 62% ($P < 0.0001$) relative reduction in relapse rate in the PO MP arm as compared to the placebo. The benefit of steroid treatment was also suggested on MRI with a trend towards reduction in mean number of new or enlarging T2 lesions and a statistically significant decrease in T2 lesion volume in the combination group. As with MECOMBINS, this trial gave some support for the hypothesis that pulse steroid may be efficacious in combination with IFNβ treatment. However, the high dropout rate in both trials in the steroid arms because of AEs may indicate that oral steroids have unacceptable tolerability profile as chronic maintenance therapy.

ACT

ACT (Avonex Combination Trial) was a randomized, multicenter, 2×2 factorial clinical trial[45] with inclusion criteria including evidence of clinical or MRI disease activity in prior 12 months, at least six months after starting IFNβ-1a (IM) therapy.[45] All participants continued IFNβ-1a (IM) through the trial and were randomized to one of four add-on regimens: weekly oral placebo, oral MTX 20 mg every week, i.v. MP 1000 mg × 3 days every two months + oral placebo, or MTX and i.v. MP (there was no i.v. placebo arm). Initially, this trial was to enroll 900 participants with primary end-points of ARR for MTX and change in brain parenchyma fraction for i.v. MP. However, because of slow recruitment, 313 participants were eventually enrolled, and the primary end-point was changed to number of new or enhancing T2 lesions for both treatments. The trial was also shortened from 24 to 12 months.

The ACT trial was not able to show any benefit from the combination of MTX and i.v. MP. There was a non-significant trend for the primary end-point with i.v. MP alone but no suggested benefit at the primary end-point for MTX alone. There was also a less impressive trend towards decreased ARR and decreased Gd-enhancing lesion in both i.v. MP + placebo arm and MTX arms. Additionally, at months 6 and 12 there was a suggestion that i.v. MP decreased prevalence of IFNβ NAbs. One criticism of this trial is that there was not a placebo for the

i.v. MP arm. Thus, participants were aware of their treatment, and this could have biased the results. Clearly, the smaller than planned numbers of this trial may have contributed to the lack of significance for any end-points.

ASA

The ASA (Avonex-Steroids-Azathioprine) study was a double-blind, placebo-controlled study with a two-year study design and an extension phase.[46] 181 participants were randomized in a 1:1:1 ratio to IFNβ-1a (IM) once weekly plus double placebo, IFNβ-1a (IM) once weekly plus AZA 50 mg once daily plus placebo, or IFNβ-1a (IM) once weekly plus AZA 50 mg once daily, plus oral prednisone 10 mg every other day. The primary end-point for the study was ARR and secondary end-points included time to sustained disability progression as well as new T2 lesion formation, and percentage change in brain volume.

At the end of two years, 147/181 patients had completed the trial on protocol. Follow-up data were available on 179/181 patients, and analysis was done as intention-to-treat. Although the dropout rate was similar in each group, the IFNβ-1a (IM)/AZA/prednisone arm had the highest retention. The most common reason for discontinuation in all arms was disease progression. There was no significant difference in ARR or time to first relapse between the three groups, although there was a trend favoring the triple combination arm. Likewise, there was no significant difference in percentage with sustained progression (although the trend favored the IFNβ-1a (IM) monotherapy group) or percentage of brain volume change between any of the groups. In fact, the only measure to reach significance in this trial was a significantly smaller increase in T2 lesion volume in the triple therapy arm vs. the double and single therapy arms. However, it is important to note that in this measure the three-year extension study and beyond did not continue to show a difference between these arms.

Cytotoxic therapies

Mitoxantrone

A number of studies have demonstrated that mitox has robust benefit on relapses, disability progression, and MRI activity in patients with active RR and SPMS. Although mitox is well tolerated in general, because of the potential for serious toxicity, including cardiotoxicity and leukemia, it would be desirable to limit the overall exposure. This could be accomplished by utilizing lower doses in combination with other agents, or through an induction therapy approach where initial therapy with mitox was followed by therapy with a standard agent. Le Page et al. studied 109 RRMS patients who were randomized in a 1:1 ratio to mitox 20 mg monthly in combination with 1000 mg i.v. MP for six months followed by IFNβ-1b for 27 months vs. IFNβ-1b for three years with monthly i.v. MP for the first six months.[57] The primary end-point of time to three-month sustained 1-point EDSS worsening was reduced by 65% in the mitox group.

ARR was reduced in this group by 61.5% as well. No serious AEs were reported.

Studies have also suggested a possible benefit with induction by mitox with subsequent GA treatment. A single-blind, randomized trial of 40 GA- and mitox-naive patients who had between 1–15 Gd-enhancing lesions on a baseline MRI were assigned to either an induction of mitox given at months 0, 1 and 2, followed by a two-week washout period and then daily subcutaneous injections of GA 20 mg ($n = 19$) vs. a group on GA for the entire 15 month study ($n = 20$).[38] This study was performed mainly to assess safety and tolerability of the mitox-GA combination vs. GA monotherapy. However, it showed a statistically significant decrease in new, Gd-enhancing lesions in the combination group compared to the monotherapy group at 6, 9, 12, and 15 months.

Cyclophosphamide

A randomized, single-blind trial enrolled 59 patients who were classified as IFNβ-1b or IFNβ-1a (IM) non-responders.[59] All patients received IFNβ-1a (IM) for the entire trial period. At baseline, every participant was given a three-day pulse of i.v. MP, 1000 mg/day. Participants were then randomized to receive either cyclophosphamide (CTX) + i.v. MP monthly for six months or i.v. MP alone. At the end of the six-month induction period, all participants continued IFNβ-1a (IM) and were followed for an additional 18 months. The CTX/i.v. MP group showed superiority in primary end-point, mean change in Gd-enhancing lesions compared to the MP group at 3, 6, and 12 months, although there was not a significant difference in change in brain parenchymal fraction or T2 lesion burden. Clinically, in the first year the CTX/i.v. MP group had a significantly lower relapse rate; however, other clinical measures were not different. Importantly, this study was troubled by a very high dropout rate of 29/59 participants. The high rate of dropout was due primarily to 23 participants with protocol-defined treatment failures, eight in the CTX/i.v. MP group and 15 in the i.v. MP group.

Combination trials with other immunomodulating agents

Daclizumab

Wynn et al. reported positive results of a Phase 2 randomized double-blind multicenter study which compared high dose daclizumab (2 mg/kg, every two weeks) and IFNβ vs. low dose daclizumab (1 mg/kg every 4 weeks) and IFNβ vs. IFNβ and placebo.[39] Eligibility criteria included diagnosis of RRMS, treatment with IFNβ >6 months, and either a clinical relapse or a Gd-enhancing lesion in the past year while on IFNβ. 230 patients were randomized to three groups, and after 24 weeks of treatment the high dose daclizumab/IFNβ group had a 72% decrease ($P < 0.004$) in new or enlarged Gd-enhancing lesion formation compared to placebo/IFNβ group. The low-dose

daclizumab/IFNβ group had a 25% decrease in lesion formation ($P = NS$). Clinically, there was a trend towards decreased ARR and time to first relapse in both daclizumab groups vs. placebo. In general, daclizumab was well tolerated in combination with IFNβ.

Teriflunomide

Teriflunomide[60] has been tested in combination in two separate randomized, double-blind, placebo-controlled Phase 2 trials with GA and IFNβ. Freedman et al. reported successful results of a 24-week trial in which 116 participants on a stable dose of IFNβ were randomized to high-dose teriflunomide (14 mg), low-dose teriflunomide (7 mg) or placebo.[40] Results revealed a relative decrease in new Gd-enhancing lesions of 56% and 81% (both $P < 0.001$) in the low-dose and high-dose groups, respectively, as compared with placebo. In a second study, 123 participants on GA were randomized in a similar fashion to high-dose teriflunomide, low-dose teriflunomide or placebo.[41] The number of new Gd-enhancing lesions was significantly reduced in the low-dose group and the Gd-enhancing lesion volume was significant reduced in the high-dose group vs. placebo. These Phase 2 studies serve as preliminary evidence that teriflunomide may be useful in combination therapy with standard platform agents.

Statins

In the past decade there has been interest in HMG-CoA reductase inhibitors, statins, as a possible agent for use in MS combination therapy, based on in vitro and in vivo evidence of immonomodulatory, anti-inflammatory and neuro-protective effects.[61] However, statin trials thus far have been small and have yielded conflicting results. Paul et al. reported an open-label trial of 41 RRMS patients that were given high-dose atorvastatin; 16/41 concurrently on IFNβ therapy.[62] There was a decrease in number of Gd-enhancing lesions ($P = 0.003$) between the sixth and ninth month on statin therapy compared with baseline. Interestingly, when those on IFNβ were analyzed separately from those not on IFNβ, the trend was much stronger for those on IFNβ ($P = 0.06$ vs. $P = 0.170$), suggesting the possibility of synergistic effect.

In contrast, Birnbaum et al. reported results of a randomized, placebo-controlled trial of RRMS patients who were stable on IFNβ-1a (SC) assigned to received either 80 mg atorvastatin ($n = 10$), 40 mg of atorvastatin ($n = 7$), or placebo ($n = 9$).[63] In this trial the patients on statin were more likely to experience disease activity, either clinical relapse or new lesion on MRI, than those on placebo ($P = 0.019$).

A post-hoc analysis of the SENTINEL trial, divided the IFNβ monotherapy arm into those who were on a statin for hyperlipidemia ($n = 40$) and those who were not taking a statin ($n = 542$).[52] This study found no significant difference in clinical or MRI measures between the two groups. It is clear from these studies, among others, that a larger Phase 3, randomized, placebo-controlled trial will be necessary to accurately define the role for statins, if any, in the treatment of MS.

Conclusions

Combination therapy is an attractive option to explore for MS treatment. Ideally, combination therapy should include at least one agent already known to be effective and for which there are substantial data concerning safety. These factors suggest that the agents to be given priority will be already-approved drugs. There have been many small studies of combination therapy for MS patients not responding to the currently approved disease-modifying drugs. Although these studies, for the most part, identified no unanticipated toxicity, and many showed promising results regarding efficacy, no definitive conclusions can be drawn from them. For that, rigorous trials with larger sample sizes and longer follow-up will be necessary. Because definitive trials of combination therapy require very large sample sizes and long follow-up as compared with trials of monotherapy versus placebo, they will be very expensive. In general, the development of combination therapy for MS may require continued research on the pathogenesis of the disease, more sensitive outcome measures in clinical trials, and novel trial designs.

References

1. Interferon beta-1b is effective in relapsing-remitting multiple sclerosis. I. clinical results of a multicenter, randomized, double-blind, placebo-controlled trial. The IFNB multiple sclerosis study group. *Neurology* 1993;43:655–61.

2. Interferon beta-1b in the treatment of multiple sclerosis: Final outcome of the randomized controlled trial. the IFNB multiple sclerosis study group and the university of British Columbia MS/MRI analysis group. *Neurology* 1995; 45:1277–85.

3. Jacobs LD, Cookfair DL, Rudick RA, *et al*. Intramuscular interferon beta-1a for disease progression in relapsing multiple sclerosis. the multiple sclerosis collaborative research group (MSCRG). *Ann Neurol* 1996; 39:285–94.

4. Randomised double-blind placebo-controlled study of interferon beta-1a in relapsing/remitting multiple sclerosis. PRISMS (prevention of relapses and disability by interferon beta-1a subcutaneously in multiple sclerosis) study group. *Lancet* 1998; 352:1498–504.

5. Johnson KP, Brooks BR, Cohen JA, *et al*. Copolymer 1 reduces relapse rate and improves disability in relapsing-remitting multiple sclerosis: Results of a phase III multicenter, double-blind placebo-controlled trial. the copolymer 1 multiple sclerosis study group. *Neurology* 1995; 45:1268–76.

6. Kurtzke JF. Rating neurologic impairment in multiple sclerosis: An expanded disability status scale (EDSS). *Neurology* 1983; 33:1444–52.

7. Kappos L, Radue EW, O'Connor P, *et al*. A placebo-controlled trial of oral fingolimod in relapsing multiple sclerosis. *N Engl J Med* 2010; 362:387–401.

8. Polman CH, O'Connor PW, Havrdova E, *et al*. A randomized, placebo-controlled trial of natalizumab for relapsing multiple sclerosis. *N Engl J Med* 2006; 354:899–910.

9. Jacobs LD, Beck RW, Simon JH, *et al*. Intramuscular interferon beta-1a therapy initiated during a first demyelinating event in multiple sclerosis. CHAMPS study group. *N Engl J Med* 2000; 343:898–904.

10. Comi G, Filippi M, Barkhof F, *et al*. Effect of early interferon treatment on conversion to definite multiple sclerosis: A randomised study. *Lancet* 2001; 357:1576–82.

11. Comi G, Martinelli V, Rodegher M, *et al*. Effect of glatiramer acetate on conversion to clinically definite multiple sclerosis in patients with clinically isolated syndrome (PreCISe study): A randomised, double-blind, placebo-controlled trial. *Lancet* 2009; 374:1503–11.

12. Confavreux C, Hutchinson M, Hours MM, Cortinovis-Tourniaire P, Moreau T. Rate of pregnancy-related relapse in multiple sclerosis. Pregnancy in multiple sclerosis group. *N Engl J Med* 1998; 339:285–91.

13. van Walderveen MA, Tas MW, Barkhof F, *et al*. Magnetic resonance evaluation of disease activity during pregnancy in multiple sclerosis. *Neurology* 1994; 44:327–9.

14. Sicotte NL, Liva SM, Klutch R, *et al*. Treatment of multiple sclerosis with the pregnancy hormone estriol. *Ann Neurol* 2002; 52:421–8.

15. Van Der Walt A, Butzkueven H, Kolbe S, *et al*. Neuroprotection in multiple sclerosis: A therapeutic challenge for the next decade. *Pharmacol Ther* 2010; 126:82–93.

16. Caminero JA, Sotgiu G, Zumla A, Migliori GB. Best drug treatment for multidrug-resistant and extensively drug-resistant tuberculosis. *Lancet Infect Dis* 2010; 10:621–9.

17. Palella FJ,Jr, Delaney KM, Moorman AC, *et al*. Declining morbidity and mortality among patients with advanced human immunodeficiency virus infection. HIV outpatient study investigators. *N Engl J Med* 1998; 338:853–60.

18. O'Dell JR. Therapeutic strategies for rheumatoid arthritis. *N Engl J Med* 2004; 350:2591–602.

19. Kuriya B, Arkema EV, Bykerk VP, Keystone EC. Efficacy of initial methotrexate monotherapy versus combination therapy with a biological agent in early rheumatoid arthritis: a meta-analysis of clinical and radiographic remission. *Ann Rheum Dis* 2010; 69:1298–304.

20. Emery P, Deodhar A, Rigby WF, *et al*. Efficacy and safety of different doses and retreatment of rituximab: A randomised, placebo-controlled trial in patients who are biological naive with active rheumatoid arthritis and an inadequate response to methotrexate (study evaluating rituximab's efficacy in MTX iNadequate rEsponders (SERENE)). *Ann Rheum Dis* 2010; 69:1629–35.

21. Williams HJ, Ward JR, Reading JC, *et al*. Comparison of auranofin, methotrexate, and the combination of both in the treatment of rheumatoid arthritis. A controlled clinical trial. *Arthritis Rheum* 1992; 35:259–69.

22. Willkens RF, Sharp JT, Stablein D, Marks C, Wortmann R. Comparison of azathioprine, methotrexate, and the combination of the two in the treatment of rheumatoid arthritis. A

forty-eight-week controlled clinical trial with radiologic outcome assessment. *Arthritis Rheum* 1995; 38:1799–806.

23. Scott DL, Dawes PT, Tunn E, *et al.* Combination therapy with gold and hydroxychloroquine in rheumatoid arthritis: A prospective, randomized, placebo-controlled study. *Br J Rheumatol* 1989; 28:128–33.

24. Zuvich RL, McCauley JL, Pericak-Vance MA, Haines JL. Genetics and pathogenesis of multiple sclerosis. *Semin Immunol* 2009; 21:328–33.

25. McCoy L, Tsunoda I, Fujinami RS. Multiple sclerosis and virus induced immune responses: autoimmunity can be primed by molecular mimicry and augmented by bystander activation. *Autoimmunity* 2006; 39:9–19.

26. Grau-López L, Raïch D, Ramo-Tello C, *et al.* Myelin peptides in multiple sclerosis. *Autoimmunity Rev* 2009; 8:650–3.

27. Zozulya AL, Wiendl H. The role of regulatory T cells in multiple sclerosis. *Nat Clin Pract Neurol* 2008; 4:384–98.

28. Harp CT, Lovett-Racke AE, Racke MK, Frohman EM, Monson NL. Impact of myelin-specific antigen presenting B cells on T cell activation in multiple sclerosis. *Clinical Immunol* 2008; 128:382–91.

29. Franciotta D, Salvetti M, Lolli F, Serafini B, Aloisi F. B cells and multiple sclerosis. *Lancet Neurol* 2008; 7:852–8.

30. Lucchinetti C, Bruck W, Parisi J, Scheithauer B, Rodriguez M, Lassmann H. Heterogeneity of multiple sclerosis lesions: Implications for the pathogenesis of demyelination. *Ann Neurol* 2000; 47:707–17.

31. Sathasivam S. Steroids and immunosuppressant drugs in myasthenia gravis. *Nat Clin Pract Neurol* 2008; 4:317 27.

32. Palace J, Newsom-Davis J, Lecky B. A randomized double-blind trial of prednisolone alone or with azathioprine in myasthenia gravis. myasthenia gravis study group. *Neurology* 1998; 50:1778–83.

33. Lublin F, Cutter G, Elont R, *et al.* A trial to assess the safety of combining therapy with interferon beta-1a and glatiramer acetate in patients with relapsing MS [Abstract]. *Neurology* 2001; 56(Suppl 3): A148.

34. Mount Sinai School of Medicine, Combination therapy in patients with relapsing-remitting multiple sclerosis (MS)CombiRx. NCT00211887 http://www.clinicaltrials.gov/ct2/show/NCT00211887(accessed Dec 29, 2010).

35. Rudick RA, Stuart WH, Calabresi PA, *et al.* Natalizumab plus interferon beta-1a for relapsing multiple sclerosis. *N Engl J Med* 2006; 354:911–23.

36. Goodman AD, Rossman H, Bar-Or A, *et al.* GLANCE: Results of a phase 2, randomized, double-blind, placebo-controlled study. *Neurology* 2009; 72:806–12.

37. EMD Serono, Phase II cladribine add-on to inteferon-beta (IFN-b) therapy in MS subjects with active disease (ONWARD). NCT00436826 http://www.clinicaltrials.gov/ct2/show/NCT00436826 (accessed Dec 29, 2010).

38. Vollmer T, Panitch H, Bar-Or A, *et al.* Glatiramer acetate after induction therapy with mitoxantrone in relapsing multiple sclerosis. *Mult Scler* 2008; 14:663–70.

39. Wynn D, Kaufman M, Montalban X, *et al.* Daclizumab in active relapsing multiple sclerosis (CHOICE study): A phase 2, randomised, double-blind, placebo-controlled, add-on trial with interferon beta. *Lancet Neurol* 2010; 9:381–90.

40. Freedman MS, Wolinsky JS, Byrnes WJ, *et al.* Oral teriflunomide or placebo to added to interferon beta for 6 months in patients with relapsing multiple sclerosis: safety and efficacy results. presented at 25th Congress of the European Committee for Treatment and Research in Multiple Sclerosis (ECTRIMS); September 11, 2009; Dusseldorf. Abstract.

41. Freedman MS, Wolinsky JS, Frangin GA, *et al.* Oral teriflunomide or placebo added to glatiramer acetate for 6 months in patients with relapsing multiple sclerosis: safety and efficacy results. presented at the Annual Meeting of the American Academy of Neurology (AAN); April 14, 2010; Toronto. Abstract.

42. Remington GM, Treadaway K, Frohman T, *et al.* A one-year prospective, randomized, placebo-controlled, quadruple-blinded, phase II safety pilot trial of combination therapy with interferon beta-1a and mycophenolate mofetil in early relapsing-remitting multiple sclerosis (TIME MS). *Ther Adv Neurol Disord* 2010; 3:3–13.

43. Ravnborg M, Sorensen PS, Andersson M, *et al.* Methylprednisolone in combination with interferon beta-1a for relapsing-remitting multiple sclerosis (MECOMBIN study): A multicentre, double-blind, randomised, placebo-controlled, parallel-group trial. *Lancet Neurol* 2010; 9:672–80.

44. Sorensen PS, Mellgren SI, Svenningsson A, *et al.* NORdic trial of oral methylprednisolone as add-on therapy to interferon beta-1a for treatment of relapsing-remitting multiple sclerosis (NORMIMS study): a randomised, placebo-controlled trial. *Lancet Neurol* 2009; 8:519–29.

45. Cohen JA, Imrey PB, Calabresi PA, *et al.* Results of the avonex combination trial (ACT) in relapsing-remitting MS. *Neurology* 2009; 72:535–41.

46. Havrdova E, Zivadinov R, Krasensky J, *et al.* Randomized study of interferon beta-1a, low-dose azathioprine, and low-dose corticosteroids in multiple sclerosis. *Mult Scler* 2009; 15:965–76.

47. University of California, Los Angeles, A Combination Trial of Copaxone Plus Estriol in Relapsing Remitting Multiple Sclerosis (RRMS) (Estriol in MS). NCT00451204 http://clinicaltrials.gov/ct2/show/NCT00451204 (accessed Dec 29, 2010).

48. Andrea Hospital Safety and Tolerability of Interferon-Beta-1a and Estroprogestins Association in MS Patients. NCT00151801 http://www.clinicaltrials.gov/ct2/show/NCT00151801(accessed Dec 29, 2010).

49. Khoury SJ, Healy BC, Kivisakk P, *et al.* A randomized controlled double-masked trial of albuterol add-on therapy in patients with multiple sclerosis. *Arch Neurol* 2010; 67:1055–61.

50. Biogen Idec. Simvastatin as an Add-on Treatment to Interferon-beta-1a for the Treatment of Relapsing–Remitting Multiple Sclerosis (SIMCOMBIN) NCT00492765. http://clinicaltrials.gov/ct2/show/NCT00492765 (accessed Dec 29, 2010).

51. Merck KGaA. Minocycline as add-on to Interferon Beta-1a (Rebif®) in Relapsing Remitting Multiple Sclerosis (RECYCLINE). NCT01134627. http://www.clinicaltrials.gov/ct2/show/NCT01134627 (accessed Dec 29, 2010).

52. Teva Pharmaceutical Industries. Safety and Efficacy Study of Copaxone Administered in Combination With Minocycline. NCT00203112. http://www.clinicaltrials.gov/ct2/show/NCT00203112(accessed Dec 29, 2010).

53. Minagar A, Alexander JS, Schwendimann RN, *et al.* Combination therapy with interferon beta-1a and doxycycline in multiple sclerosis: an open-label trial. *Arch Neurol* 2008; 65:199–204.

54. Charite University, Berlin, Germany Sunphenon Epigallocatechin-gallate (EGCg) in Relapsing-remitting Multiple Sclerosis (SuniMS Study). NCT00525668. http://clinicaltrials.gov/ct2/show/NCT00525668 (accessed Dec 29, 2010).

55. Cantonal Hospital of St. Gallen. The Neuroprotective Effect of Lamotrigine and Interferon Beta 1a in Patients With Relapsing-Remitting Multiple Sclerosis. NCT00917839..http://www.clinicaltrials.gov/ct2/show/NCT00917839 (accessed Dec 29, 2010)

56. University of California, San Francisco. Neuroprotection With Riluzole Patients With Early Multiple Sclerosis. NCT00501943. http://clinicaltrials.gov/ct2/show/NCT00501943 (accessed Dec 29, 2010).

57. Le Page E, Comi G, Filippi M, Edan G, French Italian Mitoxantrone Interferon-beta Trial Group. Comparison of two therapeutic strategies in aggressive relapsing remitting MS: mitoxantrone as induction for 6 months followed by interferon-b-1b versus interferon-b-1b. A 3-year randomized trial. *Neurology* 2008; 70(Suppl 1):A227.

58. Ramtahal J, Jacob A, Das K, Boggild M. Sequential maintenance treatment with glatiramer acetate after mitoxantrone is safe and can limit exposure to immunosuppression in very active, relapsing remitting multiple sclerosis. *J Neurol* 2006; 253:1160–4.

59. Smith DR, Weinstock-Guttman B, Cohen JA, *et al.* A randomized blinded trial of combination therapy with cyclophosphamide in patients with active multiple sclerosis on interferon beta. *Mult Scler* 2005; 117:573–82.

60. Gold R, Wolinsky JS. Pathophysiology of multiple sclerosis and the place of teriflunomide. *Acta Neurol Scand* 2010, in press.

61. Sellner J, Weber MS, Vollmar P, Mattle HP, Hemmer B, Stuve O. The combination of interferon-beta and HMG-CoA reductase inhibition in multiple sclerosis: Enthusiasm lost too soon? *CNS Neurosci Ther* 2010; 16:362–73.

62. Paul F, Waiczies S, Wuerfel J, *et al.* Oral high-dose atorvastatin treatment in relapsing-remitting multiple sclerosis. *PLoS One* 2008; 3:e1928.

63. Birnbaum G, Cree B, Altafullah I, Zinser M, Reder AT. Combining beta interferon and atorvastatin may increase disease activity in multiple sclerosis. *Neurology* 2008; 71:1390–5.

64. Rudick RA, Pace A, Rani MR, *et al.* Effect of statins on clinical and molecular responses to intramuscular interferon beta-1a. *Neurology* 2009; 72:1989–93.

Chapter

48

Dalfampridine in multiple sclerosis

Andrew D. Goodman

Introduction

People with multiple sclerosis (MS) experience a wide variety of neurological symptoms, including weakness, impaired mobility, fatigue, and spasticity. Over time, worsening of such symptoms increasingly compromises independence, quality of life, economic productivity, and the ability to function and perform activities of daily living. The eventual physical, psychological, social, and financial impact can be devastating for people with MS and their families. Although important advances with disease-modifying therapies now diminish the likelihood of developing new lesions, in general, these do not benefit those residual symptoms that accrue as a consequence of existing lesions. Gait impairment in MS patients is among the commonest and most disabling symptoms. Among 1011 people with MS surveyed, 64% experienced trouble walking at least twice weekly and, of these, 70% reported it to be the most challenging aspect of their MS.[1]

Dalfampridine, now the non-proprietary name in the United States (USA) for what was formerly known as fampridine was approved by the US Food and Drug Administration (FDA) in early 2010 as an extended release (ER) formulation of 4-aminopyridine (or "4-AP") known commercially as Ampyra.[2] This small molecule (see Fig. 48.1) administered orally is the first drug indicated to improve walking in MS patients. This review briefly considers the unique pharmacology, pharmacokinetics, history, and early clinical studies, and then focuses on the results of the clinical trials that supported the approval of dalfampridine to treat MS-related gait impairment. Finally, the use of dalfampridine in clinical practice is discussed.

Pharmacology and pharmacokinetics

Dalfampridine is a broad-spectrum voltage-gated potassium ion (K$^+$) channel blocker. It is a lipid-soluble small molecule that more readily crosses the blood–brain barrier than a similar molecule 3, 4-diaminopyridine and, therefore, its effects on the central nervous system (CNS) have been the subject of greater focus. At concentrations of 1–2 μM or less, it binds

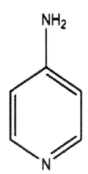

Fig. 48.1. Chemical structure of 4-aminopyridine.

multiple types of voltage-gated channels in neuron axonal membranes. Channel sensitivity to dalfampridine varies by channel type and activation state. It has a greater tendency to enter open K$^+$ channels from the cytoplasmic side and binds to a site at the intracellular opening of the pore which occludes the channel. K$^+$ channels in axons are most concentrated in the internodal regions in healthy CNS white matter. Demyelination exposes the K$^+$ channels which brings the axonal membrane potential close to the equilibrium potential of K$^+$ and impairs generation and conduction of action potentials. Slow K$^+$ channels are also uncovered, and their increased expression alters the normal regulation of hyperpolarization of action potentials.[3] Animal studies indicate that dalfampridine may act through restoration of action potential conduction in damaged, poorly myelinated nerve fibers.[4–6] Alternatively, Smith and others observed dalfampridine had prominent effects that did not involve demyelinated axons, including the potentiation of synaptic transmission and an increase in skeletal muscle twitch tension.[7] They proposed that these latter effects may be largely responsible for the beneficial action of dalfampridine in MS patients.

Early clinical studies of 4-aminopyridine in MS were carried out using immediate-release (IR) formulations with mean half-life of approximately 3.5 hours. An ER formulation was developed with the goal of optimizing pharmacokinetics and minimizing adverse effects (AEs) caused by drug peak level fluctuations. Dose-ranging studies were also used to evaluate

Multiple Sclerosis Therapeutics, Fourth Edition, ed. Jeffrey A. Cohen and Richard A. Rudick. Published by Cambridge University Press.
© Cambridge University Press 2011.

the pharmacokinetics of dalfampridine. Doses ranging from 7.5 to 25 mg every 12 hours led to longer peak concentration times (5 hours) than in IR formulations. The mean half-life was also longer (5.2 hours), and the peak plasma concentration was lower.[8]

History and early studies in multiple sclerosis

The first synthesis of the chemical, 4-aminopyridine, was accomplished in 1894 by Meyer. By 1973, the first clinical use in recovery from anesthesia was reported. By 1976 more detailed effects on K^+ channels in invertebrates had been worked out. In the 1980s the effects on demyelinated axons were described. The first clinical studies showing improvement in vision in MS were reported by Jones.[9] AEs, including seizure, were noted in these early investigations.

Davis and Stefoski reported the initial clinical studies in people with MS in 1987 through 1991.[10,11] They demonstrated through careful titration for safety, broad effects on CNS dysfunction, including improvement of weakness and visual impairment. A 1993 70-subject Dutch study in MS[12] demonstrated effects on disability assessed using the Expanded Disability Status Scale (EDSS). This suggested that dose and serum levels were related to efficacy and safety but that plasma levels were difficult to control with the IR formulation. Again, using an IR formulation in a concentration-controlled, crossover study in MS,[13] Bever et al. found a broad range of effects including improvements in such outcomes as visual contrast sensitivity, limb strength, and some aspects of the neurologic exam but no benefit on the EDSS. Seizure and acute confusional state were observed at serum levels greater than 100 ng/ml.

The results of these early clinical studies in MS suggested that IR formulations of dalfampridine were limited by: rapid rise in plasma level associated with AEs such as dizziness, nausea, parasthesias; relatively short half-life requiring frequent dosing; and a substantial effect of food on pharmacokinetics. Thus, the development of an oral ER formulation was thought to be desirable.

The first published clinical study using the ER formulation dalfampridine (Elan Corporation) utilized a randomized, placebo-controlled, crossover design in 10 subjects with MS.[14] In this trial, subjects received dalfampridine 17.5 mg or placebo twice daily for seven days prior to the crossover for an additional seven days with an intervening seven-day washout period between treatment weeks. The baseline level of disability of the subjects was in the middle to upper range of EDSS (6.0 to 7.5). A variety of quantitative measures of motor function were assessed in this pilot study. A timed gait outcome over a 25-foot (8 meter) course (timed 25-foot walk, T25FW) was significantly improved on active treatment compared to placebo and the effect of treatment was seen more frequently with this measure compared to the EDSS. Importantly, this study demonstrated that the use of quantitative outcomes were more sensitive to the therapeutic effect compared to traditional measures such as the

EDSS and, therefore, promised to be useful in other trials of symptomatic treatments for MS.[14]

Clinical development of dalfampridine in multiple sclerosis

The initial Phase 2 study was performed to determine the safety of escalating doses of dalfampridine in subjects with MS, to explore a number of outcome measures, and to examine dose-related efficacy.[15] It was a multicenter, randomized, double-blind, placebo-controlled, dose-ranging study in subjects with definite MS. Following a four-week baseline period (screening visit week, two untreated weeks, and a single-blind placebo run-in week), subjects were randomly assigned to receive dalfampridine ($n = 25$, escalating doses from 10 mg to 40 mg twice daily, increasing in 5-mg increments at weekly intervals) or placebo ($n = 11$) followed by a one-week down-titration period. A battery of assessments was performed weekly, including the MS Functional Composite (MSFC), fatigue questionnaires, lower extremity manual muscle testing, and spasticity assessment using the Ashworth scale. The most common AEs during treatment were dizziness, insomnia, paresthesia, asthenia, nausea, headache, and tremor. Five subjects discontinued dalfampridine because of AEs. Severe AEs or discontinuations occurred only at doses ≥ 25 mg twice daily, and included seizures in two subjects at doses of 30 and 35 mg twice daily. Improvements were seen in lower extremity muscle strength and walking speed (derived from the T25FW component of MSFC) in the dalfampridine group compared to placebo ($P = 0.01$ and $P = 0.03$, respectively) with the clearest evidence of a dose response in the 10–20 mg dose range. There were no significant differences between groups in the other MSFC components or fatigue scores. These results supported the idea that quantitative functional outcome measures (such as walking speed derived from timed gait and lower extremity muscle testing) were sufficiently sensitive to demonstrate efficacy. There was little if any added benefit but increased AEs at doses above 20 mg BID.

A second Phase 2 study, a double-blind, placebo-controlled, parallel-group dose comparison trial to evaluate the safety and efficacy of dalfampridine in subjects with MS, was performed next.[16] In this multicenter study, 206 subjects were randomized equally to one of four cohorts: dalfampridine 10, 15, or 20 mg bid or placebo. An initial placebo run-in period (two weeks) was followed by periods of dose escalation (two weeks), stable treatment (12 weeks), down-titration (one week), and follow-up evaluation (two weeks off drug). Eligible subjects were ages 18 to 70 years, had adequate cognitive function, and could perform required study procedures, including T25FW twice in 8–60 seconds. The primary efficacy variable was percent change from baseline in average walking speed over 25 feet. Secondary variables were Lower Extremity Manual Muscle Test (LEMMT), clinician's global impression of change, subject global impression, 9–Hole Peg Test, Paced Auditory Serial Addition Test with 3-second interstimulus interval, the Multiple Sclerosis Quality of Life Inventory, the MS Walking Scale-12 (MSWS-12, a

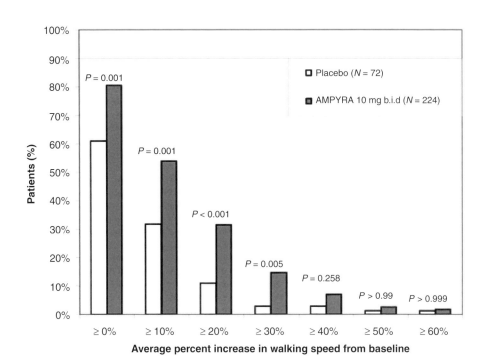

Fig. 48.2. Proportions of dalfampridine-treated subjects demonstrating varying magnitudes of walking speed improvement.[2]

P values provided at each threshold comparing AMPYRA to placebo

12-item MS walking scale that assesses subjects' perspectives on their level of ambulatory disability), and subjective global impression (SGI) scores. Safety was assessed by monitoring AEs, changes in vital signs, clinical laboratory test results, electrocardiogram, and physical examination.

In total, 195 subjects from all four groups completed the trial: dalfampridine bid 10 mg ($n = 50$), 15 mg ($n = 49$), 20 mg ($n = 51$), and placebo ($n = 45$). The T25FW demonstrated a significant effect for all dose groups compared to placebo at the first visit after up-titration. There was a strong trend toward increased walking speed during the stable dose period. LEMMT demonstrated statistically significant improvement across doses at up-titration and during stable treatment ($P = 0.007$). The AE profile was consistent with previous experience and included dizziness, insomnia, paresthesias, and nausea. Two subjects receiving 20 mg bid experienced seizures during the trial, one from an accidental overdose.

Although there was a trend toward increased walking speed during the entire stable dose period, the significance of this difference declined over time against the background variability of walking speed that was partly independent of treatment. To address this variability, a post-hoc responder analysis, based on consistency of improvement during treatment, was carried out. For the purposes of this analysis, a "responder" was defined as a subject with walking speed during at least three of the four on-drug visits faster than the maximum speed measured during the five off-drug visits (four pre-treatment, one at follow-up). In this analysis, the responder rate was significantly higher in all three active dose groups (35%, 36%, and 39%) compared to placebo (9%, $P < 0.002$ for each dose group). Responder status was not significantly related to baseline characteristics, including course, type, or severity of MS. The responder analysis applied post-hoc appeared to provide a more sensitive and representative measure of the effects of dalfampridine on ambulatory function than simply comparing average change in the timed walk.[16] Timed walk responders also showed significantly greater improvement in the MSWS-12; and SGI scores during treatment compared to non-responders.[17] This response criterion also appeared to identify a subset of subjects for whom there was a subjectively meaningful improvement of their ambulatory function and of their impression of global disability.

Based on the above results of both pre-planned and post-hoc analyses of the Phase 2 studies, two Phase 3 multicenter, parallel groups, placebo-controlled trials of dalfampridine at a dose of 10 mg bid taken orally were performed. The prospectively planned primary outcome measure used was the proportion of consistent responders (as above). In the first Phase 3 trial,[18] 301 subjects were randomized; 229 received dalfampridine and 72, placebo. A significantly greater proportion of the active treatment group were consistent responders on the T25FW compared to the placebo group (34.8 % vs. 8.3 %; $P < 0.001$). Response rates were consistently higher across all four MS disease courses. Improvement in walking speed was consistent through the 14 week treatment period among responders and significantly different from placebo ($P < 0.001$). There was significant improvement in the MSWS-12 for walking responders vs. non-responders ($P < 0.001$). The average improvement in walking speed among the dalfampridine responder group was approximately 25% above baseline for the group. AEs were largely consistent with the safety profile observed in previous studies in MS. Two serious AEs that led to discontinuation were anxiety in one subject and a seizure in another that was observed during an occurrence of urosepsis.

The second Phase 3 trial[19] was a 39 center, double-blind trial in subjects with definite MS of any course type. Participants were randomized to nine weeks of treatment with dalfampridine 10 mg twice daily ($n = 120$) or placebo ($n = 119$). Again, a response was defined as consistent improvement on the T25FW, with percentage of responders in each treatment group as the primary outcome. The last on-treatment visit provided data from 8–12 hour post-dose, to examine maintenance of effect. The proportion of responders was higher in the dalfampridine group (51/119 or 42.9%) compared to the placebo group (11/118 or 9.3%, $P < 0.0001$). The average improvement in walking speed among dalfampridine-treated responders during the 8–week efficacy evaluation period was 24.7% from baseline (95% confidence interval = 21.0–28.4%). The mean improvement at the last on-treatment visit was 25.7%, showing maintenance of effect over the inter-dosing period. Other efficacy data were largely consistent with the previous study. There were no new safety findings.

The average change in walking speed for the responders was an approximate 25% improvement over baseline as compared with a 7.5% and 4.7% in the non-responder and placebo groups, respectively. The clinical meaning of this improvement was supported by significantly greater improvement from baseline scores of responders on the MSWS-12.[17] Alternative responder analyses (see Fig. 48.2) also showed significantly greater proportions of dalfampridine-treated subjects with average increases in walking speed relative to baseline of at least 10%, 20%, 30%, or 40% compared to placebo-treated subjects (P-values < 0.05).[2]

The Phase 2 and 3 clinical trials screened subjects for pre-existing seizure disorders and administered EEGs to evaluate for any baseline abnormalities. However, in spite of these precautions, there were a small number of subjects experiencing seizures. This is not unexpected when considering the mechanism of action of dalfampridine and the increased seizure risk in MS patients. Overall, the commonest AEs were dizziness, insomnia, urinary tract infection, and paresthesia (see Table 48.1).[2]

Use of dalfampridine in practice

Based on evaluation of the above clinical trial and other data, the US FDA approved the ER formulation of dalfampridine (daily oral dose of 10 mg BID) January 22, 2010 for use in MS to improve walking.[2] Patients with a history of seizure or

Table 48.1. *Adverse events with an incidence $\geq 2\%$ of dalfampridine-treated multiple sclerosis patients, and more frequent with dalfampridine compared to placebo, in controlled clinical trials*[2]

Adverse event	Placebo ($n = 238$)	Dalfampridine 10 mg bid ($n = 400$)
Urinary tract infection	8%	12%
Insomnia	4%	9%
Dizziness	4%	7%
Headache	4%	7%
Nausea	3%	7%
Asthenia	4%	7%
Back pain	2%	5%
Balance disorder	1%	5%
MS relapse	3%	4%
Paresthesias	3%	4%
Nasopharyngitis	2%	4%
Constipation	2%	3%
Dyspepsia	1%	2%
Pharyngolaryngeal pain	1%	2%

renal insufficiency (creatinine clearance estimate < 50 ml/min) should be excluded from using it.

A practical approach to treatment is to initiate a trial period of 10 mg BID for about 2 to 4 weeks to assess tolerability and effectiveness. Effectiveness can be assessed, as with all symptomatic medications, by clinician judgment based on the patient's individual subjective experience, neurological examination, and other clinical methods such as observing gait and performing a T25FW. If the drug is determined to be ineffective or intolerable (see Table 48.1 for the most frequent side effects), it may be tapered to 10 mg daily for about a week, and then discontinued.

The FDA approval noted that the clinical impact of the drug was manifest as improved walking speed as measured by the T25FW. No stipulation regarding minimum or maximum speed based on the T25FW or the need for assistance was included. The pivotal trials required a 8 to 45 second timed walk performance for participation, based on trial design and statistical considerations alone. Some third-party payers in the USA, however, have adopted prior approval requirements for providing dalfampridine that limit the access apparently based on the trial entry requirements. These restrictions seem arbitrary as they are not stipulated in the FDA approval and as the clinical trial data, in fact, demonstrate that the spectrum of disease courses and baseline walking speeds do not predict the likelihood of timed-walk response.

References

1. http://www.nationalmssociety.org/about-multiple-sclerosis

2. http://www.accessdata.fda.gov/drugsatfda_docs/nda/2010/022250s000TOC.cfm

3. Judge SI, Bever CT Jr. Potassium channel blockers in multiple sclerosis: Neuronal Kv channels and effects of

symptomatic treatment. *Pharmacol Ther* 2006;111:224–59.

4. Sherratt RM, Bostock H, Sears TA. Effects of 4-aminopyridine on normal and demyelinated mammalian nerve fibres. *Nature* 1980;283:570–2.

5. Targ EF, Kocsis JD. 4-Aminopyridine leads to restoration of conduction in demyelinated rat sciatic nerve. *Brain Res* 1985;328:358–61.

6. Blight AR, Toombs JP, Bauer MS, Widmer WR. The effects of 4-aminopyridine on neurological deficits in chronic cases of traumatic spinal cord injury in dogs: a phase I clinical trial. *J Neurotrauma* 1991;8:103–19.

7. Smith KJ, Felts PA, John GR. Effects of 4-aminopyridine on demyelinated axons, synapses and muscle tension. *Brain* 2000;123:171–84.

8. Smith W, Swan S, Marbury T, Henney H 3rd. Single-Dose pharmacokinetics of sustained-release dalfampridine (Dalfampridine-SR) in healthy volunteers and adults with renal impairment. *J Clin Pharmacol.* 2010;50:151–9.

9. Jones RE, Heron JR, Foster DH, Snelgar RS, Mason. Effects of 4-aminopyridine in patients with multiple sclerosis. *J Neurol Sci* 1983;60:353–62.

10. Davis FA, Stefoski D, Rush J. Orally administered 4-aminopyridine improves clinical signs in multiple sclerosis. *Ann Neurol* 1990;27:186–92.

11. Stefoski D, Davis FA, Faut M, Schauf CL. 4-Aminopyridine improves clinical signs in multiple sclerosis. *Ann Neurol* 1987;21:71–7.

12. van Diemen HAM, Polman CH, van Dongen TMMM, *et al.* The effect of 4-aminopyridine on clinical signs in multiple sclerosis: a randomized, placebo-controlled, double-blind, cross-over study. *Ann Neurol* 1992;32:123–30.

13. Bever CT Jr, Young D, Anderson PA, *et al.* The effects of 4-aminopyridine in multiple sclerosis patients: results of a randomized, placebo-controlled, double-blind, concentration-controlled, crossover trial. *Neurology* 1994;44:1054–9.

14. Schwid SR, Petrie MD, McDermott MP, *et al.* Quantitative assessment of sustained-release 4-aminopyridine for symptomatic treatment of multiple sclerosis. *Neurology* 1997;48:817–21.

15. Goodman AD, Cohen JA, Cross A, *et al.* Fampridine-SR in multiple sclerosis: a randomized, double-blind, placebo-controlled, dose-ranging study. *Mult Scler* 2007;13:357–68.

16. Goodman AD, Brown TR, Cohen JA, *et al.* Dose comparison trial of extended release dalfampridine in multiple sclerosis. *Neurology* 2008;71:1134–41.

17. Hobart J, Riazi A, Lampling D, Fitzpatrick R, Thompson A. Measuring the impact of MS on walking ability. *J Neurol* 2003;60:31–6.

18. Goodman AD, Brown TR, Krupp LB, *et al.* Extended-release oral dalfampridine in multiple sclerosis: a randomised, double-blind, controlled trial. *Lancet* 2009;373:732–38.

19. Goodman AD, Brown TR, Edwards KR, *et al.* A Phase III trial of extended release oral dalfampridine in multiple sclerosis. *Ann Neurol* 2010;68:494–502.

Chapter

49

Complementary and alternative treatments in multiple sclerosis

Vijayshree Yadav, Lynne Shinto, and Dennis N. Bourdette

Introduction

Despite recent therapeutic advances, multiple sclerosis (MS) remains a chronic disabling disease with no cure. National surveys have demonstrated the widespread use of complementary and alternative medicine (CAM) among the general population in the United States, and that individuals with a variety of chronic illnesses are more likely to use CAM than the general population.[1,2] Several surveys have demonstrated that individuals with MS often explore CAM treatment options.[3–8] Neurologists have long recognized that many individuals with MS use alternative therapies but generally have taken little interest in these therapies. Individuals with MS and neurologists frequently adopt a "don't ask, don't tell" policy regarding alternative therapies. Neurologists are sometimes very negative about patient use of alternative therapies primarily for two reasons: first, they cite the lack of scientific evidence establishing efficacy for various CAM therapies; second, they focus on highly publicized therapies that are expensive, seemingly bizarre or even dangerous, such as replacement of amalgam dental fillings, magnet therapy, and bees stings, as being representative of CAM therapies and want to protect their patients from pointless expenses and risks. However, these negative attitudes are not well founded. First, despite individuals with MS reporting benefit from some alternative therapies, there has been a paucity of scientifically valid research on CAM therapies for MS. The lack of scientific evidence on efficacy does not mean that there is no benefit; we simply do not have the data to allow us to determine what works and what does not. Second, most individuals with MS who use CAM therapies tend to use affordable and low-risk treatments, such as diet therapies, nutritional supplements, herbal therapies, and mind–body therapies, such as yoga and prayer.[4–7] While there certainly are individuals with MS who make poor decisions regarding CAM use, in general, individuals with MS who use CAM seem to be sensible in their approach. Rather than ignoring the issue or adopting a universally negative attitude about CAM, neurologists should be better informed about CAM use so that they can serve as a resource for these individuals.

Table 49.1. *National Institutes of Health (NIH) classification system for alternative medicine*

Category	Examples
Alternative medical systems	Traditional Chinese medicine, ayurvedic medicine, homeopathy, naturopathic medicine
Biologically based therapies	Herbs, dietary supplements (e.g. vitamin B, fish oil), diets (e.g. low saturated fat diet)
Mind–body interventions	Meditation, prayer, hypnotherapy, relaxation, guided imagery, yoga, tai chi, qi gong, deep breathing exercises
Manipulative and body based practices	Spinal manipulation (e.g. chiropractics), massage therapy
Movement therapies	Feldenkrais, Alexander technique, pilates, Trager psychophysical integration
Other	Traditional healers, energy medicine (e.g. Reike, magnet therapy, light therapy)

Definition of CAM

One of the challenges facing neurologists is the broad spectrum of therapies that fall under the rubric of "CAM." CAM therapies are often defined as unconventional therapies that are used in addition to ("complementary") or instead of ("alternative") conventional medicine. CAM therapies are not traditionally prescribed by conventional physicians and often are not covered by health insurance. The list of practices that are considered CAM is somewhat fluid as CAM therapies that are proven safe and effective become accepted as "mainstream" healthcare practices. The National Institutes of Health has provided a useful classification scheme of CAM (Table 49.1).[9]

CAM use among individuals with MS

Several surveys have documented the high prevalence of CAM use among MS populations.[3–8,10–12] The percentages of respondents who had tried various CAM therapies in these surveys range from 50%–75%.[3–5,7,10,12,13] Interestingly, survey respondents who reported use of CAM therapies were more likely to be female, better educated, and of higher income than those not using CAM.[4,6,7,13,14] Although individuals with MS at all levels of disability use CAM, recent surveys have suggested that individuals with longer duration and higher severity of disease were more likely to use CAM therapies.[4,10,13] Individuals with MS reporting using CAM in combination with conventional medicines for their MS varied from 38% to 90%.[3,5,10]

MS individuals who use CAM generally do so because they experience improvement in their quality of life (QoL) and various MS symptoms such as fatigue, spasticity, or pain. In published surveys reasons for individuals with MS trying CAM therapies include the desire to use holistic health care, dissatisfaction with conventional medicine,[4] the attempt to find relief from physical and psychological symptoms,[3,5] and a belief that CAM is not harmful.[5]

There is a suggestion that individuals with MS who use CAM discern differential benefit among the various CAM therapies, i.e. they are able to differentiate whether a particular therapy is beneficial as compared to another. In the survey by Berkman *et al.*, 59% of respondents reported using CAM and 91% of the CAM users reported deriving benefit from CAM therapy. Only 12% felt that CAM therapies had altered their disease course and 9% reported that one or more CAM therapy had caused adverse side effects.[3] Thus, those using CAM reported benefit in symptomatic relief from some CAM therapies but generally did not think CAM therapies were altering their disease course. Our survey of MS patients living in Oregon and Clark County, Washington found that 50% of respondents rated one or more CAM therapy as being "highly beneficial" compared with 42% who rated one or more conventional disease modifying therapies as being "highly beneficial." Interestingly, the proportion of MS patients who rated 18 commonly used CAM therapies as being "highly beneficial" ranged between 13–52%, suggesting that patients perceive significant differences in efficacy among various CAM approaches.[15]

CAM therapies used commonly by individuals with MS

Mind–body therapies

Mind–body therapies include meditation, yoga, tai chi, and qi gong. Mind–body therapies incorporate self-observation of mental activity to acquire attentional control by focusing on internal and external events with non-judgmental acceptance.[16] Yoga and tai chi combine meditation with a patterned physical activity, which may have the added benefits provided by exercise.

There have been two randomized controlled trials of yoga in MS.[17,18] The study by Oken *et al.*[18] randomized 69 MS subjects into one of three groups: (1) wait-list control (*n* = 22); (2) conventional exercise on a stationary bicycle (*n* = 26) and

(3) yoga (*n* = 21). The intervention period was for six months and the primary outcome were measures of attention and alertness. After six months, there were no significant differences between groups in attention or alertness. However, a significant improvement in fatigue was found in subjects randomized to either yoga or exercise when compared wtih the wait-list control group. The study showed that both yoga and exercise interventions produced beneficial effects on measures of fatigue. The second randomized prospective 10-week study looked at the effects of sports climbing vs. yoga on spasticity, cognitive function, mood, and fatigue in 20 subjects with relapsing–remitting (RR) or progressive MS.[17] The study did not find any change in spasticity, executive function, or mood with either intervention. Subjects in the yoga group experienced a 17% increase in selective attention performance ($P = 0.005$) but no improvement in fatigue. Subjects in the sports climbing group found reduction in fatigue by 32.5% ($P = 0.015$). In both yoga studies, there were no reports of safety issues with yoga in the MS subjects.

One recent study addressed the effects of a form of meditation that does not include exercise in MS. Mindfulness-based stress reduction (MBSR) is based on Eastern meditation principles and was developed by Jon Kabat-Zinn. MBSR incorporates sitting meditation, gentle yoga exercises, body scan, and informal awareness of daily activity as a way to cultivate an ability to pay attention to daily experiences in a non-judgmental and non-reactive fashion. A study evaluating the effects of a mindfulness-based intervention (MBI), similar to MBSR, on quality of life in MS found that subjects randomized to MBI (*n* = 76) had significant improvements in quality of life, depression, and fatigue compared to those randomized to a wait-list control group (*n* = 74). A limitation of the study is that subjects randomized to MBI were only compared to a wait-list control (usual care).[19]

Tai chi is an ancient Chinese form of exercise that consists of slow, relaxed, continuous and patterned movements. Sometimes tai chi is combined with qi gong which is another example of mind–body practice with origin in ancient China. Qi gong focuses on combination of movement, meditation, and controlled breathing and intends to improve the blood flow and the flow of qi. The beneficial effects of this form of exercise have been reported in elderly people and several chronic pain syndromes.[20–22] Tai chi appears to improve flexibility, range of motion, muscle strength, and balance and thus might be beneficial for MS patients. There have been two studies evaluating tai chi in MS. The first study was a non-randomized, uncontrolled study (*n* = 19) that reported improvements in walking speed, hamstring flexibility, and subject's report of well-being after an eight-week tai chi intervention.[22] Another study included subjects (*n* = 16) randomized to a combination tai chi/qi gong intervention (*n* = 8) or control (usual care, *n* = 8).[23] This study showed no difference between groups in measures of balance. The tai chi/qi gong group reported significant improvement in balance and MS symptoms compared with the control group.

Mind–body interventions, such as yoga, mindfulness, and tai chi, show promise of benefit in MS and offer a non-pharmacologic therapy that may be effective in reducing stress, improving fatigue, and enhancing quality of life in MS.

Dietary changes and supplement use

Low fat diet

Although not specifically recommended by most neurologists, many MS patients follow low fat diets, including the Swank diet,[24] dietary recommendations of the American Heart Association (AHA), and vegetarian diets. In the survey by Nayak et al., 16% of respondents used the Swank diet and another 10% made other dietary changes for MS.[4] Stuifbergen et al. reported 45% of respondents using special diets for MS.[7] In the Oregon survey, about 59% of all respondents used some form of diet for their MS. Among these respondents, 41% followed a low fat and low cholesterol diet and 27 % used the Swank diet.[25]

The Swank diet is named after the neurologist, Dr. Roy Swank, who devised a low fat diet and advocated its use for over 40 years. The Swank diet has contributed to the popularity of low fat diet use among MS patients. This approach grew out of studies in the 1950s and then in the 1970s indicating a higher prevalence of MS among populations with diets high in saturated fat and a lower prevalence among populations with diets low in saturated fat.[26–28] Dr. Swank published a book advocating the use of a diet containing only 10–15 g/day of saturated fat supplemented with cod liver oil.[24] In 1951, Dr. Swank initiated a diet intervention study that compared the survival and neurologic disability in a cohort of 144 MS subjects, who were followed for almost 50 years. Subjects were divided into two groups: "good dieters" ($N = 70$) and "bad dieters" ($N = 74$). The "good dieters" strictly remained on a low fat diet by consuming less than 20 g/d of fat and "bad dieters" consumed more than 20 g/d of fat. Thirty-four years after the start of this study, there were 23 deaths in the "good dieters" group as compared to 58 deaths in the "bad dieters" group. Fifty years later, in 2000, Dr. Swank and colleagues contacted the subjects again and found that there were 15 survivors, all of whom were from the "good dieters" group and who had remained on the low fat diet. Most of these patients (13 of 15) were still ambulatory and found to be otherwise healthy MS patients.[29–32] This long-term uncontrolled follow-up on MS patients who followed the Swank diet suggested that those who followed the diet had a lower death rate and perhaps disability than those who did not.

Additionally, there have been epidemiological studies attempting to study the association between intake of saturated fat of animal origin and risk of developing MS that have yielded both positive[33–35] as well as negative associations.[36,37] A case-control study performed in Canada found a positive association between animal food intake and risk of MS and a protective effect of plant-derived food, such as fruits, vegetables, and grains.[35] In contrast, a large prospective case control study by Zhang et al., the Nurses Health Study, did not find any association of higher intake of saturated fat and lower intake of polyunsaturated fat with increased risk of MS.[37] The first cohort consisted of 92 422 women with 14 years of follow-up (1980–1994) and the second cohort (Nurses' Health Study II) consisted of 95 389 women with four years of follow-up (1991–1995). Thus, the role of diet in affecting the risk of developing MS is uncertain.

Weinstock-Guttman et al. conducted a double-blind, randomized clinical trial that studied whether a low fat diet intervention with omega-3 fatty acid supplementation positively affected quality of life in relapsing–remitting (RR) MS patients.[38] This one-year prospective trial included 31 patients who were randomized to one of the two dietary interventions: the Fish Oil group that received a low fat diet (15% fat) with omega-3 fish oils and the Olive Oil group that received the AHA Step I diet (fat = 30%) with olive oil supplements. The study showed clinical benefits favoring the Fish Oil group on Physical Components Summary Scale (PCS) of the Short Health Status Questionnaire (SF36) ($P = 0.05$) and Mental Health Inventory ($P = 0.05$) at six months but there were no significant differences at 12 months.

More recently, a systematic review by the Cochrane Collaboration explored the evidence supporting the use of various dietary interventions in people with MS by evaluating the studies published between 1966 and March 2006.[39] This review did not find evidence of efficacy of such interventions in MS but also indicated that poor design compromised the quality of the trials.

Although currently there is no convincing evidence that following the Swank low fat diet or any other diet has a positive effect on reducing disease activity in MS, following a diet low in saturated fat may be a common-sense approach for most individuals with MS, given the general health benefits of such a diet. In addition, a low fat diet can help with weight reduction and obesity has recently been associated with an increased risk of disability in MS.[40] Whether there is any specific benefit with regards to controlling MS progression remains unknown but may deserve further research.

Essential fatty acids

Many individuals with MS report taking essential fatty acids (EFA) as supplements. EFA supplements commonly used by people with MS include cod liver and fish oils, evening primrose oil, and flax seed oil. In the published CAM surveys in MS, evening primrose oil use by the respondents appeared to be as high as 42%–53%.[5,13]

There are two major classes of EFA, namely the omega-6 and the omega-3 fatty acids. Oils such as evening primrose oil, cod liver oil/ fish oils, and flaxseed oil contain both omega-3 and omega-6 fatty acids, although they do differ in their ratios. The omega-6 fatty acids contain linoleic acid that is converted in the body to the longer chain fatty acid, gamma linolenic acid (GLA), and then further lengthened to make arachidonic acid. Evening primrose oil is high in GLA. Sunflower seed oil contains predominantly linoleic acid. The omega-3 fatty acids contain alpha linolenic acid that is converted in the body to the longer chain fatty acid, eicosapentaenoic acid (EPA), which is further lengthened to make docosahexaenoic acid (DHA). Flaxseed oil is high in alpha linolenic acid but contains no EPA or DHA while fish and fish oils are high in EPA and DHA because the fish has converted alpha linolenic acid to these compounds.

Clinical trials treating MS patients with either EFA supplementation or increased dietary EFA have reported mixed results.[41–46] Dworkin et al., who did a re-analysis of three double-blind trials of the omega-6 EFA, linoleic acid, found that there was a suggestion of modest therapeutic benefit to supplementation with linoleic acid.[44] Among these three double-blind, controlled trials, two used sunflower seed oil as a source of linoleic acid and compared it to olive oil, which contains oleic acid, and the third trial, used a different preparation of linoleic acid. The first two trials, one by Millar et al. and the other by Bates et al., studied only patients with RR MS[41,42] whereas the third trial by Paty et al. included some patients with progressive MS.[43] These studies looked at changes in disability score, relapse severity and duration, and annual relapse rate. Although for patients with moderate to severe disability the change in disability score was not significant, patients with minimal or no disability had a suggestion of stability of their disease with linoleic acid supplementation. The possible protective role of linoleic acid was more evident on relapse severity and duration, but there was no clear benefit on the number of relapses per year. The potential protective role of linoleic acid in MS was more evident in the Millar et al. and Bates et al. trials[41,42] whereas the Paty et al. trial showed no benefit over placebo.[43]

While evening primrose oil is a popular omega-6 fatty acid, used by many individuals with MS, it contains low levels of GLA and is relatively expensive. A pilot trial in MS failed to demonstrate any significant clinical benefit[42]; hence considering its cost and low omega-6 fatty acid content, evening primrose oil appears to be of little use in treating MS.

Omega-3 fatty acid supplementation is becoming popular after recent studies in cardiovascular diseases showed potential reduction in morbidity and mortality.[47,48] There are also some data that suggest that diets enriched with essential fatty acids and supplementation with omega-3 fatty acids may have anti-inflammatory effects.[49,50] There are only a few studies that have assessed the role of omega-3 fatty acid supplementation in MS. These include the study by Weinstock-Guttman et al. discussed above,[38] one large double-blind trial in 1989 by Bates, et al.,[45] an open label pilot study by Gallai, et al.[50] and a small open-label study by Shinto et al.[51] In the Bates trial of 312 MS patients with acute RR disease, although the "treatment" group received additional omega-3 EFA supplementation, both the "control" and the "treatment" groups were advised to follow a diet that increased dietary omega-6 EFAs. Clinical analysis of duration, frequency, and severity of MS relapses as well as the number of patients who had improved or remained

unchanged was performed. There was a statistical trend favoring omega-3 treatment with 59% of patients in the "omega-3" group remaining stable or improved over 2 years compared with 46% of the "placebo" group ($P = 0.07$).[45] Gallai et al.[50] studied the immunologic responses of 20 subjects with MS and 15 age-matched healthy controls following supplementation with 6 g/day of fish oil containing 3 g EPA and 1.8 g DHA for 6 months. After three and six months of fish oil supplementation, there was a significant decrease in the levels of soluble interleukin-1β ($P < 0.03$), tumor necrosis factor-α ($P < 0.02$), interleukin-2 ($P < 0.002$), and interferon-γ ($P < 0.01$) in the both stimulated and unstimulated peripheral blood mononuclear cells from both groups. Cytokine levels returned to baseline values in both groups after a three-month washout period.

Our group assessed the effects of fish oil concentrate supplementation on matrix metalloproteinase-9 (MMP-9), which is important to T-cell migration into the central nervous system (CNS) in MS.[52] In this open-label pilot study, 10 RRMS patients received fish oil concentrate at 9.6 g per day (containing 2.9 g EPA and 1.9 g DHA) for three months. After three months there was a significant decrease in MMP-9 secreted from unstimulated peripheral blood mononuclear cells.[51] Thus, two studies have shown that omega-3 fatty acid supplementation can favorably alter immune responses in MS subjects.

Thus far, evidence appears mixed for the potential benefit of omega-6 EFA, but possibly better evidence exists for benefit of omega-3 EFA supplementation in MS. People with MS may choose to take a fish oil supplement for general health benefits, but they should be advised against potential harmful effects from high dose fish oil supplementation. The US Food and Drug Administration (FDA) considers 3 g per day of combined EPA and DHA derived from the diet and dietary supplements to be "Generally Regarded As Safe" (GRAS).[53] EPA and DHA levels in fish oil concentrate will vary depending on manufacturer, a dose range of 3–10 g per day appears to be safe.[54] A patient on a long-term dose of combined EPA and DHA above 5 g per day should be monitored for side effects which can include increased bruising and bleeding, and mild gastrointestinal upset.[53,54] In a pilot study conducted by Shinto et al. doses up to 9.6 g/day of fish oil supplementation (containing 3 grams EPA and 2 grams DHA) daily for three months appeared safe and tolerable in people with MS. In light of the emerging data about potential anti-inflammatory effects of omega-3 fatty acids, it would be worthwhile to pursue this research further in larger clinical trials as many MS patients are still taking these supplements and find them "highly beneficial."[10]

Anti-oxidants

Another promising area of CAM research is the use of natural anti-oxidants to treat MS. Oxidative and nitrogen free radicals are believed to contribute to demyelinating and axonal injury in MS.[55–58] Macrophages are the most prominent inflammatory cell in active MS plaques and are mediators of demyelination. Activated macrophages release a variety of reactive nitrogen and oxygen species, including nitric oxide, nitrite and nitrate, superoxide, and hydrogen peroxide, which may contribute to demyelination and axonal injury in MS. Natural anti-oxidants that prevent lipid peroxidation and are lipophilic may be particularly promising as therapeutic agents for MS since lipid peroxidation appears important to MS.[59] There is a long list of natural agents that have proven or postulated anti-oxidant effects, including vitamins C and E, ginkgo biloba (GB), grape seed extracts, green tea, and lipoic acid (LA). While many MS patients take one or more of these agents, only a handful of these therapies have been investigated formally as a treatment for MS.[10,60–63]

LA and its reduced form dihydrolipoic acid form a redox couple with potent anti-oxidant activity with several modes of action.[64] In humans, LA has been shown to be effective in treating diabetic polyneuropathy.[65,66] Several groups have now confirmed that LA is highly effective at suppressing and treating experimental autoimmune encephalomyelitis (EAE), an animal model of MS.[61,62,67] Our group has also conducted several studies to better understand the mechanism of action of LA as well as its potential immunological effects.[68–73] LA appears to have strong anti-inflammatory properties and its mechanism of action may involve stimulation of cAMP production in CD4+ T-cells and natural killer cells that result in protein kinase A signaling pathway activation. Additionally, LA also inhibits expression of certain key cellular adhesion molecules that are required for migration of immune cells across the blood–brain barrier.[72]

We have conducted Phase 1 pilot studies of high-dose LA in MS that demonstrated that oral LA was well tolerated and at a single dose of 1200 mg resulted in detectable serum levels of LA in almost all patients.[10,63] Importantly, despite the small sample size and relatively short duration of the pilot trial, LA appeared capable of decreasing two immunologic markers, serum MMP-9 and soluble intercellular adhesion molecule-1, which are indirectly associated with T-cell migration into the CNS.[10] We also compared different over-the-counter formulations of oral LA to better understand the variability and pharmacokinetics of these formulations and found that the 1200 mg oral LA dose, even when taken with food, gives LA levels in the serum that are comparable to those obtained in mice receiving therapeutically effective doses in EAE.[63] Hence, we believe that the 1200 mg once a day dose of LA may effectively serve as a therapeutic dose in MS. Further research on the potential therapeutic benefit of LA in MS is ongoing.

GB is a herb that has been used to treat a variety of disorders in China for thousands of years. In the past two decades, GB has gained considerable popularity in the western world as a treatment for dementia and other neurological conditions. Its biological and clinical effects are being extensively studied and in Europe it is used to treat peripheral and cerebral vascular insufficiency, memory impairment, and senile macular degeneration. In 1998, a meta-analysis of published studies suggested that GB was effective in slowing progression of Alzheimer's disease.[74] More recently, the Cochrane Collaboration conducted systematic review of the studies assessing the

efficacy and safety of GB for dementia or cognitive decline and found the evidence of efficacy of GB to be inconsistent and unreliable. This review also reported that GB appeared to be safe and showed no significant side effect as compared to placebo in clinical trials.[75,76]

The mechanisms of GB's therapeutic effects are probably multifold and mediated by its varied constituents that include flavonoids, terpenoids and organic acids. GB has both anti-platelet and anti-oxidant activities. Several recent in vitro and animal studies showed GB to be an effective lipid soluble anti-oxidant. Using a human low-density lipoprotein system, GB was shown to scavenge peroxyl radicals, which are involved in the propagation step of lipid peroxidation.[77] Furthermore, in a red blood cell system, GB was a more effective inhibitor of lipid peroxidation than vitamin C, uric acid, and reduced glutathione.[78] In rats with spinal cord injury, GB significantly decreased malondialdehyde (a marker for oxidant stress), an effect that is similar to the administration of methylprednisolone.[79]

Gingkolide B, which is a specific terpenoid compound found in ginkgo biloba extracts, is an antagonist of platelet activating factor (PAF), which has been studied in EAE.[80] After it was found to have a beneficial effect on prevention and treatment of EAE, a placebo-controlled study assessed the effect of gingkolide B as a treatment of MS relapses.[81] This trial involving 104 MS patients failed to show any efficacy of gingkolide B over placebo on relapse recovery.

Besides its antioxidant and neuroprotective effects, GB also has several compounds that could modulate neurotransmitter effects and potentially enhance cognitive function. GB extracts also enhance the release of acetylcholine, upregulate muscarinic receptors, and modulate cholinergic function by activating serotonin 5HT1A receptors.[82] Gingkolides are also glycine and GABA receptor antagonists.[83,84]

The effects of GB on cognitive performance in MS have been assessed in only a few clinical trials.[85–87] Kenney et al. conducted a six-month long, double-blind, placebo-controlled modified cross over study of subjects with mild MS ($N = 23$).[85] Subjects were randomized such that the first group received placebo for the first three months before crossing over to GB (240 mg/day) for an additional three months. The second group received GB at both three months interval. Outcome measures were conducted at baseline, three and six months and included the following battery of cognitive tests: Paced Auditory Serial Addition Test (PASAT); California Verbal Learning Test-II (CVLT-II); Delis-Kaplan Executive Measures Scale (DKEFS). Outcome measures for depression (Beck Depression Inventory), QoL (Multiple Sclerosis Quality of Life Index [MSQLI]), and fatigue (Modified Fatigue Impact Scale [MFIS]) were also done at the same time. GB-treated subjects showed a statistically significant improvement ($P = 0.04$) in performance on the PASAT at three months (mean 120.2 ± 27.1) vs. baseline (mean 105.2 ± 23.6) as compared to placebo. Perceived Deficits Questionnaire (PDQ) of the MSQLI also showed significant improvement ($P = 0.03$) in the GB-treated group. Thus, this small pilot study suggested that

GB might be beneficial for treatment of cognitive dysfunction in MS.

Lovera *et al.* conducted a double-blind, randomized, placebo controlled trial in 38 MS subjects where 120 mg of GB or placebo was given for 12 weeks.[85] The primary outcome of the study was change in performance on six neuropsychological tests, including the CVLT-II (the long delay free recall), PASAT, and the Stroop Color and Word Test (tests color-word interference condition and is a measure of attention and executive functions). While there was no significant differences in the GB and control groups on five of the cognitive tests, the GB-treated group showed a 4.5 second improvement compared with placebo (95% CI (7.6, 0.9), $P = 0.015$) on the Stroop color word test. Subjects in the study who were more impaired at baseline experienced greater improvement with the treatment group (treatment-baseline interaction, $F = 8.10$, $P = 0.008$).

Johnson *et al.* studied the effects of a ginkgo extract (EGb 761) on the functional performance in people with MS in a double-blind, placebo-controlled, parallel group design trial.[87] MS subjects ($N = 23$) were randomly assigned to receive either 240 mg per day of GB ($N = 12$) or placebo ($N = 11$) for 4 weeks. The key outcome measure included effects on depression (Center for Epidemiologic Studies of Depression Scale (CES-D)), anxiety (State-Trait Anxiety Inventory (STAI)), fatigue (MFIS); symptom severity (Symptom Inventory (SI)), and functional performance (Functional Assessment of Multiple Sclerosis (FAMS)) in the study subjects. Subjects in the GB group showed a significant improvement by mean effect size on several study measures, including the symptom severity by SI scale, functional performance by FAMS scale and fatigue by MFIS as compared to the placebo group.

These recent studies, even though limited by small sample sizes, suggest the safety of short-term use of GB in MS patients and also give a hint of efficacy on cognition as well as several other functional parameters that are of significance in MS. Further research of GB in MS appears warranted.

Vitamin C and E both are anti-oxidants and, hence, may have the potential to reduce the risk or alter the course of MS. The literature available thus far is inconsistent regarding the effect of either vitamin on MS. One case control study involving 197 newly diagnosed MS patients and 202 healthy matched controls reported a significant protective effect of vitamin C and E supplementation on the risk of MS development.[35] In contrast, another study that looked at the occurrence of definite and probable MS within two large cohorts of women followed for six to 12 years, found no relation between the use of vitamin C, vitamin E, and multivitamin supplement and risk of developing MS.[88] A small study in 24 MS patients found lower levels of vitamin C and E as compared with healthy controls during an MS attack.[89] The role of these vitamins in MS management remains to be explored, as there have been no clinical trials assessing the therapeutic benefit of vitamin C or E supplementation in MS. The role of vitamin D supplementation is discussed in another chapter.

Ginseng

Ginseng has been used in traditional Chinese medicine for centuries and is among the most extensively studied herbal product in the scientific literature. Several different members of the Araliaceae family are available as "ginseng" in the herbal market. Most share the genus Panax. Among the most popular are Asian ginseng (*Panax ginseng*, also referred to as Chinese or Korean ginseng) and American ginseng (*Panax quinquefolius*). It should be noted that another popular "ginseng" product, Siberian or Russian ginseng, is actually a more distant relative within the Araliaceae family (*Eleutherococcus senticosus*, not of the Panax genus). The active chemical constituents of the Panax genus of plants are thought to be the ginsenosides, which are non-steroidal saponins.[90] Traditionally viewed by Chinese medicine as an "adaptogen," the reported biological effects of ginseng include antioxidant activity, corticosteroidal effects, vasodilation, reduced platelet aggregation, and hypoglycemic activity. Ginseng is regarded as safe, with few demonstrable side effects when used at recommended doses.[90] Higher doses have been associated with a "ginseng abuse syndrome" characterized by hypertension, nervousness, irritability, insomnia, rash, and diarrhea.[91] There is evidence from placebo-controlled trials that ginseng reduces the effects of warfarin, and use should be avoided in patients taking anti-coagulants.[92]

Effects of ginseng on mood, cognitive function, and fatigue have been explored in a small number of clinical trials with mixed results.[93–106] In the Oregon survey of CAM use in MS patients 16% reported that they had used ginseng and more than 75% of those currently using ginseng reported benefit of the drug. No clinical trials of Asian ginseng have been reported in the MS literature, but a pilot placebo-controlled trial of American ginseng for the treatment of fatigue and found no significant differences from American ginseng compared placebo.[107]

Acupuncture

Acupuncture is a traditional form of therapy that has been used in China for at least 2500 years. According to the acupuncture theory, there are patterns of energy (Qi) that flow through the body along meridians and disturbances of the flow of Qi results in ill health. Inserting acupuncture needles into specific points along these meridians is postulated to correct the imbalances of energy flow. Although the practice of acupuncture is based on a very different model of disease than western medicine, scientific studies in animals as well as humans in the last two decades have shown that acupuncture can lead to multiple biological responses.

Acupuncture has been shown to be beneficial in controlling certain symptoms like pain and nausea in several studies.[108,109] In 1997, a National Institutes of Health panel concluded that acupuncture was effective as a treatment for some pain syndromes, addiction, asthma, and nausea.[110] Limited studies in MS also suggest that acupuncture might help a variety of MS symptoms, including pain, spasticity, insomnia, fatigue, and gait difficulties.[111] An open-label pilot study ($n = 10$) evaluated electro-acupuncture in MS patients (all types) with bladder dysfunction. Subjects received one acupuncture treatment per week over 10 weeks. A significant decrease in urge frequency and daytime leakage was reported. Acupuncture was well tolerated, and no urinary tract infections were reported.[112] A randomized pilot study evaluating Traditional Chinese Medicine ($n = 7$) vs. minimal acupuncture ($n = 7$) (needles inserted on non-acupuncture points) for QoL in MS showed no difference between groups on most QoL measures. Acupuncture/needle insertion was well tolerated in both groups.[113]

Acupuncture offers a non-pharmacologic therapy that may be beneficial for some symptoms associated with MS. The benefit of acupuncture for various symptoms in MS may warrant further investigation in controlled clinical trials.

Low-dose naltrexone

Naltrexone is an opiate receptor antagonist that has been approved by the FDA for the treatment of opiate addiction at a daily dose between 50 and 100 mg. Low-dose naltrexone (LDN) was shown in animal studies to induce beta endorphin receptors and increase intracellular beta endorphin levels in one open-label study in MS subjects.[114] LDN's ability to modulate beta endorphin levels may have a beneficial impact pain and mood in MS. There are three reported clinical studies evaluating LDN in MS. One open-label, unblinded, uncontrolled study evaluated safety and tolerability of LDN in primary progressive MS subjects ($N = 40$) over six months.[114] All subjects started with 2 mg at bedtime of LDN for two weeks, and the dose was then increased to 4 mg at bedtime until the study end (six months). The primary outcome was safety and secondary outcome measures included spasticity, pain, fatigue, depression, and QoL. The study reported five drops outs and two serious adverse events thought unrelated to LDN (renal failure from previously unrecognized polycystic kidney, and lung cancer). The remaining adverse events were mild and transient and included leukopenia, elevated liver enzymes, and mild irritability. There was a significant improvement from baseline on spasticity (assessed with Modified Ashworth Scale) at month 3 ($P < 0.001$) and month 6 (median baseline value 0.87 vs. median final value 0.5, $P < 0.01$). As compared to baseline, significant increase ($P < 0.05$) in beta endorphin levels was seen at month 3 (63.4 ± 4.8) and month 6 (76.9 ± 3.3). Pain (measured with a visual analog scale), however, showed a significant worsening at month 3 (median value 3.0; $P < 0.01$) and 6 (median value 3.0; $P < 0.05$), which did improve with treatment discontinuation. No improvements in depression, fatigue, or QoL were noted.

One double-blind, placebo-controlled study evaluated LDN at 4.5 mg (at bedtime) over eight weeks for changes in QoL in MS.[115] Eighty subjects were randomized to LDN ($n = 40$) or placebo ($n = 40$) for 8 weeks, had a one week washout, and then

crossed over to the LDN or placebo intervention for another eight weeks. Because of drop-outs and significant missing data on the QoL inventory, data were analyzed on 60 subjects. The authors reported that LDN was well tolerated and significantly improved the mental health component of the QoL measure (SF-36 short form). No serious adverse events were reported; mild adverse events in both groups included vivid dreaming (LDN $n = 10$, placebo $n = 7$), fatigue (both groups), and insomnia (placebo).

Another double-blind, placebo-controlled study evaluated LDN at 4.5 mg at bedtime for affects on QoL in MS.[116] One hundred and six subjects with either RR or secondary progressive MS were randomized to LDN ($n = 53$) or placebo ($n = 53$) for eight weeks, had a one week washout out, and crossed over to the LDN or placebo intervention for another eight weeks. The study reported no significant difference between groups on QoL. LDN appeared to be safe and well tolerated. No serious adverse events were reported. Mild and transient adverse events occurred in both groups and included nausea, stomach pain, mild irritability, and headache.

From the limited evidence, it appears that LDN at doses up to 4.5 mg at bedtime are relatively safe and well tolerated and there are mixed reports on benefit in improving spasticity, quality of life and pain. Given LDN's apparent safety and possible benefit in pilot studies, larger studies with longer invention periods may be warranted.

Cannabis

The major psychoactive constituent in cannabis is delta-9-tetrahydrocannabinol (THC). THC binds to cannabinoid receptors (CB) in the CNS and acts as a partial agonist to both CB_1 and CB_2 receptors. Cannabidol (CBD) is a non-psychoactive constituent in cannabis and is the major constituent in the plant. It is thought to decrease the clearance of THC by affecting liver metabolism. It binds to both CB_1 and CB_2 receptors in the CNS with a higher affinity to the CB_2 receptor. A review of six controlled studies evaluating a combination of THC-CBD (dornabinol or Marinol) for spasticity in MS found that THC-CBD was well tolerated and improved patient self-report of spasticity, although objective measures for spasticity such as the Ashworth score in all but one study did not show significant improvement compared with placebo.[117] Side effects were mild and reported in both treatment and placebo groups. Common side effects reported by subjects included drowsiness, dizziness, slower thinking, and dry mouth. There have been two studies evaluating THC-CBD's effect on an objective measure of cognition by administering the PASAT. One study found an improvement[118] and the other study found no difference between groups[119] suggesting that although subjects report slowed thinking, objective measures of sustained attention and processing speed are not affected by short-term THC-CBD use. Long-term use of cannabis for recreational purposes, however, showed slower processing rates on PASAT (mean reported recreational long-term use of cannabis >10

Table 49.2. *Summary of dietary supplements: biologic effects, drug interactions, contraindications*

Dietary supplement	Dose	Mechanism of action	Biologic effects	Drug interactions	Contraindications
Fish oil (ω-3)	1.7–3.0 g/day EPA and 1.4–1.9 g/day DHA	Specific mechanism unknown	Anti-inflammatory. Decreases IL-1β, TNFα, IL-2, IFNγ, MMP-9	Anticoagulants (e.g. coumadin), anti-hypertensive medications	No known
Sunflower seed oil (ω-6)	17 g/day (1.2 tablespoon)	Specific mechanism unknown	Immunomodulatory, increases TGF-β1	No known	No known
EP oil (ω-6²)	3.0 ml/day (0.6 teaspoon)	Specific mechanism unknown	Gamma linolenic acid is active constituent: immunomodulatory, anti-inflammatory	Chlorpromazine, thioridazine, trifluoperazine, fluphenazine due to an increased risk of seizure	Individuals with seizures; those taking seizure medications
Lipoic acid	1200 mg once a day	Inhibits MMP-9, increases cAMP production via prostaglandin EP2 and Ep4 receptor	Immunomodulatory and anti-inflammatory	Glucose; insulin regulating agents	No known
Ginkgo biloba	Standardized extract containing > 24% ginkgo flavone glycosides and 6% terpine lactones: 120 mg twice daily	Exact mechanism unknown	Ginkgolides are glycine and GABA receptor antagonists and can increase release of acetylcholine. Flavonoids are antioxidants and anti-inflammatory	Blood-thinning agents (e.g. coumadin), glucose and insulin-regulating agents	Pregnant and breastfeeding
Low-dose naltrexone	4–4.5 mg at bedtime	Opiate receptor antagonist	At low doses proposed to normalize endorphin levels	Opioid narcotics, immunosuppressive drugs	No known
Cannabis (Marinol)	2.5–120 mg/day	Specific mechanism unknown	Binds to cannabinoid receptors, complex CNS actions	Increased drowsiness with alcohol, barbiturates, benzodiazepines	Sensitivity to cannaboids or sesame oil

ω-3 = omega-3 fatty acid, ω-6 = omega-6 fatty acid, cAMP = cyclic adenosine monophosphate, DHA = docosahexaenoic acid, EPA = eicosapentaenoic acid, EP oil = Evening Primrose Oil, GABA = gamma amino butyric acid, IFN = interferon, IL = interleukin, MMP = matrix metalloproteinase, TGF = transforming growth factor, TNF = tumor necrosis factor.

years) compared to short-term users.[120] The scientific literature reports significant improvement in patient reported spasticity with the combination of THC-CBD and that in general THC-CBD was well tolerated in MS. As most of studies evaluating THC-CBD have been relatively short-term (2–15 weeks), longer-term studies may be necessary to better assess effects on spasticity and potential adverse effects on cognition. Unlike the dietary supplements discussed, THC-CBD (dronabinol) is a controlled substance approved by the FDA for the treatment of anorexia in AIDS patients and nausea and vomiting in cancer patients and patients undergoing chemotherapy. Table 49.2 summarizes supplements that MS patients have used.

Recommendations for future research

Despite the widespread use of CAM therapies among MS patients, most of these therapies have not been evaluated in well-designed, randomized, controlled clinical trials, the lack of which is the main reason why most neurologists do not incorporate CAM therapies into their management of MS patients. As reviewed in this chapter, controlled trials of various CAM approaches are now being conducted in MS.[18,38,86,87] While it is not practical to study every CAM therapy, there are

Table 49.3. *Resources for information about CAM*

Type of resource	
Books	Oken BS (ed). *Complementary Therapies in Neurology: An Evidence Based Approach*. New York: The Parthenon Publishing Group, 2004.
	Bowling AC. *Alternative Medicine and Multiple Sclerosis*. New York, NY: Demos Medical Publishing, 2001.
Websites	http://neurologycare.net/CAM/CAM.aspx
	http://www.nationalmssociety.org/spotlight-cam.asp(National MS Society)
	http://nccam.nih.gov/health(National Center of Complementary and Alternative Medicine – NCCAM)
	http://ods.od.nih.gov/(Office of Dietary Supplements)
	http://lpi.oregonstate.edu/infocenter/(Linus Pauling Institute micronutrient information

clearly some CAM therapies worthy of research into their efficacy in MS. There are significant differences in how MS patients rate the self-perceived benefit among specific CAM therapies, suggesting perhaps that some CAM therapies may be more effective than others. Clearly there are certain therapies, such as anti-oxidants and essential fatty acids, that have a scientific rationale for use in MS and are also supported by preclinical or pilot clinical data. Other CAM therapies, like yoga or meditation, that a high percentage of MS patients report as "highly beneficial" are also worth investigating further. Until well-designed trials of CAM therapies are performed, however, we will not know what works and what does not.

Recommendations for patients

In our MS clinics, we recommend that MS patients follow a low fat diet, exercise regularly, and learn to manage stress. For patients who are interested in incorporating CAM approaches to managing their MS, we recommend considering following the Swank low fat diet, practicing yoga or tai chi for exercise and using meditation or regular prayer for stress management. We warn patients to avoid CAM therapies that are expensive or potentially dangerous. We also provide patients with sources of information about CAM therapies (Table 49.3) and encourage patients to discuss with us CAM therapies they are considering trying or are taking.

References

1. Eisenberg DM, Kessler RC, Foster C, et al. Unconventional medicine in the United States. Prevalence, costs, and patterns of use. N Engl J Med 1993;328:246–52.

2. Eisenberg DM, Davis RB, Ettner SL, et al. Trends in alternative medicine use in the United States, 1990–1997: results of a follow-up national survey. JAMA 1998;280:1569–75.

3. Berkman C, Pignotti MG, Cavallo PF, et al. Use of alternative treatments by people with multiple sclerosis. Neurorehab Neural Repair 2003;9:461–6.

4. Nayak S, Matheis RJ, Schoenberger NE, et al. Use of unconventional therapies by individuals with multiple sclerosis. Clin Rehab 2003;17:181–91.

5. Page SA, Verhoef MJ, Stebbins RA, et al. The use of complementary and alternative therapies by people with multiple sclerosis. Chronic Diseases in Canada 2003;24:75–9.

6. Schwartz C, Laitin E, Brotman S, et al. Utilization of unconventional treatments by persons with MS: is it alternative or complementary? Neurology 1999;52:626–9.

7. Stuifbergen AK, Harrison TC. Complementary and alternative therapy use in persons with multiple sclerosis. Rehabilitation Nursing 2003;28:141–7, 158.

8. Fawcett J, Sidney JS, Hanson MJ, Riley-Lawless K. Use of alternative health therapies by people with multiple sclerosis: an exploratory study. Holist Nurs Pract 1994;8: 36–42.

9. NIH Classification of CAM, NIH

10. Yadav V, Marrracci G, Lovera J, et al. Lipoic acid in multiple sclerosis: a pilot study. Mult Scler 2005;11:159–65.

11. Esmonde L, Long AF. Complementary therapy use by persons with multiple sclerosis: benefits and research priorities. Complement Ther Clin Pract 2008;14:176–84.

12. Schwarz S, Knorr C, Geiger H, et al. Complementary and alternative medicine for multiple sclerosis. Mult Scler 2008;14:1113–19.

13. Marrie RA, Hadjimichael O, Vollmer T. Predictors of alternative medicine use by multiple sclerosis patients. Mult Scler 2003;9:461–6.

14. Hooper KD, Pender MP, Webb PM, et al. Use of traditional and complementary medical care by patients with multiple sclerosis in south-east Queensland. Int J MS Care 2001;3:3–13.

15. Shinto L, Yadav V, Morris C, et al. Demographic and health-related factors associated with complementary and alternative medicine (CAM) use in multiple sclerosis. Mult Scler 2006;12:94–100.

16. Wahbeh H, Elsas SM, Oken BS. Mind–body interventions: applications in neurology. Neurology 2008;70:2321–8.

17. Velikonja O, Curic K, Ozura A, et al. Influence of sports climbing and yoga on spasticity, cognitive function, mood and fatigue in patients with multiple sclerosis. Clin Neurol Neurosurg 2010;112:597–601.

18. Oken BS, Kishiyama S, Zajdel D, et al. Randomized controlled trial of yoga and exercise in multiple sclerosis. Neurology 2004;62:2058–64.

19. Grossman P, Kappos L, Gensicke H, et al. MS quality of life, depression, and fatigue improve after mindfulness training: a randomized trial. Neurology 2010;75:1141–9.

20. Li JX, Hong Y, Chan KM. Tai chi: physiological characteristics and beneficial effects on health. Br J Sports Med 2001;35:148–56.

21. Ross MC, Bohannon AS, Davis DC, et al. The effects of a short-term exercise program on movement, pain, and mood in the elderly. Results of a pilot study. J Holist Nurs 1999;17:139–47.

22. Husted C, Pham L, Hekking A, et al. Improving quality of life for people with chronic conditions: the example of t'ai chi and multiple sclerosis. Altern Ther Health Med 1999;5:70–4.

23. Mills N, Allen J. Mindfulness of movement as a coping strategy in multiple sclerosis. A pilot study. Gen Hosp Psychiatry 2000;22:425–31.

24. Swank RL, Dugan BB. The Multiple Sclerosis Diet Book: A Low Fat Diet for the Treatment of MS. 1987: Doubleday.

25. Yadav V, Shinto, L, Morris C, et al. Use and self reported benefit of complementary and alternative (CAM) therapies among multiple sclerosis patients. Int J MS Care 2006;8:5–10.

26. Swank RL, Lerstad O, Strom A et al. Multiple sclerosis in rural Norway its geographic and occupational incidence in relation to nutrition. N Engl J Med 1952;246:722–8.

27. Swank R. Multiple Sclerosis: a correlation of its incidence with dietary fat. Amer J Med Sci 1950;220:421–30.

28. Alter M, Yamoor M, Harshe M, Multiple sclerosis and nutrition. Arch Neurol 1974;31:267–72.

29. Swank RL. Multiple sclerosis: twenty years on low fat diet. *Arch Neurol* 1970;23:460–74.

30. Swank RL, Dugan BB. Effect of low saturated fat diet in early and late cases of multiple sclerosis. *Lancet* 1990;336:37–9.

31. Swank RL, Goodwin JW. How saturated fats may be a causative factor in multiple sclerosis and other diseases. *Nutrition* 2003;19:478.

32. Swank RL, Goodwin J. Review of MS patient survival on a Swank low saturated fat diet. *Nutrition* 2003;19:161–2.

33. Lauer K. The risk of multiple sclerosis in the U.S.A. in relation to sociogeographic features: a factor-analytic study. *J Clin Epidemiol* 1994;47:43–8.

34. Esparza ML, Sasaki S, Kesteloot H. Nutrition, latitude, and multiple sclerosis mortality: an ecologic study. *Am J Epidemiol* 1995;142:733–7.

35. Ghadirian P, Jain M, Ducuc S, et al. Nutritional factors in the aetiology of multiple sclerosis: a case-control study in Montreal, Canada. *Int J Epidemiol* 1998;27:845–52.

36. Tola MR, Granieri E, Malagu S, et al. Dietary habits and multiple sclerosis. A retrospective study in Ferrara, Italy. *Acta Neurologica* 1994;16:189–97.

37. Zhang SM, Willett WC, Hernan MA, et al. Dietary fat in relation to risk of multiple sclerosis among two large cohorts of women. *Am J Epidemiol* 2000;152:1056–64.

38. Weinstock-Guttman B, Baier M, Park Y, et al. Low fat dietary intervention with omega-3 fatty acid supplementation in multiple sclerosis patients. *Prostaglandins Leukot Essent Fatty Acids* 2005;73:397–404.

39. Farinotti M, Sims S, Di Pietrantonj C, et al. Dietary interventions for multiple sclerosis. *Cochrane Database Syst Rev* 2007;(1):CD004192.

40. Munger KL, Chitnis T, Ascherio A. Body size and risk of MS in two cohorts of US women. *Neurology* 2009;73:1543–50.

41. Millar JH, Zilkha KJ, Langman MJ, et al. Double-blind trial of linoleate supplementation of the diet in multiple sclerosis. *Br Med J* 1973;1:765–8.

42. Bates D, Fawcett PR, Shaw DA, et al. Polyunsaturated fatty acids in treatment of acute remitting multiple sclerosis. *Br Med J* 1978;2:1390–1.

43. Paty DW, Cousin HK, Read S, et al. Linoleic acid in multiple sclerosis: failure to show any therapeutic benefit. *Acta Neurol Scand* 1978;58:53–8.

44. Dworkin RH, Bates D, Millar JH, et al. Linoleic acid and multiple sclerosis: a reanalysis of three double-blind trials. *Neurology* 1984;34:1441–5.

45. Bates D, Cartlidge NE, French JM, et al. A double-blind controlled trial of long chain n-3 polyunsaturated fatty acids in the treatment of multiple sclerosis. *J Neurol Neurosurg Psychiatry* 1989;52:18–22.

46. Gallai V, Sarchielli P, Trequattrini A, et al. Supplementation of polyunsaturated fatty acids in multiple sclerosis. *Ital J Neurol Sci* 1992;13:401–7.

47. Kris-Etherton PM, Harris WS, Appel LJ. Fish consumption, fish oil, omega-3 fatty acids, and cardiovascular disease. *Circulation* 2002;106:2747–57.

48. Marchioli, R, Barzi F, Bomba E, et al. Early protection against sudden death by n-3 polyunsaturated fatty acids after myocardial infarction: time-course analysis of the results of the Gruppo Italiano per lo Studio della Sopravvivenza nell'Infarto Miocardico (GISSI)-Prevenzione. *Circulation* 2002;105:1897–903.

49. Calder PC. Dietary modification of inflammation with lipids. *Proc Nutr Soc* 2002;61:345–58.

50. Gallai V, Sarchielli P, Trequattrini A, et al. Cytokine secretion and eicosanoid production in the peripheral blood mononuclear cells of MS patients undergoing dietary supplementation with n-3 polyunsaturated fatty acids. *J Neuroimmunol* 1995;56:143–53.

51. Shinto L, Marracci G, Baldauf-Wagner S, et al. Omega-3 fatty acid supplementation decreases matrix metalloproteinase-9 production in relapsing-remitting multiple sclerosis. *Prostaglandins Leukot Essent Fatty Acids* 2009;80:131–6.

52. St-Pierre Y, Van Themsche C, Esteve PO. Emerging features in the regulation of MMP-9 gene expression for the development of novel molecular targets and therapeutic strategies. *Curr Drug Targets Inflamm Allergy* 2003;2:206–15.

53. Agency Response Letter GRAS Notice CRN 00138, FDA, Editor. 2004.

54. National Institutes of Health: Office of Dietary Supplements.. Dietary Supplement Fact Sheet: Omega-3 Fatty Acids and Health. http://ods.od.nih.gov/factsheets/ Omega3FattyAcidsandHealth./⟨τ π/⟩ Updated 10/18/2005. Accessed January 3, 2011.

55. Chia LS, Thompson JE, Moscarello MA. Disorder in human myelin induced by superoxide radical: an in vitro investigation. *Biochem Biophys Res Commun* 1983;117:141–6.

56. Arduini A, Di paola M Di Llio C, et al. Effect of lipid peroxidation on the accessibility of dansyl chloride labeling to lipids and proteins of bovine myelin. *Free Radic Res Commun* 1985;1:129–35.

57. Konat GW, Wiggins RC. Effect of reactive oxygen species on myelin membrane proteins. *J Neurochem* 1985;45:1113–18.

58. Merrill JE, Ignarro LJ, Sherman MP, et al. Microglial cell cytotoxicity of oligodendrocytes is mediated through nitric oxide. *J Immunol* 1993;151:2132–41.

59. Bagchi, D, Garg A, Krohn RL, et al. Protective effects of grape seed proanthocyanidins and selected antioxidants against TPA-induced hepatic and brain lipid peroxidation and DNA fragmentation, and peritoneal macrophage activation in mice. *Gen Pharmacol* 1998;30:771–6.

60. Bourdette D, Matejuk A, MacIntosh A, et al. Alpha lipoic acid inhibits T Cell trafficking into the spinal cord and suppresses and treats experimental autoimmune encephalomyelitis. *Neurology* 2001;56(Suppl 3):A67.

61. Marracci GH, Jones RE, McKeon GP, et al. Alpha lipoic acid inhibits T cell migration into the spinal cord and suppresses and treats experimental autoimmune encephalomyelitis. *J Neuroimmunol* 2002;131:104–14.

62. Morini M, Roccatagliata L, Dell'Eva R, et al. Alpha-lipoic acid is effective in prevention and treatment of experimental autoimmune encephalomyelitis. *J Neuroimmunol* 2004;148:146–53.

63. Yadav V, Marracci GH, Munar MY et al. Pharmacokinetic study of lipoic acid in multiple sclerosis: comparing

571

mice and human pharmacokinetic parameters. *Mult Scler* 2010;16:387–97.

64. Biewenga G, Haenen GR, Bast A. The role of lipoic acid in the treatment of diabetic polyneuropathy. *Drug Metab Rev* 1997;29:1025–54.

65. Ziegler D, Reljanovic M, Mehnert H, *et al.* Alpha-lipoic acid in the treatment of diabetic polyneuropathy in Germany: current evidence from clinical trials. *Exp Clin Endocrinol Diabetes* 1999;107:421–30.

66. Ziegler D, hanefeld M, Ruhnau KJ, *et al.* Treatment of symptomatic diabetic polyneuropathy with the antioxidant alpha-lipoic acid: a 7-month multicenter randomized controlled trial (ALADIN III Study). ALADIN III Study Group. Alpha-Lipoic Acid in Diabetic Neuropathy. *Diabetes Care* 1999;22:1296–301.

67. Schreibelt G, Musters RJ, Reijerkerk A, *et al.* Lipoic acid affects cellular migration into the central nervous system and stabilizes blood-brain barrier integrity. *J Immunol* 2006;177:2630–7.

68. Salinthone S, Yadav V, Schillace RV, *et al.* Lipoic acid attenuates inflammation via cAMP and protein kinase A signaling. *PLoS One* 2010;5.

69. Salinthone S, Schillace RV, Marracci GH, *et al.* Lipoic acid stimulates cAMP production via the EP2 and EP4 prostanoid receptors and inhibits IFN gamma synthesis and cellular cytotoxicity in NK cells. *J Neuroimmunol* 2008;199:46–55.

70. Marracci GH, McKeon GP, Marquardt WE, *et al.* Alpha lipoic acid inhibits human T-cell migration: implications for multiple sclerosis. *J Neurosci Res* 2004;78:362–70.

71. Marracci GH, Marquardt WE, Strehlow A, *et al.* Lipoic acid downmodulates CD4 from human T lymphocytes by dissociation of p56(Lck). *Biochem Biophys Res Commun* 2006;344:963–71.

72. Chaudhary P, Marracci GH, Bourdette DN. Lipoic acid inhibits expression of ICAM-1 and VCAM-1 by CNS endothelial cells and T cell migration into the spinal cord in experimental autoimmune encephalomyelitis. *J Neuroimmunol* 2006;175:87–96.

73. Schillace RV, Pisenti N, Pattamanuch N, *et al.* Lipoic acid stimulates cAMP production in T lymphocytes and NK

cells. *Biochem Biophys Res Commun* 2007;354:259–64.

74. Oken, BS, Storzbach DM, Kaye JA. The efficacy of Ginkgo biloba on cognitive function in Alzheimer disease. *Arch Neurol* 1998;55:1409–15.

75. Birks J, Grimley Evans J. Ginkgo biloba for cognitive impairment and dementia. *Cochrane Database Syst Rev* 2009:CD003120.

76. Birks J, Grimley Evans J. Ginkgo biloba for cognitive impairment and dementia. *Cochrane Database Syst Rev* 2007:CD003120.

77. Maitra I, marocci L, Droy-Lefaix MT, *et al.* Peroxyl radical scavenging activity of Ginkgo biloba extract EGb 761. *Biochem Pharmacol* 1995;49:1649–55.

78. Kose K, Dogan P, Lipoperoxidation induced by hydrogen peroxide in human erythrocyte membranes. 2. Comparison of the antioxidant effect of Ginkgo biloba extract (EGb 761) with those of water-soluble and lipid-soluble antioxidants. *J Int Med Res* 1995;23:9–18.

79. Koc RK, Akdemir H, Kurtsoy A, *et al.* Lipid peroxidation in experimental spinal cord injury. Comparison of treatment with Ginkgo biloba, TRH and methylprednisolone. *Res Exp Med* 1995;195:117–23.

80. Howat DW, Chand N, Moore AL, *et al.* The effects of platelet-activating factor and its specific antagonist BN52021 on the development of experimental allergic encephalomyelitis in rats. *Int J Immunopath Pharmacol* 1988;1:11–15.

81. Brochet B, Guinot P, Orgogozo JM, *et al.* Double blind placebo controlled multicentre study of ginkgolide B in treatment of acute exacerbations of multiple sclerosis. The Ginkgolide Study Group in multiple sclerosis. *J Neurol Neurosurg Psychiatry* 1995;58:360–2.

82. Nathan P. Can the cognitive enhancing effects of ginkgo biloba be explained by its pharmacology? *Medical Hypotheses* 2000;55:491–3.

83. Ivic L, Sands TT, Fishkin N, *et al.* Terpene trilactones from Ginkgo biloba are antagonists of cortical glycine and GABA(A) receptors. *J Biol Chem* 2003;278:49279–85.

84. Huang SH, Duke RK, Chebib M, *et al.* Ginkgolides, diterpene trilactones of Ginkgo biloba, as antagonists at recombinant alpha1beta2gamma2L

GABA A receptors. *Eur J Pharmacol* 2004;494:131–8.

85. Kenney C, Normal M, Jacobson M, *et al.* A double-blind, placebo controlled, modified crossover pilot study of the effects of gingko biloba on cognitive and functional abilities in multiple sclerosis. *Neurology* 2002;58(Suppl 3):A458.

86. Lovera J, Bagert B, Smoot K, *et al.* Ginkgo biloba for the improvement of cognitive performance in multiple sclerosis: a randomized, placebo-controlled trial. *Mult Scler* 2007;13:376–85.

87. Johnson SK, Diamond BJ, Rausch S, *et al.* The effect of Ginkgo biloba on functional measures in multiple sclerosis: a pilot randomized controlled trial. *Explore (NY)* 2006;2:19–24.

88. Zhang SM, Hernan MA, Olek MJ, *et al.* Intakes of carotenoids, vitamin C, and vitamin E and MS risk among two large cohorts of women. *Neurology* 2001;57:75–80.

89. Besler HT, Comoglu S, Okcu Z. Serum levels of antioxidant vitamins and lipid peroxidation in multiple sclerosis. *Nutr Neurosci* 2002;5:215–20.

90. Appendix 1: Chemicals and their biological activities in Panaz Ginseng Root. N.T. Program, Editor. 2004.

91. Siegel RK. Ginseng abuse syndrome. Problems with the panacea. *JAMA* 1979;241:1614–5.

92. Yuan CS, Wei G, Dey L, *et al.* Brief communication: American ginseng reduces warfarin's effect in healthy patients: a randomized, controlled trial. *Ann Intern Med* 2004;141:23–7.

93. Wiklund IK, Mattsson LA, Lindgren R, *et al.* Effects of a standardized ginseng extract on quality of life and physiological parameters in symptomatic postmenopausal women: a double-blind, placebo-controlled trial. Swedish Alternative Medicine Group. *Int J Clin Pharmacol Res* 1999;19:89–99.

94. Kennedya D, Scholeya A, Wesnes K. Dose dependent changes in cognitive performance and mood following acute administration of Ginseng to healthy young volunteers. *Nutr Neurosci* 2001;4:15.

95. Kennedy DO, Scholey AB, Wesnes KA. Modulation of cognition and mood following administration of single doses of Ginkgo biloba, ginseng, and a ginkgo/ginseng combination to healthy

young adults. *Physiol Behav* 2002;75:739–51.

96. Kennedy DO, Scholey AB, Wesnes KA. Differential, dose dependent changes in cognitive performance following acute administration of a Ginkgo biloba/Panax ginseng combination to healthy young volunteers. *Nutr Neurosci* 2001;4:399–412.

97. Kennedy, DO, Scholey AB. Ginseng: potential for the enhancement of cognitive performance and mood. *Pharmacol Biochem Behav* 2003;75:687–700.

98. Kennedy DO, Haskell CF, Wesnes KA, *et al.* Improved cognitive performance in human volunteers following administration of guarana (Paullinia cupana) extract: comparison and interaction with Panax ginseng. *Pharmacol Biochem Behav* 2004;79:401–11.

99. Ellis JM, Reddy P. Effects of Panax ginseng on quality of life. *Ann Pharmacother* 2002;36:375–9.

100. D'Angelo L, Grimaldi R, Caravaggi M, *et al.* A double-blind, placebo-controlled clinical study on the effect of a standardized ginseng extract on psychomotor performance in healthy volunteers. *J Ethnopharmacol* 1986;16:15–22.

101. Tode T, Kikuchi Y, Hirata J, *et al.* Effect of Korean red ginseng on psychological functions in patients with severe climacteric syndromes. *Int J Gynaecol Ob* 1999;67:169–74.

102. Cardinal BJ, Engels HJ. Ginseng does not enhance psychological well-being in healthy, young adults: results of a double-blind, placebo-controlled, randomized clinical trial. *J Am Dietetic Assoc* 2001;101:655–60.

103. Engels HJ, Fahlman MM, Wirth JC. Effects of ginseng on secretory IgA, performance, and recovery from

interval exercise. *Med Sci Sports Exercise* 2003;35:690–6.

104. Engels HJ, Kolokouri I, Cieslak TJ, *et al.* Effects of ginseng supplementation on supramaximal exercise performance and short-term recovery. *J Strength Cond Res* 2001;15:290–5.

105. Engels HJ, Wirth JC. No ergogenic effects of ginseng (Panax ginseng C.A. Meyer) during graded maximal aerobic exercise. *J Am Dietetic Assoc* 1997;97:1110–15.

106. Forgo I, Kayasseh L, Staub JJ. [Effect of a standardized ginseng extract on general well-being, reaction time, lung function and gonadal hormones]. *Medizinische Welt* 1981;32:751–6.

107. Kim E, Lovera J, Schaben L, *et al.* American ginseng does not improve fatigue in multiple sclerosis : a single center randomized double-blind placebo-controlled crossover pilot trial. *Mult Scler* (in press).

108. Dundee JW, Ghaly RG, Fitzpatrick KT, *et al.* Acupuncture prophylaxis of cancer chemotherapy-induced sickness. *J R Soc Med* 1989;82:268–71.

109. Patel M, Gutzwiller F, Paccaud F, *et al.* A meta-analysis of acupuncture for chronic pain. *Int J Epidemiol* 1989;18:900–6.

110. NIH Consensus Conference. Acupuncture. *J Am Med Assoc* 1998;280:1518–24.

111. Wang Y, Hashimoto S, Ramsum D, *et al.* A pilot study of the use of alternative medicine in multiple sclerosis patients with special focus on acupuncture. *Neurology* 1999;52(Suppl 2):A550.

112. Tjon Eng Soe SH, Kopsky DJ, Jongen PJ, *et al.* Multiple sclerosis patients with bladder dysfunction have decreased symptoms after electro-acupuncture. *Mult Scler* 2009;15:1376–7.

113. Donnellan CP, Shanley J. Comparison of the effect of two types of acupuncture on quality of life in secondary progressive multiple sclerosis: a preliminary single-blind randomized controlled trial. *Clin Rehab* 2008;22:195–205.

114. Gironi M, Martinelli-Boneschi F, Sacerdote P, *et al.* A pilot trial of low-dose naltrexone in primary progressive multiple sclerosis. *Mult Scler* 2008;14:1076–83.

115. Cree BA, Kornyeyeva E, Goodin DS. Pilot trial of low-dose naltrexone and quality of life in multiple sclerosis. *Ann Neurol* 2010;68:145–50.

116. Sharafaddinzadeh N, Moghtaderi A, Kashipazha D, *et al.* The effect of low-dose naltrexone on quality of life of patients with multiple sclerosis: a randomized placebo-controlled trial. *Mult Scler* 2010;16:964–9.

117. Lakhan SE, Rowland M. Whole plant cannabis extracts in the treatment of spasticity in multiple sclerosis: a systematic review. *BMC Neurol* 2009;9:59.

118. Vaney C, Heinzel-Gutenbrunner M, Jobin P, *et al.* Efficacy, safety and tolerability of an orally administered cannabis extract in the treatment of spasticity in patients with multiple sclerosis: a randomized, double-blind, placebo-controlled, crossover study. *Mult Scler* 2004;10:417–24.

119. Aragona M, Onesti E, Tomassini V, *et al.* Psychopathological and cognitive effects of therapeutic cannabinoids in multiple sclerosis: a double-blind, placebo controlled, crossover study. *Clin Neuropharmacol* 2009;32:41–7.

120. Solowij N, Stephens RS, Roffman RA, *et al.* Cognitive functioning of long-term heavy cannabis users seeking treatment. *JAMA* 2002;287:1123–31.

The role of chronic cerebrospinal venous insufficiency in multiple sclerosis

Devon Conway, Soo Hyun Kim, and Alexander Rae-Grant

Introduction

Multiple sclerosis (MS) has traditionally been thought of as a T-cell mediated autoimmune disease.[1] It is widely believed that genetically susceptible individuals develop MS after exposure to an as yet unidentified triggering environmental factor. Considerable research efforts have identified genetic and environmental risk factors,[2-5] but have failed to identify an inciting antigen. The topographic relationship between MS lesions and cerebral veins has long been recognized.[6] A classical magnetic resonance imaging (MRI) finding in MS is "Dawson fingers," which represent periventricular demyelinating lesions around the long axis of central veins.[7] Additionally, the perivenous location of MS lesions has been observed during autopsy studies.[8] A recently published case series utilized 7 tesla MRI to study two MS patients in vivo with a total of 80 lesions.[9] The high-resolution imaging allowed visualization of small venous structures and all but one lesion was found to have a central vein at its core.

Jean-Martin Charcot was the first person to recognize MS as a distinct disease. The spatial relationship between MS lesions and cerebral venous structures led Charcot to hypothesize that MS may be the result of vascular pathology.[10] This hypothesis was expanded upon in the early twentieth century.[11,12] In 1935, Tracy Putnam injected various substances into the longitudinal sinuses of 14 anesthetized dogs.[13] The intention was that the substance would run upstream and obstruct veins draining into the sinus. Autopsies were performed up to one year after the procedure, and all but two dogs were found to have cerebral lesions. Those dogs that were sacrificed at later time points were found to have MS-like demyelination with preservation of axons, leading the author to conclude that venular obstruction is an essential antecedent to MS lesion formation.

Putnam further elaborated the role of venular obstruction in MS in a 1937 post-mortem study of brains from MS patients.[14] From a sample of 17 brains, he noted the presence of thrombi within the cerebral veins of nine, and closure of vessels by fibrous plugs or endothelial cells in 14. For five of the cases, slides from other portions of the body were available. Inspection of these slides revealed that three of the five cases demonstrated thrombi in organs other than the central nervous system. This led Putnam to speculate that the primary abnormality in MS patients is likely a disorder of the blood-clotting mechanism.

In 1954, Georgio Macchi published results from a post-mortem study of four MS cases comprising 100 demyelinating plaques.[15] His observations led him to suggest that MS was not the result of venous thrombosis or of inflammation of the blood vessels, but rather secondary to slow venous drainage of the perivascular spaces. He hypothesized that stasis and congestion of venules resulted from accumulation of fat and fat-laden cells in the periadventitial spaces of vessels. Pathologic venous reflux into the skull and spine was proposed by Franz Schelling in 1986 as a possible etiology of MS.[16] The ideas of Macchi and Schelling figure prominently in the modern vascular theory of MS.

The hypothesis that MS results from venous pathology has recently been renewed by Professor Paolo Zamboni, a vascular surgeon at the University of Ferrara in Ferrara, Italy. Dr. Zamboni's group noted pathological studies suggesting excess iron accumulation within the deep gray matter of MS patients and within MS plaques.[17,18] Recent radiologic evidence has also suggested a correlation between MS disease duration and pathologic iron content.[19] Zamboni et al. hypothesized that venous stasis resulting from cerebrospinal venous insufficiency (CCSVI) leads to increased iron deposition in the brain parenchyma,[20,21] and that this iron triggers MS inflammatory activity. To investigate their hypothesis, Zamboni and colleagues evaluated venous drainage in MS patients and controls. Prior to surveying their results, a review of cerebrospinal venous drainage is essential.

Cerebral venous anatomy

Within the brain parenchyma, small venous branches arise from the capillaries.[22,23] These branches are fine channels that eventually form a plexus within the pia. From the pial plexuses, cerebral veins arise that pass through the subarachnoid space and empty into the dural venous sinuses. The dural sinuses are larger channels that exist between the meningeal and periosteal layers of the dura (Fig. 50.1). Neither the cerebral veins nor the dural sinuses contain valves.

Multiple Sclerosis Therapeutics, Fourth Edition, ed. Jeffrey A. Cohen and Richard A. Rudick. Published by Cambridge University Press.
© Cambridge University Press 2011.

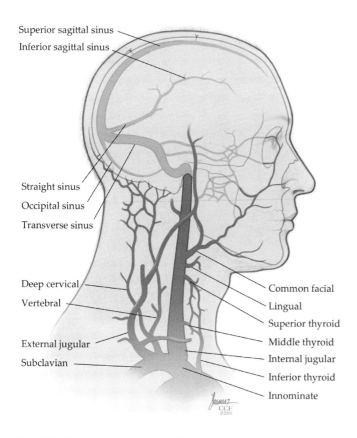

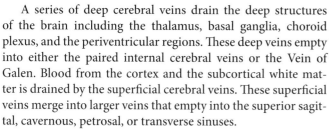

Fig. 50.1. The dural venous sinuses of the brain and the major veins of the neck.

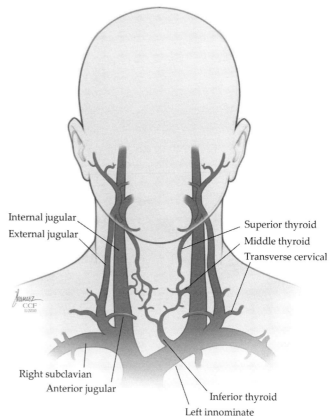

Fig. 50.2. Anterior view of the jugular system.

A series of deep cerebral veins drain the deep structures of the brain including the thalamus, basal ganglia, choroid plexus, and the periventricular regions. These deep veins empty into either the paired internal cerebral veins or the Vein of Galen. Blood from the cortex and the subcortical white matter is drained by the superficial cerebral veins. These superficial veins merge into larger veins that empty into the superior sagittal, cavernous, petrosal, or transverse sinuses.

The superior sagittal sinus runs posteriorly along the superior surface of the falx cerebri before emptying into the confluence of sinuses. The inferior sagittal sinus runs caudally along the inferior surface of the falx cerebri and then merges with the Vein of Galen to form the straight sinus, which also empties into the confluence of sinuses. The cavernous sinus is a large space adjacent to the sella turcica through which several cranial nerves and a portion of the internal carotid artery pass. The cavernous sinus communicates with the basilar venous plexus, and with the transverse sinus and internal jugular vein (IJV) by way of the petrosal sinuses. The confluence of sinuses is drained by the bilateral transverse sinuses, which proceed anteriorly before curving inferiorly as the sigmoid sinuses. The sigmoid sinuses are drained by the IJVs, which exit through the jugular foramen and merge with their respective subclavian veins to form the brachiocephalic veins (Fig. 50.2).

Cerebral venous drainage patterns differ between individuals. Doepp and colleagues examined cerebral outflow patterns in 50 healthy subjects using ultrasound and time of flight venography.[24] They found that 72% of individuals drained more than 2/3 of their global arterial cerebral blood flow (CBF) via the jugular system, 22% drained 1/3–2/3 of their CBF through the jugular system, and 6% drained less than 1/3 of the CBF via the jugular system. Thus, up to 6% of the general population may have primarily non-jugular venous drainage of the cranium without evident pathological consequences.

Spinal venous anatomy

The anterior portion of the spinal cord is drained by the anteromedian and anterolateral spinal veins, which then empty into six to eleven anterior radicular veins. The anterior radicular veins traverse the dura matter and drain into the epidural venous plexus. Similarly, the posterior portion of the spinal cord is drained by the posteromedian and posterolateral spinal veins. These veins drain into five to ten posterior radicular veins, which also empty into the epidural venous plexus. This significant variability in spinal cord vasculature was elucidated in a series of autopsy studies.[25,26]

The epidural venous plexus exists between the dura matter and the vertebral periosteum and surrounds the spinal cord.

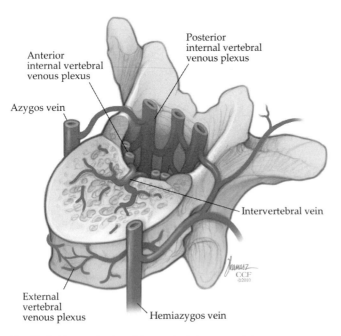

Fig. 50.3. Communication of the vertebral plexuses and the azygous system.

It ascends through the foramen magnum where it communicates with the dural sinuses and the vertebral veins. The vertebral veins also receive blood from the upper part of the back and neck before eventually draining into the brachiocephalic veins.

The epidural venous plexus communicates with the external vertebral venous plexus. The external vertebral venous plexus is divided into anterior and posterior plexuses, which surround the anterior and posterior portions of the vertebrae, respectively. The external venous plexus also is in communication with the azygous system and the lumbar veins (Fig. 50.3).[27] The azygos vein also drains the back, thoracoabdominal walls, and the mediastinal viscera. It arises from the inferior vena cava and travels along the right side of the lower eight thoracic vertebrae before eventually joining the superior vena cava. In addition, the azygos vein receives blood from the hemiazygos and accessory hemiazygos veins (Fig. 50.4).

Findings of Zamboni and colleagues

Table 50.1 summarizes results from the initial studies of CCSVI in MS. In 2009, Zamboni and colleagues published the results of venous hemodynamic studies in a cohort of MS patients and controls.[28] The study enrolled 120 patients with MS, 60 age- and gender-matched healthy controls, 80 patients older than the median age of European MS patients, and 60 subjects with other neurological diseases. Of these subjects, 11 with MS and 23 controls were excluded because of other underlying conditions that may have affected venous hemodynamics.

The subjects underwent EchoColor Doppler (ECD) to visualize the IJVs and VVs and transcranial color-coded Doppler sonography (TCCS) to assess the deep cerebral veins. Zamboni *et al.* assessed five parameters that they felt were indicative of CCSVI: (1) reflux (flow directed toward the brain for > 0.88 s)

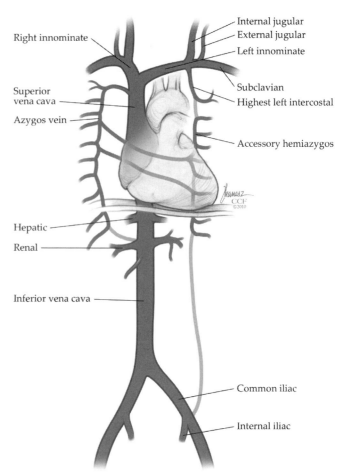

Fig. 50.4. Major veins of the thorax and abdomen, including the azygous system.

in the IJVs or VVs in the sitting and supine positions (2) reflux in the deep cerebral veins (3) evidence of IJV stenosis by high resolution B-mode analysis (4) lack of Doppler-detectable flow in the IJVs or the vertebral veins, and (5) reverted postural control of the main cerebral venous outflow pathway (meaning that the cross sectional area of the IJVs is larger in the sitting than in the supine position, which is the opposite of what is found in normal subjects). The authors found that when using the McDonald Criteria as a gold standard,[29] the first four parameters were ≥97% sensitive, and the last parameter was 74% sensitive in detecting MS, if one considers the vascular testing in a diagnostic sense. Specificity ranged from 69% to 84% among the parameters. Requiring ≥2 parameters in the same patient increased the sensitivity, specificity, positive predictive value, and negative predictive value to 100%.

In a follow-up study, Zamboni *et al.* assessed the same five ultrasound parameters in 65 MS patients and 235 healthy controls.[30] The control population included 60 healthy age- and gender-matched subjects, 82 healthy subjects who were older than the median age of MS onset, 45 participants affected by other neurological diseases, and 48 controls who had been scheduled for venography for other reasons. These 48 controls

Table 50.1. *Results from initial studies of CCSVI in MS patients and controls*

Study	Number of MS patients	Number of controls	Study findings
Zamboni[28]	120	60 age- and gender-matched healthy controls 80 controls greater than the average age of MS onset in Europe 60 controls with other neurological diseases	100% of MS patients met $\geq$2 CCSVI criteria 0% of controls met $\geq$2 CCSVI criteria
Zivadinov[33][a]	289	161 healthy controls 59 controls with other neurological diseases	56.1% of MS patients met $\geq$2 CCSVI criteria 42.3% of OND patients met $\geq$2 CCSVI criteria 38.1% of MS patients met $\geq$2 CCSVI criteria 22.7% of MS patients met $\geq$2 CCSVI criteria
Doepp[35]	56	20 age- and sex- matched healthy controls	0% of MS patients met $\geq$2 CCSVI criteria 0% of controls met $\geq$2 CCSVI criteria
Sundstrom[36]	21	20 healthy controls	No significant difference between cases and controls for total cerebral blood flow, total IJV blood flow,

MS = multiple sclerosis; CCSVI = chronic cerebrospinal venous insufficiency; OND = other neurological diseases; IJV = internal jugular vein
[a] Results are presented from the analysis with borderlines counted as "No CCSVI".

and the 65 patients with MS underwent selective venography with catheterization of the azygous and IJV systems. The physician performing the venography was not blinded to the diagnosis. Venography permitted the detection of significant stenoses (defined as venous lumen reduction greater than 50%) and manometer pressure assessments in the superior vena cava, azygous vein, and both IJVs. An odds ratio was used to determine the risk of MS in participants who had positive CCSVI ultrasound findings. The odds of MS ranged from 10 in those with reverted postural control of the IJVs to 1123 in those with IJV or VV reflux in the sitting and supine positions. The azygous vein was affected in 85% of the 65 MS patients undergoing venography and the IJVs were stenosed unilaterally or bilaterally in 91%. The MS patients were also found to have significantly higher venous pressures at the levels of stenoses as compared to adjacent open vessels. The authors were able to use flow direction data from the ultrasound studies to identify four patterns of aberrant venous return in the MS participants. The patterns were found to be significantly associated with MS disease course. For instance, 75% of the patients with primary progressive (PP) MS were found to have involvement of the azygous system at multiple segments, thereby forcing a portion of the spinal cord blood to drain upwards. Zamboni *et al.* reasoned this may explain why spinal cord involvement with spastic paraparesis is a prominent feature in PPMS.

Zamboni's group also has conducted a prospective, open-label study of angioplasty to treat CCSVI.[30] The study enrolled what appear to be the same 65 consecutive MS patients, of whom 35 had relapsing–remitting MS (RRMS), 20 had secondary-progressive MS (SPMS), and 10 had PPMS. Subjects underwent selective venography of the left renal vein, the azygous vein, and the IJVs. Anatomic obstructive abnormalities were corrected by means of compliant-type balloon angioplasty. High pressure balloons were used if the obstruction was not

relieved after the initial attempt. Vascular outcomes included: (1) the venous pressure in the superior vena cava, the azygous and the IJVs before and after angioplasty, (2) post-operative pain and the rate of post-operative complications, and (3) the rate of venous patency post-operatively as assessed by extracranial Doppler every three months, up to 18 months. Neurologic outcomes were assessed by a non-blinded neurologist and included: (1) change in the MS Functional Composite Z score,[31] (2) proportion of relapse-free patients at one year, (3) annualized relapse rate at one year compared to that during the prior two years, and (4) change in quality of life as assessed by the Quality of Life-54 questionnaire.[32]

The venous pressure in stenotic venous segments was not significantly increased compared to subjects with a normal venogram along the same segment. However, pressures following angioplasty were significantly lower than preoperative pressures in the azygous system and the IJVs. Restenosis after angioplasty was a significant problem. Post-procedural rate of venous patency in the IJVs declined to 47% at 18 months. On the other hand, patency of the azygous vein remained at over 80% after 18 months.

In a pre–post analysis, there was no significant difference in the annualized relapse rate before and after the procedure. Despite this, the authors report that the percentage of relapse-free participants was 27% in the year prior to the procedure and 50% in 18 months of post-procedural follow-up, a significant improvement. The authors also note that no relapses occurred in those participants who maintained patency of the IJVs and the azygous vein. The percentage of participants with gadolinium enhancement on MRI was 50% prior to the procedure and 12% afterward. The timing of these MRIs and how many MRIs were obtained was not described. Finally, quality of life scores were significantly improved in RRMS at 18 months, and in SPMS and PPMS at six months. This finding was not sustained at 18 months in the SPMS and PPMS participants.

Findings from other groups

Robert Zivadinov's group at the University of Buffalo recently presented interim findings from a study intended to reproduce the results of Zamboni et al.[33,34] The study plans to enroll 1700 subjects, but the initial results were from an analysis of the first 499 participants. These included 289 with MS, 21 with clinically isolated syndrome, 26 with other neurological diseases, and 163 healthy controls. Subjects were assessed by means of transcranial and extracranial venous Doppler for the five criteria of CCSVI as defined by Zamboni et al. The study noted that the chief ultrasound technologist was very experienced and had been trained for several weeks by Dr. Zamboni. Of the 499 participants, 52 fulfilled one CCSVI criteria but could not be assessed for reflux in the deep cerebral veins due to technical difficulties. These subjects were classified as having "borderline" CCSVI. When the borderline participants were excluded, the sensitivity of CCSVI in identifying MS was 62.5% and the specificity was 74.5%. With the borderline participants classified as "No CCSVI," CCSVI was detected in 56.1% of MS patients, 42.3% of patients with other neurological diseases, 38.1% of CIS patients, and 22.7% of healthy controls. Thus, the sensitivity was reduced to 56.1% and the specificity increased to 77.3%. These findings are inconsistent with those from Zamboni et al., in that CCSVI criteria were met in fewer MS patients and more control patients than expected. Dr. Zivadinov has suggested these discrepancies may be the result of the different ultrasound hardware being used in the laboratories.

Doepp et al. recently published a study that failed to confirm the findings of Zamboni et al.[35] Fifty-six patients with RRMS or SPMS and 20 age- and sex-matched healthy controls were recruited. The subjects underwent ultrasound and TCCS and were assessed for the five parameters of CCSVI as defined by Zamboni et al. In addition, measurements of global arterial cerebral blood flow (calculated as the sum of blood volume flow in the ICAs and VAs) were made. The cross-sectional area, blood flow velocity, and blood volume flow in the IJVs and VVs and the blood flow velocity and direction of flow in the intracranial veins were also assessed. Finally, the researchers assessed subjects for IJV valve incompetence by asking the participants to perform a 5 second maximal Valsalva maneuver while the IJV was insonated. Retrograde venous flow of more than 0.88 seconds was considered suggestive of incompetent valves in the IJVs. Overall, ten patients with MS (18%) met one CCSVI criterion. This included retrograde flow in the transverse sinus in one patient, lack of postural lumen reduction in the IJV in four patients, and missing flow in the VVs of five patients. Four controls (20%) met one CCSVI criterion including three with no postural lumen reduction in the IJV and one with no detectable flow in the VVs. There were no subjects who met two or more criteria for CCSVI.

Additional findings included no significant difference in mean global cerebral blood flow between MS patients and controls. With a Valsalva maneuver, 38% of patients and 30% of controls were found to have evidence of IJV valve incompetence. In the supine position, there was no difference in cross-sectional area or blood volume flow in the IJVs and VVs between patients and controls. Also, blood flow velocity in the intracranial venous structures was not significantly different between patients and controls. These results do not support those of Zamboni and colleagues. Doepp et al. suggest a number of possible explanations for the discrepancy. For instance, they note that the IJV is easily compressible and there is physiological variation in its size at different levels. As a result, compression from an ultrasound transducer or nearby anatomical structures may be misinterpreted as a stenosis. They also suggest that the color-coded duplex mode used by Zamboni and colleagues to detect blood flow in the IJVs and VVs may not have been sensitive enough to detect blood flow at low velocities. It was also suggested that pulsation artifact from the carotid arteries might be misinterpreted as reflux in the IJV.

Another study enrolled 21 patients with RRMS by McDonald diagnostic criteria and 20 healthy controls.[36] The MS subjects underwent contrast enhanced magnetic resonance angiography (MRA) with venous phase imaging to investigate the intracranial and cervical venous systems. In addition, all subjects were imaged with phase contrast MRI, which permitted assessments of blood and CSF flow. The contrast enhanced MRA examination of the MS cases revealed mid-portion IJV stenosis in three cases and no signs of venous stenosis in the other 18 cases. Total cerebral blood flow, total IJV blood flow, and the fraction of cerebral blood flow returning through both IJVs, or either of the IJVs were determined with phase contrast MRI. No significant difference was found between MS patients and controls for any of these parameters, although total cerebral blood flow tended to be lower in MS patients. Five subjects from both groups were found to have retrograde IJV flow. Finally, CSF flow stroke volume and net flow were not significantly different between the groups. The authors conclude that no evidence supporting the vascular theory of MS was found in their study. Although they found three cases of IJV stenosis among the MS patients, these results are difficult to interpret because the contrast enhanced MRA was not performed on controls. The number of cases demonstrating IJV reflux, one of the CCSVI parameters defined by Zamboni et al., was equal between cases and controls. It should be noted, however, that the authors used MRI rather than ultrasound in an attempt to detect IJV reflux, which may have influenced results.

Challenges to CCSVI

A number of authors have challenged the CCSVI hypothesis on several grounds summarized in Table 50.2:[35,37]

1. It is expected that vascular disease will worsen with increasing age. However, in one study of an MS registry containing over 17 000 cases, the peak incidence of MS in

Table 50.2. *Arguments in favor and against CCSVI as the underlying pathologic mechanism of MS*

In support of CCSVI	Against CCSVI
MS lesions tend to be oriented longitudinally along cerebral veins 100% Sensitivity, Specificity, Positive Predictive Value, and Negative Predictive Value found in the initial study	MS has genetic, immunologic, and geographic risk factors that cannot presently be explained by CCSVI
Varying patterns of aberrant venous drainage may explain the different clinical courses of MS	MS lesions are not seen in other conditions with increased venous pressure or in patients undergoing radical neck dissection
Promising pilot study data on angioplasty as a CCSVI treatment	The incidence of MS would be expected to increase rather than decline with increasing age if CCSVI was a causative factor
	There is considerable redundancy in the cerebrospinal venous system that should be able to account for stenoses
	Subsequent studies have failed to reproduce the dramatic results of Zamboni *et al.*
	Questionable methodology in the prospective angioplasty trial

women was from ages 25–29 and in men the peak occurred from ages 30–34.[38] In those over age 60, when the incidence of vascular disease would be expected to approach its peak, the incidence of MS was less than 2 per 100 000.

2. A number of neurological conditions are associated with increased cerebral venous pressures but do not result in demyelinating lesions. These include cerebral venous thrombosis,[39] which has been associated with subdural hemorrhage,[40] and subarachnoid hemorrhage,[41] but not with MS. Increased sagittal sinus pressure leading to decreased CSF absorption has been suggested as a causative mechanism in idiopathic intracranial hypertension,[42–44] but such patients have not been reported to develop MS at an increased rate. Head and neck cancers are commonly treated with a radical neck dissection, in which one or both of the IJVs are sacrificed,[45] but MS has not been reported as a complication of this procedure.

3. There is extensive redundancy of cerebrospinal venous drainage. As discussed above, drainage of the spinal cord and brain occurs through numerous intercommunicating systems.[37,46,47] The redundancy of the venous system suggests that stenosis in one region, such as the azygous vein, could easily be compensated via alternative systems without increases in venous pressure or reflux.

4. If MS is a result of CCSVI, the presence of venous structures within lesions might be expected to be a sensitive and specific marker for MS. A recent study examined the specificity of finding a central vein within white matter lesions for identifying MS patients.[48] Fifteen patients with MS and 15 patients with microangiopathic white matter lesions (mWML) were enrolled and underwent a 3-tesla MRI. No significant difference was noted in the presence of a white matter lesion between MS patients and patients with mWMLs, except for supratentorial peripheral lesions, in which the central vein was more commonly found in the mWML patients. Thus, the presence of a central vein within lesions is not a specific finding in MS.

5. Prior evidence suggests that pathologic iron accumulation in MS is due to the attraction of iron-rich macrophages to the inflammatory milieu.[17,18] If iron accumulation is secondary to inflammation rather than the cause of it, then it is unclear how CCSVI would trigger the inflammatory reaction seen in MS.

6. The methodology of Zamboni *et al.*'s treatment trial raises several issues. Neither the angiographer, examining neurologist, nor the study participants were blinded to treatment status, which may have biased all study outcomes, especially the patient self-reported quality of life. Also, the authors do not describe the definition of a clinical relapse used in the trial, specifically whether they were documented by a neurologist or based solely on patient report. The study participants appear to have had relatively active disease prior to entry, with 73% having a relapse in the prior year and 50% demonstrating gadolinium enhancement on MRI. This population's relapse rate would be subject to regression to the mean over the course of the year-long study. Finally, and perhaps most importantly, the trial lacked a control group or restriction on what other therapies patients were allowed to take. Thus, any observed benefits cannot be conclusively attributed to the endovascular procedure.

7. No data have been published regarding validation of Zamboni *et al.*'s ultrasound technique for detecting CCSVI. Inter- and intra-rater variability is unknown, and it is unclear if the ultrasound assessments yield consistent results in the same patient at different time points. Given that the results of ultrasound studies are highly dependent on the performing technician, validation of Zamboni *et al.*'s techniques should be undertaken.

Studies funded by North American MS societies

In late 2009, the National MS Society in the United States and the MS Society of Canada announced a request for grant applications to study the role of CCSVI in MS. These organizations committed more than $2.4 million, which was awarded to fund seven research projects in July 2010.[49] A group from the University of Wisconsin School of Medicine and Public Health will be studying CCSVI using quantitative time-resolved 3D MRV.[50]

This technique will allow detailed imaging of the cerebrospinal venous system and will also permit measurements of venous blood flow rates. Researchers at the Cleveland Clinic Foundation will be using Dr. Zamboni's ultrasound protocols to assess CCSVI in a group of MS patients that have been longitudinally followed for 10 years.[51] Thus, data regarding the cerebrospinal venous system in these patients can be correlated with the long-term evolution of their disease. Patients also will be assessed using MRV. Finally, with the help of an MS brain donation program, veins from autopsy will be harvested and studied, permitting an examination of CCSVI at a pathological level. A group from the Hospital for Sick Children in Toronto, Ontario will be using MRI and other non-invasive methods to assess for CCSVI in patients with pediatric MS and healthy controls.[52] Their hope is to identify early changes that may lead to CCSVI, allowing for better characterization of the disease process. Other institutions that received funding include the University of Texas Health Science Center at Houston, Ottawa Hospital, the University of British Columbia Hospital, the University of Saskatchewan, and the Foothills Medical Centre in Calgary, Alberta.

The "liberation" procedure

CCSVI has received considerable attention from the mainstream media and the lay public.[53,54] This has led to increasing pressure on physicians by patients seeking venous imaging and endovascular angioplasty, commonly referred to as the "liberation" procedure. This may lead physicians to engage in high-risk procedures that may have unforeseen consequences. For example, an interventional radiologist from Stanford Medical Center, Dr. Michael Dake, ran a program in which he placed stents in the IJVs of MS patients.[34] Two of these patients had serious complications: one died from a brain hemorrhage while being anti-coagulated after the procedure, and the other required open-heart surgery because the stent migrated to the patient's right ventricle. Endovascular treatment of MS at Stanford Medical Center has since been terminated.

The history of MS is rife with examples of uncontrolled case series of various treatments with positive results that were not confirmed by subsequent randomized trials.[55] Any treatment claims for CCSVI interventions will need to be supported by randomized trials, preferably with sham procedures or other mechanisms to reduce bias from patients, clinicians, and technicians. As an example, Albany Medical Center is currently recruiting 130 patients with MS and venous stenosis detected by ultrasound.[56] These patients will enter a double-blind, randomized study in which half of the participants will undergo venous angioplasty and the other half will serve as controls.

A major concern is the proliferation of interventions for CCSVI before such trials have been completed. The debilitating nature of MS makes the patient population highly susceptible to claims of therapeutic efficacy. Patients are often willing to undergo invasive procedures without the benefit of high-level evidence supporting their use.

Conclusions

If confirmed, the CCSVI hypothesis would represent a paradigm shift in our understanding of MS pathology. New therapeutic strategies aimed at reducing venous pressures and venous reflux could be developed and might be more effective than the immunomodulatory and immunosuppressive therapies currently being used. However, several other groups have failed to reproduce the findings of Zamboni and Zivadinov. Also, as discussed above, there are a number of challenges to the CCSVI hypothesis. If CCSVI is, in fact, associated with MS, it is not clear if it is causative or, rather, a result of MS inflammation or of the therapies used to treat MS. It is, therefore, imperative to confirm and further characterize the association of CCSVI and MS before proceeding with interventional studies and, more importantly, venous procedures in clinical practice. It is anticipated that rigorous studies such as those funded by the North American MS societies and from other investigators will clarify whether CCSVI plays a pathogenic role in MS.

References

1. McFarland HF, Martin R. Multiple sclerosis: a complicated picture of autoimmunity. *Nat Immunol* 2007; 8: 913–19.

2. Ramagopalan SV, Dobson R, Meier UC, Giovannoni G. Multiple sclerosis: risk factors, prodromes, and potential causal pathways. *Lancet Neurol* 2010; 9: 727–39.

3. Ascherio A, Munger KL. Environmental risk factors for multiple sclerosis. Part II: Noninfectious factors. *Ann Neurol* 2007; 61: 504–13.

4. Ascherio A, Munger KL. Environmental risk factors for multiple sclerosis. Part I: the role of infection. *Ann Neurol* 2007; 61: 288–99.

5. Robertson NP, Fraser M, Deans J, *et al.* Age-adjusted recurrence risks for relatives of patients with multiple sclerosis. *Brain* 1996; 119 (Pt 2): 449–55.

6. Rindfleisch E. Histologisches Detail zur grauen Degeneration von Gehirn und Ruckenmark. *Arch Pathol Anat Physiol Klin Med (Virchow)* 1863; 26: 474–483.

7. Dawson JW. The histology of disseminated sclerosis. *Trans R Soc Edin* 1916; 1: 517–40.

8. Fog T. The topography of plaques in multiple sclerosis with special reference to cerebral plaques. *Acta Neurol Scand Suppl* 1965; 15: 1–161.

9. Ge Y, Zohrabian VM, Grossman RI. Seven-Tesla magnetic resonance imaging: new vision of microvascular abnormalities in multiple sclerosis. *Arch Neurol* 2008; 65: 812–16.

10. Charcot JM. Histologie de la sclerose en plaques. *Gazette Hospital* 1868; 41: 554–6.

11. Williamson W. Review of the etiology and pathology of multiple sclerosis. *M Chron* 1903; 4: 261.

12. Putnam T. The pathogenesis of multiple sclerosis: a possible vascular factor. *N Engl J Med* 1933; 209: 786–90.

13. Putnam T. "Encephalitis" and sclerotic plaques produced by venular obstruction. *Arch Neurol Psychiatry* 1935; 33: 929–40.

14. Putnam T. Evidences of vascular occlusion in multiple sclerosis and "encephalomyelitis". *Arch Neurol Psychiatry* 1937; 37: 1298–321.

15. Macchi G. The pathology of the blood vessels in multiple sclerosis. *J Neuropathol Exp Neurol* 1954; 13: 378–84.

16. Schelling F. Damaging venous reflux into the skull or spine: relevance to multiple sclerosis. *Med Hypotheses* 1986; 21: 141–8.

17. LeVine SM. Iron deposits in multiple sclerosis and Alzheimer's disease brains. *Brain Res* 1997; 760: 298–303.

18. Craelius W, Migdal MW, Luessenhop CP et al. Iron deposits surrounding multiple sclerosis plaques. *Arch Pathol Lab Med* 1982; 106: 397–9.

19. Hammond KE, Metcalf M, Carvajal L et al. Quantitative in vivo magnetic resonance imaging of multiple sclerosis at 7 Tesla with sensitivity to iron. *Ann Neurol* 2008; 64: 707–13.

20. Zamboni P. The big idea: iron-dependent inflammation in venous disease and proposed parallels in multiple sclerosis. *J R Soc Med* 2006; 99: 589–93.

21. Singh AV, Zamboni P. Anomalous venous blood flow and iron deposition in multiple sclerosis. *J Cereb Blood Flow Metab* 2009; 29: 1867–78.

22. Parent A. *Carpenter's Human Neuroanatomy*, Ninth Edition. Media, Pennsylvania: Williams & Wilkins, 1996.

23. Burt AM. *Textbook of Neuroanatomy*. Philadelphia: WB Saunders Company, 1993.

24. Doepp F, Schreiber SJ, von Munster T, et al. How does the blood leave the brain? A systematic ultrasound analysis of cerebral venous drainage patterns. *Neuroradiology* 2004; 46:565–70.

25. Corbin JL. *Anatomie et Pathologie Arterielles de la Moelle*. Paris: Masson,1961.

26. Jellinger K. *Zur Orthologie und Pathologie der Ruckenmarksdurchblutung*. Berlin: Springer, 1966.

27. Umeoka S, Koyama T, Togashi K, et al. Vascular dilatation in the pelvis:

identification with CT and MR imaging. *Radiographics* 2004; 24: 193–208.

28. Zamboni P, Menegatti E, Galeotti R, et al. The value of cerebral Doppler venous haemodynamics in the assessment of multiple sclerosis. *J Neurol Sci* 2009; 282: 21–7.

29. Polman CH, Reingold SC, Edan G, et al. Diagnostic criteria for multiple sclerosis: 2005 revisions to the "McDonald Criteria". *Ann Neurol* 2005; 58: 840–6.

30. Zamboni P, Galeotti R, Menegatti E, et al. Chronic cerebrospinal venous insufficiency in patients with multiple sclerosis. *J Neurol Neurosurg Psychiatry* 2009; 80: 392–9.

31. Polman CH, Rudick RA. The multiple sclerosis functional composite: a clinically meaningful measure of disability. *Neurology* 2010; 74 Suppl 3: S8–15.

32. Vickrey BG, Hays RD, Harooni R, et al. A health-related quality of life measure for multiple sclerosis. *Qual Life Res* 1995; 4: 187–206.

33. Zivadinov R, Marr K, Ramanathan M, et al. *Combined Transcranial and Extracranial Venous Doppler Evaluation (CTEVD Study). Description of the Design and Interim Results of an Epidemiological Study of the Prevalence of Chronic Cerebrospinal Venous Insufficiency in MS and Related Diseases*. In 62nd AAN Annual Meeting, Edition Toronto, Ontario, Canada: 2010.

34. Qiu J. Venous abnormalities and multiple sclerosis: another breakthrough claim? *Lancet Neurol* 2010; 9: 464–5.

35. Doepp F, Paul F, Valdueza JM, et al. No cerebrocervical venous congestion in patients with multiple sclerosis. *Ann Neurol* 2010; 68: 173–83.

36. Sundstrom P, Wahlin A, Ambarki K, et al. Venous and cerebrospinal fluid flow in multiple sclerosis: a case-control study. *Ann Neurol* 2010; 68: 255–9.

37. Khan O, Filippi M, Freedman MS, et al. Chronic cerebrospinal venous insufficiency and multiple sclerosis. *Ann Neurol* 2010; 67: 286–90.

38. Koch-Henriksen N. The Danish Multiple Sclerosis Registry: a 50-year follow-up. *Mult Scler* 1999; 5: 293–6.

39. Agostoni E, Aliprandi A, Longoni M. Cerebral venous thrombosis. *Expert Rev Neurother* 2009; 9: 553–564.

40. Singh S, Kumar S, Joseph M, et al. Cerebral venous sinus thrombosis presenting as subdural haematoma. *Australas Radiol* 2005; 49: 101–103.

41. Shad A, Rourke TJ, Hamidian Jahromi A, Green AL. Straight sinus stenosis as a proposed cause of perimesencephalic non-aneurysmal haemorrhage. *J Clin Neurosci* 2008; 15: 839–41.

42. Friedman DI. Cerebral venous pressure, intra-abdominal pressure, and dural venous sinus stenting in idiopathic intracranial hypertension. *J Neuroophthalmol* 2006; 26: 61–4.

43. Johnston I, Paterson A. Benign intracranial hypertension. I. Diagnosis and prognosis. *Brain* 1974; 97: 289–300.

44. Johnston I, Paterson A. Benign intracranial hypertension. II. CSF pressure and circulation. *Brain* 1974; 97: 301–12.

45. Crile G. Excision of cancer of head and neck. *J Am Med Assoc* 1906; 47: 1780–6.

46. Lasjuanias P, *A B. Surgical neuroangiography. Part 3. Functional Vascular Anatomy of Brain, Spinal Cord and Spine*. Berlin, Germany: Springer-Verlag, 1990.

47. Van Der Kuip M, Hoogland PV, Groen RJ. Human radicular veins: regulation of venous reflux in the absence of valves. *Anat Rec* 1999; 254: 173–80.

48. Lummel N, Boeckh-Behrens T, Schoepf V, et al. Presence of a central vein within white matter lesions on susceptibility weighted imaging: a specific finding for multiple sclerosis? *Neuroradiology* 2010.

49. National Multiple Sclerosis Society. News Detail. http://www.nationalmssociety.org/news/news-detail/index.aspx?nid=3339. (Accessed August 5, 2010.).

50. National Multiple Sclerosis Society. CCSVI Study by Field Team. http://www.nationalmssociety.org/research/intriguing-leads-on-the-horizon/ccsvi/ccsvi-study-by-field-team/index.aspx. (Accessed August 5, 2010).

51. National Multiple Sclerosis Society. CCSVI Study by Fox Team. http://www.nationalmssociety.org/research/intriguing-leadsyes-on-the-horizon/ccsvi/ccsvi-study-by-fox-

team/index.aspx. (Accessed August 5, 2010).

52. National Multiple Sclerosis Society. CCSVI Study by Banwell Team. http://www.nationalmssociety.org/ research/intriguing-leads-on-the-horizon/ccsvi/ccsvi-study-by-banwell-team/index.aspx. (Accessed August 5, 2010).

53. MSNBC. New approach may mean big change in MS care. http://www. msnbc.msn.com/id/35991767/ns/ health-more_health_news/. (Accessed August 17, 2010)

54. facebook. CCSVI in Multiple Sclerosis. http://www.facebook.com/posted. php?id=110796282297&share_id= 124141330934102&comments=1#! /pages/CCSVI-in-Multiple-Sclerosis/ 110796282297?v=wall. (Accessed August 17, 2010)

55. Sibley W. *Therapeutic Claims in Multiple Sclerosis, A Guide to Treatment*, Fourth Edition. New York: Demos Vermande, 1996.

56. Albany Medical Center. Albany Med to study alternative treatment for multiple sclerosis. http://www.amc.edu/PR/ PressRelease/09_28_10_S.html. (Accessed October 4, 2010).

Chapter

51

Disease-modifying therapy for multiple sclerosis in clinical practice

Jeffrey A. Cohen and Andrew D. Goodman

Introduction

There are eight medications with regulatory approval as disease-modifying therapy (DMT) for relapsing–remitting multiple sclerosis (RRMS): interferon beta-1b (IFNβ-1b, Betaseron, Extavia), interferon beta-1a by intramuscular injection (IFNβ-1a (IM), Avonex), IFNβ-1a by subcutaneous injection (IFNβ-1a (SC), Rebif), glatiramer acetate (GA, Copaxone), mitoxantrone (Novantrone), natalizumab (Tysabri), and fingolimod (Gilenya) (Table 51.1). In addition, there are a large number of other agents that are used off-label alone or in combination to treat MS.

Neurologists managing patients with MS face the challenge of determining when to initiate therapy, deciding which agent to recommend, assessing if therapy is effective, and developing alternative therapeutic strategies when there is continued disease activity despite treatment. These decisions should be based on published and replicated data from rigorous randomized controlled clinical trials (RCTs). However, clinicians frequently are faced with individual patients who would not have been eligible for the published trials or situations for which definitive data do not exist. Ideally in such circumstances, the patient should be enrolled in a clinical trial with the hope that knowledge in the field could be advanced. Realistically, it is not feasible to enroll all such patients in clinical trials – the patient may not qualify for any trials in which the site is participating, there may be no participating sites within a reasonable distance, the time constraints may not be acceptable to the patient, etc. Rather than refusing to offer any unproven therapy, which may be unacceptable both to the patient and the clinician, a reasonable course of action must be chosen by extrapolation from the available data, the patient's disease status and activity, clinical judgment, and shared goals and expectations. Both parties need to remain cognizant that the therapeutic approach being undertaken is not guided by definitive data. Finally, the clinician must try to recognize his/her potential biases and conflicts of interest that can affect therapeutic recommendations.

This chapter outlines a practical approach to utilization of DMTs for MS in clinical practice. When the recommendations are not supported by definitive data but represent the opinions of the authors, the rationale will be provided. See the other chapters in this volume for more comprehensive reviews of the agents used to treat MS.

Goals of disease therapy and the rationale for early treatment

MS is a chronic disease with clinical manifestations that evolve over decades in most patients. In natural history studies prior to the introduction of the current DMTs, approximately 50% of patients with RRMS evolved into a secondary progressive course (SPMS) within 10 years from onset, and approximately 50% required an ambulation aid after 15 years.[1] About 10% of patients have more fulminant disease with rapid deterioration. Another 10%–20% has benign disease with mild intermittent symptoms and minimal disability decades after onset. Also, there may be recent "drift" in MS toward a more benign prognosis due to increased awareness of the disease, recognition of the benefits of early diagnosis and initiation of treatment, and widespread utilization of MRI leading to diagnosis of milder disease.[2,3] Nevertheless, the majority of patients with MS ultimately become disabled.

The principal short-term aims of DMT in RRMS are to reduce MRI activity, the frequency and severity of relapses, and accrual of residual deficits from relapses. There are robust data from RCTs supporting benefits of the currently approved DMT on these endpoints. The long-term goal is to delay or prevent evolution to SPMS and development of permanent disability. It is a reasonable assumption that the short-term actions of DMT will translate into long-term clinically meaningful benefits. The demonstrated benefit of current DMT on MRI markers of tissue injury, such as whole brain atrophy[4] and evolution of lesions into T1-hypointense "black holes",[5] supports this assumption. However, it must be recognized that this assumption is, as yet, unproven.

There now is consensus that DMT should commence early in patients with RRMS.[6,7] The rationale is summarized in Table 51.2. This recommendation is supported by the observation that patients treated with placebo in the Phase 3 RCTs and subsequently switched to active treatment in open-label extension studies continued to do less well compared with patients on

Multiple Sclerosis Therapeutics, Fourth Edition, ed. Jeffrey A. Cohen and Richard A. Rudick. Published by Cambridge University Press.
© Cambridge University Press 2011.

Table 51.1. *Currently approved disease-modifying therapies for multiple sclerosis*

Agent	Dose [a]	Approved indications [a]	Laboratory monitoring [b]	Pregnancy Category [a]
Interferon beta-1b (Betaseron/Betaferon, Extavia)	8 million IU s.c. every other day	FDA: relapsing forms of MS, CIS EMA: RRMS, SP with active disease, CIS	CBC, AST, ALT prior to therapy, at months 1, 3, 6, then every 6–12 months. Pregnancy test prior to therapy and for suspected pregnancy. NAbs after 1–2 years of therapy, particularly with ongoing activity.	C
Interferon beta-1a (Avonex)	30 mcg IM weekly	FDA: relapsing forms of MS, CIS EMA: relapsing forms of MS, CIS	CBC, AST, ALT prior to therapy, at months 1, 3, 6, then every 6–12 months. Pregnancy test prior to therapy and for suspected pregnancy. NAbs after 1–2 years of therapy, particularly with ongoing activity.	C
Interferon beta-1a (Rebif)	22 or 44 mcg s.c. 3 times per week	FDA: relapsing forms of MS EMA: MS and ≥2 relapses in prior 2 years	CBC, AST, ALT prior to therapy, at months 1, 3, 6, then every 6–12 months. Pregnancy test prior to therapy and for suspected pregnancy. NAbs after 1–2 years of therapy, particularly with ongoing activity.	C
Glatiramer acetate (Copaxone)	20 mg s.c. daily	FDA: RRMS, CIS EMA: RRMS, CIS	Pregnancy test prior to therapy and for suspected pregnancy. No monitoring required on therapy.	B
Mitoxantrone (Novantrone)	12 mg/m^2 i.v. every 3 months (Maximum: 140 mg/m^2)	FDA: SPMS and worsening RRMS EMA: varies from country to country but, in general, active RRMS or SPMS	CBC and LVEF prior to every dose. Pregnancy test prior to therapy and for suspected pregnancy.	D
Natalizumab (Tysabri)	300 mg i.v. monthly	FDA: relapsing forms of MS EMA: highly active RRMS despite treatment with IFNβ or rapidly evolving severe RRMS	AST, ALT prior to initiation, at month 3 and 6 after initiation of therapy, then every 6 months JCV serology prior to initiation Pregnancy test prior to therapy and for suspected pregnancy. NAbs after 6 months of therapy. MRI prior to therapy then every 6 months.	C
Fingolimod (Gilenya)	0.5 mg PO daily	FDA: relapsing forms of MS EMA: highly active RRMS despite treatment with IFNβ or rapidly evolving severe RRMS	CBC, AST, ALT pretreatment, and AST and AST every 6 months on treatment Pregnancy test prior to therapy and for suspected pregnancy. VZV titer in the absence of a history of chicken pox or shingles. EKG prior to treatment. Eye exam ± OCT pretreatment and after 3–4 months on treatment.	C

[a] product label. [b] author opinion.

ALT = alanine transaminase, AST = aspartate transaminase, CBC = complete blood count, CIS = clinically isolated syndrome, EKG = electrocardiogram, EMA = European Medicines Agency, FDA = United States Food and Drug Administration, IFNβ = interferon beta, IM = intramuscular, i.v. = intravenous, JCV = JC virus, LVEF = left ventricular ejection fraction, NAb = neutralizing antibodies, OCT = optical coherence tomography, RRMS = relapsing–remitting multiple sclerosis, s.c. = subcutaneous, SPMS = secondary progressive multiple sclerosis, VZV = varicella zoster virus.

Table 51.2. *The rationale for early disease therapy in relapsing forms of multiple sclerosis*

- Most cases of RRMS ultimately evolve into a SP course with some degree of permanent disability. Although benign MS exists, it is uncommon.
- The ability to predict prognosis in individual patients is limited, particularly to predict mild disease.
- The ongoing inflammatory process and resultant irreversible tissue destruction is difficult to monitor in early RRMS. Clinical features correlate poorly; much of the ongoing inflammation and tissue damage is "subclinical" at this stage. There are technical challenges in utilizing standard MRI to monitor disease progression in individual patients. Substantial evidence suggests pathology in white matter and gray matter that appears normal on standard MR imaging. Therefore, it remains difficult to be reassured that irreversible tissue damage is not accumulating.
- DMTs are available that effectively reduce disease activity and disability progression in RRMS, albeit incompletely. Extensive experience confirms that, despite troublesome side effects, these agents are safe in general.
- The available therapies are preventative and not restorative.
- Several lines of evidence demonstrate that axonal damage and atrophy accumulate from the earliest stages of the disease.
- Accumulating irreversible pathology, decreasing inflammation, and evolution of MS into a "degenerative" process limit the effectiveness of disease-modifying therapies late in the disease.
- Several studies suggest increased effectiveness of the available therapies when started early in the disease.

DMT = disease-modifying therapy, MS = multiple sclerosis, RR = relapsing–remitting, SP = secondary progressive

active treatment from the beginning of the core trial.[8,9] In general, DMT with one of the approved agents should be considered in all patients with active RRMS once the diagnosis of MS is confirmed and in selected patients with a clinically isolated demyelinating syndrome (CIS). DMT is not indicated in all patients, but the issue should be addressed.

Approved disease therapies for multiple sclerosis

The RCTs that led to approval of DMTs for MS are reviewed in detail in other chapters of this book. A brief summary of mechanisms of action, data supporting efficacy, and the adverse effects (AEs) associated with their use is presented below.

Interferon beta (see Chapter 25)

IFNβ modulates T-cell and B-cell function, decreases expression of matrix metalloproteinases reversing blood–brain barrier disruption, and alters expression of cytokines.[10] A series of double-blind, placebo-controlled Phase 3 trials in RRMS supported the benefit of IFNβ in reducing relapses (by approximately 30%), disability progression, and MRI lesion activity and accrual.[9,11–18] Slowing of whole-brain volume loss has been reported for IFNβ-1a (IM)[4,19] and for IFNβ-1a (SC) in the Early Treatment Of Multiple Sclerosis (ETOMS) study,[20] which tested 22 mcg once weekly.

Adverse effects

Although side effects are common, IFNβ generally is well tolerated. Post-injection "flu-like" symptoms (fever, chills, myalgia, fatigue, and headache) occur in ~75% of patients, probably from transient up-regulation of pro-inflammatory cytokines.[21] This reaction typically begins within six hours of injection, can last up to 24–48 hours, and usually abates within the first three months of therapy. Co-administration of acetaminophen or ibuprofen, and injection at bedtime usually adequately controls these symptoms. In some patients, initiating IFNβ at one-quarter to one-half dose and gradually up-titrating is useful.[22] Low-dose prednisone (10 mg/day) or pentoxifylline (800 mg twice per day) may be helpful for persistent, severe constitutional symptoms.[23,24]

Injection-site reactions are common with IFNβ administered by s.c. injection and typically include pain and erythema, and rarely bruising.[22] In most cases, modification of injection technique and rotation of injection sites is sufficient. Cutaneous and subcutaneous infection, and skin necrosis occur rarely and warrant antibiotics, surgical consultation, and withdrawal of IFNβ.[21,22] Cutaneous reactions are rare with IFNβ-1a (IM), although the IM injection can be more difficult or painful for some patients.

The IFNβ-1b RRMS pivotal trial[11,13] suggested increased risk of depression and suicide in IFNβ-1b-treated patients. None of the other IFNβ studies in RRMS or SPMS supported this observation.[9,14,17] Because depression is common in MS, an association with IFNβ therapy remains uncertain. Most patients who develop depression while on IFNβ can be managed with antidepressant medication or counseling. IFNβ should be discontinued in rare instances of severe or treatment-resistant depression.

The most common laboratory abnormalities with IFNβ are mild, reversible leukopenia and elevated liver enzymes.[21,22,25,28,29] In a six-year retrospective study,[28] liver function returned to normal in 74% of patients who were maintained on IFNβ therapy despite developing grade 1 or grade 2 transaminase elevation. Fulminant liver failure requiring liver transplantation has been reported in a patient treated with IFNβ-1a (SC).[30] A complete blood count and liver profile should be obtained prior to initiating IFNβ therapy, monitored regularly during the first 6 months of treatment (e.g. Months 1, 3, and 6), and checked periodically thereafter (at least yearly) in the absence of symptoms.[22]

IFNβ therapy may exacerbate pre-existing spasticity[31] and headache syndromes.[32] A variety of rare AEs have been reported with IFNβ treatment of MS, including thyroid disease,[33] psoriasis,[22] alopecia,[21] pancreatitis,[34] unmaking of autoimmune hepatitis,[35] Raynaud's phenomenon,[36] urticaria,[37] thrombocytopenic purpura-like syndrome,[38] nephrotic syndrome,[39] a capillary leak syndrome,[40] fulminant acute central nervous system (CNS) demyelinating syndrome,[41] polyneuropathy,[42] and retinopathy.[43]

Neutralizing antibodies to interferon beta

As discussed in Chapter 24, there is compelling evidence that persistent high-titer anti-IFNβ neutralizing antibodies (NAbs) abrogate the biologic actions of IFNβ and its benefit on MRI lesion activity and relapses. It seems intuitive that NAbs would also abrogate the benefit of IFNβ on disability progression; the data are consistent with this but less definitive. We agree with the published guidelines from a task force of the European Federation of Neurological Societies (EFNS) on anti-IFNβ NAbs:[44]

- The frequency of NAbs differs among IFNβ preparations. After 6–18 months of therapy, the incidence is approximately 5% with IFNβ-1a (IM), 25% with IFNβ-1a (SC), and 35% with IFNβ-1b.
- NAbs elicited by one IFNβ preparation cross-react with other IFNβs.
- NAb testing should be routinely performed 12 and 24 months after starting IFNβ, particularly if there is evidence of ongoing disease activity. Since NAbs occasionally resolve, measurement should be repeated 3–6 months later in NAb-positive patients. Since seroconversion is rare after 24 months, routine testing in previously seronegative patients after that time point generally is not necessary.
- IFNβ therapy should be discontinued in patients with persistent high-titer NAbs regardless of apparent clinical stability.

Glatiramer acetate (see Chapter 26)

GA, formerly known as copolymer-1, is a complex mixture of random synthetic polypeptides originally developed as an immunologic mimic of myelin basic protein. Recent studies suggest GA functions as an altered peptide ligand for major histocompatibility complex class II molecules and, when presented to T-cells, inhibits activation and induces regulatory cells.[45] It also may stimulate neuroprotective or repair-promoting mechanisms.[45]

Benefit of GA 20 mg administered by daily s.c. injection was reported in a pilot study[46] and confirmed in the US multicenter, randomized, placebo-controlled Phase 3 trial,[47] which like the studies of IFNβ showed an approximately 30% reduction in relapses. Prospective follow-up of these patients for 15 years showed continued efficacy and good-tolerability in those patients remaining in the study.[48] Benefit of GA on MRI lesion activity was demonstrated in a separate large-scale study.[49] MRI effects of GA appeared to be less prominent and more gradual than in studies of IFNβ. GA reduced the proportion of gadolinium (Gd)-enhancing lesions that evolved in persistent T1-hypointense lesions,[5] which are thought to represent regions of severe tissue damage.[50]

There has been minimal dose-exploration with GA. A Phase 2 study suggested an efficacy advantage of 40 mg daily over the approved 20 mg dose,[51] but a subsequent Phase 3 study demonstrated no significant differences on annualized relapse rate or MRI lesion activity.[52] Conversely, a pilot study suggested that in patients stable after one year of therapy with GA 20 mg s.c. daily, those who then switched to 20 mg two days per week had similar relapse rate, Expanded Disability Status Scale (EDSS) stability, and MRI lesion activity in the subsequent year as those maintained on daily GA.[53] Reduced dose frequency would be expected to improve tolerability and reduce development of lipoatrophy. A one-year Phase 3 study comparing GA 40 mg administered s.c. three times per week vs. placebo in RRMS is in progress.[54]

Adverse effects

In general, GA is well tolerated. Its most common side effects are injection site erythema, induration, pruritis, or tenderness.[47] Lipoatrophy, loss of cutaneous fat with scarring, is a common problem with prolonged treatment.[55] The significance is primarily cosmetic, but the skin changes usually are irreversible. Panniculitis, a more extensive subcutaneous inflammatory reaction, has been reported.[56] Lymphadenopathy and allergic reactions with rash or urticarial are rarely seen.[47]

The GA-associated immediate post-injection systemic reaction is characterized by variable combinations of flushing, diaphoresis, chest tightness, dyspnea, palpitations, and anxiety, beginning minutes after injection and resolving spontaneously in 30 minutes or less.[47] This systemic reaction is sporadic and unpredictable. It was reported at least once in 15% of patients in the pivotal trials. Typically, it occurs once in a given patient, but occasionally repeatedly. The etiology remains uncertain. It does not appear to be a hypersensitivity reaction, and there have been no reports of cardiopulmonary compromise, bronchospasm, or hypersensitivity reaction. Nevertheless, patients should be advised of this potential reaction prior to commencing treatment with GA.

In contrast to IFNβ, GA is not associated with constitutional side effects, depression, or accentuation of spasticity. It does not appear to worsen pre-existing headaches.[32,57] GA-reactive antibodies are frequently generated during GA therapy, but do not appear to affect efficacy.[58] GA is not associated with abnormalities of blood counts or liver studies. Thus, laboratory monitoring is not required.

Natalizumab (see Chapter 27)

Natalizumab is a humanized monoclonal antibody that binds α_4-integrin, blocks interaction of $\alpha_4\beta_1$ integrin on leukocytes with vascular cell adhesion molecule and fibronectin CS1 sites on vascular endothelial cells, and inhibits migration of leukocytes from the circulation into the CNS.[59] Favorable results of a Phase 2 trial[60] prompted two Phase 3 RCTs of natalizumab in RRMS. In the Natalizumab Safety and Efficacy in Relapsing–Remitting Multiple Sclerosis (AFFIRM) study,[61] natalizumab 300 mg administered by intravenous (i.v.) infusion every four weeks reduced annualized relapse rate by 68% and the risk of EDSS progression by 42% compared to placebo over two years. In the Safety and Efficacy of Natalizumab in Combination with Interferon Beta-1a in Patients with Relapsing–Remitting Multiple Sclerosis (SENTINEL) study,[62] the combination of weekly IFNβ-1a (IM) plus natalizumab 300 mg administered by intravenous (i.v.) infusion every four weeks plus reduced relapses by 55% and the risk of EDSS progression by 24% compared with IFNβ-1a (i.m.) plus placebo over two years. Both studies showed prominent benefit on MRI lesion activity.

Adverse effects

Natalizumab typically has few side effects. In the pivotal trials, side effects associated with natalizumab included fatigue, anxiety, pharyngitis, sinus congestion, peripheral edema, and infusion-related symptoms such as headache, flushing, erythema, nausea, fatigue, and dizziness,[61,62] all of which typically were mild. Very rare hepatoxicity occurs, usually at the initiation of therapy.[63] A case of pericarditis due to natalizumab therapy, with recurrence twice on re-challenge, reported.[64]

In AFFIRM, acute Type I allergic reactions occurred in 9% of natalizumab-treated subjects vs. 4% in the placebo group.[61,65] Hypersensitivity reactions, including urticaria, pruritus, anaphylaxis, and anaphylactoid syndrome, occurred in 4% of natalizumab subjects. There was a low incidence (<1%) of severe anaphylactic or anaphylactoid reactions. Type III-like reactions resembling serum sickness sometimes delayed until 1–2 weeks after infusion also were reported.[66,67] Both types of allergic reactions often can be managed with premedication with antihistamines and/or corticosteroids.

In both AFFIRM and SENTINEL, 6% of patients receiving natalizumab developed persistent anti-natalizumab NAbs, the presence of which was highly correlated to development of immediate[61,62,68] and delayed[66,67] infusion reactions (see Chapter 24). In addition, these antibodies unequivocally abrogated the benefit of natalizumab on clinical and MRI measures.[61,62,68]

The principal safety concern with natalizumab is development of progressive multifocal leukoencephalopathy (PML). As of December 31, 2010, approximately 78 800 patients received natalizumab in the world-wide post-marketing experience, and as of February 2, 2011 there were 95 confirmed cases of PML (Medical Information Services, Biogen Idec, February 23 2011). The risk is negligible in the first year of treatment, and increases in years 2 and 3. The subsequent annual risk is less precisely known, but appears not to increase substantially.

PML results from reactivation of latent JC virus (JCV). Previous estimates of the population infection prevalence were widely disparate due to assays with varying sensitivity and specificity. Assessment of JCV DNA in blood or urine does not appear to be useful for predicting PML risk or detecting incipient cases.[69] A recently developed enzyme-linked immunosorbent (ELISA) assay appears to have improved accuracy.[70] The false negative rate was estimated to be 2.5%. In patients with

natalizumab-associated PML for whom pre-PML serum samples were available, this ELISA detected anti-JCV serum antibodies in 17 of 17 specimens, which was significantly different than the 53.6% seropositivity in the overall natalizumab-treated MS population ($P < 0.0001$). Thus, this test may be able to distinguish patients with the potential to develop PML during natalizumab treatment from those with virtually no risk. The other important factor is treatment history. Prior immunosuppressive therapy increases the risk substantially in patients with positive JCV serology, to approximately 1:200 overall and 1:100 after 24 months of therapy.[71,72] Natalizumab therapy should be undertaken with great caution in such patients.

Patients receiving natalizumab require close monitoring for PML. The Tysabri Outreach: Unified Commitment to Health (TOUCH) program, which provides formal guidelines in the USA, requires direct questioning of the patient at each infusion for symptoms suggestive of PML and reauthorization every 6 months. At the Mellen Center and University of Rochester, formal clinical reassessment and MRI are performed prior to treatment initiation and every six months thereafter. Patients with a good outcome from natalizumab-associated PML have been reported,[72,73] from a combination of early detection and prompt diagnosis, accelerated removal of natalizumab with plasma exchange allowing immune reconstitution,[74] and treatment with the serotonin reuptake inhibitor mirtazapine[75,76] and the anti-malarial mefloquine.[77] Most patients develop worsening neurologic manifestations, Gd-enhancement and edema in MRI lesions, and increased CSF viral load several months after discontinuation of natalizumab or within several weeks after its removal by plasma exchange. This so-called immune-reconstitution inflammatory syndrome (IRIS), which can be life-threatening,[71] should be anticipated and treated early with a prolonged course of high-dose corticosteroids.[78]

Temporary interruption of natalizumab (i.e. a drug holiday) has been considered as an approach to allow periodic immune reconstitution to lessen the risk of PML. The duration of treatment interruption necessary to permit reinstitution of central nervous system (CNS) surveillance is unknown. Presumably, it must be at least several months to allow sufficient clearance of the monoclonal antibody and desaturation of surface α_4-integren on lymphocytes. Whether surveillance can be reinstituted to the degree necessary to lessen PML risk without recrudescence of MS inflammatory activity remains uncertain. A number of studies have reported rapid return of MS disease activity, sometimes with apparent overshoot, after discontinuation of natalizumab.[79–84] This phenomenon would not be unexpected based on typical utilization of natalizumab in highly active patients. Some of the cases had features overlapping those of IRIS, suggesting the possibility of unmasking of incipient PML.[83,84] The ongoing Treatment Interruption of Natalizumab (RESTORE) study[85] assesses the feasibility of temporary discontinuation of natalizumab.

Other opportunistic infections and neoplasms associated with generalized systemic immunosuppression have been very rare during natalizumab therapy. Single cases of ocular toxoplasmosis[86] and severe cutaneous Candida infection[87] have been reported. Mullen et al. reported two cases of melanoma,[88] and Laroni et al. recently reported a third case.[89] A single case of primary CNS B-cell lymphoma occurred in a 40-year-old man after 21 doses of natalizumab.[90] As pointed out in the accompanying editorials,[91–94] although primary CNS B-cell lymphoma is a known complication of immunosuppression, this neoplasm was unusual in not being Epstein–Barr virus related. Thus, an association with natalizumab therapy could not be confirmed or eliminated with certainty. A second case with some similar features recently was reported.[95]

Mitoxantrone (see Chapter 28)

Mitoxantrone is an anthracenedione-based chemotherapeutic agent that intercalates into DNA causing cross-linking interfering with DNA repair and RNA synthesis leading to cell cycle arrest. The US Food and Drug Administration (FDA) approved mitoxantrone in 2000 for SPMS and worsening RRMS, the only DMT specifically approved for use in SPMS by the FDA.

Several preliminary trials[96–98] and the Mitoxantrone in Multiple Sclerosis (MIMS) Phase 3 trial[99] demonstrated significant reduction of relapse rate (approximately 65%) and slowing of disability progression in patients with active RR and SPMS. Surprisingly, benefit on MRI in MIMS was not as prominent.[100] The approved dosage schedule of mitoxantrone is 12 mg/m^2 given by i.v. infusion every three months up to a maximum dose of 140 mg/m^2. An induction regimen of monthly infusions for 3–6 months sometimes is helpful for very active disease.[101,102]

Adverse effects

In general, mitoxantrone is well tolerated.[103] Common AEs include blue discoloration of sclera and urine, alopecia, nausea, and bone marrow suppression. Compared with other chemotherapeutic agents, nausea, alopecia, and bone marrow suppression typically are mild. In a large prospective case series, transient amenorrhea occurred in approximately 27% of women treated with mitoxantrone, and persistent amenorrhea in 17%.[104] The incidence of permanent amenorrhea was strongly related to age: 5% in women <35 years old and 31% in woman ≥35 years old.

The principal dose-limiting toxicity of mitoxantrone is vacuolar cardiomyopathy,[105,106] for which the risk is proportional to the lifetime total dose exposure. Thus, the cumulative dose limit is 140 mg/m^2. However, there have been several reports of decreased cardiac function with cumulative doses of mitoxantrone less than 100 mg/m^2, and several cases after only a few doses.[106–108] The overall rate of symptomatic congestive failure in large series was 0.1%–2%.[104,109] Current guidelines call for evaluation of left ventricular ejection fraction by radionuclide ventriculography or echocardiography prior to initiation of therapy and each subsequent dose.[110] It is recommended that mitoxantrone not be given to any patient with a left ventricular ejection fraction <50% or with a 10% decrease.

The other concern is multiple reports of treatment-related acute myelocytic or promyelocytic leukemia.[111–115] In two large prospective series, the estimated incidence was 0.25%–0.4%.[104,109] The cytogenetic features of treatment-related acute myeloid leukemia are distinct from those of spontaneous neoplasms.[116] In general, the response to treatment has been favorable as compared with leukemia arising de novo.[103]

Fingolimod (see Chapter 30)

Fingolimod (also known as FTY720), a sphingosine 1-phosphate receptor modulator, blocks lymphocyte egress from lymph nodes and recirculation to the CNS, and may also have direct CNS effects.[117] The FDA approved Fingolimod in September 2011 as the first oral disease therapy for RRMS. Fingolimod's efficacy in RRMS is supported by a six-month, placebo-controlled Phase 2 study;[118] a two-year, placebo-controlled Phase 3 study (FTY720 Research Evaluating Effects of Daily oral therapy in Multiple Sclerosis [FREEDOMS]);[119] a one-year Phase 3 study (Trial Assessing Injectable Interferon versus FTY720 Oral in Relapsing-Remitting Multiple Sclerosis [TRANSFORMS])[120] with an active comparator – IFNβ-1a (IM); and a >4 year Phase 2 extension.[121] These studies all demonstrated benefit of fingolimod on relapses and MRI lesion activity. FREEDOMS showed slowing of disability progression, and both Phase 3 studies showed a reduction in brain volume loss.

Adverse effects

The overall MS safety experience at the time of FDA approval of fingolimod comprised ~2600 patients and approximately ~4600 patient–years of exposure.[122] The overall safety profile was better for 0.5 mg than 1.25 mg. Given that the efficacy advantages of the two fingolimod doses over placebo and IFNβ-1a (IM) were similar, 0.5 mg appeared to have a better benefit-to-risk profile and was the dose submitted for regulatory approval.

Specific AEs associated with fingolimod included headache, influenza, diarrhea, back pain, cough, dyspnea, lower respiratory tract infection, elevation of liver enzymes, transient bradycardia and slowed atrioventricular (AV) conduction on treatment initiation, increase in blood pressure, and macular edema.[118–120,122,123] Fingolimod was generally well tolerated, and these AEs typically were mild in severity and non-serious. FDA recommendations related to fingolimod use are summarized in Table 51.1.[123]

Because fingolimod is a potent immunomodulator, increased susceptibility to infection would not be unexpected. The proportions of patients with infection AEs, severe infections, and serious infections were similar in the treatment groups in FREEDOMS and an integrated analysis of all MS studies, aside from increased lower respiratory tract infections (mainly bronchitis) across treatment groups.[122] There was one case of fatal disseminated primary varicella zoster and one case of fatal herpes simplex encephalitis in TRANSFORMS.[120] Both

Table 51.3. Limitations of approved disease-modifying therapies for multiple sclerosis

- Expense (all).

- Parenteral administration (IFNβ, GA, natalizumab, mitoxantrone).

- Side effects (all).

- Rare but serious toxicity (natalizumab, mitoxantrone, fingolimod).

- Partial effectiveness.
  – Modest potency (IFNβ, GA)
  – Development of neutralizing antibodies (IFNβ, natalizumb).
  – Immunopathological or pharmacogenetic heterogeneity among patients leading to responders and nonresponders (all?).

- Incomplete understanding of mechanism of action (all).

- Modest long-term safety and efficacy data (fingolimod)

- Data demonstrating prevention of long-term significant disability are lacking (all).

GA = glatiramer acetate, IFNβ = interferon beta.

had complicating factors, but a role for fingolimod cannot be ruled out. There have been no other opportunistic infections, including PML, with fingolimod.

Like infection, because of fingolimod's immunomodulatory and cell growth effects, there is a potential for increased risk of malignancy. In TRANSFORMS there were three cases of melanoma in the fingolimod 0.5 mg group and none in the other arms.[120] In FREEDOMS[119] and the integrated safety analysis,[122] there was no association of melanoma or other malignancy with fingolimod.

Choosing a disease-modifying therapy in relapsing–remitting multiple sclerosis

All of the available agents have been reported to reduce relapse rate, MRI lesion activity, and accumulation of disability in RRMS, although the magnitudes of benefit and the robustness of the data vary. Also, all of the currently approved DMTs for RRMS have limitations, including potential tolerability and/or safety issues (Table 51.3). Comparing the results across trials to make inferences about relative efficacy is not appropriate. The experience with the European and North American trials of IFNβ-1b in SPMS illustrates this point. Despite testing an identical therapeutic agent using very similar entry criteria and trial designs, the two trials enrolled different study populations and yielded different results. Well-designed, head-to-head studies are necessary to make valid comparisons, but only a limited number have been published. Thus, there are no definitive guidelines available to the clinician selecting therapy for RRMS.

Some investigators in the field believe that the higher dose, more frequently administered IFNβs, IFNβ-1b and IFNβ-1a (SC), are more effective than the lower dose agent administered once weekly, IFNβ-1a (IM), based on the Independent Comparison of Interferons (INCOMIN)[126] and Evidence of Interferon Dose-Response: European North American Comparative Efficacy (EVIDENCE)[127] studies. The lack of any efficacy difference

for 30 and 60 mcg doses of IFNβ-1a (i.m.) administered weekly suggests that frequency of administration is a important factor than injected dose in this dose range.[128]

The potential efficacy advantage of IFNβ-1b and IFNβ-1a (SC) has several caveats, however. First, EVIDENCE and INCOMIN were only partially blinded, which potentially could have introduced bias into the efficacy assessment. This issue is particularly relevant to outcomes based on the first relapse such as proportion of relapse-free subjects, the primary outcome in both studies. Corroboration of the benefit on relapses by MRI addresses this concern somewhat. Second, the magnitude of the efficacy advantage was modest, and in EVIDENCE superior benefit was detected predominantly in the initial six months of the study. Third, IFNβ-1a (IM)[4,19] and IFNβ-1a (SC) when administered at a dose of 22 mcg weekly[20] slowed brain volume loss but IFNβ-1a (SC) and IFNβ-1b administered as multiple doses per week did not. Fourth, side effects and laboratory abnormalities also increase with IFNβ dose. Finally, IFNβ-1b and IFNβ-1a (SC) have a substantially greater tendency to elicit NAbs.

GA tends to have fewer side effects compared with IFNβ and routine laboratory monitoring is not required, though these advantages may be offset for some patients by more frequent injection. The efficacy of GA and IFNβ on clinical measures appears to be comparable based on the Betaferon Efficacy Yielding Outcomes of a New Dose (BEYOND),[129] Betaseron vs. Copaxone in Multiple Sclerosis with Triple-Dose Gadolinium and 3-Tesla MRI Endpoints (BECOME),[130] and Rebif vs. Glatiramer Acetate in Relapsing MS Disease (REGARD)[131] studies. IFNβ reduced MRI lesion activity more rapidly and potently, suggesting IFNβ may be preferable in RRMS patients with multiple Gd-enhancing MRI lesions, but this point is unproven.

IM injection is contra-indicated in patients on anti-coagulation. A medication administered by s.c. injection should be selected for such patients. In patients with a severe pre-existing headache syndrome, depression, or spasticity, or with substantial concern about the possibility of side effects, GA may be preferable. Otherwise, taking all the issues discussed above into account, for these authors, any of three IFNβ preparations or GA is a reasonable initial therapy in most patients with RRMS.

Long-term safety and benefit of IFNβ and GA are supported by formal follow-up studies of clinical trial participants,[48,132,133] and of patients treated in clinical practice.[134] There is much less long-term experience with natalizumab, mitoxantrone, and fingolimod.

Natalizumab has good tolerability and potent efficacy. However, because of the potential for rare but significant toxicity (PML), it typically is used as a second-line agent. With the recent availability of JCV serology, use of natalizumab as initial therapy in JCV(-) patients, who have minimal risk of PML, may be reasonable.

Mitoxantrone also has been utilized primarily as a second-line agent because the potential for amenorrhea, cardiotoxicity,

Table 51.4. *Strategies to improve compliance with disease modifying therapies in multiple sclerosis*

- Therapeutic partnership between the care team and patient to decide:
  - whether to initiate therapy.
  - which agent to start.

- Comprehensive education of the patient, family, or care-givers prior to initiation of treatment concerning:
  - realistic goals for therapy.
  - medication administration.
  - side effects.
  A combination of verbal face-to-face instruction and printed material is preferable. Peer support groups and pharmaceutical company support programs also are useful.

- Anticipation, close monitoring, and aggressive management of side effects. Reassurance to patients that although side effects occur, the goal is to avoid or minimize side effects when possible.

- Regular and facilitated communication between the patient, family, and caregiver and the care team to answer questions and address concerns.

or leukemia. It is expected that, in fact, its use will decline in the future.

Fingolimod was directly compared to IFNβ-1a (IM) in TRANSFORMS and showed superior efficacy in reducing relapses, MRI lesion activity, and slowing brain volume loss.[120] It was approved by the FDA as a first-line agent but by the European Medicines Agency (EMA) as a second-line agent. Although its efficacy and oral route of administration are attractive, overall experience with fingolimod still is limited, and several potential safety issues have been identified. Therefore, the authors still present IFNβ and GA as the preferred first-line treatment options. In addition, for patients currently receiving an approved MS treatment with effective disease control and good tolerability, it seems prudent not to switch therapy routinely to fingolimod as yet. For patients with an inadequate response to previously available agents and/or intolerable side effects, fingolimod is a reasonable alternative. If the accumulating experience with fingolimod in clinical practice is favorable, early use will increase.

Managing disease therapy in relapsing–remitting multiple sclerosis

Once therapy is initiated, consistent follow-up is critical to ensure compliance (Table 51.4), monitor for tolerability and safety, and assess for ongoing efficacy.

Monitoring for tolerability and safety

Patients need to be seen on a regular basis after starting treatment to address potential side effects. We typically schedule follow-up within several months of DMT initiation to answer questions and assess tolerability. After that, the routine safety monitoring protocol depends on the agent (summarized in Table 51.1).

Monitoring for efficacy

In general, it takes at least 6–12 months to judge the efficacy of a DMT. There are no validated efficacy monitoring protocols or criteria for changing DMT, although reasonable general guidelines have been published.[135,136] In practice, it is very difficult to distinguish whether lack of apparent disease activity represents a therapeutic response or the natural history of the disease in that patient. Conversely, the presence of clinical or MRI activity on therapy can represent a therapeutic failure or partial efficacy. At present, there are no biologic markers that allow one to distinguish treatment responders, partial-responders, and non-responders. Nevertheless, a general framework can be derived from several factors:

- The overall natural history of MS.
- Previous disease course and activity in an individual patient.
- Known magnitude and kinetics of an effect of the therapeutic agent. For example, IFNβ, natalizumab, and fingolimod rapidly and potently suppress Gd-enhancing lesion activity. Continued Gd-enhancement after starting these drugs probably indicates lack of benefit. Conversely, suppression of Gd-enhancing by GA is less prominent and may take 6–9 months to fully manifest. Therefore, one should not base a determination of lack of efficacy of GA on Gd-enhancing before that time.

Measures of disease activity

In general, disease activity is assessed through a combination of interval history, clinical assessments, and imaging. Patient self-report and reports of the family or care-giver include new symptoms or change in their severity, and overall level of function. Patients differ in how observant they are and their threshold for reporting change. This sensitivity will be affected by the degree to which they are challenged at work or recreation. For example, a patient who is athletically active may detect subtle change in leg function or endurance not apparent to a more sedentary patient. Also, a patient's reporting of change will be affected by mood and effectiveness of support systems.

Relapses are an important aspect of RRMS and early SPMS. The clinician must take into account relapse frequency, severity, and degree of recovery, and how well the patient tolerates steroid therapy. Relapses are important in and of themselves; there often is some accrual of impairment as a result of incomplete recovery.[137] Relapses also are important, even if mild and with apparently complete recovery, because they indicate ongoing disease activity. Lack of reduction of relapses from the pretreatment rate is noteworthy, recognizing that relapses are not regularly spaced in time. More than one relapse per year is worrisome in any patient, even if it represents a reduction compared to a previous rate.

Worsening impairment/disability can be detected several ways in clinical practice (see Chapter 6). Traditionally, this assessment is based on the neurologic exam. However, the standard exam is primarily useful for delineating the range of neurologic deficits. It inherently is not quantitative and, thus, is not good for detecting change over time. To address this issue, a variety of rating scales have been developed. The EDSS generates a series of functional system scores and a single EDSS score that allow straightforward comparison of status over time. Based in large part on reproducibility data, a typical definition of EDSS progression in clinical trials is a 1.0-step increase sustained for three or six months. This definition is reasonable for clinical practice also. However, the EDSS is cumbersome to use and has poor responsiveness, particularly at certain levels. Therefore, most clinicians, including MS experts, do not utilize the EDSS in clinical practice.

Simple quantitative functional tests such as component tests of the MS Functional Composite (MSFC),[138] particularly the Timed 25-Foot Walk and Nine-Hole Peg Test, are well suited for clinical practice. They can be performed by nurses or trained technicians in several minutes, are well tolerated by patients, and are highly reproducible. Several studies suggest that a 10%–20% change in the time to perform the tasks represents biologic change exceeding technical variability.[139] The magnitude of change that is clinically meaningful and indicates the need to change therapy is less straightforward and depends on the context.

Cognitive impairment is a common and often disabling manifestation of MS (see Chapter 7). It can occur independent of or out of proportion to physical manifestations. The Paced Auditory Serial Addition Test, a component of the MSFC, can be used as a screening test for cognitive change, although it is somewhat more difficult to implement in standard practice than the Timed 25-Foot Walk and Nine-Hole Peg Test. In selected patients, comprehensive neuropsychological testing and targeted re-testing over time is useful to monitor disease status.

MRI is utilized in clinical practice not only to assist in making an MS diagnosis, but also to monitor disease course, both to determine the need for therapy and assess its efficacy (see Chapters 6, 55). The rationale is that much of the disease activity is subclinical in the RR phase of the disease. The scanning protocol should include axial and sagittal long TR/TE or fluid attenuated inversion recovery (FLAIR), axial proton density, and axial T1-weighted images before and after administration of Gd.[140] Precise lesion and brain volume quantification require registration and processing of images by sophisticated software that still is available only in specialized MRI reading centers. In clinical practice, the most straightforward parameters to monitor disease activity are the numbers of Gd-enhancing lesions and new or substantially enlarged T2-hyperintense lesions. Changes in overall T2-hyperintense lesion number, T1-hypointense lesion number, and degree of atrophy can be detected if they are dramatic. The technical factors that impact on utilization of MRI to monitor MS activity should not be underestimated. Apparent changes can be due to differences in scanner type, field strength, slice level or orientation, and acquisition parameters. Therefore, these factors should be standardized as much as possible

to allow valid comparison of images over time. Advanced MRI techniques, such as magnetization transfer imaging, diffusion tensor imaging, and techniques to detect cortical lesions, may have more pathologic specificity and can detect pathology not apparent on standard MRI (see chapter 10–15). However, these modalities are not available outside of specialized centers and are incompletely validated.

Optical coherence tomography is a noninvasive method providing quantitative assessment of retinal neuroanatomy (see Chapter 17).[141] The parameters most-studied in MS, macular volume and peripapillary retinal nerve fiber layer thickness, indicate the severity of optic nerve involvement. Moreover, because OCT findings correlate with whole brain atrophy measured by MRI,[142] it provides an indirect measure of brain integrity with the advantage of being a rapid (~15 minutes for the entire exam), non-invasive, and office-based procedure. OCT is increasingly utilized in MS clinical trials and routine patient management to assess disease status. In addition, OCT is the preferred method to monitor for macular edema with fingolimod therapy.

Frequency of monitoring

The efficacy monitoring protocol must be tailored to the individual patient, in large part based on his/her perceived risk of future disability. Clinical assessments should be performed at time of initiation of a DMT to serve as a baseline for that agent then every 3–6 months. After several years of stability, visit frequency can be reduced to one to two per year, with additional visits if the patient reports change. Standard office follow-up should include review of the interval history and functional status, targeted neurologic exam, and quantitative tests such as the Timed 25-Foot Walk and Nine-Hole Peg Test. MRI should be obtained at the time of initiation or major change in DMT to serve as a baseline and then every one to two years in RRMS patients. After several years of stability on a given treatment regimen, scan frequency can be decreased.

Criteria indicating need to change therapy

Determination of the need to change therapy depends on "integration" of data from a variety sources and is based on a number of considerations:

- The magnitude of ongoing activity. The clinician needs to remember that all measures have a certain amount of "noise." Also, sampling in clinical practice is intermittent and relatively infrequent. One should not be overly reassured by lack of change or modest improvement at a single visit. Conversely, the decision to make a major treatment change should not be based on modest worsening on one parameter at one visit. Change in a number of parameters and a consistent trend over time is more reliable than change in a single measure at a single visit. For patients showing changes at one visit felt insufficient to warrant change, monitoring frequency should be increased, and more data should be obtained, e.g.

MRI or cognitive testing to corroborate patient self-report of decreased functional not reflected in neurologic exam.

- Pre-existing disease burden. Patients with marked previous disease activity, significant impairment (particularly if ambulation is tenuous), or substantial MRI lesion burden or brain atrophy can be viewed as having less "reserve" and being at increased risk. Arresting ongoing activity is more imperative in such patients.

- Availability and attractiveness of other options for treatment. When patients have tried only a few agents, there may be a greater tendency to change therapy. When most options have already been tried or are contraindicated, there is a higher threshold to change therapy.

- The patient's needs and expectations. Patients differ in their willingness to change therapy.

Statistical modeling of the effects of IFNβ on MRI lesion activity suggested heterogeneity in the treatment response patterns.[143] A sizable number of studies have suggested that, in particular, development of new T2 lesions or Gd-enhancing lesions after starting IFNβ predicts a poor long-term response to treatment in RRMS.[144–148] These studies suggest that approximately 20% of patients can be defined as IFNβ non-responders within 6–12 months of treatment initiation. We advise obtaining MRI at this this time and considering changing therapy if there is unequivocal evidence of ongoing MRI activity, even if the patient appears clinically stable. Thus, in this case, a single outcome is given substantial weight.

Similar data do not yet exist for the other DMTs. Given rapid and prominent inhibition of Gd-enhancing by natalizumab and fingolimod, one would think it could be used similarly for these agents, but this has not been studied. GA tends to have a less prominent effect on MRI lesion activity that develops more gradually. Therefore, lack of an early MRI response probably does not have the same implications as for IFNβ.

Other than NAbs to IFNβ and natalizumab, there are no biomarkers that can be used to indicate or predict DMT efficacy or lack. A sizable number have been proposed, most recently interleukin-17 for IFNβ non-responsiveness,[149] but none has been validated or is available clinically. Similarly, pharmacogenetics/pharmacogenomics is an area of intense interest, but at this point has made only modest impact on routine clinical care.

Treatment options for continued disease activity

The arguments for early therapy also suggest that the goal of therapy should be to effectively suppress all detectable disease activity. However, a sizable proportion of patients had continued MRI activity, relapses, or disability progression in the active-treatment arms of all of the RCTs of all the approved DMTs, and clinical experience supports this observation. Potential explanations for partial efficacy include noncompliance with therapy, development of a superimposed pathological process, incomplete potency of available agents, pathogenic complexity, pathogenic heterogeneity between patients and in individual patients over time, development of NAbs, and pharmacogenetic/pharmacogenomic diversity.

Although continued disease activity during therapy with IFNβ or GA is a frequently encountered issue in clinical practice, the best approach remains unknown, and there are few data to guide this decision. Some clinicians switch patients with modest ongoing disease activity while on IFNβ-1a (IM) to one of the higher dose, more frequently administered IFNβ preparations. This approach should be considered only if the patient does not have anti-IFNβ NAbs. Another approach is to try a different class of agent, i.e. switch patients with ongoing activity on IFNβ to GA and vice versa. Though reasonable, there are very few data supporting the utility of this approach.

A second approach is to escalate therapy. Although natalizumab, mitoxantrone, and fingolimod appear to be more potent than IFNβ and GA, there are few definitive studies that directly compared these agents with the first-line agents and even fewer that formally assessed the utility of switching patients to them who had with continued activity on first-line agents. SENTINEL enrolled patients with at least one relapse on IFNβ-1a (IM) during the year prior to the study and showed that the combination of natalizumab and IFNβ-1a (IM) was superior to IFNβ-1a (IM) in such patients.[62] It is presumed that the potency of natalizumab accounted for this result, but this remains unproven. TRANSFORMS compared fingolimod directly to IFNβ-1a (IM) and showed it to be superior in reducing relapses, MRI lesion activity, and brain volume loss.[120] Approximately half of the study participants had previously received DMT. The magnitude of benefit of fingolimod was comparable in the two cohorts. In a 12-month extension study, patients on IFNβ-1a (IM) in the core study were re-randomized to 1.25 or 0.5 mg of fingolimod, re-demonstrating the efficacy of fingolimod in patients with continued activity on IFNβ-1a (i.m.).[150] These results provide some support the use of natalizumab or fingolimod in patients with continued disease activity on first-line agents.

Numerous other agents are used alone or in combination to treat MS, for which there are preliminary data, anecdotal reports, and clinical experience in MS and other immune-mediated diseases supporting safety and efficacy: azathioprine,[151–157] methotrexate,[158,159] regular courses of i.v. methylprednisolone (MP),[160] i.v. immunoglobulin,[161–165] i.v. cyclophosphamide,[166] mycophenolate mofetil,[167,168] and daclizumab.[169] Potent efficacy and good tolerability were demonstrated in a Phase 3 trial of oral cladribine (which currently is available only in a parenterally administered form),[170] and in Phase 2 trials of rituximab[171] and alemtuzumab.[172] These agents are discussed in detail in other chapters.

A third approach is to use DMTs in combination. As reviewed in Chapter 47 and Conway and Cohen,[173] there is a strong rationale for combination therapy in MS, and numerous preliminary studies supported the safety and efficacy of a variety of combination regimens. Only a small number of trials with sufficient sample size to provide more-definitive results have been published. The SENTINEL study showed a clear advantage of natalizumab plus IFNβ-1a (IM) compared with IFNβ-1a (IM) alone on clinical and MRI end-points.[62] However, because SENTINEL did not have a natalizumab-only arm, it remains uncertain whether the combination was more effective than natalizumab. Because two of the three initial cases of PML occurred in the combined therapy arm of SENTINEL, natalizumab has been used as monotherapy since re-introduction. The Nordic Trial of Oral Methylprednisolone as Add-on Therapy to Interferon Beta-1a for Treatment of Relapsing–Remitting Multiple Sclerosis (NORMIMS) study[174] showed benefit of monthly five-day pulses of oral methylprednisolone as add-on therapy to IFNβ-1a (SC). The Avonex Combination Trial (ACT),[175] Avonex-Steroids-Azathioprine (ASA) study,[176] and Methylprednisolone in Combination with Interferon Beta-1a for Relapsing–Remitting Multiple Sclerosis (MECOMBIN) study,[177] which studied different corticosteroid-IFNβ combination regimens, were negative. The Combination Therapy in Patients with Relapsing–Remitting Multiple Sclerosis (CombiRx) study,[178] which has completed enrollment, compares GA + IFNβ-1a (IM) vs. each agent individually in treatment-naive RRMS patients. This large, rigorously designed study should provide definitive indication of the efficacy, safety, and tolerability of GA and IFNβ-1a (IM) in combination.

Clinically isolated demyelinating syndromes

Patients with a CIS who also have multiple lesions on cranial MRI are at high risk to develop additional MRI or clinical events leading to the diagnosis of MS within 3 to 10 years.[179–181] In the revised McDonald diagnostic criteria,[182] CIS patients whose MRI shows both Gd-enhancing and non-enhancing lesions are diagnosed with RRMS. RCTs of IFNβ-1a (IM),[183] IFNβ-1a (SC),[184] IFNβ-1b,[185,186] and GA[187] initiated after a CIS all demonstrated that active treatment decreased the occurrence of a second demyelinating event leading to the diagnosis of clinically definite (CD) MS and reduced MRI activity. IFNβ-1a (IM), IFNβ-1b, and GA are approved to CIS.

Since these studies were of relatively short duration (2–3 years), it was not possible to determine definitively whether initiating treatment at the earliest phase of MS affected long-term accumulation of neurologic disability compared to initiating therapy once the diagnosis of RRMS was confirmed. For example, five years after randomization in the Controlled High-Risk Subjects Avonex Multiple Sclerosis Prevention Study (CHAMPS), there was no difference in disability in patients as a group comparing those treated with IFNβ-1a (IM) immediately and those initially randomized to placebo who started IFNβ-1a

Table 51.5. *MS features suggesting poor prognosis and need for aggressive therapy*

- Frequent relapses, particularly if severe, with incomplete recovery, and with resultant increasing impairment.

- Substantial MRI lesion burden.

- Repeatedly active MR scans with numerous gadolinium-enhancing foci or new T2-hyperintense lesions and/or increasing lesion burden.

- Continued clinical or radiographic disease activity despite treatment with a standard agent.

(IM) at the time CDMS was confirmed or at the end of the core study.[188] Thus, the clinician confronted with a patient with CIS must decide whether and when to initiate DMT. Although it is not necessary or appropriate to initiate DMT in every patient at the time of a CIS or even in some when the diagnosis of RRMS is confirmed, the issue of whether to initiate DMT needs to be considered and discussed with all patients. Patients with normal brain MRI or with fewer than two lesions are at low risk to develop early disability[179–181] and can be followed clinically and by serial MRI without immediately commencing DMT. Those with abnormal MRI with two or more lesions consistent with MS or with evidence of intrathecal antibody production on CSF examination should be considered candidates for therapy. Patients with atypical clinical or neuroimaging findings require further diagnostic evaluation before making a decision on therapy.

Fulminant multiple sclerosis

Fulminant MS manifests as frequent severe relapses that recover incompletely with rapid accrual of disability and/or continued MRI lesion activity with rapid accumulation of lesions and loss of brain volume (Table 51.5). It first is important to carefully confirm the diagnosis of MS and rule out potential mimics, to ensure that seemingly atypically active MS is not due to misdiagnosis. Once the diagnosis is confirmed, institution of effective therapy must be instituted expeditiously. There sometimes is a tendency to wait too long to escalate therapy. Although disease prognosis and responsiveness to therapy are not equivalent, standard therapies, IFNβ and GA, often are not sufficiently potent to control fulminant MS. Because these patients are at high risk of disability, they are candidates for early aggressive therapy.

The DMT currently used most often in this setting is natalizumab, either after a trial of typical first-line therapies or as initial therapy in selected patients. Mitoxantrone also is a consideration, although it is being used less often due to concerns about amenorrhea, cardiotoxicity, and leukemia. Fingolimod is a third option for such patients. A post-hoc subgroup analysis of TRANSFORMS[189] assessed patients with high disease activity despite DMT (defined as ≥1 relapse during a year of DMT and ≥1 Gd-enhancing lesion at the end of the year of DMT). In the core trial, fingolimod was superior to IFNβ-1a (i.m.) in reducing disease activity in patients who were highly active on a variety of DMTs in the year prior to the trial. In the extension study, fingolimod potently reduced disease activity in patients who had been highly active while receiving IFN-1a (i.m.) in the core trial. These results support the utility of fingolimod in highly active MS, which is the EMA-approved indication. Other available options include cyclophosphamide, rituximab, alemtuzumab, and cladribine, based on their potent immunosuppressive effects. For patients who have failed all other options, immunoablation with hematopoietic stem cell transplantation can be considered,[190] although experience remains limited to only a few centers (see Chapter 44).

Treatment of acute relapses

Many relapses are followed by substantial or complete recovery, even without therapy, due to resolution of inflammation, restoration of conduction block, and remyelination. In addition, adaptive cortical plasticity may compensate for damage to critical pathways restoring function.[191] There is a tendency not to treat very mild relapses or relapses that already are improving unless there is associated lesion activity on MRI. For relapses warranting therapy, several RCTs demonstrated that corticosteroid treatment accelerated recovery and that high-dose corticosteroids were more effective than moderate-dose regimens (see Chapter 36).[192–194] Because the Optic Neuritis Treatment Trial raised the possibility that treatment of optic neuritis with moderate doses of oral prednisone alone failed to accelerate recovery and increased the risk for a subsequent relapse,[194,195] most clinicians no longer treat MS relapses with moderate dose of oral corticosteroids alone.

A typical treatment regimen is IVMP 500–1000 mg per day for 3–7 days followed by a tapering dose of prednisone over 10–14 days. The optimal dose and duration of IVMP is unknown, as is the need for the subsequent taper. There is accumulating evidence that equivalent doses of oral corticosteroids are well tolerated[196] and have comparable bioavailability.[197] Oral administration has obvious practical and financial advantages. A number of preliminary studies failed to demonstrate a difference in efficacy.[192,198,199] However, definitive studies confirming equivalent efficacy have not yet been carried out.

For severe relapses that do not respond to high-dose corticosteroids, alternative approaches include plasma exchange (see Chapter 39)[200,201] or i.v. immunoglobulin (see Chapter 38).[202,203] These approaches also can be considered in patients who tolerate steroids poorly due to significant AEs such as severe mood disorders, gastrointestinal bleeding, severe hypertension or hyperglycemia, or allergic reactions.

Treatment of progressive multiple sclerosis

Progressive forms of MS include SPMS (progression that develops after an initial RR course), primary progressive (PP) MS (gradual progression from onset), and progressive relapsing MS (gradual progression from onset with subsequent superimposed relapses).[204] There is increasing evidence that the three forms of progressive MS have similar pathogenesis in which degenerative mechanisms predominate and inflammatory processes, most directly reflected by relapses and MRI lesion activity, are less prominent.[205,206] As a result, immunomodulatory/immunosuppressive DMTs are less effective when the disease is purely progressive.

There have been four Phase 3 RCTs of IFNβ in SPMS, the European trial of IFNβ-1b the North American trial of IFNβ-1b,[125] the Secondary Progressive Efficacy Clinical Trial of Recombinant Interferon-beta-1a in MS (SPECTRIMS) trial of IFNβ-1a (SC),[26] and the International MS Secondary Progressive Avonex Controlled Trial (IMPACT) trial of IFNβ-1a (IM) 60 mcg weekly.[27] All four trials demonstrated benefit on relapses and MRI lesion activity comparable to that seen in trials of RRMS. Only the European trial of IFNβ-1b demonstrated slowing of EDSS progression, based on which it was approved in Europe to treat SPMS. Mitoxantrone also is approved for use in SPMS. Its use is supported by data from a RCT, MIMS.[99,100] Benefit of high-dose i.v. cyclophosphamide in progressive MS was reported by the Northeast Cooperative Multiple Sclerosis Treatment Group[207] but not replicated by two other groups.[208,209] Phase 2 studies reported modest benefit of every-other-month courses of IVMP[210] and weekly low dose oral methotrexate[211] in progressive MS. Studies of GA[212] and rituximab[213] in PPMS were negative for the overall study population, although there was a suggestion of benefit in subsets of patients.

In all of these studies, patients with characteristics suggesting greater likelihood of ongoing inflammation (younger age, recent relapses, recent onset of progression, rapid decline, and MRI lesion activity) were more likely to benefit.[212–216] Thus, patients with recent relapse or MRI lesion activity superimposed on a progressive course probably can be managed like those with RRMS.

In patients with purely progressive MS, we feel it is reasonable to attempt therapy with standard agents, GA or IFNβ, in selected patients with the understanding that this approach is not based on definitive evidence and that if treatment is ineffective or side effects outweigh benefit, the medication will be discontinued. In patients with progressive MS complicated by severe spasticity, we tend to use GA. We also frequently try a course of IVMP in patients with progressive MS. If there is significant benefit and it is well-tolerated, every other month IVMP is a reasonable option in some patients. There currently is no published evidence supporting the use of natalizumab or fingolimod in progressive MS. There is an ongoing Phase 3 study of fingolimod in PPMS, and Phase 3 studies of natalizumab in SPMS and laquinimod in PPMS are planned. Because of potential toxicity, mitoxantrone, cyclophosphamide, and rituximab should be reserved for patients with rapid progression despite therapy with other agents.

Prior to initiating DMT in patients with progressive disease, it is advisable to obtain updated imaging studies to assess for the presence of active lesions to help predict the likelihood of benefit. Imaging, along with screening blood studies also is useful to rule out other treatable conditions that could be contributing to progressive disability. Health maintenance and rehabilitative approaches are of particular importance in patients with progressive MS.

Disease treatment in special populations

Pregnancy

GA is pregnancy category B; INFβ, natalizumab, and fingolimod are category C; and mitoxantrone is category D (Table 51.1). In a review of approximately 3400 patients participating in clinical trials of GA, 40 pregnancies were reported.[217] No increased risk of adverse fetal or pregnancy outcomes was identified. Two studies assessed pregnancy outcome after in utero exposure to IFNβ. Sandberg-Wollheim *et al.*[218] reviewed 69 pregnancies occurring in 3361 women participating in clinical trials of IFNβ-1a (SC). There was no difference in the rate of congenital malformations compared with that observed in 22 women who discontinued IFNβ-1a (SC) more than two weeks prior to conception. The data suggested an increased rate of spontaneous abortion. In a cohort study,[219] data on 396 pregnancies in 388 women including 88 who discontinued IFNβ less than four weeks before conception. There was no indication of increased risk of spontaneous abortion, fetal complications, malformations, or developmental abnormalities associated with exposure, although it was associated with lower birth weight and length.

Thus, the data concerning IFNβ and GA use in pregnancy are reassuring but limited. Even less information is available concerning the safety of natalizumab and fingolimod. Therefore, it remains advisable for women to practice effective contraception while on DMT, to discontinue DMT four weeks prior to attempting to become pregnant, and to discontinue DMT immediately if an unanticipated pregnancy occurs.

Children (see Chapter 54)

MS presents before age 15 in approximately 3%–5% of patients, with onset in infancy or early childhood in 0.2%–0.7% of cases.[220] More than 95% of children with MS present with a RR course.[221] Although the time from onset to development of disability is prolonged compared to adult-onset MS, the age at which disability develops is younger.[222] Thus, the rationale for disease therapy is the same in pediatric onset MS as in adults. However, none of the DMTs is approved for use in this age group. Several treatment series of IFNβ and GA have been reported.[223–229] Individual patients or small series treated with cyclophosphamide, mitoxantrone, natalizumab, monthly corticosteroids, azathioprine, i.v. immunoglobulin, and daclizumab also have been reported.[82,225,230,231] A recent review summarized the overall experience with disease treatment in

258 children.[232] In general, the efficacy and spectrum, frequency, and severity of side effects and laboratory abnormalities were similar to those seen in adults. However, the data remain limited, particularly concerning long-term safety and developmental impact.

Elderly

The rationale for disease therapy is the same in elderly patients with MS as in young adults. However, none of the Phase 3 trials of approved DMTs included elderly participants, so published experience is limited. Also, two-thirds of patients over 65 years of age have a progressive form of MS,[233] for which efficacy of the approved agents is largely unproven. Finally, the increased probability of co-morbid conditions may lessen tolerability. Thus, while age per se is not known to affect efficacy, safety, or tolerability of DMTs in this population, there are several caveats to their use.

Non-Caucasians

In general, there are no special considerations in the use of DMTs in non-Caucasian populations. Small studies suggested African-American patients may respond less well to IFNβ and GA,[234–236] but may respond better to chemotherapeutic agents such as mitoxantrone.[235] Asians with western-type MS appear to respond DMTs similar to Caucasians.[237] Because of the higher incidence of Devic's neuromyelitis optic, which appears to respond to differentially to disease therapy compared to typical RRMS, care must be taken to accurately determine diagnosis in these populations.

Conclusions

There now are eight approved DMTs for RRMS. There is a strong argument favoring early initiation of therapy. In most patients, any of the IFNβ preparations or GA is reasonable initial therapy. These agents are safe and there is extensive experience with their use. However, they are modestly effective for patients as a group and are administered by injection, which patients tend to dislike. Natalizumab, mitoxantrone, and fingolimod probably are more potent but generally are reserved for patients who have failed first-line therapy because of safety concerns and, in the case of fingolimod, limited experience. With the availability of JCV serology to quantify PML risk with natalizumab and with accumulating experience with fingolimod in clinical practice, utilization earlier in the overall treatment algorithm may increase. Ongoing monitoring for tolerability, safety, and efficacy is necessary with all of the DMTs. However, the optimal protocol for monitoring patients, criteria for changing therapy, and approach to modify therapy when efficacy is incomplete remain uncertain. This issue will become increasingly complex as additional agents are approved in the next several years.

References

1. Weinshenker BG. The natural history of multiple sclerosis. *Neurol Clin* 1995;13:119–46.

2. Marrie RA, Cutter G, Tyry T, *et al.* Changes in the ascertainment of multiple sclerosis. *Neurology* 2005;65:1066–70.

3. Tremlett HL, Paty D, Devonshire V. Disability progression in multiple sclerosis is slower than previously reported. *Neurology* 2006;66:172–7.

4. Rudick RA, Fisher E, Lee J-C, *et al.* Use of the brain parenchymal fraction to measure whole brain atrophy in relapsing-remitting MS. *Neurology* 1999;53:1698–704.

5. Filippi M, Rovaris M, Rocca MA, *et al.* Glatiramer acetate reduces the proportion of new MS lesions evolving into "black holes". *Neurology* 2001;57:731–3.

6. Goodin DS, Frohman EM, Garmany GP, *et al.* Disease modifying therapies in multiple sclerosis. Report of the Therapeutics and Technology Assessment Subcommittee of the American Academy of Neurology and the MS Council for Clinical Practice Guidelines. *Neurology* 2002;58:169–78.

7. Medical Advisory Board of the National Multiple Sclerosis Society. Disease management consensus statement. 2005; http://www.nationalmssociety.org/PRC.asp.

8. Johnson KP, Brooks BR, Ford CC, *et al.* Sustained clinical benefits of glatiramer acetate in relapsing multiple sclerosis patients observed for 6 years. *Mult Scler* 2000;6:255–66.

9. PRISMS Study Group. PRISMS-4: long-term efficacy of interferon-β-1a in relapsing MS. *Neurology* 2001;56:1628–36.

10. Dhib-Jalbut S. Mechanisms of action of interferons and glatiramer acetate in multiple sclerosis. *Neurology* 2002;58(Suppl 4):S3–S9.

11. The IFNB Multiple Sclerosis Study Group. Interferon beta-1b is effective in relapsing-remitting multiple sclerosis. I. Clinical results of a multicenter, randomized, double-blind, placebo-controlled trial. *Neurology* 1993;43:655–61.

12. Paty DW, Li DKB, the UBC MS/MRI Study Group, the IFNB Multiple Sclerosis Study Group. Interferon beta-1b is effective in relapsing-remitting multiple sclerosis. II. MRI analysis results of a multicenter, randomized, double-blind, placebo-controlled trial. *Neurology* 1993;43:662–7.

13. The IFNB Multiple Sclerosis Study Group, The University of British Columbia MS/MRI Analysis Group. Interferon beta-1b in the treatment of multiple sclerosis: Final outcome of the randomized controlled trial. *Neurology* 1995;45:1277–85.

14. Jacobs LD, Cookfair DL, Rudick RA, *et al.* Intramuscular interferon beta-1a for disease progression in relapsing multiple sclerosis. *Ann Neurol* 1996;39:285–94.

15. Rudick RA, Goodkin DE, Jacobs LD, *et al.* Impact of interferon beta-1a on neurologic disability in relapsing multiple sclerosis. *Neurology* 1997;49:358–63.

16. Simon JH, Jacobs LD, Campion M, *et al.* Magnetic resonance studies of intramuscular interferon β-1a for relapsing multiple sclerosis. *Ann Neurol* 1998;43:79–87.

17. PRISMS Study Group. Randomized double-blind placebo-controlled study of interferon β-1a in relapsing/remitting multiple sclerosis. *Lancet* 1998;352:1498–504.

18. Li DKB, Paty DW, and the UBC MS/MRI Analysis Research Group and the PRISMS Study Group. Magnetic resonance imaging results of the PRISM trial: A randomized, double-blind, placebo-controlled study of interferon-β1a in relapsing-remitting multiple sclerosis. *Ann Neurol* 1999;46:197–206.

19. Hardmeier M, Wagenpfeil S, Freitag P, *et al.* Rate of brain atrophy in relapsing MS decreases during treatment with IFNβ-1a. *Neurology* 2005;64:236–40.

20. Filippi M, Rovaris M, Inglese M, *et al.* Interferon beta-1a for brain tissue loss in patients at presentation with syndromes suggestive of multiple sclerosis: a randomised, double-blind, placebo-controlled trial. *Lancet* 2004;364:1489–96.

21. Walther EU, Hohlfeld R. Multiple sclerosis. Side effects of interferon beta therapy and their management. *Neurology* 1999;53:1622–7.

22. Lublin FD, Whitaker JN, Eidelman BH, *et al.* Management of patients receiving interferon beta-1b for multiple sclerosis: report of a consensus conference. *Neurology* 1996;46:12–8.

23. Rio J, Nos C, Bonaventura I, *et al.* Corticosteroids, ibuprofen, and acetaminophen for IFNβ-1a flu symptoms in MS. A randomized trial. *Neurology* 2004;63:525–8.

24. Rieckmann P, Weber A, Gunther A, Poser S. The phosphodiesterase inhibitor pentoxifylline reduces early side effects of interferon-β1b treatment in patients with multiple sclerosis. *Neurology* 1996;47:604.

25. European Study Group on Interferon β-1b in Secondary Progressive MS. Placebo-controlled multicentre randomized trial of interferon β-1b in treatment of secondary progressive multiple sclerosis. *Lancet* 1998;352:1491–7.

26. Secondary Progressive Efficacy Clinical Trial of Recombinant Interferon-beta-1a in MS (SPECTRIMS) Study Group. Randomized controlled trial of interferon-beta-1a in secondary progressive MS. Clinical results. *Neurology* 2001;56:1496–504.

27. Cohen JA, Cutter GR, Fischer JS, *et al.* Benefit of interferon β-1a on MSFC progression in secondary progressive MS. *Neurology* 2002;59:679–87.

28. Tremlett HL, Oger J. Elevated aminotransferases during treatment with interferon-beta for multiple sclerosis: actions and outcomes. *Mult Scler* 2004;10:298–301.

29. Tremlett HL, Yoshida EM, Oger J. Liver injury associated with the β-interferons for MS. A comparison between the three products. *Neurology* 2004;62:628–31.

30. Yoshida EM, Rasmussen SL, Steinbrecher UP, *et al.* Fulminant liver failure during interferon beta therapy of multiple sclerosis. *Neurology* 2001;56:1416.

31. Bramanti P, Sessa E, Rifici C, *et al.* Enhanced spasticity in primary progressive MS patients treated with interferon beta-1b. *Neurology* 1998;51:1720–3.

32. Pollmann W, Erasmus LP, Feneberg W, Then Bergh F, Straube A. Interferon

beta but not glatiramer acetate therapy aggravates headaches in MS. *Neurology* 2002;59:636–9.

33. Schwid SR, Goodman AD, Mattson DH. Autoimmune hyperthyroidism in patients with multiple sclerosis treated with interferon beta-1b. *Arch Neurol* 1997;57:1169–70.

34. Midgard R, Ertresvag K, Trondsen E, Spigset O. Life-threatening acute pancreatitis associated with interferon beta-1a treatment in multiple sclerosis (letter). *Neurology* 2005;65:171–2.

35. Pulicken M, Koteish A, DeBusk K, Calabresi PA. Unmasking of autoimmune hepatitis in a patient with MS following interferon beta therapy. *Neurology* 2006;66:1954–1955.

36. Linden D. Severe Raynaud's phenomenon associated with interferon-β treatment for multiple sclerosis (letter). *Lancet* 1998;352:878–9.

37. Brown DL, Login IS, Borish L, Powers PL. An urticarial IgE-mediated reaction to interferon β-1b. *Neurology* 2001;56:1416–7.

38. Herrera WG, Balizet LB, Harberts SW, Brown ST. Occurrence of a TTP-like syndrome in two women receiving beta interferon therapy for relapsing multiple sclerosis (abstract). *Neurology* 1999;52(Suppl 2):A135.

39. Auty A, Saleh A. Nephrotic syndrome in a multiple sclerosis patient treated with interferon β1a. *Can J Neurol Sci* 2005;32:366–8.

40. Schmidt S, Hertfelder HJ, von Spiegel T, *et al.* Lethal capillary leak syndrome after a single administration of interferon beta-1b. *Neurology* 1999;53:220–2.

41. Von Raison F, Abboud H, Saint Val C, Brugieres P, Cesaro P. Acute demyelinating disease after interferon β-1a treatment for multiple sclerosis (letter). *Neurology* 2000;55:1416–17.

42. Ekstein D, Linetsky E, Abramsky O, Karussis D. Polyneuropathy associated with interferon beta treatment in patients with multiple sclerosis. *Neurology* 2005;65:456–8.

43. Folden DV, Lee MS, Ryan EH. Interferon b-associated retinopathy in patients treated for multiple sclerosis. *Neurology* 2008;70:1153–5.

44. Sorensen PS, Deisenhammer F, Dudac P, *et al.* Guidelines on use of anti-IFN-β

antibody measurements in multiple sclerosis: report of an EFNS Task Force on IFN-β antibodies in multiple sclerosis. *Eur J Neurol* 2005;12:817–27.

45. Schrempf W, Ziemssen T. Glatiramer acetate: mechanisms of action in multiple sclerosis. *Autoimmunity Reviews* 2007;6:469–75.

46. Bornstein MB, Miller A, Slagle S, *et al.* A pilot trial of Cop 1 in exacerbating-remitting multiple sclerosis. *N Engl J Med* 1987;317:408–14.

47. Johnson KP, Brooks BR, Cohen JA, *et al.* Copolymer 1 reduces relapse rate and improves disability in relapsing-remitting multiple sclerosis: Results of a phase III multicenter, double-blind, placebo-controlled trial. *Neurology* 1995;45:1268–76.

48. Ford C, Goodman AD, Johnson K, *et al.* Continuous long-term immunomodulatory therapy in relapsing multiple sclerosis: results from the 15-year analysis of the US prospective open-label study of glatiramer acetate. *Mult Scler* 2010;16:342–50.

49. Comi G, Filippi M, Wolinsky JS, the European/Canadian Glatiramer Acetate Study Group. European/Canadian multicenter, double-blind, randomized, placebo-controlled study of the effects of glatiramer acetate on magnetic resonance imaging-measured disease activity and burden in patients with relapsing multiple sclerosis. *Ann Neurol* 2001;49:290–7.

50. van Walderveen MAA, Kamphorst W, Scheltens P, *et al.* Histopathologic correlate of hypointense lesions on T1-weighted spin-echo MRI in multiple sclerosis. *Neurology* 1998;50:1282–8.

51. Cohen JA, Rovaris M, Goodman AD, *et al.* Randomized, double-blind, dose-comparison study of glatiramer acetate in relapsing-remitting MS. *Neurology* 2007;68:939–44.

52. Comi G, Cohen JA, Arnold DL, *et al.* Phase III dose-comparison study of glatiramer acetate for multiple sclerosis. *Ann Neurol* 2011;69:75–82.

53. Caon C, Perumal J, Tselis A, *et al.* Twice weekly versus daily glatiramer acetate: results of a randomized, rater-blinded prospective clinical and MRI study in relapsing-remitting MS (S11.002). *Neurol India* 2010;74(Suppl 2):A193.

54. Teva Pharmaceutical Industries. GALA study NCT01067521. [cited February 25, 2011]; Available from: http://clinicaltrials.gov/ct2/show/NCT0106751?term=glatiramer ± acetate&rank=16.

55. Edgar CM, Brunet DG, Fenton P, McBride EV, Green P. Lipoatrophy in patients with multiple sclerosis on glatiramer acetate. *Can J Neurol Sci* 2004;31:58–63.

56. Ball NJ, Cowan BJ, Moore GRW, Hashimoto SA. Lobular panniculitis at the site of glatiramer acetate injections for the treatment of relapsing-remitting multiple sclerosis. *J Cutan Pathol* 2008;35:407–10.

57. Pollmann W, Erasmus LP, Feneberg W, Straube A. The effect of glatiramer acetate treatment on pre-existing headaches in patients with MS. *Neurology* 2006;66:275–7.

58. Teitelbaum D, Brenner T, Abramsky O, *et al.* Antibodies to glatiramer acetate do not interfere with its biological functions and therapeutic efficacy. *Mult Scler* 2003;592–599.

59. Ransohoff RM. Natalizumab for multiple sclerosis. *N Engl J Med* 2007;356:2622–9.

60. Miller DH, Khan OA, Sheremata WA, *et al.* A controlled trial of natalizumab for relapsing multiple sclerosis. *N Engl J Med* 2003;348:15–23.

61. Polman CH, O'Connor PW, Hardova E, *et al.* A randomized, placebo-controlled trial of natalizumab for relapsing multiple sclerosis. *N Engl J Med* 2006;354:899–910.

62. Rudick RA, Stuart WH, Calabresi PA, *et al.* Natalizumab plus interferon beta-1a for relapsing multiple sclerosis. *N Engl J Med* 2006;354:911–23.

63. Bezabeh S, Flowers CM, Kortepeter C, Avigan M. Clinically significant liver injury in patients treated with natalizumab. *Aliment Pharmacol Ther* 2010;31:1028–35.

64. Cohen M, Rocher F, Brunschwig C, Lebrun C. Recurrent pericarditis due to natalizumab treatment. *Neurology* 2009;72:1616–17.

65. Phillips JT, O'Connor PW, Havrdova E, *et al.* Infusion-related hypersensitivity reactions during natalizumab treatment. *Neurology* 2006;67:1717–18.

66. Krumbholz M, Pellkofer H, Gold R, *et al.* Delayed allergic reaction to

natalizumab associated with early formation of neutralizing antibodies. *Arch Neurol* 2007;64:1331–3.

67. Hellwig K, Schmrigk S, Fischer M, *et al.* Allergic and nonallergic delayed infusion reactions during natalizumab therapy. *Arch Neurol* 2008;65:656–8.

68. Calabresi PA, Giovannoni G, Confavreux C, *et al.* The incidence and significance of anti-natalizumab antibodies. Results from AFFIRM and SENTINEL. *Neurology* 2007;69:1391–403.

69. Rudick RA, O'Connor PW, Polman CH, *et al.* Assessment of JC virus from DNA in blood and urine from natalizumab-treated patients. *Ann Neurol* 2010;68:304–10.

70. Gorelik L, Lerner M, Bixler S, *et al.* Anti-JC virus antibodies: Implications for PML risk stratification. *Ann Neurol* 2010;68:295–303.

71. Clifford DB, DeLuca A, Simpson DM, *et al.* Natalizumab-associated progressive multifocal leukoencephalopathy in patients with multiple sclerosis: lessons from 28 cases. *Lancet Neurology* 2010;9:438–46.

72. Vermersch P, Foley J, Gold R, *et al.* Overview of clinical outcomes in cases of natalizumab-associated progressive multifocal leukoencephalopathy (oral presentation 112). *Mult Scler* 2010;16(Suppl 10):S32–3.

73. Schroder A, Lee D, Hellwig K, *et al.* Successful management of natalizumab-associated progressive multifocal leukoencephalopathy and immune reconstitution syndrome in a patient with multiple sclerosis. *Arch Neurol* 2010;67:1391–4.

74. Khatri BO, Man S, Giaovannoni G, *et al.* Effect of plasma exchange in accelerating natalizumab clearance and restoring leukocyte function. *Neurology* 2009;72:402–9.

75. Cettomai D, McArthur JC. Mirtazapine use in human immunodeficiency virus-infected patients with progressive multifocal leukoencephalopathy. *Arch Neurol* 2009;66:255–8.

76. Verma S, Cikurel K, Koralnik IJ, *et al.* Mirtazapine in progressive multifocal leukoencephalopathy associated with polycythemia vera. *J Infect Dis* 2007;196:709–11.

77. Brickelmaier M, Lugovskoy A, Kartikeyan R, *et al.* Identification and characterization of mefloquine efficacy against JC virus in vitro. *Antimicrob Agents Chemother* 2009;53:1840–9.

78. Tan K, Roda R, Ostrow L, McArthur J, Nath A. PML-IRIS in patients with HIV infection. Clinical manifestations and treatment with steroids. *Neurology* 2009;72:1458–64.

79. Vellinga MM, Castelijns JA, Barkhof F, Uitehaag BMJ, Polman CH. Postwithdrawal rebound increase in T2 lesional activity in natalizumab-treated MS patients. *Neurology* 2008;70:1150–1.

80. Killestein J, Vennegoor A, Strijbis EM, *et al.* Natalizumab drug holiday in multiple sclerosis: poorly tolerated. *Ann Neurol* 2010;68:392–5.

81. West TW, Cree BAC. Natalizumab dosage suspension: are we helping or hurting? *Ann Neurol* 2010;68:395–9.

82. Borriello G, Prosperini L, Luchetti A, Pozzilli C. Natalizumab treatment in pediatric multiple sclerosis: A case report. *Eur J Paediat Neurol* 2009;13:67–71.

83. Lenhard T, Biller A, Mueller W, *et al.* Immune reconstitution inflammatory syndrome after withdrawal of natalizumab? *Neurology* 2010;75:831–3.

84. Miravalle A, Jensen R, Kinkel RP. Immune reconstitution inflammatory syndrome in patients with multiple sclerosis following cessation of natalizumab therapy. *Arch Neurol* 2011;68:186–91.

85. Biogen Idec. Treatment interruption of natalizumab (RESTORE) NCT01071083. [cited 26 Feb 2011]; Available from: http://www.clinicatrials.gov/ct2/show/NCT01071083?term=restore&rank=11.

86. Zecca C, Nessi F, Bernasconi E, Gobbi C. Ocular toxoplasmosis during natalizumab treatment. *Neurology* 2009;73:1418–19.

87. Gutwinski S, Erbe S, Munch C, *et al.* Severe cutaneous Candida infection during natalizumab therapy in multiple sclerosis. *Neurology* 2010;74:521–3.

88. Mullen JT, Vartanian TK, Atkins MB. Melanoma complicating treatment with natalizumab for multiple sclerosis. *N Engl J Med* 2008;358:647–8.

89. Laroni A, Bedognetti M, Uccella I, Capello E, Mancardi GL. Association of melanoma and natalizumab therapy in the Italian MS population: a second case report. *Neurol Sci* 2011;32:181–2.

90. Schweisfurth H, Schioberg-Schiegnitz S, Kuhn W, Parusel B. Antiotensin I converting enzyme in cerebrospinal fluid in patients with neurological diseases. *Klin Wochenschr* 1987;65:955–8.

91. Ransohoff RM. Natalizumab, multiple sclerosis, and primary central nervous system lymphoma: enigma, wrapped in mystery, enclosed in conundrum. *Ann Neurol* 2009;66:259–61.

92. Bozic C, LaGuette J, Panzara MA, Sandrock AW. Natalizumab and central nervous system lymphoma: no clear association. *Ann Neurol* 2009;66:261–2.

93. DeAngelis LM. Natalizumab: a double-edged sword? *Ann Neurol* 2009;66:262–3.

94. Goebels N, Kappos L. Another complication of natalizumab treatment? Taking the challenge. *Ann Neurol* 2009;66:264–6.

95. Phan-Ba R, Bisig B, Deprez M, *et al.* Primary central nervous system lymphoma in a patient treated with natalizumab. *Ann Neurol* 2010;DOI:10.1002/ana.22296.

96. Millefiorini E, Gasperini C, Pozzilli C, *et al.* Randomized placebo-controlled trial of mitoxantrone in relapsing–remitting multiple sclerosis: 24-month clinical and MRI outcome. *J Neurol* 1997;244:153–9.

97. Edan G, Miller D, Clanet M, *et al.* Therapeutic effect of mitoxantrone combined with methylprednisolone in multiple sclerosis: a randomised multicentre study of active disease using MRI and clinical criteria. *J Neurol Neurosurg Psychiatry* 1997;62:112–8.

98. van de Wyngaeert FA, Beguin C, D'Hooghie MB, *et al.* A double-blind clinical trial of mitoxantrone versus methylprednisolone in relapsing, secondary progressive multiple sclerosis. *Acta Neurol Belg* 2001;101:210–6.

99. Hartung HP, Gonsette R, the MIMS Study Group. Mitoxantrone in progressive multiple sclerosis: a placebo-controlled, randomised, multicentre trial. *Lancet* 2002;360:2018–25.

100. Krapf H, Morrissey SP, Zenker O, *et al.* Effect of mitoxantrone on MRI in progressive MS. Results of the MIMS trial. *Neurology* 2005;65:690–5.

101. Le Page E, Leray E, Taurin G, *et al.* Mitoxantrone as induction treatment in

aggressive relapsing remitting multiple sclerosis: treatment response factors in 5 year follow-up observational study of 100 consecutive patients. *J Neurol Neurosurg Psychiatry* 2008;79: 52–6.

102. Vollmer T, Panitch H, Bar-Or A, *et al.* Glatiramer acetate after induction therapy with mitoxantrone in relapsing multiple sclerosis. *Mult Scler* 2008;14:663–70.

103. Cohen BA, Mikol DD. Mitoxantrone treatment of multiple sclerosis. Safety considerations. *Neurology* 2004;63(Suppl 6):S28–S32.

104. Le Page E, Leray E, Edan G, *et al.* Long-term safety profile of mitoxantrone in a French cohort of 802 multiple sclerosis patients: a 5-year prospective study. Mult Scler (in press).

105. De Castro S, Cartoni D, Millefiorini E, *et al.* Noninvasive assessment of mitoxantrone cardiotoxicity in relapsing remitting multiple sclerosis. *J Clin Pharmacol* 1995;35:627–32.

106. Ghalie RG, Edan G, Laurent M, *et al.* Cardiac adverse effects associated with mitoxantrone (Novantrone) therapy in patients with MS. *Neurology* 2002;59:909–13.

107. Strotmann JM, Spindler M, Weilbach FX, *et al.* Myocardial function in patients with multiple sclerosis treated with low-dose mitoxantrone. *Am J Cardiol* 2002;89:1222–5.

108. Avasarala JR, Cross AH, Clifford DB, *et al.* Rapid onset mitoxantrone-induced cardiotoxicity in secondary progressive multiple sclerosis. *Mult Scler* 2003;9: 59–62.

109. Rivera V, Weinstock-Guttman B, Beagan J, *et al.* Final results from Registry to Evaluate Novantrone Effects in Worsening Multiple Sclerosis study (RENEW). *Mult Scler* 2009;15:S254.

110. Marriott JJ, Miyasaki JM, Gronseth G, O'Connor PW. Evidence report: The efficacy and safety of mitoxantrone (Novantrone) in the treatment of multiple sclerosis: Report of the Therapeutics and Technology Assessment Subcommittee of the American Academy of Neurology. *Neurology* 2010;74:1463–70.

111. Vicari AM, Ciceri F, Folli F, *et al.* Acute promyelocytic leukemia following mitoxantrone as single agent for the treatment of multiple sclerosis (letter). *Leukemia* 1998;12:441–2.

112. Brassat D, Recher C, Waubant E, *et al.* Therapy-related acute myeloblastic leukemia after mitoxantrone treatment in a patient with MS. *Neurology* 2002;59:954–5.

113. Ghalie RG, Mauch E, Edan G, *et al.* A study of therapy-related acute leukaemia after mitoxantrone therapy for multiple sclerosis. *Mult Scler* 2002;8:441–5.

114. Cattaneo C, Almici C, Borlenghi E, Motta M, Rossi G. A case of acute promyelocytic leukaemia following mitoxantrone treatment of multiple sclerosis (letter). *Leukemia* 2003;17:985–6.

115. Heesen C, Bruegmann M, Gbdamosi J, *et al.* Therapy-related acute myelogenous leukaemia (t-AML) in a patient with multiple sclerosis treated with mitoxantrone (letter). *Mult Scler* 2003;9:213–14.

116. Mauritzson N, Albin M, Rylander L, *et al.* Pooled analysis of clinical and cytogenetic features in treatment-related and *de novo* adult acute myeloid leukemia and myelodysplastic syndromes based on a consecutive series in 761 patients analyzed 1976–1993 and 5093 unselected cases reported in the literature 1974–2001. *Leukemia* 2002;16:2366–78.

117. Brinkmann V. FTY720 (fingolimod) in multiple sclerosis: therapeutic effects in the immune and the central nervous system. *Br J Pharmacol* 2009;158:1173–82.

118. Kappos L, Antel J, Comi G, *et al.* Oral fingolimod (FTY720) for relapsing multiple sclerosis. *N Engl J Med* 2006;355:1124–40.

119. Kappos L, Radue E-W, O'Connor P, *et al.* A placebo-controlled trial of oral fingolimod in relapsing multiple sclerosis. *N Engl J Med* 2010;362:387–401.

120. Cohen JA, Barkhof F, Comi G, *et al.* Oral fingolimod or intramuscular interferon for relapsing multiple sclerosis. *N Engl J Med* 2010;362:402–15.

121. Montalban X, O'Connor P, Antel J, *et al.* Oral fingolimod (FTY720) shows sustained low rates of clinical and MRI disease activity in patients with relapsing multiple sclerosis: four-year results from a phase II extension (P06.128). *Neurology* 2009;72(Suppl 3):A313. abstract.

122. Collins W, Cohen J, O'Connor P, *et al.* Long-term safety of oral fingolimod (FTY720) in relapsing multiple sclerosis: integrated analyses of phase 1 and 3 studies (P843). *Mult Scler* 2010;16(Suppl 10):S295.

123. NDA 02257 FDA Approved Labeling Text for Gilenya *(fingolimod) capsules.* September 21, 2010.

124. Miller DH, Molyneux PD, Barker GJ, *et al.* Effect of Interferon-b1b on magnetic resonance imaging outcomes in secondary progressive multiple sclerosis: Results of a European multicenter, randomized, double-blind, placebo-controlled trial. *Ann Neurol* 1999;46:850–9.

125. The North American Study Group on Interferon Beta-1b in Secondary Progressive MS. Interferon beta-1b in secondary progressive MS: results from a three-year controlled study. *Neurology* 2004;63: 1788–95.

126. Durelli L, Verdun E, Barbero P, *et al.* Every-other-day interferon beta-1b versus once-weekly interferon beta-1a for multiple sclerosis: results of a 2-year prospective randomized multicentre study (INCOMIN). *Lancet* 2002;359:1453–60.

127. Panitch H, Goodin DS, Francis G, *et al.* Randomized, comparative study of interferon b-1a treatment regimens in MS. The EVIDENCE trial. *Neurology* 2002;59:1496–506.

128. Clanet M, Radue EW, Kappos L, *et al.* A randomized, double-blind, dose-comparison study of weekly interferon b-1a (Avonex) in relapsing MS. *Neurology* 2002;59:1507–17.

129. O'Connor P, Filippi M, Arnason B, *et al.* 250 mg or 500 mg interferon beta-1b versus 20 mg glatiramer acetate in relapsing-remitting multiple sclerosis: a prospective, randomised, multicentre study. *Lancet Neurology* 2009;8:889–97.

130. Cadavid D, Wolansky LJ, Skurnick J, *et al.* Efficacy of treatment of MS with IFNβ-1b or glatiramer acetate by monthly brain MRI in the BECOME study. *Neurology* 2009;72:1976–83.

131. Mikol DD, Barkhof F, Chang P, *et al.* Comparison of subcutaneous beta-1a with glatiramer acetate in patients with relapsing multiple sclerosis (the REbif

vs Glatiramer Acetate in Relapsing MS Disease [REGARD] study): a multicentre, randomised, parallel, open-label trial. *Lancet Neurology* 2008;7:903–14.

132. Kappos L, Traboulsee A, Constantinescu C, *et al*. Long-term subcutaneous interferon beta-1a therapy in patients with relapsing-remitting MS. *Neurology* 2006;67:944–53.

133. Reder AT, Ebers GC, Traboulsee A, *et al*. Cross-sectional study assessing long-term safety of interferon-β-1b for relapsing-remitting MS. *Neurology* 2010;74:1877–85.

134. Trojano M, Pellegrino F, Fuiani A, *et al*. New natural history of interferon-β-treated relapsing multiple sclerosis. *Ann Neurol* 2007;61:300–6.

135. Cohen BA, Khan O, Jeffery DR, *et al*. Identifying and treating patients with suboptimal responses. *Neurology* 2004;63(Suppl 6):S33–S40.

136. Medical Advisory Board of the National Multiple Sclerosis Society. Changing therapy in relapsing multiple sclerosis: considerations and recommendations of a task force of the National Multiple Sclerosis Society. 2005;http://www.nationalmssociety.org/PRC.asp.

137. Lublin FD, Baier M, Cutter G. Effect of relapses on development of residual deficit in multiple sclerosis. *Neurology* 2003;61:1528–32.

138. Rudick R, Antel J, Confavreux C, *et al*. Recommendations from the National Multiple Sclerosis Society Clinical Outcomes Assessment Task Force. *Ann Neurol* 1997;42:379–82.

139. Schwid SR, Goodman AD, McDermott MP, Bever CF, Cook SD. Quantitative functional measures in MS: What is a reliable change? *Neurology* 2002;58:1294–6.

140. Simon JH, Li D, Traboulsee A, *et al*. Standardized MR imaging protocol for multiple sclerosis: consortium of MS Centers consensus guidelines. *Am J NeuroRadiol* 2006;27:455–61.

141. Frohman EM, Fujimoto JG, Frohman TC, *et al*. Optical coherence tomography: a window into the mechanisms of multiple sclerosis. *Nat Clin Pract Neurol* 2008;4:664–75.

142. Gordon-Lipkin E, Chodklwski B, Reich DS, *et al*. Retinal nerve fiber layer is associated with brain atrophy in multiple sclerosis. *Neurology* 2007;69:1603–9.

143. Sormani MP, Bruzzi P, Beckmann K, *et al*. MRI metrics as surrogate endpoints for EDSS progression in SPMS patients treated with IFN β-1b. *Neurology* 2003;60:1462–6.

144. Rudick RA, Lee J-C, Simon J, Ransohoff RM, Fisher E. Defining interferon b response status in multiple sclerosis patients. *Ann Neurol* 2004;56:548–55.

145. Tomassini V, Paolillo A, Russo P, *et al*. Predictors of long-term clinical response to interferon beta therapy in relapsing multiple sclerosis. *J Neurol* 2006;253:287–93.

146. Durelli L, Barbero P, Bergui M, *et al*. MRI activity and neutralising antibody as predictors of response to interferon beta treatment in multiple sclerosis. *J Neurol Neurosurg Psychiatry* 2008;79:646–51.

147. Rio J, Rovira A, Tintore M, *et al*. Relationship between MRI lesion activity and response to IFN-beta in relapsing–remitting multiple sclerosis patients. *Mult Scler* 2008;14:479–84.

148. Prosperini L, Gallo V, Petsas N, Borriello G, Pozzilli C. One-year MRI scan predicts clinical response to interferon beta in multiple sclerosis. *Eur J Neurol* 2009;16:1202–9.

149. Axtell RC, de Jong BA, Boniface K, *et al*. T helper type 1 and 17 cells determine efficacy of interferon-b in multiple sclerosis and experimental encephalomyelitis. *Nat Med* 2010;16:406–13.

150. Khatri B, Barkhof F, Comi G, *et al*. 24-month efficacy and safety from the TRANSFORMS extension study of oral fingolimod (FTY720) in patients with relapsing–remitting multiple sclerosis(P03.125). *Neurology* 2010;74 (Suppl 2):A239.

151. British and Dutch Multiple Sclerosis Azathioprine Trial Group. Double-masked trial of azathioprine in multiple sclerosis. *Lancet* 1988;2:179–83.

152. Goodkin DE, Bailly RC, Teetzen ML, Hertsgaard D, Beatty WW. The efficacy of azathioprine in relapsing-remitting multiple sclerosis. *Neurology* 1990;41:20–5.

153. Fernandez O, Guerrero M, Mayorga C, *et al*. Combination therapy with interferon beta-1b and azathioprine in secondary progressive multiple sclerosis. A two-year pilot study. *J Neurol* 2002;249:1058–62.

154. Markovic-Plese S, Bielekova B, Kadom N, *et al*. Longitudinal MRI study. The effects of azathioprine in MS patients refractory to interferon b-1b. *Neurology* 2003;60:1849–51.

155. Lus G, Romano F, Scuotto A, Acardo C, Cotrufo R. Azathioprine and interferon b₁ₐ in relapsing–remitting multiple sclerosis patients: increasing efficacy of combined treatment. *Eur Neurol* 2004;51:15–20.

156. Pulicken M, Bash CN, Costello K, *et al*. Optimization of the safety and efficacy of interferon beta 1b and azathioprine combination therapy in multiple sclerosis. *Mult Scler* 2005;11:169–74.

157. Massacesi L, Parigi A, Barilaro A, *et al*. Efficacy of azathioprine on multiple sclerosis new brain lesions evaluated using magnetic resonance imaging. *Arch Neurol* 2005;62:1843–7.

158. Currier RD, Haerer AF, Meydrech EF. Low dose oral methotrexate treatment of multiple sclerosis. *J Neurol Neurosurg Psychiatry* 1993;56:1217–18.

159. Calabresi PA, Wilterdink JL, Rogg JM, *et al*. An open-label trial of combination therapy with interferon b-1a and oral methotrexate in MS. *Neurology* 2002;58:314–17.

160. Zivadinov R, Rudick RA, De Masi R, *et al*. Effects of IV methylprednisolone on brain atrophy in relapsing–remitting MS. *Neurology* 2001;57:1239–47.

161. Fazekas F, Deisenhammer F, Strasser-Fuchs S, *et al*. Randomized placebo-controlled trial of monthly intravenous immunoglobulin therapy in relapsing–remitting multiple sclerosis. *Lancet* 1997;349:589–93.

162. Achiron A, Gabbay U, Gilad R, *et al*. Intravenous immunoglobulin treatment in multiple sclerosis. Effect on relapses. *Neurology* 1998;50:398–402.

163. Sorensen PS, Wanscher B, Jensen CV, *et al*. Intravenous immunoglobulin G reduces MRI activity in relapsing multiple sclerosis. *Neurology* 1998;50:1273–81.

164. Achiron A, Kishner I, Sarova-Pinhas I, *et al*. Intravenous immunoglobulin treatment following the first demyelinating event suggestive of multiple sclerosis. A randomized, double-blind, placebo-controlled trial. *Arch Neurol* 2004;61:1515–20.

165. Filippi M, Rocca MA, Pagani E, et al. European study on intravenous immunoglobulin in multiple sclerosis. Results of magnetization transfer magnetic resonance imaging analysis. Arch Neurol 2004;61:1409–12.

166. Smith DR, Weinstock-Guttman B, Cohen JA, et al. A randomized blinded trial of combination therapy with cyclophosphamide in patients with active multiple sclerosis on interferon beta. Mult Scler 2005;11:573–82.

167. Ahrens N, Salama A, Haas J. Mycophenolate-mofetil in the treatment of refractory multiple sclerosis. J Neurol 2001;248:713–4.

168. Frohman EM, Brannon K, Racke MK, Hawker K. Mycophenolate mofetil in multiple sclerosis. Clin Neuropharmacol 2004;27:80–3.

169. Wynn D, Kaufman M, Montalban X, et al. Daclizumab in active relapsing multiple sclerosis (CHOICE study): a phase 2, randomised, double-blind, placebo-controlled, add-on trial with interferon beta. Lancet Neurol 2010;10.1016/S1474–4422(10)70033–8.

170. Giovannoni G, Comi G, Cook S, et al. A placebo-controlled trial of oral cladribine for relapsing multiple sclerosis. N Engl J Med 2010;362:416–26.

171. Hauser SL, Waubant E, Arnold DL, et al. B-cell depletion with rituximab in relapsing-remitting multiple sclerosis. N Eng J Med 2008;358:676–88.

172. The CAMMS223 Trial Investigators. Alemtuzumab vs. interferon beta-1a in early multiple sclerosis. N Engl J Med 2008;359:1786–801.

173. Conway D, Cohen JA. Combination therapy in multiple sclerosis. Lancet Neurology 2010;9:299–308.

174. Sorensen PS, Mellgren SI, Svenningsson A, et al. Nordic trial of oral methylprednisolone as add-on therapy to interferon beta for the treatment of relapsing remitting multiple sclerosis (NORMIMS Study): a randomised, placebo-controlled trial. Lancet Neurol 2009;8:519–29.

175. Cohen JA, Imrey PB, Calabresi PA, et al. Results of the Avonex Combination Trial (ACT) in relapsing-remitting MS. Neurology 2009;72:535–41.

176. Havrdova E, Zivadinov R, Krasensky J, et al. Randomized study of interferon beta-1a, low-dose azathioprine, and low-dose corticosteroids in multiple sclerosis. Mult Scler 2009;15:965–76.

177. Ravnborg M, Sorensen PS, Andersson M, et al. Methylprednisolone in combination with interferon beta-1a for relapsing-remitting multiple sclerosis (MECOMBIN study): a multicentre, double-blind, randomised, placebo-controlled, parallel-group trial. Lancet Neurol 2010;9:672–80.

178. Mount Sinai School of Medicine. Combination therapy in patients with relapsing-remitting multiple sclerosis (CombiRx). NCT00211887. [cited 26 February 2011]; Available from: http://www.clinicaltrials.gov/ct2/show/NCT00211887?term=combirx&rank=1.

179. O'Riordan JI, Thompson AJ, Kingsley DPE, et al. The prognostic value of brain MRI in clinically isolated syndromes of the CNS. A 10-year follow-up study. Brain 1998;121:495–503.

180. Brex PA, Ciccarelli O, O'Riordan JI, et al. A longitudinal study of abnormalities on MRI and disability from multiple sclerosis. N Engl J Med 2002;346:158–64.

181. Optic Neuritis Study Group. The 5-year risk of MS after optic neuritis. Experience of the Optic Neuritis Treatment Trial. Neurology 1997;49:1404–13.

182. Polman CH, Reingold SC, Banwell B, et al. Diagnostic criteria for multiple sclerosis: 2010 revisions to the "McDonald Criteria". Ann Neurol 2011;69: 292–302.

183. Jacobs LD, Beck RW, Simon JH, et al. Intramuscular Interferon beta-1a therapy initiated during a first demyelinating event in multiple sclerosis. N Engl J Med 2000;343:898–904.

184. Comi G, Filippi M, Barkhof F, et al. Effect of early interferon treatment on conversion to definite multiple sclerosis: a randomized study. Lancet 2001;357:1576–82.

185. Kappos L, Polman CH, Freedman MS, et al. Treatment with interferon beta-1b delays conversion to clinically definite and McDonald MS in patients with clinically isolated syndromes. Neurology 2006;67:1242–9.

186. Barkhof F, Polman CH, Radue EW, et al. Magnetic resonance imaging effects of interferon beta-1b in the BENEFIT study. Arch Neurol 2007;64:1292–8.

187. Comi G, Martinelli V, Rodegher M, et al. Effect of glatiramer acetate on conversion to clinically definite multiple sclerosis in patients with clinically isolated syndrome (PreCISe study): a randomised, double-blind, placebo-controlled trial. Lancet 2009;374:1503–11.

188. Kinkel RP, Kollman C, Glassman A, et al. Interferon beta-1a (Avonex) delays the onset of clinically definite MS over 5 years of treatment: Results from CHAMPIONS study. Neurology 2004;62(Suppl 5):A261–2.

189. Cohen J, Francis G, Meinel M, Eckert B. The benefits of fingolimod in patients with active multiple sclerosis despite previous treatment: Phase 3 results from TRANSFORMS and the TRANSFORMS extension (P04.195). Neurology 2011;TBD(Suppl TBD):TBD.

190. Burt RK, Loh Y, Cohen B, et al. Autologous non-myeloablative haemopoietic stem cell transplanatation in relapsing-remitting multiple sclerosis: a phase I/II study. Lancet 2009;8(3): 244–53.

191. Toosy AT, Hickman SJ, Miszkiel KA, et al. Adaptive cortical plasticity in higher visual areas after acute optic neuritis. Ann Neurol 2005;57:622–33.

192. LaMantia L, Eoli M, Milanese C, et al. Double-blind trial of dexamethasone versus methylprednisolone in multiple sclerosis acute relapses. Eur Neurol 1994;34:199–203.

193. Oliveri RL, Valentino P, Russo C, et al. Randomized trial comparing two different doses of methylprednisolone in MS. A clinical and MRI study. Neurology 1998;50:1833–6.

194. Beck RW, Cleary PA, Anderson MM, et al. A randomized, controlled trial of corticosteroids in the treatment of acute optic neuritis. N Engl J Med 1992;326:581–8.

195. Beck RW, Cleary PA, Trobe JD, et al. The effect of corticosteroids for acute optic neuritis on the subsequent development of multiple sclerosis. N Engl J Med 1993;329:1764–9.

196. Metz LM, Sabuda D, Hilsden RJ, Enns R, Meddings JB. Gastric tolerance of high-dose pulse oral prednisone n multiple sclerosis. Neurology 1999;53:2093–6.

197. Morrow SA, Stoian CA, Dmitrovic J, Chan SC, Metz LM. The bioavailability of IV methylprednisolone and oral prednisone in multiple sclerosis. *Neurology* 2004;63:1079–80.

198. Barnes D, Hughes RAC, Morris RW, *et al.* Randomised trial of oral and intravenous methylprednisolone in acute relapses of multiple sclerosis. *Lancet* 1997;349:902–6.

199. Alam SM, Kyriakides T, Lawden M, Newman PK. Methylprednisolone in multiple sclerosis: a comparison of oral with intravenous therapy at equivalent high dose. *J Neurol Neurosurg Psychiatry* 1993;56:1219–20.

200. Weinshenker BG, O'Brien P, Petterson TM, *et al.* A randomized trial of plasma exchange in acute central nervous system inflammatory demyelinating disease. *Ann Neurol* 1999;46:878–86.

201. Ruprecht K, Klinker E, Dintelmann T, Rieckmann P, Gold R. Plasma exchange for severe optic neuritis. Treatment of 10 patients. *Neurology* 2004;63:1081–3.

202. Soelberg Sorensen P, Haas J, Sellebjerg F, *et al.* IV immunoglobulins as add-on treatment to methylprednisolone for acute relapses in MS. *Neurology* 2004;63:2028–33.

203. Roed HG, Langkilde A, Sellebjerg F, *et al.* A double-blind, randomized trial of IV immunoglobulin treatment in acute optic neuritis. *Neurology* 2005;64:804–10.

204. Lublin FD, Reingold SC. Defining the clinical course of multiple sclerosis: Results of an international survey. *Neurology* 1996;46:907–11.

205. Cohen JA, Antel JP. Does interferon beta help in secondary progressive MS? (editorial). *Neurology* 2004;63:1768–9.

206. Trapp BD, Nave K-A. Multiple sclerosis: an immune or neurodegenerative disorder? *Annu Rev Neurosci* 2008;31:247–69.

207. Hauser SL, Dawson DM, Lehrich JR, *et al.* Intensive immunosuppression in progressive multiple sclerosis. A randomized, three-arm study of high-dose intravenous cyclophosphamide, plasma exchange, and ACTH. *N Engl J Med* 1983;308:173–80.

208. The Canadian Cooperative Multiple Sclerosis Group. The Canadian cooperative trial of cyclophosphamide and plasma exchange in progressive multiple sclerosis. *Lancet* 1991;337:441–6.

209. Likosky WH, Fireman B, Elmore R, *et al.* Intense immunosuppression in chronic progressive multiple sclerosis: the Kaiser study. *J Neurol Neurosurg Psychiatry* 1991;54:1055–60.

210. Goodkin DE, Kinkel RP, Weinstock-Guttman B, *et al.* A phase II study of IV methylprednisolone in secondary-progressive multiple sclerosis. *Neurology* 1998;51:239–45.

211. Goodkin DE, Rudick RA, Medendorp SV, *et al.* Low-dose (7.5 mg) oral methotrexate reduces the rate of progression in chronic progressive multiple sclerosis. *Ann Neurol* 1995;37:30–41.

212. Wolinsky JS, Narayana PA, O'Connor P, *et al.* Glatiramer acetate in primary progressive multiple sclerosis: results of a multinational, multicenter, double-blind, placebo-controlled trial. *Ann Neurol* 2007;61:14–24.

213. Hawker K, O'Connor P, Freedman MS, *et al.* Rituximab in patients with primary progressive multiple sclerosis. Results of a randomized double-blind placebo-controlled multicenter trial. *Ann Neurol* 2009;66:460–71.

214. Li DKB, Zhao GJ, Paty DW, the University of British Columbia MS/MRI Analysis Research Group, the SPECTRIMS Study Group. Randomized controlled trial of interferon-beta-1a in secondary progressive MS. MRI results. *Neurology* 2001;56:1505–13.

215. Weiner HL, Cohen JA. Treatment of multiple sclerosis with cyclophosphamide: critical review of clinical and immunologic effects. *Mult Scler* 2002;8:142–54.

216. Kappos L, Weinshenker B, Pozzilli C, *et al.* Interferon beta-1b in secondary progressive MS. A combined analysis of the two trials. *Neurology* 2004;63:1779–87.

217. Coyle PK, Johnson K, Pardo L, Stark Y. Pregnancy outcomes in patients with multiple sclerosis treated with glatiramer acetate (Copaxone). *Neurology* 2003;60(Suppl 1):A60.

218. Sandberg-Wollheim M, Frank D, Goodwin TM, *et al.* Pregnancy outcomes during treatment with interferon beta-1a in patients with multiple sclerosis. *Neurology* 2005;65:802–6.

219. Amato MP, Portaccio E, Ghezzi A, *et al.* Pregnancy and fetal outcomes after interferon-β exposure in multiple sclerosis. *Neurology* 2010;75:1794–802.

220. Gadoth N. Multiple sclerosis in children. *Brain Dev* 2003;25:229–32.

221. Banwell BL. Pediatric multiple sclerosis. *Current Neurology and Neuroscience Reports* 2004;4:245–52.

222. Boiko A, Vorobeychik G, Paty D, *et al.* Early onset multiple sclerosis. A longitudinal study. *Neurology* 2002;59:1006–10.

223. Tenembaum S, Martin S, Fejeman N. Disease modifying therapies in childhood and juvenile multiple sclerosis (abstract). *Mult Scler* 2001;7(Suppl 1):S57.

224. Waubant E, Hietpas J, Stewart T, *et al.* Interferon beta-1a in children with multiple sclerosis is well tolerated. *Neuropediatrics* 2001;32:211–3.

225. Kornek B, Bernert G, Balassy C, *et al.* Glatiramer acetate treatment in patients with childhood and juvenile onset multiple sclerosis. *Neuropediatrics* 2003;34:120–6.

226. Pohl D, Rostasy K, Gartner J, Hanefeld F. Treatment of early onset multiple sclerosis with subcutaneous interferon beta-1a. *Neurology* 2005;64:888–90.

227. Banwell B, Reder AT, Krupp L, *et al.* Safety and tolerability of interferon beta-1b in pediatric multiple sclerosis. *Neurology* 2006;66:472–6.

228. Ghezzi A, Amato MP, Capobianco M, *et al.* Treatment of early-onset multiple sclerosis with intramuscular interferonβ-1a:long-term results. *Neurological Science* 2007;28:127–32.

229. Mikaeloff Y, Caridade G, Tardieu M, Suissa S, on behalf of the KIDSEP study group of rhe French Neuropediatric Society. Effectiveness of early beta interferon on the first attack after confirmed multiple sclerosis: A comparative study. *Eur J Paediatric Neurol* 2008;12:205–9.

230. Huppke P, Stark W, Zurcher C, *et al.* Natalizumab use in pediatric multiple sclerosis. *Arch Neurol* 2008;65:1655–8.

231. Makhani N, Gorman MP, Branson HM, *et al.* Cyclophosphamide therapy in pediatric multiple sclerosis. *Neurology* 2009;72:2076–82.

232. Yeh EA, Chitnis T, Krupp L, *et al.* Pediatric multiple sclerosis. *Nature Reviews Neurology* 2009;5:621–31.

233. Minden SL, Frankel D, Hadden LS, Srinath KP, Perloff JN. Disability in elderly people with multiple sclerosis: An analysis of baseline data from the Sonya Slifka Longitudinal Multiple Sclerosis study. *Neurorehabilitation* 2004;19:55–67.

234. Cree BAC, Al-Sabbagh A, Bennett R, Goodin D. Response to interferon beta-1a treatment in African American multiple sclerosis patients. *Arch Neurol* 2005;62:1681–3.

235. Moore L, Kaufman M, Conway J. Response to mitoxantrone for secondary progressive multiple sclerosis in African Americans compared with whites. *Int J MS Care* 2010;12: 156–9.

236. Kister I, Chamot E, Niewczyk PM, *et al.* Rapid disease course in African Americans with multiple sclerosis. *Neurology* 2010;75:217–23.

237. Saida T, Tashiro K, Itoyama Y, *et al.* Interferon beta-1b is effective in Japanese RRMS patients. A randomized, multicenter study. *Neurology* 2005;64:621–30.

Chapter

52

Treatment for patients with primary progressive multiple sclerosis

Zhaleh Khaleeli and Alan J. Thompson

Introduction

Until recently, treatment for primary progressive multiple sclerosis (PPMS) has been a neglected area in the field of trials in multiple sclerosis (MS). This is at least partly due to the relative rarity of PPMS, but the atypical characteristics of this group have also presented difficulties for the design of and recruitment to therapeutic trials. However, many of these problems have now been addressed by the introduction of specific diagnostic criteria, a better understanding of natural history, and advances in measuring outcome. Although no treatment has yet been proved to be effective in modifying the disease course of PPMS, several randomized controlled trials have now been completed, and further Phase 3 trials are under way. This chapter reviews all the therapeutic trials in PPMS to date, but first discusses the characteristics of PPMS and the implementation of therapeutic trials in this group.

Characteristics of primary progressive multiple sclerosis

Approximately 10%–15% of patients with MS have a primary progressive course, characterized by a continuous accumulation of neurological deficit from onset, without relapse or remission.[1] The clinical presentation is most commonly motor, with progressive spastic paraparesis,[2] whereas relapsing–remitting MS (RRMS) usually has a visual or sensory presentation. Relatively more men are affected resulting in a loss of the usual female preponderance. The mean age of presentation of PPMS is later than in RRMS. Previous work has suggested that onset age is similar to that of the progressive phase in secondary progressive MS (SPMS),[3,4] but a large-scale follow-up study over 25 years has suggested that age of onset in SPMS is, in fact, significantly later.[5] Taken as a group, the rate of disease progression in patients with PPMS is similar to patients with SPMS,[3,6,7] but within the PPMS population there is a wide variation in progression rate.[8]

There are two other classifications, no longer in use, which have been applied to patients with predominantly progressive disease but in whom relapses have occurred: progressive relapsing MS (PRMS) and transitional progressive MS (TPMS).

PRMS is characterized by progressive disease from onset, with superimposed relapses.[9] TPMS has been defined as a single relapse before or after the onset of disease progression.[10] Over a quarter of patients with PPMS have been reported to experience a relapse even two or three decades after onset, although the relapse is usually mild.[11] PRMS and TPMS appear to be similar to PPMS,[10–13] and should probably be considered together with PPMS.

Magnetic resonance imaging (MRI) in PPMS shows a more marked discrepancy between the extent of MRI activity and the severity of disability than in other groups. Patients with PPMS have a paucity of focal lesions, less gadolinium (Gd)-enhancement and fewer new lesions developing over time compared with RRMS and SPMS.[14,15] However, the smaller lesions seen in PPMS may be more destructive,[16] and diffuse signal abnormality may be more common in PPMS.[17] Using quantitative MRI techniques, structural changes have been demonstrated in normal-appearing brain tissue (NABT) in PPMS. Many of these changes are similar to those seen in SPMS;[18] however, it has been suggested that changes in the spinal cord are more marked in PPMS.[19]

The MRI characteristics of PPMS are in keeping with the findings from pathological examination. White matter lesions are less numerous[20] and less inflammatory than in SPMS,[21] which may result in less acute axonal injury.[22] A unique pattern of oligodendrocyte degeneration in PPMS was postulated,[23] but this concept has been successfully challenged.[24,25] Pathological examination of normal-appearing white matter in PPMS has revealed diffuse inflammation and axonal injury, similar to that seen in SPMS, but more extensive than in RRMS.[20] Cortical demyelination is a characteristic feature in progressive MS.[26] While remyelination has been demonstrated in all MS subtypes,[27] it appears that primary progressive patients have a greater capacity for remyelination than patients with SPMS.[28] Differences in immunological and genetic characteristics have been suggested though no distinct profiles have been established.[29,30]

Whether these differences indicate that PPMS is a distinct clinical entity or just one end of the disease spectrum of MS has been a source of debate. The important question with regard to therapeutics is whether there is a fundamental difference in

Multiple Sclerosis Therapeutics, Fourth Edition, ed. Jeffrey A. Cohen and Richard A. Rudick. Published by Cambridge University Press.
© Cambridge University Press 2011.

Table 52.1. *Diagnostic criteria for primary progressive multiple sclerosis*

Clinical presentation: Insidious neurological progression suggestive of MS
1 year of disease progression AND Two out of three of the following: • Evidence for DIS in the brain based on ≥ 1 T2+ lesions in at least one area characteristic for MS • Positive spinal cord MRI (2 T2 lesions) • Positive CSF

MRI, magnetic resonance imaging; CSF, cerebrospinal fluid; DIS, dissemination in space.
Adapted from Polman, 2010[43]

the mechanisms underlying neurological deficit in a predominantly progressive disease compared with relapsing disease.[31] The pathological substrate of irreversible neurological deficit is considered to be axonal loss.[32] In RRMS the mechanism of axonal loss appears to be related to acute focal inflammatory demyelination,[33] whereas in PPMS axonal loss is associated with a mild but diffuse and chronic inflammatory process,[20] and this process in the spinal cord has been directly correlated with disability.[34] Therapeutic agents directed at axonal protection or repair may be particularly useful in PPMS, although inflammation clearly occurs and hence trials of anti-inflammatory agents are also justified.

Implementation of therapeutic trials

The atypical characteristics of PPMS have presented problems in the recruitment to and design of therapeutic trials.[35] Particular problem areas have included diagnostic criteria, sample size calculations, and choice of outcome measures. As there is no proven treatment for PPMS, it is still ethical to carry out placebo-controlled trials, and the challenges in trial design currently faced in RRMS are not yet an issue.[36]

Diagnostic criteria

Before initiating treatment in any patient group, a secure diagnosis should be made, and historically this has been difficult in PPMS. Until recently, diagnostic criteria for MS did not adequately address PPMS, and so hindered recruitment to therapeutic trials.[35,37] To facilitate the diagnosis of PPMS, specific diagnostic criteria were developed in 2000.[38] Three levels of diagnostic certainty were defined – definite, probable, and possible – based on clinical, cerebrospinal fluid (CSF), MRI, and neurophysiological findings. Evidence of intrathecal immunoglobulin (IgG) synthesis was an essential criterion for a definite diagnosis together with one of the following MRI criteria: (1) nine brain lesions, (2) two spinal cord lesions, or (3) four to eight brain lesions and one spinal cord lesion. New diagnostic criteria for MS published in 2001 incorporated the criteria for PPMS with some simplification, in that only two levels of diagnostic certainty – possible MS

and definite MS – were included.[39] Recent revisions, which have been utilized in the latest clinical trials,[40] have dropped the requirement for CSF evidence, provided that MRI criteria are met (Table 52.1).[41] However, CSF results remain crucial in the diagnosis of patients not meeting the MRI criteria. Furthermore, it has been suggested that RRMS criteria may be reliably applied in the diagnosis of PPMS if CSF findings remain an optional part of the diagnostic criteria.[42] This has been incorporated into the newly revised diagnostic criteria for PPMS which will require a progressive course, and two of the following: (1) imaging satisfying the new simplified brain MRI criteria; (2) two or more cord lesions; and (3) positive CSF.[43]

Sample size calculations and patient selection

To determine the sample size and duration of a therapeutic trial in PPMS, knowledge of the natural history of disease progression is required. Recent studies have substantially extended the available data on disease progression in PPMS.[5,44,45] Sample size tables which can be used to plan future therapeutic trials have been developed from the largest of these studies.[46] However, they confirm that large multicenter trials with several hundred patients per treatment group are required. In view of the relative rarity of PPMS, it is therefore important that treatment trials are planned according to international consensus so that patient resources are optimally utilized. Further data on which to base the design of future trials are provided by the large Phase 3 trials of glatiramer acetate and rituximab in PPMS.[40,47] These data have emphasized the importance of selecting patients in whom therapeutic gains are easier to identify. In the fingolimod study in PPMS which is currently recruiting (INFORMS; NCT00731692: see below), younger, mobile patients with shorter disease duration and evidence of recent progression are being selected, as they will be more likely to progress during the study.

Outcome measures

In any definitive therapeutic trial in MS, the primary outcome measure must be clinical, conventionally assessing relapses and disease progression.[36] In PPMS the assessment of relapses is not applicable, so clinical outcome measures must evaluate disease progression. MRI measures are widely used as surrogate markers of disease activity in MS and may be used as primary outcomes in exploratory trials or as secondary outcomes in definitive trials in RRMS and SPMS. The validity of MRI measures in PPMS has been less clear, but there is now evidence that MRI changes in the short-term are predictive of disability in the longer term in PPMS.[48,49] Changes in the NABT may provide a more sensitive alternative to conventional measures, particularly over shorter time spans.[50]

Immunological markers of disease activity may have a role in therapeutic monitoring in the future but as yet there are no well-validated immunological markers of disease progression in PPMS.

Clinical outcome measures

The most widely used measure of clinical disease progression has been the Expanded Disability Status Scale (EDSS).[51] This scale is not linear, so changes at different levels have different degrees of clinical impact.[52] A particular issue in PPMS is the poor responsiveness of the scale,[53] because disease progression is gradual and small changes may be clinically important. The Multiple Sclerosis Functional Composite (MSFC), which incorporates quantitative tests of arm, leg, and cognitive function, was developed in an attempt to provide a more responsive and multidimensional outcome measure.[54] Some studies have found the MSFC to be more sensitive than the EDSS,[54] and the timed walking test (TWT) component may be a particularly useful measure in PPMS, where limitation in mobility is often the prime indicator of progression in the early stages;[40,56] however, other studies suggest that MSFC responsiveness remains limited in PPMS, and that more extensive investigation is required.[57] Recent work has explored improving the use of the scale by defining cut-off values and worsening,[58] including a measure of vision, and standardizing the calculation of Z scores.[59] It has also been suggested that combining the TWT and EDSS could further improve responsiveness.[60]

Patient-based outcome measures have also been developed in MS.[61,62] In PPMS small changes in functioning are detectable over just nine months using the MSIS-29,[63] a scale which correlates to some extent with physician-rated measures, but may also provide complementary information.[64] The MSIS-29 has been tested in a population-based study,[65] and in clinical trial settings.[66]

Finally, a number of health-related quality of life measures have been developed for use in MS; however, to date they have been included in studies on RR and SPMS patients only.[67]

MRI outcome measures

Therapeutic trials in RRMS and SPMS conventionally assess Gd-enhancement and T2 lesions on brain imaging. Initially, it was assumed that the low level of Gd-enhancement and new lesion formation in PPMS would limit the usefulness of these measures. However, enhancement may be present in a proportion of patients, particularly early on in disease development,[68] and overall T2 lesion load is a responsive measure over one year.[69] Short-term changes in T2 lesion load have been shown to correlate with the evolution of disability over three years,[50] and to predict clinical outcome over five years,[49] although in the longer term the impact may decline.[45] The location of T2 lesions may also be important in determining progression.[70] Disappointingly, T1 lesions, which are thought to reflect more severe tissue destruction,[71] and are more common in progressive MS subtypes,[72] do not correlate with disability in PPMS.[10,73] Conventional spinal cord imaging may be expected to be more relevant as, clinically, cord involvement often predominates in PPMS, but no relationship is seen between cord lesions and disability.[10,69]

Measures of atrophy may be valid markers of disease progression in PPMS. Spinal cord cross-sectional area correlates strongly with disability in MS, and shows detectable change within one year.[69,74] Spinal cord atrophy in the short term may predict clinical outcome in the longer term and an association with clinical progression is seen over five years.[49,73] Similarly, brain atrophy is detectable within one year, and associations with disability and clinical progression are also seen.[10,73,75,76] Early changes in brain volume may be relevant to long-term disability,[45] but the relationship between brain volume loss and clinical deterioration is not linear.[50] As disease progression in PPMS may occur independently of focal lesions, MRI measures that can quantify changes in NABT may be particularly useful in this group. Such measures include magnetization transfer ratio imaging (MTR), ^{1}H magnetic resonance spectroscopy (MRS), and diffusion MRI. MTR is a robust technique that can be used to quantify diffuse tissue damage either globally or compartmentally. Abnormalities in MTR have been identified in PPMS in both brain and spinal cord.[77] MTR changes in the brain have been shown to predict disability over one year,[78] and to correlate with the evolution of disability over three years.[50] Clinically eloquent MTR changes have been localized to specific areas of the brain in PPMS.[79] Further investigation in larger natural history studies and therapeutic trials will be needed to establish the role of MTR as a therapeutic marker in PPMS.

^{1}H MRS can also be used to evaluate diffuse injury, in particular axonal damage through measurement of N-acetyl aspartate (NAA). NAA is reduced in lesions and NABT in PPMS,[80,81] but studies on the PROMiSe trial cohort did not demonstrate a relationship with clinical change over three years.[82] Abnormalities in diffusion MRI have been identified in the brain and spinal cord in PPMS,[83–85] have been shown to progress over time[86] and to correlate with clinical worsening over five years.[87]

In addition to establishing validity and responsiveness, potential therapeutic outcome measures must be proved to be reliable. This is particularly important in PPMS, as its relative rarity necessitates the involvement of multiple centers in definitive trials. MRI measures should be shown to be robust across centers, and while this process has begun for some image modalities,[88] further work is needed. Finally, using a combination of MRI parameters may be the optimal way to assess outcome, and there has been interest in creating scoring systems based on this principle.[89,90]

Therapeutic agents

Although there is no definitively proven disease-modifying treatment available for PPMS, several randomized controlled trials have now been specifically designed for this group. These include trials of all the licensed disease-modifying treatments for RRMS and SPMS (with the exception of natalizumab), the evidence for which is discussed elsewhere in this book. In addition, several trials have been carried out in progressive MS without necessarily making a clear distinction between primary and secondary progressive disease. The available treatment data specifically relating to PPMS are now reviewed.

Clinical trials in PPMS

Glatiramer acetate

The PROMiSe trial, a multi-national, double-blind, placebo-controlled trial of glatiramer acetate, is the largest trial in PPMS to date.[47] Nine hundred and forty-three patients were enrolled at centers in North America and Europe. Patients were randomized to receive subcutaneous glatiramer acetate 20 mg or placebo, in a 2:1 ratio, daily for three years. The primary end-point was the time to progression sustained over three months on the EDSS. Secondary clinical outcomes measures included the MSFC. MRI measures included cerebral lesion loads, Gd-enhancing lesions, brain volume, cervical cord atrophy, and ^{1}H MRS.

Treatment in this study was prematurely discontinued by the data safety monitoring committee as an interim analysis concluded that the study would not reach statistical significance. Patients were taken off the study medication but were given the opportunity to complete the three-year follow-up. At the time of study discontinuation, 757 patients had completed at least two years on study or terminated prematurely. No significant effect on progression was detected, and a recent Cochrane Systematic review, based on this and a study in secondary progressive MS,[91] concluded that the "therapy is not suitable for progressive MS" (http://www.ncbi.nlm.nih.gov/pubmed/14974077). However, a significant delay in progression was identified in a post-hoc subgroup analysis of treated male patients in the PROMiSe trial, perhaps detectable due to a faster background progression rate in males. A smaller increase in T2 lesion volume in the treated group was also identified.[47,92]

The PROMiSe trial also provides a large resource of data on the natural history of disease progression in PPMS. Patients with higher EDSS at entry progressed faster, and entry MSFC also predicted progression.[93] A unique feature of this study was that evidence of intrathecal IgG synthesis was sought for all subjects and was absent in approximately 20%, thus providing information about the patient characteristics according to CSF status. At study entry, patients with negative CSF had less inflammatory activity on MRI,[93] but no relationship between CSF status and treatment outcome has been mentioned in the trial results.

Rituximab

Rituximab is a monoclonal antibody that binds to CD20 antigen on B-cells and induces B-cell apoptosis. A multicenter double-blind placebo-controlled trial of rituximab in 439 patients with PPMS was recently completed.[40] Subjects were randomized to receive four two-week cycles of intravenous rituximab at a dose of 1 g, or placebo, over 96 weeks. The time to confirmed disease progression, which was the primary end-point, was increased in the treated group, but this result reached significance only in two subsets of patients: those aged less than 51, and those with

Gd-enhancing lesions identified at baseline. Secondary end-points were increase in T2 lesion load between baseline and week 96, which was significantly lower in the treated group; and change in brain volume on MRI, which did not differ between the groups. Patients in the treated arm showed significantly less mobility decline over the study period on the TWT, which was included as an exploratory outcome.

Planned clinical trials in PPMS

Fingolimod (FTY720)

Fingolimod is a sphingosine 1-phosphate receptor modulator, which inhibits migration of T-cells from lymphoid tissue into the peripheral circulation. While it is therefore primarily an anti-inflammatory agent, in vitro studies have suggested that fingolimod may also influence CNS remyelination.[94] Phase 3 studies have established the efficacy of the drug, which is administered orally, in RRMS, and a double-blind placebo-controlled trial in PPMS is currently recruiting (INFORMS; NCT00731692). It is estimated that 654 patients will be recruited and followed for three years, and the main outcome measure will be the time to sustained disability progression.

Cladribine

In a double-blind, placebo-controlled trial of subcutaneous cladribine (2-chlorodeoxyadenosine) in progressive MS, 4806159 patients enrolled had PPMS.[95] No clinical efficacy was apparent. A significant treatment effect on enhancing lesions was reported for the whole cohort, but was not seen on subgroup analysis of the primary progressive group.

In the wake of the positive Phase 3 trial of oral cladribine in RRMS (CLARITY) a similar study in early PPMS is currently being planned.

Smaller trials in PPMS

Interferon beta-1a

An exploratory double-blind, placebo-controlled study of intramuscular interferon beta-1a was the first randomized controlled trial to be specifically designed for PPMS.[96] Fifty patients were randomized to receive interferon beta-1a 30 mcg, 60 mcg, or placebo weekly for two years. The primary end-point was time to sustained progression over three months on the EDSS. Secondary clinical outcome measures included the Nine-Hole Peg Test and timed 10-Meter Walk. MRI measures included cerebral and spinal cord lesion loads, new lesions, spinal cord and cerebral atrophy, MTR, and ^{1}H MRS.

Forty-nine subjects completed follow-up. The 30 mcg dose was well tolerated but the 60 mcg dose was poorly tolerated due to flu-like reactions and raised liver enzymes. There were seven treatment withdrawals and a further seven dose reductions. No effect was seen on disease progression on the EDSS or the timed 10-Meter Walk, although there was a non-significant trend favoring interferon beta-1a 30 mcg on the Nine-Hole

Peg Test. There was also a suggestion of a treatment effect on T2 lesion load favoring interferon beta-1a 30 mcg. Subjects on interferon beta-1a 60 mcg had a worse outcome on a measure of ventricular enlargement but the results in this group were difficult to interpret due to the large proportion of treatment withdrawals. No treatment effect was seen on the other secondary MRI outcome measures. Although this study provides some evidence to support a Phase 3 study, the advisability of carrying out such a trial is unclear.

Interferon beta-1b

A double-blind, placebo-controlled trial of subcutaneous interferon beta-1b 8 MIU on alternate days for two years in 73 patients, 49 with PPMS and 24 with TPMS, was carried out.[97] The primary end-point was time to progression sustained for six months on the EDSS. Secondary clinical outcome measures included the MSFC, Ashworth scale, Beck depression scale, and Krupp fatigue scale. MRI outcome measures included cerebral lesion loads, new lesions, brain volume, cervical cord area, MTR, and ^{1}H MRS.

Seventy-three patients completed follow-up and a further three patients withdrew from treatment. There were no serious adverse events but interferon beta-1b was associated with flu-like syndrome, leukopenia, and injection-site reactions. No treatment effect was seen on EDSS progression, but there was a significant difference on the MSFC favoring interferon beta-1b. Significant differences in T2 and T1 lesion loads and new T2 lesions also favored interferon beta-1b. There was no treatment effect on spinal cord area or brain volume.

A recent Cochrane Systematic Review based on the two interferon studies concluded that the populations studied were too small to allow definitive conclusions on the efficacy of treatment, and that larger phase III studies were required (Cochrane Database Syst Rev. 2009;(1):CD006643).

Mitoxantrone

A double-blind, placebo-controlled trial of mitoxantrone 12 mg/m^2 given intravenously every three months for two years in 61 patients with PPMS, has been carried out.[98] The study examined several clinical and MRI outcomes. Preliminary analysis indicated no benefit on clinical outcomes,[99] full results have not been published. Immunological analysis of a small subgroup suggested that only two patients with Gd-enhancing lesions mounted a significant response to the drug.[100] An open label study which included seven PPMS patients suggested that mitoxantrone may halt further clinical deterioration,[101] but this was not supported by a retrospective analysis which included 25 PPMS patients treated with mitoxantrone.[102]

Riluzole

Glutamate excitotoxicity has been proposed as a mechanism of neuronal damage in MS.[103] Riluzole is a potentially neuroprotective agent which acts through inhibition of glutamate transmission. A small open-label study of riluzole was carried out in 16 patients with PPMS.[104] Subjects received no treatment for the first year and riluzole 50 mg twice a day for the second year. The primary outcome measure was cervical spinal cord area. EDSS and T1 and T2 lesion loads were secondary outcome measures. Non-significant trends for a reduction in spinal cord atrophy and T1 hypointense lesion accrual were reported. There were several limitations to this study, and further evaluation would be required to determine efficacy.

Trials which include patients with PPMS

A number of smaller exploratory studies have included patients with PPMS, but caution is required when interpreting some of these results due to methodological limitations and the small numbers involved.

A retrospective open-label study of intravenous cyclophosphamide and methylprednisolone in progressive MS included 128 patients with PPMS. While 73.5% of PPMS subjects clinically stabilized over one year,[105] the design of the study precludes any meaningful conclusions. No benefit from cyclophosphamide was reported in smaller placebo-controlled trials or open-label studies in progressive MS.[106,107] While a double-blind trial of azathioprine, which included 51 patients PPMS demonstrated a small therapeutic effect overall,[108] this benefit was not apparent in the PPMS subgroup. Twenty-two patients with PPMS were included in a retrospective observational study of autologous hematopoietic stem cell transplantation.[109] In the PPMS group progression-free survival was 66% at three years with two deaths. A larger, retrospective analysis in 178 MS patients, including 32 with PPMS, showed stabilization of neurological condition in 63% overall, with no difference in outcome in the PPMS subgroup.[110] Beneficial effects were seen in the PPMS subgroup in a double-blind, placebo-controlled trial of intravenous immunoglobulin in progressive MS.[111] However, of 231 patients in the study only 34 had PPMS, and this relatively small number prevents firm conclusions being drawn from the data. While methotrexate demonstrated a beneficial effect on progression in patients with chronic progressive MS in a double-blind, placebo-controlled trial, a significant benefit could not be demonstrated in the small subgroup of 18 patients with PPMS.[112] A small open-label study of pirfenidone also reported clinical stabilization in progressive MS over one year, but no subgroup analysis of the seven PPMS patients included was presented.[113]

A randomized, double-blind placebo controlled trial of tetrahydrocannabinol, derived from cannabis, is currently under way. The compound is postulated to be a neuroprotective agent which can prevent disability progression.[114] Four hundred and ninety-three participants with progressive MS have been recruited to the three-year study, and results are expected in 2012 (http://sites.pcmd.ac.uk/cnrg/cupid.php).

Future therapeutic approaches

Most therapeutic agents investigated to date in MS have targeted focal inflammation, and it is now emerging that anti-inflammatory medications may have a role in addressing the accumulation of disability in RRMS.[115,116] While these treatments are unlikely to have the same impact in progressive patients,[117] there may be a good rationale for treatments targeting diffuse inflammation, such as phosphodiesterase inhibitors.[116] These compounds may also act by other mechanisms to protect neurons, and their development is part of a new focus in MS therapeutics towards neuronal protection and repair. PPMS is the ideal model in which to study progression and its treatment, because disease progression appears to occur largely independently of focal inflammation.[118] A trial of idebenone, a synthetic form of coenzyme Q10 which is thought to promote remyelination, is currently recruiting patients with PPMS for a Phase 1/2 study for this reason (NCT00950248). Stem cell therapy in MS has generated a great deal of interest, and exploratory trials in progressive patients are now being considered.[119] Such strategies will be facilitated by new approaches in therapeutic monitoring and the development of markers of neural recovery. Functional MRI, which may provide information about neural adaptation and recovery in response to damage, is one potential approach. Using functional MRI, cortical reorganization has been shown to occur in the brain in PPMS,[120,121] and changes have been identified in the spinal cord,[122] although its suitability as a therapeutic marker is yet to be established. Further advances in imaging the spinal cord,[123] the use of new sequences and high field MR to study gray matter lesions,[124,125] and the optimization of clinical outcome measures, will be crucial in developing and testing treatments in PPMS.

Conclusions

Therapeutics in PPMS can no longer be considered a neglected area. Several randomized controlled trials, including Phase 3 trials of glatiramer acetate and rituximab, have now been completed. Although no treatment is yet proven to be effective, the feasibility of carrying out trials in PPMS is now well established, and common pitfalls in investigating this group are now understood. More sensitive and reliable markers of disease progression are being developed to facilitate future therapeutic trials. A better understanding of the pathophysiology of PPMS is required to guide the development of therapeutic agents to target specific pathogenic mechanisms. PPMS may be the ideal model in which to investigate disease progression and neuronal protection, and is becoming an important focus for treatment trials in these areas. It is hoped that, in future editions of this book, treatment for PPMS will not be confined to a single chapter.

References

1. Thompson AJ, Polman CH, Miller DH, et al. Primary progressive multiple sclerosis. *Brain* 1997;120(6):1085–96.

2. Miller DH, Leary SM. Primary-progressive multiple sclerosis. *Lancet Neurol* 2007;6(10):903–12.

3. Kremenchutzky M, Rice GP, Baskerville J, Wingerchuk DM, Ebers GC. The natural history of multiple sclerosis: a geographically based study 9: observations on the progressive phase of the disease. *Brain* 2006;129(Pt 3):584–94.

4. Confavreux C, Vukusic S. Age at disability milestones in multiple sclerosis. *Brain* 2006;129(Pt 3):595–605.

5. Tremlett H, Zhao Y, Devonshire V. Natural history comparisons of primary and secondary progressive multiple sclerosis reveals differences and similarities. *J Neurol* 2009;256(3):374–81.

6. Minderhoud JM, Van Der Hoeven JH, Prange AJ. Course and prognosis of chronic progressive multiple sclerosis. Results of an epidemiological study. *Acta Neurol Scand* 1988;78(1):10–15.

7. Confavreux C, Vukusic S. Natural history of multiple sclerosis: a unifying concept. *Brain* 2006;129(3):606–16.

8. Tremlett H, Paty D, Devonshire V. The natural history of primary progressive MS in British Columbia, Canada. *Neurology* 2005;65(12):1919–23.

9. Lublin FD, Reingold SC. Defining the clinical course of multiple sclerosis: results of an international survey. National Multiple Sclerosis Society (USA) Advisory Committee on Clinical Trials of New Agents in Multiple Sclerosis. *Neurology* 1996;46(4):907–11.

10. Stevenson VL, Miller DH, Rovaris M, et al. Primary and transitional progressive MS: a clinical and MRI cross-sectional study. *Neurology* 1999;52(4):839–45.

11. Kremenchutzky M, Cottrell D, Rice G, et al. The natural history of multiple sclerosis: a geographically based study. 7. Progressive–relapsing and relapsing–progressive multiple sclerosis: a re-evaluation. *Brain* 1999;122(10):1941–50.

12. Gayou A, Brochet B, Dousset V. Transitional progressive multiple sclerosis: a clinical and imaging study. *J Neurol Neurosurg Psychiatry* 1997;63(3):396–8.

13. Andersson PB, Waubant E, Gee L, Goodkin DE. Multiple sclerosis that is progressive from the time of onset: clinical characteristics and progression of disability. *Arch Neurol* 1999;56(9):1138–42.

14. Thompson AJ, Kermode AG, MacManus DG, et al. Patterns of disease activity in multiple sclerosis: clinical and magnetic resonance imaging study. *BMJ* 1990;300(6725):631–4.

15. Thompson AJ, Kermode AG, Wicks D, et al. Major differences in the dynamics of primary and secondary progressive multiple sclerosis. *Ann Neurol* 1991;29(1):53–62.

16. Meier DS, Weiner HL, Guttmann CR. MR imaging intensity modeling of damage and repair in multiple sclerosis: relationship of short-term lesion recovery to progression and disability. *Am J Neuroradiol* 2007;28(10):1956–63.

17. Nijeholt GJ, van Walderveen MA, Castelijns JA, et al. Brain and spinal cord abnormalities in multiple sclerosis. Correlation between MRI

parameters, clinical subtypes and symptoms. *Brain* 1998;121(4):687–97.

18. Filippi M, Rovaris M, Rocca MA. Imaging primary progressive multiple sclerosis: the contribution of structural, metabolic, and functional MRI techniques. *Mult Scler* 2004;10 (Suppl 1):S36–S44.

19. Agosta F, Absinta M, Sormani MP, *et al.* In vivo assessment of cervical cord damage in MS patients: a longitudinal diffusion tensor MRI study. *Brain* 2007;130(8):2211–19.

20. Kutzelnigg A, Lucchinetti CF, Stadelmann C, *et al.* Cortical demyelination and diffuse white matter injury in multiple sclerosis. *Brain* 2005;128(11):2705–12.

21. Revesz T, Kidd D, Thompson AJ, Barnard RO, McDonald WI. A comparison of the pathology of primary and secondary progressive multiple sclerosis. *Brain* 1994;117(4):759–65.

22. Bitsch A, Schuchardt J, Bunkowski S, Kuhlmann T, Bruck W. Acute axonal injury in multiple sclerosis. Correlation with demyelination and inflammation. *Brain* 2000;123(6):1174–83.

23. Lucchinetti C, Bruck W, Parisi J, Scheithauer B, Rodriguez M, Lassmann H. Heterogeneity of multiple sclerosis lesions: implications for the pathogenesis of demyelination. *Ann Neurol* 2000;47(6):707–17.

24. Barnett MH, Prineas JW. Relapsing and remitting multiple sclerosis: pathology of the newly forming lesion. *Ann Neurol* 2004;55(4):458–68.

25. Breij EC, Brink BP, Veerhuis R, *et al.* Homogeneity of active demyelinating lesions in established multiple sclerosis. *Ann Neurol* 2008;63(1):16–25.

26. Kutzelnigg A, Faber-Rod JC, Bauer J, *et al.* Widespread demyelination in the cerebellar cortex in multiple sclerosis. *Brain Pathol* 2007;17(1):38–44.

27. Patrikios P, Stadelmann C, Kutzelnigg A, Rauschka H, Schmidbauer M, Laursen H, *et al.* Remyelination is extensive in a subset of multiple sclerosis patients. *Brain* 2006;129(12):3165–72.

28. Bramow S, Frischer JM, Lassmann H, *et al.* Demyelination versus remyelination in progressive multiple sclerosis. *Brain* 2010;133(10):2983–98.

29. Neuhaus O, Hartung HP. In search of a disease marker: the cytokine profile of

primary progressive multiple sclerosis. *Mult Scler* 2001;7(3):143–4.

30. Stankovich J, Butzkueven H, Marriott M, *et al.* HLA-DRB1 associations with disease susceptibility and clinical course in Australians with multiple sclerosis. *Tissue Antigens* 2009;74(1):17–21.

31. Thompson A. Overview of primary progressive multiple sclerosis (PPMS): similarities and differences from other forms of MS, diagnostic criteria, pros and cons of progressive diagnosis. *Mult Scler* 2004;10 (Suppl 1):S2–S7.

32. Trapp BD, Peterson J, Ransohoff RM, Rudick R, Mork S, Bo L. Axonal transection in the lesions of multiple sclerosis. *N Engl J Med* 1998;338(5):278–85.

33. Ferguson B, Matyszak MK, Esiri MM, Perry VH. Axonal damage in acute multiple sclerosis lesions. *Brain* 1997;120(3):393–9.

34. Tallantyre EC, Bo L, Al-Rawashdeh O, *et al.* Clinico-pathological evidence that axonal loss underlies disability in progressive multiple sclerosis. *Mult Scler* 2010;16(4):406–11.

35. Leary SM, Stevenson VL, Miller DH, Thompson AJ. Problems in designing and recruiting to therapeutic trials in primary progressive multiple sclerosis. *J Neurol* 1999;246(7):562–8.

36. McFarland HF, Reingold SC. The future of multiple sclerosis therapies: redesigning multiple sclerosis clinical trials in a new therapeutic era. *Mult Scler* 2005;11(6):669–76.

37. McDonnell GV, Hawkins SA. Application of the Poser criteria in primary progressive multiple sclerosis. *Ann Neurol* 1997;42(6):982–3.

38. Thompson AJ, Montalban X, Barkhof F, *et al.* Diagnostic criteria for primary progressive multiple sclerosis: a position paper. *Ann Neurol* 2000;47(6):831–5.

39. McDonald WI, Compston A, Edan G, *et al.* Recommended diagnostic criteria for multiple sclerosis: guidelines from the International Panel on the diagnosis of multiple sclerosis. *Ann Neurol* 2001;50(1):121–7.

40. Hawker K, O'Connor P, Freedman MS, *et al.* Rituximab in patients with primary progressive multiple sclerosis: results of a randomized double-blind placebo-controlled multicenter trial. *Ann Neurol* 2009;66(4):460–71.

41. Polman CH, Reingold SC, Edan G, *et al.* Diagnostic criteria for multiple sclerosis: 2005 revisions to the "McDonald Criteria". *Ann Neurol* 2005;58(6):840–6.

42. Montalban X, Sastre-Garriga J, Filippi M, *et al.* Primary progressive multiple sclerosis diagnostic criteria: a reappraisal. *Mult Scler* 2009;15(12): 1459–65.

43. Polman CH, Reingold SC, Banwell B, *et al.* Diagnostic Criteria for Multiple Sclerosis: 2010 Revisions to the "McDonald Criteria *Ann Neurol* 2011;69:292–302.

44. Degenhardt A, Ramagopalan SV, Scalfari A, Ebers GC. Clinical prognostic factors in multiple sclerosis: a natural history review. *Nat Rev Neurol* 2009;5(12):672–82.

45. Khaleeli Z, Ciccarelli O, Manfredonia F, *et al.* Predicting progression in primary progressive multiple sclerosis: a 10-year multicenter study. *Ann Neurol* 2008;63(6):790–3.

46. Cottrell DA, Kremenchutzky M, Rice GP, Hader W, Baskerville J, Ebers GC. The natural history of multiple sclerosis: a geographically based study. 6. Applications to planning and interpretation of clinical therapeutic trials in primary progressive multiple sclerosis. *Brain* 1999;122(4):641–7.

47. Wolinsky JS, Narayana PA, O'Connor P, *et al.* Glatiramer acetate in primary progressive multiple sclerosis: results of a multinational, multicenter, double-blind, placebo-controlled trial. *Ann Neurol* 2007;61(1):14–24.

48. Stevenson VL, Ingle GT, Miller DH, Thompson AJ. Magnetic resonance imaging predictors of disability in primary progressive multiple sclerosis: a 5-year study. *Mult Scler* 2004;10(4):398–401.

49. Sastre-Garriga J, Ingle GT, Rovaris M, *et al.* Long-term clinical outcome of primary progressive MS: predictive value of clinical and MRI data. *Neurology* 2005;65(4):633–5.

50. Khaleeli Z, Altmann DR, Cercignani M, Ciccarelli O, Miller DH, Thompson AJ. Magnetization transfer ratio in gray matter: a potential surrogate marker for progression in early primary progressive multiple sclerosis. *Arch Neurol* 2008;65(11):1454–9.

51. Kurtzke JF. Rating neurologic impairment in multiple sclerosis: an

expanded disability status scale (EDSS). *Neurology* 1983;33(11):1444–52.

52. Twork S, Wiesmeth S, Spindler M, *et al.* Disability status and quality of life in multiple sclerosis: non-linearity of the Expanded Disability Status Scale (EDSS). *Health Qual Life Outcomes* 2010;8:55.

53. Hobart J, Freeman J, Thompson A. Kurtzke scales revisited: the application of psychometric methods to clinical intuition. *Brain* 2000;123(5):1027–40.

54. Cutter GR, Baier ML, Rudick RA, *et al.* Development of a multiple sclerosis functional composite as a clinical trial outcome measure. *Brain* 1999;122(5):871–82.

55. Cohen JA, Cutter GR, Fischer JS, *et al.* Use of the multiple sclerosis functional composite as an outcome measure in a phase 3 clinical trial. *Arch Neurol* 2001;58(6):961–7.

56. Montalban X. Overview of European pilot study of interferon beta-Ib in primary progressive multiple sclerosis. *Mult Scler* 2004;10 (Suppl 1):S62–4.

57. Kragt JJ, Thompson AJ, Montalban X, *et al.* Responsiveness and predictive value of EDSS and MSFC in primary progressive MS. Neurology 2008;70: 1084–91.

58. Bosma LV, Kragt JJ, Brieva L, *et al.* Progression on the Multiple Sclerosis Functional Composite in multiple sclerosis: what is the optimal cut-off for the three components? *Mult Scler* 2010;16(7):862–7.

59. Polman CH, Rudick RA. The multiple sclerosis functional composite: a clinically meaningful measure of disability. *Neurology* 2010;74 (Suppl 3):S8–15.

60. Bosma LV, Kragt JJ, Brieva L, *et al.* The search for responsive clinical endpoints in primary progressive multiple sclerosis. *Mult Scler* 2009;15(6):715–20.

61. Hobart J, Lamping D, Fitzpatrick R, Riazi A, Thompson A. The Multiple Sclerosis Impact Scale (MSIS-29): a new patient-based outcome measure. *Brain* 2001;124(5):962–73.

62. Hobart JC, Riazi A, Lamping DL, Fitzpatrick R, Thompson AJ. Measuring the impact of MS on walking ability: the 12-Item MS Walking Scale (MSWS-12). *Neurology* 2003;60(1):31–6.

63. Hobart JC, Riazi A, Lamping DL, Fitzpatrick R, Thompson AJ. How

responsive is the Multiple Sclerosis Impact Scale (MSIS-29)? A comparison with some other self report scales. *J Neurol Neurosurg Psychiatry* 2005;76(11):1539–43.

64. Costelloe L, O'Rourke K, McGuigan C, Walsh C, Tubridy N, Hutchinson M. The longitudinal relationship between the patient-reported Multiple Sclerosis Impact Scale and the clinician-assessed Multiple Sclerosis Functional Composite. *Mult Scler* 2008;14(2):255–8.

65. Gray O, McDonnell G, Hawkins S. Tried and tested: the psychometric properties of the multiple sclerosis impact scale (MSIS-29) in a population-based study. *Mult Scler* 2009;15(1):75–80.

66. Giordano A, Pucci E, Naldi P, *et al.* Responsiveness of patient reported outcome measures in multiple sclerosis relapses: the REMS study. *J Neurol Neurosurg Psychiatry* 2009;80(9):1023–8.

67. Miller D, Rudick RA, Hutchinson M. Patient-centered outcomes: translating clinical efficacy into benefits on health-related quality of life. *Neurology* 2010;74 (Suppl 3):S24-35.

68. Khaleeli Z, Ciccarelli O, Mizskiel K, Altmann D, Miller DH, Thompson AJ. Lesion enhancement diminishes with time in primary progressive multiple sclerosis. *Mult Scler* 2010;16(3):317–24.

69. Stevenson VL, Miller DH, Leary SM, *et al.* One year follow up study of primary and transitional progressive multiple sclerosis. *J Neurol Neurosurg Psychiatry* 2000;68(6):713–18.

70. Bodini B, Battaglini M, De SN, *et al.* T2 lesion location really matters: a 10 year follow-up study in primary progressive multiple sclerosis. *J Neurol Neurosurg Psychiatry* 2010;82:72–7.

71. van Walderveen MA, Kamphorst W, Scheltens P, *et al.* Histopathologic correlate of hypointense lesions on T1-weighted spin-echo MRI in multiple sclerosis. *Neurology* 1998;50(5):1282–8.

72. van Walderveen MA, Lycklama ANG, Ader HJ, *et al.* Hypointense lesions on T1-weighted spin-echo magnetic resonance imaging: relation to clinical characteristics in subgroups of patients with multiple sclerosis. *Arch Neurol* 2001;58(1):76–81.

73. Ingle GT, Stevenson VL, Miller DH, Thompson AJ. Primary progressive

multiple sclerosis: a 5-year clinical and MR study. *Brain* 2003;126(11): 2528–36.

74. Losseff NA, Webb SL, O'Riordan JI, *et al.* Spinal cord atrophy and disability in multiple sclerosis. A new reproducible and sensitive MRI method with potential to monitor disease progression. *Brain* 1996;119(3):701–8.

75. Fox NC, Jenkins R, Leary SM, *et al.* Progressive cerebral atrophy in MS: a serial study using registered, volumetric MRI. *Neurology* 2000;54(4):807–12.

76. Sastre-Garriga J, Ingle GT, Chard DT, *et al.* Grey and white matter volume changes in early primary progressive multiple sclerosis: a longitudinal study. *Brain* 2005;128(6):1454–60.

77. Rovaris M, Judica E, Sastre-Garriga J, *et al.* Large-scale, multicentre, quantitative MRI study of brain and cord damage in primary progressive multiple sclerosis. *Mult Scler* 2008;14:455–64.

78. Khaleeli Z, Sastre-Garriga J, Ciccarelli O, Miller DH, Thompson AJ. Magnetisation transfer ratio in the normal appearing white matter predicts progression of disability over 1 year in early primary progressive multiple sclerosis. *J Neurol Neurosurg Psychiatry* 2007;78(10):1076–82.

79. Khaleeli Z, Cercignani M, Audoin B, Ciccarelli O, Miller DH, Thompson AJ. Localized grey matter damage in early primary progressive multiple sclerosis contributes to disability. *Neuroimage* 2007;37(1):253–61.

80. Suhy J, Rooney WD, Goodkin DE, *et al.* 1H MRSI comparison of white matter and lesions in primary progressive and relapsing-remitting MS. *Mult Scler* 2000;6(3):148–55.

81. Sastre-Garriga J, Ingle GT, Chard DT, *et al.* Metabolite changes in normal-appearing gray and white matter are linked with disability in early primary progressive multiple sclerosis. *Arch Neurol* 2005;62(4):569–73.

82. Sajja BR, Narayana PA, Wolinsky JS, Ahn CW. Longitudinal magnetic resonance spectroscopic imaging of primary progressive multiple sclerosis patients treated with glatiramer acetate: multicenter study. *Mult Scler* 2008;14(1):73–80.

83. Agosta F, Benedetti B, Rocca MA, *et al.* Quantification of cervical cord pathology in primary progressive MS

using diffusion tensor MRI. *Neurology* 2005;64(4):631–5.

84. Ciccarelli O, Werring DJ, Wheeler-Kingshott CA, *et al.* Investigation of MS normal-appearing brain using diffusion tensor MRI with clinical correlations. *Neurology* 2001;56(7):926–33.

85. Filippi M, Cercignani M, Inglese M, Horsfield MA, Comi G. Diffusion tensor magnetic resonance imaging in multiple sclerosis. *Neurology* 2001; 56(3):304–11.

86. Rovaris M, Gallo A, Valsasina P, *et al.* Short-term accrual of gray matter pathology in patients with progressive multiple sclerosis: an in vivo study using diffusion tensor MRI. *Neuroimage* 2005;24(4):1139–46.

87. Rovaris M, Judica E, Gallo A, *et al.* Grey matter damage predicts the evolution of primary progressive multiple sclerosis at 5 years. *Brain* 2006;129(10):2628–34.

88. Barker GJ, Schreiber WG, Gass A, *et al.* A standardised method for measuring magnetisation transfer ratio on MR imagers from different manufacturers–the EuroMT sequence. *MAGMA* 2005;18(2):76–80.

89. Bakshi R, Neema M, Healy BC, *et al.* Predicting clinical progression in multiple sclerosis with the magnetic resonance disease severity scale. *Arch Neurol* 2008;65(11):1449–53.

90. Poonawalla AH, Datta S, Juneja V, *et al.* Composite MRI scores improve correlation with EDSS in multiple sclerosis. *Mult Scler* 2010;16(9):1117–25.

91. Bornstein MB, Miller A, Slagle S, *et al.* A placebo-controlled, double-blind, randomized, two-center, pilot trial of Cop 1 in chronic progressive multiple sclerosis. *Neurology* 1991;41(4):533–9.

92. Wolinsky JS, Shochat T, Weiss S, Ladkani D. Glatiramer acetate treatment in PPMS: why males appear to respond favorably. *J Neurol Sci* 2009;286(1–2):92–8.

93. Wolinsky JS. The PROMiSe trial: baseline data review and progress report. *Mult Scler* 2004;10(Suppl 1): S65–71.

94. Miron VE, Jung CG, Kim HJ, Kennedy TE, Soliven B, Antel JP. FTY720 modulates human oligodendrocyte progenitor process extension and survival. *Ann Neurol* 2008;63(1):61–71.

95. Rice GP, Filippi M, Comi G. Cladribine and progressive MS: clinical and MRI outcomes of a multicenter controlled trial. Cladribine MRI Study Group. *Neurology* 2000;54(5):1145–55.

96. Leary SM, Miller DH, Stevenson VL, Brex PA, Chard DT, Thompson AJ. Interferon beta-1a in primary progressive MS: an exploratory, randomized, controlled trial. *Neurology* 2003;60(1):44–51.

97. Montalban X, Sastre-Garriga J, Tintore M, *et al.* A single-center, randomized, double-blind, placebo-controlled study of interferon beta-1b on primary progressive and transitional multiple sclerosis. *Mult Scler* 2009;15(10):1195–205.

98. Stuve O, Kita M, Pelletier D, *et al.* Mitoxantrone as a potential therapy for primary progressive multiple sclerosis. *Mult Scler* 2004;10 (Suppl 1):S58–61.

99. Kita M, Cohen JA, Fox RJ. A phase II trial of mitoxantrone in patients with primary progressive multiple sclerosis. *Neurology* 2004. 62(Suppl 5):A99.

100. Pelfrey CM, Cotleur AC, Zamor N, Lee JC, Fox RJ. Immunological studies of mitoxantrone in primary progressive MS. *J Neuroimmunol* 2006;175(1–2):192–9.

101. Hellwig K, Schimrigk S, Lukas C, *et al.* Efficacy of mitoxantrone and intrathecal triamcinolone acetonide treatment in chronic progressive multiple sclerosis patients. *Clin Neuropharmacol* 2006;29(5):286–91.

102. Debouverie M, Taillandier L, Pittion-Vouyovitch S, Louis S, Vespignani H. Clinical follow-up of 304 patients with multiple sclerosis three years after mitoxantrone treatment. *Mult Scler* 2007;13(5):626–31.

103. Pitt D, Werner P, Raine CS. Glutamate excitotoxicity in a model of multiple sclerosis. *Nat Med* 2000;6(1):67–70.

104. Kalkers NF, Barkhof F, Bergers E, van SR, Polman CH. The effect of the neuroprotective agent riluzole on MRI parameters in primary progressive multiple sclerosis: a pilot study. *Mult Scler* 2002;8(6):532–3.

105. Zephir H, de SJ, Duhamel A, *et al.* Treatment of progressive forms of multiple sclerosis by cyclophosphamide: a cohort study of 490 patients. *J Neurol Sci* 2004;218(1–2):73–7.

106. Weiner HL, Cohen JA. Treatment of multiple sclerosis with cyclophosphamide: critical review of clinical and immunologic effects. *Mult Scler* 2002;8(2):142–54.

107. Schwartzman RJ, Simpkins N, Alexander GM, *et al.* High-dose cyclophosphamide in the treatment of multiple sclerosis. *CNS Neurosci Therap* 2009;15(2):118–27.

108. Double-masked trial of azathioprine in multiple sclerosis. *British and Dutch Multiple Sclerosis Azathioprine Trial Group. Lancet* 1988;2(8604):179–83.

109. Fassas A, Passweg JR, Anagnostopoulos A, *et al.* Hematopoietic stem cell transplantation for multiple sclerosis. A retrospective multicenter study. *J Neurol* 2002;249(8):1088–97.

110. Saccardi R, Kozak T, Bocelli-Tyndall C, *et al.* Autologous stem cell transplantation for progressive multiple sclerosis: update of the European Group for Blood and Marrow Transplantation autoimmune diseases working party database. *Mult Scler* 2006;12(6):814–23.

111. Pohlau D, Przuntek H, Sailer M, *et al.* Intravenous immunoglobulin in primary and secondary chronic progressive multiple sclerosis: a randomized placebo controlled multicentre study. *Mult Scler* 2007;13(9):1107–17.

112. Goodkin DE, Rudick RA, VanderBrug MS, *et al.* Low-dose (7.5 mg) oral methotrexate reduces the rate of progression in chronic progressive multiple sclerosis. *Ann Neurol* 1995;37(1):30–40.

113. Bowen JD, Maravilla K, Margolin SB. Open-label study of pirfenidone in patients with progressive forms of multiple sclerosis. *Mult Scler* 2003;9(3):280–3.

114. Zajicek JP, Sanders HP, Wright DE, *et al.* Cannabinoids in multiple sclerosis (CAMS) study: safety and efficacy data for 12 months follow up. *J Neurol Neurosurg Psychiatry* 2005;76(12):1664–9.

115. Jones JL, Anderson JM, Phuah CL, *et al.* Improvement in disability after alemtuzumab treatment of multiple sclerosis is associated with neuroprotective autoimmunity. *Brain* 2010;133(8):2232–47.

116. Barkhof F, Hulst HE, Drulovic J, Uitdehaag BM, Matsuda K, Landin R. Ibudilast in relapsing–remitting

multiple sclerosis: a neuroprotectant? *Neurology* 2010;74(13):1033–40.

117. Coles A, Deans J, Compston A. Campath-1H treatment of multiple sclerosis: lessons from the bedside for the bench. *Clin Neurol Neurosurg* 2004;106(3):270–4.

118. Matthews PM. Primary progressive multiple sclerosis takes centre stage. *J Neurol Neurosurg Psychiatry* 2004;75(9):1232–3.

119. Martino G, Franklin RJ, Van Evercooren AB, Kerr DA. Stem cell transplantation in multiple sclerosis: current status and future prospects. *Nat Rev Neurol* 2010;6(5):247–55.

120. Ciccarelli O, Toosy AT, Marsden JF, *et al.* Functional response to active and passive ankle movements with clinical correlations in patients with primary progressive multiple sclerosis. *J Neurol* 2006;253(7):882–91.

121. Ceccarelli A, Rocca MA, Valsasina P, *et al.* Structural and functional magnetic resonance imaging correlates of motor network dysfunction in primary progressive multiple sclerosis. *Eur J Neurosci* 2010;31(7):1273–80.

122. Agosta F, Valsasina P, Absinta M, Sala S, Caputo D, Filippi M. Primary progressive multiple sclerosis: tactile-associated functional MR

activity in the cervical spinal cord. *Radiology* 2009;253(1):209–15.

123. Bakshi R, Thompson AJ, Rocca MA, *et al.* MRI in multiple sclerosis: current status and future prospects. *Lancet Neurol* 2008;7(7):615–25.

124. Calabrese M, Rocca MA, Atzori M, *et al.* Cortical lesions in primary progressive multiple sclerosis: a 2-year longitudinal MR study. *Neurology* 2009;72(15):1330–6.

125. Gilmore C, Geurts J, Evangelou N, *et al.* Spinal cord grey matter lesions in multiple sclerosis detected by post-mortem high field MR imaging. *Mult Scler* 2009;15(2):180–8.

Chapter

53

Diagnosis, pathogenesis, and treatment of neuromyelitis optica (NMO) spectrum disorders

Sean J. Pittock

NMO and the evolving spectrum of water channel autoimmunity

Water channels are a newly recognized target for central nervous system (CNS), inflammatory autoimmune demyelinating diseases. Neuromyelitis optica (NMO; aka optic spinal multiple sclerosis) is a devastating disease that disproportionally affects non-Caucasians. It is characterized by recurrent episodes of optic neuritis and transverse myelitis, which may result in blindness and paraplegia. It is frequently misdiagnosed as multiple sclerosis (MS). NMO is the first MS-like disease for which a specific antigen has been identified – the astrocytic water channel aquaporin-4 (AQP4). This discovery represents a seismic shift from historic emphasis on the oligodendrocyte and myelin to the astrocyte. An autoantibody specific for AQP4 (NMO/AQP4-IgG) is a clinically validated serum biomarker that distinguishes relapsing NMO from MS. MS has no distinguishing biomarker and calls for different therapies.

The traditional view-Devic's disease

In 1894, Devic reported a case of combined optic neuritis and myelitis that was fatal and provided a review of 16 similar cases from the literature.[1] The syndrome that Devic described was a monophasic illness characterized by both bilateral optic neuritis and transverse myelitis occurring at the same time. The lack of involvement of the brain was emphasized. Over the following 100 years, many investigators reported single cases or case series of patients with variations on this theme. It became increasingly recognized that patients may have (1) unilateral rather then bilateral optic neuritis, and (2) interval of weeks to years between attacks of optic neuritis and myelitis rather then simultaneous onset. Subsequently it was recognized that NMO was a relapsing disease in at least 80% of cases. Investigators put forward diagnostic criteria for NMO, all of which emphasized restriction of clinical symptoms and signs to the optic nerves and spinal cord and a normal brain MRI.[2–4] Longitudinally extensive T2 signal abnormalities spanning three or more vertebral segments were reported to be characteristic of NMO, a situation rarely found in MS where lesions (at least in adults) are generally asymmetric and short. Over this period of time, NMO or Devic's syndrome was considered by most to be a variant of MS.

The new perspective-NMO and water channel autoimmunity

In 2004, Lennon and colleagues discovered a novel biomarker for NMO.[5] This biomarker, an autoantibody named "NMO-IgG" was reported to be 73% sensitive and 91% specific for NMO as defined by the 1999 Wingerchuk criteria.[4,5] Discovery that the target antigen of NMO-IgG, defining a clinical spectrum of NMO-related disorders was AQP4 the most abundant water channel in the CNS, indicated a new direction in CNS demyelinating disease research.[6] Since then a combination of clinical, pathological, radiological, and serological observations in the last six years have clearly distinguished NMO and its partial or inaugural forms (constituting a spectrum of NMO-related disorders) from classical MS and other MS variants for which no specific biomarkers are recognized. The NMO of today represents a relapsing spectrum of disease that is not necessarily restricted to the optic nerves and spinal cord and is very different from the monophasic disorder in which near simultaneous bilateral optic neuritis and transverse myelitis occur as was originally described by Devic.[1,7] These differences are further highlighted by the contrasting prevalences of NMO-IgG in relapsing (>80%) vs. monophasic (<13%) NMO.[8] Perhaps relapsing NMO and the monophasic illness described by Devic are in fact different diseases?

Epidemiology and genetics

Patients who have NMO are often initially misdiagnosed and treated as "severe MS" (Mayo NMO Consortium, unpublished observations). NMO, however, is a discrete relapsing demyelinating disease with clinical, neuroimaging, and laboratory findings that distinguish it from MS (Table 53.1). Relapsing NMO affects women nine times more frequently than men. The median age of onset is 39, about 10 years older than for MS. NMO also occurs in very young and very elderly patients. The prevalence of NMO spectrum disorders

Multiple Sclerosis Therapeutics, Fourth Edition, ed. Jeffrey A. Cohen and Richard A. Rudick. Published by Cambridge University Press.
© Cambridge University Press 2011.

Table 53.1. *Definitions and characteristics of multiple sclerosis and neuromyelitis optica*

	Multiple sclerosis	**Neuromyelitis optica**
Definition	Central nervous system symptoms and signs indicating involvement of the white matter tracts. Evidence of dissemination in space and time on the basis of clinical or MRI findings. No better explanation	Transverse myelitis and optic neuritis. At least two of the following: brain MRI, non-diagnostic for MS; spinal cord lesion extending over three or more vertebral segments; or seropositive for NMO-IgG.
Clinical onset and course	85% relapsing–remitting 15% primary-progressive Not monophasic	Onset always with relapse 80–90% relapsing course 10–20% monophasic course
Median age of onset (years)	29	39
Sex (F:M)	2:1	9:1
Secondary progressive course	Common	Rare
MRI: brain	Periventricular white matter lesions	Usually normal or non-specific white matter lesions; 10% unique hypothalamic, corpus callosal, periventricular, or brain stem lesions
MRI: spinal cord	Short-segment peripheral lesions	Longitudinally extensive ($\geq$3 vertebral segments) central lesions
CSF white blood cell number and differential count	Mild pleocytosis Mononuclear cells	Occasional prominent pleocytosis Polymorphonuclear cells and mononuclear cells
CSF oligoclonal bands	85%	15–30%

From: Wingerchuk DM, Lennon VA, Lucchinetti CF, Pittock SJ, Weinshenker BG. The spectrum of neuromyelitis optica. [Review.] *Lancet Neurol* 2007; 6:805–15.[7]

Table 53.2. *Comparison of 1999 and 2006 diagnostic criteria for NMO*

Absolute criteria (all required)	
1999	2006 "New"
1. Optic neuritis	1. Optic neuritis
2. Acute myelitis	2. Acute myelitis
3. No clinical disease outside of optic nerve and spinal cord	

Diagnosis additionally requires	
One major *or* two minor	At least two of three supportive criteria

Supportive criteria	
Major	
1. Negative brain MRI at disease onset	1. Negative brain MRI at onset
2. Spinal cord MRI with contiguous T2 weighted signal abnormality $\geq$ 3 vertebral segments	2. Spinal cord MRI with contiguous T2 weighted signal abnormality extending over 3 or more vertebral segments
3. CSF pleocytosis >50x10^6 leukocytes or >5x10^6 neutrophils/L	3. NMO IgG seropositivity
Minor	
1. Bilateral optic neuritis	
2. Severe optic neuritis with fixed visual acuity worse than 20/200 in at least one eye.	
3. Severe, fixed, attack-related weakness (MCR grade $\leq$ 2 in 1 or more limbs)	

From: Pittock SJ. Neuromyelitis optica: a new perspective. *Semin Neurol* 2008; 28(1):95–104.[9]

is currently unknown. In North America, a majority of recognized NMO cases are Caucasian, but by comparison with the MS population, non-Caucasian ethnicities (African, Hispanic, Asian, American Indian) are significantly over-represented.[7,9] In Japan, NMO is known as "optic-spinal multiple sclerosis" (OSMS), and accounts for 20%–30% of all "MS" cases.[10–15] In a French Afro-Caribbean natural history study of CNS demyelinating disease on the island of Martinique, 17.3% of cases had an NMO phenotype.[16] A Nigerian hospital-based study (1957 to 1969) identified 95 cases of NMO and only 2 cases of MS; the investigators estimated the prevalence of NMO to be 43/100 000 of the general Nigerian population.[17] This extraordinary report that NMO accounts for 98% of CNS demyelinating disorders encountered in Africa warrants contemporary re-investigation. In São Paulo, Brazil, a study of 67 consecutive patients diagnosed with MS reported that 30% actually had NMO.[18] These

frequencies are likely an under-representation of the true frequency of NMO because they are based on outdated clinical and radiologic criteria,[4] more restrictive than applied in contemporary diagnosis of NMO spectrum disorders (Table 53.2).[19] Ethnic differences in the frequency of NMO spectrum disorders support the importance of genetic predisposing factors.[7]

The reported familial cases are mainly restricted to siblings (mostly sisters).[20–23] Familial cases account for at least 3% of NMO. A recent report of 12 multiplex NMO pedigrees with a total of 25 affected individuals found familial NMO was more common than would be expected from its frequency in the general population and was indistinguishable clinically and serologically from sporadic NMO.[24] Taken together, these data suggest complex genetic susceptibility in NMO. Reported major histocompatibility complex (MHC) associations of NMO are not persuasive. The high frequency of the HLA DPB1*0501 allele in the general population of Japan makes it difficult to interpret the significance of this haplotype's high frequency in Asian NMO.[13] A recent study reported a negative association between the presence of HLA-DRB1* 1501 and NMO (odds ratio 0.57) which was in contrast to the positive association in MS (OR 3.93).[25] These data suggest different MHC-based genetic susceptibilities for NMO and MS, but larger more definitive studies are required.

A recent study reported screening of 110 NMO cases (106 NMO-IgG positive) for potential coding mutations in AQP4. They detected mutations at Arg19 in 1.8% of NMO patients but not in controls subjects. The authors speculated that this missense mutation may augment formation of AQP4 macromolecular aggregates through alteration of AQP4 M1 isoform properties.[26]

Clinical features, course; and prognosis

NMO is a severe, inflammatory, demyelinating disorder characterized by recurrent attacks of optic neuritis (single > bilateral) or longitudinally extensive transverse myelitis which may occur either simultaneously sequantially, or in isolation.[7] The course of the disease can be monophasic (20%) or relapsing (80%).[4] Approximately 60% of patients have a relapse within the first year after onset and 90% after 3 years.[19]

Relapses of NMO (optic neuritis and longitudinally extensive transverse myelitis) have onset over days and then slowly improve over weeks to months. Unlike MS, recovery from attacks is usually incomplete and patients develop incremental attack-related disability. The prognosis of untreated NMO is significantly worse than that of MS. Fifty percent of patients with NMO are blind in one or both eyes or have paraplegia requiring the need for a wheelchair within five years of disease onset.[4] A poor prognosis is associated with frequent early attacks.[7] In contrast to MS, where most disability results from the progressive phase of the illness, disability in NMO is attack related and a secondary progressive course is rare.[27] About 30% of untreated NMO patients will be dead within five years from onset. Death occurs most commonly from neurogenic respiratory failure due to a high cervical cord/lower medullary lesion.[7] With early diagnosis followed by immediate initiation of immunosuppressant or antibody depleting agents, it is likely that a more favorable outcome, than the natural history described above, can be expected. Clinical features relating to brain involvement in NMO is discussed under the "Neuroimaging (Brain)" section.

NMO AQP4-IgG

First biomarker for any form of inflammatory CNS demyelinating disease

NMO (AQP4)-IgG selectively binds to the abluminal face of CNS microvessels (Fig. 53.1(a)), and colocalizes with the extracellular matrix protein laminin, Fig. 53.1(b)), pia (Fig. 53.1(c)) and subpia (Fig. 53.1(c)) in a distribution that paralleled the immunocomplex deposition previously reported by Lucchinetti and colleagues in spinal cord NMO lesions.[29] Within two years of Lennon and colleagues' *Lancet* paper, multiple independent international investigators confirmed these observations and validated NMO-IgG as a highly specific biomarker with specificities between 91% and 100% for distinguishing NMO or NMO spectrum disorders from MS and other inflammatory CNS diseases.[29–34] The inclusion of NMO-IgG in the 2006 revised diagnostic criteria for NMO (Table 53.2) was justified on the basis of these findings.

The distribution of immunoreactivity of NMO-IgG in distal collecting tubules of the kidney (Fig. 53.1(d)) and in the basolateral membranes of gastric mucosal epithelium (Fig. 53.1(e)) led to the identification of potential candidate antigens, including the water channel protein AQP4. Subsequent experiments confirmed AQP4 to be the target of NMO-IgG. These experiments included demonstration of (1) NMO-IgG colocalization with AQP4 in mouse tissues by dual staining (Fig. 53.1(c), (d), and (e)), (2) lack of immunoreactivity of patients' serum (containing NMO-IgG) on tissues from a AQP4 transgenic knockout mouse, (3) demonstration that NMO-IgG bound selectively to membranes of AQP4-transfected cells, and (4) NMO-IgG immunoprecipitates green fluorescent protein-AQP4 but not related dystroglycan complex proteins.[6]

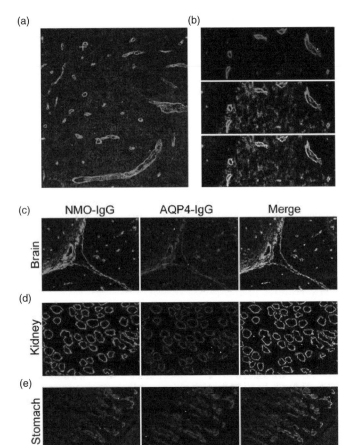

Fig. 53.1. (From Hinson *et al.*, *Neuroscience* 2010; 168: 1009–18 with permission).
Pattern of NMO–IgG binding to mouse tissues. Dual immunofluorescence staining of mouse tissues. (a) Spinal cord: NMO–IgG (green) in a patient's serum binds to the abluminal face of microvessels; endothelium binds rabbit-IgG-specific for factor VIII (red) (× 400). (b) Cerebellar cortex: NMO–IgG (green) colocalizes with extracellular matrix protein laminin (red) around microvessels (i.e. at the blood–brain barrier), and also binds to astrocytic mesh in the granular layer (Lennon *et al.*, 2004[5]). Colocalization of NMO–IgG (green) and AQP4 (red) in brain (c), in distal renal collecting tubules (d) and gastric parietal cells (e) (Lennon *et al.*, 2005[6]) (see also color plate section).

AQP4-the immune target in NMO

AQP4 is widely distributed in multiple organ systems and is the most abundant water channel in the CNS.[36] AQP4, a homotetrameric protein, is anchored by the dystroglycan protein complex in the plasma membrane of astrocytes and is highly concentrated in their foot processes abutting microvessels at the blood–brain barrier (BBB), surrounding synapses and nodes of Ranvier.[36,37] It is also highly expressed in the subpial and subependymal zones[38] and in the hypothalamus. AQP4 protein is expressed as two major polypeptides of 30 and 32 kDa in length, which arise from two different translation-initiating methionines, M23 and M1. Multiple tetramers of AQP4 assemble in the plasma membrane in a well-organized structure called orthogonal arrays of particles (OAPs).[39] Freeze–fracture studies demonstrated that the expression ratio of M1 and M23 isoforms is the major determinant of the size of OAPs. Formation of stable and large OAPs requires the expression of AQP4-M23 whereas coexpression of the M1 and M23 isoforms leads to OAPs of different sizes, depending on the ratio of the two isoforms.[40] M1 does not form OAPs alone and expression of M1 limits OAP formation. The immunobiologic implications of NMO-IgG binding to these different AQP4 combinations remains to be elucidated but is likely important in understanding NMO pathogenesis.

AQP4 is involved in the development, function, and integrity of the interface between the brain and blood and between the brain and cerebrospinal fluid.[41] It plays a critical role in controlling the extracellular environment through regulation of water movement accompanying potassium (K^+) fluxes and perisynaptic glutamate homeostasis.[36,42] It is involved in brain edema formation in the context of trauma, water intoxication, ischemia, infection, and tumor.[36,38,43,44]

NMO-IgG detection-immunoassays

In current clinical practice, the indirect immunofluorescence assay test is approximately 60% sensitive for both adults and children with relapsing NMO,[5,8,45] 25% sensitive for relapsing optic neuritis, and 52% sensitive for recurrent longitudinally extensive myelitis.[5] Several international groups have confirmed the specificity of the NMO/AQP4-IgG biomarker (defined by immunofluorescence on mammalian tissue substrates) for distinguishing NMO spectrum disorders from other acquired CNS demyelinating disorders (MS spectrum).[32,34,46,47] Recent clinical correlative studies have reported application of alternative tests employing the specific AQP4 protein, either green fluorescent protein-tagged in dual fluorescence imaging of transfected cell lines or solubilized in immunoprecipitation assays (green fluorescent protein-tagged or radiolabeled).[48] Some investigators have reported higher sensitivities for immunoprecipitation, cell-binding assays and enzyme-linked immunosorbent assay compared with tissue-based immunofluorescence assays.[49–51] There is little doubt that as assay methodologies for detection of NMO-IgG are improved, the frequency of "seronegative NMO" will drop. It will be important to maintain high specificity. The true rate of seronegative NMO awaits optimization of these assays.

The prognostic value of NMO-IgG

NMO-IgG predicts a high likelihood of relapse

In addition to its use as a diagnostic tool, NMO-IgG also is useful as a prognostic tool. NMO-IgG is detected in up to 40% of patients with a single episode of longitudinally extensive transverse myelitis. Weinshenker and colleagues reported that five of nine seropositive patients with longitudinally extensive transverse myelitis had either a relapse of longitudinally extensive transverse myelitis or developed optic neuritis (and thus NMO) within a year of their initial attack.[52] This was in sharp contrast to the 14 NMO-IgG seronegative longitudinally extensive transverse myelitis patients, none of whom relapsed in the follow–up period. A similar finding was reported for both recurrent and isolated optic neuritis.[53,54] Matiello and colleagues reported that the frequency of NMO-IgG in a consecutive clinic based series of patients with first time optic neuritis, in whom NMO-IgG was ordered, was low at 5.5%.[53] For six patients with isolated optic neuritis who were positive for NMO-IgG, 50% developed relapse (one had optic neuritis, and two had longitudinally extensive transverse myelitis) a median of 18 months after their initial attack. Only one of 22 NMO-IgG-negative patients (4.5%) had a further event during the follow–up period, and this patient was subsequently diagnosed as MS. A multicenter European study recently reported a seropositive rate of 5.8% in acute monosymptomatic optic neuritis and an identical rate of relapse of 50% in seropositive patients.[55]

NMO-IgG and disease severity

Few available data correlate NMO/AQP4-IgG serum levels and disease severity. Studies published to date are based on low numbers of patients, all evaluated serologically by minimally validated academic laboratory-based methodologies, and clinically by disease severity scales designed for MS, not NMO. Consistent with a report by Tanaka and colleagues[56] we found that the final visual score for a cohort of NMO/AQP4-IgG-positive patients with recurrent optic neuritis was worse than that of NMO/AQP4-IgG-negative patients ($P = 0.02$).[54] Takahashi et al. reported that the AQP4-transfected cell binding immunofluorescence assay was more sensitive than the tissue-based immunofluorescence.[35] He reported higher NMO/AQP4-IgG values in six cases with blindness compared with 15 cases without blindness and noted a correlation between titer and extensive or large cerebral lesions on MRI. The lengths of spinal cord MRI lesions

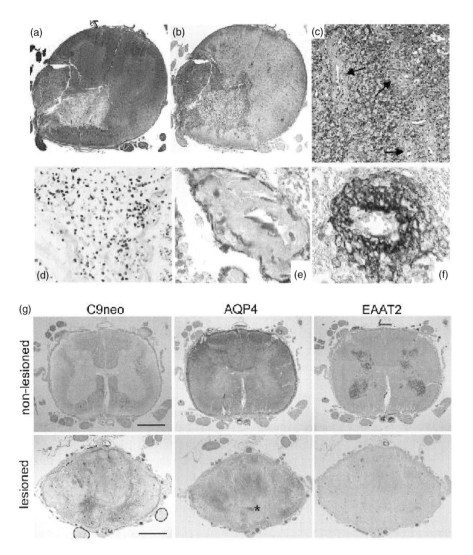

Fig. 53.2. (From Hinson *et al.*, *Neuroscience* 2010; 168: 1009–18 with permission) Histopathological characteristics of NMO lesions. (a) Spinal cord cross-sections demonstrate extensive demyelination involving both grey and white matter (Luxol fast blue and PAS myelin stain, mag 10 ×) and (b) infiltration of macrophages (KiM1p, pan-macrophage stain). (c) Thickened hyalinized blood vessels are prominent. (d) Eosinophils are prominent in the inflammatory infiltrate (haematoxylin-eosin, mag 100 ×). The terminal membrane attack complex of complement (C9neo antigen) is deposited around blood vessels in a "rim" (e) and "rosette" (f) pattern (Lucchinetti *et al.*, 2002[29]; Roemer *et al.*, 2007[59]). (g) Spinal cord sections from a single NMO–IgG-positive patient. Above: non-lesioned tissue, lumbar cord. Note lack of complement deposition (C9neo) and prominent AQP4 (brown stain) in both gray and white matter. EAAT2 (brown stain) is highly expressed in gray matter. Below: lesioned tissue, thoracic cord. Note prominence of C9neo deposition (brick red) in gray matter, corresponding to regions of AQP4 and EAAT2 loss in adjacent sections (Hinson *et al.*, 2008[48]). Asterisk indicates central canal. Scale bar = 200 μm (see also color plate section).

correlated positively with NMO/AQP4-IgG levels at peak exacerbation. However, despite median titers being different there was significant overlap in values raising concern for specificity. Another study reported that AQP4-IgG levels correlated with clinical disease activity in eight patients but high AQP4-IgG levels were not always associated with clinical relapse.[57] A recent Japanese paper reported detection of NMO/AQP4-IgG by ELISA assay with 71% sensitivity for NMO.[51] Correlation between NMO/AQP4-IgG level and disability (measured by the Expanded Disability Status Scale [EDSS])[58] was not persuasive (r squared 0.15, $P = 0.07$). We have not observed a strong correlation between NMO-AQP4-IgG titer and disease activity, but a preliminary study found that a functional assay measuring the % AQP4-tranfected cells lesioned by complement was a better predictor of attack severity ($P = 0.005$) than antibody titer ($P = 0.09$).[28] Systematic study of large numbers of clinically well-characterized patients using clinically validated assays are currently under way and will help identify which laboratory-based measures of NMO-IgG levels or their functional effects are most predictive of disease severity.

Pathogenesis: Evidence that NMO-IgG is pathogenic

Immunopathology

Detailed immunopathologic evaluation of autopsied and biopsied CNS tissues from patients with NMO or NMO spectrum have shown significant difference when compared with MS. Prior to the identification of NMO-IgG, Lucchinetti and colleagues described the following immunopathological hallmarks of NMO: extensive demyelination and necrosis extending over multiple cord segments involving both gray and white matter (Fig. 53.2(a)); thickened and hyalinized intralesional blood vessels (Fig. 53.2(c)); active lesions with a vasculocentric deposition of immunoglobulin (IgG and IgM) and products of complement activation in a NMO typical "rim" (Fig. 53.2(e)) and "rosette" (Fig. 53.2(f)) pattern (where AQP4 is highly expressed at astrocytic endfeet); parenchymal edema and infiltration by lymphocytes, plasma cells, macrophages (Fig. 53.2(b)) as well as eosinophils (Fig. 53.2(d))

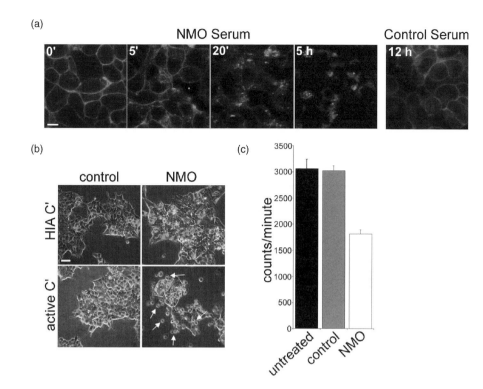

(a)

NMO Serum   Control Serum

0'   5'   20'   5 h   12 h

(b)

control   NMO

HIA C'

active C'

(c)

Fig. 53.3. (a) and (b) from Hinson *et al.*, Neurology 2007; 69:2221–31[42] with permission; (c) provided by Hinson and Lennon, Mayo Clinic (same image submitted for article in Continuum: Lifelong Learning in Neurology series on Autoimmune Myelopathy). Functional effects of NMO-IgG binding to the extracellular domain of AQP4 in living cell membranes. (a) Time-Lapse imaging of GFP tagged AQP4 in transfected HEK293 cells during 12 hours of exposure to NMO serum reveals reorganization and internalization, but not in control serum where AQP4 remains linear on the membrane. (b) Complement activation by NMO-IgG binding to AQP4 expressing HEK293 cells. Cells expressing GFP-AQP4 are shown in green. Untransfected (AQP4 deficient) cells are shown in gray. In the presence of control or NMO serum and heat-inactivated complement (HIA C'), cells remain in a monolayer. Addition of active complement (active C' in the presence of NMO, but not control, serum induces cell death indicated by rounding up and floating morphology (arrows). Only cells that express the GFP-AQP4 (green) are killed by NMO-IgG and complement. (c) Glutamate uptake is reduced in primary astrocytes after treatment with NMO patient serum. Untreated (black bar) and control (gray bar) treated cells uptake radiolabelled glutamate at approximately 3000 counts/minute. Treating the cells with NMO serum reduces glutamate uptake by approximately 50% (white bar) (see also color plate section).

and neutrophils.[29] These findings were interpreted by the authors to suggest a pathogenic role for humoral immunity with a target antigen in the perivascular area.

More recently, Roemer and colleagues' immunopathologic study of nine NMO cases showed that all had a unique pattern of AQP4 loss (Fig. 53.2(g)), middle) that was independent of stage of demyelination, site of lesion or degree of tissue necrosis.[60] In addition to AQP4 loss, there was also a striking loss of the excitatory amino acid transporter 2 (EAAT2, Fig. 53.2(g)). These changes precede demyelination. In contrast to NMO, in the early MS lesion AQP4 and EAAT2 are up-regulated.[59,60] The NMO typical immunopathologic findings recognized in the spinal cord lesions are identical to that seen in NMO brain lesions.[59]

In vitro evidence: AQP4 down-regulation, complement activation, EAAT2 down-regulation and blood–brain barrier disruption

In vitro data support a pathophysiological role for NMO-IgG as the principal effector of NMO.[42,48] Hinson *et al.* initially demonstrated the pathogenic potential of NMO/AQP4-IgG using non-neural cells transgenically expressing AQP4.[42] NMO patient serum IgG, but not IgM, bound to the extracellular domain of AQP4 and reversibly down-regulated its plasma membrane expression (Fig. 53.3(a)).[42] In the presence of complement, selective binding of patient IgG to surface AQP4 initiated robust complement activation and rapid loss of the target

membrane's integrity (Fig. 53.3(b)).[42] These findings were subsequently confirmed in cultured astrocytes.[48]

In addition to effects on the AQP4 protein itself, binding of NMO patient's IgG to surface epitopes of AQP4, in the absence of complement, caused EAAT2 (GLT–1), translocation from the cell surface to the endolysosomal pathway and reduced Na^+-dependent glutamate uptake by approximately 50% (Fig. 53.3(c)).[48] This was a very important finding as EAAT2 accounts for >90% reuptake of extracellular glutamate in the CNS.[61] Disruption of glutamate homeostasis by IgG would have greater excitotoxic potential for surrounding neurons and oligodendrocytes than for astrocytes which are relatively tolerant of increased glutamate concentrations. Focally increased glutamate levels secondary to IgG-induced down-regulation of AQP4-associated EAAT2 may be sufficient to injure or kill oligodendrocytes expressing Ca^{2+}–permeable glutamate receptors in the paranodal processes.[62,63] Modest elevation of extracellular glutamate concentration renders oligodendrocytes susceptible to immunoglobulin-independent (alternative pathway) complement attack.[64]

Using flow cytometry, Vincent *et al.* demonstrated that sera from NMO-IgG-positive patients reacted with CNS-derived human fetal astrocytes, whereas sera from MS patients did not.[65] Using an in vitro model of the BBB in which human fetal astrocytes were grown above a monolayer of human BBB-derived endothelial cells, they showed that NMO-IgG binding to astrocytes alters AQP4 polarized expression and increases permeability of a human BBB endothelium/astrocyte barrier. They showed that NK cells co–cultured with human fetal

Table 53.3. *Summary of study methods and outcomes*

Study methods	Post-IgG outcome	Control findings	Reference
NMO-serum injected four times intraperitoneally into rats at EAE[d] onset (MBP[c] immunization)	**Day 4:** • EAE[d] augmented • AQP4 and GFAP immunoreactivity loss, prominent around vessels • Deposition of human-IgG and rat complement products • Astrocyte damage/loss • Massive inflammation (macrophages, neutrophils, eosinophils) in gray matter	• No effect with IgG$_{MS}$ or IgG$_{normal}$	Kinoshita *et al.*[66]
AQP4-IgG$^+$ serum injected once intraperitoneally into rats at EAE[d] onset (intravenous MBP[c] T cells)	**Day 1:** • EAE[d] augmented • Loss of AQP4, GFAP[a] and S100β[a] around vessels • Deposition of human-IgG and rat complement • Mature astrocyte damage/loss • Lesional granulocytes and macrophages (not eosinophils) greatly increased	• Minor effect with IgG$_{NMO-AQP4-absorbed}$ • No effect with: IgG$_{seronegative-NMO}$ IgG$_{MS}$ IgG$_{other neurologic disorders}$ IgG$_{NMO}$ plus nonpathogenic T cells	Bradl *et al.*[67]
rAb$_{AQP4-specific}$[b], injected once intravenously into rats at EAE[d] onset (MBP[c] peptide immunization)	**Day 1.25:** • No EAE[d] augmentation recorded • Perivascular deposition of human IgG and rat-complement • Astrocyte depletion, myelin vacuolization	• No effect with: rAb$_{measles-specific}$ rAb$_{human-AQP4-specific}$	Bennett *et al.*[68]
AQP4-IgG$^+$ serum plus human complement injected 1–3 times into the right cerebral hemisphere in mice	**Hour 12:** • Ipsilateral AQP4 loss • Perivascular deposition of complement products • Myelin breakdown • Glial swelling • Axonal injury • Polymorphonuclear cells in vessels **Day 7:** • Contralateral visual-field neglect • Massive macrophage infiltration, extensive demyelination, reactive astrocyte loss, neuronal death, and perilesional gliosis	• No effect with: IgG$_{non-NMO control}$ IgG$_{NMO}$ into AQP4-null mice • Minor inflammation with IgG$_{NMO}$ plus complement inhibitor	Saadoun *et al.*[69]

[a] GFAP/S100β = astrocytic proteins.
[b] rAb$_{AQP4-specific}$ = recombinant monoclonal IgG derived from cerebrospinal fluid plasma cell in a patient with NMO.
[c] MBP = myelin basic protein.
[d] EAE = experimental autoimmune encephalomyelitis.
From: Lennon VA. (2010). Mini–Review Article: The role of immunoglobulin G in neuromyelitis optica: Does IgG play a causal role in the pathology of neuromyelitis optica? J *Watch Neurol*, 2010; 12: 52–3.

astrocytes degranulate in the presence of NMO-IgGs, and astrocyte death ensues. Finally, they demonstrated that the addition of NMO patient serum, but not MS patient serum to this culture system promoted migration of granulocytes across the endothelial cell layer and this was dependent on the presence of fresh complement-thus indicating complement-dependent granulocyte attraction. These studies provide new insights into BBB breakdown, loss of AQP4 immunoreactivity, and perivascular granulocyte infiltration described in active NMO lesions.

In vivo evidence – animal models

Animal model data have been reported from four independent groups (Table 53.3) supporting a role for AQP4-specific IgG as an effector of the inflammatory demyelinating pathology of NMO: (1) Kinoshita and colleagues used IgG prepared from NMO patients' plasma (therapeutic plasmapheresis) to develop an animal model by passive transfer of IgG in rats recently immunized with myelin basic protein and adjuvant.[66] The rats developed active CNS lesions that exhibited immunohistopathological characteristics similar to those of NMO, marked by astrocytic loss and perivascular deposition of IgG and complement; (2) Bradl and colleagues showed that NMO-IgG augments clinical disease in myelin oligodendrocyte glycoprotoin-T–cell mediated experimental autoimmune encephalomyelitis (EAE) and induces superimposed CNS lesions that are characteristic of NMO;[67] (3) Bennett and colleagues showed that administration of an AQP4-specific recombinant antibody (derived from cerebrospinal fluid plasma

(a) (b) (c)

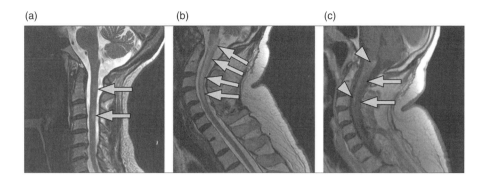

Fig. 53.4. Sagittal MRI of cervical spinal cord in MS and NMO (from Wingerchuk *et al.*, 2007[7] with permission) (a) T2-weighted image shows typical dorsal, short-segment signal abnormalities (arrows) characteristic of MS. (b) T2-weighted image from a patient with acute myelitis and neuromyelitis optica shows a typical longitudinally extensive, expansile, centrally located cord lesion that extends into the brainstem (arrows). (c) enhancement with intravenous gadolinium administration (arrowheads), indicative of active inflammation.

cells from an NMO patient) to rats with EAE, induced NMO-like immunopathology with perivascular astrocyte depletion, myelinolysis, and complement and Ig deposition;[68] (4) Saadoun and colleagues injected NMO-IgG with human complement into a living mouse brain at days 0, 3, and 5. At killing on day 7, the mouse had CNS lesions that were pathologically similar to those reported in NMO patients.[69]

Neuroimaging
Spinal cord: The longitudinally extensive lesion

In NMO, the most characteristic finding on spinal cord imaging is a longitudinally extensive T2-weighted signal abnormality involving at least three vertebral segments (Fig. 53.4(b)) and (c).[7,19] This finding in a patient presenting with myelitis for the first time should raise suspicion for an NMO spectrum disorder. During an acute relapse of myelitis, the spinal cord lesion may enhance, though the enhancement may be patchy and may be shorter than the more extensive T2 signal abnormality. In Wingerchuk's 2006 article proposing new diagnostic criteria for NMO (Table 53.2), analysis of individual components of those criteria revealed that the longitudinally extensive (≥3 vertebral levels) T2-weighted signal abnormality on MRI cord lesion had a specificity of 83% and sensitivity of 98% for NMO compared with other clinical, laboratory, and brain MRI findings.[19]

Longitudinally extensive lesions are exceedingly rare in adult North American MS patients in whom the cord lesions are usually short in length, asymmetric and well-circumscribed (Fig. 53.4(a)). Scott *et al.* identified only 1 of 22 patients, with acute partial transverse myelitis (short lesions on MRI) as seropositive for NMO-IgG.[70] This patient, however, subsequently developed recurrent episodes of longitudinally extensive transverse myelitis consistent with an NMO spectrum disorder. Caution must be urged, however, when interpreting the length of the lesion in formulating a differential diagnosis as the timing of the MRI may be important. If the MRI is performed too early or late in the evolution of the myelitis, it may miss the active inflammatory lesion at its maximum length.

In the first study of NMO-IgG in children with CNS demyelinating disorders, Banwell reported that a majority of children with relapsing–remitting MS had short, asymmetric spinal lesions as seen in adult MS.[8] However, 14% of children

with relapsing remitting MS had longitudinally extensive spinal cord lesions, exceedingly rare in adult North American MS patients.[8] Thus, a longitudinally extensive spinal cord lesion does not exclude the diagnosis of MS in a child and such a lesion is less predictive for a NMO-spectrum disorder than in adult patients.[8]

As discussed above, seropositivity for NMO-IgG in a patient with a single episode of longitudinally extensive transverse myelitis predicts relapse of longitudinally extensive transverse myelitis or development of optic neuritis and, thus, NMO. Patients seropositive for NMO-IgG with single episode or recurrent episodes of longitudinally extensive transverse myelitis in whom the optic nerves are spared are considered NMO spectrum disorders and fall under the umbrella term of "aquaporin-4 autoimmunity."

Brain

Recent studies have reported a high frequency of brain MRI abnormalities in NMO spectrum disorders. In a review of 60 NMO patients, brain lesions were identified in 60% of patients.[71] The majority were non-specific. "MS-like" brain lesions were identified in six patients (10%) and four of these fulfilled Barkof criteria for MS within three years of symptom onset. "Atypical" brain lesions were observed in five (8%) patients and included diencephalic (thalamic or hypothalamic) lesions in three and extensive cerebral white matter signal abnormality associated with encephalopathy in two. Hypothalamic involvement, some with associated hypothalamic endocrinopathies, is a recognized association of NMO.[72,73] In 2006, an analysis of brain MRIs from 120 NMO-IgG positive patients described "NMO typical" brain lesions as being localized at sites of high AQP4 expression at the astroglial foot processes, particularly located in the subpial and subependymal zones around the ventricles, most commonly around the third and fourth ventricles (Fig. 53.5).[74]

In 2005 Misu and colleagues reported that 17% of Japanese NMO patients had intractable hiccups and nausea and MRI brain detected linear medullary lesions involving the perical region, the area postrema, and the nucleus tractus solitarius.[75] In Caucasian patients hiccups, seem to be less frequent than in Japanese patients. A recent paper reported that 12% of AQP4

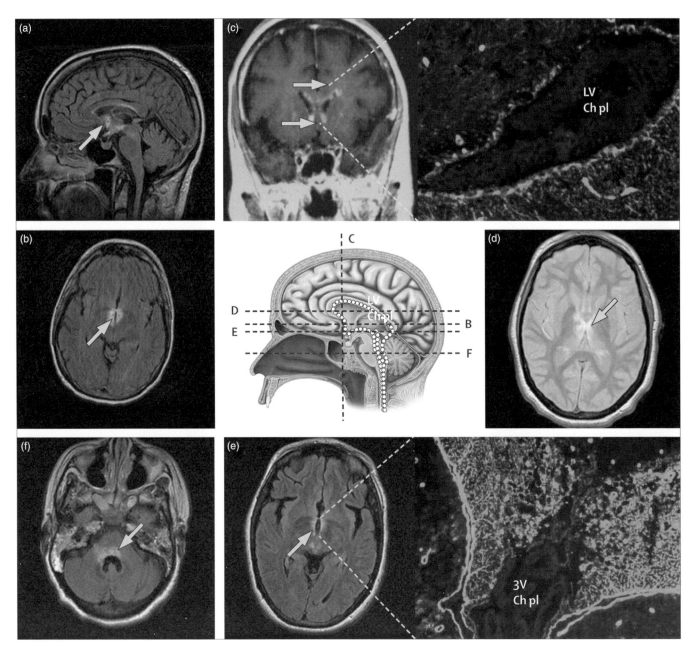

Fig. 53.5. NMO typical brain lesions (Wingerchuk *et al.*, 2007[7] with permission) NMO typical brain lesions localize at the sites of high aquaporin 4 expression (white dots on centre picture). In center picture dashed black lines show the anatomical level of MRI in the diagram; arrows show abnormality on fluid-attenuated inversion recovery (FLAIR), T2-weighted signal or after being given gadolinium Patient 1: FLAIR signal abnormality around the 3rd ventricle [image (a) (sagittal) and image (b) (axial)] with extension into the hypothalamus. Patient 2: Post-contrast T1-weighted image has subependymal enhancement along the frontal horns bilaterally and in the adjacent white matter [image C (coronal)]. The immunofluorescence photomicrograph linked to image (c) shows the binding pattern of the serum IgG from a patient with NMO in a mouse brain (400x). Intense immunoreactivity of basolateral ependymal cell membranes lining the lateral ventricle (LV) and extending into the subependymal astrocytic mesh coincides with aquaporin 4 immunoreactivity; the choroid plexus (Ch pl) is unstained. Patient 3 has contiguous signal abnormality throughout the periventricular tissues: diencephalon (image (d); axial T2-weighted), third ventricle (image (e); axial, FLAIR), and 4th ventricle (image (f); axial FLAIR). Immunofluorescence photomicrograph linked to image (e) shows the binding pattern of the serum IgG from a patient with neuromyelitis optica in a mouse brain (400x), with intense staining of periventricular tissues (third ventricle, 3V); choroid plexus (Ch pl) is unstained (see also color plate section).

antibody-positive patients had intractable vomiting as their initial presenting symptom of NMO, and 75% of these patients initially presented to a gastroenterologist.[76] In this paper neuroimaging revealed signal abnormalities in the area postrema and immunopathology of autopsy brain tissues showed loss of AQP4 in the area postrema of an NMO patient. These observations suggest the AQP4-rich area postrema may be a first point of attack in NMO. Both Japanese patients with intractable hiccups and nausea and Caucasian patients with intractable vomiting had beneficial response to corticosteroid therapy. The complete reversibility of hiccups, nausea and vomiting suggests a different immunopathogenesis for the area postrema lesion in NMO compared to the destructive lesions seen in the optic nerves or spinal cord. Roemer and colleagues described a novel NMO lesion phenotype in the medullary floor of the fourth ventricle (including the area postrema) that exhibits loss of AQP4 and contains inflammatory cells, but lacks demyelination or necrosis.[59]

In a systematic study of 88 consecutive NMO-IgG seropositive children evaluated at Mayo Clinic's neuroimmunology laboratory, 26 (45%) had episodic cerebral symptoms (encephalopathy, ophthalmoparesis, ataxia, seizures, intractable vomiting, or hiccups).[77] Thirty-eight (68%) had brain MRI abnormalities including (1) clinically silent lesions limited to the immediate periventricular regions; (2) hypothalamic, thalamic, and diencephalic lesions; (3) long spindle or tentacle-like white matter signal change extending from the lateral ventricles into the cerebrum (unlike the short, pericallosal-confined "Dawson's fingers" of MS); (4) white matter abnormalities, extensive and confluent, or discrete juxtaposed to or extending from the lateral ventricles; (5) brain stem and cerebellar lesions adjacent to the aqueduct of Sylvius and fourth ventricle. Eight NMO-IgG seropositive children in that study had clinical and radiologic features overlapping with criteria proposed for diagnosis of acute disseminated encephalomyelitis (ADEM): initial polysymptomatic encephalopathy accompanied by focal or multifocal hyperintense lesions predominantly affecting white matter.[78]

Cerebrospinal fluid

Cerebrospinal fluid testing in the setting of an acute longitudinally extensive transverse myelitis may reveal a prominent pleocytosis (often with a predominance of polymorphonuclear cells (including neutrophils and eosinophils) of 50–1000 × 10^6 white blood cells/l). This finding differs from that encountered in classical MS where pleocytosis is rarely above 50×10^6 white blood cells/L.[3,4,79–81] Oligoclonal bands are present in up to 90% of MS patients.[82,83] In contrast, they are uncommon in NMO (about 25%).[3,4,84,85]

NMO-IgG testing in CSF

In our experience, it is rare that NMO-IgG is detected in cerebrospinal fluid but not in serum. Klawiter *et al.* reported three patients who had an NMO spectrum disorder, but were seronegative for NMO-IgG. It is reasonable to test CSF for NMO-IgG if serum testing is negative and there is a high suspicion for an NMO spectrum disorder.[86]

Cytokine and chemokines

The role of cytokines and chemokines in the pathogenesis of MS has been investigated extensively. There have been only

a few studies investigating their role in the pathogenesis of NMO. To date, cerebrospinal fluid levels of interferon-gamma, inducible protein–10 (IP–10), thymus and activation-regulated chemokines (TARC), interleukin (IL)–1b, IL–1 receptor antagonists, IL–6, IL–8, IL–13, and granulocyte colony-stimulating factor have been reported to be increased.[87–90] Uzawa and colleagues showed that IL-10 and interferon-gamma-inducible protein-10 were elevated in both NMO and MS.[87] In serum analyses, only the IL-6 level showed significant elevation in NMO. Uzawa reported that the CSF IL-6 level had a significant correlation with the CSF glial fibrillary acidic protein (GFAP) level and CSF cells, and only a weak correlation with anti-AQP4 antibody titers.[87] These results emphasize the difference in CSF cytokine and chemokine levels in patients with NMO compared with MS, supporting the view that NMO is immunopathologically distinct from MS. Overall, the IL–6 pathway may be a potential therapeutic target for NMO treatment in the future.

GFAP

Misu and colleagues reported that the CSF-GFAP levels during relapse in NMO were several thousand times higher than in MS and considerably higher than those in spinal infarct and ADEM.[91] The levels returned close to normal along with clinical improvement soon after corticosteroid therapy in NMO. The authors subsequently reported a strong correlation between the CSF-GFAP (and S100B) levels and attack severity or length of the lesion on MRI in NMO. CSF-GFAP (and S100B) may be clinically useful biomarkers in NMO.[92] The marked elevations implicate astrocytic damage as a primary and early event in the acute phase of NMO.

NMO, other autoimmune disorders, and cancer

Non-organ specific

Patients with NMO spectrum disorders commonly have co-existing non-organ-specific autoantibodies and multisystem autoimmune diseases. In 78 patients fulfilling diagnostic criteria for NMO, non-organ-specific autoantibodies were detected with the following frequencies: antinuclear antibody, 53%; anti-double-stranded DNA, 11.5%; antibodies to extractable nuclear antigen, 17% (SSA [8 %], SSB [4%] U1-RNP [1%], Scl-70[1%], Jo [1%]); rheumatoid factor, 3%.[93] The prevalence of co-existing non-organ-specific autoantibodies in patients with recurrent longitudinally extensive transverse myelitis was similar.[93] Though the vast majority of these patients do not fulfill diagnostic criteria for a specific connective tissue disorder such as systemic lupus erythematosis or Sjögren's syndrome, there is an increased frequency of co-existing autoimmune diseases. In the Mayo Clinic study 5 of 153 patients with NMO spectrum disorders fulfilled clinical classification criteria for Sjögren's syndrome or systemic lupus erythematosis. Two

Table 53.4. *Neural autoantibodies found in 177 neuromyelitis optica patients, 77 multiple sclerosis patients, and 173 healthy subjects*

Autoantibody (Ab) detected[a] median nmol/L (range)	NMO (N = 177) N positive (%) median nmol/l (range)	Healthy controls (N = 173) N positive (%) median nmol/l (range)	MS controls (N =77) N positive (%) median nmol/l (range)	P value[b]
NMO-IgG	148 (83)	0	0	< 0.0001
Acetylcholine receptor Ab				
Muscle-type normal ≤ 0.02 nmol/l	19 (11) 0.39 (0.05–6.1)	0	0	<0.0001
Ganglionic-type normal ≤ 0.02 nmol/l	11 (6) 0.07 (0.03–0.18)	1 (0.6) 0.17	1 (1.3) 0.04	0.0019
Glutamic acid decarboxylase Ab, normal ≤ 0.02 nmol/l	26 (15) 0.09 (0.03–0.41)	5 (3) 0.08 (0.03–42.1)	1(1.3) 225[c]	<0.0001
Collapsin response- mediator protein (CRMP)-5 IgG (by Western blot)	2 (1)[d]	0	0	< 0.0001
Voltage-gated potassium channel Ab normal ≤ 0.02 nmol/l	9 (5) 0.10 (0.03–0.30)	4 (2) 0.05 (0.04–0.09)	0	0.02
Voltage-gated calcium channel Ab				
P/Q-type normal ≤ 0.02 nmol/l	3 (2) 0.06 (0.03–0.07)	0	1 (1.3) 0.33	0.30
N-type normal ≤ 0.03 nmol/l	7 (4) 0.09 (0.07–0.54)	1 (0.6) 0.05	4 (5) 0.07 (0.04–0.25)	0.52
≥ 1 autoantibody detected (excluding NMO-IgG)	61 (34)	11 (6)	7 (9)	< 0.0001

[a] With the exception of NMO-IgG detection, immunofluorescence testing was negative in all cases.
[b] Calculated using data from healthy and MS controls combined.
[c] No history of stiff-man syndrome or other GAD65 antibody associated disorders, including type 1 diabetes mellitus.
[d] Thymic carcinoma was detected in 1 patient.
From: McKeon A, Lennon VA, Jacob A, *et al.* Coexistence of myasthenia gravis and serological markers of neurological autoimmunity in neuromyelitis optica. *Muscle Nerve* 2009;39: 87–90.

patients had rheumatoid arthritis and one had Raynaud phenomenon.

Patients presenting with transverse myelitis who have co-existing non-organ-specific autoantibodies are customarily classified as having "disease-associated" acute transverse myelitis regardless of whether or not symptoms or signs of Sjögren syndrome or SLE are present. The etiology of these myelitis attacks have been considered to represent complications, perhaps vasculitic, of non-organ-specific autoimmune diseases.[94–101] An alternative hypothesis to the presumption of a direct contribution of Sjögren syndrome or SLE to the pathogenesis is the coexistence of an NMO spectrum disorder (AQP4 autoimmunity) with the non-organ-specific autoimmune disorders. Recent data have demonstrated the specificity of NMO-IgG for a discrete "NMO spectrum" of CNS inflammatory demyelinating disorders, which includes limited forms of NMO with and without evidence of connective tissue disorders. NMO-IgG is not detected in patients with Sjögren's syndrome or SLE without an NMO spectrum disorder. The association of non-organ-specific antibodies in patients with an NMO spectrum disorder (and seropositivity for NMO-IgG) likely reflect the co-existence of two autoimmune disorders.[93] NMO-IgG seropositive optic neuritis or myelitis are unlikely to represent a vasculitic complication of Sjögren syndrome or SLE, but rather co-existing NMO spectrum disorder.

Organ specific

Organ-specific autoimmune diseases also commonly co-exist with NMO and include in reducing order of frequency: hypothyroidism (19%), pernicious anemia (6%), myasthenia gravis (2%), ulcerative colitis (2%), primary sclerosing cholangitis (2%), and idiopathic thrombocytopenic purpura (2%).[4,102] In a systematic study of the frequency of neural autoantibodies in 177 patients with NMO, 61 patients had one or more coexisting neural autoantibodies including in decreasing frequency: muscle acetylcholine receptor antibody, 11%; glutamic acid decarboxylase antibody, 15%; ganglionic acetylcholine receptor antibody, 6%; voltage-gated potassium channel complex autoantibodies, 5%; voltage gated calcium channel complex autoantibodies-N type (4%) and PQ type (2%), and collapsin response-mediator protein (CRMP)–5 IgG, 2% (Table 53.4). Given the high frequency of muscle acetylcholine receptor antibody in NMO patient serum, a diagnosis of co-existent MG should be considered in any NMO patient who has respiratory compromise.

Paraneoplastic NMO

Thymoma and thymic carcinoma have previously been reported as sporadic accompaniments of NMO.[103] In 2008, the concept of paraneoplastic NMO was reported where NMO-IgG was associated temporally with cancer in nine patients (seven with an NMO-spectrum disorder).[104] Breast carcinoma was the most common cancer observed in 33%. NMO-IgG was detected in two patients whose neurological symptoms were attributable to CNS metastases of breast and lung carcinomas, but who lacked NMO like symptoms or signs. Tissue microarray analyses have revealed AQP4 immunoreactivity in multiple cancer types.[104] Prospective studies are needed to investigate the frequency of AQP4 autoantibodies in patients with cancer.

Treatment

This can be divided into three parts: (1) treatment of the acute attack, (2) attack prevention, and (3) symptomatic treatment (beyond the scope of this chapter).

Acute attack

In NMO, attacks of optic neuritis or transverse myelitis are frequently severe. Acute optic neuritis is often associated with significant loss of vision. Longitudinally extensive transverse myelitis may be associated with paraparesis or paraplegia. These attacks warrant treatment.

The first line of treatment in the management of either an acute attack of optic neuritis or myelitis is intravenous corticosteroids. The usual dose given is 1000 mg of methylprednisolone intravenously daily for five consecutive days.[9] Prednisone taper is often used after this course of intravenous methylprednisolone and, in fact, as will be discussed in the *Attack Prevention Section of Treatment*, a low dose daily or alternate day prednisone is often required over the longer term in the management of patients with NMO. It is important to note that there have been no clinical trials that have specifically addressed treatment of an acute NMO attack. The use of corticosteroids in the treatment of optic neuritis has been supported by a randomized controlled trial comparing oral prednisone treatment alone vs. placebo. Patients who received corticosteroid recovered faster.[105]

The goal of corticosteroids during the acute phase of longitudinally extensive transverse myelitis is to stop worsening and reduce inflammation thereby increasing rate of recovery. There have been no randomized controlled trials of corticosteroids in transverse myelitis. Evidence supporting the use of intravenous methylprednisolone as first-line therapy in the management of acute NMO relapse is mainly supported from case series or by extrapolation from clinical trials involving MS patients.[106] Patients should be informed of the potential side effects of intravenous methylprednisolone, which include hypertension, hyperglycemia, increased appetite, weight gain, agitation, anxiety, psychosis, heartburn, gastritis, headache, electrolyte disturbance, and avascular necrosis of the hip.

In our experience, the earlier the intravenous methylprednisolone can be commenced the better. Patients with NMO spectrum disorders may often get early indication of a potential attack; for example, they may note onset of back pain or tingling numbness in the lower extremities and if they have a known diagnosis of NMO spectrum disorder intravenous methylprednisolone or high-dose oral prednisone should be initiated as soon as possible. In cases where patients have developed disability and have not responded to intravenous methylprednisolone, plasmapheresis should be used as a second line of treatment. Again, it is important to note that there have been no randomized controlled trials of plasmapheresis in NMO spectrum disorders alone and much of what we know relates to studies that have included patients with myelitis secondary to a heterogeneous group of inflammatory demyelinating disorders.

Weinshenker and colleagues reported in a small, randomized controlled trial of patients with paraplegia or quadriplegia occurring in the setting of idiopathic CNS demyelinating disease that 42% of patients treated with plasmapheresis showed meaningful benefit compared with 6% of patients in the sham-treated group.[107] It was noted that, among this heterogeneous group of patients, the NMO patients were the most likely to respond to treatment.

A subsequent retrospective review of Mayo Clinic patients treated with plasmapheresis for acute severe attacks of CNS demyelination reported that male sex, preserved reflexes and early treatment were associated with a greater likelihood of improvement. Of note, 10 of the 59 patients included in this study had NMO and clinically significant improvements were seen in 60% of these patients within days of commencement of plasmapheresis.[108]

Watanabe *et al.* reported that three of six patients with NMO acute attacks, refractory to corticosteroids, responded to plasmapheresis.[109] Given the strong evidence that NMO is an antibody mediated disease and that NMO IgG is the pathogenic antibody, it is likely that the underlying etiology of transverse myelitis is similar to that of optic neuritis. Though plasmapheresis has been mainly reported as a treatment for transverse myelitis, it is likely that this treatment would also work for severe episodes of optic neuritis. For patients with NMO attacks, the likelihood of a clinically significant response to plasmapheresis reduces with increasing delay from attack onset to treatment. Rarely, patients may have improvement in vision or lower extremities symptoms after as long a delay from attack onset as three to six months. The plasmapheresis regimen that is recommended is seven exchanges of approximately 55 ml/kg with each exchange. This is administered every other day for 14 days. Patients may require a central line for this treatment.

Attack prevention

Disability in NMO accrues incrementally with repeated attacks. In contrast to patients with MS in whom disability usually occurs during the progressive rather than the relapsing phase of the disease, a progressive phase of disease is rare in NMO.[27] Disability in NMO is attack related. It is likely that early initiation of immunotherapy with combined successful attack prevention will likely have a greater impact on the natural history of NMO compared with MS. In contrast to MS, there is a growing

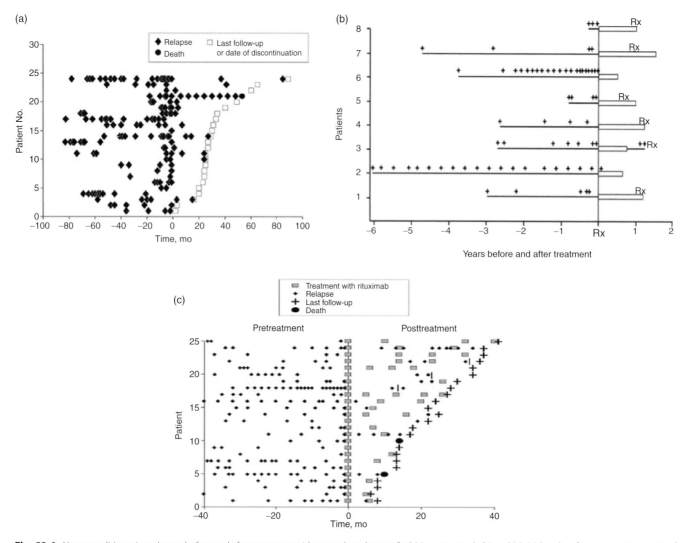

Fig. 53.6. Neuromyelitis optica relapses before and after treatment with mycophenolate mofetil (a), or rituximab (b) and (c). (a) Results of a retrospective study of mycophenolate mofetil in 24 NMO patients. 0 on the x-axis indicates the start date of treatment. Each interrupted line on the y-axis represents a patient. (Jacob *et al.*, 2009,[113] with permission) (b) Results of an open-label treatment trial of rituximab in NMO. *History of pre- and post-rituximab exacerbations for each patient.* + = *Exacerbations of transverse myelitis or optic neuritis; Rx = rituximab retreatment; open bars = B-cell depletion. (Cree et al., 2005[114] with permission)* (c) Results of a retrospective study of rituximab in NMO (Jacob *et al.*, 2009,[115] with permission)

literature suggesting that interferon-beta drugs have no effect or increase relapse rate in NMO.[110–112] Currently, immunosuppression is the mainstay of treatment in NMO. Unfortunately, there have been no randomized controlled trials of any medication in this disorder.

Throughout the USA, the most commonly used immunosuppressant medication in the treatment of NMO is azathioprine, though there has been a recent increase in usage of mycophenolate and rituximab in recent years. Azathioprine is generally used either alone or combined with oral prednisone in varying doses. The use of azathioprine is based upon. Mandler and colleagues' paper in which he reported seven patients who remained relapse-free for 18 months and had significant improvement in their EDSS scores with a combination of long-term prednisone (approximately 10 mg per day) and azathioprine (75–100 mg per day).[79]

Due to the relatively high frequency of thiopurine methyltransferase deficiency, or an inability of the patient to tolerate azathioprine (elevated liver enzymes), other immunosuppression medications may need to be considered. Mycophenolate mofetil is a reasonably safe medication and appears to be effective in the prevention of NMO relapses. In a recent retrospective study of 24 patients with NMO spectrum disorders, the efficacy and safety of mycophenolate mofetil therapy was evaluated.[113] The median dose of mycophenolate mofetil used in the study was 2000 mg per day and nine of the 24 patients were also receiving prednisone. The median follow–up after commencement of mycophenolate mofetil was 28 months (range of 18–89 months). Eighty percent of patients were continuing mycophenolate mofetil treatment at the end of the study period. Figure 53.6(a) depicts the timing of relapses before and after treatment. The median annualized post-treatment relapse rate was 0.09

(range of 0.0–1.5), which was statistically significantly lower than the pretreatment rate of 1.3 (range of 0.23–11.8). In addition, it was noted that the median EDSS score at the start of treatment was 6 (range of 0–8) and the median EDSS score at last follow-up was 5.5 (range of 0–10). Overall the EDSS score remained unchanged in 15 of the patients and, in fact, improved in seven patients. One patient died after being bed-bound for 54 months. Mycophenolate mofetil is considerably more expensive than azathioprine, and there has been no head-to-head studies comparing these medication options.

Prednisone is often required on an ongoing basis to maintain remission. The dose required in combination with immunosuppressant medications is often low, as low as 20 mg on alternate days. Patients may relapse when the dose is dropped to lower than 20 mg on alternate days. If the patient has been relapse free on a combination of low dose oral prednisone and mycophenolate mofetil for a year then it may be reasonable at that point to wean the patient off prednisone in an attempt to maintain the patient on oral steroid-sparing immunosuppressant medication alone.

It is important to inform patients of the potential toxicities of mycophenolate mofetil. Progressive multifocal leukoencephalopathy has been reported in transplant patients and in systemic lupus erythematosus where mycophenolate mofetil has been used in combination with other immunosuppressant medications. Concern has been raised regarding the potential risk for lymphoma.[113] Patients receiving mycophenolate mofetil should have their blood counts checked weekly for the first month, twice monthly for the second and third month, and then monthly thereafter as the white blood cell count may drop and should be monitored. Gastrointestinal symptoms are probably the most common side effect reported by patients using mycophenolate mofetil.

Cree and colleagues in 2005 reported the results of an open label study of the effects of rituximab in eight NMO patients (Fig. 53.6(b)).[114] The median attack rate declined from 2.6 attacks per patient/year to zero attacks per patient/year. Seven of eight patients experienced improvement of neurologic function with dramatic recovery in some cases. Despite these promising results, unfortunately, a randomized controlled trial has not yet been undertaken to investigate this medication further. A retrospective study of rituximab in 25 patients was reported by Jacob and colleagues in 2008 (Fig. 53.6(c)).[115] Of these 25

patients, 23 patients had experienced relapses despite use of other immunosuppressant medications. The authors reported that at a median follow-up of 19 months, the median annualized pre-treatment relapse rate dropped from 1.7 (range of 0.5–5.0) to a post-treatment relapse rate of 0 (range of 0.0–3.2), $P = 0.001$. In addition, disability appeared to improve or stabilize in 80% of patients. The frequency of use of concomitant immunotherapies was lower than in the mycophenolate mofetil study. In the retrospective rituximab study other immunotherapies were used in five patients – azathioprine with prednisone in one, prednisone alone in three and interferon beta in one.

Overall, these recent studies provide optimism and indicate likely "true benefit" from these medications in terms of relapse rate reduction. For patients that continue to have relapses despite these approaches, other therapies could be considered. Some investigators in the field consider mitoxantrone of benefit, especially in more severe cases of NMO. Unfortunately, however, data are lacking on the use of this medication. In a small perspective study of five patients with relapsing NMO, mitoxantrone hydrochloride given monthly for six months followed by infusions every three months for further three treatments appeared beneficial.[116] During the two years of mitoxantrone treatment, two of five patients had a single relapse within the initial five months of treatment, though improvements were seen clinically and on MRI in four patients. Further study of this medication is likely warranted. In 2004 Bakker and colleagues reported intravenous gamma globulin therapy in two patients with NMO and reported that monthly infusions of IVIG resulted in relapse prevention and neurologic recovery.[117]

Conclusions

Advanced serological interpretive insights, coupled with increased understanding of the pathogenic inpact of binding of NMO-IgG to AQP4 on the astrocytic end foot (complement activation, AQP4 down-regulation and coupled glutamate transporter down-regulation) as well as future identification of novel pathogenic mechanisms will lead to formulation of individual patient-specific NMO therapies. Potential therapeutic approaches might include: inhibition of complement activation; inhibition of cytokine mediated events such as IL-6: small molecules that bind NMO-IgG or prevent its binding to AQP4; drugs that inhibit glutamate toxicity.

References

1. Devic E. Myélite aiguë compliquée de névrite optique. *Bull Med* 1894; 8: 1033–4.

2. Mandler RN, Davis LE, Jeffery DR, Kornfeld M. Devic's neuromyelitis optica: a clinicopathological study of 8 patients. *Ann Neurol* 1993; 34: 162–8.

3. O'Riordan JI, Gallagher HL, Thompson AJ, *et al*. Clinical, CSF, and MRI findings in Devic's neuromyelitis optica. *J Neurol Neurosurg Psychiatry* 1996; 60: 382–7.

4. Wingerchuk DM, Hogancamp WF, O'Brien PC, Weinshenker BG. The clinical course of neuromyelitis optica

(Devic's syndrome). *Neurology* 1999; 53: 1107–14.

5. Lennon VA, Wingerchuk DM, Kryzer TJ, *et al*. A serum autoantibody marker of neuromyelitis optica: distinction from multiple sclerosis. *Lancet* 2004; 364: 2106–12.

6. Lennon VA, Kryzer TJ, Pittock SJ, Verkman AS, Hinson SR. IgG marker of optic-spinal multiple sclerosis binds to the aquaporin-4 water channel. *J Exp Med* 2005; 202: 473–7.

7. Wingerchuk DM, Lennon VA, Lucchinetti CF, Pittock SJ, Weinshenker BG. The spectrum of neuromyelitis optica. *Lancet Neurol* 2007; 6: 805–15.

8. Banwell B, Tenembaum S, Lennon VA, *et al.* Neuromyelitis optica-IgG in childhood inflammatory demyelinating CNS disorders. *Neurology* 2008; 70: 344–52.

9. Pittock SJ. Neuromyelitis optica: a new perspective. *Semin Neurol* 2008; 28: 95–104.

10. Fukazawa T, Yamasaki K, Ito H, *et al.* Both the HLA-CPB1 and -DRB1 alleles correlate with risk for multiple sclerosis in Japanese: clinical phenotypes and gender as important factors. *Tissue Antigens* 2000; 55: 199–205.

11. Kira J. Multiple sclerosis in the Japanese population. *Lancet Neurol* 2003; 2: 117–27.

12. Nakashima I, Fujihara K, Takase S, Itoyama Y. Decrease in multiple sclerosis with acute transverse myelitis in Japan. *Tohoku J Exp Med* 1999; 188: 89–94.

13. Yamasaki K, Horiuchi I, Minohara M, *et al.* HLA-DPB1*0501-associated opticospinal multiple sclerosis: clinical, neuroimaging and immunogenetic studies. *Brain* 1999; 122: 1689–96.

14. Kinaka S, McAlpine D, Miyagawa K. Multiple sclerosis in northern and southern Japan. *World Neurol* 1960; 1: 22–42.

15. Okinaka S, Tsubaki T, Kuroiwa Y, Toyokura Y, Imamura Y, Yoshikawa M. Multiple sclerosis and allied diseases in Japan. *Neurology* 1958; 8: 756–63.

16. Cabre P, Heinzlef O, Merle H, *et al.* MS and neuromyelitis optica in Martinique (French West Indies). *Neurology* 2001; 56: 507–14.

17. Osuntokun BO. The pattern of neurological illness in tropical Africa. Experience at Ibadan, Nigeria. *J Neurol Sci* 1971; 12: 417–42.

18. Lana-Peixoto MA, Lana-Peixoto MI. Is multiple sclerosis in Brazil and Asia alike? *Arq Neuropsiquiatr* 1992; 50: 419–25.

19. Wingerchuk DM, Lennon VA, Pittock SJ, Lucchinetti CF, Weinshenker BG. Revised diagnostic criteria for neuromyelitis optica. *Neurology* 2006; 66: 1485–9.

20. Keegan M, Weinshenker B. Familial Devic's disease. *Can J Neurol Sci* 2000; 27: S57–8.

21. Ch'ien L, Medeiros M, Belluomini J, Lemmi H, Whitaker J. Neuromyelitis optica (Devic's syndrome) in two sisters. *Clin Electroencephalogr* 1982; 13: 36–9.

22. McAlpine D. Familial neuromyelitis optica: its occurrence in identical twins. *Brain* 1938; 61: 430–48.

23. Yamakawa K, Kuroda H, Fujihara K, *et al.* Familial neuromyelitis optica (Devic's syndrome) with late onset in Japan. *Neurology* 2000; 55: 318–20.

24. Matiello M, Kim HJ, Kim W, *et al.* Familial neuromyelitis optica. *Neurology* 2010; 75: 310–15.

25. Matiello M, Schaefer-Klein J, Brum DG, Atkinson EJ, Kantarci OH, Weinshenker BG. HLA-DRB1*1501 tagging rs3135388 polymorphism is not associated with neuromyelitis optica. *Mult Scler* 2010; 16: 981–4.

26. Matiello M, Schaefer-Klein J, Hebrink D, Kingsbury D, Lennon VA, Weinshenker BG. Two different Arg19 mutations in the N-terminus of aquaporin-4 suggest a molecular mechanism for susceptibility to neuromyelitis optica. *Neurology* 2009; 72: A119–20.

27. Wingerchuk DM, Pittock SJ, Lucchinetti CF, Lennon VA, Weinshenker BG. A secondary progressive clinical course is uncommon in neuromyelitis optica. *Neurology* 2007; 68: 603–5.

28. Hinson SR, McKeon A, Fryer JP, Apiwattanakul M, Lennon VA, Pittock SJ. Prediction of neuromyelitis optica attack severity by quantitation of complement-mediated injury to aquaporin 4-expressing cells. *Arch Neurol* 2009; 66: 1164–7.

29. Lucchinetti CF, Mandler RN, McGavern D, *et al.* A role for humoral mechanisms in the pathogenesis of Devic's neuromyelitis optica. *Brain* 2002; 125: 1450–61.

30. Zuliani L, Lopez de Munain A, Ruiz Martinez J, Olascoaga J, Graus F, Saiz A. NMO-IgG antibodies in neuromyelitis optica: a report of 2 cases. *Neurologia* 2006; 21: 314–17.

31. Littleton E, Jacob A, M B, Palace J. An audit of the diagnostic usefulness of the NMO-IgG assay for neuromyelitis optica. *Mult Scler* 2006; 12: S156.

32. Marignier R, De Seze J, Durand-Dubief F. NMO-IgG: a French experience. *Mult Scler* 2006; 12: S4.

33. Akman-Demir G. Probably NMO-IgG in Turkish patients with Devic's disease and multiple sclerosis. *Mult Scler* 2006; 12: S157.

34. Jarius S, Franciotta D, Bergamaschi R, *et al.* NMO-IgG in the diagnosis of neuromyelitis optica. *Neurology* 2007; 68: 1076–7.

35. Takahashi T, Fujihara K, Nakashima I, *et al.* Anti-aquaporin-4 antibody is involved in the pathogenesis of NMO: a study on antibody titre. *Brain* 2007; 130: 1235–43.

36. Amiry-Moghaddam M, Frydenlund D, Ottersen O. Anchoring of aquaporin-4 in brain: molecular mechanisms and implications for the physiology and pathophysiology of water transport. *Neuroscience* 2004; 129: 999–1010.

37. Rash JE, Davidson KG, Yasumura T, Furman CS. Freeze-fracture and immunogold analysis of aquaporin-4 (AQP4) square arrays, with models of AQP4 lattice assembly. *Neuroscience* 2004; 129: 915–34.

38. Lehmann GL, Gradilone SA, Marinelli RA. Aquaporin water channels in central nervous system. *Curr Neurovasc Res* 2004; 1: 293–303.

39. Rash JE, Yasumura T, Hudson CS, Agre P, Nielsen S. Direct immunogold labeling of aquaporin-4 in square arrays of astrocyte and ependymocyte plasma membranes in rat brain and spinal cord. *Proc Natl Acad Sci USA* 1998; 95: 11981–6.

40. Furman CS, Gorelick-Feldman DA, Davidson KG, *et al.* Aquaporin-4 square array assembly: opposing actions of M1 and M23 isoforms. *Proc Natl Acad Sci USA* 2003; 100: 13609–14.

41. Nicchia GP, Nico B, Camassa LM, *et al.* The role of aquaporin-4 in the blood-brain barrier development and integrity: studies in animal and cell culture models. *Neuroscience* 2004; 129: 935–45.

42. Hinson SR, Pittock SJ, Lucchinetti CF, *et al.* Pathogenic potential of IgG binding to water channel extracellular

domain in neuromyelitis optica. *Neurology* 2007; 69: 2221–31.

43. Aoki K, Uchihara T, Tsuchiya K, Nakamura A, Ikeda K, Wakayama Y. Enhanced expression of aquaporin 4 in human brain with infarction. *Acta Neuropathol (Berl)* 2003; 106: 121–4.

44. Warth A, Mittelbronn M, Wolburg H. Redistribution of the water channel protein aquaporin-4 and the K+ channel protein Kir4.1 differs in low- and high-grade human brain tumors. *Acta Neuropathol (Berl)* 2005; 109: 418–26.

45. McKeon A, Fryer J, Apiwattanakul M, *et al.* Diagnosis of neuromyelitis spectrum disorders: comparative sensitivities and specificities of immunohistochemical and immunoprecipitation assays. *Arch Neurol* 2009; 66: 1134–8.

46. Nakashima I, Fujihara K, Miyazawa I, *et al.* Clinical and MRI features of Japanese patients with multiple sclerosis positive for NMO-IgG. *J Neurol Neurosurg Psychiatry* 2006; 77: 1073–5.

47. Takahashi T, Fujihara K, Nakashima I, *et al.* Establishment of a new sensitive assay for anti-human aquaporin-4 antibody in neuromyelitis optica. *Tohoku J Exp Med* 2006; 210: 307–13.

48. Hinson SR, Roemer SF, Lucchinetti CF, *et al.* Aquaporin-4-binding autoantibodies in patients with neuromyelitis optica impair glutamate transport by down-regulating EAAT2. *J Exp Med* 2008; 205: 2473–81.

49. Waters P, Jarius S, Littleton E, *et al.* Aquaporin-4 antibodies in neuromyelitis optica and longitudinally extensive transverse myelitis. *Arch Neurol* 2008; 65: 913–19.

50. Jarius S, Probst C, Borowski K, *et al.* Standardized method for the detection of antibodies to aquaporin-4 based on a highly sensitive immunofluorescence assay employing recombinant target antigen. *J Neurol Sci* 2010; 291: 52–6.

51. Hayakawa S, Mori M, Okuta A, *et al.* Neuromyelitis optica and anti-aquaporin-4 antibodies measured by an enzyme-linked immunosorbent assay. *J Neuroimmunol* 2008; 196: 181–7.

52. Weinshenker BG, Wingerchuk DM, Vukusic S, *et al.* Neuromyelitis optica IgG predicts relapse after longitudinally extensive transverse myelitis. *Ann Neurol* 2006; 59: 566–9.

53. Matiello M, McKeon A, Pittock S, Weinshenker B. Frequency and prognostic value of NMO-IgG seropositivity in isolated optic neuritis. *Neurology* 2010; 74: A156.

54. Matiello M, Jacob A, Pittock S, *et al.* NMO-IgG predicts the outcome of recurrent optic neuritis. *Neurology* 2008; 70: 2197–200.

55. Jarius S, Frederikson J, Waters P, *et al.* Frequency and prognostic impact of antibodies to aquaporin-4 in patients with optic neuritis. *J Neurol Sci* 2010; 298: 158–62.

56. Tanaka M, Tanaka K, Komori M, Saida T. Anti-aquaporin 4 antibody in Japanese multiple sclerosis: the presence of optic-spinal multiple sclerosis without long spinal cord lesions and anti-aquaporin 4 antibody. *J Neurol Neurosurg Psychiatry* 2007; 78: 990–2.

57. Jarius S, Aboul-Enein F, Waters P, *et al.* Antibody to aquaporin-4 in the long-term course of neuromyelitis optica. *Brain* 2008; 131: 3072–80.

58. Kurtzke J. Rating neurologic impairment in multiple sclerosis: an expanded disability status scale (EDSS) *Neurology* 1983; 33: 1444–52.

59. Roemer SF, Parisi JE, Lennon VA, *et al.* Pattern-specific loss of aquaporin-4 immunoreactivity distinguishes neuromyelitis optica from multiple sclerosis. *Brain* 2007; 130:1194–205.

60. Vallejo-Illarramendi A, Domercq M, Perez-Cerda F, Ravid R, Matute C. Increased expression and function of glutamate transporters in multiple sclerosis. *Neurobiol Dis* 2006; 21: 154–64.

61. Zeng X, Sun X, Gao L, Fan Y, Ding J, Hu G. Aquaporin-4 deficiency down-regulates glutamate uptake and GLT-1 expression in astrocytes. *Mol Cell Neurosci* 2007; 34: 34–9.

62. Salter M, Fern R. NMDA receptors are expressed in developing oligodendrocyte processes and mediate injury. *Nature* 2005; 438: 1167–71.

63. Smith T, Groom A, Zhu B, Turski L. Autoimmune encephalomyelitis ameliorated by AMPA antagonists. *Nat Med* 2000; 6: 62–6.

64. Alberdi E, Sanchez-Gomez M, Torre I, *et al.* Activation of kainite receptors sensitizes oligodendrocytes to complement attack. *J Neurosci* 2006: 3220–8.

65. Vincent T, Saikali P, Cayrol R, *et al.* Functional consequences of neuromyelitis optica-IgG astrocyte interactions on blood-brain barrier permeability and granulocyte recruitment. *J Immunol* 2008; 181: 5730–7.

66. Kinoshita M, Nakatsuji Y, Kimura T, *et al.* Neuromyelitis optica: Passive transfer to rats by human immunoglobulin. *Biochem Biophys Res Commun* 2009; 386: 623–7.

67. Bradl M, Misu T, Takahashi T, *et al.* Neuromyelitis optica: pathogenicity of patient immunoglobulin in vivo. *Ann Neurol* 2009; 66: 630–43.

68. Bennett JL, Lam C, Kalluri SR, *et al.* Intrathecal pathogenic anti-aquaporin-4 antibodies in early neuromyelitis optica. *Ann Neurol* 2009; 66: 617–29.

69. Saadoun S, Waters P, Bell BA, Vincent A, Verkman AS, MC P. Intra-cerebral injection of neuromyelitis optica immunoglobulin G and human complement produces neuromyelitis optica lesions in mice. *Brain* 2010; 133: 349–61.

70. Scott TF, Kassab SL, Pittock SJ. Neuromyelitis optica IgG status in acute partial transverse myelitis. *Arch Neurol* 2006; 63: 1398–400.

71. Pittock SJ, Lennon VA, Krecke K, Wingerchuk DM, Lucchinetti CF, Weinshenker BG. Brain abnormalities in neuromyelitis optica. *Arch Neurol* 2006; 63: 390–6.

72. Vernant JC, Cabre P, Smadja D, *et al.* Recurrent optic neuromyelitis with endocrinopathies: a new syndrome. *Neurology* 1997; 48: 58–64.

73. Poppe AY, Lapierre Y, Melancon D, *et al.* Neuromyelitis optica with hypothalamic involvement. *Mult Scler* 2005; 11: 617–21.

74. Pittock SJ, Weinshenker BG, Lucchinetti CF, Wingerchuk DM, Corboy JR, Lennon VA. Neuromyelitis optica brain lesions localized at sites of high aquaporin 4 expression. *Arch Neurol* 2006; 63: 964–8.

75. Misu T, Fujihara K, Nakashima I, Sato S, Itoyama Y. Intractable hiccup and nausea with periaqueductal lesions in

neuromyelitis optica. *Neurology* 2005; 65: 1479–82.

76. Apiwattanakul M, Popescu BF, Matiello M, *et al.* Intractable vomiting as the initial presentation of neuromyelitis optica. *Ann Neurol* 2010; 68: 757–61.

77. McKeon A, Lennon VA, Lotze T, *et al.* CNS aquaporin-4 autoimmunity in children. *Neurology* 2008; 71: 93–100.

78. Tenembaum S, Chitnis T, Ness J, Hahn JS. Acute disseminated encephalomyelitis. *Neurology* 2007; 68: S23–36.

79. Mandler RN, Ahmed W, Dencoff JE. Devic's neuromyelitis optica: a prospective study of seven patients treated with prednisone and azathioprine. *Neurology* 1998; 51: 1219–20.

80. Milano E, Di Sapio A, Malucchi S, *et al.* Neuromyelitis optica: importance of cerebrospinal fluid examination during relapse. *Neurol Sci* 2003; 24: 130–3.

81. McDonald WI, Compston A, Edan G, *et al.* Recommended diagnostic criteria for multiple sclerosis: guidelines from the International Panel on the diagnosis of multiple sclerosis. *Ann Neurol* 2001; 50: 121–7.

82. Ebers GC, Paty DW. CSF electrophoresis in one thousand patients. *Can J Neurol Sci* 1980; 7: 245–80.

83. McLean BN, Luxton RW, Thompson EJ. A study of immunoglobulin G in the cerebrospinal fluid of 1007 patients with suspected neurological disease using isoelectric focusing and the Log IgG-Index. A comparison and diagnostic applications. *Brain* 1990; 113: 1269–89.

84. de Seze J, Stojkovic T, Ferriby D, *et al.* Devic's neuromyelitis optica: clinical, laboratory, MRI and outcome profile. *J Neurol Sci* 2002; 197: 57–61.

85. Bergamaschi R, Tonietti S, Franciotta D, *et al.* Oligoclonal bands in Devic's neuromyelitis optica and multiple sclerosis: differences in repeated cerebrospinal fluid examinations. *Mult Scler* 2004; 10: 2–4.

86. Klawiter EC, Alvarez E, 3rd, Xu J, *et al.* NMO-IgG detected in CSF in seronegative neuromyelitis optica. *Neurology* 2009; 72: 1101–3.

87. Uzawa A, Mori M, Arai K, *et al.* Cytokine and chemokine profiles in

neuromyelitis optica: significance of interleukin-6. *Mult Scler* 2010; 16: 1443–52.

88. Narikawa K, Misu T, Fujihara K, Nakashima I, Sato S, Itoyama Y. CSF chemokine levels in relapsing neuromyelitis optica and multiple sclerosis. *J Neuroimmunol* 2004; 149: 182–6.

89. Yanagawa K, Kawachi I, Toyoshima Y, *et al.* Pathologic and immunologic profiles of a limited form of neuromyelitis optica with myelitis. *Neurology* 2009; 73: 1628–37.

90. Uzawa A, Mori M, Ito M, *et al.* Markedly increased CSF interleukin-6 levels in neuromyelitis optica, but not in multiple sclerosis. *J Neurol* 2009; 256: 2082–4.

91. Misu T, Takano R, Fujihara K, Takahashi T, Sato S, Itoyama Y. Marked increase in cerebrospinal fluid glial fibrillar acidic protein in neuromyelitis optica: an astrocytic damage marker. *J Neurol Neurosurg Psychiatry* 2009; 80: 575–7.

92. Takano R, Misu T, Takahashi T, Sato S, Fujihara K, Itoyama Y. Astrocytic damage is far more severe than demyelination in NMO: a clinical CSF biomarker study. *Neurology* 2010; 75: 208–6.

93. Pittock SJ, Lennon VA, de Seze J, *et al.* Neuromyelitis optica and non organ-specific autoimmunity. *Arch Neurol* 2008; 65: 78–83.

94. April RS, Vansonnenberg E. A case of neuromyelitis optica (Devic's syndrome) in systemic lupus erythematosus. Clinicopathologic report and review of the literature. *Neurology* 1976; 26: 1066–70.

95. Kinney EL, Berdoff RL, Rao NS, Fox LM. Devic's syndrome and systemic lupus erythematosus: a case report with necropsy. *Arch Neurol* 1979; 36: 643–4.

96. Mochizuki A, Hayashi A, Hisahara S, Shoji S. Steroid-responsive Devic's variant in Sjogren's syndrome. *Neurology* 2000; 54: 1391–2.

97. de Seze J, Stojkovic T, Breteau G, *et al.* Acute myelopathies: clinical, laboratory and outcome profiles in 79 cases. *Brain* 2001; 124: 1509–21.

98. Krishnan AV, Halmagyi GM. Acute transverse myelitis in SLE. *Neurology* 2004; 62: 2087.

99. Tellez-Zenteno JF, Remes-Troche JM, Negrete-Pulido RO, Davila-Maldonado L. Longitudinal myelitis associated with systemic lupus erythematosus: clinical features and magnetic resonance imaging in six cases. *Lupus* 2001; 10: 851–56.

100. Im CY, KIM SS, Kim HK. Bilateral optic neuritis as first manifestation of systemic lupus erythematosus. *Korean J Ophthalmol* 2002; 16: 52–8.

101. Hummers LK, Krishnan C, Casciola-Rosen L, *et al.* Recurrent transverse myelitis associated with anti-Ro (SSA) autoantibodies. *Neurology* 2004; 62: 147–9.

102. McKeon A, Lennon VA, Jacob A, *et al.* Coexistence of myasthenia gravis and serological markers of neurological autoimmunity in neuromyelitis optica. *Muscle Nerve* 2009; 39: 87–90.

103. Antoine JC, Camdessanche JP, Absi L, Lassabliere F, Feasson L. Devic disease and thymoma with anti-central nervous system and antithymus antibodies. *Neurology* 2004; 62: 978–80.

104. Pittock S, Lennon V. Aquaporin-4 autoantibodies in a paraneoplastic context. *Arch Neurol* 2008; 65: 629–32.

105. Beck RW, Cleary PA, Anderson MM, Jr., Keltner JL, Shults WT, Kaufman DI, Buckley EG, Corbett JJ, Kupersmith MJ, Miller NR, *et al.* A randomized, controlled trial of corticosteroids in the treatment of acute optic neuritis. The Optic Neuritis Study Group. *N Engl J Med* 1992; 326: 581–8.

106. Frohman EM, Wingerchuk DM. Clinical practice. Transverse myelitis. *N Engl J Med* 2010; 363: 564–72.

107. Weinshenker BG, O'Brien PC, Petterson TM, *et al.* A randomized trial of plasma exchange in acute central nervous system inflammatory demyelinating disease. *Ann Neurol* 1999; 46: 878–86.

108. Keegan M, Pineda AA, McClelland RL, Darby CH, Rodriguez M, Weinshenker BG. Plasma exchange for severe attacks of CNS demyelination: predictors of response. *Neurology* 2002; 58: 143–6.

109. Watanabe S, Nakashima I, Misu T, *et al.* Therapeutic efficacy of plasma exchange in NMO-IgG-positive patients with neuromyelitis optica. *Mult Scler* 2007; 13: 128–32.

110. Palace J, Leite MI, Nairne A, Vincent A. Interferon Beta treatment in

neuromyelitis optica: increase in relapses and aquaporin 4 antibody titers. *Arch Neurol* 2010; 67: 1016–17.

111. Shimizu J, Hatanaka Y, Hasegawa M, *et al.* IFNbeta-1b may severely exacerbate Japanese optic-spinal MS in neuromyelitis optica spectrum. *Neurology* 2010; 75: 1423–7.

112. Tanaka M, Tanaka K, Komori M. Interferon-beta(1b) treatment in neuromyelitis optica. *Eur Neurol* 2009; 62: 167–70.

113. Jacob A, Matiello M, Weinshenker BG, *et al.* Treatment of neuromyelitis optica with mycophenolate mofetil: retrospective analysis of 24 patients. *Arch Neurol* 2009; 66: 1128–33.

114. Cree BA, Lamb S, Morgan K, Chen A, Waubant E, Genain C. An open label study of the effects of rituximab in neuromyelitis optica. *Neurology* 2005; 64: 1270–2.

115. Jacob A, Weinshenker BG, Violich I, *et al.* Treatment of neuromyelitis optica with rituximab: retrospective analysis of 25 patients. *Arch Neurol* 2008; 65: 1443–8.

116. Weinstock-Guttman B, Ramanathan M, Lincoff N, *et al.* Study of mitoxantrone for the treatment of recurrent neuromyelitis optica (Devic disease). *Arch Neurol* 2006; 63: 957–63.

117. Bakker J, Metz L. Devic's neuromyelitis optica treated with intravenous gamma globulin (IVIG). *Can J Neurol Sci* 2004; 31: 265–7.

Chapter

54

Management of pediatric multiple sclerosis

E. Ann Yeh and Bianca Weinstock-Guttman

Introduction

Pediatric multiple sclerosis (MS), defined as MS with an onset before 18 years of age, comprises 2–5% of MS cases.[1-3] Increasing information regarding specific clinical characteristics and treatment options for this young population has emerged in recent years. We will review these topics, with specific attention to the management of MS in children and adolescents.

Definitions

According to the International Pediatric MS Study Group (IPMSSG) definitions, published in 2007,[4] pediatric MS may be diagnosed at any age below 18 following two clinical inflammatory-demyelinating episodes of the central nervous system (CNS), which are not classified as acute disseminated encephalomyelitis (ADEM), that are separated by at least 30 days. In addition, as in adult MS, brain MRI criteria (Barkhof criteria) can be used to meet the requirement for dissemination in space.[5] The combination of an abnormal CSF (at least two oligoclonal bands (OCB) and/or an elevated IgG index) and two lesions on MRI, of which one must be in the brain, can also meet the dissemination in space criteria. The MRI may also be used to satisfy the criteria for dissemination in time following the initial clinical event, even in the absence of a new clinical demyelinating event; new T2-bright or gadolinium (Gd)-enhancing foci that must develop three or more months following the initial clinical event (McDonald criteria).

These definitions are operational and are currently under review in the pediatric population. For example, the adult MRI criteria mentioned above have been found to have low sensitivity in pediatric MS.[6] Because of this, several groups have proposed new MRI diagnostic criteria primarily related to the dissemination in space requirements for pediatric MS. According to one set of criteria, more than two of the following criteria must be satisfied: ≥5 T2 lesions, two periventricular lesions, or one brainstem lesion.[7] The same group has proposed the following MRI criteria for differentiating MS from ADEM, an entity known to be self-limited. The criteria require two or more of the following: absence of diffuse bilateral lesion pattern, presence of black holes not associated with Gd-enhancement, or more than two periventricular lesions.[8,9] These MRI criteria have been found to be highly sensitive (99%) and relatively specific (75%) in differentiating MS from ADEM when evaluated in an independent cohort of children with known MS.[7]

Clinical presentation and clinical course

The initial clinical course in the vast majority of patients with pediatric MS is relapsing–remitting, characterized by acute relapses followed by remission of neurological symptoms in 85.7% to 100% of cases, rates that are somewhat higher than for adults.[2,10,11] Relapses have been reported to be more frequent in pediatric onset MS than adult onset MS, occurring at a rate of 1.13/yr vs. 0.40/yr. ($P < 0.001$).[12] The first interattack interval is less than one year, particularly in the younger population (<10 years of age).[13]

Although the rate of disability progression varies from individual to individual regardless of the age at onset, a consistent finding in most retrospective pediatric MS studies is lower disability scores compared to adult MS patients when controlling for disease duration. Despite its known limitations, the Kurtzke Expended Disability Status Scale (EDSS) is also used in the pediatric population to monitor disability status, as in the adult population.[13,14] Median time to reach an EDSS of 4 (defined as visible, often irreversible neurologic deficit in a patient who is still able to ambulate at least 500 meters without assistance) is approximately 20 years for pediatric MS vs. 10 years for adult MS.[3]

Similar data were obtained from a large European database (EDMUS) that identified 394 patients who were less than 16 years of age at MS onset. These patients were compared to a cohort of 1775 patients with adult onset MS.[11] The median times from onset to disability scores of 4 (visible neurological deficit but still able to walk unassisted at least 500 meters), 6 (need for unilateral assistance/cane to walk 100 meters), and 7 (ability to walk no more than 10 meters) were 20, 29.9, and 37 years, respectively, approximately 10 years longer than in the adult MS population. Nevertheless, after reaching a DSS/EDSS

Multiple Sclerosis Therapeutics, Fourth Edition, ed. Jeffrey A. Cohen and Richard A. Rudick. Published by Cambridge University Press.
© Cambridge University Press 2011.

of 4, the time to reach a higher level of disability was similar in the pediatric and adult groups: the time to worsen from DSS 4 to DDS 6 was 6 years in the pediatric onset group vs. 5.7 in the adult onset group.[11] Although the time it takes from onset to reach irreversible disability in childhood-onset MS is 10 years longer than in adult-onset MS, pediatric MS patients reach these disability milestones when they are about 10 years younger than their adult MS counterparts (i.e. 34.6, 42.2, 50.5 to reach DSS of 4, 6, and 7, respectively).

Despite a relatively slow physical decline in this young population, the neurocognitive outlook of pediatric MS is not benign. A cross-sectional study has shown deficits in cognition in over 1/3 of children, while another cross-sectional study showed deficits in visuomotor integration, general cognition, language, and visual memory.[15,16] Follow-up data on 50 patients with pediatric-onset MS and 50 healthy controls demonstrated cognitive impairment (failure on three neuropsychological tests) in 70% of patients after two years, and deterioration in 75%.[17] Another study suggested that, although there was no difference between children with pediatric MS and controls on measures of general intelligence and language, specific deficits on tests of visual processing speed and memory can be seen in this population in comparison to controls.[14]

Pediatric onset MS is also characterized by greater MRI disease burden both early in the disease and at later stages,[18,19] with evidence for accelerated disease burden in comparison to the adult population. Specifically, children with MS have a higher T1 lesion volume on brain MRI, higher T1 lesion volume to brain parenchymal volume ratio, and lower magnetization transfer in T2 lesions as well as in normal appearing gray and white matter when compared to adults with similar disease duration.

Treatment of relapses
Steroids

Randomized, controlled trials of therapies for acute MS relapses have not been conducted in children. Clinical practice in the pediatric population is, therefore, based largely on adult practices. Importantly, not all children experiencing episodes of acute demyelination receive treatment for the relapses. If symptoms are mild and do not cause impairment, the decision to provide only supportive care may be made by some practitioners.[20]

Evidence in adult MS suggests that i.v. steroids are beneficial in hastening the recovery from an acute attack and may lead to decreased risk for the development of MS in the first two years after an initial episode of optic neuritis (ON).[21,22] The relative superiority of i.v. steroids over oral steroids for acute MS relapses has been the subject of debate.[23] Some have argued that the two may be equivalent, although heterogeneity between outcome measures and patient populations limit confidence in this conclusion.[24] In adults with MS, a standard dosing

recommendation of methylprednisolone (IVMP) 1 g i.v. daily for 3 to 5 days is commonly used. In the pediatric population, a survey of US practitioners suggests that many adhere to the treatment regimen of IVMP 20–30 mg/kg/day (up to 1 g/day) for three to five days for acute MS relapses.[20] The literature in adult MS does not support the need for a steroid taper after completion of pulse steroid therapy, but no evidence is available for the pediatric population. According to a survey of practitioners specializing in the treatment of pediatric demyelinating disorders, steroid tapers were considered by a majority of respondents in optic neuritis (62%), transverse myelitis (58%), ADEM (56%), and MS relapse (50%).[20] Recurrent or worsening symptomatology after discontinuation of i.v. steroids may raise the possible need for an oral taper as well as re-evaluation of the diagnosis, especially in atypical cases and in very young children.

Intravenous immunoglobulin

The use of Intravenous Immunoglobulin (IVIg) for acute MS relapses in adults has only been evaluated in two trials (as an adjunct to IVMP), where superiority was not demonstrated.[25,26] However, it may be of benefit in the treatment of corticosteroid refractory acute optic neuritis in adults.[27] In the pediatric MS population, individual case reports of treatment with IVIg in refractory cases of acute demyelination in children have been published, suggesting possible improvement, although these cases are limited to children with optic neuritis and ADEM[28–30] Anecdotally, practitioners may use IVIg first-line in febrile children or in children in whom an infectious process is not fully ruled out. The dose is 2 g/kg given over 2–5 days.

Plasma exchange

Successful use of plasma exchange (PLEX) for severe episodes of corticosteroid-resistant acute demyelination has been described in the adult population.[31,32] One case report and one case series described a decrease in relapses and clinical improvement in three of four children with pediatric MS who had severe relapses and were treated with PLEX.[33,34] Often PLEX is reserved for use in severe relapses that don't respond well to steroids or IVIG.

Disease-modifying therapies
First-line disease-modifying therapies

As noted above, pediatric onset MS has been associated with frequent early relapses, significant cognitive impairment[16,35] and lesion burden on MRI.[19] Early intervention with disease modifying therapies (DMT) in pediatric MS has been demonstrated to result in a decreased likelihood of a third clinical relapse.[36]

Seven therapies have been approved for treatment of relapsing–remitting (RR) MS in the adult population, including four first line (glatiramer acetate (GA), intramuscular (IM) and

Table 54.1 *Tolerability and response to different disease-modifying therapies in patients with pediatric MS*

	IFNβ-1a IM	IFNβ-1a s.c.	IFNβ-1b	GA
First therapy	*n* = 92	*n* = 76	*n* = 32	*n* = 53
Remained on first therapy	45%	63%	31%	64%
Poor tolerance or compliance	19%	21%	25%	15%
Refractory disease	36%	16%	44%	21%
Time to second drug, years	1.3 ± 1.5	1.1 ± 0.7	1.4 ± 1.5	1.1 ± 0.7
Total follow-up time, years	4.8 ± 3.4	2.9 ± 2.0	3.9 ± 2.2	3.6 ± 2.5
Second therapy	*n* = 12	*n* = 31	*n* = 8	*n* = 33
Remained on second therapy	33%	77%	38%	61%
Poor tolerance or compliance	42%	7%	37%	18%
Refractory disease	25%	16%	25%	21%

Reproduced with permission from.[57] GA = glatiramer acetate, IFNβ = interferon beta, IM = intramuscular, s.c. = subcutaneous.

subcutaneous (s.c.) interferon beta-1a IFNβ-la, and s.c., and two second-line therapies (mitoxantrone (MITO) and natalizumab), and the first oral therapy, fingolimod (all covered in other chapters in this book). In addition, therapies such as alemtuzumab, rituximab, daclizumab, and cyclophosphamide (CTX) have been evaluated in Phase 2 trials as have add-on therapies such as repeated cycles of IVMP and IVIg especially in breakthrough disease patients.[37–42] Additional oral therapies are under investigation, including cladribine that is awaiting Food and Drug administration (FDA) approval.[43–45] In the sections below, we will review currently available evidence for the use of these agents in children with MS.

Interferon beta

IFNβ is thought to act in MS via inhibition of proinflammatory cytokines, induction of anti-inflammatory mediators, reduction of cellular migration, and inhibition of autoreactive T-cells.[46,47] Large Phase 3 studies showed that chronic administration of recombinant IFNβ reduced the number of relapses and slowed progression of physical disability in adult patients with RRMS. These studies demonstrated an approximately 30% reduction in exacerbation (relapse) rate in patients treated for 2–4 years compared with placebo.[48]

Several retrospective case series have described the use of IFNβ-1a in the pediatric population. Follow-up in these studies ranged from 12 to 48 months. Although the majority of reports are of children over 10 years of age, Tenembaum *et al.*[49] included eight children under the age of 10 at first injection in their series. Apart from four patients with relapsing-SPMS reported in Tenembaum's paper, all patients had RRMS. Specific information regarding outcomes and response to therapy in children with SPMS is not available in this paper.

With respect to efficacy, there have been no randomized control trials evaluating the efficacy of IFNβ in the pediatric population. However, in a prospective, open-label study, Ghezzi *et al.*[50] followed 52 patients with pediatric-onset

MS who were treated with IM IFNβ-1a, and reported a reduction in annualized relapse rate from 1.9 pre-treatment to 0.4 after an average of 42 months on therapy. Similarly, Mikaeloff *et al.*, reporting on 197 children with RRMS on IFNβ followed for a mean of 5.5 years, found a reduction in risk of MS attack in both the first year of treatment with IFNβ (hazard ratio = 0.31, 95% confidence interval: 0.13–0.72) as well as over the first two years of treatment (hazard ratio = 0.40, 95% confidence interval: 0.20–0.83). After four years of follow-up, the annualized relapse rate remained lower, but the 95% confidence interval was broader due to the smaller sample size, as not all patients had such a long follow-up (hazard ratio = 0.57, 95% confidence interval 0.30–1.10).[36]

No data are available on whether IFNβ slows the progression of disability in children. It is important to keep in mind the limited value of using natural history data without placebo control groups.[51] Furthermore, no data on the MRI effect of these medications in children are available.

IFNβ-1a and 1b appear to be safe and well tolerated in this population, although discontinuation rates are 30%–50%.[52–57] A review of 258 pediatric MS patients found that approximately 20%–25% discontinued IFNβ due to poor tolerance or non-compliance, and up to 44% were switched from IFNβ due to breakthrough disease after IFNβ treatment as first therapy. These switches occurred at an average of 1.1 to 1.4 years after initiating therapy (see Table 54.1).[57]

Many children on IFNβ (35%–65%) report flu-like symptoms. Other relatively frequently observed side effects include leukopenia (8%–27%), thrombocytopenia (16%), anemia (12%) and transient elevation in transaminases (10%–62%).[49,52,53,55] Abnormalities in liver function tests (LFTs) may be more pronounced in younger children taking IFNβ. In one study, 25% of children (average age of initiation of medication 14.6 years, range 8.1–17.9 years) taking IFNβ-1a s.c. were found to have elevated LFTs. Information regarding the dosing (22 vs. 44 mcg) was not discussed in the paper. None of these children required discontinuation of therapy. Over two-thirds of these elevations occurred in the first six months of therapy.[55] Similarly, in another study evaluating IFNβ-1b, eight of 43 patients experienced elevation of LFTs (> two times the upper limit of normal). Five of the 8 (62.5%) were under 10 years of age. Two of these children were on full adult doses (8 MIU), two were on half of the adult dose (4 MIU), and one on one-quarter of the adult dose (2 MIU). By contrast, only 10% (3/30) of children over 10 years of age had elevated LFTs in the first six months of treatment with IFNβ-1b.[53,55] Temporary interruption of IFN treatment appears to lead to normalization of LFTs with safe reintroduction of IFNβ therapy.[53,55] Given these results, we recommend close LFT monitoring on all children on IFNβs, particularly for younger patients in the first six months of treatment.

Over 2/3 of children taking the s.c. formulation of IFNβ-1a have reported injection site reactions. The injection site reactions occur throughout the treatment course in equal proportions. Pohl *et al.* reported that, after a mean follow-up of 1.8 years, children were equally likely to report injection site reactions early on (0–6 months) and later.[55] Six percent of children on IFNβ-1a s.c. experienced abscess and 6% injection-site necrosis over an average follow-up of 1.8 years.[55] Of those on IFN beta-1b, only 20% over 10 years of age and 25% under 10 years of age experienced mild injection site reactions (average follow-up of 33.8 months) that did not lead to discontinuation of therapy.[53]

Dosing of IFNβ is not established in this population. However, most patients tolerate doses titrated following adult protocols, or gradual titration to 30 mcg once weekly for IM IFNβ-1a and 22 mcg TIW or 44 mcg TIW for s.c. IFNβ-1a. Children over the age of 10 tolerate full doses of IFNβ-1b, though decreased tolerance may exist in the younger population. In one study, two of eight children who initiated IFNβ-1b at 25%–50% of adult doses did not tolerate escalation to full adult doses. Both were under 10 years of age.[53]

It has been noted widely in the adult literature that neutralizing antibodies (NAB) may appear after a patient has been treated with IFNβ. In the adult population, NAB are more likely to occur with s.c. IFNβ preparations, which are given multiple times weekly.[58] Sustained, high titers of NAB have been associated with decreased biological activity as well as decreased clinical benefit in adult MS[59–62] (Chapter 24). Knowledge regarding the frequency of NAB in the pediatric population, however, is limited. Although no systematically evaluations of NAB in the pediatric MS population exist, preliminary data suggest a lower frequency in the pediatric MS population treated with IFNβ.[63]

Glatiramer acetate

Glatiramer acetate (GA) is postulated to induce myelin-specific response of suppressor T-lymphocytes and to inhibit specific effector T-cells (Chapter 26).[64] In the pivotal Phase 3 trial of GA in adult RRMS patients, active treatment reduced the number of relapses by 29% compared with placebo.[65] GA has also

been shown to reduce MRI activity in a randomized, controlled trial of adults treated with GA vs. placebo.[66] Recent studies in adults have suggested that GA and IFNβ have similar efficacy on clinical and MRI activity.[67]

Only three retrospective studies have been published evaluating the use of GA in pediatrics.[68–70] Kornek *et al.*[70] followed seven patients with pediatric onset RRMS for 24 months and reported that GA was well tolerated. Children were aged 9–16 at the time of GA initiation. Only 2/7 patients were relapse free over the 24-month treatment period and EDSS was stable in only 3/7 of the children. In two separate papers, Ghezzi *et al.* described nine and 11 patients on GA. GA was found to be relatively well tolerated, with three of 11 patients experiencing side effects (injection site reactions in two and chest pain in one).[68] The mean annualized relapse rate decreased from 2.8 to 0.25.[69] The data, although limited by the small number of patients, studied suggest similar benefits as seen in adult population.

Second-line therapies

Treatment failure

Treatment failure is a concern in the pediatric MS population. Of 258 children with MS who were followed by a network of six US Pediatric MS Centers of Excellence, 48% were switched from their first therapy, and 4% quit therapy altogether (see Fig. 54.1). Non-compliance and side effects accounted for a significant proportion of these cases: 42 (16%) changed therapies due to non-compliance or side effects, whereas 72 (28%) changed due to breakthrough disease. Nine (4%) discontinued therapy entirely after the first agent.[57]

Although the definition of treatment failure is challenging, it is generally accepted that at least six months of observation on a given treatment is necessary prior to deciding that a treatment is suboptimal. At present, our practice is to follow these guidelines and observe all patients for six months after initiation of therapy before deciding to change therapies.

There are no consensus criteria for breakthrough disease in pediatric MS. Some have proposed criteria including lack of decrease in relapse rate, occurrence of new MRI lesions, or worsening of cognitive or motor disability.[57,71,72] Limitations include the lack of adequate observational time to gauge whether an individual's relapse rate has decreased. Some advocate clinical evaluation every 3–6 months and an annual MRI in the adult population in order to monitor response to therapy closely. Given the more frequent relapses seen in the pediatric population,[12] our practice is to perform MRI scans of the brain on a semi-annual basis with clinical visits every three months for the first year after diagnosis. Population studies in adults have shown that the disease course during the first five years of disease is an excellent predictor of future deficits. Therefore, more frequent follow-up in the early course of the disease is warranted.

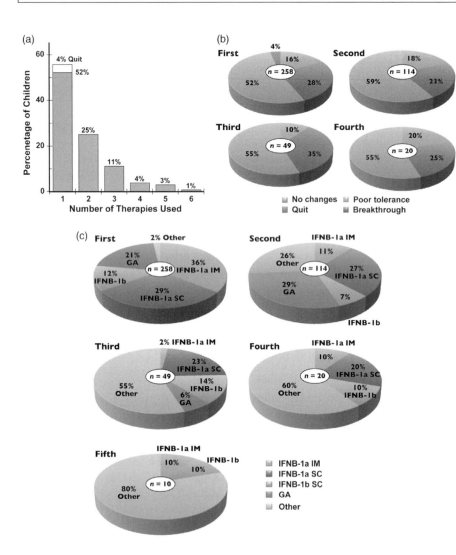

Fig. 54.1. The majority of children with pediatric MS are successfully treated with first-line therapies. 52% used only one therapy (4% quit therapy), and an additional 25% used two therapies (a). (b) shows the reasons for switching therapy in pediatric MS. The proportion of treated patients with breakthrough disease is shown in green and the proportion with poor tolerance or compliance is in red. The value labels indicate the percentage of children. The sample size is indicated at the center of the pie chart). (c) shows distribution of the types of therapies required at each stage of therapy. The value labels indicate the percentage of children. The sample size is indicated at the center of the pie chart. Reproduced with permission from reference [57].

As with adults, there is no generally accepted algorithm for management of breakthrough disease in the pediatric MS population. However the following options may be considered:

1. Increase the frequency of IFNβ therapy (i.e. switching from once a week to three times a week or every other day injections). While some data support a short-term advantage of more frequent dosing on relapses, the magnitude of the advantage is small.[73,74] This small potential advantage must be weighed against the disadvantages associated with frequent s.c. doses vs. IM once a week dose regimens, as more frequent dosing has been associated with a higher frequency of IFNβ NAB.[75,76]

2. Switch from one monotherapy to another. Switching from IFNβ to GA appears most rationale in the presence of IFNβ NAB with sustained titers ≥20. Even in the absence of IFNβ NAB, switching from IFNβ to GA is reasonable, although there are no class 1 data supporting this. Switching from GA to IFNβ is also an option, particularly given the rapid and robust effect of IFNβ on inflammatory activity as measured by MRI.[77]

3. Add agents to the "platform" IFNβ or GA therapy, including other immunomodulatory or cytotoxic agents.

The next section of this chapter will be devoted to immunomodulatory and cytotoxic agents that have been used in treatment-resistant cases. The discussion will be limited to agents whose use in pediatric MS has been described, including natalizamab, CTX, MITO, and rituximab.

Natalizumab

Natalizumab, a recombinant, humanized monoclonal antibody binds the α4 subunit of α4β1 (very late antigen-4, VLA-4) and α4 β7 integrins (adhesion molecules) interfering with the interaction between VLA-4 and its counter-receptor, vascular endothelial adhesion molecule-1 (VCAM-1) (Chapter 27). Two pivotal, randomized, placebo-controlled Phase 3 clinical trials demonstrated that natalizumab is an effective therapy for RRMS.[78,79] Both trials confirmed the efficacy of natalizumab treatment in reducing relapse rate, disease progression, and occurrence of new MRI lesions in MS. Natalizumab was well tolerated. Importantly, cases of progressive multifocal leukoencephalopathy (PML), a rare, often fatal CNS infection caused by the JC polyomavirus, occurred in association with natalizumab therapy in combination with IFNβ, prompting its withdrawal.[80–82] After extensive review, the US FDA approved the re-introduction of natalizumab for treating MS. Its use currently requires patient and prescriber registration and compliance, following specific guidelines using a risk map (TOUCH program).

There have been four published papers describing the use of natalizamab in the pediatric population; one is a case report of a 12-year-old child with first-line agent-resistant disease who responded well to natalizumab.[83] A German group reported three patients who were selected for natalizumab therapy either because they suffered from poorly controlled disease or adverse effects from first-line therapies. The medication was well tolerated by these children. Follow-up MRI scans, performed every six months, showed no new or Gd-enhancing lesions in these patients.[84]

In another case series, Ghezzi *et al.* described nineteen patients with pediatric MS treated with natalizumab. Average age at treatment initiation was 14.6 years with an average number of previous relapses of 5.2. Follow up was for an average of 15 months (range 6–26 months); all children remained on therapy for the duration of the follow up period. Although two children developed new T2 lesions at month 6, further lesions did not develop in these children. The number of Gd-enhancing lesions was significantly reduced, from an average of 4.1 at initiation of therapy to zero at follow-up evaluation ($P = 0.008$). Transient side effects occurred in eight children (42%), but these did not result in discontinuation of the medication. Median EDSS decreased from 2.5 to 2.0 at the last visit ($P < 0.001$).[85]

Finally, pediatric patients treated with natalizumab were described in a larger retrospective study of the treatment of refractory pediatric MS.[57] Of 258 patients with pediatric MS followed at the US Pediatric MS Centers of Excellence, 26 were treated with natalizamab for breakthrough disease.[86] The medication appeared to be well tolerated, and, further, seemed to result in improved disease control. Of children started on natalizumab, only three changed therapies subsequently: one experienced hypersensitivity reaction in the presence of anti-natalizumab antibodies (after being previously exposed to one infusion before the medication was suspended from the market), one was discontinued due to breakthrough disease one month after initiation, and one discontinued the medication due to GI side effects. There have been no reports to date of PML in association with this young population, although only a few patients to date were treated for more than 24 months.

Mitoxantrone

MITO is an anthracendione cytotoxic agent with immuno-suppressive properties. Safety and efficacy studies have been performed.[87,88] Based on the results of a Phase 3 study of 194 patients randomized to two treatment groups (MITO 12 mg/m^2 vs. 5 mg/m^2) and one placebo group, MITO was approved in the

USA and Europe for the treatment of worsening RR and secondary progressive (SP) MS in adults.[89] MITO is structurally related to anthracycline agents, with well-known cardiotoxicity. Long-term clinical use of MITO requires caution; the lifetime cumulative dosage should not exceed 140 mg/m.^{2} LVEF evaluation (MUGA or ECHO) should be performed before each MITO infusion and close monitoring of blood counts should be performed regularly because of an increased risk for treatment-related acute leukemia. Importantly, recent data point to a higher than previously reported dose-dependent risk for acute leukemia in patients who have received MITO, with greatest risk in patients receiving >60 mg/m^2.[90,91] Twelve of 258 patients followed at the US Pediatric MS Centers of Excellence received mitoxantrone.[57] No major side effects have been noted to date. However, we suggest caution with its use, given the potential for major side effects, including leukemia.

Rituximab

B-cells, immunoglobulins, and complement are increasingly being implicated in the pathogenesis of MS.[92] Rituximab is a B-cell-depleting chimeric monoclonal antibody that recognizes the B-cell surface receptor CD20. It was originally used in the treatment of non-Hodgkin's lymphoma. It has been used with success in multiple autoimmune diseases such as rheumatoid arthritis, Idiopathic thrombocytopenia purpura (ITP), lupus, and Sjögren's, among others.

A Phase 2 double-blind placebo-controlled trial evaluating response in adult-onset RRMS to two infusions of rituximab, given on days 1 and 15, showed convincing evidence for decreased inflammatory brain lesions and clinical relapses over a 48-week period. At 24 weeks, 14.5% of patients in the rituximab group had relapses vs. 40% in the placebo group. At week 48, the number was 20% vs. 40%. Side effects were more common in the rituximab than placebo groups (98% of patients on rituximab vs. 35% on placebo). The number of patients experiencing serious adverse events was similar in the placebo (14.3%) and rituximab (13.0%) groups. It is therefore a promising therapy for patients with active RRMS.[37,38] The future of CD20 antibody therapy will depend on studies of the humanized CD20 monoclonal antibody ocrelizumab, and full assessment of the safety profile. The FDA recently issued a warning about rituximab after two patients with lupus developed PML while on therapy with rituximab.

In the pediatric MS population, only one case report of rituximab has been published; a dramatic decrease in relapse number was reported in an adolescent with severe RRMS. The effect lasted for two years from the time therapy was initiated.[93]

Cyclophosphamide

CTX, an alkylating agent with potent cytotoxic and immuno-suppressive effects, has been studied in controlled, unblinded trials using high-doses i.v. as an induction therapy or in repeated cycles; these regimens have shown benefit in patients with SPMS in some, but not all studies.[87,88] CTX, has multiple side effects including leukopenia, myocarditis, hemorrhagic cystitis, infertility, and alopecia. Therefore, some consider CTX to be a treatment for adult RRMS patients with active disease who have failed less toxic therapies or have a rapidly progressive course. One case series described a cohort of 17 children with highly inflammatory and aggressive RRMS in whom CTX was initiated.[94] All children experienced multiple relapses (average annualized relapse rate 3.8) in the year prior to CTX, despite being treated with a first-line therapy. Physical disability in this cohort was marked; almost 25% of the cohort had an EDSS of 6.0 or higher. Half of the children who received CTX in this study later required combination therapy or treatment with another second-line agent. Only one-third of the children were able to go back to a first-line therapy. With regards to tolerability, almost all children receiving CTX experienced side effects, some of which were serious, including ITP, infertility, osteoporosis, and transitional cell bladder carcinoma. This therapy should, therefore, be used with caution in this population. Long-term safety data are not available.

Oral agents: fingolimod and cladribine

Phase 3 clinical trials have been published on two oral agents in adult MS: fingolimod and cladribine.[44,45,95] Both of these agents target lymphocytes through different mechanisms of action. Fingolimod is a sphingosine 1-phosphate-receptor modulator that was approved by the FDA in 2010 for use in adult patients with RRMS. It prevents the egress of lymphocytes from lymph nodes. Two pivotal Phase 3 randomized controlled trials, one a placebo-controlled trial and the other a comparison of fingolimod to IM IFNβ-1a, showed efficacy of oral fingolimod over placebo at doses of 0.5 mg or 1.25 mg daily. The placebo-controlled trial showed a significant reduction in annualized relapse rate (0.18 (0.5 mg), 0.16 (1.25 mg), 0.4 (placebo), $P <$ 0.001), risk of disability progression, and MRI measures of atrophy and lesion count in patients on fingolimod.[45] In the trial comparing fingolimod to IFNβ-1a IM, patients on fingolimod had a significantly lower annualized relapse rate than those on IFN (0.2 (1.25 mg), 0.16 (0.5 mg) vs. 0.33 (IFNβ-la), $P <$ 0.001). Adverse events in both trials included elevated LFTs, macular edema, skin cancer, herpes virus infections (including two fatal infections at the 1.25 mg dose), hypertension and cardiac arrhythmias (bradycardia, atrioventricular conduction block).[43,45]

Cladribine is an immunomodulatory agent that targets lymphocyte subsets. Two dosing regimens were evaluated in a pivotal Phase 3 trial: 3.5 mg and 5.25 mg per kilogram body weight. In this large, randomized, placebo-controlled double-blind trial, in comparison to patients on placebo, patients on cladribine were found to have a significant reduction in annualized relapse rate (0.14 (3.5 mg/kg), 0.15 (5.25 mg/kg), 0.33 (placebo), $P < 0.001$)) and MRI lesion count. Patients on cladribine were also found to have higher relapse-free rate than those on placebo (79.7% (3.5 mg/kg), 78.9% (5.25 mg), 60.9% (placebo), $P < 0.001$)). The most significant complications were those of lymphocytopenia and herpes zoster.[44]

No studies of the use of these agents in the pediatric population have been published. However, given the serious adverse events reported in association with these agents in the adult population, including cancer and lethal herpetic infections, caution should be taken before adopting these therapies for the pediatric population.

IVIg

Monthly IVIg therapy to prevent MS relapses in adults has been evaluated in several trials.[96–100] In 1997, a randomized, double blind, placebo controlled trial of 150 adults with RR MS suggested benefit of monthly IVIg at a dose of 0.15–0.2 g/kg when compared to placebo.[42] Patients on IVIg had a drop in EDSS scores (−0.23 (−0.43 to −0.03)). Nevertheless, a dose-finding placebo controlled trial published in 2008 suggested no benefit of either IVIg at 0.2 or 0.4 grams/kg/month in comparison to placebo in relapsing patients.[100] Similarly, controversial data on IVIg effectiveness in progressive patients raise the consideration of disease heterogeneity. A large study on SPMS patients (318 patients) did not show clinical benefit of IVIg,[101] although a delay in progression of disease in patients with primary progrossive MS, and a trend in favor of IVIg treatment in patients with primary progressive MS was shown in a more recent study.[102] In a retrospective review of 258 children followed by the US Network of Pediatric MS Centers, 9/258 received monthly IVIg therapy as an add-on therapy for breakthrough disease. It was well tolerated and deemed beneficial.[57]

Repeated IVMP cycles

Conflicting data regarding the role of chronic steroid administration in preventing MS disease progression exist. One Phase 2, double-blind study of two doses of pulse IVMP in patients with relapsing–progressive MS showed benefit on delaying the time to sustained progression of disability,[103] and a randomized, controlled, single-blind, five-year, Phase 2 clinical trial of IVMP in patients with RRMS demonstrated that chronic administration of pulse IVMP may limit clinical and MRI markers of disease progression.[104] Six of 258 pediatric patients of the US Network of Pediatric MS Centers received monthly steroids for refractory disease, which was deemed beneficial and well tolerated.[57]

Psychosocial aspects of care and symptomatic therapies

Cognitive decline, fatigue and affective disorders (e.g. depression) have been found at increased rates in children with MS.[15–17,35,105,106] Frequently, children with pediatric MS will require additional symptomatic therapies directed at these issues. Unfortunately, no clinical trials for these symptoms have been conducted specifically in pediatric MS. Rather, treatment decisions aimed at symptomatic relief are based on ancillary evidence in children with other underlying conditions, e.g. cerebral palsy. Below, we outline some approaches to frequently encountered psychosocial problems and symptoms in pediatric MS.

Educational support

Almost 75% of patients with pediatric MS fulfilled criteria for cognitive impairment, with 75% of those cases showing deteriorating cognitive performance, according to an Italian follow-up study.[17] The most prominent areas affected include verbal memory, complex attention, verbal fluency, and receptive language.[17] For these reasons, a key element of the care of children with MS includes involvement of a social worker together with a neuropsychologist, occupational therapist, and physical therapist. This team can assess the child and advise individualized educational plans, 504 plans (for school-based accommodations), and can serve as a liaison for other school-based services.

Mobility

Although irreversible motor disability is reported to appear decades after disease onset in pediatric MS patients, children with MS frequently encounter mobility problems after an acute relapse. These children should be assessed by a physical therapist, not only to improve mobility and balance, but also for assistive devices, including ankle-foot orthoses, unilateral and bilateral assistive devices, and wheelchairs. These devices are commonly only needed temporarily, but the often temporary nature of the impairment should not deter one from seeking physical therapy evaluation.

Dalfampridine extended release (Ampyra), a potassium channel blocker was recently approved by the FDA for use in improving gait in adults with MS.[107,108] This medication has not been studied in the pediatric population. Pediatric dosing, efficacy, and tolerability in this population are, therefore, unknown.

Spasticity

Mild to moderate spasticity, manifested clinically as impaired gait or focal muscle pain, occurs frequently in pediatric MS. Practice parameters regarding the use of drugs for spasticity in children with cerebral palsy exist,[109] and can be used as a guideline for pediatric MS. Agents used for spasticity in children are similar to those used in the adult MS population and include diazepam, baclofen, tizanidine, and dantrolene. These drugs may provide significant symptom relief. Evidence for the effectiveness of diazepem in childhood spasticity in patients with cerebral palsy patients exists,[109] but sedation and risk of habituation or withdrawal limit the use of benzodiazepines in pediatric MS. Oral baclofen has been available for the treatment of spasticity since the mid-1970s,[110] and its efficacy in adult MS is well established.[111,112] Only one publication has documented significant effectiveness for reducing spasticity in

children with cerebral palsy aged 2–16; functional improvement varies.[113] Side effects of baclofen include muscle weakness, somnolence, and reduced seizure threshold. Dosing starts at 5–10 mg/day divided three times a day. Of note, because abrupt discontinuation of the therapy may result in hallucinations, hyperthermia, and seizures, gradual tapering of the medication is recommended.[114–118]

Intrathecal (IT) baclofen, widely used in the adult MS population, has also been studied in the pediatric population. A study of 17 children with spastic cerebral palsy who were randomized to immediate or delayed treatment with IT baclofen showed significant differences at six months between children who received the IT baclofen compared with children in whom treatment had not yet initiated therapy.[119] Follow-up (mean 18 months, range 12–24 months).[120]

Tizanadine has been found to be efficacious for the treatment of spasticity in adult MS, and may be associated with greater tolerability and less weakness than diazepam or baclofen.[121] Side effects associated with tizanidine include weakness, somnolence, and gastrointestinal side effects. Children are reported to have significantly fewer side effects than adults, with fewer serious side effects in children as well (19.2% vs. 45.9%).[122] Transient liver transaminase elevations have been reported in a small number of children.[122] One small study of the use of tizanidine (patients $n = 10$, controls $n = 30$) reported a significant reduction in spasticity in children at a dose of 0.05 mg/kg/day.[123]

Dantrolene has been evaluated only in one small double-blind study of 20 children with spasticity secondary to cerebral palsy. A decrease in spasticity was found with dantrolene compared to placebo, but no functional improvement was seen in this population.[124] Liver function abnormalities have been reported after several months of therapy.[125] The side effect profile and lack of clear evidence for efficacy limit its clinical utility.

Botulinum toxin-A has been evaluated for the focal treatment of spasticity in children. Although it provides temporary improvement in spasticity, a two-year placebo-controlled trial of 64 children with cerebral palsy receiving up to 30 μ/kg every three months showed only temporary benefit of the therapy.[126] Doses of 15–22 U /kg body weight in children <45 kg and 800 to 1200 U in young adults have been reported to be safe in a retrospective study of 94 children and 14 adults with spasticity.[127]

Affective disorders and depression

Affective disorders have been noted in almost 1/3 of children with MS.[17] As such, when symptoms of depression appear, involvement of psychiatrists and counselors with special expertise in childhood psychiatry is essential. Interventions for these children include counseling and, when necessary, treatment with antidepressants, such as selective serotonin reuptake inhibitors (SSRIs), or tricyclic antidepressants.

In 2003, the FDA administered a black box warning regarding an increase in suicidality in children treated with SSRIs, which resulted in a marked decrease in both diagnoses of depression and SSRI prescriptions across the country.[128] The FDA recommended that introduction of pharmacologic intervention for depression in this group is accompanied by increased and close supervision (seven contacts in three months).[129] Following these guidelines, we recommend close involvement of a psychiatric team in children with MS who have affective disorders.

Fatigue

Fatigue has been reported in children/adolescents with MS,[17,35,105,106] with rates ranging from 21% in an Italian study using a standardized measure of adult fatigue in MS (fatigue severity scale (FSS))[17] to 73% when levels of fatigue were compared to healthy controls using the same cohort of Italian children.[35] The etiology of fatigue may be multifactorial and related not only to the underlying disease process, but also to affective disorders and neurologic dysfunction (e.g. spasticity, weakness). It is suggested that the underlying etiology of the fatigue be treated with appropriate psycho-social and medical interventions, including school-based accommodations, psychiatric intervention, counseling, assistive devices, and amelioration of sleep-related difficulties.

An adult MS randomized trial should improvement in fatigue, quality of life and depression in 150 patients (intervention $n = 76$ vs. usual care ($n = 74$)) using a structured eight-week program of "mindfulness training." Mindfulness training is identified as being based on "concepts of mental training that propose that nonjudgmental awareness of moment-to-moment experience may positively affect accuracy of perception, acceptance of intractable health-related changes, realistic sense of control, and appreciation of available life experiences." Practically speaking, the training includes interviews, goal setting, and specific exercises.[130] These techniques have not been evaluated in the pediatric MS population.

In the adult MS population, modafinil has been evaluated for treatment of fatigue in randomized placebo-controlled and open-label trials.[131–134] Open-label trials have suggested improvement in the FSS, as has a single-blind Phase 2 study.[133] However, one five-week double-blind, placebo-controlled parallel group study, which enrolled 115 patients with MS, found no differences in the Modified Fatigue Impact Scale (MFIS) between patients on modafinil and placebo after treatment.[134] The mechanism of action of modafinil has not been elucidated, but it acts as a stimulant. It is FDA approved for the treatment of narcolepsy, but has not been approved for fatigue associated with MS. Pharmacologic agents for fatigue in MS, including modafinil, have not been tested in pediatric MS. Modafinil has been shown to be well tolerated and efficacious in children with attention deficit hyperactivity disorder.[135,136]

Conclusions

A growing body of literature has helped to provide better guidelines for the diagnosis and treatment of pediatric MS. Pediatric MS has been shown to carry a greater disease burden than adult MS, both in terms of annualized relapse rate and MRI parameters. First-line therapies currently used in the adult population appear to be safe in children with pediatric MS. Breakthrough disease requiring a change in therapy is relatively common in this population. Current second-line therapies used in the adult population have been used in a small number of children with pediatric MS and appear to be well tolerated. Oral agents have not been evaluated in children with MS. Fatigue, spasticity, and depression are frequently seen in this population. Studies of symptomatic interventions in the pediatric MS population have not been published. Treatment of these symptoms is, therefore, based on available evidence in children with similar symptomatic issues. Future studies evaluating the role of acute, symptomatic and preventative therapies already approved for use in the adult MS population in children with MS are necessary. International registries monitoring benefit and long-term safety in pediatric MS population are being organized for these purposes.

References

1. Chitnis T, Glanz B, Jaffin S, Healy B. Demographics of pediatric-onset multiple sclerosis in an MS center population from the Northeastern United States. *Mult scler* 2009;15(5): 627–31.

2. Boiko A, Vorobeychik G, Paty D, Devonshire V, Sadovnick D. Early onset multiple sclerosis: a longitudinal study. *Neurology* 2002;59(7): 1006–10.

3. Simone IL, Carrara D, Tortorella C, *et al.* Course and prognosis in early-onset MS: comparison with adult-onset forms. *Neurology* 2002; 59(12):1922–28.

4. Krupp LB, Banwell B, Tenembaum S. Consensus definitions proposed for pediatric multiple sclerosis and related disorders. *Neurology* 2007;68(16 Suppl 2):S7–12.

5. Barkhof F, Filippi M, Miller DH, *et al.* Comparison of MRI criteria at first presentation to predict conversion to clinically definite multiple sclerosis. *Brain* 1997;120 (11):2059–69.

6. Hahn CD, Shroff MM, Blaser SI, Banwell BL. MRI criteria for multiple sclerosis: Evaluation in a pediatric cohort. *Neurology* 2004;62(5): 806–8.

7. Ketelslegers IA, Neuteboom RF, Boon M, Catsman-Berrevoets CE, Hintzen RQ. A comparison of MRI criteria for diagnosing pediatric ADEM and MS. *Neurology* 2010;74(18):1412–15.

8. Callen DJ, Shroff MM, Branson HM, *et al.* Role of MRI in the differentiation of ADEM from MS in children. *Neurology* 2009;72(11):968–73.

9. Callen DJ, Shroff MM, Branson HM, *et al.* MRI in the diagnosis of pediatric

multiple sclerosis. *Neurology* 26 2009; 72(11):961–7.

10. Duquette P, Murray TJ, Pleines J, *et al.* Multiple sclerosis in childhood: clinical profile in 125 patients. *J Pediat* 1987; 111(3):359–63.

11. Renoux C, Vukusic S, Mikaeloff Y, *et al.* Natural history of multiple sclerosis with childhood onset. *N Engl J med* 2007;356(25):2603–13.

12. Gorman MP, Healy BC, Polgar-Turcsanyi M, Chitnis T. Increased relapse rate in pediatric-onset compared with adult-onset multiple sclerosis. *Arch neurol* 2009;66(1): 54–59.

13. Ruggieri M, Polizzi A, Pavone L, Grimaldi LM. Multiple sclerosis in children under 6 years of age. *Neurology* 1999;53(3):478–84.

14. Smerbeck A, Parrish J, Serafin D, *et al.* Visual-cognitive processing deficits in pediatric multiple sclerosis. *Mult Scler* 2011;17(4):449–56.

15. Banwell BL, Anderson PE. The cognitive burden of multiple sclerosis in children. *Neurology* 2005;64(5): 891–4.

16. MacAllister WS, Belman AL, Milazzo M, *et al.* Cognitive functioning in children and adolescents with multiple sclerosis. *Neurology* 2005;64(8):1422–5.

17. Amato MP, Goretti B, Ghezzi A, *et al.* Cognitive and psychosocial features in childhood and juvenile MS: two-year follow-up. *Neurology* 75(13):1134–40.

18. Waubant E, Chabas D, Okuda DT, *et al.* Difference in disease burden and activity in pediatric patients on brain magnetic resonance imaging at time of multiple sclerosis onset vs adults. *Arch Neurol* 2009;66(8):967–71.

19. Yeh EA, Weinstock-Guttman B, Ramanathan M, *et al.* Magnetic resonance imaging characteristics of children and adults with paediatric-onset multiple sclerosis. *Brain* 2009;132(12):3392–400.

20. Waldman A, Gorman M, Rensel M, *et al.* Pediatric CNS Demyelinating Disorders: Survey of US Practice Patterns. *J Child Neurol* 2011;26(6): 675–82.

21. Brusaferri F, Candelise L. Steroids for multiple sclerosis and optic neuritis: a meta-analysis of randomized controlled clinical trials. *J Neurol* 2000;247(6): 435–42.

22. Beck RW. The optic neuritis treatment trial: three-year follow-up results. *Arch Ophthalmol* 1995;113(2):136–7.

23. Alam SM, Kyriakides T, Lawden M, Newman PK. Methylprednisolone in multiple sclerosis: a comparison of oral with intravenous therapy at equivalent high dose. *J Neurol Neurosurg Psychiatry* 1993;56(11):1219–20.

24. Burton JM, O'Connor PW, Hohol M, Beyene J. Oral versus intravenous steroids for treatment of relapses in multiple sclerosis. *Cochrane Database Syst Rev.* 2009(3):CD006921.

25. Visser LH, Beekman R, Tijssen CC, *et al.* A randomized, double-blind, placebo-controlled pilot study of i.*v.* immune globulins in combination with i.*v.* methylprednisolone in the treatment of relapses in patients with MS. *Mult Scler* 2004;10(1):89–91.

26. Sorensen PS, Haas J, Sellebjerg F, Olsson T, Ravnborg M. IV immunoglobulins as add-on treatment to methylprednisolone for acute relapses in MS. *Neurology* 2004; 63(11):2028–33.

27. Tselis A, Perumal J, Caon C, *et al.* Treatment of corticosteroid refractory optic neuritis in multiple sclerosis patients with intravenous immunoglobulin. *Eur J Neurol* 2008;15(11):1163–7.

28. Straussberg R, Schonfeld T, Weitz R, Karmazyn B, Harel L. Improvement of atypical acute disseminated encephalomyelitis with steroids and intravenous immunoglobulins. *Pediat Neurol* 2001;24(2):139–43.

29. Spalice A, Properzi E, Lo Faro V, Acampora B, Iannetti P. Intravenous immunoglobulin and interferon: successful treatment of optic neuritis in pediatric multiple sclerosis. *J Child Neurol* 2004;19(8):623–6.

30. Shahar E, Andraus J, Savitzki D, Pilar G, Zelnik N. Outcome of severe encephalomyelitis in children: effect of high-dose methylprednisolone and immunoglobulins. *J Child Neurol* 2002;17(11):810–14.

31. Rodriguez M, Karnes WE, Bartleson JD, Pineda AA. Plasmapheresis in acute episodes of fulminant CNS inflammatory demyelination. *Neurology* 1993;43(6):1100–4.

32. Llufriu S, Castillo J, Blanco Y, *et al.* Plasma exchange for acute attacks of CNS demyelination: Predictors of improvement at 6 months. *Neurology* 2009;73(12):949–53.

33. Schilling S, Linker RA, Konig FB, *et al.* [Plasma exchange therapy for steroid-unresponsive multiple sclerosis relapses: clinical experience with 16 patients]. *Nervenarzt* 2006;77(4): 430–8.

34. Takahashi I, Sawaishi Y, Takeda O, Enoki M, Takada G. Childhood multiple sclerosis treated with plasmapheresis. *Pediat Neurol* 1997; 17(1):83–7.

35. Amato MP, Goretti B, Ghezzi A, *et al.* Cognitive and psychosocial features of childhood and juvenile MS. *Neurology* 2008;70(20):1891–7.

36. Mikaeloff Y, Caridade G, Tardieu M, Suissa S. Effectiveness of early beta interferon on the first attack after confirmed multiple sclerosis: a comparative cohort study. *Eur J Paediatr Neurol* 2008;12(3):205–9.

37. Hauser SL, Waubant E, Arnold DL, *et al.* B-cell depletion with rituximab in relapsing-remitting multiple sclerosis. *N Eng j Med* 2008;358(7):676–88.

38. Bar-Or A, Calabresi PA, Arnold D, *et al.* Rituximab in relapsing-remitting multiple sclerosis: a 72-week, open-label, phase I trial. *Ann Neurol* 2008;63(3):395–400.

39. Bielekova B, Richert N, Howard T, *et al.* Humanized anti-CD25 (daclizumab) inhibits disease activity in multiple sclerosis patients failing to respond to interferon beta. *Proc Natl Acad Sci USA* 2004;101(23):8705–8.

40. Krishnan C, Kaplin AI, Brodsky RA, *et al.* Reduction of disease activity and disability with high-dose cyclophosphamide in patients with aggressive multiple sclerosis. *Arch Neurol* 2008;65(8):1044–51.

41. Then Bergh F, Kumpfel T, Schumann E, *et al.* Monthly intravenous methylprednisolone in relapsing-remitting multiple sclerosis – reduction of enhancing lesions, T2 lesion volume and plasma prolactin concentrations. *BMC Neurol.* 2006;6:19.

42. Fazekas F, Deisenhammer F, Strasser-Fuchs S, Nahler G, Mamoli B. Randomised placebo-controlled trial of monthly intravenous immunoglobulin therapy in relapsing-remitting multiple sclerosis. Austrian Immunoglobulin in Multiple Sclerosis Study Group. *Lancet* 1997;349(9052):589–93.

43. Cohen JA, Barkhof F, Comi G, *et al.* Oral fingolimod or intramuscular interferon for relapsing multiple sclerosis. *N Engl J Med*; 362(5): 402–15.

44. Giovannoni G, Comi G, Cook S, *et al.* A placebo-controlled trial of oral cladribine for relapsing multiple sclerosis. *N Engl J Med*; 362(5):416–26.

45. Kappos L, Radue EW, O'Connor P, *et al.* A placebo-controlled trial of oral fingolimod in relapsing multiple sclerosis. *N Engl J Med*; 362(5):387–401.

46. Group IMSS. Interferon beta-1b is effective in relapsing-remitting multiple sclerosis. I Clinical results of a multicenter, randomized, double blind, placebo-controlled trial. *Neurology*. 1993;43(4):655–661.

47. Jacobs L, Cookfair D, Rudick R, *et al.* Intramuscular interferon beta-1a for disease progression in relapsing multiple sclerosis. *Ann Neurol.* 1996;39:285–94.

48. Group PRISMS. Randomized double-blind placebo-controlled study of interferon β-1a in relapsing/remitting multiple sclerosis. *Lancet* 1998;352:1498–504.

49. Tenembaum SN, Segura MJ. Interferon beta-1a treatment in childhood and juvenile-onset multiple sclerosis. *Neurology* 2006;67(3):511–13.

50. Ghezzi A, Amato MP, Capobianco M, *et al.* Treatment of early-onset multiple sclerosis with intramuscular interferonbeta-1a: long-term results. *Neurol Sci* 2007;28(3):127–32.

51. Pittock SJ, McClelland RL, Mayr WT, *et al.* Clinical implications of benign multiple sclerosis: a 20-year population-based follow-up study. *Ann Neurol* 2004;56(2):303–6.

52. Mikaeloff Y, Moreau T, Debouverie M, *et al.* Interferon-beta treatment in patients with childhood-onset multiple sclerosis. *J Pediat* 2001;139(3):443–6.

53. Banwell B, Reder AT, Krupp L, *et al.* Safety and tolerability of interferon beta-1b in pediatric multiple sclerosis. *Neurology* 2006;66(4):472–6.

54. Bykova OV, Kuzenkova LM, Maslova OI. [The use of beta-interferon-1b in children and adolescents with multiple sclerosis]. *Zh Nevrol i psikhiatrii imeni S.S.* 2006;106(9):29–33.

55. Pohl D, Rostasy K, Gartner J, Hanefeld F. Treatment of early onset multiple sclerosis with subcutaneous interferon beta-1a. *Neurology* 2005;64(5): 888–90.

56. Waubant E, Hietpas J, Stewart T, *et al.* Interferon beta-1a in children with multiple sclerosis is well tolerated. *Neuropediatrics* 2001;32(4):211–13.

57. Yeh E, Waubant E, Krupp L, *et al.* MS therapies in pediatric MS patients with refractory disease. *Arch Neurol.* 2010;68(4):437–44.

58. Malucchi S, Sala A, Gilli F, *et al.* Neutralizing antibodies reduce the efficacy of betaIFN during treatment of multiple sclerosis. *Neurology* 2004;62(11):2031–7.

59. Perini P, Calabrese M, Biasi G, Gallo P. The clinical impact of interferon beta antibodies in relapsing-remitting MS. *J Neurol* 2004;251(3):305–9.

60. Bertolotto A, Gilli F, Sala A, *et al.* Persistent neutralizing antibodies abolish the interferon beta bioavailability in MS patients. *Neurology* 2003;60(4):634–9.

61. Rudick RA, Simonian NA, Alam JA, *et al.* Incidence and significance of neutralizing antibodies to interferon beta-1a in multiple sclerosis. Multiple Sclerosis Collaborative Research Group (MSCRG). *Neurology* 1998;50(5):1266–72.

62. Neutralizing antibodies during treatment of multiple sclerosis with interferon beta-1b: experience during the first three years. The IFNB Multiple Sclerosis Study Group and the University of British Columbia MS/MRI Analysis Group. *Neurology* 1996;47 (4):889–94.

63. Yeh E, Heim R, Karpinski M, Ray J, Weinstock-Guttman B. Neutralizing antibodies to interferon in children with MS on interferon treatment. *American Academy of Neurology.* Abstract Annual Meeting. Toronto, ON2010.

64. Dhib-Jalbut S. Sustained immunological effects of Glatiramer acetate in patients with multiple sclerosis treated for over 6 years. *J Neurol Sci.* 2002;201:71–7.

65. Johnson KP, Brooks BR, Cohen JA, *et al.* Copolymer 1 reduces relapse rate and improves disability in relapsing-remitting multiple sclerosis: results of a phase III multicenter, double-blind placebo-controlled trial. The Copolymer 1 Multiple Sclerosis Study Group. *Neurology* 1995;45(7): 1268–76.

66. Comi G, Filippi M, Wolinsky JS. European/Canadian multicenter, double-blind, randomized, placebo-controlled study of the effects of glatiramer acetate on magnetic resonance imaging – measured disease activity and burden in patients with relapsing multiple sclerosis. European/Canadian Glatiramer Acetate Study Group. *Ann Neurol* 2001;49(3): 290–7.

67. Cadavid D, Wolansky LJ, Skurnick J, *et al.* Efficacy of treatment of MS with IFNbeta-1b or glatiramer acetate by monthly brain MRI in the BECOME study. *Neurology* 2009;72(23): 1976–83.

68. Ghezzi A. Immunomodulatory treatment of early onset multiple sclerosis: results of an Italian Co-operative Study. *Neurol Sci* 2005;26 (Suppl 4):S183–6.

69. Ghezzi A, Amato MP, Capobianco M, *et al.* Disease-modifying drugs in childhood-juvenile multiple sclerosis: results of an Italian co-operative study. *Mult Scler* 2005;11(4):420–4.

70. Kornek B, Bernert G, Balassy C, Geldner J, Prayer D, Feucht M. Glatiramer acetate treatment in patients with childhood and juvenile onset multiple sclerosis. *Neuropediatrics* 2003;34(3):120–6.

71. Cohen BA, Khan O, Jeffery DR, *et al.* Identifying and treating patients with suboptimal responses. *Neurology* 2004;63(12 Suppl 6):S33–40.

72. Ghezzi A, Banwell B, Boyko A, *et al.* The management of multiple sclerosis in children: a European view. *Mult Scler* 2010;16(10):1258–67.

73. Panitch H, Goodin D, Francis G, *et al.* Randomized, comparative study of interferon beta-1a treatment regimens in MS; The EVIDENCE Trial. *Neurology* 2002;359:1453–60.

74. Durelli L, Verdun E, Barbero F, *et al.* Every other day interferon beta-1b versus once-weekly interferon beta-1a for multiple sclerosis; results of a 2-year prospective randomized multicenter study (INCOMIN). *Lancet* 2002; 359:1453–60.

75. Group. IMSSGatUoBCMMA. Neutralizing antibodies during treatment of multiple sclerosis with interferon beta-1b: experience during

the first 3 years. *Neurology* 1996;47:889–94.

76. Sorensen P, Ross C, Clemmesen K, *et al.* Clinical importance of neutralizing antibodies against interferon beta in patients with relapsing remitting multiple sclerosis. *Lancet* 2003;302:1184–91.

77. Calabresi PA, Stone LA, Bash CN, Frank JA, McFarland HF. Interferon beta results in immediate reduction of contrast-enhanced MRI lesions in multiple sclerosis patients followed by weekly MRI. *Neurology* 1997;48(5):1446–8.

78. Rudick RA, Stuart WH, Calabresi PA, *et al.* Natalizumab plus interferon beta-1a for relapsing multiple sclerosis. *N Engl J Med* 2006;354(9):911–23.

79. Polman CH, O'Connor PW, Havrdova E, *et al.* A randomized, placebo-controlled trial of natalizumab for relapsing multiple sclerosis. *N Engl J Med* 2006;354(9):899–910.

80. VanAssche G, Ranst MV, Sciot R, *et al.* Progressive multifocal leukoencephalopathy after natalizumab therapy for Crohn's disease. *N Engl J Med* 2005;353:362–8.

81. Langer-Gould A, Atlas S, Green A, *et al.* Progressive multifocal encephalopathy in a patient treated with natalizumab. *N Engl J Med* 2005;353:375–81.

82. Kleinschmidt-DeMasters B, Tyler K. Progressive multifocal leukoencphalopathy complicating treatment with natalizumab and interferon beta-1a for multiple sclerosis *N Engl J Med.* 2005;353:369–74.

83. Borriello G, Prosperini L, Luchetti A, Pozzilli C. Natalizumab treatment in pediatric multiple sclerosis: A case report. *Eur J Paediatr Neurol* 2009;13(1):67–71.

84. Huppke P, Stark W, Zurcher C, Huppke B, Bruck W, Gartner J. Natalizumab use in pediatric multiple sclerosis. *Arch Neurol* 2008;65(12):1655–8.

85. Ghezzi A, Pozzilli C, Grimaldi LM, *et al.* Safety and efficacy of natalizumab in children with multiple sclerosis. *Neurology*; 75(10):912–7.

86. Yeh E, Kuntz N, Chabas D, *et al.* Use of natalizumab in pediatric MS: a collaborative network study. *Child Neurology Society.* Meeting Abstract, Louisville, KY 2009.

87. Weiner H, ackin G, Orav E, *et al.* Intermittent cyclophosphamide pulse therapy in progressive multiple sclerosis: final report of the Northeast Cooperative Multiple Sclerosis Treatment Group. *Neurology* 1993;43:910–18.

88. Group TCcMS. The Canadian cooperative trial of cyclophosphamide and plasma exchange in progressive multiple sclerosis. *Lancet* 1991;337:441–6.

89. Hartung H, Gonsette R, Konig N, *et al.* Group tM-S. Mitoxantrone in progressive multiple sclerosis: a placebo-controlled, double-blind, randomized, multicenter trial. *Lancet* 2002;360:2018–25.

90. Ellis R, Boggild M. Therapy-related acute leukaemia with Mitoxantrone: what is the risk and can we minimise it? *Mult Scler* 2009;15(4):505–8.

91. Pascual AM, Tellez N, Bosca I, *et al.* Revision of the risk of secondary leukaemia after mitoxantrone in multiple sclerosis populations is required. *Mult Scler* 2009;15(11):1303–10.

92. Lucchinetti C, Bruck W, Parisi J, Scheithauer B, Rodriguez M, Lassmann H. Heterogeneity of multiple sclerosis lesions: implications for the pathogenesis of demyelination. *Ann Neurol* 2000;47(6):707–17.

93. Karenfort M, Kieseier BC, Tibussek D, Assmann B, Schaper J, Mayatepek E. Rituximab as a highly effective treatment in a female adolescent with severe multiple sclerosis. *Dev Med Child Neurol* 2009;51(2):159–61.

94. Makhani N, Gorman MP, Branson HM, Stazzone L, Banwell BL, Chitnis T. Cyclophosphamide therapy in pediatric multiple sclerosis. *Neurology* 2009;72(24):2076–82.

95. Chun J, Hartung HP. Mechanism of action of oral fingolimod (FTY720) in multiple sclerosis. *Clin Neuropharmacol* 2010;33(2):92–101.

96. Fazekas F, Deisenhammer F, Strasser-Fuchs S, Nahler G, Mamoli B. Treatment effects of monthly intravenous immunoglobulin on patients with relapsing–remitting multiple sclerosis: further analyses of the Austrian Immunoglobulin in MS study. *Mult Scler* 1997;3(2):137–41.

97. Sorensen PS, Wanscher B, Schreiber K, Blinkenberg M, Jensen CV, Ravnborg M. A double-blind, cross-over trial of intravenous immunoglobulin G in multiple sclerosis: preliminary results. *Mult Scler.* Apr 1997;3(2):145–8.

98. Achiron A, Gabbay U, Gilad R, *et al.* Intravenous immunoglobulin treatment in multiple sclerosis. Effect on relapses. *Neurology* 1998;50(2):398–402.

99. Sorensen PS, Fazekas F, Lee M. Intravenous immunoglobulin G for the treatment of relapsing-remitting multiple sclerosis: a meta-analysis. *Eur J Neurol* 2002;9(6):557–63.

100. Fazekas F, Lublin FD, Li D, *et al.* Intravenous immunoglobulin in relapsing-remitting multiple sclerosis: a dose-finding trial. *Neurology* 2008;71(4):265–71.

101. Hommes OR, Sorensen PS, Fazekas F, *et al.* Intravenous immunoglobulin in secondary progressive multiple sclerosis: randomised placebo-controlled trial. *Lancet* 2004;364(9440):1149–56.

102. Pohlau D, Przuntek H, Sailer M, *et al.* Intravenous immunoglobulin in primary and secondary chronic progressive multiple sclerosis: a randomized placebo controlled multicentre study. *Mult Scler* 2007;13(9):1107–17.

103. Goodkin DE, Kinkel RP, Weinstock-Guttman B, *et al.* A phase II study of i.*v.* methylprednisolone in secondary-progressive multiple sclerosis. *Neurology* 1998;51(1):239–45.

104. Zivadinov R, Zorzon M, De Masi R, Nasuelli D, Cazzato G. Effect of intravenous methylprednisolone on the number, size and confluence of plaques in relapsing-remitting multiple sclerosis. *J Neurol Sci* 2008;267(1–2):28–35.

105. MacAllister WS, Boyd JR, Holland NJ, Milazzo MC, Krupp LB. The psychosocial consequences of pediatric multiple sclerosis. *Neurology* 2007;68(16 Suppl 2):S66–9.

106. MacAllister WS, Christodoulou C, Troxell R, *et al.* Fatigue and quality of life in pediatric multiple sclerosis. *Mult Scler* 2009;15(12):1502–8.

107. Goodman AD, Brown TR, Krupp LB, *et al.* Sustained-release oral fampridine in multiple sclerosis: a randomised, double-blind, controlled trial. *Lancet* 2009;373(9665):732–8.

108. Goodman AD, Brown TR, Edwards KR, *et al.* A phase 3 trial of extended release oral dalfampridine in multiple sclerosis. *Ann Neurol* 68(4):494–502.

109. Delgado MR, Hirtz D, Aisen M, *et al.* Practice parameter: pharmacologic treatment of spasticity in children and adolescents with cerebral palsy (an evidence-based review): report of the Quality Standards Subcommittee of the American Academy of Neurology and the Practice Committee of the Child Neurology Society. *Neurology* 74(4): 336–43.

110. Brogden RN, Speight TM, Avery GS. Baclofen: a preliminary report of its pharmacological properties and therapeutic efficacy in spasticity. *Drugs* 1974;8(1):1–14.

111. Feldman RG, Kelly-Hayes M, Conomy JP, Foley JM. Baclofen for spasticity in multiple sclerosis. Double-blind crossover and three-year study. *Neurology* 1978;28(11):1094–8.

112. Bass B, Weinshenker B, Rice GP, *et al.* Tizanidine versus baclofen in the treatment of spasticity in patients with multiple sclerosis. *Can J Neurol Sci* 1988;15(1):15–19.

113. Milla PJ, Jackson AD. A controlled trial of baclofen in children with cerebral palsy. *J Int Med Res* 1977;5(6):398–404.

114. Lees AJ, Clarke CR, Harrison MJ. Hallucinations after withdrawal of baclofen. *Lancet* 1977;1(8016):858.

115. Hyser CL, Drake ME, Jr. Status epilepticus after baclofen withdrawal. *J Natl Med Assoc* 1984;76(5):533, 537–8.

116. Chawla JM, Sagar R. Baclofen-induced psychosis. *Ann Pharmacother* 2006; 40(11):2071–3.

117. D'Aleo G, Cammaroto S, Rifici C, *et al.* Hallucinations after abrupt withdrawal of oral and intrathecal baclofen. *Funct Neurol* 2007;22(2):81–8.

118. Malhotra T, Rosenzweig I. Baclofen withdrawal causes psychosis in otherwise unclouded consciousness. *J Neuropsychiatry Clin Neurosci* 2009; 21(4):476.

119. Hoving MA, van Raak EP, Spincemaille GH, Palmans LJ, Becher JG, Vles JS. Efficacy of intrathecal baclofen therapy in children with intractable spastic cerebral palsy: a randomised controlled trial. *Eur J Paediatr Neurol* 2009; 13(3):240–6.

120. Hoving MA, van Raak EP, Spincemaille GH, *et al.* Safety and one-year efficacy of intrathecal baclofen therapy in children with intractable spastic cerebral palsy. *Eur J Paediatr Neurol* 2009;13(3):247–56.

121. Groves L, Shellenberger MK, Davis CS. Tizanidine treatment of spasticity: a meta-analysis of controlled, double-blind, comparative studies with baclofen and diazepam. *Adv Ther* 1998;15(4):241–51.

122. Henney HR, 3rd, Chez M. Pediatric safety of tizanidine: clinical adverse event database and retrospective chart assessment. *Paediatr Drugs* 2009; 11(6):397–406.

123. Vasquez-Briceno A, Arellano-Saldana ME, Leon-Hernandez SR, Morales-Osorio MG. [The usefulness of tizanidine. A one-year follow-up of the treatment of spasticity in infantile cerebral palsy]. *Rev Neurol* 2006; 43(3):132–6.

124. Joynt RL, Leonard JA, Jr. Dantrolene sodium suspension in treatment of spastic cerebral palsy. *Dev Med Child Neurol* 1980;22(6):755–67.

125. Chan CH. Dantrolene sodium and hepatic injury. *Neurology* 1990; 40(9):1427–32.

126. Moore AP, Ade-Hall RA, Smith CT, *et al.* Two-year placebo-controlled trial of botulinum toxin A for leg spasticity in cerebral palsy. *Neurology* 2008; 71(2):122–8.

127. Goldstein EM. Safety of high-dose botulinum toxin type A therapy for the treatment of pediatric spasticity. *J Child Neurol* 2006;21(3):189–92.

128. Libby AM, Brent DA, Morrato EH, Orton HD, Allen R, Valuck RJ. Decline in treatment of pediatric depression after FDA advisory on risk of suicidality with SSRIs. *Am J Psychiatry* 2007; 164(6):884–91.

129. Morrato EH, Libby AM, Orton HD, *et al.* Frequency of provider contact after FDA advisory on risk of pediatric suicidality with SSRIs. *Am J Psychiatry* 2008;165(1):42–50.

130. Grossman P, Kappos L, Gensicke H, *et al.* MS quality of life, depression, and fatigue improve after mindfulness training: a randomized trial. *Neurology* 75(13):1141–9.

131. Zifko UA, Rupp M, Schwarz S, Zipko HT, Maida EM. Modafinil in treatment of fatigue in multiple sclerosis. Results of an open-label study. *J Neurol* 2002;249(8):983–7.

132. Rammohan KW, Lynn DJ. Modafinil for fatigue in MS: a randomized placebo-controlled double-blind study. *Neurology* 2005;65(12):1995–7; author reply 1995–7.

133. Rammohan KW, Rosenberg JH, Lynn DJ, Blumenfeld AM, Pollak CP, Nagaraja HN. Efficacy and safety of modafinil (Provigil) for the treatment of fatigue in multiple sclerosis: a two centre phase 2 study. *J Neurol Neurosurg Psychiatry* 2002;72(2):179–83.

134. Stankoff B, Waubant E, Confavreux C, *et al.* Modafinil for fatigue in MS: a randomized placebo-controlled double-blind study. *Neurology* 2005;64(7):1139–43.

135. Biederman J, Swanson JM, Wigal SB, *et al.* Efficacy and safety of modafinil film-coated tablets in children and adolescents with attention-deficit/ hyperactivity disorder: results of a randomized, double-blind, placebo-controlled, flexible-dose study. *Pediatrics* 2005;116(6):e777–84.

136. Kahbazi M, Ghoreishi A, Rahiminejad F, Mohammadi MR, Kamalipour A, Akhondzadeh S. A randomized, double-blind and placebo-controlled trial of modafinil in children and adolescents with attention deficit and hyperactivity disorder. *Psychiatry Res* 2009;168(3):234–7.

55

Use of MRI in the clinical management of multiple sclerosis

J. Theodore Phillips and Lael A. Stone

Introduction

Magnetic resonance imaging (MRI) has revolutionized the diagnosis of multiple sclerosis (MS), to the point where most clinicians would not be comfortable making the diagnosis of the MS in the absence of characteristic MRI findings. MRI has also provided key insights to the pathophysiology of MS and has proven vital to the performance of MS clinical trials. There is tremendous variability though, in the use of MRI in the routine clinical management of MS. In this chapter, we will provide retrospective and current views on the use of MRI in assisting the clinical management of MS from initial presentation with a clinically isolated syndrome (CIS), diagnosis of MS, and throughout the course of the disease.

History of MRI in the diagnosis of MS

The first formal clinical diagnostic MS criteria were established in 1954 by Allison and Millar,[1] nearly 30 years before the routine use of clinical MRI. These early criteria focused on three categories of MS: early, probable, and possible disseminated sclerosis (i.e. MS). These criteria recognized the importance of dissemination of disease events in time (DIT), but dissemination of disease events in space (DIS) was not formally required. During the 1960s, the need for more structured criteria to provide standardized classifications for research and clinical guidance was recognized. In 1965, Schumacher and colleagues published what are commonly called the "Schumacher criteria." These criteria were the first to require both dissemination of disease events in space *and* time.[2] DIS required objective evidence by clinical examination of two or more neuroanatomically separate sites of central nervous system (CNS) damage. DIT was met by clinical symptoms lasting ≥ 24 hours, and two CNS events separated by at least 30 days. Based on natural history studies, the average frequency of relapses is 1.1/year.[3] Therefore, individuals could go several years without formal diagnosis using the Schumacher criteria. In that era, however, where preventative treatment was unavailable, this delay in diagnosis was deemed of limited clinical consequence, and was not necessarily considered a shortcoming of the diagnostic criteria.

Although the first human MRI scans occurred in 1977, the general availability of MRI scanning was still limited in the early 1980s. Thus, in 1983, another expert panel introduced new diagnostic criteria, commonly known as the "Poser criteria," which while including the use of paraclinical data (computed tomography scans, evoked potentials, and cerebrospinal fluid (CSF) analysis), did not include MRI criteria.[4] In 1986, Paty and colleagues discussed the role of MRI in the diagnosis of MS,[5] and these concepts were partially integrated into the existing Poser criteria for dissemination in time and space, and published in 1987.[6] However, the Poser criteria were designed primarily for research protocols and included many different categories of clinically or laboratory-supported, probable or definite MS. Unfortunately, this extensive categorization of supported, probable, and definite MS was confusing and cumbersome for use in the clinical setting.

Although the Poser criteria were not readily adopted outside of the research arena, the clinical use of MRI became increasingly common, and by the 1990s assumed a prominent place in the diagnosis of MS. Parallel to the increasing ease of MS diagnosis, disease-modifying treatments (DMTs) came to the market place in 1993. Indeed, MRI was a critical component of the evidence supporting approval of the first DMT in 1993. In late 2010, there were eight Regulatory-approved therapies for the treatment of MS, all of which have included MRI assessments in the clinical trial process. Each of these therapies reduce clinical and MRI manifestations of the disease.[7-15] These therapeutic successes Reinforce the need for early diagnosis and treatment of MS patients to limit neurological symptoms and potential long-term disability.

With these issues in mind, the International Panel on the Diagnosis of MS, set out to re-evaluate then current Poser diagnostic criteria and create new criteria that could be used both by the practicing neurologist, and by the researcher.[16] These criteria, commonly cited as the McDonald criteria, in honor of the late panel member Professor Ian McDonald, were published in 2001 and had three important changes from previous criteria. The first change was the simplification of the diagnostic categories; now limited to only "MS, possible MS, and not MS." The many different probable MS categories of the earlier Poser criteria were eliminated. The second change was formal inclusion of MRI criteria to establish DIT, allowing for earlier diagnostic certainty and treatment. The panel recognized that MRI

Multiple Sclerosis Therapeutics, Fourth Edition, ed. Jeffrey A. Cohen and Richard A. Rudick. Published by Cambridge University Press.
© Cambridge University Press 2011.

changes are common in other neurologic diseases and in order to avoid incorrect diagnosis, the McDonald MRI criteria specified stringent specificity and sensitivity requirements based on findings of Barkhof *et al.*[17] and Tintore *et al.*[18] The third change was inclusion of new criteria for the often-challenging diagnosis of primary progressive (PP) MS. Although the panel's foremost intent was applicability to everyday clinical practice, the McDonald criteria have become a mainstay in MS research as well.

Since the introduction of the original 2001 McDonald criteria, further revisions in these criteria have occurred.[19] The latest version of the McDonald criteria (Polman *et al.*, 2011) incorporates recent recommendations from the international Magnetic Imaging in MS (MAGNIMS) committee.[20] These more simplified criteria are also intended to apply to patients with typical CIS (aged 15–50 years, after differential diagnostic considerations have been applied) thereby accommodating even earlier diagnosis of MS. DIS is established by ≥ 1 asymptomatic T2 lesion in each of ≥2 characteristic locations – periventricular, juxtacortical, posterior fossa, or spinal cord. DIT is established by: (1) simultaneous presence of asymptomatic gadolinium (Gd)-enhancing and non-enhancing T2 lesion(s) at any time; *or* (2) new T2 and/or Gd-enhancing lesion(s) on follow-up MRI irrespective of timing of the baseline scan.

MRI and the differential diagnosis of MS

The differential diagnosis of MS includes an extensive list of possibilities that have been well reviewed elsewhere.[21–23] Many alternative diagnoses can be excluded based on the clinical history and simple laboratory testing alone. MRI can be helpful in securing the diagnosis of MS when findings are typical and have a characteristic interval evolution on subsequent MRI scans. Typical MRI changes seen in MS include ovoid, sub-centimeter, white matter T2 hyperintense lesions with little or no mass effect or edema, located in the intracranial, infratentorial, and spinal cord (especially cervical) areas mentioned in the previous paragraph. Lesion configuration is also an important characteristic. For instance, in comparing MRI features of MS and CNS vasculitis, the presence of perpendicular periventricular T2 lesions (in MS) was found statistically different and reliable in distinguishing these two entities.[24] In other circumstances, the MRI may lead to erroneous concern about MS when the MRI demonstrates unexpected T2 abnormalities, especially in the absence of a suitable clinical history or neurological exam findings. MRI changes, specifically T2 changes, are often non-specific or age related, and can occur in a variety of other neurologic and systemic diseases (Table 55.1). Indeed, the gradual accumulation of T2 hyperintense foci appears to be a normal, expected age-related finding in healthy populations, as demonstrated in the Framingham cohort.[25] Therefore, MRI alone is never sufficient to make the diagnosis of MS, and care must be taken to interpret MRI white matter changes in the appropriate clinical context. The typical MRI features of MS lesions have been reviewed and discussed by several authors.[18,26–28]

Table 55.1. *Differential considerations for MRI white matter abnormalities*

Autoimmune	Multiple sclerosis Neuromyelitis optica spectrum Behçet disease Sjögren Syndrome Systemic lupus erythematosis Anti-phospholipid antibody syndrome Collagen vascular disorders
Inflammatory	Acute disseminated encephalomyelitis Sarcoidosis
Infectious	Lyme disease Syphilis JC virus (progressive multifocal leukoencephalopathy) HIV Human T-lymphotrophic virus I/II
Genetic	Cerebral autosomal dominant arteriopathy, subcortical infarcts and leukoencephalopathy Leukodystrophy (adrenoleukodystrophy, metachromatic leukodystrophy)
Vascular	Ischemic optic neuropathy Migraine Stroke Susac disease Vascular malformations Vasculitis
Metabolic	Copper deficiency Vitamin B12 deficiency
Neoplasm	Glioma Meningioma Lymphoma
Miscellaneous	Age-related white matter changes Cervical spondylosis or stenosis Celiac disease

The MRI guidelines originally chosen by the International Panel in 2001[16] were chosen to balance both sensitivity and specificity, therefore establishing these diagnostic guidelines as generally useful in determining the significance and potential etiology of white matter lesions seen on MRI scans. The newest revision of the McDonald criteria (Polman *et al.* 2011) further simplifies MRI diagnostic guidelines while preserving this high degree of sensitivity and specificity.

MRI and the evaluation of the clinically isolated syndrome (CIS)

The first clinically apparent episode of MS is typically referred to as a CIS. The most common of these involve the optic nerve, spinal cord, or brainstem/cerebellar structures. However, some instances of CIS never recur, and are not indicative of underlying MS or other chronic, recurring process. As reviewed, there has been a gradual evolution of our concept of MS, to the point where the 2010 McDonald criteria allow for many patients previously classified as CIS to be reassigned as MS, with criteria for DIS and DIT being met by MRI evaluation. However, much of the background literature upon which our current diagnostic conclusions are based relies on the original "CIS" terminology,

Table 55.2. *Conversion of clinically isolated syndrome patients based on baseline MRI characteristics*

	5 yrs (mean 5.3)[34]		10 yrs (mean 9.7)[37]		14 yrs (mean 14.1)[36]		20 yrs (mean 20.2)[35]	
MRI at baseline	Normal	Abnormal	Normal	Abnormal	Normal	Abnormal	Normal	Abnormal
Clinically definite MS[a]	1/32 (3%)	37/57 (65%)	3/27 (11%)	45/54 (83%)	4/21 (19%)	44/50 (88%)	7/34 (21%)	60/73 (82%)
MRI changes	10/32 (31%)	48/57 (84%)	9/27 (33.3)	37/40 (93%)	8/21 (38%)	Not reported	Not reported	Not reported
Multiphasic disease-clinical and/or MRI changes	Not reported	Not reported	10/27 (37%)	47/54 (87%)	8/21 (38%)	49/50 (98%)	Not reported	Not reported

[a] By Poser Criteria.[4]

which distinguishes a one-time, isolated clinical inflammatory demyelinating event (CIS) from the clinically multiphasic (by definition) condition MS.

Indeed, current evidence strongly supports the early treatment of individuals with CIS who are at "high risk" for conversion to MS in order to prevent later disability.[29–32] Individuals "at risk" have been defined by longitudinal studies of CIS cohorts. Studies report that between 50%–80% of patients with CIS have abnormal brain MRI at baseline.[33–35] In an ongoing landmark study, 107 out of 143 original patients from the United Kingdom with CIS (optic neuritis, spinal cord syndromes, and brainstem syndromes, e.g. diplopia, vertigo) have been followed for over 20 years. Rates of conversion to CDMS (clinically definite MS; originally defined by Poser criteria at study initiation) have been reported at approximately 1, 5, 10, 14, and 20 years (Table 55.2). At all five time intervals, patients with abnormal brain MRI at baseline ($\geq$1 T2 white matter lesions typical of MS) were more likely convert to CDMS. The rate of conversion increased incrementally over time with 82% of patients with CIS and abnormal MRI brain at baseline having established CDMS (Poser criteria) by 20 years.[35] If MRI changes in the absence of a discrete second clinical event are included, 98% of subjects demonstrated multiphasic, evolving disease by 14 years.[36] Surprisingly, even among those with CIS and a normal brain MRI at baseline, multiphasic disease (clinical or MRI changes) were found in >35% at both 14 and 10 years post-presentation.[36,37] Optic neuritis presentation of CIS in individuals with abnormal baseline MRI had the highest rate of conversion (65%), compared to brainstem syndromes (60%) and spinal cord syndromes (61%) at 20 years.[35] In reviewing these studies, it should be recalled that these baseline MRI studies were done in the mid-1980s using a Picker 0.5 T scanner with 10 mm thick axial slices,[34] and, thus, were less capable of detecting white matter lesions than today's routine higher field strength/thinner slice scans. Thus, some of the scans classified initially as "normal" may have had lesions that were missed. Therefore, the rate of conversion among those with "normal" scans may in fact be an over-estimation, and the rate of CDMS conversion among those with truly normal initial scans may be lower than originally estimated. Subsequent analyses at years 10, 14, and 20 were performed with a more sensitive 1.5 T scanner with a more sensitive 5 mm slice thickness.[35]

In addition to the number and distribution of T2 changes, CIS patients with Gd-enhancing lesions at presentation are at an increased risk of conversion to CDMS.[38–40] Compared to T2 brain MRI changes, Gd-enhancing lesion(s) appear to have the greatest positive predictive value of MS conversion (70%); however, this is at the cost of lower sensitivity (39%).[39] In the CHAMPS study of patients with CIS treated with intramuscular interferon β-1a, one or more Gd-enhancing lesions at baseline were the best predictor of CDMS conversion over the next 2 years. Among patients with $\geq$ 2 Gd-enhancing lesions at baseline, 52% developed CDMS compared with 24% CDMS in those with 0–1 Gd-enhancing lesion.[40]

Among CIS patients, the original 2001 McDonald MRI criteria have a 75% positive predictive value and 83% accuracy of clinical conversion to MS.[41] Tintore and colleagues evaluated the 2001 McDonald criteria and found that 80% of patients fulfilling them developed a second clinical event with a mean follow-up period of 49 months. One year after symptom onset, more than three times as many patients with CIS were diagnosed with MS using these diagnostic criteria incorporating MRI results, compared with older criteria.[42]

In 2003, the Therapeutics and Technology Assessment Subcommittee of the American Academy of Neurology argued for a re-consideration of the 2001 McDonald criteria particularly with regard to the CIS patient, recommending a less stringent approach to early MS diagnosis.[43] Subsequently in 2005, the International Panel revised the McDonald criteria to simplify the criteria for both MRI-determined DIT and diagnosis of PPMS, and to clarify the diagnostic role of spinal cord imaging.[19] The new criteria for DIT allowed a Gd-enhancing lesion at least three months after onset of the initial clinical event and not at the site of the original clinical event, or a new T2 lesion at any time compared to a reference scan done at least 30 days after onset of the initial clinical event.

In 2006, in an effort to improve sensitivity of the 2005 McDonald criteria, Swanton and colleagues suggested modification of the McDonald criteria to use a less stringent definition for DIS (at least one T2 lesion in at least two of four locations – juxtacortical, periventricular, infratentorial, or spinal) and to allow a new T2 lesion after three months as evidence of DIT.[44] These criteria were compared to the original 2001 and 2005 McDonald criteria in a large cohort of CIS patients to assess their relative performances regarding conversion to CDMS.[45] The specificity and sensitivity of MRI criteria for CDMS after three years was assessed in 208 patients. The specificity of all criteria for CDMS was high (2001 McDonald, 91%; 2005 McDonald, 88%; 2006 Swanton, 87%). Sensitivity of the 2006 Swanton (72%) and 2005 McDonald (60%) criteria were higher than the 2001 McDonald criteria (47%). A Cox proportional hazards model showed a higher conversion risk for all three criteria in those with both DIS and DIT than in those with either DIS or DIT alone. The authors concluded that the newly modified criteria were simpler than the 2005 McDonald criteria without compromising specificity and accuracy. These observations were subsequently incorporated and formalized into new recommended MRI criteria specifically for determination of MS in CIS patients, and was published in 2010 by the international Magnetic Imaging in MS (MAGNIMS) committee.[20] As reviewed above, these criteria were included in the revised 2010 McDonald criteria.

Spinal MRI, particularly of the cervical cord, can at times be extremely helpful in defining dissemination in time and space in the evaluation for MS, as well as in evaluating the patient's presenting symptoms. However, care should be taken to obtain these MRIs in the technically most sophisticated manner due to the high incidence of both false-positive and false-negative examinations in technically inadequate spinal MRIs. Reference to the Consortium of MS Centers (CMSC) MRI Protocols (revised 2009);[46] can be particularly helpful in this regard. Particular note should also be made of the usefulness of spine MRI in distinguishing Devic's disease (neuromyelitis optica) cases that have multiple (longitudinally extensive) segments of often necrotizing demyelination in the spinal cord. While symptoms and serological testing usually distinguish these patients from MS patients, confirmatory MRI is useful as the overall treatment and management of these patients is quite different owing to a pathophysiology different from MS (Chapter 53).

Radiologically isolated syndrome (RIS)

With the widespread use of MRI in most developed countries, occasionally patients are encountered who have an MRI highly suggestive of MS in the complete absence of a relevant clinical history or abnormal neurological examination. Some have designated this group as radiologically isolated syndrome (RIS). There is still a fair amount of debate regarding both the use of the term as well as the management of this situation. Many practitioners would look for characteristics generally felt to be worrisome for overall prognosis, such as one or more Gd-enhancing lesions, T1 hypointensities, and high T2 lesion burden. These patients could be managed as CIS or early RRMS accordingly, while electing for periodic yearly clinical and MRI monitoring of those patients deemed to be at lesser risk. One recently published study indicated that about 30% of RIS patients develop MS within two years.[47] Regardless of the remaining unanswered questions regarding the ultimate

significance of RIS, we believe that it is currently prudent to carefully monitor RIS patients over at least 2–5 years for additional MRI changes indicative of DIT or clinical changes consistent with early MS.

Follow-up MRI and monitoring of MS by MRI

The timing of a follow-up MRI after the diagnosis of MS depends primarily on what clinical question is being asked. Some of the potential reasons are discussed above in the cases of CIS and RIS, but several other indications exist including: (1) baseline MRI before initiating or changing a therapeutic intervention; (2) monitoring a patient while on therapy for therapeutic response or lack thereof; (3) monitoring of patients who decline DMT, and (4) investigation of symptoms/signs in MS patients which are not typical of MS. Any type of follow-up MRI recommendation is predicated on the ability to compare serial scans. Therefore, serial scans should be, where possible, obtained on the same magnet using the same acquisition sequences to allow for appropriate comparison. The revised CMSC acquisition protocol for MRIs is available on the MSCARE.org website, and provides optimization suggestions for scanning of MS patients.[46]

We do not generally obtain an MRI of the brain or spinal cord during an MS relapse if the symptoms and signs are consistent with MS and there are no other worrisome features. However, if the patient has an altered level of consciousness or other atypical or concerning symptoms suggestive of other possible etiologies, such as stroke or mass lesion, we would obtain a contrasted MRI as an important part of a more comprehensive evaluation.

The interest in monitoring patients while on disease modifying treatments arose from longitudinal MRI studies of MS patients that demonstrated active MRI changes during periods of clinical stability.[48,49] This has to the concept that the clinical course of a patient can be only the "tip of the iceberg" regarding true underlying, but clinically inapparent, ongoing disease activity. That is, a patient can appear to be stable, but in fact can be having extensive MRI activity, including new Gd-enhancing lesions. With increasing, albeit at times inconsistent, evidence that the extent for MRI T2 lesion burden/disease correlates to long-term prognosis, the degree of MRI activity is generally thought to be clinically relevant. Although one should use caution in relying only on MRI changes or so-called "treating the MRI," the degree of MRI activity over time can be responsibly used to guide treatment decisions. We do not view these discrepancies between MRI and apparent clinical status as merely a limitation of conventional MRI technologies; rather, we consider MRI and clinical assessments as two complementary views of an MS patient's current (and perhaps future) status.

Studies of early CIS patients at risk for MS demonstrated benefit of early treatment with the standard MS therapies. However, some patients and clinicians may decide to delay initiating therapy until the diagnosis of MS can be made with absolute certainty. In this circumstance, the MRI can be utilized to augment clinical monitoring that would demonstrate DIT (and/or DIS) and secure the earliest diagnosis of MS (as demonstrated in the 2010 McDonald criteria).

While, in general, early treatment of MS patients is favored, there does appear to be a subgroup of MS patients with a relatively benign course.[50] In this population, the use of the currently available therapies may have limited effect on the natural history of the disease, but may have undesired side effects and risk in excess of possible benefit. Other patients may, despite recommendations for treatment, decline therapy at the time of diagnosis. In these untreated MS patients, MRI monitoring can be a useful adjunct to clinical monitoring to evaluate the character of their disease over time. Brain MRI every 12–24 months may be generally appropriate for monitoring these two groups of patients. In patients with minimal T2 lesion burden and stable findings over time, continued monitoring might be appropriate without necessarily utilizing a DMT. However, if such a patient begins to have increased number or frequency of Gd-enhancing lesions or T2 lesion burden, we believe that treatment should be instituted, even in the absence of clinically apparent change. Due to the sporadic nature of Gd-enhancing lesions, T2 lesion accumulation is a more reliable measure of disease progression as almost all Gd-enhancing lesions leave a T2 lesion footprint. The absence of Gd-enhancing lesions alone on any randomly obtained MRI study can therefore be falsely reassuring in the setting of marked T2 changes.

Although comparison of serial MRI's is the most direct way to assess DIT and changes in disease activity, the practicality of this procedure can be fraught with difficulty. MRI scans are often obtained on different machines resulting in varying quality. For instance, one scan may have 5 mm cuts with gaps and resultant volume averaging, while another may have been obtained with contiguous images. A reportedly "new" lesion detected on the latter scan may instead be old, and only newly visible compared to the former scan. When comparing studies, it is also important to compare images from similar sequences, e.g. T2 to T2, and fluid attenuated inversion recovery (FLAIR) to FLAIR. Additionally, T2-weighted imaging is preferred when looking for potential posterior fossa changes due to the lesser sensitivity of FLAIR imaging in this region.

All of the current MS therapies reduce the relapse rate and MRI activity in RRMS patients. However, there are treated patients who continue to have MRI or clinical disease activity; so-called "breakthrough" disease. The onset of treatment effect also varies among the approved therapies, and appears different for clinical versus MRI measurements, which makes the monitoring of treated patients more challenging. For example, studies suggest that the interferon beta (IFNβ) products have an earlier onset of anti-inflammatory effects compared to glatiramer acetate. Both IFNβ-1a preparations have a demonstrated effect on MRI as early as 24 weeks.[51] MRI effects of glatiramer appear slower to occur; Gd and T2 effects are seen at nine months after treatment onset.[52] In general, MRI at 9–12 months after treatment initiation is useful to evaluate disease activity and

potential response to therapy. In treated patients with established RRMS, the presence of Gd-enhancing or new (or enlarging) T2 lesions is associated with a relatively poor outcome. Rudick and colleagues examined this relationship in the context of the Phase 3 trial of intramuscular IFNβ-1a in order to evaluate criteria for "treatment response."[53] Patients were classified as responders or non-responders using (1) the number of relapses during the two-year trial; (2) the number of new T2 lesions after two years; and (3) the number of Gd-enhancing lesions at year 1 and year 2 on-study. Outcomes included two-year change in the EDSS, Multiple Sclerosis Functional Composite (MSFC), and brain parenchymal fraction (BPF). Subgroups with high on-study relapses had more disease progression, but differences between responder subgroups were similar in the IFNβ-1a and placebo arms. In contrast, subgroups with high numbers of new MRI lesions had significantly more disease progression only in the IFNβ-1a arm. Baseline characteristics failed to account for differential outcome. The authors concluded that new MRI lesion activity during IFNβ-1a treatment correlates with poor response to IFNβ-1a and that follow-up MRI classification for patients starting IFNβ may facilitate rational therapeutic decisions. A number of other studies have confirmed that Gd-enhancing lesions and new T2 lesions predict relapses and disability progression.[54] The risk of having a suboptimal response to treatment with IFNβ increased eight[55,56] to ten-fold[57] in patients who had as little as a single active lesion after one year of treatment. Durelli and colleagues found that an active scan (a scan with either a Gd-enhancing lesion or a new T2 lesion) in the first 3–6 months of treatment had a predictive value of 60%–70% for new clinical activity over the subsequent 18 months.[58] Inflammatory activity on the MRI also predicts brain atrophy in treated patients, which in turn predicts disability.[59]

Thus, MRI evidence of disease activity while on DMT may warrant re-examination of therapeutic options, given direct MRI evidence of lack of optimal response, even in the relative absence of clinically evident worsening. In this regard, the character and extent of new MRI activity is important. Minimal T2 change in the first year of treatment may be cautiously tolerated, while extensive increase in T2 lesion burden or new Gd-enhancing lesions, may prompt treatment change. Also to be considered, a standard course of pulse corticosteroids may affect contrast enhancement for as long as 6–8 weeks, during which time current enhancement will usually resolve. For this reason, some practitioners delay an MRI by 8–10 weeks after a steroid-treated relapse to look for persisting, or new silent or subclinical MRI activity before considering whether to change disease-modifying therapy.

The decision to change or add therapies is a complicated one and beyond the scope of this chapter. Freedman *et al.* published a guideline for treatment optimization that includes the integration of clinical relapses, disease progression, and MRI changes to guide treatment decisions.[60] In some circumstances, neither MRI nor clinical changes alone may be sufficient to guide treatment decisions, and an integrated approach is often needed.

Current research in the augmentation of traditional medications is ongoing and will hopefully provide information about the benefits and drawbacks of these approaches.

There is no current rationale for monitoring patients with progressive MS with MRI, except in certain, specific instances. In patients with secondarily progressive MS (SPMS), MRI activity as assessed by white matter T2 lesion burden is dissociated from disability progression, particularly in patients who no longer have clinical or MRI evidence of active focal white matter inflammation.[61] This observation appears to be due to the fact that the majority of the progression in these patients results from a different pathogenesis that does not involve focal inflammatory lesions in the white matter.[62,63] As currently available DMTs for MS have their primary mode of action against inflammation, treatment options in these patients are limited. However, there are two reasons to obtain follow-up MRI scans in patients with progressive MS. First, Gd-enhancing enhancing lesions may form the rationale for therapy with an approved MS DMT. Second, MRI may be needed to address the possibility of non-MS processes (e.g. cervical stenosis, herniated disc, etc.) causing or contributing to neurological deterioration.

MRI safety

In general, Gd contrast agents are considered safe, and MRI of the brain or spinal cord with a Gd-chelated contrast agent for most MS-related questions is preferred. These agents allow detection of some measure of inflammatory activity in MS, as well as assisting to ensure that alternative diagnoses are addressed. However, recent safety concerns have arisen relative to the use of these agents in the setting of renal compromise due to the risk of nephrogenic systemic fibrosis (NSF) in patients with kidney disease.[64] NSF is characterized by thickening and hardening of the skin on the trunk and limbs as well as marked expansion of the dermis in association with CD34 positive fibrocytes. While the skin findings are characteristic, some patients have developed fibrosis of deeper structures including muscle, fascia, lungs, and heart. NSF occurs exclusively in patients with kidney failure; therefore, it is recommend that a serum creatinine level be obtained according to American College of Radiology guidelines,[65] generally for those above age 60, and for anyone with a history of renal problems, including diabetes. Each institution will have policies for hydration and use of Gd in patients based on age, estimated glomerular filtration rate and presence of risk factors such as diabetes, known renal disease, or other potentially mitigating factors.

The indications for obtaining an MRI in pregnancy are few and essentially none for the use of a contrast agent. Breast feeding women generally should express breast milk and discard it for at least 24 hours after a Gd-enhanced MRI, and many practitioners would simply delay obtaining the MRI until after weaning has occurred.

While patients with spinal cord stimulators, deep brain stimulators, and bladder stimulators (and, of course, cardiac pacemakers) cannot be routinely scanned in the current generation of MRI scanners, patients with intrathecal pumps can be scanned by special arrangement, whereby the pump is turned off before the scan and turned back on afterwards by experienced personnel.

Magnetic field strength

Most currently utilized clinical MRI scanners are 1.5 T units and, as mentioned, we recommend the CMSC revised guidelines[46] for obtaining clinical scans in MS patients. However, some patients are claustrophobic or exceed weight limits for these scanners, and need to be scanned on low field or "open" magnets. Extreme care should be taken in the interpretation of these low field scans, particularly in the spine, as the scanner results are quite prone to artifact. Patients should also be counseled that the "open" scanners are not completely open and that these scanners may also require significantly longer scan acquisition times. It is hoped that with hardware improvements with larger bore magnets in higher field strength scanners and improved software these issues will become less problematic, particularly with the growing problem of obesity in the USA and elsewhere. While the research literature in MS increasingly contains more elegant data from high-field 7 T magnets, whether or not these will see clinical usage in the next 10 years is unclear. Higher field strength magnets (i.e. 3 T and above) allow not only for better definition of structures, but also for the application of other techniques such as magnetic resonance spectroscopy (MRS), magnetization transfer imaging (MTI), and functional connectivity (fMRI).

Future directions

There has been considerable lag time between the research application of newer techniques to expand our understanding of the pathophysiology of MS and their routine clinical applications. While other chapters will cover these techniques in more detail, it may be worth noting why they are not included in this clinical chapter. Although MRS, MTI, and fMRI techniques have been available for a number of years, it is not anticipated that they will have application in routine clinical scans due to three main factors (a) the need to acquire the data on a higher field magnet such as a 3 T scanner; (b) the complicated and rather variable nature of the software needed; and (c) the extensive and time-consuming post-acquisition processing of data that is required. Also, other areas requiring considerable post-acquisition processing include the use of quantitative techniques for MRI parameters such as atrophy, quantitative T2 lesion burden, T1 hypointensity volume, and others. While utilized extensively in clinical research trials, and some commercially available software for analysis is available, the practical clinical applicability of these considerably more advanced techniques remains to be demonstrated. Newer MR techniques to study the gray matter pathology and also axonal/myelin integrity will also be useful clinically, given that many authors, as expressed in other chapters of this book, believe that gray matter lesions are at least as, if not more, important in the pathophysiology and progressive clinical features of MS. Indeed, MRI evaluation of intracortical gray matter lesions may contribute to the next iteration of MS diagnostic criteria.[66]

Conclusions

Conventional, widely available MRI technologies have considerable impact on the early diagnosis of MS, and therefore affect meaningful treatment decisions with agents that improve the long-term outcome of the disease. MRI examines a different, but complimentary aspect of MS compared to our clinical assessments. At this time, conventional MRI assessments appear most sensitive in detecting subclinical inflammatory activity (and therefore therapeutic effect of most currently available DMTs), and perhaps less sensitive in detecting MRI correlates of slow, irreversible clinical disease progression. Newer MRI technologies are targeting the less inflammatory (or non-inflammatory) aspects of MS, and hopefully will provide additional, reliable, and non-invasive measures of disease progression in the future.

References

1. Allison RS, Millar JH. Prevalence of disseminated sclerosis in Northern Ireland. *Ulster Med J* 1954; 23:1–27.

2. Schumacher GA, Beebe G, Kibler RF, *et al.* Problems of experimental trials of therapy in multiple sclerosis: report by the panel on the evaluation of experimental trials of therapy in multiple sclerosis. *Ann NY Acad Sci* 1965; 122:552–68.

3. Patzold U, Pocklington PR. Course of multiple sclerosis. First results of a prospective study carried out of 102 MS patients from 1976–1980. *Acta Neurol Scand* 1982; 65:248–66.

4. Poser CM, Paty DW, Scheinberg L, *et al.* New diagnostic criteria for multiple sclerosis: guidelines for research protocols. *Ann Neurol* 1983; 13:227–31.

5. Paty DW, Asbury AK, Herndon RM, *et al.* Use of magnetic resonance imaging in the diagnosis of multiple sclerosis. *Neurology* 1986; 36:1575.

6. Poser CM. Diagnostic criteria for multiple sclerosis: an addendum. *Ann Neurol* 1987; 22:773.

7. IFNB Multiple Sclerosis Study Group. Interferon beta-1b in the treatment of multiple sclerosis: final outcome of the randomized controlled trial. *Neurology* 1995; 45:1277–85.

8. Johnson KP, Brooks BR, Cohen JA, *et al.* Copolymer 1 reduces relapse rate and improves disability in relapsing-remitting multiple sclerosis: results of a phase III multicenter, double-blind placebo-controlled trial. *Neurology* 1995; 45:1268–76.

9. Ge Y, Grossman RI, Udupa JK, *et al.* Glatiramer acetate (Copaxone) treatment in relapsing–remitting MS: quantitative MR assessment. *Neurology* 2000; 54:813–17.

10. Jacobs LD, Cookfair DL, Rudick RA, *et al.* Intramuscular interferon beta-1a for disease progression in relapsing multiple sclerosis. *Ann Neurol* 1996; 39:285–94.

11. PRISMS Study Group. Randomised double-blind placebo-controlled study of interferon beta-1a in relapsing/remitting multiple sclerosis. *Lancet* 1998; 352:1498–504.

12. Hartung HP, Gonsette R, Konig N, *et al.* Mitoxantrone in progressive multiple sclerosis: a placebo-controlled, double-blind, randomised, multicentre trial. *Lancet* 2002; 360:2018–25.

13. Krapf H, Morrissey SP, Zenker O, *et al.* Effect of mitoxantrone on MRI in progressive MS: results of the MIMS trial. *Neurology* 2005; 65:690–5.

14. Miller DH, Soon D, Fernando KT, *et al.* MRI outcomes in a placebo-controlled trial of natalizumab in relapsing MS. *Neurology* 2007; 68:1390–401.

15. Kappos L, Radue EW, O'Connor P, *et al.* A placebo-controlled trial of oral fingolimod in relapsing multiple sclerosis. *N Engl J Med* 2010; 362:387–401.

16. McDonald WI, Compston A, Edan G, *et al.* Recommended diagnostic criteria for multiple sclerosis: guidelines from the International Panel on the diagnosis of multiple sclerosis. *Ann Neurol* 2001; 50:121–7.

17. Barkhof F, Filippi M, Miller DH, *et al.* Comparison of MRI criteria at first presentation to predict conversion to clinically definite multiple sclerosis. *Brain* 1997; 120:2059–69.

18. Tintore M, Rovira A, Martinez MJ, *et al.* Isolated demyelinating syndromes: comparison of different MR imaging criteria to predict conversion to clinically definite multiple sclerosis. *Am J Neuroradiol* 2000; 21:702–6.

19. Polman CH, Reingold SC, Edan G, *et al.* Diagnostic criteria for multiple sclerosis: 2005 revisions to the "McDonald Criteria". *Ann Neurol* 2005; 58:840–6.

19A. A Polman CH, Reingold SC, Banwell B, *et al.* Diagnostic criteria for multiple sclerosis: 2010 revisions to the McDonald criteria *Ann Neurol* 2011; 69(2):292–302.

20. Montalban X, Tintore M, Swanton J, *et al.* MRI criteria for MS in patients with clinically isolated syndromes. *Neurology* 2010; 74:427–34.

21. Miller AE, Bourdette DN, Cohen JA, *et al.* Differential diagnosis of multiple sclerosis. *Continuum Lifelong Learning Neurol* 1999; 5:58–70.

22. Miller DH, Compston A. The differential diagnosis of multiple sclerosis. In: Compston A, *et al.*, ed. *McAlpine's Multiple Sclerosis*: Elsevier; 2006, 389–437.

23. Cree BAC. Diagnosis and differential diagnosis of multiple sclerosis. *Continuum Lifelong Learning Neurol* 2010; 16:19–36.

24. Kim SS, Richman DP, Johnson WO, *et al.* Limited applicability of Barkhof's MRI criteria in distinguishing multiple sclerosis from diseases mimicking multiple sclerosis. *Neurology.* [Meeting Abstract] 2005; 64:S26.006.

25. Atwood LD, Wolf PA, Heard-Costa NL, *et al.* Genetic variation in white matter hyperintensity volume in the Framingham study. *Stroke* 2004; 35:1609–13.

26. Paty D, Oger J, Kastrukoff L, *et al.* MRI in the diagnosis of MS: a prospective study with comparison of clinical evaluation, evoked potentials, oligoclonal banding, and CT. *Neurology* 1988; 38:180–5.

27. Fazekas F, Offenbacher H, Fuchs S, *et al.* Criteria for an increased specificity of MRI interpretation in elderly subjects with suspected multiple sclerosis. *Neurology* 1988; 38:1822–5.

28. Fazekas F, Barkhof F, Filippi M, *et al.* The contribution of magnetic resonance imaging to the diagnosis of multiple sclerosis. *Neurology* 1999; 53:448–56.

29. Jacobs LD, Beck RW, Simon JH, *et al.* Intramuscular Interferon beta-1a therapy initiated during a first demyelinating event in multiple sclerosis. *N Engl J Med* 2000; 343:898–904.

30. Comi G, Filippi M, Barkhof F, *et al.* Effect of early interferon treatment on conversion to definite multiple sclerosis: a randomized study. *Lancet* 2001; 357:1576–82.

31. Kappos L, Polman CH, Freedman MS, *et al.* Treatment with interferon beta-1b delays conversion to clinically definite and McDonald MS in patients with clinically isolated syndromes. *Neurology* 2006; 67:1242–9.

32. Comi G, Martinelli V, Rodegher M, *et al.* Effect of glatiramer acetate on conversion to clinically definite multiple sclerosis in patients with clinically isolated syndrome (PreCISe study): a randomised, double-blind, placebo-controlled trial. *Lancet* 2009; 374:1503–11.

33. Ford B, Tampiere D, Francis G. Long-term follow-up of acute partial transverse myelopathy. *Neurology* 1992; 42.

34. Morrissey SP, Miller DH, Kendall BE, *et al.* The significance of brain magnetic resonance imaging abnormalities at presentation with clinically isolated syndromes suggestive of multiple sclerosis. A 5-year follow-up study. *Brain* 1993; 116:135–46.

35. Fisniku LK, Brex PA, Altmann DR, *et al.* Disability and T2 MRI lesions: a 20-year follow-up of patients with relapse onset of multiple sclerosis. *Brain* 2008; 131:808–17.

36. Brex PA, Ciccarelli O, O'Riordan JI, *et al.* A longitudinal study of abnormalities on MRI and disability from multiple sclerosis. *N Engl J Med* 2002; 346:158–64.

37. O'Riordan J, Thompson, AJ, Kingsley, DP. The prognostic value of brain MRI in clinically isolated syndromes of the CNS: a 10-year follow-up. *Brain* 1998; 121:495–503.

38. Brex PA, O'Riordan JI, Miszkiel KA, *et al.* Multisequence MRI in clinically isolated syndromes and the early development of MS. *Neurology* 1999; 53:1184–90.

39. Brex PA, Miszkiel KA, O'Riordan JI, *et al.* Assessing the risk of early multiple sclerosis in patients with clinically isolated syndromes: the role of a follow-up MRI. *J Neurol Neurosurg Psychiatry* 2001; 70:390–3.

40. CHAMPS Study Group. MRI predictors of early conversion to clinically definite MS in the CHAMPS placebo group. *Neurology* 2002; 59:998–1005.

41. Dalton CM, Brex PA, Miszkiel KA, *et al.* Application of the new McDonald criteria to patients with clinically isolated syndromes suggestive of multiple sclerosis. *Ann Neurol* 2002; 52:47–53.

42. Tintore M, Rovira A, Rio J, *et al.* New diagnostic criteria for multiple sclerosis: application in first demyelinating episode. *Neurology* 2003; 60:27–30.

43. Frohman EM, Goodin DS, Calabresi PA, *et al.* The utility of MRI in suspected MS: report of the Therapeutics and Technology Assessment Subcommittee of the American Academy of Neurology. *Neurology* 2003; 61:602–11.

44. Swanton JK, Fernando K, Dalton CM, *et al.* Modification of MRI criteria for multiple sclerosis in patients with clinically isolated syndromes. *J Neurol Neurosurg Psychiatry* 2006; 77:830–3.

45. Swanton JK, Rovira A, Tintore M, *et al.* MRI criteria for multiple sclerosis in patients presenting with clinically isolated syndromes: a multicentre retrospective study. *Lancet Neurol* 2007; 6:677–86.

46. CMSC MRI Working Group. Consortium of MS centers MRI protocol for the diagnosis and followup of MS: 2009 revised guidelines. 2009 [cited 2011 Jul 1]; Available from: http://www.mscare.org/cmsc/images/pdf/MRIprotocol2009.pdf.

47. Lebrun C, Bensa C, Debouverie M, *et al.* Association between clinical conversion to multiple sclerosis in radiologically isolated syndrome and magnetic resonance imaging, cerebrospinal fluid, and visual evoked potential: follow-up of 70 patients. *Arch Neurol* 2009; 66:841–6.

48. Isaac C, Li DK, Genton M, *et al.* Multiple sclerosis: a serial study using MRI in relapsing patients. *Neurology* 1988; 38:1511–5.

49. Willoughby EW, Grochowski E, Li DK, *et al.* Serial magnetic resonance scanning in multiple sclerosis: a second prospective study in relapsing patients. *Ann Neurol* 1989; 25:43–9.

50. Pittock S, McClelland R, Mayr W, *et al.* Clinical implications of benign multiple sclerosis: a 20-year population-based follow-up study. *Ann Neurol* 2004; 56:303–6.

51. Panitch H, Goodin DS, Francis G, *et al.* Randomized, comparative study of interferon b-1a treatment regimens in MS. The EVIDENCE trial. *Neurology* 2002; 59:1496–506.

52. Ge Y, Grossman RI, Udupa JK, *et al.* Glatiramer acetate (Copaxone) treatment in relapsing-remitting MS. quantitative MR assessment. *Neurology* 2000; 54:813–17.

53. Rudick RA, Lee JC, Simon J, *et al.* Defining interferon beta response status in multiple sclerosis patients. *Ann Neurol* 2004; 56:548–55.

54. Kappos L, Moeri D, Radue EW, *et al.* Predictive value of gadolinium-enhanced magnetic resonance imaging for relapse rate and changes in disability or impairment in multiple sclerosis: a meta-analysis. *Lancet* 1999; 353:964–9.

55. Rio J, Rovira A, Tintore M, *et al.* Relationship between MRI lesion activity and response to IFN-beta in relapsing-remitting multiple sclerosis patients. *Mult Scler* 2008; 14:479–84.

56. Tomassini V, Paolillo A, Russo P, *et al.* Predictors of long-term clinical response to interferon beta therapy in relapsing multiple sclerosis. *J Neurol* 2006; 253:287–93.

57. Prosperini L, Gallo V, Petsas N, *et al.* One-year MRI scan predicts clinical response to interferon beta in multiple sclerosis. *Eur J Neurol* 2009; 16:1202–9.

58. Durelli L, Barbero P, Bergui M, *et al.* MRI activity and neutralising antibody as predictors of response to interferon beta treatment in multiple sclerosis. *J Neurol Neurosurg Psychiatry* 2008; 79:646–51.

59. Fisher E, Rudick RA, Simon JH, *et al.* Eight-year follow-up study of brain atrophy in patients with MS. *Neurology* 2002; 59:1412–20.

60. Freedman MS, Patry DG, Maison FG, *et al.* Treatment optimization in multiple sclerosis. *Can J Neurol Sci* 2004; 31:157–68.

61. Kappos L. Effect of drugs in secondary disease progression in patients with multiple sclerosis. *Mult Scler* 2004; 10 Suppl 1:S46–54; discussion S-5.

62. Frischer JM, Bramow S, Dal-Bianco A, *et al.* The relation between inflammation and neurodegeneration in multiple sclerosis brains. *Brain* 2009; 132:1175–89.

63. Bramow S, Frischer JM, Lassmann H, *et al.* Demyelination versus remyelination in progressive multiple sclerosis. *Brain* 2010; 133: 2983–98.

64. Kuo PH, Kanal E, Abu-Alfa AK, *et al.* Gadolinium-based MR contrast agents and nephrogenic systemic fibrosis. *Radiology* 2007; 242:647–9.

65. American College of Radiology Committee on Drugs and Contrast Media. ACR Manual on Contrast Media: Chapter 11 – Nephrogenic Systemic Fibrosis. 2010 [updated 2010; cited 2011 Jul 1]; Version 7: Available from: http://www.acr.org/Secondary MainMenuCategories/quality_safety/ contrast_manual.aspx.

66. Filippi M, Rocca MA, Calabrese M, *et al.* Intracortical lesions: relevance for new MRI diagnostic criteria for multiple sclerosis. *Neurology* 2010; 75:1988–94.

Chapter

56
Multiple sclerosis-associated fatigue

Lauren B. Krupp and Dana J. Serafin

Introduction

Fatigue, the most common symptom of multiple sclerosis (MS),[1] can also occur among healthy individuals and in other medical disorders.[2] The challenge is to understand how fatigue interacts with other MS symptoms, to define and measure fatigue, understand its pathogenesis, and implement effective therapies. Interest in MS fatigue occurred early in the history of fatigue studies[3,4] most likely due to its high frequency in MS and the focus of MS practitioners on symptomatic management prior to the availability of disease modifying therapies. There has been progress in defining neuroanatomical correlates of fatigue with neuroimaging, but fatigue's pathophysiology still remains elusive. Non-pharmacologic interventions show promise, and the methodology for testing pharmacologic therapies is improving. Still, better treatments are needed. Here, we review fatigue's clinical features, its possible pathogenic mechanisms, and therapeutic approaches.

Definition

Fatigue is typically viewed as a subjective feeling experienced by an individual,[5] but it can also be conceptualized as fatigability consisting of either a motor or cognitive behavioral performance decrement over time. The definition according to the 1998 Multiple Sclerosis Council for Clinical Practice Guidelines is a "subjective lack of physical and mental energy that is perceived by the individual or caregiver to interfere with usual and desired activities."[6] The Council divided fatigue into primary or secondary causes depending on the relations to chronic illness factors such as depression, concurrent medications, or poor sleep. While this classification is of theoretical interest, fatigue most often is multi-factorial comprising aspects intrinsic to the MS disease process and features influenced by comorbid cofactors or symptoms.

Clinical characteristics of MS fatigue
General features

Fatigue can be severe and disabling.[3] It can be particularly intense during relapses,[7] lead to unemployment,[8-10] and can result in reduced quality of life (QoL).[11-13] MS fatigue differs from the fatigue experienced by healthy individuals due to its deleterious effects on daily functioning such as meeting one's responsibilities and being able to sustain prolonged physical functioning. Another core MS fatigue feature distinct from other conditions is its extreme sensitivity to heat.[3,14] Relative to the fatigue of healthy adults, fatigue in MS is frequent[3] and is more likely to persist. For example, in a one year longitudinal study of 2768 MS outpatients, persistence of fatigue correlated with baseline pain, severity of baseline fatigue, mood and neurological impairment.[15]

The adverse effects on QoL[11,16,17] associated with fatigue have socio-economic consequences. Severely fatigued MS patients relative to those with less fatigue are at increased risk to retire early[18] or decrease their work hours from full-time to part-time.[8,9,18] Use of health care services is increased among those with severe fatigue, including more frequent outpatient visits.[19]

The relations between specific demographic factors and MS fatigue vary across studies.[10,16,20-24] Older age has been linked to increased fatigue in some studies,[10,22,23] but not in others.[16,24] Similar inconsistencies have been found for gender, with some finding that males are more likely to have severe fatigue,[10] while others have not found any gender association.[22-24] What has been consistently observed is that fatigue is more severe in those with less education.[10,23,24]

MS subtypes

Fatigue occurs among patients of all MS subtypes, but it is somewhat more frequent in those with secondary progressive MS[15] and more pronounced in individuals with greater mobility impairment,[10] although in one study, controlling for depression, fatigue no longer correlated with disability.[17] People with relapsing disease and accumulating impairment tend to be more fatigued than those with a relapsing but stable disease course.[10]

Effects of concurrent medication

One concern for individuals with MS is whether their disease modifying therapies or other MS-related treatments contribute to fatigue. In an analysis of disease-modifying therapies and fatigue among 320 consecutive patients, no relation was noted between severe fatigue and use of immunosuppressive or immunomodulating medications.[20] Similarly, of 9205 MS respondents to a North American Research Committee on Multiple Sclerosis (NARCOMS) survey, no differences in fatigue severity were identified between individuals on different disease modifying therapies. However, respondents noting medication changes in the prior six months reported lower fatigue levels after changing from interferon beta to glatiramer acetate.[10] Another study evaluated fatigue levels in 220 MS patients, prior to taking any disease-modifying therapy and then again at 3, 6, 9, and 12 months after starting glatiramer acetate. Results showed that fatigue decreased after 12 months of treatment.[25] The degree to which symptomatic treatments cause fatigue is less clear. Changes in anti-spasticity medication can occasionally cause increased fatigue or sleepiness, and a careful history can often uncover such an association. Nonetheless, fatigue can persist even after doses of concurrent medications are modified.

Depression

Between 20% and 50% of individuals with MS experience depression,[21,26,27] and depressed mood is clearly associated with fatigue.[15,28–35] Depression can predict fatigue and anxiety, and anxiety and fatigue can predict later depression.[28] Manifestations of depression such as lack of motivation, inability to complete tasks, and sleep disturbance are frequent in fatigued MS patients. As with depression, MS fatigue is associated with a low sense of control over one's symptoms or environment.[31,36–39] The association between fatigue and depression persists even when fatigue-related items are removed from depression scales.[24,40] In general, MS fatigue worsens as the day progresses whereas depression-related fatigue is more often severe upon awakening. Rest sometimes lessens fatigue but is less likely to improve depressive symptoms. Despite the strong association between depression and fatigue, there are many MS patients who experience severe fatigue without depressive symptomatology. For example, one can identify, for trials, fatigued patients who lack severe depressive symptoms.[41]

Anxiety

Anxiety is another affective disorder common in MS.[42] However, its relation to fatigue has not received as much attention as depression. The available data support a relatively consistent relation between anxiety and fatigue.[24,34,38,43,44] Anxiety may be more strongly related to mental fatigue as opposed to physical fatigue.[34,38]

Sleep disturbances

Sleep disorders occur frequently in MS and include insomnia, sleep apnea, narcolepsy, rapid eye movement (REM) sleep behavior disorder,[45] periodic limb movements of sleep, restless leg syndrome, and sensory alveolar hypoventilation syndrome.[45–48] Objective measures of poor sleep, including lower sleep efficiency, wake time after sleep onset, and arousal index occur more frequently among patients with severe fatigue compared to those without.[49,50] Restless leg syndrome is another common sleep problem that can be linked to fatigue.[47,51] While the exact relation between sleep dysfunction and fatigue remains unclear, when polysomnography was performed on 66 MS patients, those with severe fatigue had over twice the frequency of sleep disorders than those without severe fatigue.[52] What still needs to be determined is the extent to which fatigue improves once sleep disorders have been identified and treated.

Even in the absence of an identifiable sleep disorder, night time sleep can be disrupted from nocturia, pain, or muscle spasms.[45,53] A study of 60 patients evaluated with a fatigue scale, sleep diary, and the Epworth Sleepiness Scale, found that insomnia in the middle of the night was significantly correlated with fatigue.[54] Exploring possible medical reasons for disrupted sleep is another strategy in fatigue management.

Pain

MS patients may experience neuralgias, dysesthesias, and painful muscle spasms in addition to other pain-related problems. Pain contributes to physical deconditioning, and worsens depression. Physical pain compounded by fatigue may result in a progressive loss of functioning.[38,54] Although pain and fatigue can be linked,[15] pain is most strongly associated with depression.[55]

Cognition and cognitive fatigability

Despite the intuitive link between the experience of fatigue and cognitive difficulties, self-reported fatigue does not correlate well with routine neuropsychological testing or with many experimental measures of cognitive functioning.[56–62] However, slowed cognitive processing speed has been associated with self-reported fatigue.[61–63] Computerized measures of executive control have also been linked to fatigue and show an interaction distinct from the association between executive function and depressive symptoms.[64] It is possible that self-reported fatigue reflects, in part, greater effort by individuals with MS to maintain their level of cognitive performance, as compared to healthy individuals.[65,66] For example, individuals with MS display greater brain activation on functional MRI (fMRI) often including regions of the right prefrontal cortex during the execution of cognitive tasks, possibly indicating that they require greater cerebral resources and effort relative to healthy controls.[67–71]

Cognitive fatigability, defined as a decrement in mental performance over time, can be demonstrated in MS but is distinct from self-reported fatigue. When performance on neuropsychological tests was assessed before and after a continuously effortful cognitive task,[58] cognitive function declined on neuropsychological testing among MS patients compared to controls, but the changes did not correlate well with self-reported fatigue scales, nor was there a significant difference in performance among those with high and low fatigue levels.[58] Cognitive fatigability in MS has also been demonstrated with ongoing tasks of vigilance or working memory, in which performance declines with continuous testing.[72,73]

Motor function and motor fatigability

Similar to the concept of cognitive fatigability, patients with MS often suffer from motor fatigability defined as a decrement in force generation over time. Motor fatigability does not consistently correspond to self-reported fatigue. Deficits in the ability to sustain muscle contraction, recruit motor pathways efficiently, maintain normal levels of muscle metabolites during exertion, and abnormalities in motor unit firing rates are well documented in MS but are disassociated from perceived fatigue.[74–81] Although the motor component of a multidimensional fatigue scale[82] was associated with distance walked in six minutes, both healthy controls and MS subjects were involved in the analysis,[83] limiting interpretation of the findings.

A study involving electroencephalography recordings indicated that the sensorimotor areas of MS patients with fatigue were hyperactive during the execution of a movement and failed to become inhibited after the movement was terminated.[84] The electrophysiological correlates of self-reported fatigue in MS have also been explored with transcranial magnetic stimulation testing.[85] When MS patients performed a fatiguing handgrip exercise, reduced motor cortical inhibition was noted in those with fatigue compared to the patients without fatigue and to normal controls. The findings were interpreted as showing an exercise-induced reduction of membrane excitability in the motor cortex. However, such changes may not be specific to MS.[85]

Fatigue measurement

Perceived fatigue in contrast to cognitive or motor fatigability is typically assessed with structured questionnaires or scales that target the patient's subjective experience.[6] Measures can be subscales of more comprehensive QoL assessments or can be specific to fatigue. The QoL measure, the SF-36, includes a vitality subscale that is inversely correlated with fatigue.[86,87] Other examples of QoL scales that include a fatigue component are the Profile of Mood States, which has a fatigue-inertia subscale,[88] and the Sickness Impact Profile[89] which has a sleep-rest subscale.

Self-report measures specific to fatigue vary from single item visual analog scales[14] to longer multi-item instruments.[90,91] An extensive review of fatigue measurement is available elsewhere.[65,91] However, some examples of MS fatigue specific scales include the Fatigue Scale for Motor and Cognitive Functions,[92] the Wurzburg Fatigue Inventory for MS, which contains subscores for cognitive and physical fatigue,[7] the MS-specific Fatigue Severity Scale (MFSS),[90] and the Fatigue Descriptive Scale, which identifies three modalities of fatigue by distinguishing asthenia (fatigue at rest), from fatigability, and worsening symptoms with exercise.[93]

Among the more commonly used self-report scales in MS are the Fatigue Severity Scale (FSS)[14] and the Modified Fatigue Impact Scale (MFIS).[6] Both are relatively short, have good psychometric properties, and appear responsive to changes in fatigue due to disease progression or treatment.[91] The FSS was designed as a unidimensional scale. A Rasch analysis of the FSS indicated that the removal of some items improved its psychometric properties.[94,95] The MFIS uses a multidimensional approach with cognitive, physical, and psychosocial components. It, too, has been subjected to a Rasch analysis.[96] The physical dimension is most associated with measures of motor impairment such as the Expanded Disability Status Scale (EDSS).[97] In contrast, neuropsychological measures do not correlate well with the cognitive dimension. Aside from the FSS and the MFIS, the Fatigue Scale[57,98] is of interest in that it was responsive to the improved fatigue levels among MS participants following a cognitive behavioral therapy trial aimed at fatigue reduction.[99]

A variety of newer scaling techniques have developed using a combination of qualitative interviews and quantitative psychometric procedures. One tool incorporating these methods is the Neurological Fatigue Index (NFI-MS),[100] created through patient interviews, item generation, factor analysis, and Rasch analysis followed by testing in an evaluative and then validation sample. The summary 10-item scale includes items from physical and cognitive subscales. The NFI-MS might be helpful because it includes some of the requirements that the US Food and Drug Administration has posted for self-reported outcomes.[101]

Another measurement approach comes from a National Institutes of Health funded effort to improve the quality of patient reported outcomes.[102–105] Development of a fatigue measure from this initiative involved patient interviews, review of over 1000 fatigue items from published scales, and independent input from a fatigue expert.[106] Ultimately, an item bank of 95 items was developed which can be used to select specific fatigue measures of varying lengths for different purposes. The items are listed on the web at http://www.nihpromis.org/default.aspx. Despite these methodological improvements in fatigue scale development, challenges remain. All self-report measures suffer from recall bias and respondents can be influenced by the context within which fatigue is evaluated. Nonetheless, fatigue scales are readily available, can be quickly administered, and can easily be incorporated into clinical trials.

Pathogenesis

Neuroimaging has helped our understanding of the mechanisms which might underlie fatigue. Studies of the brain using measures of global and regional atrophy, lesion burden, MR spectroscopy (MRS), diffusion tensor imaging (DTI), positron emission tomography (PET), and fMRI have each contributed to the definition of neural pathways which might underlie fatigue.

Structural neuroimaging

Fatigue is not easily localizable to a single area of the central nervous system and early studies found little association with lesion burden,[107,108] atrophy,[107] or enhancing lesions.[109] However, more modern methods of MRI analysis have revealed that MS patients with fatigue compared to those without fatigue have more atrophy of the gray and white matter.[110] In a longitudinal study, brain atrophy was noted to have a positive association between global measures of fatigue.[111] Measures of gray and white matter atrophy as well as overall T2 lesion burden and T1 volume, correlate with a subscale of fatigue and thinking from a larger QoL inventory.[112] However, not all studies demonstrate a difference between fatigued and non-fatigued patients relative to total lesion volume.[113] On the other hand, lesion volume in specific regions has been linked to fatigue. For example, one investigation demonstrated an association between fatigue and lesion volume in the right parietal-temporal region and frontal white matter, areas associated with complex attention.[114] Gray matter atrophy involving the frontal and parietal lobes is also associated with fatigue.[113,114] While there is some variability among studies regarding which regions are most correlated with fatigue, the assumption is that regions underlying attentional processes are most important.

Abnormalities of the thalamus and basal ganglia have also been implicated in fatigue and support the theory that pathways between the basal ganglia, thalamus, limbic system, and cortex underlie the generation of fatigue symptoms.[115] In addition to the thalamus and caudate, the hypothalamus has been linked to fatigue.[113,116-118] These studies have shown either atrophy, decreased blood flow, or increased T1 relaxation times in these specific regions.[116,117,119] Other modalities studied in MS include MRS and DTI. Fatigue correlated with measures of diffuse axonal injury on MRS.[120] This association has been interpreted as suggesting that decreased mitochondrial function might be a contributing factor.[120] DTI has demonstrated disruption of frontal–striatal, frontal–frontal, frontal–limbic, and frontal–occipital pathways.[121] Such findings are possibly related to deficits in frontal networks and could affect motor planning as well as attention.[122]

Functional neuroimaging

The role of fMRI in elucidating fatigue in medical and neurological disorders is reviewed elsewhere.[123] Here we highlight only a few studies. For example, fMRI has shown that cortical functional reorganization occurs in MS.[124] When MS patients and healthy controls performed a repetitive motor task, there was increased cortical activation in both the ipsilateral and contralateral regions in fatigued vs. non-fatigued MS patients as well as in MS patients compared to healthy controls.[125] In another investigation of brain activation with fMRI, MS patients compared to controls showed limits in the degree to which brain activation occurred during a fatiguing hand grip exercise.[126] When MS patients performed a motor task and

fMRI, before and after undergoing a mentally fatiguing task of working memory (the Paced Auditory Serial Addition Test, PASAT), activation was increased in brain regions subserving motor function. In contrast, controls showed decreases in activation.[127] The challenge with fMRI changes is that coactivation may be a transient phenomenon which disappears as the disease progresses and neural connections disappear.

PET scanning has also uncovered interesting findings. Fatigued vs. non-fatigued MS patients showed decreases in glucose utilization in specific brain regions including the brainstem, basal ganglia, thalamus, limbic system, and prefrontal cortex.[128] Overall, both PET and fMRI have the potential to further delineate pathophysiological mechanisms.

Neuroimmune mechanisms

Fatigue is a common feature of many different autoimmune disorders, including systemic lupus erythematosus and rheumatoid arthritis. It is reasonable to consider that immune dysregulation contributes to fatigue. The observation that administration of medications with predominant effects on immune function can produce fatigue (e.g. interferon betas) further supports the link between immune regulation, cytokines, and fatigue. Another line of evidence suggesting a role for the immune system is the observation that elevations in some circulating immune parameters are found in fatiguing disorders such as chronic fatigue syndrome, cancer, and viral infections,[129-132] as well as in some but not all studies of MS.[133-135]

Neuroendocrine mechanisms

There appears to be hyperactivity as well as dysregulation of the hypothalamic–pituitary–adrenal (HPA) axis in MS[136] supported by the finding of significantly elevated adrenocorticotrophic hormone levels among 31 MS patients with fatigue relative to a non-fatigued group.[136] This dysregulation was postulated to be due to elevation of pro-inflammatory cytokines producing impairment of corticoid receptor signaling. Low circulating levels of dehydroepiandrosterone (DHEA) and its sulphated conjugate (DHEAS) were identified in fatigued relative to non-fatigued MS patients.[137] Low levels of DHEA could further activate the HPA axis through a positive feedback mechanism as well as lead to pro-inflammatory cytokines. Despite these intriguing links between the HPA axis and fatigue, not all studies point to such an association.[135]

Autonomic nervous system dysregulation

It has been theorized that symptoms of cardiovascular autonomic dysregulation, such as dizziness, generalized weakness, and neurocognitive complaints, bear similarities to the symptoms described in MS-related fatigue. Among fatigued MS patients, 20% had co-existing signs of autonomic failure.[138] Another study of autonomic tests and measures of heart rate variability in 60 MS patients with fatigue found impairment in the hypoadrenergic orthostatic response, a finding attributed to impaired sympathetic vasomotor activity.[139] However, the association between fatigue severity and autonomic dysfunction has been inconsistent.[140]

Physical deconditioning

Without adequate exercise MS patients may become physically deconditioned and subsequently more fatigued. This can lead to a pattern of further avoidance of exercise resulting in increased weakness. In patients who are severely disabled, respiratory function may become compromised. Physical reconditioning should always be a priority in treatment.[141]

Evaluation

Fatigue should be investigated with a comprehensive history and examination. Self-report measures can be helpful in distinguishing fatigue from depression or excessive sleepiness. The patient should be questioned as to possible triggers such as heat, stress, concurrent medications, and mood. Attention to co-existent factors is important as depression is often under-recognized and under-treated.[142,143] At least at some time during the evaluation, routine labs should be performed to rule out other causes of fatigue, such as infection, anemia, thyroid disease, or other metabolic abnormalities.

Treatment

Non-pharmacologic approaches

The first issue in management is to address the degree to which other MS symptoms such as depression, pain, or sleep disturbance are contributing factors. If present, depression should first be treated. Similarly, if a patient is unable to sleep because of frequent nocturia, addressing the bladder problems and improving sleep could lead to improved energy. In some cases, sleep disorders, such as sleep apnea, need treatment. Nonetheless, fatigue is frequently due to the MS itself and requires a more directed intervention. Table 56.1 summarizes some treatment strategies. Exercise can reduce fatigue[144-147] and show a treatment effect up to six months. Exercise programs that involve more than 90 minutes per week and are aerobic rather than involving resistance training appear most effective.[148]

Despite some encouraging findings, some studies show only a trend towards improvement with exercise and a meta-analysis concluded that exercise is only mildly beneficial on QoL.[159] One factor to avoid during exercise is excessive heat. In fact, using cooling jackets has been found to decrease fatigue.[158,160] In addition to exercise, energy conservation strategies have been tried. When patients were taught energy-conserving techniques, their fatigue improved relative to a wait-listed control group.[147] Another treatment strategy is to include rest breaks in an individual's daily schedule.

Table 56.1. *Treatment of fatigue*

Fatigue Treatments	Studies in MS	Comments
Physical exercise	144	Negative, positive effect on quality of life but not on fatigue
	145	Positive
	146	Positive
Energy conservation	147	Positive
Cognitive behavior therapy	99	Positive
Mindfullness	148	Positive
Fatigue Group ("Fatigue take control" program)	149	Positive
	150	Positive
	151	Positive, small study with only ten participants.
Amantadine	152	Concludes studies do not demonstrate clear substantial evidence of a treatment effect
	41	Positive
Modafinil	154	Positive, but weakness derived from cross-over design, and surprising dose effect (only 200 mg and not 400 mg) limits the interpretation
	168	Negative
Aspirin	155	Positive
Carnitine	157	Negative
Prokarin	170	Positive, small pilot study, only seven people in placebo group, never replicated

An exciting development in the non-pharmacologic management of fatigue has been the beneficial application of a mindfulness-based intervention.[148] This treatment program involves training participants to have non-judgmental awareness of moment-to-moment experiences. The goals are to improve perception, accept health-related challenges, enhance a realistic sense of control, and increase the appreciation of life's positive experiences. The program that showed positive effects with a mindfulness intervention relative to usual care required a clear commitment including weekly classes in mindfulness practices, homework assignments, and group meetings.[148] Using this approach the intervention showed improvements in overall QoL, fatigue, depression, and anxiety.

Other fatigue interventions aim primarily to empower the patient. One program improved fatigue and taught self-efficacy through formal group training. Patients also watched DVDs, did homework, participated in group discussions designed to improve knowledge about fatigue, and learned management strategies such as goal setting and environmental modifications.[161] In contrast, other multidisciplinary interventions with similar goals, but requiring less input from the participants, have not been as effective.[162]

Cognitive behavioral therapy (CBT) can help MS fatigue[99] as well as the fatigue associated with chronic fatigue syndrome.[163-165] In one trial, CBT and relaxation training both lessened fatigue in MS patients and healthy controls. However, CBT was more effective, lowering patient fatigue levels to that of the healthy control group.[99] The positive effects of CBT were sustained six months after treatment. CBT also was helpful in decreasing depression, anxiety, and stress.[99] Such results are encouraging; however, a better definition of the details of what constitutes a successful intervention is needed since not all fatigue management programs are effective.[162]

Medications

Often non-pharmacologic interventions are either not available or are not sufficiently successful. In these situations medication should be considered. As shown in Table 56.1, many medications have been tried in MS fatigue with either unclear benefit or have been found to be effective in only small studies that have yet to be replicated. The most frequently studied medication is modafinil, currently used for sleep disorders. Other medications that can be used to supplement non-pharmacologic interventions include amantadine and methylphenidate. One study noted some benefit with aspirin. The treatment approach should consider the occasional treatment success as a victory and to monitor the response including consideration of drug holidays since occasionally with time benefits become attenuated.

Amantadine was the first medication tried for MS fatigue. Although often used for the flu,[166] this medication has dopaminergic effects and acts on glutamate receptors. Four randomized clinical trials showed positive results using different fatigue outcome assessments.[41,150,151,167] Unfortunately, as covered in a recent Cochrane review, the studies all had limitations in design or analysis complicating the interpretation of the treatment effect.[152]

Modafinil is the most frequently prescribed fatigue treatment as reported by patients participating in the NARCOMS registry.[10] Modafinil has dual noradrenergic and dopaminergic properties, but is not a classic sympathomimetic. A small randomized controlled trial of modafinil showed that while on treatment patients had dramatic improvements in fatigue, focused attention, and dexterity.[153] However, results of other controlled trials have been mixed. In one trial with a cross-over design, the modafinil relative to the placebo group improved on the FSS. However, it is not clear why only the 200 mg dose, but not the 400 mg dose, was effective.[154] In contrast, a randomized placebo-controlled trial of modafinil using a parallel group design was negative and there were more adverse events involving insomnia and gastrointestinal problems in the modafinil group.[168] Among 39 patients treated with open-label modafinil in an outpatient center between 2000 and 2007, 46% reported fatigue reduction one month after beginning therapy but the positive effect was lost in 17% by 4½ years. One possible explanation for the variety of outcomes in different fatigue trials are the diverse contributors to fatigue. For example, among the 39 patients treated in the open-label study, responders were more likely to have concurrent sleepiness compared to those for whom the drug was not helpful.[169] Overall, while the data in

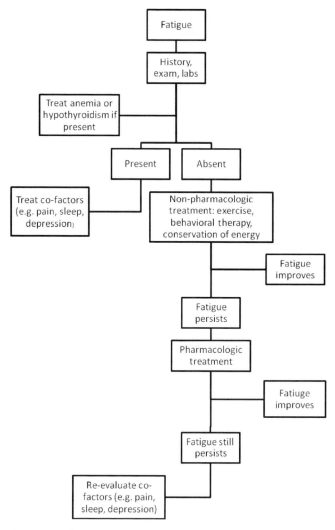

Fig. 56.1. Evaluation and treatment of fatigue in MS patients.

aggregate are weak for modafinil, a subgroup of patients seems to respond favorably to treatment.

Other treatments have not been extensively studied. Aspirin showed a positive effect on fatigue in a randomized trial, but some have argued that pain reduction may have been responsible for the observed benefit.[155,156] Carnitine has been tried to treat fatigue, but a randomized controlled trial included amantadine as a comparator and showed a very weak relative benefit. Further, the cross-over design for this study introduced problems in interpretation since changes in fatigue over time and carry over effects could have influenced the observed outcome.[157] Prokarin was studied in a small trial and showed a benefit over placebo.[170] However, the placebo group included only seven patients and there have not been additional published studies with this agent.[170] Methylphenidate is used by some clinicians for MS-associated fatigue but has not been subjected to any clinical trials. However, methylphenidate did improve attention as measured by the PASAT in a small randomized placebo-controlled trial of 26 MS subjects.[171]

Table 56.2. Major features of MS-related fatigue

- Fatigue is the most common symptom in MS.
- Fatigue adversely affects quality of life and socio-economic functioning.
- Anxiety, depression, pain, and disrupted sleep are cofactors.
- Generic as well as MS specific rating scales can measure fatigue.
- Atrophy of the gray and white matter is associated with increased fatigue.
- Functional MRI shows increased activation in fatigued vs. non-fatigued MS patients.
- Non-pharmacologic treatment includes exercise, energy conservation, mindfulness, and cognitive behavioral therapy.
- Occasionally patients respond to amantadine or modafinil.
- More research is needed to uncover the pathophysiology and identify more effective therapies.

Overall, no clearly effective medication emerges as the best option. Nonetheless, some patients report benefit.[169] Due to the multi-factorial nature of fatigue and the strong placebo effect, it is not surprising that the results of treatment studies have been so variable. As shown in Fig. 56.1, fatigue management includes consideration of the cofactors or secondary causes of fatigue. Non-pharmacologic interventions and in some patients selected medications could be incorporated into a treatment plan. However, when all interventions fail, it can be helpful to re-evaluate for depression as a co-factor.

Implications for practice

Major features of fatigue, including implications for practice, are summarized in Table 56.2. With new-onset fatigue, the evaluation should assess for a relapse; and explore the potential contributions of pain, sleep anxiety, and depression; and reassess symptomatic therapies. A stepwise treatment approach, as shown in Fig. 56.1, is best. Non-pharmacological interventions, as well as helping patients allocate their energy to their most pressing concerns, can be helpful. While clinical trials with medications have yielded conflicting results, individual patients may show benefit from specific treatments such as modafinil or amantadine.

Implications for research studies

Our understanding of MS fatigue has grown from a primarily descriptive analysis to a clearer definition of pathogenic mechanisms with the help of neuroimaging, and from the fields of sleep research, neuroimmunology and neuroendocrinology. Examination of the psychological aspects of fatigue has led to enhanced non-pharmacologic interventions which are likely to become more standardized with time. Along with a better sense of the pathophysiology of fatigue, which hopefully will lead to potential therapies, there is a clearer path to identifying more sound psychometric measurement tools, developments which could yield better clinical trial designs for pharmacologic therapies.

References

1. Minden, SL, Frankel D, Hadden L, Perloff J, Srinath KP, Hoaglin DC. The Sonya Slifka Longitudinal Multiple Sclerosis Study: methods and sample characteristics. *Mult Scler* 2006;12:24–38.

2. DeLuca J, ed. *Fatigue as a Window to the Brain*. Cambridge, MA: MIT Press, 2005; 336.

3. Krupp, LB, Alvarez LA, LaRocca NG, Scheinberg LC. Fatigue in multiple sclerosis. *Arch Neurol* 1988;45:435–7.

4. Freal, JE, Kraft GH, Coryell JK. Symptomatic fatigue in multiple sclerosis. *Arch Phys Med Rehabil* 1984;65:135–8.

5. Wessely S, Hotopf M, Sharpe D. *Chronic Fatigue and its Syndromes*. New York: Oxford University Press, 1988.

6. Fatigue and Multiple Sclerosis: Evidence-based management strategies for fatigue in multiple sclerosis. Multiple Sclerosis Council for Clinical Practice Guidelines, ed. M.S.C.F.C.P. Guidelines. Washington DC: Paralyzed Veterans Association of America, 1998.

7. Flachenecker P, Meissner H. Fatigue in multiple sclerosis presenting as acute relapse: subjective and objective assessment. *Mult Scler* 2008;14:274–7.

8. Smith MM, Arnett PA. Factors related to employment status changes in individuals with multiple sclerosis. *Mult Scler* 2005;11:602–9.

9. Julian, LJ, Vella L, Vollmer T, *et al.* Employment in multiple sclerosis. Exiting and re-entering the work force. *J Neurol* 2008;255:1354–60.

10. Hadjimichael O, Vollmer T, Oleen-Burkey M. Fatigue characteristics in multiple sclerosis: the North American Research Committee on Multiple Sclerosis (NARCOMS) survey. *Health Qual Life Outcomes* 2008;6:100.

11. Amato MP, Ponziani G, Rossi F, *et al.* Quality of life in multiple sclerosis: the impact of depression, fatigue and disability. *Mult Scler* 2001;7:340–4.

12. Aronson KJ. Quality of life among persons with multiple sclerosis and

their caregivers. *Neurology* 1997;48:74–80.

13. Janardhan V, Bakshi R. Quality of life in patients with multiple sclerosis: the impact of fatigue and depression. *J Neurol Sci* 2002;205:51–8.

14. Krupp LB, LaRocca NG, Muir-Nash J, Steinberg AD. The fatigue severity scale. Application to patients with multiple sclerosis and systemic lupus erythematosus. *Arch Neurol* 1989;46:1121–3.

15. Patrick E, Christodoulou C, Krupp LB. Longitudinal correlates of fatigue in multiple sclerosis. *Mult Scler* 2009;15:258–61.

16. Flachenecker P, Kumpfel T, Kallmann B, *et al.* Fatigue in multiple sclerosis: a comparison of different rating scales and correlation to clinical parameters. *Mult Scler* 2002;8:523–6.

17. Bakshi R, Shaikh ZA, Miletich RS, *et al.* Fatigue in multiple sclerosis and its relationship to depression and neurologic disability. *Mult Scler* 2000;6:181–5.

18. Edgley K, Sullivan MJ, Dehoux E. A survey of multiple sclerosis: II Determinants of employment status. *Can J Rehabil* 1991;4:127–32.

19. Johansson S, Ytterberg C, Gottberg K, *et al.* Use of health services in people with multiple sclerosis with and without fatigue. *Mult Scler* 2009;15:88–95.

20. Putzki N, Katsarava Z, Vago S, Diener HC, Limmroth V. Prevalence and severity of multiple-sclerosis-associated fatigue in treated and untreated patients. *Eur Neurol* 2008;59:136–42.

21. Patten SB, Beck CA, Williams JV, Barbui C, Metz LM. Major depression in multiple sclerosis: a population-based perspective. *Neurology* 2003;61:1524–7.

22. Colosimo C, Millefiorini E, Grasso MG, *et al.* Fatigue in MS is associated with specific clinical features. *Acta Neurol Scand* 1995;92:353–5.

23. Lerdal A, Celius EG and Moum T. Fatigue and its association with sociodemographic variables among multiple sclerosis patients. *Mult Scler* 2003;9:509–14.

24. Chwastiak LA, Gibbons LE, Ehde DM, *et al.* Fatigue and psychiatric illness in a large community sample of persons with multiple sclerosis. *J Psychosom Res* 2005;59:291–8.

25. Ziemssen T, Hoffman J, Apfel R, Kern S. Effects of glatiramer acetate on fatigue and days of absence from work in first-time treated relapsing-remitting multiple sclerosis. *Health Qual Life Outcomes* 2008;6:67.

26. Feinstein A. The neuropsychiatry of multiple sclerosis. *Can J Psychiatry* 2004;49:157–63.

27. Sadovnick AD, Remick RA, Allen J, *et al.* Depression and multiple sclerosis. *Neurology* 1996;46:628–32.

28. Brown RF, Valpiani EM, Tennant CC, *et al.* Longitudinal assessment of anxiety, depression, and fatigue in people with multiple sclerosis. *Psychol Psychother* 2009;82:41–56.

29. Johansson S, Ytterberg C, Hillert J, Widen Holmqvist L, von Koch L. A longitudinal study of variations in and predictors of fatigue in multiple sclerosis. *J Neurol Neurosurg Psychiatry* 2008;79:454–7.

30. Bol Y, Duits AA, Hupperts RM, Vlaeyen JW, Verhey FR. The psychology of fatigue in patients with multiple sclerosis: a review. *J Psychosom Res* 2009;66:3–11.

31. Schwartz CE, Coulthard-Morris L, Zeng Q. Psychosocial correlates of fatigue in multiple sclerosis. *Arch Phys Med Rehabil* 1996;77:165–70.

32. Kroencke DC, Lynch SG, Denney DR. Fatigue in multiple sclerosis: relationship to depression, disability, and disease pattern. *Mult Scler* 2000;6:131–6.

33. Fisk JD, Pontefract A, Ritvo PG, Archibald CJ, Murray TJ. The impact of fatigue on patients with multiple sclerosis. *Can J Neurol Sci* 1994;21:9–14.

34. Ford H, Trigwell P, Johnson M. The nature of fatigue in multiple sclerosis. *J Psychosom Res* 1998;45:33–8.

35. Moller A, Wiedemann G, Rohde U, Backmund H, Sonntag A. Correlates of cognitive impairment and depressive mood disorder in multiple sclerosis. *Acta Psychiatr Scand* 1994;89:117–21.

36. Vercoulen JH, Swanink CM, Galama JM, *et al.* The persistence of fatigue in chronic fatigue syndrome and multiple sclerosis: development of a model. *J Psychosom Res* 1998;45:507–17.

37. Van Der Werf SP, Evers A, Jongen PJ, and Bleijenberg G. The role of helplessness as mediator between neurological disability, emotional instability, experienced fatigue and depression in patients with multiple sclerosis. *Mult Scler* 2003;9:89–94.

38. Trojan DA, Arnold D, Collet JP, *et al.* Fatigue in multiple sclerosis: association with disease-related, behavioural and psychosocial factors. *Mult Scler* 2007;13:985–95.

39. Jopson NM, Moss-Morris R. The role of illness severity and illness representations in adjusting to multiple sclerosis. *J Psychosom Res* 2003;54:503–11; discussion 513–14.

40. Vercoulen JH, Hommes OR, Swanink CM, *et al.* The measurement of fatigue in patients with multiple sclerosis. A multidimensional comparison with patients with chronic fatigue syndrome and healthy subjects. *Arch Neurol* 1996;53:642–9.

41. Krupp LB, Coyle PK, Doscher C, *et al.* Fatigue therapy in multiple sclerosis: results of a double-blind, randomized, parallel trial of amantadine, pemoline, and placebo. *Neurology* 1995;45:1956–61.

42. Feinstein A, O'Connor P, Gray T, Feinstein K. The effects of anxiety on psychiatric morbidity in patients with multiple sclerosis. *Mult Scler* 1999;5:323–6.

43. Skerrett TN, Moss-Morris R. Fatigue and social impairment in multiple sclerosis: the role of patients' cognitive and behavioral responses to their symptoms. *J Psychosom Res* 2006;61:587–93.

44. Iriarte J, Subira ML, Castro P. Modalities of fatigue in multiple sclerosis: correlation with clinical and biological factors. *Mult Scler* 2000;6:124–30.

45. Fleming WE, Pollak CP. Sleep disorders in multiple sclerosis. *Semin Neurol* 2005;25:64–8.

46. Tachibana N, Howard RS, Hirsch NP, *et al.* Sleep problems in multiple sclerosis. *Eur Neurol* 1994;34:320–3.

47. Brass SD, Duquette P, Proulx-Therrien J, Auerbach S. Sleep disorders in patients with multiple sclerosis. *Sleep Med Rev* 2010;14:121–9.

48. Ferini-Strambi L, Filippi M, Martinelli V, *et al.* Nocturnal sleep study in multiple sclerosis: correlations with clinical and brain magnetic resonance imaging findings. *J Neurol Sci* 1994;125:194–7.

49. Kaynak H, Altintas A, Kaynak D, *et al.* Fatigue and sleep disturbance in multiple sclerosis. *Eur J Neurol* 2006;13:1333–9.

50. Attarian HP, Brown KM, Duntley SP, Carter JD, Cross AH. The relationship of sleep disturbances and fatigue in multiple sclerosis. *Arch Neurol* 2004;61:525–8.

51. Moreira, NC, Damasceno RS, Medeiros CA, *et al.* Restless leg syndrome, sleep quality and fatigue in multiple sclerosis patients. *Braz J Med Biol Res* 2008;41:932–7.

52. Veauthier C, Radbruch H, Gade G, *et al.* Polysomnographic investigation of frequency of sleep disorders in consecutive unselected fatigued and non-fatigued multiple sclerosis patients. *Neurology* 2010;74(Suppl 2):A99.

53. Amarenco G, Kerdraon J, Denys P. [Bladder and sphincter disorders in multiple sclerosis. Clinical, urodynamic and neurophysiological study of 225 cases]. *Rev Neurol* (Paris) 1995;151:722–30.

54. Stanton BR, Barnes F, Silber E. Sleep and fatigue in multiple sclerosis. *Mult Scler* 2006;12:481–6.

55. Brochet B, Deloire MS, Ouallet JC, *et al.* Pain and quality of life in the early stages after multiple sclerosis diagnosis: a 2-year longitudinal study. *Clin J Pain* 2009;25:211–17.

56. Johnson SK, Lange G, DeLuca J, Korn LR, Natelson B. The effects of fatigue on neuropsychological performance in patients with chronic fatigue syndrome, multiple sclerosis, and depression. *Appl Neuropsychol* 1997;4:145–53.

57. Paul RH, Beatty WW, Schneider R, Blanco CR, Hames KA. Cognitive and physical fatigue in multiple sclerosis: relations between self-report and objective performance. *Appl Neuropsychol* 1998;5:143–8.

58. Krupp LB, Elkins LE. Fatigue and declines in cognitive functioning in multiple sclerosis. *Neurology* 2000;55:934–9.

59. Parmenter BA, Denney DR, Lynch SG. The cognitive performance of patients with multiple sclerosis during periods of high and low fatigue. *Mult Scler* 2003;9:111–18.

60. Bailey A, Channon S, Beaumont JG. The relationship between subjective fatigue and cognitive fatigue in advanced multiple sclerosis. *Mult Scler* 2007;13:73–80.

61. Beatty WW, Goretti B, Siracusa G, *et al.* Changes in neuropsychological test performance over the workday in multiple sclerosis. *Clin Neuropsychol* 2003;17:551–60.

62. Urbanek C, Weinges-Evers N, Bellmann-Strobl J, *et al.* Attention Network Test reveals alerting network dysfunction in multiple sclerosis. *Mult Scler* 2010;16:93–9.

63. Andreasen AK, Spliid PE, Andersen H, Jakobsen J. Fatigue and processing speed are related in multiple sclerosis. *Eur J Neurol* 2010;17:212–18.

64. Holtzer R, Foley F. The relationship between subjective reports of fatigue and executive control in multiple sclerosis. *J Neurol Sci* 2009;281:46–50.

65. Christodoulou C. The assessment and measurement of fatigue. In *Fatigue as a Window to the Brain*. DeLuca J, ed. New York: MIT Press, 2005; 19–35.

66. DeLuca J. Fatigue, cognition, and mental effort. In *Fatigue as a Window to the Brain*. DeLuca J, ed. New York: MIT Press, 2005 37–57.

67. Hillary FG, Chiaravalloti ND, Ricker JH, *et al.* An investigation of working memory rehearsal in multiple sclerosis using fMRI. *J Clin Exp Neuropsychol* 2003;25:965–78.

68. Staffen W, Mair A, Zauner H, *et al.* Cognitive function and fMRI in patients with multiple sclerosis: evidence for compensatory cortical activation during an attention task. *Brain* 2002;125:1275–82.

69. DeLuca J, Genova HM, Hillary FG, Wylie G. Neural correlates of cognitive fatigue in multiple sclerosis using functional MRI. *J Neurol Sci* 2008;270:28–39.

70. Chiaravalloti N, Hillary F, Ricker J, *et al.* Cerebral activation patterns during working memory performance in multiple sclerosis using FMRI. *J Clin Exp Neuropsychol* 2005;27:33–54.

71. Christodoulou C, DeLuca J, Ricker JH, *et al.* Functional magnetic resonance imaging of working memory impairment after traumatic brain injury. *J Neurol Neurosurg Psychiatry* 2001;71:161–8.

72. Kujala P, Portin R, Revonsuo A, Ruutiainen J. Attention related performance in two cognitively different subgroups of patients with multiple sclerosis. *J Neurol Neurosurg Psychiatry* 1995;59:77–82.

73. Schwid SR, Tyler CM, Scheid EA, *et al.* Cognitive fatigue during a test requiring sustained attention: a pilot study. *Mult Scler* 2003;9:503–8.

74. Sharma KR, Kent-Braun J, Mynhier MA, Weiner MW, Miller RG. Evidence of an abnormal intramuscular component of fatigue in multiple sclerosis. *Muscle Nerve* 1995;18:1403–11.

75. Sheean GL, Murray NM, Rothwell JC, Miller DH, Thompson AJ. An electrophysiological study of the mechanism of fatigue in multiple sclerosis. *Brain* 1997;120:299–315.

76. Kent-Braun JA, Sharma KR, Miller RG, Weiner MW. Postexercise phosphocreatine resynthesis is slowed in multiple sclerosis. *Muscle Nerve* 1994;17:835–41.

77. Latash M, Kalugina E, Nicholas J, *et al.* Myogenic and central neurogenic factors in fatigue in multiple sclerosis. *Mult Scler* 1996;1:236–41.

78. Schwid SR, Thornton CA, Pandya S, *et al.* Quantitative assessment of motor fatigue and strength in MS. *Neurology* 1999;53:743–50.

79. Djaldetti R, Ziv I, Achiron A, Melamed E. Fatigue in multiple sclerosis compared with chronic fatigue syndrome: a quantitative assessment. *Neurology* 1996;46:632–5.

80. Krupp LB, Pollina DA, Mechanisms and management of fatigue in progressive neurological disorders. *Curr Opin Neurol* 1996;9:456–60.

81. Schubert M, Wohlfarth K, Rollnik JD, Dengler R. Walking and fatigue in multiple sclerosis: the role of the corticospinal system. *Muscle Nerve* 1998;21:1068–70.

82. Fisk JD, Ritvo PG, Ross L, *et al.* Measuring the functional impact of fatigue: initial validation of the fatigue impact scale. *Clin Infect Dis* 1994;18(Suppl 1):S79–83.

83. Goldman MD, Marrie RA, Cohen JA. Evaluation of the six-minute walk in multiple sclerosis subjects and healthy controls. *Mult Scler* 2008;14:383–90.

84. Leocani L, Colombo B, Magnani G, *et al.* Fatigue in multiple sclerosis is associated with abnormal cortical activation to voluntary movement–EEG evidence. *Neuroimage* 2001;13: 1186–92.

85. Liepert J, Mingers D, Heesen C, Baumer T, Weiller C. Motor cortex excitability and fatigue in multiple sclerosis: a transcranial magnetic stimulation study. *Mult Scler* 2005;11:316–21.

86. Ware JE Jr, Sherbourne CD. The MOS 36-item short-form health survey (SF-36). I. Conceptual framework and item selection. *Med Care* 1992;30:473–83.

87. Ware JE Jr. SF-36 health survey update. *Spine (Phila Pa 1976)*, 2000;25: 3130–9.

88. McNair DM, Lorr M, Droppleman LF. *Profile of Mood States Manual.* 1971, San Diego: Educational and Industrial Testing Service.

89. Gilson BS, Gilson JS, Bergner M, *et al.* The sickness impact profile. Development of an outcome measure of health care. *Am J Public Health* 1975;65:1304–10.

90. Schwartz JE, Jandorf L, Krupp LB. The measurement of fatigue: a new

instrument. *J Psychosom Res* 1993;37:753–62.

91. Whitehead L. The measurement of fatigue in chronic illness: a systematic review of unidimensional and multidimensional fatigue measures. *J Pain Symptom Mgmt* 2009;37:107–28.

92. Penner IK, Raselli C, Stocklin M, *et al.* The Fatigue Scale for Motor and Cognitive Functions (FSMC): validation of a new instrument to assess multiple sclerosis-related fatigue. *Mult Scler* 2009;15:1509–17.

93. Iriarte J, Katsamakis G, de Castro P. The Fatigue Descriptive Scale (FDS): a useful tool to evaluate fatigue in multiple sclerosis. *Mult Scler* 1999;5:10–6.

94. Mills R, Young C, Nicholas R, Pallant J, Tennant A. Rasch analysis of the Fatigue Severity Scale in multiple sclerosis. *Mult Scler* 2009;15:81–7.

95. Lerdal A, Johansson S, Kottorp A, von Koch L. Psychometric properties of the Fatigue Severity Scale: Rasch analyses of responses in a Norwegian and a Swedish MS cohort. *Mult Scler* 2010;16:733–41.

96. Mills RJ, Young CA, Pallant JF, Tennant A. Rasch analysis of the Modified Fatigue Impact Scale (MFIS) in multiple sclerosis. *J Neurol Neurosurg Psychiatry* 2010;81:1049–51.

97. Kurtzke JF. Rating neurologic impairment in multiple sclerosis: an expanded disability status scale (EDSS). *Neurology* 1983;33:1444–52.

98. Chalder T, Berelowitz G, Pawlikowska T, *et al.* Development of a fatigue scale. *J Psychosom Res* 1993;37:147–53.

99. van Kessel K, Moss-Morris R, Willoughby E, *et al.* A randomized controlled trial of cognitive behavior therapy for multiple sclerosis fatigue. *Psychosom Med* 2008;70:205–13.

100. Mills RJ, Young CA, Pallant JF, Tennant A. Development of a patient reported outcome scale for fatigue in multiple sclerosis: The Neurological Fatigue Index (NFI-MS). *Health Qual Life Outcomes* 2010;8:22.

101. Administration, US FDA, Draft guidance for industry on patient reported outcome measures: use in medicinal product development to support labeling claims. (Docket 2006D-0044). *Fed Register* 2006;71:5862–5863.

102. Reeve BB, Hays RD, Bjorner JB, *et al.* Psychometric evaluation and calibration of health-related quality of life item banks: plans for the Patient-Reported Outcomes Measurement Information System (PROMIS). *Med Care* 2007;45(5 Suppl 1):S22–31.

103. Cella D, Yount S, Rothrock N, *et al.* The Patient-Reported Outcomes Measurement Information System (PROMIS): progress of an NIH Roadmap cooperative group during its first two years. *Med Care* 2007;45(5 Suppl 1):S3–S11.

104. DeWalt DA, Rothrock N, Yount S, Stone AA. Evaluation of item candidates: the PROMIS qualitative item review. *Med Care* 2007;45(5 Suppl 1):S12–21.

105. Christodoulou C, Junghaenel DU, DeWalt DA, Rothrock N, Stone AA. Cognitive interviewing in the evaluation of fatigue items: Results from the patient-reported outcomes measurement information system (PROMIS). *Qual Life Res* 2008;17:1239–1246.

106. Riley WT, Rothrock N, Bruce B, *et al.* Patient-reported outcomes measurement information system (PROMIS) domain names and definitions revisions: further evaluation of content validity in IRT-derived item banks. *Qual Life Res* 2010;19:1311–21.

107. Bakshi R, Miletich RS, Henschel K, *et al.* Fatigue in multiple sclerosis: cross-sectional correlation with brain MRI findings in 71 patients. *Neurology* 1999;53:1151–3.

108. Van Der Werf SP, Jongen PJ, Lycklama a Nijeholt GJ, *et al.* Fatigue in multiple sclerosis: interrelations between fatigue complaints, cerebral MRI abnormalities and neurological disability. *J Neurol Sci* 1998;160:164–70.

109. Mainero C, Faroni J, Gasperini C, *et al.* Fatigue and magnetic resonance imaging activity in multiple sclerosis. *J Neurol* 1999;246:454–8.

110. Tedeschi G, Dinacci D, Lavorgna L, *et al.* Correlation between fatigue and brain atrophy and lesion load in multiple sclerosis patients independent of disability. *J Neurol Sci* 2007;263:15–9.

111. Marrie RA, Fisher E, Miller DM, Lee JC, Rudick RA. Association of fatigue and brain atrophy in multiple sclerosis. *J Neurol Sci* 2005;228:161–6.

112. Mowry, EM, Beheshtian A, Waubant E, *et al.* Quality of life in multiple sclerosis is associated with lesion burden and brain volume measures. *Neurology* 2009;72:1760–5.

113. Andreasen AK, Jakobsen J, Soerensen L *et al.* Regional brain atrophy in primary fatigued patients with multiple sclerosis. *NeuroImage* 2010;50:608–15.

114. Sepulcre J, Masdeu JC, Goni J, *et al.* Fatigue in multiple sclerosis is associated with the disruption of frontal and parietal pathways. *Mult Scler* 2009;15:337–44.

115. Chaudhuri A, Behan PO, Fatigue in neurological disorders. *Lancet* 2004;363:978–88.

116. Inglese M, Park SJ, Johnson G, *et al.* Deep gray matter perfusion in multiple sclerosis: dynamic susceptibility contrast perfusion magnetic resonance imaging at 3T. *Arch Neurol* 2007;64:196–202.

117. Niepel G, Tench CR, Morgan PS, *et al.* Deep gray matter and fatigue in MS: a T1 relaxation time study. *J Neurol* 2006;253:896–902.

118. Zellini F, Niepel G, Tench CR, Constantinescu CS. Hypothalamic involvement assessed by T1 relaxation time in patients with relapsing–remitting multiple sclerosis. *Mult Scler* 2009;15:1442–9.

119. Gallo P, Rinaldi F, Grossi P, Favaretto A, Calabrese M. Magnetic resonance evidence of the involvement of the striatal-thalamic-frontal cortex system in determining fatigue in multiple sclerosis. *Neurology* 2010;74(Suppl 2):A508.

120. Tartaglia MC, Narayanan S, Francis SJ, *et al.* The relationship between diffuse axonal damage and fatigue in multiple sclerosis. *Arch Neurol* 2004;61:201–7.

121. Filippi M, Rocca MA. Toward a definition of structural and functional MRI substrates of fatigue in multiple sclerosis. *J Neurol Sci* 2007;263:1–2.

122. Pardini M, Bonzano L, Mancardi GL, Roccatagliata L. Frontal networks play a role in fatigue perception in multiple sclerosis. *Behav Neurosci* 2010;124:329–36.

123. DeLuca J, Genova HM, Capili EJ, Wylie GR. Functional neuroimaging of fatigue. *Phys Med Rehabil Clin N Am* 2009;20:325–37.

124. Rocca MA, Agosta F, Colombo B, *et al.* fMRI changes in relapsing-remitting multiple sclerosis patients complaining of fatigue after IFNbeta-1a injection. *Hum Brain Mapp* 2007;28:373–82.

125. Filippi M, Rocca MA, Colombo B, *et al.* Functional magnetic resonance imaging correlates of fatigue in multiple sclerosis. *Neuroimage* 2002;15:559–67.

126. White AT, Lee JN, Light AR, Light KC. Brain activation in multiple sclerosis: a BOLD fMRI study of the effects of fatiguing hand exercise. *Mult Scler* 2009;15:580–6.

127. Tartaglia MC, Narayanan S, Arnold DL. Mental fatigue alters the pattern and increases the volume of cerebral activation required for a motor task in multiple sclerosis patients with fatigue. *Eur J Neurol* 2008;15:413–19.

128. Roelcke U, Kappos L, Lechner-Scott J, *et al.* Reduced glucose metabolism in the frontal cortex and basal ganglia of multiple sclerosis patients with fatigue: a 18F-fluorodeoxyglucose positron emission tomography study. *Neurology* 1997;48:1566–71.

129. Bower JE, Ganz PA, Aziz N, Fahey JL. Fatigue and proinflammatory cytokine activity in breast cancer survivors. *Psychosom Med* 2002;64:604–11.

130. Kerr JR, Barah F, Mattey DL, *et al.* Circulating tumour necrosis factor-alpha and interferon-gamma are detectable during acute and convalescent parvovirus B19 infection and are associated with prolonged and chronic fatigue. *J Gen Virol* 2001;82:3011–19.

131. Kurzrock R. The role of cytokines in cancer-related fatigue. *Cancer* 2001;92(6 Suppl):1684–8.

132. Patarca R. Cytokines and chronic fatigue syndrome. *Ann NY Acad Sci* 2001;933:185–200.

133. Giovannoni G, Thompson AJ, Miller DH, Thompson EJ. Fatigue is not associated with raised inflammatory markers in multiple sclerosis. *Neurology* 2001;57:676–81.

134. Flachenecker P, Bihler I, Weber F, *et al.* Cytokine mRNA expression in patients with multiple sclerosis and fatigue. *Mult Scler* 2004;10:165–9.

135. Heesen C, Nawrath L, Reich C, *et al.* Fatigue in multiple sclerosis: an example of cytokine mediated sickness behaviour? *J Neurol Neurosurg Psychiatry* 2006;77:34–9.

136. Gottschalk M, Kumpfel T, Flachenecker P, *et al.* Fatigue and regulation of the hypothalamo-pituitary-adrenal axis in multiple sclerosis. *Arch Neur* 2005;62:277–80.

137. Tellez N, Comabella M, Julia E, *et al.* Fatigue in progressive multiple sclerosis is associated with low levels of dehydroepiandrosterone. *Mult Scler* 2006;12:487–94.

138. Merkelbach S, Dillmann U, Kolmel C, Holz I, Muller M. Cardiovascular autonomic dysregulation and fatigue in multiple sclerosis. *Mult Scler* 2001;7:320–6.

139. Flachenecker P, Rufer A, Bihler I, *et al.* Fatigue in MS is related to sympathetic vasomotor dysfunction. *Neurology* 2003;61:851–3.

140. Egg R, Hogl B, Glatzl S, Beer R, Berger T. Autonomic instability, as measured by pupillary unrest, is not associated with multiple sclerosis fatigue severity. *Mult Scler* 2002;8:256–60.

141. Foglio K, Clini E, Facchetti D, *et al.* Respiratory muscle function and exercise capacity in multiple sclerosis. *Eur Respir J* 1994;7:23–8.

142. Krupp LB. *Fatigue in Multiple Sclerosis: A Guide to Diagnosis and Management.* Demos Medical Publishing, 2004.

143. Mohr DC, Hart SL, Goldberg A. Effects of treatment for depression on fatigue in multiple sclerosis. *Psychosom Med* 2003;65:542–7.

144. Petajan JH, Gappmaier E, White AT, *et al.* Impact of aerobic training on fitness and quality of life in multiple sclerosis. *Ann Neurol* 1996;39:432–41.

145. Oken BS, Kishiyama S, Zajdel D, *et al.* Randomized controlled trial of yoga and exercise in multiple sclerosis. *Neurology* 2004;62:2058–64.

146. McCullagh R, Fitzgerald AP, Murphy RP, Cooke G. Long-term benefits of exercising on quality of life and fatigue in multiple sclerosis patients with mild disability: a pilot study. *Clin Rehabil* 2008;22:206–14.

147. Sauter C, Zebenholzer K, Hisakawa J, Zeitlhofer J, Vass K. A longitudinal study on effects of a six-week course for energy conservation for multiple sclerosis patients. *Mult Scler* 2008;14:500–5.

148. Grossman P, Kappos L, Gensicke H, *et al.* MS quality of life, depression, and fatigue improve after mindfulness

training: a randomized trial. *Neurology* 2010;75:1141–19.

149. Hugos C, Copperman L, Fuller B, *et al.* Clinical trial of a formal group fatigue program in multiple sclerosis. *Mult Scler* 2010;16:724–32.

150. The Canadian MS Research Group. A randomized controlled trial of amantadine in fatigue associated with multiple sclerosis. *Can J Neurol Sci* 1987;14:273–8.

151. Rosenberg GA, Appenzeller O. Amantadine, fatigue, and multiple sclerosis. *Arch Neurol* 1988;45: 1104–6.

152. Pucci E, Branas P, D'Amico R, *et al.* Amantadine for fatigue in multiple sclerosis. *Cochrane Database Syst Rev* 2007:CD002818.

153. Lange R, Volkmer M, Heesen C, Liepert J. Modafinil effects in multiple sclerosis patients with fatigue. *J Neurol* 2009;256:645–50.

154. Rammohan KW, Rosenberg JH, Lynn DJ, *et al.* Efficacy and safety of modafinil (Provigil) for the treatment of fatigue in multiple sclerosis: a two centre phase 2 study. *J Neurol Neurosurg Psychiatry* 2002;72:179–83.

155. Wingerchuk DM, Benarroch EE, O'Brien PC, *et al.* A randomized controlled crossover trial of aspirin for fatigue in multiple sclerosis. *Neurology* 2005;64:1267–9.

156. Schwid SR, Murray TJ, Treating fatigue in patients with MS: one step forward, one step back. *Neurology* 2005;64:1111–12.

157. Tejani AM, Wasdell M, Spiwak R, Rowell G, Nathwani S. Carnitine for fatigue in multiple sclerosis. *Cochrane Database Syst Rev* 2010:CD007280.

158. Mostert S, Kesselring J. Effects of a short-term exercise training program on aerobic fitness, fatigue, health perception and activity level of subjects with multiple sclerosis. *Mult Scler* 2002;8:161–8.

159. Motl RW, McAuley E, Snook EM. Physical activity and multiple sclerosis: a meta-analysis. *Mult Scler* 2005;11:459–63.

160. Geisler M, Sliwinski M, Coyle PK, *et al.* LB, Cooling and multiple sclerosis: cognitive and sensory effects. *J Neurol Rehab* 1996;10:17–22.

161. Hugos CL, Copperman LF, Fuller BE, *et al.* Clinical trial of a formal group

fatigue program in multiple sclerosis. *Mult Scler* 2010;16:724–32.

162. Kos D, Duportail M, D'Hooghe M, Nagels G, Kerckhofs E. Multidisciplinary fatigue management programme in multiple sclerosis: a randomized clinical trial. *Mult Scler* 2007;13:996–1003.

163. Deale A, Chalder T, Marks I, Wessely S. Cognitive behavior therapy for chronic fatigue syndrome: a randomized controlled trial. *Am J Psychiatry* 1997;154:408–14.

164. Prins JB, Bleijenberg G, Bazelmans E, *et al.* Cognitive behaviour therapy for chronic fatigue syndrome: a

multicentre randomised controlled trial. *Lancet* 2001;357:841–7.

165. Sharpe M, Hawton K, Simkin S, *et al.* Cognitive behaviour therapy for the chronic fatigue syndrome: a randomized controlled trial. *BMJ* 1996;312:22–6.

166. Hayden FG. Combination antiviral therapy for respiratory virus infections. *Antiviral Res* 1996;29:45–8.

167. Cohen RA, Fisher M. Amantadine treatment of fatigue associated with multiple sclerosis. *Arch Neurol* 1989;46:676–80.

168. Stankoff B, Waubant E, Confavreux C, *et al.* Modafinil for fatigue in MS: a randomized placebo-controlled

double-blind study. *Neurology* 2005;64:1139–43.

169. Littleton ET, Hobart JC, Palace J. Modafinil for multiple sclerosis fatigue: does it work? *Clin Neurol Neurosurg* 2010;112:29–31.

170. Gillson G, Richard TL, Smith RB, Wright JV. A double-blind pilot study of the effect of Prokarin on fatigue in multiple sclerosis. *Mult Scler* 2002;8:30–5.

171. Harel Y, Appleboim N, Lavie M, Achiron A. Single dose of methylphenidate improves cognitive performance in multiple sclerosis patients with impaired attention process. *J Neurol Sci* 2009;276:38–40.

Chapter

57

Management of spasticity

Francois A. Bethoux and Matthew Sutliff

Introduction

Spasticity is defined as a velocity-dependent increase in resistance to passive muscle stretching due to the exaggeration of tonic stretch reflexes.[1] Spasticity is frequently encountered in multiple sclerosis (MS), often with significant subjective and objective consequences. In a prevalence study of 301 MS patients, 52% reported cramps, and 57% had increased muscle tone on examination.[2] In a more recently published survey of over 20 000 individuals with MS, only 16% of responders reported no spasticity, and approximately 1/3 reported moderate or severe spasticity (although a majority received ongoing symptomatic treatment).[3] Disease-modifying therapies usually do not provide relief of spasticity-related symptoms, and there are reports of increased spasticity with interferon beta.[4] Although the pathophysiology of spasticity is incompletely understood, a wide array of symptomatic therapies are available to the clinician.

Pathophysiology

The main end mechanism leading to spasticity is the hyperexcitability of alpha motor neurons, caused by decreased descending inhibitory signals secondary to damage to the central nervous system (CNS).[5] The lack of inhibition of intramedullary oligo- or polysynaptic pathways, physiologically mediated by the neurotransmitter gamma amino butyric acid (GABA), results in hyperactivity of the stretch reflex. Two clinical models have been described. In the spinal model, reflex activity builds up more slowly, suggesting predominant involvement of polysynaptic pathways. In the cerebral model, monosynaptic pathways could be responsible for a more rapid increase in reflex activity.[6] Spasticity from MS is often considered to be of spinal origin, although the presence of diffuse lesions throughout the neuraxis suggests a mixed pathophysiology.

Clinical features

The upper motor neuron (UMN) syndrome can be divided into positive (increased muscle tone, exaggerated tendon reflexes, spread of stretch reflex, clonus, synergy patterns, extensor plantar response), and negative (loss of dexterity, weakness) signs and symptoms, which most often co-exist in the individual patient, and in MS are often associated with deficits of other neurologic systems (e.g. ataxia and sensory deficits).

Consequences of spasticity reported by patients and/or caregivers are muscle stiffness, spasms, pain or discomfort, loss of extremity function, difficulty maintaining standing or sitting postures, and interference with self-care (e.g. difficulty performing intermittent catheterization due to adductor spasticity). Objective signs include exaggerated stretch reflexes, clonus, spasms, synergy patterns, co-contraction of agonist and antagonist muscles, increased resistance to passive movement with or without "clasp-knife" phenomenon, decreased range of motion, and abnormal posture. Dynamic phenomena (abnormal movements) are related to reflex hyperexcitability, and static phenomena (decreased range of motion) are caused by changes in the rheologic properties of musculoskeletal structures. Spasticity often contributes to limitations in the ability to perform activities and to fulfill familial and societal roles, along with other neurologic impairments. Spasticity increases with stress and noxious stimuli (e.g. pain, decubiti, urinary tract infection, ingrown toenail), and usually exhibits spontaneous fluctuations (typically increasing at night). Variations in ambient and core body temperature have been reported anecdotally to affect spasticity.

It is important to remember that spasticity can also have beneficial consequences. For example, a patient may use extensor tone to stand and perform pivot transfers, which would otherwise be compromised by severe paraparesis. It is also believed that, in some situations, spasticity decreases the risk of deep venous thrombosis and pressure ulcers by maintaining muscle tone in paralyzed muscles.

Assessment of spasticity
Clinical evaluations
Spasticity-related impairment

The most common way to evaluate spasticity is to record the symptoms and signs listed above during a standard neurologic examination, sometimes quantified using the Expanded Disability Status Scale (EDSS), which includes assessment of

Multiple Sclerosis Therapeutics, Fourth Edition, ed. Jeffrey A. Cohen and Richard A. Rudick. Published by Cambridge University Press.
© Cambridge University Press 2011.

spasticity within the Pyramidal Functional System Score or as a separate subscore. Passive and active range of motion (ROM) measurement, as well as manual muscle testing, should be performed as part of a comprehensive spasticity assessment. These methods usually are sufficient for routine clinical practice. However, for research purposes and clinical trials, more standardized, quantitative, and reliable measures are needed.

- The *Ashworth scale*, in its standard[7] or modified (Modified Ashworth Scale [MAS])[8,9] versions, is an ordinal measure of resistance to passive movement in the extremities. Variable inter- and intra-rater reliability in trained evaluators has been reported. The Ashworth scale exhibits low sensitivity to change, and addresses only one aspect of spasticity. Despite several publications reporting on the limitations of the Ashworth scale,[10,11] it continues to be widely used in clinical trials of interventions for spasticity.

- The *Tardieu scale*[12] is an ordinal rating of resistance to passive mobilization, and is most frequently used in its modified version.[13] Testing is performed at three different angular velocities (as slow as possible = V1, at the speed of the limb falling under gravity = V2, and as fast as possible = V3). Two angles are measured: R1 corresponds to the first point of resistance (catch) to a quick stretch, and R2 corresponds to the passive ROM with a slow stretch. R1 represents a measure of dynamic (active) tone, whereas R2 is more representative of rheologic changes in the tissue (passive tone).

Spasticity-related activity limitation

Improving or preserving function is an important goal of spasticity management. Therefore, it is useful to incorporate functional measures when evaluating the consequences of spasticity and treatment outcomes. However, these instruments may lack sensitivity and specificity in the context of spasticity management, therefore results should be interpreted with caution. Potentially useful instruments include:

- Generic (e.g. Functional Independence Measure [FIM™], Barthel Index) or MS-specific (e.g. Incapacity Status Scale) global activity limitation scales.
- Measures of walking performance (e.g. Timed 25-ft Walk, Ambulation Index, Timed Up & Go Test, Dynamic Gait Index).
- Measures of upper extremity motor function (e.g. Nine-Hole Peg Test, Box and Blocks Test).

Quantitative tests

Quantitative tests are designed to be more reliable and sensitive than clinical measures. Generally, they are too cumbersome to be used in routine clinical practice. They do not always correlate well with clinical measures. Quantitative tests to assess spasticity include:

- The *Pendulum Test*[14] requires the use of an electrogoniometer to quantify the number of swings and the degree of excursion at the knee after the leg of the

patient is dropped from maximum extension. Additional data can be gathered by combining video or electromyography (EMG) recordings, and isokinetic dynamometry.
- The *Vibration Inhibitory Index* consists of comparing the amplitude of the H-reflex before and after application of 60-Hz vibration to the Achilles tendon. This test is based on the observation that vibration inhibits the H-reflex in healthy nonspastic subjects.[15]
- The *H-reflex* and *Hmax/Mmax* ratio are measures of the excitability of motor neurons at rest via EMG. The H-reflex is decreased with exposure to baclofen, particularly when administered intrathecally (intrathecal baclofen, ITB) and has been proposed as a useful complement to clinical measures in assessing the response to ITB.[16]

Patient-reported outcomes

Several patient self-report measures exist to assess spasticity.

- The *Spasm Frequency Scale*[17] assesses the frequency of spasms over a 24-hour period, and whether spasms occur with stimulation or spontaneously. It is easy to use and has shown sensitivity to treatment effect, even though it does not assess spasm severity or spasm-related pain.
- A spasticity *Numeric Rating Scale* (NRS) from 0 to 10 was recently proposed, and in two separate publications, demonstrated satisfactory test-retest reproducibility and significant correlations with more traditional measures of spasticity severity.[18,19] An absolute change of −1.27 in the raw score or relative change of −29.5% was proposed by Farrar *et al.*[18] as being clinically significant.
- A 10-cm Visual Analog Scale or other self-report measures can be used to evaluate the pain related to spasticity, directly (e.g. painful spasms) or indirectly (e.g. joint pain exacerbated by spasticity).
- Hobart *et al.* developed the 88-item *Multiple Sclerosis Spasticity Scale (MSSS-88)*, using both qualitative methods for item development and Rasch analysis for item selection, to fully capture the impact of spasticity on MS patients.[20] Although the length of the questionnaire raises concerns regarding responder burden in both clinical and research settings, this scale is the only validated self-report instrument available for use in clinical trials.[21]
- Generic (e.g. Medical Outcomes Study 36-item Short Form [SF-36 Sickness Impact Profile) or disease-specific (e.g. Multiple Sclerosis Quality of Life Inventory, MS Quality of Life-54) *quality of life measures* may be used for spasticity management, with the same caveats noted above for activity limitation scales.

Treatment of spasticity
General considerations

The goals of spasticity management are to relieve symptoms, improve function and/or ease of care, improve posture, and prevent long-term complications such as fixed contractures. The treatment plan should address both the dynamic and the static components of spasticity. In addition, the interaction with other neurologic deficits, the role of extraneous factors (e.g. noxious stimuli, medications), and the balance between deleterious and beneficial effects of spasticity on function should be taken into account. Complementary treatment modalities can be combined, following an integrated care model. The Multiple Sclerosis Council for Clinical Practice Guidelines published evidence-based recommendations for the management of spasticity in MS.[22]

Rehabilitation and exercise

The rationale for the use of rehabilitation in the management of spasticity is mostly empirical. Although rehabilitative interventions (primarily physical therapy and occupational therapy) alone are not always sufficient, they should be part of the plan of care at all stages. In mild-to-moderate spasticity, therapists can educate the patient about consequences of spasticity, teach a home stretching and exercise program, recommend ankle–foot orthoses or other devices as appropriate, and evaluate and treat functional consequences of spasticity. In severe spasticity with contractures, improvement of ROM and posture will be sought through aggressive stretching, splinting, and serial casting, usually in combination with medications and sometimes surgical interventions (see below). A single-blind, randomized, controlled pilot study showed added benefit on spasticity from combining physical therapy with botulinum toxin (BT) injections, compared to BT therapy alone.[23]

A pilot study of locomotor training in four MS patients using body weight support showed encouraging results on spasticity, walking speed, and balance.[24] Unloaded leg cycling exercise (and to a lesser degree arm cycling) was demonstrated to result in short-term reduction of H-reflex and MAS scores.[25] However, a randomized controlled trial of four weeks of unloaded leg cycling exercise (30 minutes per session three times per week) conducted by the same research team showed more limited results, with a significant improvement of MSSS-88 scores, but no significant change in H-reflex or MAS scores.[21]

Physical treatments such as electrical stimulation and application of cold-packs may help, although the benefit is usually short lived. They can be used at the beginning of a therapy session, to facilitate the exercises. A multicenter, randomized, placebo-controlled crossover trial of a cooling garment (single session, immediate effect) in 43 MS patients with heat sensitivity showed significant improvement of patient-reported symptoms of spasticity, but not of MAS scores.[26] A randomized controlled trial of whole-body vibration and exercise in MS showed a significant improvement of muscle spasms as reported in the MSSS-88, but no significant change in MAS scores.[27]

Oral medications

Oral anti-spasticity medications are widely used, although a systematic review of the literature showed limited evidence supporting their efficacy and tolerability in MS.[28] Monotherapy, in association with stretching, is usually effective in mild-to-moderate spasticity. When spasticity is severe, drugs can be combined, with tolerability being the main limiting factor. Most anti-spasticity medications can cause CNS sedation, which is of particular concern in MS patients, a majority of whom complain of chronic fatigue. Therefore, they are usually started at a low dose, with a gradual dose titration.

Baclofen

Baclofen (Lioresal®), a structural analog of GABA, binds to pre- and post-synaptic GABA-b receptors. Pre-synaptic binding results in membrane hyperpolarization, reduced influx of calcium, and decreased endogenous transmitter release. Post-synaptic binding increases potassium conductance and enhances presynaptic inhibition. Activation of GABA-b receptors may also inhibit gamma motor neuron activity and decrease muscle spindle sensitivity. Baclofen is rapidly absorbed after oral administration with a mean elimination half-life of 3.5 hours. Most of the drug is directly excreted by the kidney (15% is metabolized in the liver). As a consequence, the dosage should be reduced in patients with impaired renal function, and periodic monitoring of liver function is recommended. Side effects mainly consist of CNS depression (sedation, drowsiness, fatigue), confusion, and dizziness. Baclofen can potentiate the effect of antihypertensive agents. Abrupt discontinuation of treatment can result in a withdrawal syndrome with severe muscle stiffness, paresthesias, hallucinations, confusion, fever, and seizures. Overdose of baclofen can produce hypotonia, respiratory depression, hypotension, and coma. Another common problem is the development or worsening of muscle weakness with baclofen, probably both by direct action of the medication and indirectly through unmasking of underlying weakness. Treatment is usually initiated at 5–10 mg daily, and increased by 5–10 mg increments until the desired effect is obtained or undesirable side effects occur. The recommended maximum total dose is 80 mg per day in 3–4 divided doses, but daily doses above 100 mg have been used.

Early trials showed that baclofen is effective in reducing spasticity in MS patients, with a more prominent benefit on spasms.[29,30] Brar et al. studied the effect of low-dose oral baclofen and muscle stretching, alone or combined, compared to placebo, in 30 MS patients with mild-to-moderate spasticity, using a double-blind cross-over design.[31] There was significant improvement of spasticity with baclofen compared to stretching or placebo; adding stretching to baclofen resulted in a nonsignificant trend for further improvement. A more recent double-blind cross-over trial of oral baclofen vs. placebo in 13 mild-to-moderately disabled MS patients showed no significant improvement of muscle tone or gait characteristics with treatment.[32]

Tizanidine

Tizanidine (Zanaflex®), an imidazoline derivative, is a central alpha-2 adrenergic receptor agonist. Tizanidine inhibits the release of excitatory amino-acids from the pre-synaptic spinal interneurons and may facilitate the action of glycine. It is well absorbed and undergoes extensive first-pass hepatic metabolism. Therefore, tizanidine should be used with caution in patients with liver dysfunction, and monitoring of liver function is recommended. The usual starting dose is 2–4 mg per day. The maximum recommended dose is 36 mg per day in 3–4 divided doses. Sedation and drowsiness are frequently reported by patients. Other side effects include dry mouth, dizziness, hypotension, elevated liver enzymes, and hallucinations. Combination with antihypertensive agents should be avoided or done with caution due to the risk of potentiation of blood pressure lowering effects.

Tizanidine has been shown to be effective in relieving spasticity in MS, although functional improvement was not demonstrated.[33] Both the anti-spasticity effect and side effects of tizanidine correlate with drug plasma concentration.[34] Its efficacy appears comparable to that of baclofen,[35-37] though weakness was reported less often with tizanidine than with baclofen.[38] Results of a double-blind placebo-controlled trial in 187 MS patients published by the United Kingdom Tizanidine Study Group[39] showed significant reduction of Ashworth scores in the treatment group, with no significant between-group difference in muscle strength. Again, no effect was seen on measures of disability. The use of sublingual tizanidine at bedtime has been explored in MS in a double-blind, double-dummy, randomized, three-treatment, two-way crossover clinical trial versus placebo and oral tizanidine,[40] with improvement in next-day spasticity (up to 14 hours) and less sleepiness.

Benzodiazepines

Benzodiazepines act by decreasing mono- and polysynaptic reflexes in the spinal cord. This effect is mediated by the functional coupling of a benzodiazepine – GABA-a receptor – chloride ionophore complex. Long-acting benzodiazepines: diazepam (Valium), clonazepam (Klonopin), chlordiazepoxide (Librium) and short-acting benzodiazepines: (oxazepam (Serax), lorazepam (Ativan) differ by the production of pharmacologically active metabolites in the former. Diazepam is the oldest anti-spasticity medication. It is well absorbed and reaches a peak blood level within one hour, is 98% protein-bound, and has elimination half-life is 20–80 hours. Its hepatic metabolism produces active metabolites (nordazepam, oxazepam). It crosses the placental barrier and is excreted into breast milk. CNS depression is the main adverse effect, and is potentiated by alcohol. Overdose can lead to coma and respiratory depression. Abrupt discontinuation can result in a withdrawal syndrome with anxiety, tremor, agitation, insomnia, and possibly psychotic manifestations and seizures. The severity of withdrawal symptoms is dose-dependent.

A study by From et al. comparing baclofen and diazepam with a double-blind cross-over design in 17 MS patients[41] showed no difference in efficacy between the two agents, sedation was more frequently reported with diazepam. Deterioration of gait performance due to weakness was observed in one out of two ambulatory patients, both with diazepam and baclofen. An open trial comparing baclofen (n = 33, 80% MS), clonazepam (n = 25, 100% MS), and placebo (n = 10, 100% MS) showed comparable efficacy of both active drugs, but patients with more severe spasticity at baseline appeared to respond better to baclofen.[42] Because of the risk of sedation, benzodiazepines are often prescribed at bed to relieve nocturnal spasms, at a low dosage, and in combination with other anti-spasticity agents.

Gabapentin

Gabapentin (Neurontin®) was introduced in 1994 as an add-on therapy for patients with refractory partial seizures. Its structure is similar to GABA, but it does not bind to conventional CNS receptors. It is well absorbed, and reaches peak serum concentration after 2–3 hours. It is not bound to proteins, and is excreted in its original form in the urine. Adverse effects including nystagmus, diplopia, somnolence, ataxia, and dizziness, have been reported in a small percentage of patients. There is no evidence of toxicity on any major organ system. Dosages up to 3600 mg per day (in divided doses) have been used. Gabapentin is also used to treat subjective sensory symptoms (paresthesias, neuropathic pain).

Dunevsky and Perel reported improvement of Ashworth scores and functional status in two MS patients treated with gabapentin at the dose of 400 mg per day.[43] A recent double-blinded placebo-controlled trial of gabapentin in 21 veterans with MS (19 men) showed statistically significant improvements in subjective and objective impairment in the treatment group. There was no significant difference in disability measured by the EDSS between the two groups, but EDSS is not likely to be very sensitive to changes in functional performance related to spasticity relief.[44]

Dantrolene sodium

Dantrolene sodium (Dantrium®), a hydantoin derivative, acts peripherally by reducing the action potential-induced release of calcium from the sarcoplasmic reticulum of skeletal muscle fibers. This results in partial excitation-contraction uncoupling, which appears to be more prominent on fast-twitch extrafusal fibers. Dantrolene sodium is absorbed approximately 70%, achieves a peak serum concentration after 3–6 hours, and is largely metabolized by the liver leading to production of an active metabolite 5-hydroxydantrolene. The molecule is lipophilic and, therefore, easily crosses cell membranes. In particular, it crosses the placental barrier. Side effects include CNS sedation (usually mild), GI symptoms, and hepatotoxicity, which can be severe with necrosis of the liver. The incidence of fatal hepatitis is 0.3%. Therefore, liver function should be tested before treatment and periodically after treatment initiation. Dantrolene sodium is also used to treat malignant hyperthermia and the neuroleptic malignant syndrome. Toxicity, the risk of weakness, and modest efficacy in early clinical trials[45,46] explain the limited use of dantrolene sodium in MS.

Clonidine

Clonidine (Catapres®) acts as an alpha-2 adrenergic agonist throughout the CNS. It is primarily used as an antihypertensive agent. The effect of clonidine on blood pressure appears to be mediated by inhibition of neurons in the locus coeruleus, resulting in decreased sympathetic outflow. The medication is readily absorbed, and peak plasma concentration is reached after 3–5 hours. It is both metabolized by the liver and excreted unchanged in the urine, in equal proportions. Side effects include bradycardia, hypotension, drowsiness, dry mouth, constipation, dizziness, pedal edema, and depression.

Trials of clonidine, mostly in patients with spinal cord injury, showed a positive effect on spasticity.[47,48] Clonidine usually is combined with other medications such as baclofen. Poor tolerance is a concern, particularly the risk of hypotension in MS patients with dysautonomia. The transdermal patch appears to be as effective as the oral form on spasticity, and may decrease the occurrence and severity of side effects.[49]

Cannabinoids

Cannabinoids have been reported to improve tremor and spasticity, both in animal models of MS[50] and in MS patients.[51] Nabiximols (Sativex) has been approved in some countries to treat MS-related pain and spasticity. Nabiximols is a cannabis extract administered as an oromucosal spray containing mainly delta(9)-tetrahydrocannabinol and cannabinol. A multicenter randomized placebo-controlled parallel group trial of naxibimols in 337 MS patients showed a nonsignificant improvement is spasticity NRS scores in favor of the active treatment in the intention-to-treat analysis, while the per protocol population analysis and responder analysis both showed a statistically significant treatment effect.[52] A meta-analysis of three randomized, placebo-controlled trials involving 666 patients, showed a significantly higher rate of responders and a significantly greater improvement in spasticity NRS scores in the active treatment group.[53] Adverse events were frequent, most of them mild-to-moderate, and all drug-related serious adverse events were reported to have resolved.

Cyproheptadine

Cyproheptadine (Periactin®), a histamine and serotonin antagonist, was found to be effective on clonus in an open trial of patients with spasticity of spinal origin.[54] Side effects mainly consist of CNS sedation and anticholinergic symptoms.

Low-dose naltrexone

Statistically significant improvement of MAS scores was reported in a pilot open-label uncontrolled trial of low-dose naltrexone, an opiate antagonist, on 40 patients with primary progressive MS.[55]

Local treatments

Local treatments are used to provide short- or long-term relaxation of specific muscles or muscle groups, to facilitate stretching and ROM exercises, to improve comfort, and in some cases to improve function. If the spasticity involves an entire limb or several limbs, as is usually the case in MS, local treatments are usually administered in combination with systemic agents.

Anesthetic agents

Local anesthetic agents, such as lidocaine, eitdocaine, or bupivacaine, can be injected via perineural or intramuscular injection. They exert a blocking action on sensory and motor nerves, muscle fibers, and at the neuromuscular junction. Small nerve fibers, and fibers that have been recently and repetitively stimulated, are more sensitive to the anesthetic block. Onset of action is rapid, usually within minutes, and duration varies according to the lipid solubility and protein affinity of the anesthetic, usually a few hours. Systemic side effects include CNS stimulation, cardiovascular depression, and rare hypersensitivity reactions. Therefore, resuscitation equipment should be available. Intensive use of local anesthetic should be avoided in individuals with liver failure, since they are metabolized by the liver. Due to their short duration of action, local anesthetics are used to evaluate the potential benefit of more long-lasting local procedures, or to facilitate physical therapy.

Chemical neurolysis

Chemical neurolysis produces a nerve block by damaging nerve structures. Phenol and ethyl alcohol are the two chemical agents used for these procedures, and work by denaturing proteins and causing tissue necrosis. The destruction is non-selective and depends upon the concentration of the chemical administered. Regrowth of axons is expected and accounts for the reversibility of the effect. However, damage to the microcirculation may result in fibrosis impairing nerve regeneration. The main side effects are local, and consist of pain during the injection or chronic dysesthesias. Onset of effect is rapid. Duration of effect is highly variable, usually several months (up to 36 months). Both perineural and intramuscular injections can be performed. Injection of purely or largely motor nerves (e.g. obturator nerve for adductor spasticity) is preferred, to minimize the risk of chronic dysesthesias.

Botulinum toxin

BT is widely used in various indications, including spasticity. BT is a very potent toxin produced by the anaerobic organism *Clostridium botulinum* that blocks the release of acetylcholine by presynaptic terminals at the neuromuscular junction. Of the seven known serotypes of BT, only BT-A and BT-B are available in preparation for injections. Onabotulinum toxin A was recently approved in the United States for the treatment of focal upper extremity spasticity in adults, while various formulations of BT-A have been approved for spasticity in other countries.

BT is injected into the muscle, and diffuses approximately 30 mm around the injection site. EMG or electrical stimulation can be used to locate small and deep muscles, particularly in the distal upper extremity. The therapeutic effect appears after 24–72 hours, peaks at 2–4 weeks, and usually lasts 12 weeks or more. The reversibility of the effect of BT is due to nerve sprouting and the creation of new neuromuscular junctions. Repetition of the injection usually produces an identical or better effect. Muscle atrophy is commonly observed. Partial muscle weakness is a logical consequence of BT injection, therefore target muscles should be determined with caution to avoid negative functional consequences. Systemic side effects of BT are rare. They can be minor but severe reactions leading to hospitalization and death have been reported. BT should be used with caution in patients with disorders of the neuromuscular junction, and in patients taking aminoglycosides, which also may interfere with neuromuscular transmission. Cost can be an issue, since the injections must be repeated to maintain a long-term effect.

The development of antibodies to BT-A can lead to resistance to therapy, and has been linked to higher doses of toxin injected, frequent injections, and higher protein load in the preparation.[56] For this reason, it is recommended to administer a maximum dose of 600 U per visit, and to repeat injections no more frequently than every three months. The frontalis test can be used to detect resistance to BT-A clinically. It consists of injecting 15 U of BT in the corrugator muscle on one side, and evaluating the ability to move this muscle after two weeks. Several types of assays are available to detect antibodies to BT-A in the serum. These antibodies are not expected to cross-react with BT-B.

The Therapeutics and Technology Assessment Subcommittee of the American Academy of Neurology published an evidence-based review of the use of BT in spasticity management, and concluded that, in adults, BT is effective on upper and lower limb spasticity in reducing muscle tone and improving passive function (Level A recommendation), and probably effective in improving active function (Level B recommendation).[57] Published evidence on the efficacy and safety of BT in MS is scarce, as most of the clinical trials were conducted in post-stroke survivors. A double-blind, placebo-controlled trial in ten non-ambulatory MS patients studied BT or placebo injected in the thigh adductor muscles with cross-over injection at three months.[58] There was significant improvement of spasticity scores and ease of care with BT. Kerty and Stein reported improvement of adductor spasticity in two of five patients with advanced MS.[59] Borg-Stein *et al.* noted improvement of spasticity and function in two MS patients treated with BT.[60] Controlled studies with standardized evaluation of functional outcomes are needed to further evaluate the indications of BT in MS.

Neuro-orthopedic interventions

Neuro-orthopedic interventions are considered when contractures resulting from severe spasticity are present. Procedures include tendon lengthening (e.g. Achilles tendon), tendon transfer, neurectomy (e.g. obturator neurectomy for adductor spasticity), and less frequently intramuscular lengthening. Due to the risks related to surgery, indications should be evaluated with caution, and post-surgical care should be carefully planned. It is recommended to perform these interventions during periods of disease stability, and expectations, in terms of ease of care, posturing, or function, must be realistic. Surgery is usually followed by aggressive stretching, serial casting, or splinting, to avoid recurrence of contractures. MS patients are often reluctant to consider such interventions, by fear of complications or because of their destructive character, but they can be very helpful in select cases.

Intrathecal medication

Intrathecal baclofen

ITB is approved by the US Food and Drug Administration for the treatment of severe spasticity of spinal or cerebral origin refractory to oral anti-spastic medications. The medication is delivered directly into the intrathecal space via a programmable infusion system, consisting of a battery-powered pump implanted subcutaneously or subfascially in the lower abdominal wall, and an intraspinal catheter tunneled subcutaneously to the pump catheter port. The catheter tip is usually placed at the lower thoracic level, providing relief of spasticity in the low back and legs. Higher catheter placement has been reported to treat upper extremity spasticity, particularly in stroke, cerebral palsy, and spinal cord injury patients.

The pump contains a reservoir for the medication, which can be accessed for refills through a port. The maximum interval between refills is 180 days, to ensure that the medication remains stable. The pump can be interrogated and programmed non-invasively through an external computer, which exchanges information with the pump via telemetry. Safety features include a low reservoir volume and a low battery alarm to prevent withdrawal. ITB administration allows effective cerebrospinal fluid (CSF) concentrations to be achieved with much smaller doses of baclofen, and resultant plasma concentrations 100 times less than those occurring with oral administration. The lumbar-cisternal CSF concentration gradient is estimated at 4:1, accounting for the reduced incidence of CNS sedation compared to oral baclofen. It is required to perform a test injection of ITB before pump implantation. The dose injected usually varies between 25–100 mcg. The effect of ITB on lower extremity spasticity and weakness is evaluated periodically over the following 4–8 hours. Vital signs and any adverse effects are monitored during the same period.

There are few contra-indications to ITB therapy: known hypersensitivity to baclofen, active infection at the time of screening injection or surgery, and all severe concomitant pathologies which would preclude surgery. Potentially life-threatening complications of ITB therapy include overdosing and abrupt withdrawal, which have been discussed earlier in this chapter. Overdose is generally related to procedural errors. Abrupt withdrawal can be related to procedural errors, empty reservoir, catheter malfunction, or pump malfunction. Other complications include infections, wound dehiscence, seroma, and CSF leak. Causes of catheter malfunction include catheter fracture, subdural migration, dislodgement, and fibrosis or granulomata at the tip of the catheter. Cranial migration of the intrathecal catheter with associated subarachnoid hemorrhage was reported in one patient. Pump malfunctions are rare, and include unexpected battery failure, and rotor lock. Specific procedures are followed for patient management and troubleshooting of complications and malfunctions. Other drawbacks of ITB therapy are cost, the need for periodic refills and adjustments, and the need to undergo repeat surgery for battery end-of-life (usually every five years). A pregnancy with delivery of a healthy infant was reported in an MS patient treated with ITB.[61]

A publication reported the frequency of adverse effects and complications of ITB therapy from a survey of 40 centers (936 pump placements).[51] The most common side effects after screening intrathecal injection of baclofen were nausea and vomiting, sedation, hypotension, and urinary retention. The most common complications during hospitalization after pump implantation were constipation, headache, and CSF leak or collection. The most frequent long-term complication was infection, which was also the most common reason for early pump replacement. The catheter had to be replaced for malfunction in 7% of cases.

ITB has been used for over 10 years in the treatment of refractory lower extremity spasticity in MS and other pathologies of the CNS, and several studies have demonstrated its efficacy.[62–66] Improvement of bladder function has also been reported, but is never a primary indication for ITB. ITB is traditionally used in non-ambulatory MS patients with severe spasms. In this population, ITB has been shown to provide relief of discomfort and pain related to spasticity, greater ease of care, improved posture, and improved ability to transfer.[67,68] A survey of 198 MS patients using ITB found significantly lower levels of spasticity compared to a group of 315 patients using oral medications, despite the fact that the ITB group reported significantly higher levels of disability.[3] ITB patients also reported a higher level of satisfaction with the results of treatment compared to oral therapy patients. Zahavi *et al.* reported on a five-year observational study of ITB therapy in 21 patients with spasticity of spinal origin (53% with MS) and noted a good long-term clinical control of spasticity and high level of patient satisfaction, but no significant improvement on global disability and subjective health status measures.[69] Bensmail *et al.* found significant improvement of sleep quality and no adverse effect on respiratory function with ITB therapy in patients with MS and spinal cord injury.[70] Interestingly, an increase in upper extremity motor evoked potential amplitude was reported in a sample of 11 patients with severe spastic quadriparesis treated with ITB

(compared to pre-ITB testing), but the authors did not indicate if this was correlated with changes in upper extremity spasticity, strength, or function.[71]

More recently, ITB has been increasingly used in ambulatory MS patients.[72,73] This represents a more challenging patient subgroup, in particular because of the potential risk of loss of function from increased lower extremity weakness. On the other hand, these patients have a greater potential for reduction of disability and/or handicap from ITB, because they are more likely to be involved in household- or work-related activities. New outcomes measures, particularly easy-to-use measures of gait performance, need to be validated for this purpose. Preliminary data suggest that satisfactory control of spasticity can be achieved in ambulatory patients without loss of function.[74]

Other intrathecal medications

Opiates and clonidine have also been used intrathecally to treat intractable pain and spasticity in MS, alone or more frequently in combination with baclofen.[75,76] A recent publication reported significant improvement of bladder function in spinal cord injury patients treated with i.t. clonidine.[77] The authors recommended combining clonidine with baclofen to achieve better tolerance.

Neurosurgical interventions

Historically, stereotactic electrocoagulation of different parts of the brain (globus pallidus, thalamus, cerebellum), cerebellar stimulation, cordectomy, and myelotomy have been performed, but are not currently warranted in the treatment of spasticity. Selective posterior rhizotomy has been used with some success, particularly in cerebral palsy. The rationale for posterior rhizotomy is to decrease afferent signals to the spinal cord, disrupting the reflex arc involved in dynamic phenomena related to spasticity. Indications, contra-indications, and surgical techniques have been refined over the years. For many reasons, this treatment modality is not commonly used in MS, although positive results have been published.[78]

Conclusions

The scarcity of scientific evidence in MS, as well as the unpredictability and heterogeneity of the disease, make it difficult for the clinician to design treatment algorithms for spasticity management that take into account all of the available modalities. Nevertheless, recently published clinical guidelines can be a helpful resource for the clinician. Training, interests, anecdotal experience, and the proximity of specialized centers heavily influence practice habits. Education of the patients and prevention of long-term complications are essential, and oral medications are often helpful. More invasive and costly interventions, such as ITB therapy, are probably underused, and should be considered earlier instead of as a "last resort," but their success requires thorough assessments and a realistic treatment plan, which will ideally involve a multidisciplinary team.

References

1. Lance J. Symposium synopsis. In Feldman RG, Young RR, Koella WP, eds. *Spasticity: Disordered Motor Control.* Chicago: Year Book Medical Publishers, 1980;485–94.

2. Matthews B. Symptoms and signs of multiple sclerosis. In Compston A, Ebers G, Lassmann H, McDonald I, Matthews B, Wekerle H, eds. *McAlpine's Multiple Sclerosis.* London: Churchill Livingstone, 1998.

3. Rizzo M, Hadjimichael O, Preiningerova J, Vollmer T. Prevalence and treatment of spasticity reported by multiple sclerosis patients. *Mult Scler* 2004;10:589–95.

4. Walther E, Hohlfeld R. Multiple sclerosis: side effects of interferon beta therapy and their management. *Neurology* 1999;53:1622–7.

5. Young R. Spasticity: a review. *Neurology* 1994;44:S12–20.

6. Herman R, Freedman W, Meeks S. Physiological aspects of hemiplegic and paraplegic spasticity. In Desmedt J, ed. *New Developments in Electromyography and Clinical Neurophysiology.* Basel: Karger, 1973.

7. Ashworth B. Preliminary trial of carisoprodol in multiple sclerosis. *Practitioner* 1964;192:540–2.

8. Bohannon R, Smith M. Inter-rater reliability of a modified Ashworth scale of muscle spasticity. *Phys Ther* 1987; 67:206–7.

9. Ghotbi N, Ansari NN, Naghdi S, *et al.* Inter-rater reliability of the Modified Ashworth Scale in assessing lower limb muscle spasticity. *Brain Injury* 2009; 23:815–19.

10. Pandyan AD, Johnson GR, Price CIM, *et al.* A review of the properties and limitations of the Ashworth and Modified Ashworth Scales as measures of spasticity. *Clin Rehab* 1999;13: 373–83.

11. Fleuren JF, Voerman GE, Erren-Wolters CV, *et al.* Stop using the Ashworth Scale for the assessment of spasticity. *J Neurol Neurosurg Psychiatry* 2010;81:46–52.

12. Tardieu G, Shentoub S, Delarue R. A la recherche d'une technique de mesure de la spasticite. *Rev Neurol* 1954;91: 143–4.

13. Love S, Valentine J, Blair E, *et al.* The effect of botulinum toxin type A on the functional ability of the child with spastic hemiplegia a randomized controlled trial. *J Neurol* 2001;8 (Suppl 5):50–8.

14. Bajd T, Vodovnik L. Pendulum testing of spasticity. *J Biomed Eng* 1984;6:9–16.

15. Delwaide P. Human monosynaptic reflexes and presynaptic inhibition: an interpretation of spastic hyperreflexia. In Desmedt J, ed. *New Developments in Electromyography and Clinical Neurophysiology.* Basel: Karger, 1973.

16. Stokic D, Yablon S, Hayes A. Comparison of clinical and neurophysiologic responses to intrathecal baclofen bolus administration in moderate-to-severe spasticity after acquired brain injury. *Arch Phys Med Rehab* 2005;86:1801–6.

17. Penn RD, Savoy SM, Corocs D, *et al.* Intrathecal baclofen for severe spinal spasticity. *N Engl J Med* 1989;320: 1517–21.

18. Farrar JT, Troxel AB, Stott C, Duncombe P, Jensen MP. Validity, reliability, and clinical importance of change in a 0–10 numeric rating scale measure of spasticity: a post hoc analysis of a randomized, double-blind, placebo-controlled trial. *Clin Ther* 2008;30:974–85.

19. Anwar K, Barnes MP. A pilot study of a comparison between a patient scored numeric rating scale and clinician scored measures of spasticity in multiple sclerosis. *Neurorehabilitation* 2009;24:333–40.

20. Hobart JC, Riazi A, Thompson AJ, *et al.* Getting the measure of spasticity in multiple sclerosis: the Multiple Sclerosis Spasticity Scale (MSSS-88). *Brain* 2006;129:224–34.

21. Sosnoff J, Motl RW, Snook EM, Wynn D. Effect of a 4-week period of unloaded leg cycling exercise on spasticity in multiple sclerosis. *Neurorehabilitation* 2009;24:327–31.

22. Multiple Sclerosis Council for Clinical Practice Guidelines. *Spasticity management in multiple sclerosis.* Consortium of Multiple Sclerosis Centers, 2003.

23. Giovannelli M, Borriello G, Castri P, Prosperini L, Pozzilli C. Early physiotherapy after injection of botulinum toxin increases the beneficial effects on spasticity in patients with multiple sclerosis. *Clin Rehab* 2007;21:331–7.

24. Giesser, Beres-Jones J, Budovitch A, Herlihy E, Harkema S. Locomotor training using body weight support on a treadmill improves mobility in persons with multiple sclerosis: a pilot study. *Mult Scler* 2007;13:224–31.

25. Sosnoff JJ, Motl RW. Effect of acute unloaded arm versus leg cycling exercise on the soleus H-reflex in adults with multiple sclerosis. *Neurosci Lett* 2010;479:307–11.

26. Nilsagard Y, Denison E, Gunnarsson LG. Evaluation of a single session with cooling garment for persons with multiple sclerosis-a randomized trial. *Disabil Rehab Assist Technol* 2006;1: 225–33.

27. Schyns F, Paul L, Finlay K, Ferguson C, Noble E. Vibration therapy in multiple sclerosis: a pilot study exploring its effects on tone, muscle force, sensation and functional performance. *Clin Rehab* 2009;23:771–81.

28. Shakespeare D, Young C, Boggild M. Anti-spasticity agents for multiple sclerosis. *Cochrane Database Syst Rev* 2000;4(CD-ROM)

29. Pinto O, Polikar M, Debono G. Results of international clinical trials with Lioresal. *Postgrad Med J* 1972;48:18–23.

30. Feldman R, Kelly-Hayes M, Conomy J, Foley J. Baclofen for spasticity in multiple sclerosis: double-blind crossover and three year study. *Neurology* 1978;28:1094–8.

31. Brar S, Smith M, Nelson L, Franklin G, Cobble N. Evaluation of treatment protocols on minimal to moderate spasticity in multiple sclerosis. *Arch Phys Med Rehab* 1991;72:186–9.

32. Orsnes G, Sorensen P, Larsen T, Ravnborg M. Effect of baclofen on gait in spastic MS patients. *Acta Neurol Scand* 2000;101:244–8.

33. Lapierre Y, Bouchard S, Tansey C, *et al.* Treatment of spasticity with tizanidine in multiple sclerosis. *Can J Neurol Sci* 1987;14:513–17.

34. Nance P, Sheremata W, Lynch S, *et al.* Relationship of the antispasticity effect of tizanidine to plasma concentration in patients with multiple sclerosis. *Arch Neurol* 1997;54:731–6.

35. Smolenski C, Muff S, Smolenski-Kautz S. A double-blind comparative trial of a

new muscle-relaxant, tizanidine (DS102–282), and baclofen in the treatment of chronic spasticity in multiple sclerosis. *Curr Med Res Opin* 1981;7:374–83.

36. Stein R, Nordal H, Oftedal S, Slettebo M. The treatment of spasticity in multiple sclerosis: a double-blind clinical trial of a new anti-spasticity drug tizanidine compared with baclofen. *Acta Neurol Scand* 1987;75: 190–4.

37. Hoogstraten M, Van Der Ploeg R, Van Der Burg W, *et al.* Tizanidine versus baclofen in the treatment of multiple sclerosis patients. *Acta Neurol Scand* 1988;77:224–30.

38. Bass B, Weinsheker B, Rice G. Tizanidine versus baclofen in the treatment of spasticity in patients with multiple sclerosis. *J Neurol Sci* 1988; 15:15–19.

39. The United Kingdom Tizanidine Study Group. A double-blind placebo-controlled trial of tizanidine in the treatment of spasticity caused by multiple sclerosis. *Neurology* 1994;44: 70–9.

40. Vakhapova V, Auriel E, Karni A. Nightly sublingual tizanidine HCl in multiple sclerosis: clinical efficacy and safety. *Clin Neuropharmacol* 2010;33: 151–4.

41. From A, Heltberg A. A double-blind trial with baclofen and diazepam in spasticity due to multiple sclerosis. *Acta Neurol Scand* 1975;51:158–66.

42. Cendrowski W, Sobczyk W. Clonazepam, baclofen, and placebo in the treatment of spasticity. *Eur Neurol* 1977;16:257–62.

43. Dunevsky A, Perel A. Gabapentin for relief of spasticity associated with multiple sclerosis. *Am J Phys Med Rehab* 1998;77:451–4.

44. Cutter N, Scott D, Johnson J, Whiteneck G. Gabapentin effect of spasticity in multiple sclerosis: a placebo-controlled, randomized trial. *Arch Phys Med Rehab* 2000;81: 164–9.

45. Gelenberg A, Poskanzer D. The effect of dantrolene sodium on spasticity in multiple sclerosis. *Neurology* 1973; 23:1313–15.

46. Tolosa E, Soll R, Loewenson R. Treatment of spasticity in multiple sclerosis with dantrolene (letter). *J Am Med Assoc* 1975;233:1046.

47. Donovan W, Carter R, Rossi C, Wilkerson M. Clonidine effect on spasticity: a clinical trial. *Arch Phys Med Rehab* 1988;69:193–4.

48. Nance P, Shears A, Nance D. Clonidine in spinal cord injury. *Can Med Assoc J* 1985;133:41–2.

49. Yablon S, Sipski M. Effect of transdermal clonidine on spinal spasticity: a case series. *Am J Phys Med Rehabil* 1993;72:154–7.

50. Baker D, Pryce G, Croxford J, *et al.* Cannabinoids control spasticity and tremor in a multiple sclerosis model. *Nature* 2000;404:84–7.

51. Petro D, Ellenberger C. Treatment of human spasticity with delta-9-tetrahydrocannabinol. *J Clin Pharmacol* 1981;21:413S–16S.

52. Collin C, Ehler E, Waberzinek G, *et al.* A double-blind, randomized, placebo-controlled, parallel-group study of Sativex in subjects with symptoms of spasticity due to multiple sclerosis. *Neurol Res* 2010;32:451–9.

53. Wade DT, Collin C, Stott C, Duncombe P. Meta-analysis of the efficacy and safety of Sativex (nabiximols) on spasticity in people with multiple sclerosis. *Mult Scler* 2010;16:707–14.

54. Barbeau H, Richards C, Bedard B. Action of cyproheptadine in spastic paraparetic patients. *J Neurol Neurosurg Psychiatry* 1982;45:923–6.

55. Gironi M, Martinelli-Boneschi F, Sacerdote P, *et al.* A pilot trial of low-dose naltrexone in primary progressive multiple sclerosis. *Mult Scler* 2008;14:1076–83.

56. Brin M. Botulinum toxin: chemistry, pharmacology, toxicity, and immunology. *Muscle Nerve* 1997;Suppl 6:S146–68.

57. Simpson DM, Gracies JM, Graham HK, *et al.* Assessment: Botulinum neurotoxin for the treatment of spasticity (an evidence-based review): report of the Therapeutics and Technology Assessment Subcommittee of the American Academy of Neurology. *Neurology* 2008;70:1691–8.

58. Snow B, Tsui J, Bhatt M, *et al.* Treatment of spasticity with botulinum toxin: a double-blind study. *Ann Neurol* 1990;28:512–15.

59. Kerty E, Stein R. Treatment of spasticity with botulinum toxin. *Tidsskr Nor Laegeforen* 1997;117:2022–4.

60. Borg-Stein J, Pine Z, Miller J, Brin M. Botulinum toxin for the treatment of spasticity in multiple sclerosis. *Am J Phys Med Rehab* 1993;72:364–8.

61. Dalton CM, Keenan E, Jarrett L, Buckley L, Stevenson VL. The safety of baclofen in pregnancy: intrathecal therapy in multiple sclerosis. *Mult Scler* 2008;14:571–2.

62. Abel N, Smith R. Intrathecal baclofen for treatment of intractable spinal spasticity. *Arch Phys Med Rehab* 1994;75:54–8.

63. Azouvi P, Mane M, Thiebaut J, *et al.* Intrathecal baclofen administration for control of severe spinal spasticity: functional improvement and long-term follow-up. *Arch Phys Med Rehab* 1996;77:35–9.

64. Becker W, Harris C, Long M, *et al.* Long term intrathecal baclofen therapy in patients with intractable spasticity. *Can J Neurol Sci* 1995;22:208–17.

65. Nance P, Schryvers O, Schmidt B, *et al.* Intrathecal baclofen therapy for adults with spinal spasticity: therapeutic efficacy and effect on hospital admissions. *Can J Neurol Sci* 1995; 22:22–9.

66. Ordia J, Fischer E, Adamski E, Spatz E. Chronic intrathecal delivery of baclofen by a programmable pump for the treatment of severe spasticity. *J Neurosurg* 1996;85:452–7.

67. Stempien L, Tsai T. Intrathecal baclofen pump use for spasticity. *Am J Phys Med Rehab* 2000;79:536–41.

68. Jarrett L, Siobhan M, Porter B, *et al.* Managing spasticity in people with multiple sclerosis: a goal-oriented approach to intrathecal baclofen therapy. *Int J MS Care* 2001;3:10–21.

69. Zahavi A, Geertzen JHB, Middel B, Staal M, Rietman JS. Long term effect (more than five years) of intrathecal baclofen on impairment, disability, and quality of life in patients with severe spasticity of spinal origin. *J Neurol Neurosurg Psychiatry* 2004;75:1553–7.

70. Bensmail D, Quera Salva MA, Roche N, *et al.* Effect of intrathecal baclofen on sleep and respiratory function in patients with spasticity. *Neurology* 2006;67:1432–6.

71. Auer C, Siebner H, Dressnandt J, Conrad B. Intrathecal baclofen increases corticospinal output to hand muscles in multiple sclerosis. *Neurology* 1999;52:1298–9.

72. Sadiq SA, Wang GC. Long-term intrathecal baclofen therapy in ambulatory patients with spasticity. *J Neurol* 2006;253:563–9.

73. Bethoux F, Gogol D, Schwetz K, Kinkel R. Use of a registry of intrathecal baclofen therapy in a large multiple sclerosis center: analysis of data on 82 patients and proposed changes (letter). *Arch Phys Med Rehab* 2001;82:1329.

74. Bethoux F, Stough D, Sutliff M. Treatment of severe spasticity with intrathecal baclofen therapy in ambulatory multiple sclerosis patients: 6-month follow-up. *Arch Phys Med Rehab* 2004;84:A10.

75. Delehanty L, Sadiq S. Use of combination intrathecal baclofen and morphine in MS patients with intractable pain and spasticity. *Neurology* 2001;56:A99.

76. Masterson M, Sadiq S. Use of intrathecal clonidine infusion alone, or in combination with intrathecal baclofen, for relief of intractable pain syndromes. *Neurology* 2001;56:A351.

77. Denys P, Chartier-Kastler E, Azouvi P, Remy-Neris O, Bussel B. Intrathecal clonidine for refractory detrusor hyperreflexia in spinal cord injured patients: a preliminary report. *J Urol* 1998;160:2137–8.

78. Sindou M, Millet M, Mortamais J, Eyssette M. Results of selective posterior rhizotomy in the treatment of painful and spastic paraplegia secondary to multiple sclerosis. *Appl Neurophysiol* 1982;45: 335–40.

Chapter

58

Management of bladder and sexual dysfunction in multiple sclerosis

Natasha Frost, Jessica Szpak, Scott Litwiller, and Alexander Rae-Grant

Introduction

Many multiple sclerosis (MS) patients have symptoms of lower urinary tract (bladder and urethral) dysfunction (LUTD) or sexual dysfunction early in their course.[1] More than 96% of patients with the disease for 10 years will have had urological manifestations.[2-7] The effects of MS on the genitourinary tract can range from minor bladder and urethral symptoms to incontinence and impotence. Consequently, genitourinary symptoms are a major sources of frustration and distress for people with MS.[8] Patients with bladder dysfunction have lower scores on quality of life scales.[9] Therefore, a working knowledge of the anatomy, pathophysiology, evaluation, and treatment of these conditions is essential for the MS specialist, who is often called upon to care for these symptoms.

Neural control of voiding

The peripheral nervous system has direct inputs that affect voiding: these are parasympathetic, sympathetic, and somatic in nature.[10] Parasympathetic preganglionic neurons in the sacral parasympathetic nucleus (sacral 2–4 spinal cord segments) send cholinergic axons to the peripheral ganglia and postganglionic neurons in the bladder wall and pelvis plexus. The noradrenergic sympathetic nerves begin in the lumbar spinal cord (cord levels thoracic 10– lumbar 2) cause relaxation of the bladder and contraction of the bladder outlet and urethra causing retention of urine. Somatic efferent fibers originate in Onuf's nucleus in the lateral ventral horn and travel via the pelvic and pudendal nerves to innervate the urethral and anal sphincters the pelvic floor and perineal muscles, and are connected via the pudendal nerve to the S2–4 spinal cord. These control voluntary voiding and sphincter closure. Afferents from the bladder and sphincters travel in pelvic, hypogastric, and pudendal nerves via A-delta and C-fibers. They provide conscious and unconscious information about bladder fullness.

Urinary continence is achieved by urethral closure at a pressure above intravesicular pressure. During micturition, urethral pressure is relaxed and intravesicular pressure increases. Intravesicular pressure is mediated by the detrusor muscle, while urethral closure pressure is mediated by internal and external urethral sphincters.[11]

Supranuclear control of bladder function occurs at multiple central nervous system (CNS) levels (spinal cord, brain stem, subcortical, cortical). Disease in various areas may affect conscious control of micturition by altering input signal (delayed awareness of need to void), changing reflex timing of micturition, and affecting the control of voiding (incontinence). Some studies have suggested a correlation between lesion site and bladder dysfunction type but due to the multiplicity of MS lesions throughout the neuraxis such correlations are problematic.[12]

Neurological effects on the urinary tract

MS plaques can occur anywhere in the CNS, including cortical, subcortical, brainstem, and spinal cord.[13-17] Involvement of the corticospinal and reticulospinal tracts in the spinal cord is common and important for voiding, as these tracts innervate of the detrusor muscle and external urethral sphincter.[18-28] Overall, due to varying functional effects of lesions and the multiplicity of lesions in MS patients, the distribution of lesions in an individual patient cannot be used to predict or treat bladder dysfunction.

Sacral cord effects

The frequency of lower motor neuron lesions affecting bladder function in MS patients varies widely depending on the series.[9] An autopsy study showed sacral cord plaques in 18% of cases.[24] The clinical importance of sacral cord lesions is unclear as spinal cord imaging results may vary and multiple lesions are seen throughout the neuraxis in most patients.[21-23] Prolonged reflex latencies, which may suggest sacral nerve dysfunction, have been documented in MS, but their relationship with bladder dysfunction is uncertain.[26-29]

Suprasacral spinal cord effects

Autopsy series show involvement of the spinal cord above the sacral region in up to 80% of MS patients,[29] which can cause loss of descending inhibition of autonomous bladder contractions resulting in detrusor hyperactivity (detrusor hyperreflexia, DH). Spinal lesions affecting reticulospinal pathways from the pons alter synergistic integration of urethral sphincter

Multiple Sclerosis Therapeutics, Fourth Edition, ed. Jeffrey A. Cohen and Richard A. Rudick. Published by Cambridge University Press.
© Cambridge University Press 2011.

and detrusor activity.[29] Such disruption can cause three main abnormalities: detrusor sphincter dyssynergia (DSD), incomplete sphincteric relaxation (ISR), or sphincter paralysis.[30]

Intracranial plaques

Most patients with MS have involvement above the spinal cord.[29,31–33] Disease in the brain and brain stem can cause urological dysfunction by various mechanisms. In one study of 90 MS patients, there was no correlation between cranial MRI findings and any urodynamic parameter.[34] Other studies indicate a correlation of bladder symptoms with midbrain lesions.[35,36]

Clinical presentations

Symptoms of LUTD in MS include frequency, urgency, incontinence, hesitancy, and urinary retention.[13–17] The frequency of these symptoms varies depending on the series, but frequent urination and urgency are more common than urinary retention or incontinence.[13–17] Although the incidence of urinary symptoms ranges between 52 and 97%, the presence or absence of symptoms is an unreliable indicator of the extent or type of bladder dysfunction.[37] For example, in one study only 47% of patients with an elevated post-void residual (PVR) had a sensation of incomplete emptying.[21] In one study all those with urological symptoms had evidence of LUTD, but 52% of those without symptoms also had LUTD.[5] A study in 297 patients at an MS clinic who underwent PVR testing showed that there was no correlation with scores on the Expanded Disability Status Scale, Bladder/Bowel Functional System Scale, or the Guy's Neurological Disability Scale.[38] The authors of the latter study recommended PVR scanning in every patient with MS regardless of clinical symptoms. A systematic literature review found that on average detrusor or sphincter dysfunction occurs six years after onset of MS.[8]

Several studies have shown a correlation between the presence of LUTD and disease duration, age, degree of sensory and motor disturbance, and disability measures. Awad et al.[23] found that the presence of pyramidal tract dysfunction was most closely related to LUTD. Secondary progressive MS has the highest prevalence of LUTD.[5]

In patients with MS, particularly those with more disability, urinary tract infections (UTIs) can cause a worsening of MS symptoms, a so-called "pseudo-exacerbation." UTI should be specifically sought when MS patients develop new or increased neurological symptoms, particularly in the setting of fever or malaise.[11]

Urinary symptoms may be age-related and follow a bimodal distribution. Patients under age 40 are most bothered by bladder storage and voiding symptoms, although these findings may be related to the inherent expectations of younger patients as compared with their older counterparts. Patients over the age of 50 are also greatly bothered by bladder symptoms, which may be related to their longer duration of disease or the cumulative effect of other causes of bladder dysfunction, such as benign

Table 58.1. *Medications with urologic adverse effects*

Medicine	Mechanism	Potential adverse effect
Tricyclic antidepressants	Anticholinergic	Urine retention
Oxybutynin	Anticholinergic	Urine retention
Tolteridine	Antimuscarinic	Urine retention
Doxazocin, terazocin	a adrenergic antagonists	Incontinence
Cyclophosphamide	Chemotherapy	Bladder cancer, delayed
Corticosteroids	Immunomodulatory	Increased risk of urinary tract infection

prostatic hyperplasia (BPH) in men or genuine stress incontinence in women.[39] Although increasing duration of disease is linked to increased frequency of overall symptoms, no one urological symptom is more prevalent in patients with long-standing disease. No significant relationship has been found between the incidence of overall symptoms and gender. However, men with MS report a higher incidence of obstructive symptoms compared to women, which may be linked to age-related changes in the prostate or the severity of DSD in males.[5] As a result of LUTD and urinary stasis, patients may develop bladder calculi, renal calculi, and frequent UTIs, often involving atypical organisms.[40]

Evaluation of voiding dysfunction

History

The history of having MS itself should raise the issue of urological dysfunction, particularly in view of the often asymptomatic nature of voiding dysfunction. Patients with more severe MS, longer duration of disease, and significant physical disability should be evaluated fully for bladder symptoms. Patient should be asked questions about frequency, nocturia, urgency, urge or stress incontinence, hesitancy, and ease of micturition. The use of protective devices (e.g. pads) should be determined. There are incontinence-specific quality of life measures available to assess the overall daily impact of these urinary symptoms.[41–43] A United Kingdom consensus panel recommended the assessment of all patients with MS who complain of lower urinary tract symptoms by a suitably trained health care professional.[44]

Patients with MS often self-manage bladder symptoms by reducing daily fluid intake. This potentially could cause hyperconcentration of urine leading to more irritative symptoms. A fluid intake and voiding diary may be useful. Current and past medicines should be evaluated as many medications used in MS have urologic adverse effects (Table 58.1).

Surgical history is also important. A history of gynecological procedures, perineal region surgery, multiple births, rectocele, cystocele, vaginal prolapse, or prior stress incontinence may raise the suspicion of concurrent anatomical factors affecting continence. Chronic constipation may affect urological function both from mechanical compression and sacral nerve feedback.

Physical examination

The general physical exam may be of assistance in the assessment for urological dysfunction. Abdominal and perineal examination is useful to note prior urological, gynecological, or major abdominal surgery. Rectal tone should be assessed as well as bulbocavernosus reflex (S2–4) as these may indicate sacral reflex dysfunction. Assessment for fecal impaction and (in men) prostate hypertrophy may also be helpful. In women the vaginal examination is helpful in assessing coexisting vaginal pathology such as cystocele, rectocele, atrophic vaginitis, etc. Patients managed with an indwelling catheter may have specific issues of urethral erosion.

Neurological examination should be generalized, but also focused on L1-S4 cord segments. Thus, deep tendon reflex examination in the legs (patellar L4, hamstring L5, and Achilles S1), and dermatomal sensory exam (L1 groin, L2 upper anterior thigh, L3 knee, L4 medial shin, L5 dorsal foot, S1 lateral foot, S2 upper posterior thigh, S3–5 perianal sensation and groin) should be performed. The plantar response reflects pyramidal tract integrity. The cremasteric reflex in males assesses L1 root integrity. Internuclear ophthalmoplegia[21] and sensory loss in lower extremities, particularly vibration sensation loss,[45] correlate with bladder dysfunction. Upper extremity examination for strength, coordination, and sensation is important if patients will need to perform procedures such as self-catheterization.

Urinalysis

Urinalysis is an integral part of the urological evaluation. In most instances, a multicomponent dip-stick suffices for screening. The method of collection is of prime importance, as many patients are treated inappropriately because of a falsely contaminated specimen. Theoretically, a suprapubic aspiration is the best method as it avoids contamination by urethral commensal organisms.[46] However, this is clinically difficult and impractical due to the invasive nature of this test. Straight catheter technique is the next best but still has cost, comfort, and practical issues that preclude its use in uncomplicated situations.[46] Urine should be collected as a mid-stream, clean-catch specimen. However, because of spasticity or obesity, many patients are unable to provide an uncontaminated specimen. In these instances, or in patients with repeated infections, sterile catheterization provides the most reliable way to ensure proper specimen collection. The urine should be transported as rapidly as possible to reduce false-positives.[47]

Leukocyte esterase and nitrite are good screening tests for UTI. Leukocyte esterase is based on hydrolysis of ester substrates by proteins with esterolytic activity. Human neutrophils produce many proteins with these activities.[46] These react with esters to produce alcohols and acids which show a color change

proportional to the amount of esterase. False-positives for these tests include presence of vaginal fluid, and when there is Trichomonas or eosinophils in urine.[48] The nitrite test is based on biochemical reactions associated with the family *Enterobacteriaceae* which are the most common pathogens causing UTIs. The usefulness of the nitrite test is limited because nitrite production is not associated with *S. saprophyticus*, *Pseudomonas* species, or enterococci.[49] This test also requires that a first morning urine be tested as it requires four or more hours for bacteria to convert nitrate to nitrite at levels that are reliably detected. The sensitivity of these tests is fairly high; UTI is rare in the setting of negative results. Urine specific gravity is a useful test to determine the state of hydration, as many patients with MS restrict their fluids in an attempt to control incontinence and frequency. The presence of blood in the urine, although often seen with infection, is a worrisome sign, and raises suspicion of a bladder stone or tumor, especially in the patient who has had multiple courses of cyclophosphamide.

Post-void residual measurement

PVR using non-invasive suprapubic ultrasonography is a simple and easily obtainable office procedure. In one systematic review it was recommended that all MS patients, irrespective of urinary symptoms, should undergo a measure of PVR by this technique.[8] This approach addressed the group of patients with asymptomatic bladder dysfunction who might, otherwise, progress to more severe dysfunction. If PVR was negative, the authors suggested a simple survey after this initial evaluation assessing urinary symptoms. The UK consensus panel suggested a simple testing paradigm for patients with urgency and frequency,[44] consisting of testing for UTI with reagent strips for urinalysis, then measuring PVR. If >100 ml, the panel recommended teaching clean intermittent self-catheterization (CIC). If <100 ml, they recommended treatment with antimuscarinics and in both cases retesting after intervention.

Upper urinary tract imaging

Baseline radiographic assessment of the MS patient might be an important part of the initial urological evaluation useful but is rarely undertaken in the absence of symptoms. In a review of 14 series comprising 2076 patients, Koldewijn *et al.*[5] found the incidence of hydronephrosis or renal complication to be 0.34%. All seven affected patients had DSD. Progression to upper tract deterioration is unusual in MS[5,25,39,50–53] and linked to several risk factors: (1) DSD in the male and (2) the presence of an indwelling catheter (1.7%).[4,20,31] In these high-risk patients, a baseline renal sonogram is advisable, as it may diagnose clinically silent calculi, identify parenchymal scarring and provide comparison for longitudinal monitoring.

Lower urinary tract imaging

In the incontinent or otherwise symptomatic woman, an initial lateral voiding cystourethrogram or videourodynamics

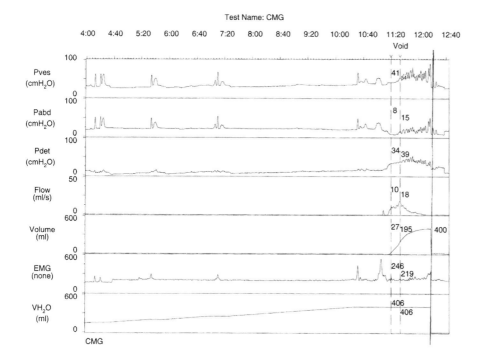

Fig. 58.1. Normal urodynamic tracing. Note how the bladder accommodates a large volume at a very low pressure. P_{ves} = total bladder pressure (vesical pressure, cm H_2O) and is a measured value from the dual lumen urethral catheter. P_{abd} = abdominal pressure (cm H_2O) and is measured value derived from a rectal catheter. P_{det} is calculated by subtracting ($P_{ves} - P_{abd}$) and represents the true detrusor pressure (cm H_2O) in the absence of abdominal effects. Flow = the rate of urinary flow (ml/second). V_{H2O} = the volume infused (ml). Volume = volume voided (ml). EMG = electromyographic muscle activity of the pelvic floor and external sphincter.

(urodynamic evaluation performed with concomitant fluoroscopic bladder imaging) may aid in the assessment of bladder neck support, urethral hypermobility, and bladder diverticuli. As patients in this age group may have competing symptomatologies, such as genuine stress incontinence and urge incontinence, this type of imaging may be beneficial in determining the relative contribution of anatomical factors (urethral hypermobility or cystocele) to voiding dysfunction or incontinence. Videourodynamics may also be of benefit in the more accurate determination of DSD. In the patient with no stress incontinence or with good pelvic floor support on physical examination, lower tract radiological imaging may not be necessary.

Urodynamic evaluation

Numerous studies have shown that the clinical symptoms of MS vesicourinary dysfunction are poorly correlated with specific urinary pathophysiology. This argues for the use of urodynamics (Fig. 58.1) to allows proper identification of any underlying bladder and sphincteric abnormalities and direct individualized management.[8] During this study, the bladder is filled via a small (5–7 French) multilumen catheter. Measurements of bladder pressure are continuously made during both filling and voiding. Concomitant rectal manometry is performed to correct for the effect of intra-abdominal contents on bladder pressure. Electromyography (EMG) monitoring of the external sphincter is performed during the study to assess bladder and sphincteric coordination.

Numerous series of urodynamic findings in MS have been published (Table 58.2). Blaivas *et al.*[18] found that 73% of MS patients without urodynamic evaluation were treated inappropriately. Indeed, 73% of patients with symptoms suggestive of

obstruction were found to have detrusor areflexia. In equivocal cases, urodynamic evaluation may lend support to a suspected diagnosis of MS in 10%–14% of patients.[2,21,39] Within the MS patient population, the incidence of abnormal urodynamic findings is as high as 100% in some series.[4] In a meta-analysis of 22 series and 1882 patients, the incidence of normal urodynamic findings was only 9%. However, because most published series deal with symptomatic patients referred specifically for urological evaluation, there has been a significant reporting bias toward patients with advanced disease and pyramidal dysfunction. To date, there are few prospective studies dealing with asymptomatic bladder dysfunction. In one prospective study, 52% of patients (21/40) demonstrated silent urodynamic abnormalities. The incidence of positive urodynamic findings in patients with lower urinary tract complaints was 98%.[31] Once a urodynamic diagnosis is rendered, therapy may be tailored to each patient's storage and emptying function, thereby eliminating a trial and error method of management.

Detrusor hyperreflexia (also known as neurogenic detrusor hyperactivity) is defined as bladder over activity due a disturbance of nervous control mechanisms, and is the most commonly encountered urodynamic abnormality seen in MS (Fig. 58.2). The incidence of DH varies directly with the level of the neurological lesion.[32] That is, patients with a higher predominance of cervical plaques have a higher incidence of DH. In 22 published series evaluating primarily symptomatic MS patients, 62% of patients (1194 of 1882) were found to have DH as their primary urodynamic diagnosis. This is not surprising, given the high incidence of cervical and intracranial plaques in MS.[18,27,28,39] Commonly, DH is manifested as urgency, frequency, and generalized irritative symptoms. Among patients

Table 58.2. *Published series of urodynamic findings in multiple sclerosis*

Series	Sample Size	DH n (%)	DSD n (%)	Hyporeflexia n (%)	Normal n (%)
Andersen[3]	52	33 (63)	16 (31)	21 (40)	2 (4)
Awad[23]	57	38 (66)	30 (52)	12 (21)	7 (12)
Beck[54]	46	40 (87)	–	6 (13)	–
Betts[21]	70	63 (90)	–	0	7 (10)
Blaivas[16]	41	23 (56)	12 (30)	16 (40)	2 (4)
Bradley[55]	99	58 (60)	20 (20)	40 (40)	1 (1)
Bradley[4]	302	127 (62)	–	103 (34)	10 (24)
Eardley[29]	24	15 (63)	6 (25)	3 (13)	6 (25)
Goldstein[2]	86	65 (76)	57 (66)	16 (19)	5 (6)
Gonor[56]	64	40 (78)	8 (12)	13 (20)	1 (2)
Hinson[25]	70	44 (63)	15 (21)	20 (28)	6 (9)
Koldwijn[5]	212	72 (34)	27 (13)	32 (8)	76 (36)
Mayo[22]	89	69 (78)	5 (6)	5 (6)	11 (12)
McGuire[20]	46	33 (72)	21 (46)	13 (28)	0
Peterson[57]	88	73 (83)	36 (41)	14 (16)	1 (1)
Philip[24]	52	51 (99)	16 (37)	0	1 (2)
Piazza[58]	31	23 (74)	9 (47)	2 (6)	3 (9)
Schoenberg[59]	39	27 (69)	20 (5)	2 (6)	6 (15)
Sirls[60]	113	79 (70)	15 (28)	17 (15)	7 (6)
Summers[61]	50	26 (52)	6 (12)	6 (12)	9 (18)
Van Poppel[40]	160	105 (66)	38 (24)	38 (24)	16 (10)
Weinstein[62]	91	64 (70)	16 (18)	15 (16)	11 (12)
Total	1882	1194 (62)	373/1464 (25)	394 (20)	188 (10)

DH = detrusor hyperreflexia, DSD = detrusor sphincter dyssynergia.

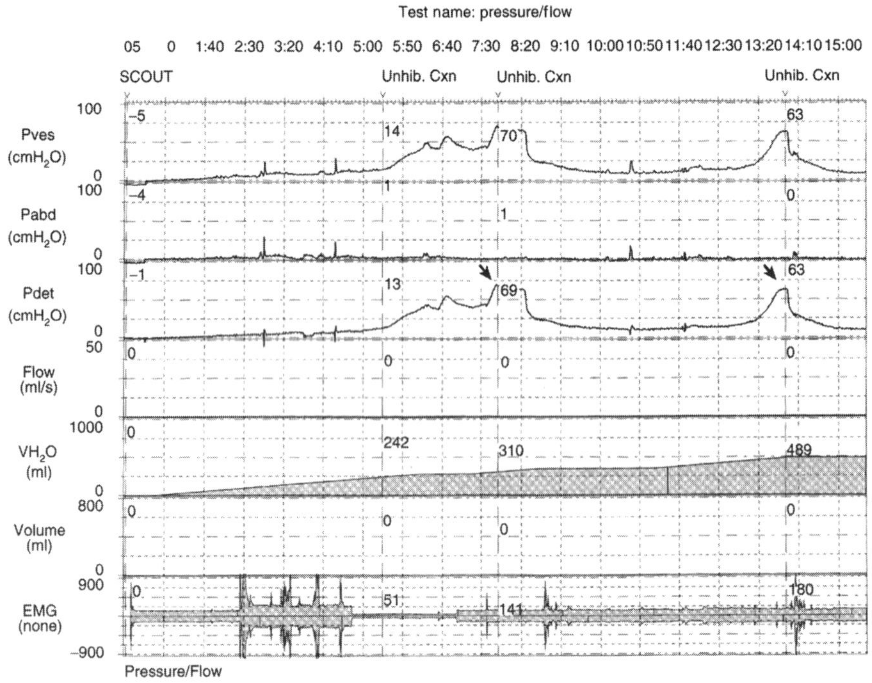

Fig. 58.2. Detrusor Hyperreflexia in a 50-year-old woman with MS and severe urinary urgency. Note the rise in bladder pressure and detrusor pressure in the absence of abdominal pressure. The sphincter is quiet during these contractions, denoting the absence of detrusor sphincter dyssynergia. This patient was effectively treated with oral anticholinergic medication.

(a)

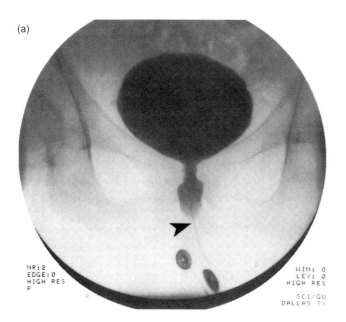

Fig. 58.3. Detrusor sphincter dyssynergia (DSD). This cystourethrogram (a) demonstrates DSD in a 40-year-old man with relapsing remitting MS who presented with poor bladder emptying. Note the columnation of the radiographic contrast down to the external sphincter (arrowhead). The two round densities at the bottom of the screen are electromyograph leads. In the accompanying urodynamic tracing (b), sphincter activity increases dramatically and is accompanied by attempted voiding at a detrusor pressure of over 45 cm H_2O. Note the virtual absence of flow and near complete retention.

(b)

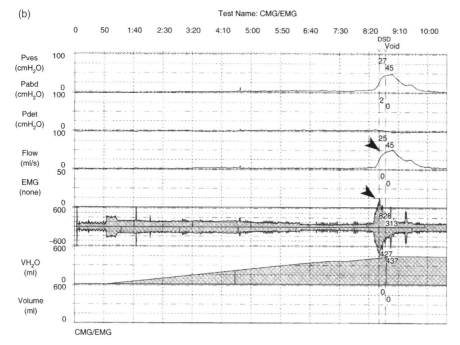

with DH, 67% display synergic voiding, and 43% display DSD.[63] Patients in the latter group may suffer from both storage and emptying failure, complicating their management.

Detrusor hypocontractility can be seen in up to 63% of patients with or without associated hyperreflexia. True areflexia is only seen in 20% of patients, and may be associated with hesitancy and elevated PVR. Hypocontractility may be related to cerebellar plaque involvement, lack of cortical facilitory input, or sacral cord involvement,[4,21,29] Some evidence suggests that areflexia is a temporary condition that progresses to hyperreflexia in 57%–100% of patients.[2,57]

Urethral dysfunction, ISR, and DSD represent a continuum, which may be seen in 12%–84% (mean 25.4%) of patients

(Fig. 58.3)[18,21,29] Consequently, a variety of clinical effects may be seen, including hesitancy, retention, or incontinence. DSD is correlated with cervical plaques as well as with increased levels of cerebrospinal fluid myelin basic protein.[2,5,32] Most commonly, DSD presents with incomplete emptying and stranguria (straining to urinate), symptoms also seen with hypocontractility. DSD is the most extreme defect in this continuum and is seen when a detrusor voiding contraction is accompanied by concomitant internal or external sphincter contraction.[18] In sharp contrast to the dyssynergia seen in spinal cord injury patients, DSD seen in the MS population is rarely associated with upper tract dysfunction, but rather with local symptoms of incomplete emptying, elevated PVR, bladder calculi, and infection.[5,18,29,51,54,56] This may be due to the fact that despite the presence of DSD, voiding detrusor pressures are usually not significantly elevated above normal levels.[64] Alternatively, the degrees of DH and external sphincter spasm seen in MS may be less severe than that seen in spinal cord injury.[29,56,57]

Although the diagnosis of DSD is most commonly made by EMG, the optimal criteria for the diagnosis of DSD are unclear, including utility of urethral versus anal EMG, wire or patch electrodes, urethral pressure gradients and videourodynamic urethral assessment.[18,19,56–62,65] The necessity for sphincteric assessment and diagnosis of DSD has been questioned.[18,20,31,32] Sirls et al.[39] found sphincteric evaluation by EMG unhelpful in the management of 15 patients with DSD. ISR is similar to DSD but of lesser magnitude and less commonly associated with lower urinary tract complications. Rather, ISR may be manifested by a weak force of stream or stranguria. Sphincteric paralysis (flaccidity) is seen in less than 15% of patients and may manifest as sphincteric incontinence.[3]

Stability of urodynamic findings. As MS is a dynamic disease characterized by exacerbations, remissions, and progression, changes in lower urinary tract function over time and in response to therapy can occur. In studies of selected patients, 15%–55% of patients demonstrate changes on repeat urodynamic testing.[55] Of note, once DSD is observed on urodynamic evaluation, it rarely resolves.[18,55] However, there have been few longitudinal studies following individual MS patients over time with or without disease treatment or evaluating the natural progression of urological findings in patients who are mildly symptomatic or asymptomatic.

Management of urinary symptoms in MS patients

In low-risk patients (those without indwelling catheters or DSD), there is a low incidence of renal complications and upper tract deterioration,[5,23,39,45] supporting a conservative approach to upper tract management. Routine upper tract monitoring should be considered in high-risk patients, patients with changing urological symptoms, or those with progression of disease.[21,25,39,66] Aggressive surgical management for mild hydronephrosis, as practiced in the past, has largely been replaced by CIC.[50,67] Although pyelonephritis is rare, its treatment may be complicated by atypical organisms (34% *Pseudomonas* spp., 31% *Proteus* spp., 25% *Providencia* spp.).[40]

Treatment decisions should take into account the patient's level of disability, ability to function independently, manual dexterity, competing medical problems, and social support networks. A team approach involving the patient's treating neurologist, urologist, and rehabilitation specialist is essential to optimize patient care. An empirical trial and error method is discouraged, as it may be time consuming and costly, and leave many patients improperly treated and at risk for potential complications.[18,31] Rather, an accurate understanding of each patient's underlying pathology should be established based on objective parameters such as flow rate, residual urine and urodynamic evaluation. For treatment purposes, patients may be separated into those with storage problems, emptying problems, or both. In most patients, conservative measures are an effective means of primary management (Table 58.3).

Conservative therapy for failure to store urine

Symptoms arising from storage disorders (frequency, urgency, nocturia, and incontinence) are the most common cause for urological consultation. As nearly two-thirds of patients suffer from DH, treatment usually involves pharmacological therapy to suppress uninhibited bladder contractions. Traditionally, the use of atropine-like drugs which competitively bind the acetylcholine receptor, thereby blocking muscarinic effects, represented the cornerstone of treatment. A variety of drugs can be used.[35,68–76] Dosages of these drugs are titrated to therapeutic response or until anticholinergic side-effects become intolerable.[72] The use of imipramine in MS may be tempered by its α-agonistic properties, thus impairing bladder emptying in patients with DSD.[69] The concomitant use of other antidepressants in the MS population also limits the effective use of imipramine. When monotherapy fails to improve DH, medications with pure anticholinergic properties (propantheline) may be combined with those having additional direct smooth-muscle relaxant properties (oxybutynin, flavozate).[68,69,77–80] A recent Cochrane review of the use of anticholinergics for urinary symptoms found that there was not enough evidence to advocate the use of these medicines in MS.[81] This was primarily due to methodological deficiencies in studies in this specific disease and results in the three included trials which precluded conclusions about efficacy. Most of the evidence for use of the medicines comes from anecdote and extrapolation from studies of overactive bladder in mixed populations.[81]

Oxybutynin chloride (Ditropan™) is one of the most widely prescribed of these medications, and has shown fair to good response in 67%–80% of MS patients. Anticholinergic side effects (decreased salivation, blurred vision, and constipation) occur in 57%–94% of patients, and can have a significant effect on patient compliance. Attrition rates of up to 50% have been reported in long-term studies.[69–71] These side effects are especially troublesome in the MS population, as blurry vision may be mistaken for deterioration due to optic neuritis, and constipation is a frequent problem in MS patients.[72] The once-a-day preparation of this medication (Ditropan XL™) has similar efficacy to conventional oxybutynin but with a reduction of anticholinergic side effects and increased patient compliance. In one study, the twice-weekly oxybutynin transdermal (Oxytrol™) patch significantly improved quality of life in patients with hyperactive bladders.[82] By avoiding hepatic and gastrointestinal metabolism it undergoes less conversion to the active metabolite, *N*-desthyloxybutynin. This metabolite is thought to be responsible for some of the anticholinergic side effects. Phase 3 studies in overactive bladder demonstrated similar efficacy to the oral preparations, and a further decrease in

Table 58.3. *Pharmacotherapy for bladder dysfunction*

Drug	Drug class	How supplied	Typical dose	Key side effects
Detrusor hyperreflexia				
Hyoscyamine	Anticholinergic	SL ER	0.125 mg q 4 h 0.375 mg q 12 h	Dry mouth, blurred vision, constipation, dizziness, nausea, urinary retention
Oxybutinin	Anticholinergic	PO ER Intravesical Transdermal	2.5–5 mg q 8 h 5–30 mg q day 5–10 mg q 8–12 h 1 patch twice/week	
Tolterodine	Antimuscarinic	PO	2 mg q 12 h	
Solifenacin	Antimuscarinic	PO	5–10 mg q 24 h	
Darifenacin	Antimuscarinic	PO	7.5–15 mg q 24 h	
Trospium	Antimuscarinic	PO	20 mg q 12 h	
Imipramine	Tricyclic antidepressant	PO	25 mg q 8 h or 50 mg qhs	Anticholinergic side effects, orthostasis, drowsiness, asthenia, weakness
Nocturia				
DDAVP	Vasopressin analog	Intranasal PO	1–2 puffs qhs 0.05–0.2 mg q 12 h	Edema, hyponatremia, headache, weight gain
Sphincter dyssynergia				
Doxazocin	α_1 adrenergic antagonist	PO	4–12 mg qhs	Orthostatic hypotension, asthenia, incontinence
Terazocin	α_1 adrenergic antagonist	PO	8 mg q 8 h	
Tizanidine	α_2 adrenergic agonist	PO	4–8 mg q 6–8 h	Asthenia, weakness, somnolence, orthostatic hypotension

DDAVP = 1-desamino-8-D-vasopressin, ER = extended release, PO = oral, SL = sublingual.

the incidence of dry mouth. There was a small incidence of cutaneous reactions with patch application.[73,83,84]

The selective muscarinic receptor blockers tolterodine (Detrol™ and Detrol LA™) and trospium chloride (Sanctura™) also are moderately effective in controlling urgency and frequency, with a lower incidence of anticholinergic side effects.[76,85–89] Quality of life improved in a community based cohort of patients with overactive bladder syndrome using trospium.[90] Trospium is thought to have fewer CNS side effects because it is less lipid-soluble, but this also decreases its bioavailability when taken with food.[76] Two mucarinic (M3) subtype-specific receptor blockers are available: solifenacin succinate (VESIcare™) and darifenacin (Enablex™). M3 selectivity is the proposed mechanism for fewer CNS (M1-mediated) and cardiovascular (M2-mediated) side effects observed in initial trials.[74,83,89,91] Again, patient compliance is enhanced and side effects are lessened, thereby providing a more favorable drug treatment profile. Sativex was compared with placebo in a randomized controlled trial for DH in MS.[92] The study did not meet its primary end-point of reduced daily incontinence episodes but showed trends to improvement on other measures. At present, this is not approved for this indication. There are few head-to-head trials of the newer bladder medications.

In some patients, CIC can be combined with anticholinergic therapy, and may be especially beneficial in patients with both storage and emptying failure. In these patients, urinary retention is promoted by anticholinergics, thus alleviating storage problems, while emptying is accomplished by CIC.

In an attempt to avoid anticholinergic side effects from oral medications, intravesical administration of a variety of medications (verapamil, lidocaine, oxybutynin) has been tested for DH.[93–98] These agents are crushed, suspended, and instilled into the bladder via sterile catheterization. The most commonly used intravesical agent is oxybutynin. The therapeutic response to intravesical oxybutynin in MS patients has exceeded 86% in selected studies. However, the inconvenience of this route of administration has contributed to a high attrition rate, and has tempered enthusiasm for this treatment method.[99] Nevertheless, in a select group of patients already on CIC, intravesical oxybutynin may lead to a significant improvement in continence with fewer side effects.[99–105]

The intravesical medications, resiniferatoxin and capsaicin, also show promise. These compounds exert a selective action on C sensory fiber axons, which are thought to play an important role in bladder reflex pathways following spinal cord insult. When instilled intravesically, capsaicin exerts a neurotoxic effect on afferent C fiber axons, causing the depletion of substance P and calcitonin gene-related peptide.[106–113] In a study of 18 patients by Fowler *et al.*,[110] 61% of patients treated with capsaicin demonstrated excellent results and 17% demonstrated clinical improvement. The duration of patient response ranged from 3–6 months. Optimism for capsaicin has been tempered by its pain on instillation. Resiniferatoxin lacks these side-effects, and is 1000-fold more potent. Thus, it may represent a more attractive form of intravesical therapy. In studies evaluating the effect of resiniferatoxin, the mean bladder volume at initial urge was not affected, although total bladder capacity was increased by an average of 105 cm^3.[107] These preliminary results suggest a difference in the urodynamic effect between resiniferatoxin and capsaicin that merits further evaluation. As capsaicin and resiniferatoxin are not regulatory-approved drugs, their use at the present time is limited to investigational protocols.

DH (especially nocturia) can also be treated by decreasing urine production. In multiple placebo-controlled trials evaluating MS patients, DDAVP nasal spray (1-desamino-8-D-vasopressin) has shown significant efficacy in reducing the incidence of nocturia and enuresis, and increasing sleep time.[114–116] The use of DDAVP can be especially helpful in the management of patients with DH who cannot tolerate anticholinergic medication, or have concomitant emptying failure due to DSD or hypocontractility. In a Phase 1 trial, doses of 10–20 μg were found to provide a significant decrease in nocturnal urinary volumes, without hyponatremia.[115] Increased dosages to 60 μg were no more efficacious, and were accompanied by a trend toward lower serum sodium. Recently, DDAVP has become available in a tablet preparation, which is more convenient for some patients.

Botulinum toxin type A (Botox^{TM} or DYSPORT^{TM}) or type B (MyoBloc^{TM} or NeuroBloc^{TM}) injection into the detrusor muscle can be used to treat urinary incontinence secondary to DH. Botulinum toxin prevents presynaptic acetylcholine release at the neuromuscular junction, and thus limits synaptic transmission and muscle contraction. Studies of patients with neurological causes of DH have included small numbers of patients with spinal cord injury or meningomyelocele, and very few with MS.[117–118] These studies have shown an improvement in subjective measures, a decrease in the number of incontinence episodes and decreased detrusor pressure measurements. Injection effects typically last 3–9 months, and can be performed transurethrally or transperineally. A possible side effect of botulinum toxin includes detrusor paralysis and the need for CIC until effects subside. There have also been rare reports of distal weakness, flu-like illness, malaise, and dry mouth. Large randomized controlled trials are needed to determine who will best benefit from this more invasive treatment.

Recent work using percutaneous posterior tibial nerve stimulation in MS patients with neurogenic bladder dysfunction showed increased bladder capacity at first involuntary detrusor contraction. However, clinical and quality of life parameters were not measured to see if this effect was translated into a clinically meaningful outcome.[119]

Conservative therapy for emptying failure

In addition to DH, 42% of MS patients also suffer from emptying difficulties due to DSD, unsustained voiding contractions, or detrusor hypocontractility. In a select group of

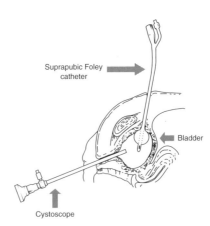

Fig. 58.4. Suprapubic tube placed percutaneously using cystoscope. From reference 124.

MS patients, timed voiding or double voiding may be sufficient for adequate emptying. However, in most patients, intervention is required to prevent infection, calculi, or overflow incontinence. Attempts to manage these patients conservatively with α_1 adrenergic blocking agents (prazosin, terazosin, doxazosin) and muscle relaxants (diazepam, baclofen, dantrolene) have had mixed results.[120–121] Anecdotal success has been reported with the use of tizanidine (Zanaflex^{TM}), a spasmolytic with centrally acting α_2 adrenergic properties. The use of α blockers and muscle relaxants in patients with emptying failure should be limited to patients with urodynamically proven DSD and not detrusor hypocontractility.

CIC is the primary means of management for patients with inadequate emptying, and has been shown possibly to aid in bladder rehabilitation.[122] Urodynamic evaluation may facilitate the decision for CIC by defining bladder storage capabilities and selecting the optimum catheterization interval. A randomized controlled trial of a multifaceted, individualized bladder rehabilitation program in patients with MS, found that treated patients scored better on a variety of measures of bladder disability after the treatment program.[123] This reinforces the benefit of a comprehensive program of bladder management in such patients.

Surgical management of bladder dysfunction

When a conservative approach fails in the management of LUTD, more aggressive surgical options may be entertained. A variety of factors should be considered, including degree of manual dexterity, social support systems, disability status, life expectancy of 20–50 additional years, and urodynamic parameters. Thus, short-term solutions may need to be dismissed in favor of a more comprehensive long-term approach. Surgical options include suprapubic cystostomy, sphincterotomy, sphincteric stents (Urolume^{TM}; American Medical Systems, Minnetonka, MN), augmentation cystoplasty (surgical enlargement using an intestinal patch) with or without a catheterizable limb, incontinent vesicostomy, supravesical diversion, and electrical stimulation techniques.[125–128]

Suprapubic cystostomy (Fig. 58.4) may be an attractive initial plan for patients who fail conservative management. It

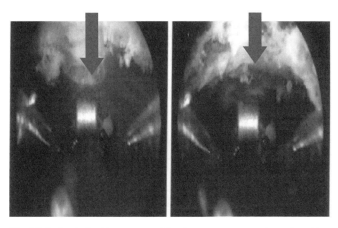

Fig. 58.5. Surgical sphincterotomy. The electroresectoscope is used to ablate the external sphincter at the 12:00 position.

has several distinct advantages over a conventional indwelling catheter. Urethral erosion, often seen in the patient with chronic Foley catheterization is avoided. Personal hygiene and catheter care are simplified, as the catheter position is readily accessible and remote from vaginal or perineal soilage. Commonly, the tube can be placed percutaneously under local anesthesia. This is often done in the operating room, especially for larger catheter sizes, and should be done in the operating room if there has been prior abdominal surgery. This therapeutic approach is reversible; the tube may be removed without difficulty, and the site will heal in 1–2 days. Suprapubic cystostomy may not be a good long-term option for younger patients because of the risk of bladder calculi, infection, and the development of squamous cell carcinoma.[129–131]

In the male patient with high detrusor pressers and outlet obstruction who cannot be managed by conservative measures, an outlet-reducing procedure such as a sphincterotomy (endoscopically cutting the external sphincter, Fig. 58.5) or urethral stent (Urolume, Fig. 58.6) may facilitate bladder emptying. With both, a condom catheter may be necessary to manage the resulting incontinence. These procedures are best reserved for patients with limited hand function, for whom CIC is not an option. The documentation of adequate detrusor contractility is imperative, as patients with hypocontractile bladders may carry an unacceptably high residual level even after the procedure.[127–128]

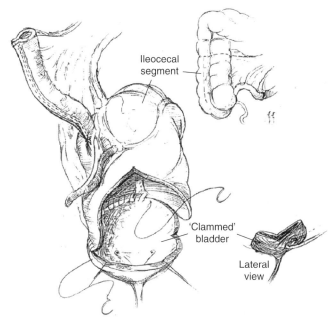

Fig. 58.7. Catheterizable augmentation cystoplasty using ileocecal segment. An ileocecal segment is used, not only to augment the existing bladder but to provide an alternate access to the bladder via a efferent stoma. This allows the patient to catheterize while sitting or fully clothed. From reference 132.

Surgical bladder augmentation for detrusor dysfunction is usually reserved for patients in whom all other conservative options have been exhausted. As the course of MS is by nature dynamic and progressive, permanent procedures using intestinal segments should be undertaken only after careful consideration of the current course of disease and overall prognosis. Patients undergoing augmentation cystoplasty should be assessed for manual dexterity, as most will continue to require some degree of CIC.[126] In most cases, surgical augmentation is combined with a catheterizable abdominal stoma, which allows easy catheterization especially in the chair-bound patient, the patient with lower-extremity spasticity or the patient with poor dexterity who cannot perform urethral catheterization (Fig. 58.7).

When neither the patient nor a family member nor caregiver can perform CIC, and conservative management has failed, cutaneous ileovesicostomy has been used quite successfully for both storage and emptying abnormalities in MS

(i)

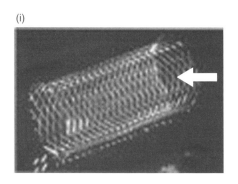

(ii)

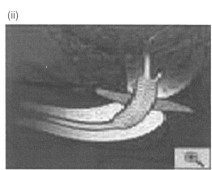

Fig. 58.6. Urolume prosthesis (American Medical Systems). Urolume bridging the external sphincter thereby preventing detrusor sphincter dyssynergia.

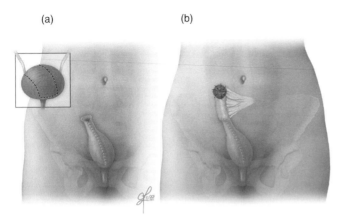

(a) (b)

Fig. 58.8. (a) and (b) Ileovesicostomy. The ileovesicostomy allows the bladder to be tubularized and brought toward the abdominal wall. As the bladder will rarely reach the skin on its own, an interposed segment of ileum is used to bridge this gap. The bladder is allowed to drain freely, and a relatively maintenance-free appliance is placed on the skin.

patients (Fig. 58.8). In this procedure, a segment of ileum is used to construct a chimney from the bladder to allow cutaneous drainage to an external collection device.[126] The advantages of this procedure over supravesical diversion are preservation of the bladder and ureterovesical junctions (if competent), lack of a defunctionalized bladder, and decreased blood loss. Although some patients are reluctant to proceed with major surgical intervention, often it improves quality of life and daily management of incontinence.

Electrical stimulation devices are used directly to stimulate the bladder, peripheral nerves, nerve roots, and the conus medullaris. Application ranges from the transcutaneous application of an electrical current to the surgical placement of internal electrical leads and generators. Techniques include intravesical electrostimulation, direct bladder stimulation, transvaginal stimulation, selective pudendal nerve stimulation, transcutaneous electrical nerve stimulation, stimulation of the sacral spine and roots (Medtronic InterStim™), sacral anterior root stimulation after dorsal rhizotomy, electrical stimulation of the thigh muscle and electrical stimulation of the tibial nerve.[125,133,134] There are no long-term data regarding the use of any of these techniques in MS patients. In addition, outcome data for electrical stimulation have not used standardized patient characteristics or outcome measures. Long-term randomized studies are needed to evaluate better the utility of the multiple available electrical stimulation modalities and to determine the most efficacious technique in MS. The benefits of implantable bladder stimulators must also be weighed against inability to obtain future MRIs to follow the disease.

Surgical management of urethral incompetence

The treatment of urethral incompetence includes the use of injectable bulking agents (collagen, fat, polytetrafluoroethylene, calcium hydoxyylapatite (Coaptite™ Boston Scientific),

urethral inserts, conventional bladder-suspension procedures and compressive slings.[135,136] In women with urethral incompetence or destruction due to indwelling catheterization, transvaginal bladder-neck closure and suprapubic drainage may serve as a minimally invasive way to deal with intractable incontinence. Surgical intervention for urethral insufficiency should consider a variety of factors such as voiding efficiency, ability to perform CIC, stability of disease and general overall health. Patients should be informed of the risk of post-surgical urinary retention, which may adversely affect the amount of nursing care required and their quality of life. The artificial urinary sphincter has had a limited role in the management of incontinence in MS. This is primarily due to the significant incidence of DH in MS and its association with upper tract deterioration in patients undergoing artificial urinary sphincter placement.[137] Before any outlet-enhancing procedure is performed, adequate bladder storage and voiding function should be confirmed, as patients with poorly sustained voiding contractions are at risk for on the skin postoperative urinary retention.

Sexual dysfunction

As MS affects young adults, sexual dysfunction may become an important factor in determining quality of life. MS adversely affects sexual functioning in up to 91% of males and 72% of females. In 64% of males and 39% of females, sexual activity ceases, or is unsatisfactory,[6,138–148] Foley and Iverson[149] proposed a model for sexual issues in MS which include primary, secondary, and tertiary sexual dysfunction. Primary sexual dysfunction refers to symptoms directly due to CNS lesions of MS. This may include altered genital sensation, problems with arousal and orgasm, decreased libido, decreased vaginal lubrication, and difficulties with erections. Secondary sexual dysfunction stems from non-sexual physiological changes that can impair sexual responses. This includes typical MS symptoms such as fatigue, spasticity, bladder/bowel problems, tremor, and pain. Tertiary sexual dysfunction refers to psychosocial, emotional and cultural issues that can interfere with sexual functioning e.g. depression, role changes, negative self image, or communication difficulties.[150] For example, Mattson et al.[142] found associated marital relationship problems in 71% of MS patients, with complaints of primary sexual dysfunction. The frequency of primary sexual dysfunction varies between types of MS. Primary sexual dysfunction was present 77% of patients with relapsing–remitting MS, 77% of secondary progressive patients, and 100% with primary progressive.[150] The frequency and extent of symptoms of sexual dysfunction in MS patients increase over time.[150]

Imaging studies have correlated sexual dysfunction with parietal lesions, increased lateral ventricle size, and total lesion burden. Two studies totaling 94 MS patients found that sexual dysfunction was specifically correlated with pontine atrophy and overall lesion burden.[151,152] Neither study found whole-brain or frontal-lobe atrophy or lesion load to be predictors of sexual dysfunction. In 31 of these patients, cervical spine MRI measures, urodynamic properties and cortical evoked potentials were also determined, and did not correlate with sexual dysfunction.[151,152] Neither of these studies included imaging of the spine below the cervical level and, therefore, could not exclude the role of more caudal cord lesions. Larger imaging studies are needed to define the anatomic correlates of sexual function in MS.

Male sexual dysfunction

Men with MS report a variety of sexual symptoms, including erectile dysfunction, decreased sensation, fatigue, and decreased libido resulting in orgasmic dysfunction.[138] The onset of erectile dysfunction typically occurs 3.7–9 years after diagnosis.[139,140] Yet, despite impotence rates as high as 80%, more than 75% of patients report a continued interest in sexual activity.[135] In some studies, sexual dysfunction parallels the level of overall disability.[136,137] However, other studies demonstrated erectile dysfunction to be independent of disability, and more closely related to bladder and pyramidal dysfunction alone.[141,142] In a study by Betts *et al.*,[140] 100% of 48 patients with erectile dysfunction were found to have concomitant bladder dysfunction. However, the absence of bladder or pyramidal dysfunction does not ensure adequate sexual function, as up to 50% of patients without pyramidal symptoms suffer from sexual impairment.[138]

Several authors have studied the physiological basis of erectile dysfunction using pudendal reflex latencies and tibial, pudendal, and cortical evoked potentials. These studies have shown consistent deficits in cortical and pudendal evoked potentials, without consistent changes in sacral reflex latencies (bulbocavernosis).[18] Thus, it is thought that MS-related impotence is related to suprasacral mechanisms. Abnormal pudendal evoked potentials are also predictive of ejaculatory dysfunction.[142] In addition to neurophysiological abnormalities, nocturnal penile tumescence studies demonstrated a significant psychogenic component in over 50% of patients.[143]

Evaluation of male sexual dysfunction

The evaluation of sexual dysfunction should begin with a thorough sexual and urological history. Patients should be questioned about a variety of topics (see the "Appendix"). A number of patients complain of decreased libido. However, close questioning may discriminate patients who have a physiologically decreased desire for sex from those in whom MS has made sexual activity an anxiety-laden burden. If morning erectile activity is normal, it confirms erectile integrity. Erections which spontaneously detumesce may indicate a venous leak or steal phenomenon. Spasticity and fatigue are often severely limiting factors for sexual activity, and can play a role in both patient positioning and desire for sex. The presence of an understanding stable partner cannot be overestimated, making it preferable to have them present for this portion of the office visit. Physiological evaluation for erectile dysfunction has centered around the use of penile Doppler flow evaluation and nocturnal penile tumescence monitoring. Although these are helpful in selected patients, many physicians have used a more practical approach for a number of reasons. These tests are expensive, and carry a variable degree of false-positives and negatives. They may not accurately reproduce what happens in a patient's sexual encounter at home. Finally, the options for management are often not altered by the results of the testing. The one clear benefit to these tests is their ability to discern psychogenic impotence from physiological dysfunction.

Treatment options for male sexual dysfunction

Treatment options are summarized in Table 58.4 and Fig. 58.9. Treatment decisions should take into account a variety of factors, including degree of manual dexterity, stability of the patient's current relationship, degree of disability, and course of disease. The approach to treatment should be one involving the neurologist, rehabilitation physician, and urologist. An initial course of sexual counseling may aid in the treatment of any psychological factors and also help to develop a better understanding between partners, thereby promoting intimacy. There are few studies involving impotence treatment specifically in the MS patient, and much of what is known is extrapolated from general studies involving neurogenic impotence.[128,129] Although the possibility for recovery of erectile activity is low (2%), non-surgical options, such as oral agents, vacuum erection devices, and intracorporal injection therapy (prostaglandin E_1 or papaverine), play a more prominent role than prosthetic implantation, as most patients are reluctant to undergo surgery for impotence.[145]

Oral therapy for impotence, although receiving a recent increase in popularity, is not a new concept. Probably the oldest oral treatment option available is yohimbine, which first saw clinical use in the 1950s. Since that time, a number of clinical studies have produced varied results. In a meta-analysis by Ernst and Pittler,[153] yohimbine was found to be slightly superior to placebo (odds ratio 3.85, 95% confidence interval 2.2–6.7). Side effects include anxiety (18%), headache (13%), urinary frequency (32%) and vertigo (14%).[154,155] The American Urological Association's guidelines panel on erectile dysfunction recommended that yohimbine should not be used as treatment for organic erectile dysfunction.[134] The use of yohimbine in MS patients has never been tested. With the recent advent of newer oral therapy for erectile dysfunction, most patients will elect to pursue this option first.

There are currently three oral phosphodiesterase-5 inhibitors available for erectile dysfunction. These include sildenafil (Viagra^{TM}), vardenafil (Levitra^{TM}), and tadalafil (Cialis^{TM}).[156–159] All of these agents require psychological or tactile stimulation to achieve affect. A placebo-controlled study of oral sildenafil in men with MS reported an 89% improvement

Table 58.4. *Treatment options for sexual dysfunction*

Option	Gender	Cost	Insurance coverage	Pros	Cons
Sexual counseling	M/F	$50–100/hr	No	Promotes a healthy relationship, helps partner, fosters intimacy.	None.
Vibratory stimulation	M/F	$25–350	No	Inexpensive.	None.
Yohimbine	M	$100/month		Natural, spontaneous.	Poor efficacy in organic erectile dysfunction.
Sildenafil	M/??F	~$10/dose	Sometimes	Spontaneous, convenient.	Cost, contraindication in patients taking nitrates or with cardiac issues, may need vibratory assistance.
Vardenafil	M/??F	~$10/dose	Sometimes	Spontaneous, convenient.	Cost, contraindication in patients taking nitrates or with cardiac issues, may need vibratory assistance.
Tadalafil	M/??F	~$10/dose	Sometimes	Spontaneous, convenient, long half-life.	Cost, contraindication in patients taking nitrates or with cardiac issues, may need vibratory assistance.
Vacuum erection devices	M	~$300/unit	Usually	One-time cost, safe.	Penis may feel cool and may look blue, less spontaneous, may need partner assistance.
Injection pharmacotherapy	M	$10–20/dose	Usually	Provides a reliable, firm erection	Penile fibrosis, priapism, pain, may need partner assistance, high attrition rate (50–80%).
Penile prosthesis	M	~$10,000	Usually	High patient and partner satisfaction, reliable	Risk of infection or mechanical failure, may require partner assistance, precludes reversion to other therapies.

F = female, M = male.

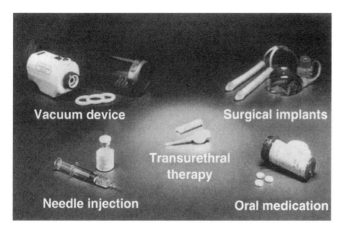

Fig. 58.9. Examples of treatment for erectile dysfunction.

in erectile function (vs. 24% with placebo) and improved quality of life scores.[160] Studies in the spinal cord injury population have also shown a nearly 70% success rate when sildenafil is used in combination with vibratory stimulation.[161] Sildenafil (50–100 mg) and vardenafil (2.5–20 mg) are taken one hour prior to intercourse. Tadalafil (5–20 mg) has a longer half-life (greater than 17 hours), and its effect can last up to 36 hours. This increases the window of opportunity for spontaneous sexual activity.[159] In 2008, Tadalafil was approved by the US Food and Drug Administration to be used for once daily dosing at dosage 2.5 mg.[162] This allows greater spontaneity and potentially less side effects for patients. Caution should

be exercised with the use of phosphodiesterase-5 inhibitors as there are a number of potential drug interactions (macrolide antibiotics, antihypertensive agents, cimetidine, and oral antifungal agents). Their use in patients with known cardiac disease or on topical or oral nitrate therapy is contraindicated. Side effects are similar with all three agents, and are usually limited to headache (most common), nasal congestion, flushing, and dyspepsia.[156,157,159,160]

Although studies in men with MS are lacking, vibratory stimulation may be utilized as an adjunct to virtually any type of erectile therapy, and has been well studied in the spinal cord injury population.[163] Vibratory stimulation may enhance erections, and may be used to decrease the orgasmic threshold for both men and women.

Vacuum erection devices (Fig. 58.10) have been used successfully in a variety of patients with erectile dysfunction, including in MS.[164] When using this form of therapy, a plastic tube is placed over the penis, and a pump is used to create a vacuum, drawing blood into the penis. A silicone or latex ring is then slipped over the base of the penis to maintain the erection. Although results in some studies are promising, the attrition rate may be high in improperly selected patients. Many patients feel that the use of vacuum erection devices makes their penis feel cold, is painful, and is less natural than other options. Patients may require partner assistance in operating the device, as some degree of dexterity is needed. Vacuum erection devices are, however, relatively inexpensive and have few associated risks.

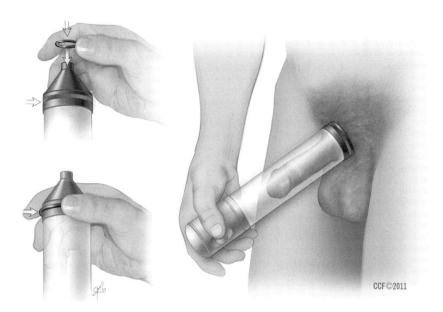

Fig. 58.10. The vacuum erection device. When using a vacuum erection device, a constriction ring is first placed on the base of the vacuum tube. The tube is then placed over the penis and the manual or battery operated vacuum pump is activated, drawing blood into the penis. The elastic ring (arrow) is then slipped off the tube to constrict the base of the penis and prevent egress of blood. After intercourse, the constriction ring is removed allowing detumescence.

CCF©2011

The introduction of vasoactive substances into the penis has been in use for nearly 20 years, and may take one of two forms, intraurethral suppositories (prostaglandin E_1) and injected suspensions (prostaglandin E_1 or papavarine). These medications, although fairly reliable, carry with them a risk of pain, priapism (a painful prolonged erection accompanied by corporal hypoxia), and chronic penile fibrosis (0.5%).[165] Despite a better than over 95% initial success rate with injection therapy, the attrition rate at two years in MS patients is 39%–80%.[166,167]

Penile prostheses in MS patients have been used for over 20 years,[165–168] and may take one of two forms, inflatable and semi-rigid or malleable prostheses. Although the inflatable prosthesis provides a more natural esthetic erection, it requires manual dexterity by either the patient or partner to activate its use. Infection rates range from 1.2%–1.8%, and the need for revision ranges from 4.5%–7.7%.[168–170] A five-year comparison was made of patients undergoing penile prosthesis with those undergoing injection therapy. Patients undergoing prosthesis insertion had sex twice as often as patients who used injection therapy. There were also significantly higher patient (77% vs. 70%) and partner satisfaction rates (88% vs. 67%) with prostheses.[171]

Female sexual dysfunction

Although the majority of women with MS wish to remain sexually active, sexual dysfunction is a significant problem for 56%–72%.[138,139,172,173] The most common reasons include fatigue (68%), decreased sensation (48%), decreased or absent orgasm (72%), difficulty with arousal (35%), and frequent UTIs (21%). Fatigue is a symptom of secondary sexual dysfunction that is

more significantly common in women than in men.[150] Vaginal dryness also is a frequently reported complaint, and may be exacerbated by anticholinergic medications.

Evaluation of female sexual dysfunction

The evaluation of the female MS patient with sexual dysfunction should begin with a thorough sexual history. It is important to remember to discuss sexual dysfunction early, even with the newly diagnosed MS patient, as 35% of these patients may have sexual dysfunction.[174] Patients should be questioned about their sexual activity and sexual satisfaction before MS, as well as present symptoms and their current methods of coping. As the sexual response in the female is less dependent on the mechanics of erection or sexual performance and more dependent on the relationship dynamics, therefore sufficient time should be spent discussing the ways that patients and partners relate both sexually and non-sexually. Often, a helpful way to assess the female sexual response is with the use of a validated questionnaire.[173] This may allow the practitioner to appreciate better physiological and psychosocial factors involved in the sexual response. A complete medication history is of prime importance, as a number of drugs (especially serotonin reuptake inhibitors) used in the MS population may have adverse effects on sexual functioning, especially libido and orgasm.

The physical examination of the female with sexual dysfunction remains an integral part of the overall evaluation. As sexual dysfunction may be closely associated with bladder dysfunction,[173] a careful vaginal and pelvic examination is important to rule out the coexistence of urogenital pathology such as cystocele, enterocele, rectocele, or urethral diverticulum. Perineal and perianal sensation should also be assessed as decreased sensation may be reported by up to half of patients.[172]

The laboratory evaluation of these patients is limited. Although normal values for testosterone have been established in healthy females, the use of testosterone as an adjunct to diagnosis and treatment of sexual dysfunction is not established and remains unsupported.

Treatment options for female sexual dysfunction

Treatment for female sexual dysfunction may take many forms (Table 58.4). First and foremost, is to ensure the presence of a loving and supportive partner. In nearly all relationships, sexual dysfunction can be a major stressor. For that reason, sexual counseling by a registered therapist can prove invaluable. Symptomatic treatment is also of great benefit. Vaginal dryness can be effectively treated with water-soluble vaginal moisturizers or lubricants. For patients with orgasmic dysfunction, vibratory stimuli may aid in decreasing the orgasmic threshold. In patients with decreased mobility, sexual positioning may be altered to aid in patient comfort. Involvement of the patient's neurologist and careful attention to overall systemic treatment can alleviate many somatic symptoms related to sexual dysfunction (such as fatigue and spasticity).

Historically, oral or parenteral testosterone has been used in an effort to improve libido and sexual response. However, the female sex drive is not testosterone dependent, and few patients benefit from this type of therapy. Testosterone supplementation also is not without risk and side effects. Patients may note mood swings and the growth of facial or body hair. Systemic complications of testosterone therapy include hepatic or renal damage, increased risk for stroke and suppression of the hypothalamic axis. In the majority of cases, loss of libido is more closely related to frustration and feelings of hopelessness over relationship issues and lack of sexual responsiveness than to physiologically decreased sexual desire.

Two small studies have looked at oral phosphodiesterase-5 inhibitors, specifically sildenafil, in women with neurological disease and sexual dysfunction.[176,177] The basis for phosphodiesterase-5 inhibitor use lies in the homologous nature of the male and female genitalia, and the presence of type 5 phosphodiesterase activity in the genital tissues of both sexes.[158] A single double-blind trial of 19 women with MS and sexual dysfunction[176] showed a statistically significant improvement only in the lubrication domain of sexual dysfunction. There was no change in quality of life. A study in 19 women with spinal cord injury and sexual dysfunction showed improved subjective arousal following sildenafil.[177] These studies provide the only data on the use of these medications in women with neurological diseases, and definitive conclusions cannot be drawn from these small numbers.

Conclusions

The majority of patients with MS will manifest lower urinary tract symptoms or sexual dysfunction at some point. Although these symptoms are rarely life threatening, they nonetheless have a significant impact on quality of life. Consequently, the neurologist may be called upon to assist in the care of these patients. To treat these problems effectively and intelligently, the neurologist must have a fundamental working knowledge of the disease process itself and its effects on the genitourinary system. Using this knowledge, a logical and individualized treatment plan can be formulated.

Appendix
Sexual questionnaire

Males and females

- How was your sexual functioning before multiple sclerosis? Please explain.
- How has multiple sclerosis changed your sexual functioning? Please explain.
- Describe your level of libido (desire for sex).
- Are you able to have orgasms? Do they occur sooner or later than you would like?
- How understanding is your partner of your sexual dysfunction? Are they willing to alter the way you have sex in order to make it more satisfying for you?
- Does fatigue or spasticity limit your sexual functioning? How?
- Do you have decreased genital sensation?

Males only

- Do you wake up with morning erections? How firm are they? Do you have erections with masturbation or oral sex?
- Are your erections, with stimulation, firm enough for penetration?
- Do you lose your erection soon after penetration?

Females only

- Is intercourse painful for you?
- Do you have a problem with vaginal dryness during intercourse?

References

1. Nakipoglu GF, Kaya AZ, Orhan G, *et al*. Urinary dysfunction in multiple sclerosis. *J Clin Neurosci* 2009;16:1321–4.

2. Goldstein I, Siroky MB, Sax DS, Krane RJ. Neurologic abnormalities in multiple sclerosis. *J Urol* 1982;128:541–5.

3. Andersen JT, Bradley WE. Abnormalities of detrusor and sphincter function in multiple sclerosis. *Br J Urol* 1976;43:193–8.

4. Bradley WE. Urinary bladder dysfunction in multiple sclerosis. *Neurology* 1978;29:52–8.

5. Koldewijn EL, Hommes OR, Lemmens WA, *et al.* Relationship between lower urinary tract abnormalities and disease-related parameters in multiple sclerosis. *J Urol* 1995;154:169–73.

6. Hennessey A, Robertson NP, Swingler R, Compston DA. Urinary, faecal and sexual dysfunction in patients with multiple sclerosis. *J Neurol* 1999;246:1027–32.

7. DasGupta R, Fowler CJ. Sexual and urological dysfunction in multiple sclerosis: better understanding and improved therapies. *Curr Opin Neurol* 2002;15:271–8.

8. De Seze M., Ruffion A, Denys P, *et al.* The neurogenic bladder in multiple sclerosis: review of the literature and proposal of management guidelines. *Mult Scler* 2007;13:915–28.

9. Nortvedt MW, Riise T, Frugaard J, *et al.* Prevalence of bladder, bowel and sexual problems among multiple sclerosis patients two to five years after diagnosis. *Mult Scler* 2007;13:106–12.

10. Brazis PW, Masdeu JC, Biller J. *Localization in Clinical Neurology.* Philadelphia: Lippincott, Williams and Wilkins, 2007.

11. Hockel M. Basic neuroanatomy and neurophysiology of the urethrovesical function with special reference to extended hysterectomy. *CME J Gynecologic Oncol* 2002;7:32–5.

12. Araki I, Matsui M, Ozawa K, Takeda M, Kuno S. Relationship of bladder dysfunction to lesion site in multiple sclerosis. *J Urol* 2003;169:1384–7.

13. Fog T. Topographic distribution of plaques in the spinal cord in multiple sclerosis. *Arch Neurol Psychol* 1950;63:382–414.

14. Oppenheimer DR. The cervical cord in multiple sclerosis. *Neuropathol Appl Neurobiol* 1978;4:151–62.

15. Nathan PW, Smith MC. The centrifugal pathway for micturition within the spinal cord. *J Neurol* 1958;21:177–89.

16. Blaivas JG, Barbalias GA. Detrusor external sphincter dyssynergia in men with multiple sclerosis: an ominous urologic condition. *J Urol* 1984;131:91–4.

17. Blaivas JG. The neurophysiology of micturition: a clinical study of 550 patients. *J Urol* 1982;127:958–63.

18. Blaivas JG, Bhimani G, Labib KB. Vesicourethral dysfunction in multiple sclerosis. *J Urol* 1979;122:342–7.

19. Siroky MB, Krane RJ. Neurologic aspects of detrusor-sphincter dyssynergia, with reference to the guarding reflex. *J Urol* 1982;127:953–7.

20. McGuire EJ, Savastano JA. Urodynamic findings and long term outcome management of patients with multiple sclerosis-induced lower urinary tract dysfunction. *J Urol* 1984;132:713–15.

21. Betts CD, D'Mellow MT, Fowler CJ. Urinary symptoms and the neurological features of bladder dysfunction in multiple sclerosis. *J Neurol Neurosurg Psych* 1993;56:245–50.

22. Mayo ME, Chetner MP. Lower urinary tract dysfunction in multiple sclerosis. *Urology* 1992;39:67–70.

23. Awad SA, Gajewski JB, Sogbein SK, *et al.* Relationship between neurologic and urologic status in patients with multiple sclerosis. *J Urol* 1984;139:499–502.

24. Philip T, Read DJ, Higson RH. The urodynamic characteristics of multiple sclerosis. *Br J Urol* 1981;53:672–5.

25. Hinson JL, Boone TB. Urodynamics and multiple sclerosis. *Urol Clin North Am* 1996;23:475–81.

26. Kruse MN, Mallory BS, Noto HL, *et al.* Modulation of the spinobulbospinal micturition reflex in cats. *Am J Physiol* 1992;262:478–84.

27. Kruse MN, Mallory BS, Noto H. Properties of the descending limb of the spinal-bulbospinal reflex pathway in the cat. *Brain Res* 1991;556:6–12.

28. Andersen JT, Bradley WF. Bladder and urethral innervation in multiple sclerosis. *Br J Urol* 1976;48:239–43.

29. Eardley I, Nagendran K, Lecky B, *et al.* Neurophysiology of the striated sphincter muscle in multiple sclerosis. *Br J Urol* 1991;68:81–8.

30. Chancellor MB, Anderson RU, Boone TB. Pharmacotherapy for neurogenic detrusor overactivity. *Am J Phys Med Rehabil* 2006;85:536–45.

31. Bemelmans BL, Hommes OR, Van Kerrebroeck PE, *et al.* Evidence for early lower urinary tract dysfunction in multiple sclerosis. *J Urol* 1991;145:1219–24.

32. Francis GS, Evans AC, Arnold DL. Neuroimaging in multiple sclerosis. *Neurol Clin* 1995;13:147–71.

33. Filippi M, Miller DH. Magnetic resonance imaging in the differential diagnosis and monitoring of the treatment of multiple sclerosis. *Curr Opin Neurol* 1996;9:178–86.

34. Kim YH, Goodman C, Omessi E, *et al.* The correlation of urodynamic findings with cranial magnetic resonance imaging findings in multiple sclerosis. *J Urol* 1998;159:972–6.

35. Pozzilli C, Grasso MG, Bastianello S, *et al.* Structural correlates of neurourologic abnormalities in multiple sclerosis. *Eur Neurol* 1992;32:228–30.

36. Stevens JC, Kinkel WR, Polachini I. Clinical correlation in 64 patients with multiple sclerosis. *J Neurol* 1986;43:1145–8.

37. Rao SM, Leo GJ, Haughton VM, *et al.* Correlation of magnetic resonance imaging with neuropsychological testing in multiple sclerosis. *Neurology* 1989;39:161–6.

38. Kragt JJ, Hoogervorst LJ, Uitdehaag MJ, Polman CH. Relation between objective and subjective measures of bladder dysfunction in multiple sclerosis. *Neurology* 2004;63:1716–18.

39. Sirls LT, Zimmern PE, Leach GE. Role of limited evaluation and aggressive medical management in multiple sclerosis: a review of 113 patients. *J Urol* 1994;151:946–50.

40. Van Poppel H, Baert L. Treatment of multi-resistant urinary infections in patients with multiple sclerosis. *Pharmacol Weekly* 1987;9(Suppl): 76–7.

41. Shumaker SA, Wyman JF, Uebersax JS, *et al.* Health related quality of life measures for women with urinary incontinence: the Incontinence Impact Questionnaire and the Urogential Distress Inventory. *Qual Life Res* 1994;3:291–306.

42. Raz S, Erickson DR. SEAPI QMM incontinence classification system. *Neurourol Urodyn* 1992;11:187–99.

43. Bonniaud V, Bryant D, Parratte B, Guyatt G. Qualiveen, a urinary-disorder specific instrument: 0.5 corresponds to the minimal important difference. *J Clin Epid* 2008;61:505–10.

44. Fowler CJ, Panicker JN, Drake M, *et al.* A UK consensus on the management of the bladder in multiple sclerosis. *J Neurol Neurosurg Psychiatry* 2009;80:470–7.

45. Fowler CJ. Bladder dysfunction in multiple sclerosis: causes and treatment. *Int Mult Scler J* 1996;1:431–40.

46. Wilson ML, Gaido L. Laboratory diagnosis of urinary tract infections in adult patients. *Med Microbiol* 2004;38:1150–7.

47. Jefferson H, Dalton HP, Escobar MR, Allison MJ. Transportation delay and the microbiological quality of clinical specimens. *Am J Clin Pathol* 1975;64:689–93.

48. Reller ML, Gaido L. Laboratory diagnosis of urinary tract infections in adult patients. *Med Microbiol* 2004;38:1150–8.

49. Pappas PG. Laboratory in the diagnosis and management of urinary tract infections. *Med Clin N Am* 1991;75:313–25.

50. Samellas W, Rubin B. Management of upper urinary tract complications of multiple sclerosis by means of urinary diversion to an ileal conduit. *J Urol* 1965;93:169.

51. Franz DA, Towler MA, Edlich RF, Steers WD. Functional urinary outlet obstruction causing urosepsis in a male multiple sclerosis patient. *J Emerg Med* 1992;10:281–4.

52. Onal B, Siva A, Buldu I, *et al.* Voiding dysfunction due to multiple sclerosis: a large scale retrospective analysis. *Int Braz J Urol* 2009;35:326–33.

53. Krhut J, Hradilek P, Zalpetalova O. Analysis of the upper urinary tract function in multiple sclerosis patients. *Acta Neurol Scand* 2008;118:115–19.

54. Beck RP, Warren KG, Whitman P. Urodynamic studies in female patients with multiple sclerosis. *Am J Obstet Gynecol* 1981;139:273–6.

55. Bradley WE, Logothetis JL, Timm GW. Cystometric and sphincter abnormalities in multiple sclerosis. *Neurology* 1973;23:1131–9.

56. Gonor SE, Carroll DJ, Metcalfe JB. Vesical dysfunction in multiple sclerosis. *Urology* 1985;128:541–5.

57. Peterson T, Pederson J. Neurourodynamic evaluation of voiding dysfunction in multiple sclerosis. *Acta Neurol Scand* 1984;69:402–11.

58. Piazza DH, Diokno AC. Review of neurogenic bladder in multiple sclerosis. *Urology* 1979;14:33–5.

59. Schoenberg HW, Gutrich K, Banno J. Urodynamic patterns in multiple sclerosis. *J Urol* 1979;122:648–50.

60. Sirls LT, Weese D, Zimmern PE. Intravesical oxybutynin for refractory detrusor overactivity. *Presented at the Annual Meeting of the Urodynamics Society*, San Antonio, TX, 1993.

61. Summers JL. Neurogenic bladder in the women with multiple sclerosis. *J Urol* 1978;120:555–6.

62. Weinstein MS, Cardenas DD, O'Shughnessy EJ, Catanzaro ML. Carbon dioxide cystometry and postural changes in patients with multiple sclerosis. *Arch Phys Med Rehabil* 1988;69:923–7.

63. Litwiller SE, Frohman EM, Zimmern PE. Multiple sclerosis and the urologist. *J Urol* 1999;161:743–57.

64. Lemack GE, Frohman E, Ramnarayan P. Women with voiding dysfunction secondary to bladder outlet dyssynergia in the setting of multiple sclerosis do not demonstrate significantly elevated intravesical pressures. *Urology* 2007;69:893–897.

65. Chancellor MB, Blaivas JG. Multiple sclerosis and diabetic neurogenic bladder. In Blaivas JG, Chancellor MB, eds. *Atlas of Urodynamics*, 1st edn. Philadelphia PA: Lippincott Williams & Wilkins, 1996, 187–9.

66. Bakke A, Myhr KM, Gronning M, Nyland H. Bladder, bowel and sexual dysfunction in patients with multiple sclerosis: a cohort study. *Scand J Urol Nephrol* 1996;179(Suppl):61–6.

67. Webb RJ, Lawson AL, Neal DE. Clean intermittent self-catheterization in 172 adults. *Br J Urol* 1990;65:20–3.

68. Hebjorn S. Treatment of detrusor hyperreflexia in multiple sclerosis: a double blind cross over clinical trial comparing methantheline bromide (Banthine), flavoxate chloride (Uripas) and meladrazine tartarate (Lisidonil). *Urol Int* 1977;32:209–17.

69. Rabey JM, Moriel EZ, Farkas A, *et al.* Detrusor hyperreflexia in multiple sclerosis. Alleviation by combination of imipramine and propantheline, a clinico-laboratory study. *Eur Neurol* 1979;18:33–7.

70. Schoenberg HW, Gutrich JM. Management of vesical dysfunction in multiple sclerosis: the role of drug therapy. *Urology* 1980;16:444–7.

71. Awad SA, Wilson JW, Fenemore J, Kiruluta HG. Dysfunction of the detrusor and urethra in multiple sclerosis: the role of drug therapy. *Can J Surg* 1982;25:259–62.

72. Blaivas JG, Kaplan SA. Urologic dysfunction in patients with multiple sclerosis. *Semin Neurol* 1988;8:159–65.

73. Dmochowski RR, Sand PK, Zinner NR, *et al.* Comparative efficacy and safety of transdermal oxybutynin and oral tolterodine versus placebo in previously treated patients with urge and mixed urinary incontinence. *Urology* 2003;62:237–42.

74. Cardozo L, Lisec M, Millard R, *et al.* Randomized, double blind placebo controlled trial of the once daily antimuscarinic agent solifenacin succinate in patients with overactive bladder. *J Urol* 2004;172:1919–24.

75. Chapple C, Steers W, Norton P, *et al.* A pooled analysis of three phase III studies to investigate the efficacy, tolerability and safety of darifenacin, a muscarinic M3 selective receptor antagonist, in the treatment of overactive bladder. *BJU Int* 2005;95:993–1001.

76. Cardozo L, Chapple CR, Toozs-Hobson P, *et al.* Efficacy of trospium chloride in patients with detrusor instability: a placebo controlled, randomized, double blind, multicenter clinical trial. *BJU Int* 2000;85:659–64.

77. Blaivas JG, Sinha HP, Zayed AA, Labib KB. Detrusor-external sphincter dyssynergia. *J Urol* 1981;125:542–4.

78. Dibenedetto M, Yalla SV. Electrodiagnosis of striated urethral sphincter dysfunction. *J Urol* 1978;122:361–5.

79. Miklos JR, Sze EH, Karram MM. A critical approach of the methods of measuring leak point pressures in women with stress incontinence. *Obstet Gynecol* 1995;86:349–52.

80. Miller H, Simpson CA, Yeates WK. Bladder dysfunction in multiple sclerosis. *Br Med J* 1965;1:1265–9.

81. Nicholas RS, Friede T, Hollis S, Young CA. Anticholinergics for urinary

symptoms in multiple sclerosis. *Cochrane Database Syst Rev* 2009, Issue 1. Art. No.: CD004193. DOI: 10.1002/14651858.CD004193.pub2

82. Sand PK, Goldberg RP, Dmochowski RR, McIlwain M, Dahl NV. The impact of the overactive bladder syndrome on sexual function: a preliminary report from the Multicenter Assessment of Transdermal Therapy in Overactive Bladder with Oxybutynin trial. *Am J Obstet Gynecol* 2006;195:1730–5.

83. Appell RA, Chancellor MB, Zobrist RH, *et al.* Pharmacokinetics, metabolism, and saliva output during transdermal and extended-release oral oxybutynin administration in healthy subjects. *Mayo Clin Proc* 2003;78:696–702.

84. Davila GW. Transdermal oxybutynin: a new treatment for overactive bladder. *Expert Opin Pharmacol* 2003;4:2315–24.

85. Wein AJ. Pharmacologic approaches to the management of bladder dysfunction. *J Contin Educ Urol* 1979;18:17.

86. Diokno AC, Lapides J. Oxybutynin: a new drug with analgesic and anticholinergic properties. *J Urol* 1972;108:307–9.

87. Nilvebrant L, Hallen B, Larsson G. Tolterodine – a new bladder selective muscarine receptor antagonist: preclinical pharmacological and clinical data. *Life Sci* 1997;60:1129–36.

88. Jonas U, Hofner K, Madersbacher H, Holmdahl TH. Efficacy and safety of two doses of tolterodine versus placebo in patients with detrusor over activity and symptoms of frequency, urge incontinence and urgency: urodynamic evaluation. *World J Urol* 1997;15:144–51.

89. Haab F, Cardozo L, Chapple C, *et al.* Long-term open-label solifenacin treatment associated with persistence with therapy in patients with overactive bladder syndrome. *Eur Urol* 2005;47:376–84.

90. Dmochowski RR, Rosenberg MT, Zinner NR, Staskin DR, Sand PK. Extended-release trospium chloride improves quality of life in overactive bladder. *Value Health*. 2010;13(2): 251–7.

91. Yamanishi T, Chapple CR, Chess-Williams R. Which muscarinic receptor is important in the bladder? *World J Urol* 2001;19:299–306.

92. Kavia RBC, de Ridder D, Constantinescu CS, Stott CG, Fowler CJ. Randomized controlled trial of Sativex to treat detrusor overactivity in multiple sclerosis. *Mult Scler* 2010;16:1349–59.

93. Tompson IM, Lauvetz R. Oxybutynin in bladder spasms, neurogenic bladder and enuresis. *Urology* 1976;8: 452–4.

94. Brooks ME, Braf ZF. Oxybutynin chloride (Ditropan) clinical uses and applications. *Paraplegia* 1980;18:64–8.

95. Moisey CU, Stephenson TP, Brendler CB. The urodynamic and subjective results of treatment of detrusor instability with oxybutynin chloride. *Br J Urol* 1980;52:472–5.

96. Thuroff JW, Bunke B, Ebner A, *et al.* Randomized, double-blind multicenter trial on treatment of frequency, urgency and incontinence related to detrusor hyperactivity: oxybutynin versus propantheline versus placebo. *J Urol* 1991;145:813–17.

97. Tapp AJ, Cardozo LD, Versi E, Cooper D. The treatment of detrusor instability in post menopausal women with oxybutynin hydrochloride, a double blind placebo controlled study. *Br J Obstet Gynaecol* 1990;97:521–6.

98. Fowler CJ, Van Kerrebroeck PE, Nordenbo A, Van Poppel H. Treatment of lower urinary tract dysfunction in patients with multiple sclerosis. *J Neurol* 1992;55:986–9.

99. Madersbacher H, Jilg G. Control of detrusor hyperreflexia by the intravesical instillation of oxybutynin hydrochloride. *Paraplegia* 1991;28:84–90.

100. Greenfield SP, Fera M. Intravesical oxybutynin in children with neurogenic bladder. *J Urol* 1991;146:532–4.

101. Mohler JL. Relaxation of intestinal bladders by intravesical oxybutynin chloride. *Neurourol Urodyn* 1990;9:179–82.

102. Brendler CB, Radelbaugh LC, Mohler JL. Topical oxybutynin chloride for relaxation of dysfunctional bladders. *J Urol* 1989;141:350–2.

103. Higson RH, Smith JC, Hills W. Intravesical lidocaine and detrusor instability. *Br J Urol* 1979;51:500–3.

104. Mattiasson A, Ekstrom B, Anderson KE. Effects of instillation of verapamil into patients with detrusor

hyperactivity. *Neurourol Urodyn* 1987;6:253–6.

105. Wees DL, Rosenkamp DA, Zimmern PE. Intravesical oxybutynin: experience with 42 patients. *Urology* 1993;41:527–30.

106. Sharkey KA, Williams RG, Schultzberg WM. Sensory substance P-innervation of the urinary bladder: possible site of action of capsaicin in causing urinary retention in rats. *Neuroscience* 1983;10:861–8.

107. Szallasi A, Blumberg P. Resiniferatoxin and its analogs provide novel insights into the pharmacology of the vanilloid (capsaicin) receptor. *Life Sci* 1990;47:1339–408.

108. Maggi CA, Barbanti G, Santicioli P, *et al.* Cystometric evidence that capsaicin sensitive nerves modulate the afferent branch of the micturition reflex in humans. *J Urol* 1989;142:150–4.

109. De Ridder D, Chandiramani V, Dasgupta P, *et al.* Intravesical capsaicin as a treatment for refractory detrusor hyperreflexia: a dual center study with long term follow-up. *J Urol* 1997;158:2087–92.

110. Fowler CJ, Beck RO, Gerrard S, *et al.* Intravesical capsaicin for the treatment of detrusor hyperreflexia. *J Neurol Neurosurg Psychiatry* 1994;57: 169–73.

111. Fowler CJ, Jewkes D, McDonald WI, *et al.* Intravesical capsaicin for neurogenic bladder dysfunction. *Lancet* 1992;339:1239.

112. Lazzeri M, Beneforti P, Turini D. Urodynamic effects of intravesical resiniferatoxin in humans: preliminary results in stable and unstable detrusor. *J Urol* 1997;158:2093–6.

113. Hilton P, Hertogs K, Stanton SL. The use of desmopressin for nocturia in women with multiple sclerosis. *J Neurol Neurosurg Psychiatry* 1983;46:854–5.

114. Kinn AC, Larsson PO. Desmopressin: a new principle for symptomatic treatment of urgency and incontinence in patients with multiple sclerosis. *Scand J Urol Nephrol* 1990;24:109–12.

115. Eckford SD, Carter PG, Jackson SR, *et al.* An open in-patient incremental safety study of desmopressin in women with multiple sclerosis and nocturia. *Br J Urol* 1995;76:459–63.

116. Valiquette G, Herbert J, D'Alisera PM. Desmopressin in the management of

nocturia in patients with multiple sclerosis. *Arch Neurol* 1996;53:1270–5.

117. Schurch B, de Seze M, Denys P, *et al.* Botulinum toxin type A is a safe and effective treatment for neurogenic urinary incontinence: results of a single treatment, randomized, placebo controlled 6-month study. *J Urol* 2005;174:196–200.

118. Sahai A, Khan M, Fowler CJ, Dasgupta P. Botulinum toxin for the treatment of lower urinary tract symptoms: a review. *Neurourol Urodyn* 2005;24:2–12.

119. Kabay S, Kabay SC, Yucel M, Ozden H, Yilmaz Z, Aras O, Aras B. The clinical and urodynamic results of a 3-month percutaneous posterior tibial nerve stimulation treatment in patients with multiple sclerosis-related neurogenic bladder dysfunction. *Neurourol Urodyn.* 2009;28:964–8.

120. Nordling J. Alpha blockers and urethral pressure in neurological patients. *Urol Int* 1978;33:304–9.

121. O'Roirdan JI, Doherty C, Javed M, *et al.* Do alpha blockers have a role in lower urinary tract dysfunction in multiple sclerosis? *J Urol* 1995;153:1114–16.

122. Kornhuber HH, Schutz A. Efficient treatment of neurogenic bladder disorders in multiple sclerosis with intermittent catheterization and ultrasound controlled training. *Eur J Neurol* 1990;30:260–7.

123. Khan F, Pallant JF, Pallant JI, Brand C, Kilpatrick TJ. A randomized controlled trial: outcomes of bladder rehabilitation in persons with multiple sclerosis. *J Neurol Neurosurg Psychiatry* 2010;81:1033–8.

124. Hollander JB, Diokno AC. Urinary diversion and reconstruction in the patient with spinal cord injury *Urol Clin North Am* 1993;20:465–74.

125. Van Balken MR, Vergunst H, Bemelmans BLH. The use of electrical devices for the treatment of bladder dysfunction: a review of methods. *J Urol* 2004;172:846–51.

126. Schwartz SL, Kennelly MJ, McGuire EJ, Faerber GJ. Incontinent ileo-vesicostomy urinary diversion in the treatment of lower urinary tract dysfunction. *J Urol* 1994;152:99–102.

127. Juma S, Niku SD, Brodak PP, Joseph AC. Urolume urethral wall stent in the treatment of detrusor sphincter dyssynergia. *Paraplegia* 1994;32:616–21.

128. Sauerwein D, Gross AJ, Kutzenberger J, Ringert RH. Wallstents in patients with detrusor sphincter dyssynergia. *J Urol* 1995;154:495–7.

129. Maruf NJ, Godec CJ, Strom RL, Cass AS. Unusual therapeutic response of massive squamous cell carcinoma of the bladder. *J Urol* 1982;128:1313–15.

130. Broecher BH, Klein FA, Hackler RH. Cancer of the bladder in spinal cord injury patients. *J Urol* 1981;125:196–7.

131. Bejany EC, Lockhart JL, Rhamy RK. Malignant vesical tumors following spinal cord injury. *J Urol* 1987;138:1390–2.

132. Sutton MA, Hinson JL, Nickell KG, Boone TB. Continent ileocecal augmentation cystoplasty. *Spinal Cord* 1998;36:246–51.

133. Appell RA. Electrical stimulation for the treatment of urinary incontinence. *Urology* 1998;51(Suppl 2A):24–6.

134. Siegel SW, Catanzaro F, Dijkema HE, *et al.* Longterm results of a multicenter study on sacral nerve stimulation for treatment of urinary urge incontinence, urgency-frequency, and retention. *Urology* 2000;56(Suppl 1):87–91.

135. Haab F, Zimmern PE, Leach GE. Female stress incontinence due to intrinsic sphincter deficiency: recognition and management. *J Urol* 1996;165:3–17.

136. Winters JC, Appell R. Periurethral injection of collagen in the treatment of intrinsic sphincteric deficiency in the female patient. *Urol Clin North Am* 1995;22:673–8.

137. Light JK, Pietro T. Alteration in detrusor behavior and the effect on renal function following insertion of the artificial urinary sphincter. *J Urol* 1986;136:632–5.

138. Lilius HG, Valtonen EJ, Wikstrom J. Sexual problems in patients suffering from multiple sclerosis. *J Chron Dis* 1976;29:643–7.

139. Vas CJ. Sexual impotence and some autonomic disturbances in men with multiple sclerosis. *Acta Neurol Scand* 1969;45:166–82.

140. Betts CD, Jones SJ, Fowler CG, Fowler CJ. Erectile dysfunction in multiple sclerosis. Associated neurologic deficits, and treatment of the condition. *Brain* 1994;117:1303–10.

141. Ghezzi A, Malvestitti GM, Baldini S, *et al.* Erectile impotence in multiple sclerosis: a neurophysiological study. *J Neurol* 1995;242:123–6.

142. Mattson D, Petrie M, Srivastava DK, McDermott M. Multiple sclerosis. Sexual dysfunction and its response to medications. *Arch Neurol* 1995;52:862–8.

143. Valleroy ML, Kraft GH. Sexual dysfunction in multiple sclerosis. *Arch Phys Med Rehabil* 1984;65:125–8.

144. Lundberg PO. Sexual dysfunction in patients with multiple sclerosis. *Sex Disabil* 1978;1:218–22.

145. Kirkeby HJ, Poulsen EU, Derup J. Erectile dysfunction in multiple sclerosis. *Neurology* 1988;38:1366–74.

146. Zorzon M, Zivandinov R, Bosco A, *et al.* Sexual dysfunction in multiple sclerosis: a case-control study. I. Frequency and comparison of groups. *Mult Scler* 1999;5:418–27.

147. Zorzon M, Zindinov R, Monti Bragadin L, *et al.* Sexual dysfunction in multiple sclerosis: a 2-year follow-up study. *J Neurol Sci* 2001;187:1–5

148. Borello-France D, Leng W, O'Leary M, *et al.* Bladder and sexual function among women with multiple sclerosis. *Mult Scler* 2004;10:455–61.

149. Foley FW, Iverson J. Sexuality and multiple sclerosis. In Kalb RC, Scheinberg LC eds., *Multiple Sclerosis and the Family*. New York: Demos, 1992; 63–82.

150. Demirkiran M, Sarica Y, Uguz S, Yerdelen D, Aslan K. Multiple sclerosis patients with and without sexual dysfunction: are there any differences? *Mult Scler* 2006;12:209–14.

151. Zorzon M, Zivadinov R, Locatelli L, *et al.* Correlation of sexual dysfunction and brain magnetic resonance imaging in multiple sclerosis. *Mult Scler* 2003;9:108–10

152. Zivadinov R, Zorzon M, Locatelli L, *et al.* Sexual dysfunction in multiple sclerosis: a MRI, neurophysiological and urodynamic study. *J Neurol Sci* 2003;210:73–6.

153. Ernst R, Pittler MH. Yohimbine for erectile dysfunction: a new systematic review and meta-analysis of randomized clinical trials. *J Urol* 1998;159:433–6.

154. Teloken C, Rhoden EL, Sogari P, *et al.* Therapeutic effects of high dose yohimbine hydrochloride on organic

erectile dysfunction. *J Urol* 1998;159:122–4.

155. Montague DK, Barada JH, Belker AM, *et al.* Clinical guidelines panel on erectile dysfunction: summary report on the treatment of organic erectile dysfunction. *J Urol* 1996;156:2007–11.

156. Hellstrom WJ, Gittelman M, Karlin G, *et al.* Sustained efficacy and tolerability of vardenafil, a highly potent selective phosphodiesterase type 5 inhibitor, in men with erectile dysfunction: results of a randomized, double blind, placebo controlled pivotal trial. *Urology* 2003;61(Suppl 1):8–14.

157. Giuliano F, Donatucci C, Montorsi F, *et al.* Vardenafil is effective and well-tolerated for treating erectile dysfunction in a broad population of men, irrespective of age. *BJU Int* 2005;95:110–16.

158. Goldstein I, Lue TF, Padma-Nathan H, *et al.* Oral sildenafil in the treatment of erectile dysfunction. *N Engl J Med* 1998;338:1397–404.

159. Skoumal R, Chen J, Kula K, *et al.* Efficacy and treatment satisfaction with on-demand tadalafil (Cialis) in men with erectile dysfunction. *Eur Urol* 2004;46:362–9.

160. Fowler CG, Miller JR, Sharief MK, *et al.* A double blind randomized study of sildenafil citrate for erectile dysfunction in men with multiple sclerosis. *J Neurol Neurosurg Psychiatry* 2005;76:700–5.

161. Derry F, Gardner BP, Glass C, *et al.* Sildenafil (Viagra): a double-blind, placebo-controlled, single-dose, two-way crossover study in men with erectile dysfunction caused by

traumatic spinal cord injury [Abstract]. *J Urol* 1997;157(Suppl):181.

162. Washington SL, Shindel AW. A once-daily dose of tadalafil for erectile dysfunction: compliance and efficacy. *Drug Des Devel Ther* 2010;4:159–71.

163. Sonksen J, Biering-Sorensen F, Kristensen JK. Ejaculation induced by penile vibratory stimulation in men with spinal cord injuries. The importance of the vibratory amplitude. *Paraplegia* 1994;32:651–60.

164. Heller L, Keren O, Aloni, R, Davidoff G. An open trial of vacuum penile tumescence constriction therapy for neurological impotence. *Paraplegia* 1992;30:550–3.

165. Hirsch JH, Smith RL, Chancellor MB, *et al.* Use of intracavernous injection of prostaglandin E1 for neuropathic erectile dysfunction. *Paraplegia* 1994;32:661–4.

166. Flynn RJ, Williams G. Long term follow-up of patients with erectile dysfunction commenced on self-injection with intracavernosal papaverine with or without phentolamine. *Br J Urol* 1996;78:628–31.

167. Weiss JN, Badlani GH, Ravalli R, Brettschneider N. Reasons for high drop-out rate with self injection therapy for impotence. *Int J Impot Res* 1994;6:171–4.

168. Massey EW, Pleet AB. Penile prosthesis for impotence in multiple sclerosis. *Ann Neurol* 1978;5:451–4.

169. Goldstein I, Newman L, Baum N, *et al.* Safety and efficacy of Mentor alpha-1

inflatable penile prosthesis implantation for impotence treatment. *J Urol* 1997;157:833–9.

170. Randrup E, Wilson S, Mobley D, *et al.* Clinical experience with Mentor alpha 1 inflatable penile prosthesis. *Urology* 1993;42:305–8.

171. Sexton WJ, Benedict JF, Jarow JP. Comparison of long term outcomes of penile prosthesis and intracavernosal injection therapy. *J Urol* 1998;159:811–15.

172. Minderhoud JM, Leemhuis JG, Kremer J, *et al.* Sexual disturbances arising from multiple sclerosis. *Acta Neurol Scand* 1984;70:299–306.

173. Hudson WW, Harrison DF, Crosscup PC. A short form scale to measure sexual discord in dyadic relationships. *J Sex Res* 1981;17:157–74.

174. Tzortzis V, Skriapas K, Hadjigeorgiou G *et al.* Sexual dysfunction in newly diagnosed multiple sclerosis women. *Mult Scler* 2008;14:561–3.

175. Langworthy OR. Disturbances in micturition associated with disseminated sclerosis. *Nerv Ment Disord* 1938;88:760–70.

176. Dasgupta R, Wiseman OJ, Kanabar G, *et al.* Efficacy of sildenafil in the treatment of female sexual dysfunction due to multiple sclerosis. *J Urol* 2004;171:1189–93.

177. Sipski ML, Rosen RC, Alexander CJ, Hamer RM. Sildenafil effects on sexual and cardiovascular response in women with spinal cord injury. *Urology* 2000;55:812–15.

Depression in multiple sclerosis

Adam I. Kaplin and Ryan E. Stagg

Introduction

Current estimates suggest the prevalence of multiple sclerosis (MS) may be approximately 600 000 people in the United States.[1] Although attention is typically focused on the physical disability associated with MS, the profound impact of mood disorders on the presentation and prognosis has recently begun to be appreciated.[2–6] Depression as an early and important clinical manifestation of MS is not a new observation, although it has taken over a century for systematic investigations to be undertaken.

Recently, more efforts have been made by providers to treat depression as part of the comprehensive and holistic approach provided to patients with various general medical conditions. The prevalence and impact of comorbid depression in patients with MS cannot be ignored; notably, of all the mental state changes that could potentially occur with MS, depression is the most common by far. Independent of the premorbid prevalence of depression in patients diagnosed with MS, numerous reports have found that the incidence of depression after the onset of MS remarkably elevated four-fold.[7] The profound impact that depression can have on a patient with MS necessitates its ascertainment and intervention.

Epidemiology and impact of depression on MS

From its earliest characterization, depression was among the first symptoms recognized as being associated with MS. Jean-Martin Charcot (1825–1893) was the first individual to provide an accurate and comprehensive clinicopathological description of MS, which he termed disseminated sclerosis.[8] Charcot noted early on that grief, vexation, and adverse changes in social circumstance were related to the onset of MS. Even from its initial description, depression has been recognizable as a serious and potentially life-threatening component of MS.

Depression is extremely common in MS, with a point prevalence of major depression in MS clinic patients of 15%–30%, and a lifetime prevalence of 40%–60%.[9] This rate of depression is three to ten times that of the general population, and depression is more common in MS than in other chronic illnesses, including other neurologic disorders.[10] Depression in MS patients not only causes great personal suffering, but it can dramatically affect a patient's function, quality of life, and longevity. Multiple studies have demonstrated that depression is the primary determining factor in a patient's self-reported quality of life, with a greater impact than other variables investigated including physical disability, fatigue, and cognitive impairment.[11–13] MS patients with depression and/or anxiety disorders have been shown to be almost five times more likely to have difficulty with adherence to MS treatment.[14]

Function

Compared to other major causes of chronic disability in the general medical outpatient population, depression is second only to coronary artery disease in the degree of functional impairment it causes.[15] The level of depression in patients with MS is the primary determining factor in the quality of their primary relationships when rated both by the patients and significant others,[16] which has important long-term implications for the ability of MS patients to maintain their stable social support systems. In MS patients, depression is associated with increased time lost from work, disruption of social support, and decreased adherence to neuromedical treatment regimens for MS.[4]

Cognition

Some degree of impaired cognitive functioning occurs in 50% of MS patients in epidemiologic studies of community samples, even when patients with depression are excluded.[17] Although quite varied, the most common cognitive impairments in MS involve memory recall, information processing speed, executive functioning, and working memory. These cognitive deficits are also common in depressed individuals. Although the association between depression and cognitive dysfunction in MS is complex, generating mixed findings in the literature, recent work suggests that performance in depressed MS patients may be less impaired on routine tasks than on tasks that demand effortful attention.[18] Treating depression has been found to improve cognitive functioning in many affected MS patients.

Multiple Sclerosis Therapeutics, Fourth Edition, ed. Jeffrey A. Cohen and Richard A. Rudick. Published by Cambridge University Press.
© Cambridge University Press 2011.

Fatigue

Depression is strongly associated with the impact of fatigue on the lives of MS patients. Fatigue is a common symptom of both MS and depression. MS patients with depression are six times more likely to report disabling fatigue.[19] When mental fatigue and physical fatigue are measured separately, depression is more strongly correlated with mental fatigue ($r = 0.54$, $P < 0.0001$) than with physical fatigue ($r = 0.31$, $P < 0.01$).[19] Recently, a study of a large community sample of MS patients investigated disabling fatigue, defined as fatigue that often or almost always interferes with activities.[20] Subjects with clinically significant depressive symptoms were six times more likely to report disabling fatigue, and the presence of disabling fatigue had a sensitivity and specificity of 70% for predicting clinically significant levels of depression. Moreover, it has been shown that treatment of depression leads to reduction of fatigue in MS patients in proportion to the improvement in their mood, with an efficacy comparable to the effectiveness of treatments that directly target the symptoms of fatigue.[21]

Suicide

There is a 30% lifetime incidence of suicidal intent in patients with MS, defined as a desire to kill oneself, and, overall, an astounding 6%–12% of MS patients make a suicide attempt.[6,20] It is, therefore, not surprising that studies have suggested that suicide, the most acutely grave consequence of severe depression, occurs in MS at a rate 7.5 times that of the age-matched general population.[22] In a Maryland-based forensics study, suicide (8%) was second only to cardiovascular disease (18%) among the leading causes of unexpected death of 50 autopsies.[23] In a large Canadian study, suicide was found to be the third leading cause of death, accounting for 15% of all deaths during this 16-year period.[22] Patients dying from suicide were considerably younger and less disabled compared to the other two leading causes in this cohort. A Danish MS study found an elevated rate of suicide compared to the general population, with overall 2.12-fold more suicides in MS patients.[24] The elevated rate of suicide continued to be twice the anticipated rate even 20–45 years after the MS diagnosis. In a separate study of MS outpatients, suicidal intent was *not* related to gender, employment status, disease duration, physical disability, or cognitive status.[25] The three most important variables for predicting suicidal intent were severity of major depression, living alone, and alcohol abuse, which in combination had an 85% predictive accuracy for suicidal intent. The lack of association between suicidal intent and physical disability strongly argues against this being merely a reaction to the stress of adverse circumstances associated with MS, but rather a lethal outcome of the comorbid depression associated with this disease.

Based on its profound impact on patients' quality of life, function, and longevity, depression represents what is perhaps the most treatable cause of morbidity and mortality in patients with MS. Despite this important impact, depression in MS is frequently under-diagnosed and under-treated. In 2005, the Goldman Consensus stated that despite the severe negative impact depression can have on the course of MS, many cases remain undiagnosed and untreated, leading the group to encourage better screening and treatment by neurologists of depression in their MS patients.[4]

Demoralization

Sometimes an individual's capacity to adapt is overwhelmed by the stresses with which he is confronted, and he becomes discouraged, bewildered, and overwhelmed. This is state is called demoralization. Demoralization has been defined[26] as a state of helplessness, hopelessness, confusion, subjective incompetence, isolation, and diminished self-esteem. The subjective experience of demoralization involves feeling incapable of meeting both internal and external expectations, feelings of being trapped and powerless to change or escape, and feelings of being unique and, therefore, not understood. The combined effect usually leads to frustration, bewilderment, and isolation.

A study of MS patients whose average time since diagnosis was nine years, examined their subjective experiences and the psychosocial consequences of their disease.[27] The results of this study are very instructive, in that they demonstrate that even though autoimmune neurologic diseases can be difficult to adapt to acutely, most patients appreciate, over time, that there are beneficial as well as detrimental effects of their illness on their lives.[27]

What is depression?
Criteria for major depression:

The Diagnostic and Statistical Manual (DSM)-IV criteria for major depression require the presence of five or more of the following symptoms during the same two-week period accompanied by functional impairment:

1. insomnia or hypersomnia
2. loss of interest or pleasure (anhedonia)
3. feelings of worthlessness or inappropriate/excessive guilt
4. fatigue or loss of energy
5. depressed mood
6. diminished ability to think or concentrate, or indecisiveness
7. significant weight loss when not dieting or weight gain, or decrease or increase in appetite
8. psychomotor agitation or retardation
9. recurrent thoughts of death or suicide

In order to meet criteria for major depression, at least one of the five or more symptoms that are present must either be depressed mood or loss of interest/pleasure.[28]

Diagnosing depression in MS patients

Recognizing depression in MS patients can be challenging because of the overlap of symptoms between these psychiatric and neurologic illnesses. For example, fatigue, cognitive impairment, poor appetite, and insomnia occur in many non-depressed MS patients, making reliance on these symptoms difficult in making a diagnosis of depression. Nonetheless, certain symptoms, such as feelings of self-blame, guilt, and self-recrimination are not common reactions to a medical illness, but are almost always found to some degree in depression.[29] The pervasiveness of symptoms can also suggest depression. Low mood most of the time or loss of pleasure in activities that require skills that are made more difficult because of neurologic deficits can occur commonly in MS. This is particularly true during the first few weeks of adjustment to this disease, as this is a period wrought with uncertainty and the conception of loss of health. However, persistent low mood and lack of pleasure in all activities should raise suspicion for depression. Similarly, failure to progress beyond the acute shock of being diagnosed with MS after many months or years should raise questions about a supervening depression. If an individual was progressing well initially in terms of recovery from his neurologic deficits, but suddenly stopped improving and, in fact, began to lose ground, the possibility of depression as a cause should be entertained.[30] Finally, suicidal thoughts should prompt an urgent assessment by a trained physician or mental health professional, because the rate of suicide in MS depression appears at least as great, if not greater, compared with other medical conditions.[22] Suicide is universally considered the most extreme consequence of depressive illness; concern for suicide in a patient with a medical condition presents a major health care priority to identify and treat an underlying affective illness.

Several points need to be considered when making the diagnosis of depression in MS patients. First, there are common presentations of these symptoms that may suggest one condition over the other. Early morning awakening, for example, is commonly seen in patients with depression whereas difficulty initiating or maintaining sleep is more prevalent in MS related insomnia.[31] Diurnal variation in patient's mood and energy level is common in depression, with patients progressively improving during the course of the day.[32] MS patients more commonly report worsening fatigue in the latter half of the day. Debilitating fatigue that almost always interferes with a patient's activities should be considered a symptom likely made worse by an underlying depression until proven otherwise.[20] Cognitive impairment in depression is often characterized by a fluctuating course and a tendency on the part of patients to highlight their difficulties and put forth poor effort on testing because of limited motivation.[33] Effort and attention are commonly affected by depression. MS cognitive impairment, by contrast, typically is stable when present, and patients tend to conceal their difficulties and provide good effort on testing. With experience, the different qualities of these overlapping symptoms in depression and MS can become apparent to the clinician practiced in mental status examination.

The second consideration in diagnosing depression in MS patients is that frequently these symptoms can be multifactorial. Clinically, it is common for patients who become depressed to have a dramatic worsening in their pre-existing fatigue and concentration problems, which may improve substantially with effective treatment of their depression.[17,21,34] Because depression is currently often far more responsive to treatment than are the other comorbid symptoms of MS such as fatigue and cognitive impairment, clinicians should not miss the opportunity to alleviate these symptoms by treating a suspected underlying depression.

The third consideration is the observation that symptom-guided pharmacologic treatments can occasionally worsen the patient's other conditions. For instance, a patient with a missed underlying depression who is presumed to be suffering solely from MS-related fatigue might be given modafinil, which can exacerbate insomnia, prompting the addition of a benzodiazepine, which worsens cognition, leading to donapezil, which worsens appetite and in turn lowers energy and increases fatigue. If an underlying depression was responsible for a significant portion of the patient's fatigue and concentration difficulties, then the use of an antidepressant would likely prove much more efficacious.

Fourth and perhaps most important in correctly diagnosing depression is to resist the temptation to attribute a patient's distress as solely a reaction to environmental stressors, and miss a possible endogenous contribution. As mentioned earlier, although demoralization is common in many medical conditions, depression is a separate entity, the devastating manifestations of which should not be underappreciated. The presence or severity of depression in MS does not correlate well with the degree of physical disability, suggesting that involvement of the brain and not the degree of stress is paramount in precipitating depression.[25,35,36] Stress alone is not sufficient to precipitate depression, although it may play a role in its genesis in vulnerable individuals. A patient's mood state should not be dismissed as solely a reaction to stressful circumstances.

Causes of depression in MS

Mounting evidence suggests that depression in MS is immune-mediated and the result of brain inflammation rather than the patient's environmental situation (Table 59.1). The existing evidence is consistent with a cytokine-mediated pathogenesis of depression in MS, with these same mediators of inflammatory damage to the central nervous system (CNS) causing perturbations in mood regulation.[44–46,50] Taken from this vantage point, depression can be viewed as both a pathophysiological complication as well as a clinical symptom of MS. This would suggest that the management of depression is an integral part of the general management of MS, entirely analogous to the treatment of other disease-related disabilities involving motor, sensory, and autonomic dysfunction, with potential prognostic implications for the overall course of the disease progression.

Treating MS depression

Unlike depression in the general population that resolves spontaneously in roughly 75% of patients over an average of 6–12 months, MS depression generally is unremitting and tends

Table 59.1. *Evidence for immune-mediated depression in multiple sclerosis (MS)*

Observations in the literature

- No correlation between severity of depression and physical disability.[25,35,36]
- Risk studies suggest that genetic contribution to the development of depression in MS is small compared to the effects of MS itself.[37]
- Potentially mood destabilizing effects of steroid treatment of MS patients requires careful monitoring during management of neurologic exacerbations.[38]
- Increased rate of suicide at times of relapse.[39–41]
- Neuroimaging shows differences in hippocampal size in depressed MS patients vs. controls.[42]
- Differences in presence/location of lesions and brain atrophy identified with MRI in patients with depression.[43]

Models for immune mediation

- Cytokine model: Well documented role in autoimmune diseases; cytokines have been shown to be elevated in depressed patients and correlate with treatment outcome.[44–48]
- Role of interferons: Identified as contributing to development of depression in patients with hepatitis C infection and possibly MS.[49]
- Role of glucocorticoids: Shown to have a plethora of neuropsychiatric effects including producing symptoms of depression, mania, psychosis, and delirium.[4,38]

to worsen without therapeutic intervention.[51] The literature on the treatment outcomes in depressed MS patients is limited and largely anecdotal (Table 59.2). The first randomized double-blind placebo-controlled trial of an antidepressant to treat MS depression involved five weeks of desipramine compared to placebo.[52] Patients treated with desipramine improved significantly more than the placebo group, but side effects limited desipramine dosage in half of the treated patients. A three-month open-label study of fluvoxamine 200 mg to treat MS depression found 79% of patients achieved response, and the drug was well tolerated.[54] Two separate open-label design three-month trials of either sertraline or meclobemide demon-

strated positive responses in 90% of subjects.[55,58] A more recent double-blinded placebo trial of paroxetine showed a trend towards improvement in symptoms compared to placebo. However, most of the end-points were not statistically significant.[53]

Empirical studies have examined several types of psychotherapy to treat MS depression, including cognitive behavioral, relaxation, and supportive group therapies. Psychotherapy with an emphasis on coping skills have been found more likely to be effective than insight oriented therapy in treating depression in MS patients.[51] Cognitive Behavioral Psychotherapy (CBT) has been found to be particularly effective in treating MS depression, and there are a number of small studies – some of them randomized – demonstrating the short- and long-term efficacy of this form of treatment. Because many MS patients with mobility impairments have difficulty attending a clinic on a regular basis, researchers conducted a 16-week randomized, controlled study of telephone administered CBT compared to supportive emotion-focused therapy.[56] Improvements in MS patients' depression using telephone administered CBT was significantly greater in the active treatment group. Adherence to disease-modifying treatments was improved in subjects who received telephone CBT compared to subjects in the usual care conditions. A new study looking at the use of cognitive rehabilitation showed improvements in attention, executive functioning, and information processing in MS patients.[57]

Currently, there are studies underway looking at the benefits of physical activity on mood in MS patients. Ehde and Bombardier reviewed the potential benefits of exercise as an adjunct treatment for MS depression.[3] Exercise has been shown to have many functional benefits in patients with MS, including improving mood, sexual function, pain, and fatigue. In the general population, even moderate exercise (e.g. 20 minutes per day at 60% maximum heart rate) has shown benefit in decreasing anxiety and stress components of depression. The two limitations of this intervention are motivating depressed patients to begin a new schedule of exercise, and the rapid loss of efficacy for depression if regular exercise is terminated.

Table 59.2. *Current evidence for the efficacy of depression treatment in multiple sclerosis (MS)*

Antidepressant	Class	Conclusions	Reference
Desipramine (Norpramin)	TCA	Double-blind, placebo-controlled. Improved significantly over placebo.	52
Paroxetine (Paxil)	SSRI	Double-blind, placebo-controlled. Improved but not statistically significant	53
Fluvoxamine (Luvox)	SSRI	79% of participants improved and tolerated dosage	54
Sertraline (Zoloft)	SSRI	90% improvement rate	55
Cognitive Behavioral Therapy	Therapy	Adherence to disease-modifying treatments was improved in subjects who received telephone CBT compared to subjects given usual care. Cognitive rehabilitation showed improvements in attention, executive functioning, and information processing in MS patients	56,57
Alternative Medicines	CAM	Studies are needed to evaluate the potential benefits of CAM in the treatment of depression in MS patients	N/A

CAM = complementary and alternative medicines, CBT = cognitive behavioral therapy, SSRI = selective serotonin reuptake inhibitor, TCA = tricyclic antidepressant.

Antidepressant selection in treating MS depression

There are three general strategies that can be applied to selecting an antidepressant to treat an MS patient suffering from depression. First, try to minimize the patient's side effect and potential drug–drug interactions, as these patients are often taking multiple medications. Escitalopram and sertraline are distinguished by their relatively low side effect burden and little to no clinically significant risk of drug–drug interactions.[59,60] These medications are serotonin selective reuptake inhibitors (SSRIs) that have no significant anticholinergic (e.g. sedation, dry mouth, constipation, urinary hesitancy), antihistaminergic (sedation, weight gain), or antiadrenergic (orthostatic hypotension) side effects. Their primary drawback for patients with MS is that, like the other SSRIs, they cause sexual side effects in up to 30%–60% of patients.[51] Bupropion by contrast is devoid of any sexual side effects but does lower seizure threshold.[62] Although there is a theoretical concern that patients with MS are at an increased risk of seizures, there are no reports of bupropion-related seizures in patients with MS, and we have found it quite effective in many MS patients.

The second approach is to tailor the side effects of medication to alleviate the patient's depressive symptoms. For example, bupropion, fluoxetine, and venlafaxine tend to be activating and can partially ameliorate MS fatigue in some patients. Desipramine, mirtazepine, and paroxetine by contrast are sedating and stimulate appetite, which is useful for patients with insomnia and loss of appetite. Although there is the theoretical potential for tricyclics to interfere with cognition,[63] it has been our experience that they are well tolerated when dosed correctly in MS patients (i.e. start low, and go slow during the initial dose escalation).

The third approach is to select an antidepressant that is useful in simultaneously treating depression and also the comorbid symptoms related to the MS separate from the depression. Tricyclic antidepressants can help with detrussor hyperactivity urinary urgency (because they are anticholinergic) as well as treat neuropathic pain, both of which are common in MS patients.[64] Duloxetine also is effective in treating neuropathic pain, in addition to treating depression.[65] The possibility of preventing polypharmacy through the use of a single medication for multiple symptoms (such as nortiptyline for depression, neuropathic pain, urinary urgency, and insomnia) is often ideal for the appropriate MS patients.

Potential impact of treating depression on MS disease course

Depression can have a profound impact on varied aspects of MS. Depression is associated with immune dysregulation, including elevated proinflammatory cytokines.[47] Depression is also associated with adverse CNS changes, as evidenced by reports from several studies that have shown a reduction in hippocampal volume that is more severe in patients with multiple previous depressive episodes and longer durations of depression without any antidepressant treatment.[66] The posterior segment of the hippocampus appears primarily reduced in volume in depressed patients, which is consistent with cognitive studies that showed that learning and memory are altered in patients with a major depressive disorder.[67] Recent MRI studies have shown that MS patients have smaller hippocampi when compared to controls, and increased cortisol levels were found in MS patients with depressive symptoms.[42] Because of immune activation and brain dysfunction, it would be plausible that depression could lead to worse neurologic outcomes in MS patients.

The idea that psychological states could trigger disease activity was originally described by Charcot, who speculated that grief, vexation, and adverse changes in social circumstances were related to the onset of MS.[8] Depression is a state of extreme, prolonged psychological stress, and there has been a growing consensus in the literature that specific types of chronic stress are linked to increased risk for clinical relapse as well as accrual of disability.[68] A recent prospective study tracked number of stressful life events per week and found up to a five-fold increased risk of MS relapse in patients with three or more stressful life events during a four-week period.[69] A meta-analysis found a significantly elevated risk of relapse associated with stressful life events in 13 of 14 investigations.[70] The degree that stress increased the risk of MS relapse in this meta-analysis was on average 60% greater than the magnitude of beneficial treatment effect of interferon-beta (IFNβ) treatment, suggesting that a therapy that completely prevented relapses in response to stress would be more effective than IFNβ in MS.

The effects of treating depression on MS disease course was more directly investigated in a longitudinal study demonstrating that treatment-related reductions in depression in MS patients are associated with reductions in T-cell production of interferon-gamma (IFNγ).[71] IFNγ is an important proinflammatory cytokine produced by activated T-cells and is thought to be a key player in MS pathogenesis, particularly in lesion formation and clinical relapse. T-cells isolated from depressed MS patients were found to be primed to produce twice the levels of IFNγ than T-cells from non-depressed controls. Reductions in depression with sertraline or psychotherapy were paralleled by declines in T-cell IFNγ production, which returned to control levels in the MS patients who showed a mood response to either treatment. This study suggested that treatment for depression can have a highly specific effect on immune mechanisms involved in MS pathogenesis.

Barriers to seeking and accepting treatment for MS depression

Rehabilitation and recovery from the disability associated with MS relapses or progression can constitute a painstaking and laborious journey. Depression can derail this process of adjustment. Unfortunately, classic symptoms of depression, such as hopelessness and loss of interest or motivation, are commonly interpreted as "giving up" and equated with being "weak" or "lazy" rather than interpreted as symptoms of an illness that needs to be treated. Moreover, laypeople sometimes equate being depressed and seeking treatment for depression with being "crazy" and so avoid seeking evaluation and treatment for fear of being stigmatized.

Preconceptions and myths about antidepressants also represent common barriers to accepting treatment for depression. Antidepressants specifically target and treat changes in the brains of patients who are suffering from depression, but they have no mood-elevating effects on individuals who are not depressed. As a result, antidepressants are not addicting, unlike drugs of abuse that induce euphoria, and they have no street value. Antidepressants do not give people "fake" feelings or make them feel things they would not normally feel. Instead, antidepressants restore the normal cycle of ups and downs, in response to life's rewards and stresses that is lost in individuals suffering from depression. Finally, individuals occasionally refrain from using antidepressants based on a perception that they do not want to "end up like a zombie" based on knowing or having heard of someone who was not the same once they started taking medication. The fallacy in this argument is that depression is far more likely to make someone appear impaired than is the medication that treats their mood disorder. While it is true that many medications including those used to treat mental illness *can* produce noticeable side effects, such as over-sedation, the judicious use of antidepressants by trained professionals results in a return to previous functioning in patients in whom depression is responsible for changed behavior. The goal with antidepressant therapy is to return affected individuals to the helm of their own ships, and allow them to better chart the course of their thoughts, emotions, and behaviors as they regain control of the direction their life is taking. Rather than develop noticeable side effects that suggest a person is being treated for depression with medication, the only thing that other people notice is that the person being treated seems "more like their old self." However, the biggest barrier to seeking and accepting treatment for depression, bar none, is the effects of depression itself, which makes people hopeless, unmotivated, and unable to imagine that things could get better.

Standard of care for neurologists diagnosing and treating MS depression

The Goldman Algorithm, as presented by Schiffer *et al.* based upon evidence presented at the Goldman Consensus Conference,[4,72] aims to establish a standard of care for neurologists to identify and treat major depression in MS patients (Table 59.3). Key steps in the algorithm include regularly screening for the presence of depressive symptoms in all MS patients, diagnosing major depression when present, establishing the functional impact of the depression, and screening for the presence of suicidality. If a severe depression is diagnosed

and causes severe impairment, referral to a psychiatrist is in order. If the patient does not have significant depression, or the patient does not wish to receive psychiatric treatment in the setting of minimal to moderate impairment, treatment by the neurologist is recommended with future regular reassessments.

Shoring up support: who cares for the caregivers?

There are both positive and negative aspects of being a caregiver; being able to care for the people whom we love in their time of need is both a privilege and a burden. Caregivers are dramatically impacted by both MS and depression in the people for whom they care. The majority of caregivers report that the demands of care giving disrupt their other obligations to friends, family, and career.[90] Caregivers often feel unable to leave the care-recipient alone, which leads to a perception of confinement.[51] Frequently MS patient's perception about the degree of their caregiver's burden is less than that reported by the caregiver.[91] Caregivers, patients, and health-care providers usually focus virtually all of their attention on the well-being of the MS patient, often to the neglect of concerns for the caregiver who usually functions as the patient's primary source of support. This occurs despite the fact that the well-being of the patient is often vitally dependent on the continued efforts and support from the caregiver, which can best be furnished by a healthy individual.

Poor social support and living alone are both associated with significantly higher rates of suicide in MS patients.[91] Poor social support also has been implicated as a factor in increasing the rate of MS relapses.[92] Conversely, social support acts as a buffer in the relationship between depression and immune activation.[93] As noted previously, depression is associated with worsening MS disease course possibly related to increased IFNγ production from T-cells. The effect of depression on T-cell production of IFNγ was significantly moderated by social support. Specifically, the relationship between depression and IFNγ production was particularly strong among patients with low levels of support, but was virtually non-existent among patients with high social support. This suggests that maximizing social support might buffer the effects of stress and depression on MS pathogenesis and be a crucial part of the treatment of MS patients.

Four considerations can be recommended for caregivers to keep in mind while caring for their loved ones without neglecting themselves. First, caregivers should enhance their problem-focused coping skills. This usually involves recognizing what can and cannot be changed, and trying different solutions to the problems that arise until the right one is found. Second, education is crucial because what caregivers do not know about MS and depression will increase their anxiety and prevent them from being able to efficiently problem solve. Peer education opportunities are often invaluable for both information and support. Third, care givers must remember to take care of their own needs, which should not be viewed as being in conflict with

Table 59.3. *Diagnosing and treating in multiple sclerosis (MS) depression*

Step		Details and clinical recommendations
Screen for presence of depression	Problem	Our present care in the US fails to identify over half of the MS patients with depressive disorders.[4,72]
	Diagnostic and Statistical Manual IV	Screening for the presence of depression in MS with DSM-IV is complicated by the fact that four of the nine symptoms of depression laid out by DSM-IV are also symptoms of MS – fatigue, psychomotor retardation, decreased concentration, and sleep disturbance. Experienced physicians agree that depression can still be distinguished from MS associated symptoms with the DSM-IV criteria during a clinical interview.
	Beck Depression Inventory[73]	The BDI is the most commonly used depression scale in MS-associated depression. It is a self-report scale with 21 items. Using the BDI with a 13-point cut-off score screens for about 70% of MS patients with significant depression.[79,80] The BDI-Fast Screen has also been developed to select for the most sensitive items in relation to MS patients.[81]
	Center for Epidemiologic Studies – Depression Scale[74]	CES-D is a scale that has gained visibility in several large World Health Organization epidemiologic studies. It has been shown to be a fairly consistent scale that screens positive for about 30% of MS patients at any visit. On a year to year basis, only about 5% of the patients increase scores dramatically (by more than 10 points).[82]
	Multi-Scale Depression Inventory[75]	MDI is a screening device that has subscales to help separate depressive symptoms that are vegetative and physical from those that are affective and cognitive.
	Inventory of Depressive Symptomatology[76]	IDS is a scale that has the advantage of having both clinician-rated and self-report versions.
	Patient Health Questionnaire-9[77]	PHQ-9 consists of the nine DSM-IV items and rates them on a four-point scale on the extent to which patients have been bothered by the symptom over the past two weeks.
	Hospital Anxiety and Depression Scale[78]	A recent study of HADS showed that a threshold score of 8 on the depression subscale resulted in 90% sensitivity in screening MS patients for depression.[83]
	Suicidality	Most important acute consideration. Obtaining this history should not wait for referral to psychiatrist, but rather should be elicited immediately by the treating neurologist. If present, emergent psychiatric evaluation in an emergency room is advised.
Consider level of impairment presented by depression		Patients who meet screening thresholds for depression or endorse suicidal ideations should be actively assessed for severity and quality of depression. They should be considered for follow-up treatment recommendations and referred to a psychiatrist for moderate to severe depression.
Consider and discuss treatment options with patient	Problem	When depressed MS patients are identified, many are not properly treated.[4,72]
	Psychotherapy	A variety of psychotherapeutic treatments used in group settings have been shown to be effective in reducing depression severity in MS groups.[84] Individual psychotherapy using a cognitive-behavioral approach has also been shown to lower self-report measures of depression compared to other neuromedical treatments.[85]
	Pharmacotherapy	Multiple studies have shown the effectiveness of antidepressants in treating depression in MS patients.[52,55,86] In one study, setraline and CBT were both shown to be roughly equal in their effectiveness of treating depression in MS patients.[87]
	Integrated Biopsychosocial Treatment	The treatment of depression in a complex matter and should be individualized for each person. According to the Goldman Consensus Group, an integrated approach involving both psychotherapy and medication should be the gold standard to be used, at least for the more severe depression.[4,72,88]
Maintenance or surveillance	Psychotherapy	Psychotherapy should continue as long as the patient benefits.
	Pharmacotherapy	With little to no history of depressive episodes, medication can be tapered and discontinued after about a year of use. If the patient relapses, medication should be restarted. For patients with history of chronic depression, or more than three depressive episodes, indefinite continuation of medications is recommended, although the dose may be reduced.[89]

BDI = Beck Depression Inventory, CBT = cognitive behavioral therapy, CES-D = Center for Epidemiologic Studies – Depression Scale, DSM = *Diagnostic and Statistical Manual*, HADS = Hospital Anxiety and Depression Scale, IDS = Inventory of Depressive Symptomatology, MDI = Multi-Scale Depression Inventory, MS = multiple sclerosis, PHQ-9 = Patient Health Questionnaire-9.

the care recipient's needs. Knowing how to get additional help is often critical to the well-being of both parties. And fourth, care givers and care recipients must not lose sight of the fact that they share common struggles and rewards together. Coping strategies must, therefore, be complementary. There are often multiple solutions to the same problems, so a premium should be placed on maintaining enough flexibility to maximize the benefits for both care recipients and caregivers.

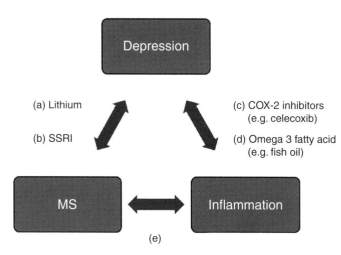

Fig. 59.1. The association of multiple sclerosis (MS), depression, and inflammation.

(a) Lithium has been shown to be protective and beneficial in studies of experimental autoimmune encephalomyelitis.[94] It has been postulated to affect inflammatory signaling, including decreasing activity of COX-1 and COX-2 as well as decreasing one of their prostaglandin products in rats.[95]

(b) Antidepressants (selective serotonin reuptake inhibitors (SSRI) and tricyclics) have been shown to improve symptoms of MS including fatigue, cognition, and overall morbidity. Current evidence suggests an anti-inflammatory effect of these medications, including decreased production of interferon-gamma[96] and effects on the arachidonic pathway.[95]

(c) Studies demonstrate superior efficacy in treatment of depressive disorders with concominant use of antidepressants and COX-2 inhibitors suggesting a role for anti-inflammatory agents in treating mood disorders.[97]

(d) Studies suggest that omega 3 fatty acids (N-3 polyunsaturated fatty acids) improve mood as well as have significant effects in the prostaglandin production pathways, again implying a role for anti-inflammatory agents in treating mood disorders.[98]

(e) As more agents become available which target inflammation in MS specifically, it may be possible to further evaluate the effects of decreased inflammation on the symptoms of depression.

Conclusions

The importance of making the appropriate and timely diagnosis of depression in MS patients cannot be overestimated. Often, what is most debilitating is not the requirement for assistance with walking or adaptations to disability that must be endured, but the depression that leads to difficulty getting out of bed, social isolation, and lowered pain tolerance. Routinely for MS patients with depression, the majority of the functional impact of their disability is due to the depression, and treatment usually leads to a dramatic increase in their function. Fortunately, depression is one of the most treatable comorbidities of MS, with the usual expectation that individuals who receive adequate treatment will make a complete recovery. What is required to achieve this result is often the same level of aggressive management that MS patients routinely invest in managing other aspects of the effects of their disease, such as injecting immunomodulatory treatments to curb inflammation, physical therapy and rehabilitation to enhance ambulation, or urologic management for urinary incontinence.

Before depression can be adequately treated, however, it must be properly recognized, diagnosed, and comprehensively managed. It is imperative to consider the impact that MS and depression have on both patients and their loved ones, because successful management will ultimately be measured by how well individuals are functioning in the context of their families and their collective lives together.

More work is needed to thoroughly explore the bidirectional influence that MS and depression exert on one another, and the impact of inflammation in mediating this influence (Fig. 59.1). We have reviewed here evidence that MS causes depression and that depression worsens MS. Elucidation of the degree to which treatment of MS protects affected patients from co-morbid depression, and treatment of depression helps to ameliorate the inflammation and progression of MS, awaits further study.

References

1. Kaplin AI, Williams M. How common are the "common" neurologic disorders? *Neurology* 2007;69:410.

2. Mohr DC, Cox D. Multiple sclerosis: empirical literature for the clinical health psychologist. *J Clin Psychol* 2001;57:479–99.

3. Ehde DM, Bombardier CH. Depression in persons with multiple sclerosis. *Phys Med Rehabil Clin N Am* 2005;16: 437–48.

4. Goldman Consensus Group. The Goldman Consensus statement on depression in multiple sclerosis. *Mult Scler* 2005;11:328–37.

5. Siegert RJ, Abernethy DA. Depression in multiple sclerosis: a review. *J Neurol Neurosurg Psychiatry* 2005;76:469–75.

6. Feinstein A. The neuropsychiatry of multiple sclerosis. *Can J Psychiatry* 2004;49:157–63.

7. Feinstein A. *The Clinical Neuropsychiatry of Multiple Sclerosis* 2nd edn.: Cambridge University Press, 2007.

8. Butler MA, Bennett TL. In search of a conceptualization of multiple sclerosis: a historical perspective. *Neuropsychol Rev.* 2003;13:93–112.

9. Caine ED, Schwid SR. Multiple sclerosis, depression, and the risk of suicide. *Neurology* 2002;59:662–3.

10. Lobentanz IS, Asenbaum S, Vass K, *et al.* Factors influencing quality of life in multiple sclerosis patients: disability, depressive mood, fatigue and sleep quality. *Acta Neurol Scand* 2004;110: 6–13.

11. Benedict RH, Wahlig E, Bakshi R, *et al.* Predicting quality of life in multiple sclerosis: accounting for physical disability, fatigue, cognition, mood disorder, personality, and behavior change. *J Neurol Sci* 2005;231:29–34.

12. Fruehwald S, Loeffler-Stastka H, Eher R, Saletu B, Baumhackl U. Depression and quality of life in multiple sclerosis. *Acta Neurol Scand* 2001;104:257–61.

13. Provinciali L, Ceravolo MG, Bartolini M, Logullo F, Danni M. A multidimensional assessment of multiple sclerosis: relationships between disability domains. *Acta Neurol Scand* 1999;100:156–62.

14. Bruce JM, Hancock LM, Arnett P, Lynch S. Treatment adherence in multiple sclerosis: association with emotional status, personality, and cognition. *J Behav Med* 2010;33:219–27.

15. Wells KB, Stewart A, Hays RD, *et al.* The functioning and well-being of depressed patients. Results from the Medical Outcomes Study. *J Am Med Assoc* 1989;262:914–19.

16. King KE, Arnett PA. Predictors of dyadic adjustment in multiple sclerosis. *Mult Scler* 2005;11:700–7.

17. Bagert B, Camplair P, Bourdette D. Cognitive dysfunction in multiple sclerosis: natural history, pathophysiology and management. *CNS Drugs* 2002;16:445–55.

18. Arnett PA. Longitudinal consistency of the relationship between depression symptoms and cognitive functioning in multiple sclerosis. *CNS Spectrum* 2005;10:372–82.

19. Ford H, Trigwell P, Johnson M. The nature of fatigue in multiple sclerosis. *J Psychosom Res* 1998;45(1 Spec No):33–8.

20. Chwastiak LA, Gibbons LE, Ehde DM, *et al.* Fatigue and psychiatric illness in a large community sample of persons with multiple sclerosis. *J Psychosom Res* 2005;59:291–8.

21. Mohr DC, Hart SL, Goldberg A. Effects of treatment for depression on fatigue in multiple sclerosis. *Psychosom Med* 2003;65:542–7.

22. Sadovnick AD, Eisen K, Ebers GC, Paty DW. Cause of death in patients attending multiple sclerosis clinics. *Neurology* 1991;41:1193–6.

23. Riudavets MA, Colegial C, Rubio A, *et al.* Causes of unexpected death in patients with multiple sclerosis: a forensic study of 50 cases. *Am J Forens Med Pathol* 2005;26:244–9.

24. Bronnum-Hansen H, Stenager E, Nylev Stenager E, Koch-Henriksen N. Suicide among Danes with multiple sclerosis. *J Neurol Neurosurg Psychiatry* 2005;76:1457–9.

25. Feinstein A. An examination of suicidal intent in patients with multiple sclerosis. *Neurology* 2002;59:674–8.

26. Frank JD FJ. *Persuasion and Healing: A Comparative Study of Psychotherapy.* 3rd edn ed. Baltimore: Johns Hopkins University Press; 1991.

27. Mohr DC, Dick LP, Russo D, *et al.* The psychosocial impact of multiple sclerosis: exploring the patient's perspective. *Health Psychol* 1999;18:376–82.

28. *Diagnostic and Statistical Manual of Mental Disorders*: DSM-IV-TR. Revised 4th Edition ed. Association AP, editor. Washington, DC: American Psychiatric Publishing, Inc, 2000.

29. Silverstone PH, Salsali M. Low self-esteem and psychiatric patients: Part I – The relationship between low self-esteem and psychiatric diagnosis. *Ann Gen Hosp Psychiatry* 2003;2:2.

30. Yorkston KM, Johnson KL, Klasner ER. Taking part in life: enhancing participation in multiple sclerosis. *Phys Med Rehabil Clin N Am* 2005;16:583–94.

31. Fleming WE, Pollak CP. Sleep disorders in multiple sclerosis. *Semin Neurol* 2005;25:64–8.

32. Hasler G, Drevets WC, Manji HK, Charney DS. Discovering endophenotypes for major depression. *Neuropsychopharmacology* 2004;29:1765–81.

33. Lamberty GJ, Bieliauskas LA. Distinguishing between depression and dementia in the elderly: a review of neuropsychological findings. *Arch Clin Neuropsychol* 1993;8:149–70.

34. MacAllister WS, Krupp LB. Multiple sclerosis-related fatigue. *Phys Med Rehabil Clin N Am* 2005;16:483–502.

35. McGuigan C, Hutchinson M. Unrecognised symptoms of depression in a community-based population with multiple sclerosis. *J Neurol* 2006;253:219–23.

36. Patten SB, Metz LM. Depression in multiple sclerosis. *Psychother Psychosom* 1997;66:286–92.

37. Sadovnick AD, Remick RA, Allen J, *et al.* Depression and multiple sclerosis. *Neurology* 1996;46:628–32.

38. Sirois F. Steroid psychosis: a review. *Gen Hosp Psychiatry* 2003;25:27–33.

39. Kroencke DC, Denney DR, Lynch SG. Depression during exacerbations in multiple sclerosis: the importance of uncertainty. *Mult Scler* 2001;7:237–42.

40. Dalos NP, Rabins PV, Brooks BR, O'Donnell P. Disease activity and emotional state in multiple sclerosis. *Ann Neurol* 1983;13:573–7.

41. Fassbender K, Schmidt R, Mossner R, *et al.* Mood disorders and dysfunction of the hypothalamic-pituitary-adrenal axis in multiple sclerosis: association with cerebral inflammation. *Arch Neurol* 1998;55:66–72.

42. Gold SM, Kern KC, O'Connor MF, *et al.* Smaller cornu ammonis 2–3/dentate gyrus volumes and elevated cortisol in multiple sclerosis patients with depressive symptoms. *Biol Psychiatry*; 68:553–9.

43. Feinstein A, Roy P, Lobaugh N, *et al.* Structural brain abnormalities in multiple sclerosis patients with major depression. *Neurology* 2004;62:586–90.

44. Schiepers OJ, Wichers MC, Maes M. Cytokines and major depression. *Prog Neuropsychopharmacol Biol Psychiatry* 2005;29:201–17.

45. Anisman H, Merali Z, Poulter MO, Hayley S. Cytokines as a precipitant of depressive illness: animal and human studies. *Curr Pharm Des* 2005;11:963–72.

46. Miller DB, O'Callaghan JP. Depression, cytokines, and glial function. *Metabolism* 2005;54(5 Suppl 1):33–8.

47. Pucak ML, Kaplin AI. Unkind cytokines: current evidence for the potential role of cytokines in immune-mediated depression. *Int Rev Psychiatry* 2005;17:477–83.

48. Imitola J, Chitnis T, Khoury SJ. Cytokines in multiple sclerosis: from bench to bedside. *Pharmacol Ther* 2005;106:163–77.

49. Van Gool AR, Kruit WH, Engels FK, *et al.* Neuropsychiatric side effects of interferon-alfa therapy. *Pharm World Sci* 2003;25:11–20.

50. Pucak ML, Kaplin AI. Unkind cytokines: current evidence for the potential role of cytokines in immune-mediated depression. *Int Rev Psychiatry* 2005;17:477–83.

51. Mohr DC, Cox D. Multiple sclerosis: empirical literature for the clinical health psychologist. *J Clin Psychol* 2001;57:479–99.

52. Schiffer RB, Wineman NM. Antidepressant pharmacotherapy of depression associated with multiple sclerosis *Am J Psychiatry* 1990;147:1493–7.

53. Ehde DM, Kraft GH, Chwastiak L, *et al.* Efficacy of paroxetine in treating major depressive disorder in persons with multiple sclerosis. *Gen Hosp Psychiatry* 2008;30:40–8.

54. Benedetti F, Campori E, Colombo C, Smeraldi E. Fluvoxamine treatment of major depression associated with multiple sclerosis. *J Neuropsychiatry Clin Neurosci* 2004;16:364–6.

55. Scott TF, Nussbaum P, McConnell H, Brill P. Measurement of treatment response to sertraline in depressed multiple sclerosis patients using the Carroll scale. *Neurol Res* 1995;17: 421–2.

56. Mohr DC, Hart SL, Julian L, *et al.* Telephone-administered psychotherapy for depression. *Arch Gen Psychiatry* 2005;62:1007–14.

57. Mattioli F, Stampatori C, Bellomi F, *et al.* Neuropsychological rehabilitation in adult multiple sclerosis. *Neurol Sci* 2010;31(Suppl 2):S271–4.

58. Barak Y, Ur E, Achiron A. Moclobemide treatment in multiple sclerosis patients with comorbid depression: an open-label safety trial. *J Neuropsychiatry Clin Neurosci* 1999;11:271–3.

59. Murdoch D, Keam SJ. Escitalopram: a review of its use in the management of major depressive disorder. *Drugs* 2005;65:2379–404.

60. Hansen RA, Gartlehner G, Lohr KN, Gaynes BN, Carey TS. Efficacy and safety of second-generation antidepressants in the treatment of major depressive disorder. *Ann Intern Med* 2005;143:415–26.

61. Taylor MJ, Rudkin L, Hawton K. Strategies for managing antidepressant-induced sexual dysfunction: systematic review of randomised controlled trials. *J Affect Disord* 2005;88:241–54.

62. Jefferson JW, Pradko JF, Muir KT. Bupropion for major depressive disorder: pharmacokinetic and formulation considerations. *Clin Ther* 2005;27:1685–95.

63. Gray SL, Lai KV, Larson EB. Drug-induced cognition disorders in the elderly: incidence, prevention and management. *Drug Safety* 1999;21: 101–22.

64. Arroll B, Macgillivray S, Ogston S, *et al.* Efficacy and tolerability of tricyclic antidepressants and SSRIs compared with placebo for treatment of depression in primary care: a meta-analysis. *Ann Fam Med* 2005; 3:449–56.

65. Wernicke JF, Gahimer J, Yalcin I, Wulster-Radcliffe M, Viktrup L. Safety and adverse event profile of duloxetine. *Expert Opin Drug Safety* 2005;4:987–93.

66. Saylam C, Ucerler H, Kitis O, Ozand E, Gonul AS. Reduced hippocampal volume in drug-free depressed patients. *Surg Radiol Anat* 2006;4:1–6.

67. Neumeister A, Wood S, Bonne O, *et al.* Reduced hippocampal volume in unmedicated, remitted patients with major depression versus control subjects. *Biol Psychiatry* 2005;57:935–7.

68. Mohr DC, Pelletier D. A temporal framework for understanding the effects of stressful life events on inflammation in patients with multiple sclerosis. *Brain Behav Immun* 2006; 20:27–36.

69. Mitsonis CI, Zervas IM, Mitropoulos PA, *et al.* The impact of stressful life events on risk of relapse in women with multiple sclerosis: a prospective study. *Eur Psychiatry* 2008;23:497–504.

70. Mohr DC, Hart SL, Julian L, Cox D, Pelletier D. Association between stressful life events and exacerbation in multiple sclerosis: a meta-analysis. *BMJ* 2004;328:731.

71. Mohr DC, Goodkin DE, Islar J, Hauser SL, Genain CP. Treatment of depression is associated with suppression of nonspecific and antigen-specific T(H)1 responses in multiple sclerosis. *Arch Neurol* 2001;58:1081–6.

72. Schiffer RB. Depression in neurological practice: diagnosis, treatment, implications. *Semin Neurol* 2009;29: 220–33.

73. Beck AT, Ward CH, Mendelson M, Mock J, Erbaugh J. An inventory for measuring depression. *Arch Gen Psychiatry* 1961;4:561–71.

74. Verdier-Taillefer MH, Gourlet V, Fuhrer R, Alperovitch A. Psychometric properties of the Center for Epidemiologic Studies-Depression scale in multiple sclerosis. *Neuroepidemiology* 2001;20:262–7.

75. Nyenhuis DL, Rao SM, Zajecka JM, *et al.* Mood disturbance versus other symptoms of depression in multiple sclerosis. *J Int Neuropsychol Soc* 1995;1:291–6.

76. Rush AJ, Gullion CM, Basco MR, Jarrett RB, Trivedi MH. The Inventory of Depressive Symptomatology (IDS): psychometric properties. *Psychol Med* 1996;26:477–86.

77. Kroenke K, Spitzer RL, Williams JB. The PHQ-9: validity of a brief depression severity measure. *J Gen Intern Med* 2001;16:606–13.

78. Zigmond AS, Snaith RP. The hospital anxiety and depression scale. *Acta Psychiatr Scand* 1983;67:361–70.

79. Sullivan MJ, Weinshenker B, Mikail S, Bishop SR. Screening for major depression in the early stages of multiple sclerosis. *Can J Neurol Sci* 1995;22:228–31.

80. Sullivan MJ, Weinshenker B, Mikail S, Edgley K. Depression before and after diagnosis of multiple sclerosis. *Mult Scler* 1995;1:104–8.

81. Benedict RH, Fischer JS, Archibald CJ, *et al.* Minimal neuropsychological assessment of MS patients: a consensus approach. *Clin Neuropsychol* 2002; 16:381–97.

82. Patten SB, Berzins S, Metz LM. Challenges in screening for depression in multiple sclerosis. *Mult Scler* 2010;16:1406–11.

83. Honarmand K, Feinstein A. Validation of the Hospital Anxiety and Depression Scale for use with multiple sclerosis patients. *Mult Scler* 2009;15: 1518–24.

84. Larcombe NA, Wilson PH. An evaluation of cognitive-behaviour therapy for depression in patients with multiple sclerosis. *Br J Psychiatry* 1984;145:366–71.

85. Foley FW, Bedell JR, LaRocca NG, Scheinberg LC, Reznikoff M. Efficacy of stress-inoculation training in coping with multiple sclerosis. *J Consult Clin Psychol* 1987;55:919–22.

86. Wallin MT, Wilken JA, Turner AP, Williams RM, Kane R. Depression and multiple sclerosis: Review of a lethal combination. *J Rehabil Res Dev* 2006;43:45–62.

87. Mohr DC, Goodkin DE, Islar J, Hauser SL, Genain CP. Treatment of depression is associated with suppression of nonspecific and antigen-specific T(H)1 responses in multiple sclerosis. *Arch Neurol* 2001;58:1081–6.

88. Havelka M, Lucanin JD, Lucanin D. Biopsychosocial model–the integrated

approach tohealth and disease. *Coll Anthropol* 2009;33:303–10.

89. Schiffer RB. Depression in neurological practice: diagnosis, treatment, implications. *Semin Neurol* 2009;29: 220–33.

90. O'Brien MT. Multiple sclerosis: health-promoting behaviors of spousal caregivers. *J Neurosci Nurs* 1993;25: 105–12.

91. Aronson KJ, Cleghorn G, Goldenberg E. Assistance arrangements and use of services among persons with multiple sclerosis and their caregivers. *Disabil Rehabil* 1996;18:354–61.

92. Warren S, Warren KG, Cockerill R. Emotional stress and coping in multiple sclerosis (MS) exacerbations. *J Psychosom Res* 1991;35:37–47.

93. Mohr DC, Genain C. Social support as a buffer in the relationship between treatment for depression and T-cell production of interferon gamma in patients with multiple sclerosis. *J Psychosom Res* 2004;57:155–8.

94. De Sarno P, Axtell RC, Raman C, *et al.* Lithium prevents and ameliorates experimental autoimmune encephalomyelitis. *J Immunol* 2008; 181:338–45.

95. Rao JS, Rapoport SI. Mood-stabilizers target the brain arachidonic acid cascade. *Curr Mol Pharmacol* 2009;2: 207–14.

96. Kubera M, Lin AH, Kenis G, *et al.* Anti-Inflammatory effects of antidepressants through suppression of the interferon-gamma/interleukin-10 production ratio. *J Clin Psychopharmacol* 2001;21:199–206.

97. Pucak ML, Carroll KA, Kerr DA, Kaplin AI. Neuropsychiatric manifestations of depression in multiple sclerosis: neuroinflammatory, neuroendocrine, and neurotrophic mechanisms in the pathogenesis of immune-mediated depression. *Dialogues Clin Neurosci* 2007;9: 125–39.

98. Su KP. Biological mechanism of antidepressant effect of omega-3 fatty acids: how does fish oil act as a 'mind-body interface'? *Neurosignals* 2009;17:144–52.

60

Assessment and treatment of pain disorders in multiple sclerosis

Jahangir Maleki and Amy Sullivan

Introduction

Pain is a common complaint in individuals with multiple sclerosis (MS); however estimates of its prevalence vary widely, from 29% to 86%.[1,2] The extreme variability may be due to the wide range of research methodologies used to define and measure pain type, location, severity, duration, and impairment; unreliable data collection; variation in the study population (e.g. clinic vs. community); and sampling methods. Although MS patients usually describe their pain as widespread, chronic, severe, and disabling, pain in MS may be either acute or chronic in nature, may originate in different bodily sites, and may or may not be related to the MS disease process.[3–6]

Pain is classified as acute or chronic; each has separate causes, treatment modalities, and therapeutic goals. *Acute pain* is generally provoked by a specific injury or disease process, is usually time limited, well localized, and constant. For the most part, acute pain in MS is brief and paroxysmal, described as sharp, intermittent spasms that are spontaneous in onset. In acute pain, when the tissue injury resolves, the pain resolves. Treatment of acute pain is focused on its underlying cause. In contrast, *chronic pain* lasts longer than six months, persists beyond the apparent healing process of injury or damaged tissue, and may be considered as an independent disease state. Chronic pain may result from injury or dysfunction of the central or peripheral nervous system. Chronic pain persists regardless of disease duration or process. Chronic pain is debilitating in many ways, as it contributes to decreased quality of life through physical, social, and psychological losses. Moreover, nearly half of individuals with chronic pain acknowledge coexisting symptoms of anxiety and depression, further complicating the treatment of this disorder.[6] In MS patients, chronic pain can result from a variety of factors associated with the disease process. Little is known regarding the complex relationship between the MS disease processes and chronic pain. Stenager *et al.* conducted the only published longitudinal study of pain in MS, and found that the prevalence of chronic pain increased dramatically in MS patients over a five-year period of time.[7] Specifically, it was found that chronic back pain doubled and extremity pain tripled. Notably, the prevalence of chronic pain increased with worse Expanded Disability Status Scale (EDSS) scores.

Complexities and putative mechanisms of pain in MS patients

The presence of chronic pain in isolation or in conjunction with MS poses a major diagnostic and management challenge. In particular, an underlying diagnosis of MS adds considerably to the diagnostic and treatment complexity in patients presenting with a pain disorder. MS not only gives rise to a variety of sensory-perceptual disturbances and neuropathic pain phenomena, but also MS complicates the course of pain syndromes, and conversely, pain influences the course of MS.

Independent from MS-related neuropathic pain and other sensory-perceptual symptoms, MS-related disabilities themselves – difficulty with coordination, motor weakness, abnormal postural reflexes, visual disturbance, and the like – predisposes the individual to physical injury. Thus, MS patients have a higher incidence of injury-related acute pain. At the same time, MS-related neurological deficits impede recovery from injury, thus making the pain more likely to become chronic. Similarly, pain in and of itself results in abnormal segmental reflexes, worsening muscle spasm, contributing to disuse weakness, and may influence variety of sensory phenomena, all of which can influence the clinical findings in MS patients. Despite the increased prevalence of injury-related pain in MS patients, little is known about the interaction between pain and MS at the systemic and cellular levels. Therefore, irrespective of the underlying pathophysiologic mechanisms, the addition of pain to other symptoms of MS augments and may perpetuate the physical and psychological burden of illness.

It is very difficult to estimate the risk of common musculoskeletal pain syndromes in MS patients. However, the prevalence of chronic pain in the general population is high (e.g. lower back pain is estimated to affect ∼ 20 million people in the USA each year). It is therefore assumed that the risk of musculoskeletal pain syndromes is very high in MS as well. It is often difficult to ascertain whether low back pain, for example, is due to MS or to an independent cause. In experimental models of pain, the presence of ongoing afferent nociceptive input results in maladaptive changes across the entire neuraxis. Multiple associated peripheral and central nervous system pathophysiologic mechanisms have been identified as potentially

Multiple Sclerosis Therapeutics, Fourth Edition, ed. Jeffrey A. Cohen and Richard A. Rudick. Published by Cambridge University Press.
© Cambridge University Press 2011.

maintaining maladaptive changes such as central and peripheral sensitization, altered descending inhibition, or sympathetic sprouting. To what extent these chronic changes alter and influence overall MS symptom expression is unclear. Nevertheless, one should consider this possibility in patients who are experiencing pain symptoms, particularly when the pain does respond to pain management. Increasing disability from pain does not imply failure of MS immunomodulatory therapy.

The close reciprocal relationship and interaction between the immune system and pain-processing pathways are relevant to pain syndromes in MS. It is well known that immune- and injury-mediated inflammation are closely related to nociceptor activation, which results in neurogenic inflammation in the periphery, whereas immune-mediated glia interactions within the CNS help maintain pain at a central level. Pain-related alterations in immune and endocrine responses are also well-documented neurohumoral pituitary and adrenal stress responses. Thus, corticosteroids form the cornerstone of interventional pain management (e.g. epidural steroid injections).

The complex interactions between MS symptoms and pain make each patient unique, requiring an individualized comprehensive assessment and plan of care. Flare-up of pain symptoms commonly accompanies an MS relapse. Relapses accompanied by pain may be attributed to different causes, depending on where the patient is seen. If the evaluation is done in a pain clinic, symptom worsening might be attributed entirely to uncontrolled pain. If a neurologist sees the patient, it may be attributed entirely to the MS relapse itself. In reality, MS relapses and pain are inextricably tied together. A relatively common example is the development of lower back pain occurring in the presence of worsening weakness, spasticity, deconditioning, and impaired mobility. The back pain ensues as a result of a maladaptive and complex symptom interaction occurring in a patient with incomplete MS symptom remission. Although the patient may transiently benefit from a spinal steroid injection, not addressing other MS symptoms adequately means the pain treatment will ultimately fail. Similarly, complete resolution of symptoms is unlikely if the patient is treated only with i.v. methylprednisolone. Opiates are also frequently used as a "short-term fix" by both pain and neurology specialists. Regardless, because the underlying cause of the symptom and pain exacerbation has not been established, the patient most likely will develop additional physical and psychosocial dysfunction, increased suffering, and overall disability. Under these circumstances, collaboration between health care providers may improve outcome.

Psychological aspects of pain

Further complicating the treatment of pain is that nearly half of individuals with chronic pain acknowledge coexisting symptoms of depression, anxiety, or both.[6] Depression and anxiety may even contribute to the emergence of chronic pain in selected populations. Epidemiologic studies suggest that depression is twice as prevalent in patients with chronic medical conditions as in those without.[8]

The psychological aspects of pain are clearly included in the definition of pain, as identified by the International Association for the Study of Pain, "… an unpleasant sensory and emotional experience associated with actual or potential tissue damage or described in terms of such damage".[9] That pain "is an unpleasant sensory and emotional experience," clearly acknowledges that individuals not only physically feel pain, but also often place pain in an emotional context. For example, individuals may describe pain as not only sharp, aching, or burning but also as miserable, intolerable, agonizing, or other emotionally laden terms. Further, "…associated with actual or potential tissue damage," indicates how tissue damage is not necessary to perceive pain, but instead the mind may influence the perception of pain. Therefore, if an individual believes there is a potential for harm and, in particular, has previously experienced the harm, the pain can be perceived as quite severe.

In contrast to the general literature on psychological aspects of pain, little research has been done on the psychological aspects of pain in the MS population. A few studies have reported that psychological distress was higher among MS patients with pain than among those without.[3] As with the general pain literature, research suggests that psychosocial variables in the MS population better predict pain severity and disability than do biological or disease severity variables.[5,6] Greater pain severity is also associated with increased disability, poorer psychological functioning, female sex, increased age, non-stable MS, lower education, poorer overall health, longer duration of pain, and more health care utilization.[5,10,11] Each of these variables is also associated strongly with depression.

Consistent reports in the MS literature have shown a higher prevalence of depression, anxiety, or both in the MS population, with studies indicating that at least 50% of patients with MS experience depression at some point in their disease process.[12] This number is four times as high as that of the general, non-MS population, and three times that reported for other chronic illnesses with comparable disability (e.g. rheumatoid arthritis).[13,14] Depression and anxiety are, therefore, common and of significant clinical importance in patients with MS.

The diagnosis of depression and anxiety in the MS population is somewhat difficult to establish, as many symptoms of MS mirror or overlap several of the cardinal symptoms of depression and anxiety. Sleeping difficulties, fatigue, reduced concentration, irritability, anxiety, and depression itself are common MS symptoms. Little research has been done on anxiety in MS, and in depression, although studies have been preformed, methodological problems exist related to ascertainment of depression in this population, including lack of blinding, patient selection criteria, diagnostic criteria, and selection of appropriate control groups.[15] In addition, Minden and Schiffer showed that DSM-IV-TR criteria may not be appropriate for diagnosing depression in MS because depression in MS patients may include symptoms such as anger, irritability, worry, and discouragement, which are not symptoms associated with depression in the DSM-IV-TR.[16,17]

MS patients with psychological symptoms tend to have shorter disease duration and greater disability, as measured by the EDSS.[18] Depression can also amplify an individual's pain experience and suffering, compounding functional impairment. In addition to the high prevalence of psychosocial factors, profound physical deconditioning frequently occurs as a result of both the disease process and sedentary life. This deconditioning is characterized by a lowered exercise tolerance (e.g. walking on a treadmill) and quicker fatigue with usual daily activities (e.g. using the vacuum cleaner). Pain-related fear and avoidance are major contributors to the overall suffering, dysfunction, and disability of chronic pain.[19,20,21] As pain perception, anxiety, and inactivity increase, so does deconditioning.[22,23] Physical and psychological factors both strongly correlate with future disability, deconditioning, and use of health care services.[19] Thus, the appropriate diagnosis and treatment of both is unquestionably important, as these symptoms are reported to be among the most disabling and, thus, substantially influence the disease process and quality of life in patients with MS.

Treatment approaches for pain and associated symptoms

A comprehensive individualized plan of care is the ultimate goal for a successful functional recovery, stabilization, and prevention of relapse prevention for both MS and pain. Although short-term and unimodal treatment measures can be very effective in treating obvious and occasional pain flare-ups, recurrent and complex symptoms may necessitate a multidisciplinary assessment before a treatment plan is established. For example, infrequent pain flare-ups that are associated with other signs, and symptoms of MS relapse in general respond to treatment of the underlying MS relapse and rarely require long-term pain management. Indeed, the pain relief can even precede the remission of other MS symptoms. Long-term use of pain medications is usually unnecessary in patients with MS, but chronic non-painful sensory motor symptoms such as spasticity and dysesthesia can be a therapeutic target in a rehabilitation setting.

Similarly a pain flare-up that occurs without MS relapse can be potentially managed by adjusting previous medications or prescribing physical therapy or psychological counseling. A biopsychosocial frame of reference is very helpful when assessing a patient's underlying dysfunction and formulating a specific treatment strategy. Clearly, high-dose intravenous steroid infusion is inappropriate for every pain flare-up. Thus, identification and effective management of the primary pain generator is essential in improving patient outcome and limiting unnecessary side effects.

Patients with MS frequently have muscle spasms that increase disability, and these spasms can occur as a result of MS

but are often aggravated by pain. It is important to note that not all muscle spasms are the same and so they require detailed evaluation. Table 60.1 outlines suggested treatment strategies for some of the common spasm-related clinical conditions. Arbitrarily, one can differentiate between the following pathophysiologic mechanisms:

- *MS-related muscle spasm.* Muscle spasm commonly occurs in patients with MS in association with spasticity syndromes affecting the extremity or paraspinal muscles. Spasms may be mild, described as only an "annoyance," or can interfere with activities of daily living or sleep, limit range of motion, slow mobility, or delay activation of protective postural reflexes. Irrespective of the pain, spasticity tends to promote deconditioning, adding to pre-existing weakness and, thus, increasing the risk that the patient will fall and that recovery will be delayed from resulting injuries.

- *Pain-induced muscle spasm.* Pain, especially pain of musculoskeletal origin, is frequently associated with muscle spasm. However, in cases of acute trauma, the muscle spasm may also further irritate the injured site, serving as an independent pain generator. Muscle spasm is also frequently encountered in the myotomal distribution of an injured and/or entrapped proximal nerve such as occurs in radiculopathy. Pain-related chronic maladaptive posture and deconditioning also decrease soft tissue mobility and increase the possibility for muscle spasm.

- *Central sensitization.* Irrespective of the source of pain, i.e. whether it is MS-related or of peripheral origin, chronic pain has the capacity to generate and maintain additional pain and spasm because it facilitates central pain processing and development of what is known as "central sensitization (CS)." CS is a frequent finding in patients with fibromyalgia syndrome or complex regional pain syndrome. It leads to altered sensory processing and is frequently associated with the spread of pain in a non-dermatomal fashion. Patients commonly report spontaneous muscle pain and soreness and have an altered sensory threshold to evoked thermal and mechanical stimuli. Clinically, it can be very difficult to isolate whether it is MS or the presence of chronic pain that gives rise to CS. Nevertheless when CS is present, ongoing pain and spasms are significantly amplified, profoundly adding to the individual's overall disability. For example, patients complain more commonly of "non-painful" symptoms such as fatigue, or insomnia, while they describe the extremities as heavy and previously nonpainful movements and spasms as now being painful.

- *Muscle spasm and psychosocial comorbidity.* While the sources of pain-related muscle spasm can be multiple, the concomitant presence of spasticity from MS, along with psychological factors such as stress-induced muscle tension, pain behaviors, and somatization disorder add to the complexity of the clinical presentation.

Table 60.1. *Treatment of musculoskeletal pain syndromes in MS*

Pathomechanism of spasm	Treatment options	Examples
MS-related spasticity	Muscle relaxants	Baclofen, tizanidine
Trauma-related muscle spasm	Combination of muscle relaxants with nonsteroidal anti-inflammatory drugs and/or opiates	Cyclobenzaprine, Ibuprofen with or without narcotic analgesic
Focal dystonia	Chemodenervation	Botulinum toxin injection
Myofascial pain	Trigger point injection	In conjunction with other measures blocks performed with local anesthetic +/− steroids can provide significant and immediate relief, thus limiting deconditioning and facilitating recovery.
Radiculopathy	Selective nerve root block	
Facet syndrome with paraspinal spasm or arthritis related periarticular spasm ("en bloc movement")	Intra-articular extremity and/or paraspinal joint injection	
Maladaptive stress-induced muscle tension	Education and self- management techniques	Relaxation, biofeedback, improved coping skills, self- hypnosis
Deconditioning with maladaptive posture, muscle tension, and restricted soft tissue mobility	Education and physical therapy and home exercise program	Behavioral modification, active exercise, myofascial release +/− passive thermal modalities
Somatization disorder	Education and psychotherapy	Cognitive behavioral therapy

Most monophasic symptoms can be safely treated by considering a specific treatment modality similar to those for musculoskeletal pain syndromes as outlined in Table 60.1. In contrast to occasional symptom flare-ups, recurrent, frequent, or progressive episodes require a more in-depth assessment and often multidisciplinary management. This is particularly true when multiple symptoms from the physical and psychosocial domains are simultaneously present, when symptoms are not directly associated with identifiable structural pathology, or when symptoms that originate from a structural lesion but become chronic beyond the time required for healing. Due to complex interactions between different symptoms and the presence of pre- and co-existing medical and psychosocial conditions, identification of underlying pain generators and their mechanisms may not be straightforward. Under such circumstances, a biopsychosocial approach is more likely to reveal the complicated nature of the symptom expression and its underlying mechanisms.

As such, symptom management along with physical and psychosocial rehabilitation builds the basis for a successful recovery; thus educating patients about psychophysical consequences of recurrent symptoms at any point can only improve the outcome. While balancing the risks and benefits, and based on findings in clinical assessment, one may consider symptomatic management by using one or a combination of the following pharmacotherapy approaches.

In treating neuropathic pain, classically the trigeminal neuralgia has been treated with carbamazepine. Other neuropathic pain phenomena associated with dysesthesia, paresthesia, hyperesthesia, allodynia, hyperalgesia, and hyperpathia are best treated by initiating therapy with one of the newer generation antiepileptic drugs (e.g. gabapentin). Occasionally, one may need to add a second antiepileptic drug, which should be done once other aspects of pain management are addressed, rather than just relying on one modality of treatment and/or one class of drugs.

Management of spasticity is a cornerstone of treatment. Muscle spasm may be intermittent, interfering with the activities of daily living, such as resting, ambulation, and or sleep. It may be also present as the result of any of the above neuropathic symptoms, or it can result in generation of a variety of neuropathic symptoms by compressing upon peripheral neural structures. Frequently, ongoing "painless" muscle spasm, especially across the paraspinal muscle groups, can give rise to chronic maladaptive posture and secondary musculoskeletal pain disorders. If findings point toward intermittent or ongoing muscle spasm, adequate management of the spasm in conjunction with the neuropathic symptoms is a reasonable approach.

Familiarity with the pharmacology of neurotropic medications is essential for initiating and maintaining a safe and effective treatment protocol. As an example, treatment with gabapentin can be started at a dose of 100 to 300 mg at night with gradual titration to three times daily followed by an increase to 600 or 900 and eventually 1200 mg twice daily. Rarely, patients may not be able to tolerate this titration, in which case the liquid form (50 mg/ml) is preferred and a slower titration schedule should be adopted. Similarly, tizanidine can be initiated at the lowest dose of 1 to 2 mg at night (i.e. one-quarter to one-half tablet of a 4 mg tablet) to prevent daytime somnolence (a major side effect) while improving sleep. The dose can than be increased gradually up to 4 to 8 mg at night, if necessary. Once the upper dose is tolerated, one can also add a lower dose during the daytime.

Additional application of topical agents such as lidocaine (Lidoderm patch) can potentiate the effect of gabapentin if the epicenter of the pain is more localized or if superficial cutaneous hypersensitivity and signs of CS and neuropathic symptoms are present. Other topical alternatives used off-label includes ketamine and doxepin cream. Topical diclofenac (Flector patch) may also prove to be effective, especially if one suspects an

Table 60.2. *List of commonly used medication in management of neuropathic pain*

	Medication	Initial dose (mg)	Effective dose (mg)	Comments
Anti-epileptics	Gabapentin	100 tid	300–1200 tid	Approved for treatment of PHN and DPNP
	Pregabalin	50 bid	150 bid-tid	Approved for treatment of PHN, DPNP & Fibromyalgia
	Levetiracetam	250 bid	750 bid-tid	Available as i.v. and ER formulations
	Carbamazepine	100 bid	300–600 bid	Approved for TGN; Available in ER form
	Valproate	250 bid	500–750 tid	Available as i.v. and ER formulations
	Topiramate	25 bid	150 bid	Risk of kidney stone, hypoglycemia and possible hyperchloremic, non-anion gap metabolic acidosis
Antidepressants*	Doxepin	10–20 hs	100 hs	Possible anticholinergic side effects and orthostatic hypotension; assessment of patients for ischemic heart disease, heart failure and arrhythmias including an EKG for conduction abnormalities prior to the initiation of therapy is recommended
	Nortriptyline	10–25 hs	50–150 hs	
	Amitriptyline	10–25 hs	50–150 hs	
	Duloxetine	20 qd	60 qd	Approved for PHN, DPNP and musculoskeletal pain
	Venlafaxine	37.5 qd	150–225 qd	Multiple studies show potential benefit
	Milnacipran	12.5 qd	50 bid	Approved for fibromyalgia
Muscle Relaxants	Baclofen	5 bid-tid	10–20 tid	Also available as intrathecal preparation
	Tizanidine	1–2 hs	4–8 tid	Slow titration; Elevation of LFTs in <5%.
	Cyclobenzaprine	5 tid	10 tid	Available in ER formulation
	Metaxalone	400 tid	800 tid-qid	Relatively weak but may be used as an adequate alternative in sensitive patients
	Methocarbamol	500 tid	500–750 tid-qid	
Miscellaneous	Lidocaine Patch	I-III Patches	III per 12 hrs	Topical 5% patch approved for PHN
	Lidocaine IV	1.5–2 mg/KG	1 mg/KG/hr	Lidocaine infusion requires close cardiac monitoring
	Capsaicin Cream	0.025% tid	0.075% tid-qid	Requires several weeks of therapy for effectiveness
	Ketamine Cream	50 tid	100 tid	Topical ketamine requires compounding

Abbreviations: PHN = Post herpetic neuralgia; TGN = Trigeminal neuralgia; DPNP = Diabetic peripheral neuropathy; qd = once a day; bid = twice a day; tid = three times a day; hs = every night; IV = intravenous; LFT = Lever enzyme test; ER = Extended release. * Additional risks of increased suicide in young individuals. Doses are guidelines only. Dosage recommendations listed in this table are attributable to published literature, manufacturers' package inserts, and adjustments from adult-dosing guidelines; some dosages reflect clinical practice experiences. Actual dose requirements may vary based on clinical indication, age, and patient weight. Doses should be individualized and titrated based on clinical response and adverse effects.
Adapted from: Lussier D, Huskey AG, Portenoy RK. Adjuvant analgesics in cancer pain has management. *Oncologist*, 2004; 9: 571–91.
Miaskowski C. American Pain Society, Clinical Practice Guideline Development Committee (2008). *Principles of Analgesics Use in the Treatment of Acute Pain and Cancer Pain*. 6th edn.

underlying inflammatory process, such as that following blunt trauma (Table 60.2).

When used in the right setting, such as post-operative pain, cancer pain, acute pain conditions, or to bridge a treatment gap, opiates are excellent drugs to consider. Morphine's analgesic effect is exceptional when compared to that of NSAIDs. In general, knowledge gained from the treatment of cancer pain has prompted an enormous growth in opiate prescription for non-malignant pain over the past 15 to 20 years. Unfortunately, despite this growth, there has been not only no decline but rather a reported growth in the number of patients with chronic pain. During the same time, a major increase in drug diversion and illegal marketing of opiates has occurred, which has

resulted in major sanctions and much debate across pain organizations, state medical boards, and the Food and Drug Administration.

Except for situations when one is dealing with acute pain or there is a transient need, the long-term use of opiates and benzodiazepines can be very complicated and may result in long-term treatment failure. Due to the psychotropic effects of these medications, it is very likely that comorbid psychopathology such as chronic depression and anxiety are not properly managed, resulting in administration of escalating doses of narcotics and eventually treatment-refractory pain. Indeed, in patients who have become tolerant to high doses of narcotics, the effect of other neurotropic medications is extremely limited. As such, opiates raise the possibility not only of the development of tolerance but also cross-resistance to at least some other neurotropic medications. To our knowledge, no research has addressed this aspect of opiate therapy. We suggest that practitioners who would like to prescribe long-term opiates in exceptional MS cases familiarize themselves in depth with effects, side effects, interactions, the different formulations, risk assessment and mitigation, including the use of an opiate contract, documentation and regulatory restrictions, and reporting guidelines.

Effective treatment of depression associated with pain

With the high psychological and pain comorbidities noted in the MS population, treatment should include assessment, diagnosis, and attention to the myriad of symptoms an MS patient is likely experiencing. Effective treatment of psychological conditions generally includes both psychopharmacology and psychotherapy. To date, only two randomized blinded trials of antidepressant therapy have been conducted in the MS population, leaving little evidence guiding treatment decisions in this population. Schiffer studied desipramine in 24 patients with MS in a double-blinded trial with psychotherapy. There was a trend toward modest "benefit," but this study was likely underpowered to show an effect.[15] Ehde et al. did a parallel, placebo-controlled, double-blinded study of paroxetine in 42 patients and showed depression decreased as measured by the Hamilton Depression Rating Scale vs. controls, but this difference was not statistically significant.[24]

Proper diagnosis and adequate treatment of depression are key to a successful outcome. While one may consider using tricyclic antidepressants or duloxetine (Cymbalta) for management of depression and pain, if the depression is severe, it should be addressed by a psychiatrist. Indeed, treating the different aspects of mood disorder and providing adequate psychosocial support is beyond the scope of a routine neurological or pain management clinic. Similarly, use of neuroleptics to potentiate antidepressant efficacy or to improve various aspects of psychopathology should be managed within a mental health practice. Similarly, the use of benzodiazepines should be limited to short-term symptomatic treatment of mood and anxiety disorders.

Regarding psychotherapy approaches, a referral to a health/medical psychologist who is specifically trained in the management of chronic illness and disease is warranted. Several approaches are employed to treat depression and comorbid pain in patients with MS. The effectiveness of cognitive behavioral therapy has been well examined in the MS literature[25] and thus several principles are utilized in MS treatment. In addition, behavioral strategies,[26] such as relaxation training, assertiveness training, and fear hierarchies can be appropriately used for pain management, couples therapy, and depression and anxiety management. Lazarus and Folkman's[27] coping literature, motivational interviewing,[28] as well as methods from interpersonal theories can all be utilized. The goals of health psychology are appropriate coping and adjustment to MS and the disease process, improved functioning in several domains, and an emotionally and physically healthy lifestyle.

In addition to psychotropics and psychotherapy, exercise has been found to be effective for managing pain and mood. In a study by Sullivan, Covington, and Scheman, a 10-minute exercise protocol led to significant immediate improvements in both anxiety and depression, and over a three-week span in an intensive outpatient chronic pain program, pain significantly improved.[29]

For patients who show severe functional and psychological impairments, effective treatment requires awareness of, and attention to, both physical and psychological factors. With the high level of psychological comorbidity, treatment in an interdisciplinary pain rehabilitation program is considered the premier treatment for patients with MS and chronic pain.[30-33] Such programs have been found to markedly increase physical activity in formerly sedentary patients.[30] In a few weeks' time, individuals involved in endurance training (e.g. walking, biking) begin to perform physical and daily living activities comfortably and for prolonged periods at exercise intensities that they did not maintain prior to the training. Treatment in interdisciplinary pain rehabilitation programs improves pain, function, and mood in severely impaired individuals with pain.[30-32]

References

1. Clifford DB, Trotter JL. Pain in multiple sclerosis. *Arch Neurol* 1984; 41(12): 1270–72.

2. Stenager E, Knudsen L, Jensen K. Acute and chronic pain syndromes in multiple sclerosis: A 5 year follow-up study. *Ital Neurol Sci* 1995; 16: 629–32.

3. Ehde DM, Gibbons LE, Chwastiak L, et al. Chronic pain in a large community sample of persons with multiple sclerosis. *Mult Scler* 2003; 9(6): 605–11.

4. Ehde DM, Osborne TL, Jensen MP. Chronic pain in persons with multiple sclerosis. *Phys Med Rehabil Clin N A* 2005; 16(2): 503–12.

5. Ehde DM, Osborne TL, Hanley MA, et al. The scope and nature of pain in persons with multiple sclerosis. *Mult Scler* 2006; 12(5): 629–38.

6. Marcus D. Treatment of nonmalignant chronic pain. *Am Fam Physician* 2000; 61(5): 1331–46.

7. Stenager E., Knudsen L., Jensen K. Acute and chronic pain syndromes in multiple sclerosis: a 5 year follow-up study. *Ital J Neurol Sci* 1995; 16: 629–32.

8. Goldmann Consensus Group. Goldmann consensus statement on depression in multiple sclerosis: *Mult Scler* 2005; 11: 3328–37.

9. IASP Pain Terminology: International Association for the Study of Pain. 1973. http://www.iasp-pain.org/AM/Template.cfm?Section=

General_Resource_Links&Template=
/CM/HTMLDisplay.cfm&ContentID=
3058#Pain. (Accessed September 17,
2010.)

10. Osborne TL, Raichle KA, Jensen MP, *et al.* The reliability and validity of pain interference measures in persons with multiple sclerosis. *J Pain Symptom Manage* 2006; 32(3): 217–29.

11. O'Connor AB, Schwid SR, Herrmann DN, *et al.* Pain associated with multiple sclerosis: systematic review and proposed classification. *Pain* 2008; 137(1): 96–111.

12. Sadovnick AD, Remick RA, Allen J, *et al.* Depression and multiple sclerosis. *Neurology* 1996; 46: 628–32.

13. Wilhelm K, Mitchell P, Slade T, *et al.* Prevalence and correlates of DSM-IV major depression in an Australian national survey. *J Affect Disord* 2003; 75:155–62.

14. Pincus T, Griffith J, Pearce S, *et al.* Prevalence of self-reported depression in patients with rheumatoid arthritis. *Br J Rheumatol* 1996; 35: 879–83.

15. Schiffer RB, Wineman NM. Antidepressant pharmacotherapy of depression associated with multiple sclerosis. *Am J Psychiatry* 1990; 147: 11.

16. Minden SL, Schiffer B. Depression and mood disorders in multiple sclerosis. *Neuropsychiatry Neuropsychol Behav Neurol* 1991; 4(1): 62–77.

17. American Psychiatric Association. *Diagnostic and Statistical Manual of Mental Disorders* (4th edn, text revision). Washington, DC: APA, 2000.

18. Chwastiak L, Ehde DM, Gibbons LE, *et al.* Depressive symptoms and severity of illness in multiple sclerosis: epidemiologic study of a large community sample. *Am J Psychiatry* 2002; 159: 1862–8.

19. Carragee E. Persistent low back pain. *N Engl J Med* 2005; 352: 1891–8.

20. Crombez G, Vlaeyen JW, Heuts PH, *et al.* Fear of pain is more disabling than the pain itself: further evidence on the role of pain-related fear in chronic back pain disability. *Pain* 1999; 80: 529–39.

21. Turk DC, Okifuji A. Psychological factors in chronic pain: evolution and revolution. *J Consulting Clin Psych* 2002; 70(3): 678–90.

22. Brox J, Sorensen R, Friis A, *et al.* Randomized clinical trial of lumbar instrumented fusion and cognitive intervention and exercise in patients with chronic low back pain and disc degeneration. *Spine* 2003; 28(17): 1913–21.

23. Turner-Stokes L, Erkeller-Yuksel F, Miles A, *et al.* Outpatient cognitive behavioral pain management programs: a randomized comparison of a group-based multidisciplinary versus an individual therapy model. *Arch Phys Med Rehabil* 2003; 84: 781–8.

24. Ehde DM, Kraft GH, Chwastiak L, *et al.* Efficacy of paroxetine in treating major depressive disorder in persons with multiple sclerosis. *Gen Hosp Psychiatry* 2008; 30(1): 40–8.

25. Mohr DC, Boudewyn AC, Goodkin DE, *et al.* Comparative outcomes for individual cognitive-behavioral therapy, supportive-expressive group therapy, and sertraline for the treatment of depression in multiple sclerosis. *J Consulting Clin Psych* 2001; 69: 942–9.

26. Wolpe J, Lazarus A. *Behavior Therapy Techniques: A Guide to the Treatment of Neuroses.* Oxford: Pergamon Press, 1966.

27. Lazarus R, Folkman S. *Stress, Appraisal, and Coping.* New York: Springer Publishing Co., 1984

28. Emmons KM, Rollnick S. Motivational interviewing in health care settings: Opportunities and limitations. *Am J Preventative Med* 2001; 20(1): 68–74.

29. Sullivan AB, Covington E, Scheman J. Immediate benefits of a brief 10-minute exercise protocol in a chronic pain population: a pilot study. *Pain Med* 2010; 11(4): 524–9.

30. Flor H, Fydrich T, Turk D. Efficacy of multidisciplinary pain treatment centers: a meta-analytic review. *Pain* 1992; 49(2): 221–30.

31. Gatchel R, Okifuji A. Evidence-based scientific data documenting the treatment and cost-effectiveness of comprehensive pain programs for chronic nonmalignant pain *J Pain* 2006; 7(11): 779–93.

32. Friedrich M, Gittler G, Arendasy M, *et al.* Long-term effect of a combined exercise and motivational program on the level of disability of patients with chronic low back pain *Spine* 2005; 30: 995–1000.

Management of medical comorbidities in patients with multiple sclerosis

John R. Scagnelli and Myla D. Goldman

Introduction

Multiple sclerosis (MS), a chronic debilitating disease of the central nervous system (CNS), typically presents in individuals during the second to fourth decade of life. Traditionally thought to occur in otherwise healthy individuals, little was known about the incidence and relevance of comorbidities in persons living with MS. Emerging research has broadened our understanding about the relationship between comorbidities, general medical health maintenance, MS disease progression, and MS treatment modalities. These comorbid conditions may impact time to diagnosis, lessen patients' well-being, contribute towards further disability as MS patient's age, and affect immune-targeted therapy choice. In this chapter we discuss the prevalence, diagnosis, and management of medical comorbidities seen in patients with MS. We review what is known about how other medical conditions impact the natural history of MS. Lastly, we discuss the management of disease-modifying medications in MS patients with other medical conditions.

Immunization

While the exact causative agent in MS is unknown, current evidence suggests that environmental factors coupled with genetic susceptibility results in disease expression. Potential environmental triggers have been extensively researched; one debate has been the practice of population-based immunization protocols and the risk for MS.

Vaccinations are important for overall health, but may also be beneficial for MS patients by preventing infection. The American Academy of Neurology (AAN) states that "there is definitive evidence for an increased risk of MS relapses during the weeks around an infectious episode (Level A Recommendation)" in their 2002 summary statement on *Immunization and MS*.[1] In a study of 34 patients, 48% of MS relapses were associated with infections and 40% of infections were associated with MS relapses.[2] MS relapses have been linked to time periods around influenza infection, nasopharyngeal infections, and the common cold.[3]

Vaccination during relapse

In individuals with MS, recommendations for vaccination are generally consistent with those put forth by the Centers for Disease Control (CDC) for patients with chronic neurologic illnesses.[1] One exception is during times of MS relapse. Although the literature does not support increases in relapse following vaccination, the potential for febrile episodes following vaccination has the potential to worsen or delay functional recovery during times of relapse. When there is no medical contraindication for delaying vaccination (e.g. tetanus vaccination following a wound), vaccination should be delayed for 4–6 weeks following relapse.[1]

Live-attenuated vaccines

Live-attenuated vaccines are created by reducing the virulence of a pathogen but still keeping it in a living and active state. Currently available live-attenuated vaccines include measles, mumps and rubella vaccine (MMR), varicella zoster vaccine, oral polio vaccine (Sabin), and the nasal-spray flu vaccine. Below, we discuss varicella infection and vaccination. See Table 61.1 for information regarding the other live-attenuated vaccines.

Varicella

Varicella Zoster Virus (VZV) is a human herpes virus that causes the clinical syndromes of chicken pox and shingles. Exposure to VZV is nearly ubiquitous by adolescence in developed countries. Complications of infection in immune-competent patients include rash, post-herpetic neuralgia, ocular complications such as uveitis, motor neuropathy, and meningitis.[5] In the immune-compromised host, which includes MS patients currently taking immunosuppressive drugs, the complications can be more severe including encephalitis, transverse myelitis, and disseminated zoster which recently contributed to the death of an MS patient in a Phase 3 clinical trial of fingolimod (Gilenya).[6]

There has been much interest regarding VZV infection as a potential etiologic agent for MS. Patients with both

Multiple Sclerosis Therapeutics, Fourth Edition, ed. Jeffrey A. Cohen and Richard A. Rudick. Published by Cambridge University Press.
© Cambridge University Press 2011.

Table 61.1. *CDC vaccination recommendations*[4]

Vaccine	Type	Immunocompetent with chronic neurologic disease	Immunocompromized/ immunosuppressed	Pregnant
Hepatitis B	Inactivated	3 dose series recommended if another risk factor is present (i.e. health care worker, HIV infection, sexual risk factors)		
HPV	Inactivated	3 doses for females up to age 26		Not recommended
Influenza	Inactivated	Annual vaccination for all patients >6 months of age		
Influenza (oral)	Attenuated	Contraindicated	Contraindicated	Contraindicated
Measles, mumps, rubella	Attenuated	2 doses	Contraindicated	Contraindicated
Meningococcal	Inactivated	Recommended only if another risk factor is present	Recommended only if another risk factor is present	Recommended only if another risk factor is present
Pneumococcal	Inactivated	Recommended only if another risk factor is present	Recommended	Recommended only if another risk factor is present
TDaP/TD	Inactivated	TDaP once, then TD booster every 10 years (Tdap contraindicated in pregnancy)		
Varicella	Attenuated	2 doses	Contraindicated	Contraindicated
Zoster	Attenuated	2 doses when >60 years of age	Contraindicated	Contraindicated

CDC = Centers for Disease Control, HIV = Human immunodeficiency virus, HPV = human papilloma virus, TDaP = tetanus diphtheria acellular pertussis.

relapsing–remitting (RR) and primary progressive MS have significantly increased titers of VZV in lymphocytes as well as in the CNS.[7] In RRMS, the presence of VZV particles in cerebrospinal fluid is greatly increased around the time of MS relapse. In one study, VZV DNA was found in 95% of MS patients during times of relapse.[8] While this does not prove causation, the association between VZV infection and MS relapse warrants further investigation.

VZV vaccination has been shown to reduce the incidence of VZV infection by 51%.[9] Not only does the vaccine appear to be safe, with almost no serious side effects of vaccination, including autoimmune reactions,[10] but also evidence that VZV vaccination may actually be protective in MS has been reported.[11] In a study of VZV vaccination in MS patients with a 12-month follow-up, 27% of patients had improvement in their clinical status. Vaccination is recommended for all patients without previous VZV infection. For the newly approved medication, fingolimod, VZV titers and vaccination for those with insufficient titers, prior to onset of therapy is recommended.[12]

Inactivated vaccines

Inactivated vaccines are those that contain virus particles that have been killed. The virus is not living. However, viral proteins contained within can be recognized by the immune system. Currently available inactivated vaccines include: Hepatitis B (Hep B), influenza, tetanus, and polio vaccine (Salk). Hep B, influenza and tetanus are discussed in detail as they have been studied most in MS. For information regarding other inactivated vaccines refer to Table 61.1.

Hepatitis B

Hep B vaccine is effective in preventing chronic infection in over 95% of vaccinated patients.[13] Hepatitis B infection can result in acute liver failure and chronic infection has been associated

with hepatocellular cancer; the public health impact of vaccination is of great importance.

There has been concern regarding the safety of the Hep B vaccine in both population-based programs and in MS patients specifically. The concern originated in France when over 200 cases of CNS demyelination were reported shortly after the 1996 vaccine season.[14] The French government suspended the Hep B vaccine program shortly thereafter. Since that time, there have been many studies investigating Hep B vaccination and the risk of subsequent demyelination. Ascherio *et al.* studied a large cohort subgroup from the Nurse's Health Study to evaluate the risk of MS after Hep B vaccination.[15] This study along with many others found no association between vaccination and the incidence of MS. Based on cumulative available evidence, the AAN panel for clinical guidelines recommended Hep B vaccinations for those individuals at risk, including health care workers, inmates, family members of Hep B patients, and unvaccinated adolescents.[1] Following these recommendations, Hernan *et al.* reported on the relationship between Hep B vaccination and MS symptom onset. They found a 3.1-fold risk for MS symptom onset within three years of vaccination compared to the non-vaccinated population.[16] Thus, the question regarding Hep B vaccination and the risk for MS remains unanswered; however the potential benefits from vaccination are likely to outweigh the risks of vaccination.

Influenza

Each year, health care providers are faced with decisions about whether to recommend influenza vaccination to MS patients. In a placebo-controlled trial of influenza vaccination, safety was established with no increase in MS relapse or pseudorelapse associated with vaccine administration.[17] Additionally, there was no change in disease course in patients who were vaccinated during the six months following vaccination. The

Table 61.2. *Drugs during pregnancy and lactation*[24]

Drug	FDA class	Use during pregnancy	Presence in Milk	Use during breast feeding
Cyclophosphamide	D	Not recommended	Yes	Not recommended
Dalfampradine	C	Not recommended	Unknown	Not recommended
Fingolimod	C	Not recommended	Unknown	Not recommended
Glatiramer acetate	B	Probably safe	Yes	Not recommended
Interferon beta 1a and 1b	C	Not recommended	Unknown	Not recommended
Intravenous immunoglobulin	C	Probably Safe	Yes	Probably safe
Methotrexate	X	Contraindicated	Yes	Contraindicated
Methylprednisolone	C	Yes	Yes	Probably safe
Mitoxantrone	D	Not recommended	Yes	Not recommended
Natalizumab	C	Not recommended	Unknown?	Not recommended

Immunization Panel of the Multiple Sclerosis Council for Clinical Practice Guidelines recommends influenza vaccination citing "strong evidence for an increased risk of MS relapse during the weeks around an infectious episode".[1] As of March 2010, the CDC recommended the influenza vaccine for all people over the age of six months and particularly for groups at high risk for complications of influenza infection. Patients with neurologic illnesses, including MS, are amongst the groups in this high-risk category.[18]

Tetanus

Administration of the tetanus–diphtheria–acellular pertussis (TDaP) vaccine is routinely recommended in children, with a tetanus–diphtheria (TD) booster recommended at 11 to 12 years of age and at 10-year intervals throughout life.[19] Despite this recommendation, studies have shown the actual immunity among adults in the United States to be only 43%.[20]

Tetanus immunity has been linked with a risk reduction for the development of MS. Hernan *et al.* report an odds ratio of 0.67 for developing MS in those who have received the tetanus vaccine.[21] The mechanism for protection of the tetanus vaccine is not clear but it may relate to the inclusion of a peptide that can bind to MHC class II epitopes. This may lead to a shift from a Th1 to a Th2 biological response.[21] It remains unclear whether tetanus vaccination is beneficial for the overall disease course of MS; however, it is clear that MS patients should receive vaccination per CDC guidelines.

Immunization and MS disease treatment

Immunization in the setting of immune-targeted medications raises concerns about vaccine effectiveness. Interferon beta (IFNβ) does not affect the ability to mount titers after vaccination.[22] It is assumed that glatiramer acetate (GA, Copaxone) similarly does not affect titer formation after vaccination, although this is not known. There is not much known about the effectiveness of vaccines in MS patients on immunosupressants; however, there is evidence from the bone marrow transplant literature that patients with severe levels of

immunosupression may not mount an antibody response after vaccination.[22] Patients being treated with immunosuppressants should not be immunized with live, attenuated vaccines such as VZV or MMR as this could potentiate the expression of the actual infectious disease.[17] In the recent trial with fingolimod there was a death in the treatment arm of disseminated Zoster.[5] For patients on immunosupressants, the effectiveness of inactivated vaccines may be decreased and there may be a safety concern with the use of live, attenuated vaccinations. If possible, both types of vaccines should be administered prior to initiation of these therapies.[11]

Reproductive issues

MS occurs in greatest numbers among woman of child-bearing age. The prevalence and natural history of pregnancy and MS is covered elsewhere in this book. Herein, we will focus on the management of MS before, during, and after pregnancy.

Immunomodulatory management of MS in pregnancy

See Table 61.2 for complete listing.

Interferon beta

None of the four IFNβ preparations approved as MS therapy (Avonex, Betaseron, Extavia, Rebif) has been formally studied in pregnancy, and, therefore, all are Class C medications. There are, however, data from clinical trials in which patients became pregnant while receiving drug. A study published in 2005 pooled pregnancy data on IFNβ-1a from eight clinical trials.[25] This included 41 pregnancies that occurred within two weeks of the last medication injection. The incidence of spontaneous abortion was 22% compared to an average rate of spontaneous abortion in recognized pregnancies of about 15%.[26] Another investigation of 23 IFNβ-exposed pregnancies[27] revealed a significant increase in spontaneous abortions when compared to unexposed MS patients and healthy women. All MS patients discontinued therapy in the first trimester of pregnancy.

Additionally, there was an increased risk for lower birth weight amongst infants exposed to IFNβ. Because of the increased risk of spontaneous abortion, it is recommended that women of child-bearing age who are taking IFNβ therapy use birth control and discontinue drug before attempting pregnancy. Women with unplanned pregnancies should be advised to discontinue drug at the time of pregnancy discovery. Elective pregnancy termination is not advised. A pregnancy registry is available for each of the IFNβ drugs. Information about these registries can be found at clinicaltrials.gov.

Glatiramer acetate

Neurologists' practice patterns show a preference for GA in pregnancy.[28] GA has been studied in pregnancy.[27] It is a pregnancy Class B medication. In a case series of 13 women with MS, there were 14 pregnancies and 13 live births.[27] Nine infants were exposed to GA at conception, pregnancy, and delivery. Mean birth weight was in the normal range. There does not appear to be an increased risk of spontaneous abortions or poor fetal outcomes with GA. In the above study and in other observational studies the risk of spontaneous abortion appears to be consistent with that of healthy, untreated pregnancies. In the post-marketing surveillance the miscarriage rate was 17% amongst 277 known pregnancies.[28]

Natalizumab

Natalizumab (Tysabri) is a pregnancy Class C medication. It has not been studied in humans but has been shown to decrease fertility in animal models.[29] The preliminary results from the Tysabri Pregnancy Exposure Registry revealed no increase in miscarriages among natalizumab-exposed patients compared to the general population.[30] Women receiving natalizumab are advised not to get pregnant and to use birth control to avoid pregnancy. If patients become pregnant on natalizumab, the medication should be discontinued. The Tysabri Pregnancy Exposure Registry can be accessed at clinicaltrials.gov.

Fingolimod

Fingolimod is a pregnancy Class C medication. It has not been studied in humans; however, it has been associated with teratogenicity and spontaneous abortions in animal models.[12] Fingolimod has a long half-life, requiring up to two months to be eliminated from the body. Women should use birth control to avoid pregnancy during fingolimod therapy and for two months following discontinuation. There is a Gilenya pregnancy registry which can be accessed at clinicaltrial.gov.

Management of MS relapse in pregnancy

Relapses tend to occur less frequently in pregnancy. The risk of relapse is higher in the first and second trimester, annualized relapse rate 0.5 compared to the 0.2 in the third trimester.[31] Intravenous methylprednisolone (IVMP) is a pregnancy Class C medication. There is no evidence that IVMP is directly harmful to the fetus.[24] In patients with disease activity during pregnancy, thought should be given to the effects of high-dose steroids on the mother including but not limited to cataracts, an increased incidence of infection, bone loss, glucose intolerance, hypertension, premature rupture of membranes, and preeclampsia.[24] Intravenous gamma globulin (IVIg) is a pregnancy Class C medication. IVIg has not been approved as a treatment for MS but it has been studied in pregnancy to prevent relapses.[32] IVIg was administered to pregnant women for five consecutive days every six weeks. Annualized relapse rate in this group was 0.43 in the first trimester, 0.15 in the second trimester and 0.00 in the third trimester, significantly reduced compared to no IVIg. No severe adverse events were associated with IVIg treatment in mothers or fetuses either during the pregnancy or post-partum period.

Breast feeding

The risk for MS relapse is higher in the post-partum period.[31] Many new mothers would like to breast feed, and there is certainly much known about the positive long-term consequences of breast feeding on children. Patients with MS who deliver and would like to breast feed will often worry about the risk of breast feeding and post-partum relapses. Additionally, they may be concerned about immunomodulatory medications (see Table 61.2) and breast feeding.

Recent data suggest that breast feeding may have a protective effect on the risk of post partum relapse. Women who breast fed exclusively for two months following pregnancy were five times less likely to relapse compared with women who did not exclusively breast feed.[33] The reason for this is unclear, but it has been postulated to be related to prolonged return of menses in these women. Based on this study, it appears safe and perhaps preferable for patients to breast feed their infants as long as they will be breast feeding exclusively.

Hormonal therapy

The dichotomy of disease activity intrapartum and post-partum is theorized to be related to shifts of sex hormones during these times.[30] Similarly, an increase in MS-related symptoms around the time of menses has been described.[34]

Estrogen

Estrogen has powerful immunomodulatory effects that can be seen in a variety of animal models.[35] Estrogen levels are increased throughout pregnancy and then decrease in the postpartum period, which may in part relate to the decrease relapse rate during the former and the increased rate during the latter.[35] A study of exogenous estrogen in the form of estriol in MS women showed decreased gadolinium-enhancing lesions on MRI in patients treated with estriol; when the hormone was discontinued, enhancing lesions were increased.[36] There currently are no clinical data regarding the long-term use of estrogen in patients with MS. However, there are three trials currently enrolling to investigate the effects of exogenous

Table 61.3. *Medications that reduce the efficacy of oral contraception*[38]

1. Broad spectrum antibiotics
2. Carbamezapine (Tegretol)
3. Dantrolene
4. Modafinil (Provigil)
5. Phenytoin (Dilantin)
6. Topiramate (Topamax)

estrogen on MS disease course and more information can be found at clinicaltrials.gov.

Oral contraception

Although estrogen replacement may decrease disease activity in MS, oral contraceptive use does not affect the risk of developing MS or change the disease course.[37] The frequency of contraceptive use is unknown in the MS population. Studies have shown that in those patients who use contraceptives, 86% prefer oral hormonal contraceptives.[28] There are, however, concerns regarding oral contraception in MS patients. The effectiveness of oral contraception can be reduced with many medications used commonly in the MS population (see Table 61.3). Patients taking these medications should be advised to add an additional form of contraception or switch to a non-hormonal form of primary contraception. Additionally, oral contraceptives raise the risk of deep venous thrombosis and caution should be used in MS patients with impaired mobility in which the risk of deep vein thrombosis is also increased.[38]

Hormone-assisted reproduction

Data suggest that MS alone does not affect ability to conceive;[31] however, in the USA infertility impacts 10% of the female population.[4] Some MS patients will therefore seek reproductive counseling for hormonal therapy to achieve pregnancy. Therapies that may be used include anti-estrogen techniques (clomiphene, citrate, etc.), gonadotropin techniques, gonadotrophin releasing hormone (GnRH) agonists or antagonists. In a retrospective analysis of in vitro fertilization (IVF) in six MS patients, a significant increase in relapse rate was seen in the three months following treatment in patients who received GnRH agonists, but not antagonists.[39] All patients had stopped their immunomodulatory therapies one year prior to fertility treatment and none of the patients had MS relapse during the three months before treatment. This pilot study provides preliminary evidence that IVF, depending on the approach used may induce MS activity. Until more is known about this, decisions regarding IVF therapy should be discussed on a case-by-case basis with a reproductive specialist.

Bone health
Osteoporosis and osteopenia

Osteopenia and osteoporosis are common diseases in the general population; the risk is greatest in Caucasian woman after the onset of menopause.[40] Osteopenia and osteoporosis are similar diseases on a spectrum of bone loss disorders.

Table 61.4. *Risk factors for osteoporosis and fracture*[41]

Major risk factors	Minor risk factors
• Personal history of fracture as an adult	• Impaired vision[a]
• History of fracture in a first degree relative	• Estrogen deficiency at an early age
• Low body weight	• Dementia[a]
• Current smoking	• Poor health or frailty[a]
• Use of daily oral corticosteroids[a]	• Recent falls[a]
	• Low calcium intake
	• Low physical activity[a]
	• >2 alcoholic drinks per day

[a] Risk factors associated with multiple sclerosis.

Osteopenia is defined as a bone mineral density (BMD) of greater than 1.0 standard deviation (SD) below the reference mean; osteoporosis is defined as a bone density greater than 2.5 SD below the reference mean.[41] This is an important distinction as the relative risk of hip fracture is 2.6 for every 1 SD decrease in BMD as measured by the Z score.[42] The National Osteoporosis Foundation has published risk factors for osteoporosis and fracture (Table 61.4).

MS predisposes patients to bone loss and eventually to fragility fractures. Patients with MS have an increased likelihood to have corticosteroid exposure, impaired vision, cognitive impairment, poor health, falls, and low physical activity, all of which are independent risk factors for bone loss and fracture. In a large cross-sectional study of bone health in MS, Marrie *et al.* report about fractures and risk factors for fracture.[43] They found that 32% of patients reported bone loss (15% osteoporosis, 17% osteopenia). Osteoporosis was linearly associated with age and disability level. Risk factors for fracture were common in the MS population with 55% reporting falls in the last year, 26% reporting fracture, and 57% with three or more fracture risk factors.

Screening and prevention of bone loss are not well implemented in the MS population.[43] Slightly >50% have formal BMD testing; patients with low socioeconomic status and education level are at particular risk for not being screened. Treatment is insufficiently given, with bisphospohanate use in only 14.3%, calcium supplementation in 49%, and vitamin D supplementation in 66.3%.[43]

In MS patients, BMD and total body bone mass are linearly associated with age, severity of MS and ambulatory status. MS patients have a 2–3.4-fold increased risk for fracture compared to age-matched controls. Over 50% of MS patients have insufficient vitamin D levels, and over 25% have deficient vitamin D levels. BMD is significantly lower in those with deficient vitamin D levels compared to those with adequate vitamin D levels.[44]

Vitamin D

Vitamin D has received much interest in the past decade as a link to many systemic diseases including immune disorders.

Vitamin D exerts its effect on the immune system through the vitamin D receptor present on CNS glial cells and antigen presenting cells throughout the body. Downstream, vitamin D has been linked to a variety of immunoregulatory functions such as inhibiting T-cell activation, suppressing Th1 cells and promoting Th2 cells.[45] Vitamin D supplementation has been linked to a significantly lower risk of developing MS.[46] MS risk has been found to be highest in individuals with levels of 6–25 ng/ml and lowest in individuals with levels of 40–61 ng/ml.[47]

In practice, vitamin D levels should be routinely checked on patients with MS and supplements should be prescribed to bring levels of vitamin D to the appropriate range (>30 ng/ml). Additionally, all patients despite their current vitamin D level should take at a minimum the current US Food and Drug Administration-recommended level of vitamin D, 400–800 IU daily.

Vascular disease

Patients with MS have the same prevalence of vascular comorbidities as the general population.[48] Fifty percent of patients have one vascular comorbidity, 16% have two comorbidities, 4.4% three comorbidities, and 1% four comorbidities.[48] Diagnosis and management of MS can be made more difficult by vascular comorbidities such as dyslipidemia, peripheral vascular disease, hypertension, diabetes, and smoking. The delayed diagnosis of MS can lead to a greater level of disability at the time of diagnosis.[49] Vascular disease can result in cerebral T2 hyperintensities on MRI that can have similar appearance to demyelination which may delay time to diagnosis of MS and delay treatment with disease-modifying medication. The damage from intra-cerebral vascular disease comorbid with MS can have additive effects on neurologic disability.

Patients with vascular comorbidities may present to physicians later due to misattribution of MS symptoms. For example, blurred or double vision may be interpreted as related to a patient's known hypertension or diabetes. Additionally, physicians may misinterpret the patient's symptoms, exam features or radiographic findings as being related to the patients' known vascular disease. Lastly, other neurological diseases related to vascular diseases such as peripheral neuropathy may alter the physical examination and lead to an assumption of one neurologic diagnosis where two may exist.

Vascular comorbidity has a great impact on functional ability in MS patients. Having MS and one vascular risk factor is associated with a 50% increase in ambulatory disability. When MS patients have two vascular risk factors, the increase in ambulatory disability soars to 228% above those with no risk factors.[49]

Obesity has been linked to an increased likelihood of developing MS. In a retrospective questionnaire that looked at body mass index (BMI) at age 18 and other putative MS risk factors (Scandinavian descent, smoking, northern latitude) and development of MS, women classified as obese (BMI >30) at age 18 had a 2.25-fold increased risk of MS when compared to normal weight women. Outside of adolescence, no association was found between obesity and MS; further highlighting importance of this period of time in the risk of developing MS.[47] Obese individuals have a decreased level of vitamin D metabolites and obesity is associated with a low-level chronic inflammatory state.[47] Additionally, obese women are more likely to smoke. Therefore, it may not be obesity itself that causes MS, but rather common features between obese adolescents and MS patients.

Smoking

In the MS population, the prevalence of smoking is similar to the general population. Seventeen percent of MS patients currently smoke and 54.2% ever smoked cigarettes.[50] Smoking cigarettes has a particular concern when it comes to MS. Tobacco smoking not only contributes to vascular disease, but also is teratogenic and oncogenic. There is also evidence that smoking tobacco contributes to a worsened course of MS.[51]

Cessation of tobacco has the potential to prevent conversion from the first demyelinating event (clinically isolated syndrome, CIS) to clinically definite (CD) MS. During a three-year follow-up of 129 patients with a CIS, 75% of smokers developed CDMS while only 51% of non-smokers developed CDMS.[52] Thus, the number needed to harm with tobacco smoking for conversion from CIS to CDMS is 4. In comparison, the number needed to treat with IM IFNβ-1a to prevent conversion from CIS to CDMS is 6.[53] Smokers have a significantly shorter time interval to their second relapse.[52]

Once patients have developed CDMS, smoking cessation can still have an impact on disease course. In a comparison between smokers and non-smokers, patients were followed for MRI changes and clinical changes regarding relapse rates and disability progression. The mean Expanded Disability Status Scale score for smokers was 3.0, while the mean for non-smokers was 2.5. Additionally smokers were at increased risk for gadolinium-enhancing lesions, increased T2 and T1 lesion volumes, and progression of global and central atrophy.[51]

Patients with MS often ask what they can do to ensure a more favorable disease course. Cessation of tobacco smoking is an important way for patient to take part in the prevention of disease progression. CIS and MS patients who currently smoke tobacco should be counseled to stop as soon as possible. They should also be counseled to not begin smoking if they do not currently smoke.

Thyroid disease

Thyroid disorders are common in MS patients. Women with MS are three-times more likely to have thyroid disease than healthy controls.[53] Hypothyroidism accounts for the majority of thyroid disease in the MS population with Hashimoto's thyroiditis as the most likely etiology of thyroid dysfunction.[54] Thyroid disease and MS can have similar symptoms, particularly fatigue or asthenia. Screening for hypothyroidism is therefore advisable in MS patients with these symptoms to ensure thyroid replacement may not ameliorate these symptoms.

Interferon beta therapy and thyroid dysfunction

IFNβ therapy is associated with increased incidence of thyroid dysfunction, occurring in 24% of patients in one study.[55] Thyroid dysfunction occurs particularly within the first year of treatment. Thyroid dysfunction is most commonly subclinical. While the most common thyroid abnormality in IFNβ-treated patients is hypothyroidism,[55] autoimmune thyroid dysfunction, particularly the development of thyroid peroxidase antibodies is also increased.[56] Thyroid function assessment should be performed within the first year of IFNβ therapy. After this serum TSH measurement should be checked in patients with clinical symptoms consistent with thyroid dysfunction or in those with known thyroid disease.

Alemtuzumab

In the clinical trials of alemtuzumab, a monoclonal antibody therapy being investigated for use in MS, 22% of patients were noted to develop auto-immune thyroid disease in addition to other autoimmune diseases such as immune thrombocytopenic purpura and anti-glomerular basement membrane disease.[58] Thyroid disease was not limited to the period immediately after therapy and one affected patient was discovered 30 months post-treatment. Subclinical as well as clinical thyroid dysfunction will need to be monitored closely in patients if alemtuzumab is approved to treat MS.

Sleep disorders

Fatigue is common in MS patients, and evidence suggests the causes of fatigue are multi-factorial. Investigating fatigue in the MS patient requires a focus on sleep behaviors and characteristics. One of the main sources of fatigue is the lack of restorative sleep that many patients with MS experience. Sleep disorders are reported to occur in 25%–54% of MS patients.[59] The disorders are varied and include insomnia, sleep disordered breathing, restless leg syndrome, narcolepsy, and rapid eye movement (REM) sleep disorder. Sleep dysfunction is linked with increases mortality, cardiac disease, obesity and diabetes as well as contributing to depression, pain, and fatigue.[59] Many medications used to modulate the immune system or treat the symptoms of MS can have potential effects on sleep and fatigue (see Table 61.5). With the high prevalence of fatigue and sleep disorders in MS patients, those who report daytime fatigue should be thoroughly evaluated for concurrent sleep disorders.

Insomnia

Insomnia is very common in patients with MS. Most insomnia in MS is secondary to MS-related symptoms such as pain, anxiety, and nocturia. Insomnia occurs in three categories: initial insomnia, middle insomnia, and terminal insomnia. The causes and successful treatments of these are often different. Initial insomnia is defined as difficulty initiating sleep. The most

Table 61.5. *Medications used for MS and their potential impact on sleep and fatigue*[59]

Medication	Side effects	Impact on polysomnogram
Amantadine	Insomnia	Unknown
Baclofen	Sedation	Total sleep time increased, wake after sleep onset reduced
Clonazepam	Somnolence	Total sleep time increased, REM reduced, sleep latency reduced
Dalfampridine	Insomnia	Unknown
Gabapentin	Somnolence	Decreased stage I sleep, increased stage III sleep, increased REM
Interferon beta	Fatigue, hyper somnolence, insomnia	Unknown
Methylphenidate	Insomnia	REM suppressed
Methylprednisolone	Insomnia	Decreased REM
Modafinil	Insomnia	Reduced sleep latency
Oxybutinin	Sedation	Decreased REM sleep
Tizanidine	Daytime drowsiness	Improved sleep induction and maintenance

common causes of initial insomnia in MS patients are pain and anxiety.[60] Alleviating pain and anxiety at night can be helpful in managing initial insomnia. Additionally, patients with MS often have poor sleep hygiene and other behavioral sleep disorders that can lead to initial insomnia. For these patients, sleep behavioral therapy is a therapeutic option. Middle insomnia is defined as initially obtaining sleep, but then waking at least twice in the middle of the night. Patients most often awake at night to urinate. Some patients with MS may awaken multiple times per night to use the bathroom.[60] Treatment with anticholinergics, limiting evening fluid intake, and scheduled urination prior to getting in bed are helpful strategies for managing middle insomnia due to nocturia. Middle insomnia has the strongest association with daytime fatigue.[60] Terminal insomnia refers to awakening prior to the desired wake time. Typically patients will awaken in the early morning hours and then will need to get out of bed because they cannot fall back to sleep. This is also often caused by nocturia which can be managed as above. Additionally, external factors such as sunlight, household noise, pets, and children can contribute to terminal insomnia.

Narcolepsy

Narcolepsy is a sleep disorder that is associated with daytime fatigue, frequent sleep attacks, sleep paralysis, hypnagogic/hypnapopic hallucinations, cataplexy, and abnormal REM sleep. MS is the fourth most common cause of narcolepsy due to a medical condition, after head injury, inherited disorders, and brain tumors.[61] Genetically, 50% of MS patients and 95% of narcoleptic patients are DR2 positive and there is also a relation to DQB1*0602.[62] There are reported cases of narcolepsy in MS associated with hypothalamic lesions.[62] Narcolepsy can be quite disabling and should be screened for in patients with MS who report fatigue. The daytime sleepiness associated with narcolepsy can be treated with stimulants such as modafinil or methylphenidate.

Sleep disordered breathing

Sleep disordered breathing includes both central and obstructive sleep apnea (OSA). Central sleep apnea (CSA) refers to apneas that occur without respiratory effort while OSA occurs when apneas are associated with respiratory effort. Sleep apnea leads to daytime fatigue, decreased concentration, mood changes. Sleep apnea can also lead to comorbid vascular disease which as stated above can lead to increased risk for disability accrual in MS patients. OSA has been reported to be increased in the MS population.[63] Given the high occurrence of OSA in the general population, patients with MS who complain of fatigue and snoring should be screened for possible OSA. The medications that are used to treat symptoms of MS (i.e. baclofen) could also lead to or exacerbate OSA through relaxation of the pharyngeal musculature.[59] CSA has been demonstrated in MS patients as part of the central alveolar hypoventilation syndrome or "Ondine's Curse." This is the result of the failure of unconscious respiratory drive. This has been associated with MS plaques at the cervico-medullary junction.[64]

REM sleep behavior disorder

REM sleep behavior disorder (RSBD) is a parasomnia in which patients do not develop muscle atonia during REM sleep and will move during sleep as if they are "acting out" their dreams. RSBD in MS has been demonstrated to be linked to a pontine lesion, in the area of the pedunculopontine nucleus which through the pontine reticular formation is felt to be responsible for muscle atonia during REM sleep.[65] MS patients with RSBD can be effectively treated with clonazepam at bedtime. RSBD can be exacerbated by tricyclic antidepressants and these should be prescribed with caution in patients with known RSBD.

Restless legs syndrome

Restless legs syndrome (RLS) is defined as an urge to move the legs usually from an uncomfortable sensation in the legs. Movement of the legs improves the urge and symptoms are worse at rest and in the evening. RLS can disrupt sleep and lead to daytime fatigue. RLS is two times more common in MS patients compared to the general population.[66] In the Italian REMS study,[67] certain risk factors for RLS in the MS population included older age, leg jerks before sleep onset, and PPMS. MS patients with RLS were more likely to use pharmacologic sleep aids compared with those who did not suffer from RLS. Lastly, MS patients experienced more severe RLS than non-MS controls. After screening for iron deficiency, RLS should be treated with a dopamine agonist as first-line therapy.

References

1. Rutschmann O, McCrory D, Matchar D, et al. Immunization and MS: A summary of published evidence and recommendations. Neurology 2002; 59: 1837–1843.

2. Sibley W, Foley J. Infection and immunization. Mult Scler 1965; 122: 457–68.

3. De Keyser J, Zwanikken C, Boon M. Effects of influenza vaccination and influenza illness on exacerbations in multiple sclerosis. J Neurol Sci 1998; 159: 51–53.

4. Centers for Disease Control and Prevention. 2010. Available at: http://www.cdc.gov/mmwr/preview/mmwrhtml/rr5515a1.htm#tab1 [cited 2010 3 Nov]

5. Galil K, Choo PW, Donahue JG, et al. The sequelae of herpes zoster. Arch Intern Med 1997; 157: 1209–13.

6. Cohen JA, Barkhof F, Comi G, et al. Oral fingolimod or intramuscular interferon for relapsing multiple sclerosis. N Engl J Med 2010; 362: 402–15.

7. Ordoñez G, Martinez-Palomo A, Corona T, et al. Varicella zoster virus in progressive forms of multiple sclerosis. Clin Neurol Neurosurg 2010; 112: 653–7.

8. Sotelo J, Martínez-Palomo A, Ordoñez G, et al. Varicella-zoster virus in cerebrospinal fluid at relapses of multiple sclerosis. Ann Neurol 2008; 63: 303–11.

9. Oxman MN, Levin MJ, Johnson GR, et al. A vaccine to prevent herpes zoster and postherpetic neuralgia in older adults. N Engl J Med 2005; 352: 2271–84.

10. Galea SA, Sweet A, Beninger P, et al. The safety profile of varicella vaccine: a 10-year review. J Infect Dis 2008; 1: 197.

11. Ross RT, Nicolle LE, Cheang M. The varicella zoster virus: a pilot trial of a potential therapeutic agent in multiple sclerosis. J Clin Epidemiol 1997; 50: 63–8.

12. Stein NP. Gilenya Package Insert. 2010.

13. Kane M. Hepatitis B. In Jamison DT. Disease Control Priorities in Developing Countries. Oxford, UK: Oxford University Press; 1993, 321–330.

14. Gout O. Central nervous system demyelination after recombinant hepatitis B vaccination: report of 25 cases. Neurology. 1997: Suppl:A424.

15. Ascherio A, Zhang SM, Hernán MA, et al. Hepatitis B vaccination and the risk of multiple sclerosis. N Engl J Med. 2001; 344: 327–32.

16. Hernán MA, Jick SS, Olek MJ, et al. Recombinant hepatitis B vaccine and the risk of multiple sclerosis. Neurology 2004: 838–42.

17. Miller AE, Morgante LA, Buchwald LY, et al. A multicenter, randomized, double-blind, placebo-controlled trial of influenza immunization in multiple sclerosis. Neurology 1997; 48: 312–14.

18. Centers for Disease Control and Prevention. Available from: HYPERLINK "http://www.cdc.gov/flu/" http://www.cdc.gov/flu/ [cited 2010 October 25]

19. Centers for Disease Control and Prevention. 2010. Available from: HYPERLINK "http://www.cdc.gov/vaccines/vpd-vac/tetanus/default.htm"

http://www.cdc.gov/vaccines/vpd-vac/tetanus/default.htm. [cited 2010 November 3]

20. McQuillan GM, Kruszon-Moran D, Deforest A, et al. Serologic immunity to diphtheria and tetanus in the United States. *Ann Intern Med* 2002; 136: 660–6.

21. Hernán MA, Alonso A, Hernández-Díaz S. Tetanus vaccination and the risk of multiple sclerosis: a systematic review. *Neurology* 2006: 212–15.

22. Schwid SR, Decker MD, Lopez-Bresnahan M, et al. Immune response to influenza vaccine is maintained in patients with multiple sclerosis receiving interferon beta-1a. *Neurology* 2005; 65: 1964–6.

23. Avetisyan G, Ragnavölgyi E, Toth GT, et al. Cell-mediated immune responses to influenza vaccination in healthy volunteers and allogenic stem cell transplant recipients. *Bone Marrow Transplant* 2005; 36: 411–15.

24. Ostensen M, Ramsey-Goldman R. Treatment of Inflammatory Rheumatic Disorders in Pregnancy. *Drug Safety* 1998; 19: 389–410.

25. Sandberg-Wollheim M, Frank D, Goodwin TM, et al. Pregnancy outcomes in patients receiving IFN beta-Ia for treatment of multiple sclerosis. *Neurology* 2005; 65: 807–11.

26. Boskovic R, Wide R, Wolpin J, et al. The reproductive effects of beta interferon in pregnancy. *Neurology* 2005; 65: 807–11.

27. Salminen HJ, Leggett H, Boggild M. Glatiramer acetate exposure in pregnancy: preliminary safter and birth outcomes. *J Neurol Sci* 2010; 81: 38–41.

28. Coyle PK, Christie S, Fodor P, et al. Multiple sclerosis gender issues: clinical practices of women neurologists. *Mult Scler* 2004; 10: 582–8.

29. Wehner NG, Skov M, Shopp G, et al. Effects of natalizumab, an alpha4 integrin inhibitor, on fertility in male and female guinea pigs. *Birth Defects Res B Dev Reprod Toxicol* 2009; 86: 108–16.

30. LM Cristiano, Biogen Idec, Inc., *Cambridge, MA. Preliminary Evaluation of Pregnancy Outcomes from the TYSABRI®* (Natalizumab) Pregnancy Exposure Registry; 2010; Toronto.

31. Confavreux C, Hutchinson M, Hours MM, et al. Rate of pregnancy-related relapse in multiple sclerosis. *N Engl J Med* 1998; 339: 285–91.

32. Achiron A, Kishner I, Dolev M, et al. Effect of intravenous immunoglobulin treatment on pregnancy and postpartum-related relapses in multiple sclerosis. *J Neurol* 2004; 251: 1133–7.

33. Langer-Gould A, Huang S, Van Den Eeden SK, et al. Exclusive breastfeeding and the risk of postpartum relapses in women with multiple sclerosis. *Arch Neurol* 2009; 66: 958–63.

34. Zorgdrager A, De Keyser J. The premenstrual period and exacerbations in multiple sclerosis. *Eur Neurol* 2002; 48: 204–6.

35. Gold SM, Voskuhl RR. Estrogen treatment in multiple sclerosis. *J Neurol Sci* 2009; 286: 99–103.

36. Soldan SS, Alvarez Retuerto AI, Sicotte NL, et al. Immune modulation in multiple sclerosis patients treated with the pregnancy hormone estriol. *J Immunol* 2003; 171: 6267–74.

37. Hernán MA, Hohol MJ, Olek MJ, et al. Oral contraceptives and the incidence of multiple sclerosis. *Neurology*. 2000; 55: 848–54.

38. Dwosh E, Guimond C, Sadovnick AD. Reproductive counselling for MS: a rationale. *Int MS J* 2003; 10: 52–9.

39. Laplaud DA, Lefrère F, Leray E, et al. Increased risk of relapse in multiple sclerosis patients after ovarian stimulation for in vitro fertilization. *Gynecol Obstet Fertil* 2007; 35: 1047–50.

40. National Osteoporosis Foundation. [Online]; 2010 [cited 2010 11 3. Available from: HYPERLINK "http://www.nof.org/" http://www.nof.org/

41. Khosla S, Melton LJ. Osteopenia. *N Engl J Med* 2007; 356: 2293–300.

42. Marshall D, Johnell O, Wedel H. Meta-analysis of how well measures of bone mineral density predict occurrence of osteoporotic fractures. *BMJ* 1996; 312: 1254–9.

43. Marrie RA, Cutter G, Tyry T, et al. A cross sectional study of bone health in multiple sclerosis. *Neurology* 2009; 73: 1394–8.

44. Nieves J, Cosman F, Herbert J, et al. High prevalence of Vitamin D deficiency and reduced bone mass in

multiple sclerosis. *Neurology* 1994; 44: 1687–92.

45. Solomon AJ, Whitham RH. Multiple sclerosis and vitamin D: a review and recommendations. *Curr Neurol Neurosci Rep* 2010; 10: 389–96.

46. Munger KL, Zhang SM, O'Reilly E, et al. Vitamin D intake and incidence of multiple sclerosis. *Neurology* 2004; 62: 60–5.

47. Munger KL, Chitnis T, Ascherio A. Body size and risk of MS in two cohorts of US women. *Neurology* 2009; 73: 1543–50.

48. Marrie R, Horwitz R, Cutter G, et al. High frequency of adverse health behaviors in multiple sclerosis. *Multe Scler* 2009; 15: 105–13.

49. Marrie RA, Horwitz R, Cutter G, et al. Comorbidity delays diagnosis and increases disability at diagnosis in MS. *Neurology* 2009; 72: 117–24.

50. Marrie RA, Rudick R, Horwitz R, et al. Vascular comorbidity is associated with more rapid disability progression in multiple sclerosis. *Neurology* 2010; 74: 1041–7.

51. Zivadinov R, Weinstock-Guttman B, Hashmi K, et al. Smoking is associated with increased lesion volumes and brain atrophy in multiple sclerosis. *Neurology* 2009; 73: 504–10.

52. Di Pauli F, Reindl M, Ehling R, et al. Smoking is a risk factor for early conversion to clinically definite multiple sclerosis. *Mult Scler* 2008; 14: 1026–30.

53. CHAMPS Study Group. The Controlled High Risk Avonex® Multiple Sclerosis Trial. *J Neuroophthalmol* 2001; 21: 292–5.

54. Karni A, Abramsky O. Association of multiple sclerosis with thyroid disorders. *Neurology* 1999; 53: 883–5.

55. Niederwieser G, Buchinger W, Bonelli RM, et al. Prevalence of autoimmune thyroiditis and non-immune thyroid disease in multiple sclerosis. *J Neurol Sci* 2003; 250: 672–5.

56. Caraccio N, Dardano A, Manfredonia F, et al. Long-term follow-up of 106 multiple sclerosis patients undergoing interferon-beta 1a or 1b therapy: predictive factors of thyroid disease development and duration. *J Clin Endocrinol Metab* 2005; 90: 4133–7.

57. Rotondi M, Oliviero A, Profice P, et al. Occurrence of thyroid autoimmunity

and dysfunction throughout a nine-month follow-up in patients undergoing interferon-beta therapy for multiple sclerosis. *J Endocrinol Invest* 1998: p. 748–52.

58. Coles AJ, Compston DA, *et al.* Alemtuzumab versus interferon betal-1a in early multiple sclerosis. *New Engl J Med* 2008; 359: 1786–801.

59. Brass SD, Duquette P, Proulx-Therrien J, *et al.* Sleep disorders in patients with multiple sclerosis. *Sleep Med Rev* 2010; 14: 121–9.

60. Stanton BR, Barnes F, Silber E. Sleep and fatigue in multiple sclerosis. *Mult Scler* 2006; 12: 481–6.

61. Nishino S. Narcolepsy: pathophysiology and pharmacology. *J Clin Psychiatry* 2007; 68: 9–15.

62. Nishino S, Kanbayashi T. Symptomatic narcolepsy, cataplexy and hypersomnia, and their implications in the hypothalamic hypocretin/orexin system. *Sleep Med Rev* 2005; 9: 269–310.

63. Ajayi OF, Chang-McDowell T, Culpepper II WJ, *et al.* High prevalence of sleep disorders in veterans with multiple sclerosis. *Neurology* 2008; 50: 141.

64. Auer RN, Rowlands CG, Perry SF, *et al.* Multiple sclerosis with medullary plaques and fatal sleep apnea (Ondine's curse). *Clin Neuropathol* 1996; 15: 101–5.

65. Plazzi G, Montagna P. Remitting REM sleep behavior disorder as the initial sign of multiple sclerosis. *Sleep Med* 2002; 3: 437–9.

66. Deriu M, Cossu G, Molari A, *et al.* Restless legs syndrome in multiple sclerosis: A case-control study. *Mov Disord.* 2009; 24: 697–701.

67. Manconi M, Ferini-Strambi L, Filippi M, *et al.* Multicenter case–control study on restless legs syndrome in multiple sclerosis: the REMS study. *Sleep* 2008; 31: 944–52.

Chapter

62

Rehabilitation in multiple sclerosis

Francois A. Bethoux and Matthew Sutliff

Background

Rehabilitation is defined by the World Health Organization (WHO) as "a proactive and goal-oriented activity to restore function and/or to maximize remaining function to bring about the highest possible level of independence, physically, psychologically, socially, and economically. It involves combined and coordinated use of medical, nursing, and allied health skills, along with social, educational, and vocational services, to provide individual assessment, treatment, regular review, discharge planning, and follow-up. Rehabilitation is concerned, not only with physical recovery, but also with psychological and social recovery and reintegration (or integration) of the person into the community". As illustrated by this definition, the concept of rehabilitation seeks a broad, comprehensive approach of the person in relation to his/her environment, which is not contradictory, but rather complementary to the traditional biomedical model.[1] To target these ambitious goals, inpatient and outpatient rehabilitation programs usually rely on a multidisciplinary team, which can comprise physiatrists, nurses and physician assistants, physical therapists, occupational therapists, speech-language therapists, neuropsychologists, psychologists, social workers, recreation therapists, and other rehabilitation professionals. Rehabilitative interventions can impact significantly on the consequences of central nervous system (CNS) damage due to multiple sclerosis (MS).

Conceptual framework

The most widely used theoretical framework in rehabilitation was introduced by the WHO in the International Classification of Functioning, Disability and Health (ICF).[2] Definitions of basic ICF concepts are presented in Table 62.1. The relevance of the ICF to the description of the consequences of MS has been demonstrated.[3]

In addition, there is an increasing interest for patient-reported outcomes (PRO) such as perceived health status, symptom severity, and quality of life (QoL). The WHO definition of QoL reflects the complexity of this concept, and its relevance to rehabilitative interventions: "…an individual's perception of their position in life in the context of the

Table 62.1. *International classification of functioning terminology*

In the context of a health condition…

Impairment: loss or abnormality of body structure or of a physiological or psychological function.

Activity: nature and extent of functioning at the level of the person. Activities may be limited in nature, duration, and quality.

Participation: nature and extent of a person's involvement in life situations in relation to impairment, activities, health conditions and contextual factors. Participation may be limited in nature, duration, and quality.

culture and value systems in which they live and in relation to their goals, expectations, standards and concerns."[4]

The National Institute of Neurological Disorders and Stroke (NINDS) recently funded a multi-center study to develop Neuro-QoL, a set of self-report measures assessing the health-related QoL of adults and children with neurological disorders, including MS.[5]

Difficulties in implementing rehabilitation in individuals with MS

The Medical Advisory Board of the National Multiple Sclerosis Society published recommendations for the use of rehabilitation in persons with MS, based on a thorough review of the literature and expert opinion.[6] Although rehabilitation is recognized as an important component of the plan of care for persons with MS, its exact role and modalities are not as clearly defined as in other pathologies of the CNS, such as spinal cord injury, stroke, or traumatic brain injury. The relatively low incidence of MS, the progression of disability over time observed in many patients, and the generally low tolerance of MS patients for exertion, may explain this situation. Additionally, the attention of patients, families, and health professionals has been focused on an increasing number of disease-modifying therapies, which aim at preventing the development of disability over time. Environmental and economic obstacles also limit the access to rehabilitation for individuals with MS. The more disabled patients have difficulty getting to MS centers or to larger rehabilitation facilities with experience in neurorehabilitation. Third-party payers are tightening the rules to qualify patients

---

Multiple Sclerosis Therapeutics, Fourth Edition, ed. Jeffrey A. Cohen and Richard A. Rudick. Published by Cambridge University Press.
© Cambridge University Press 2011.

for rehabilitation, and often allow an insufficient number of sessions. In response to these limitations, community neurorehabilitation and tele-rehabilitation services are being developed in some areas.[7,8]

Neuroplasticity and rehabilitation in MS

It is commonly acknowledged that rehabilitative interventions, particularly in neurorehabilitation, do not affect the underlying disease process. However, the concept of neural plasticity opens the possibility of helping recovery at the cellular level through rehabilitation. Plasticity is defined as the tendency of synapses and neuronal circuits to change because of activity".[9] "Fast" short-term plasticity is related to down-regulation of gamma aminobutyric acid, while "slow" long-term plasticity involves structural changes and long-term potentiation. Assessment of plasticity can be performed at the microscopic level, but in the clinical setting, non-invasive procedures such as functional imaging and transcranial magnetic stimulation are obviously preferred. Most of the literature on plasticity and rehabilitation deals with stroke and spinal cord or brain injury,[10,11] and plasticity may be limited in MS by the presence of multiple lesions and ongoing disease process.[12] Recent publications have shown improvement of walking performance in stable MS patients, both with conventional and robot-assisted gait training, providing preliminary clinical evidence in support of the existence of plasticity in MS.[13,14] Similarly, a pilot-uncontrolled study of robot-assisted upper extremity training in seven MS patients showed improvement of performance on the Nine-Hole Peg Test.[15] Imaging studies have also shown functional reorganization in the brain in relation to cognitive impairments.[16]

Measuring functional limitations and the results of rehabilitation in MS

To better understand the rehabilitation literature, it is necessary to possess a minimal knowledge of the language and tools used in rehabilitation practice and research. Evidence-based medicine was introduced relatively recently in the field of Physical Medicine and Rehabilitation (PM&R). Other medical specialties often have well-defined interventions (e.g. medications, surgical interventions, as opposed to a multidisciplinary individualized rehabilitation program), focused outcomes (e.g. mortality, biological indicators, defined medical events such as exacerbations, stroke or myocardial infarction, as opposed to performance in activities of daily life), and rehabilitative interventions do not lend themselves easily to double blinding and placebo interventions. However, methodological standards for PM&R have now been published,[17] and the development of specific concepts and derived assessment tools has set the basis for the development of methodologically sound clinical research. In addition, concepts that are familiar to rehabilitation professionals, such as disability and quality of life, are increasingly used as efficacy measures in the evaluation of traditional surgical and medical interventions.

Valid and reliable outcomes scales were developed, often based on the WHO concepts defined above. It is beyond the scope of this chapter to present all outcomes measures available for MS. Detailed information can be obtained elsewhere in this book or in other publications.[18] We will discuss a few instruments which have often been used in publications on MS rehabilitation:

Disease-specific measures

- The Minimal Record of Disabilities (MRD) for MS, developed under the auspice of the International Federation of Multiple Sclerosis Societies, includes the Expanded Disability Status Scale (EDSS), the Incapacity Status Scale (ISS), and the Environmental Status Scale (ESS).[19] The EDSS combines an evaluation of neurologic impairments (Functional Systems) and disability (walking, transfers, etc.). Despite well-known limitations,[18,20] the EDSS remains widely used in the MS field. In rehabilitation research, the EDSS is often used as a measure of neurologic status at baseline and/or an indicator of clinical disease progression.[21–24] In most cases, EDSS average scores either remain stable or worsen slightly during the course of prospective rehabilitation studies, which seems to support the absence of effect of rehabilitation on the disease process. The ISS associates traditional assessment of disability (ambulation, self-care, sphincter control) with observed or reported severity of common MS symptoms (e.g. visual symptoms, fatigue). Although validated and potentially more informative than generic measures of disability, the ISS has been seldom used by rehabilitation professionals. This is also true of the ESS, which is a measure of the consequences of MS on participation. A self-administered version of the MRD was developed and validated.[25]

- The UK (Guy's) Neurological Disability Scale (UKNDS) is a patient-report measure of disability used in MS, which contains 67 items exploring 12 domains of disability.[26] The UKNDS has demonstrated satisfactory psychometric properties.

- The Multiple Sclerosis Impact Scale (MSIS-29) is a 29-item questionnaire focused on the consequences of MS on activities of daily life, which has been validated.[27,28]

- The Multiple Sclerosis Functional Composite (MSFC), which comprises the Timed 25-Foot (7.62 meter Walk) Walk (T25FW), the Nine-Hole Peg Test, and the Paced Auditory Serial Addition Test, appears as a promising tool for therapeutic trials in MS, but its relevance to MS rehabilitation remains to be evaluated.[29]

- Disease-specific measures of perceived health status and QoL are discussed elsewhere in this book.

Measures of walking performance

Previously described disability scales, such as the EDSS, the UKNDS, the MSIS-29, and the MSFC, include some objective or patient-reported evaluation of walking.

The T25FW is simple and quick to administer, and exhibits sound psychometric properties, but the clinical significance of changes in performance is not completely understood. The T25FW was used as a primary outcome measure in clinical trials of dalfampridine, a recently approved symptomatic medication to improve walking in patients with MS.[30] Other measures of walking speed on a short distance have been proposed, such as the 10-meter walk.[31]

The six-minute walk test is a test of walking endurance, initially designed for patients with cardiovascular and respiratory disorders and recently validated in patients with MS.[32] The two-minute walk test appears to have similar properties to the six-minute walk test, while being more feasible and less burdensome for patients.[33]

The Timed Up and Go Test (TUG) is a simple and easily reproducible timed test that involves basic components of mobility – standing from a chair, walking 3 meters, turning 180 degrees, walking back to the chair, and returning to a seated position.[34]

The Dynamic Gait Index (DGI) provides a more thorough measure of walking performance as it incorporates various challenges to gait that may be seen in real life ambulation.[35]

The Ambulation Index (AI)[36] was developed for clinical trials in MS. It gives a score from 0 to 9 based on quality of gait, use of a walking aid, and the time to walk 25 feet.

The Mellen Center Gait Test was developed as an attempt to bridge this gap by providing a relatively simple, yet more complete test that can be administered in an outpatient or inpatient rehabilitation setting. The gait course includes: 25 foot walk on carpeted floor, ascend and descend four six inch stairs with one railing, ascend a four foot ramp onto a platform, turn 180 degrees and descend the same ramp, walk five feet on carpet, and then walk 10 feet over a simulated grassy surface. A time is provided for patients who complete the whole course. In addition, ordinal scores are given for completion and quality of gait. This test has not been yet validated.

The MS Walking Scale (MSWS-12)[37] is a 12-item patient-reported outcome measure exploring walking performance in usual activities. This scale has been well validated, and showed concurrent score improvements in subjects defined as responders, based on sustained improvement on the T25FW, in clinical trials of dalfampridine.

Generic scales

- *Impairments.* The EDSS gives a global picture of neurologic impairments in a given individual, but is not very useful for the evaluation of treatments focused on a specific impairment. Validated generic scales or instrumented measurements will usually be preferred, such as the Manual Muscle Testing or dynamometry for muscle strength, or the Modified Ashworth scale or H-reflex for spasticity.

- *Activity limitations.* The Functional Independence Measure (FIM^{TM}) has established itself as the "gold standard" for the evaluation of disability in rehabilitation settings, at least in North America. More precisely, the FIM^{TM} is a measure of dependence, which correlates well with burden of care in MS patients.[38] In general, the FIM^{TM} is sensitive to change for inpatient rehabilitation, and this appears to be true in particular for the MS population.[39] Its performance in an outpatient setting, where MS patients get most of their care, is not well established. The Rehabilitation Institute of Chicago Functional Assessment Scale (RIC-FAS) has been used in a prospective study of outpatient rehabilitation in MS.[40]

- *Perceived health status.* Different authors have used either the SF-36,[41,42] or the Sickness Impact Profile (SIP),[43] to evaluate the results of rehabilitative interventions in MS. Freeman *et al.* observed that the SF-36 may not be the most sensitive measure of subjective health status in a rehabilitation setting, due to marked floor effect in several subscales,[41] and questioned the validity and usefulness of adding disease-specific items to the SF-36, after observing no change in measurement properties between the SF-36 and the MSQOL-54 in 150 patients with MS (44 evaluated prospectively for responsiveness).[44] The recently developed Neuro-QOL battery, which combines cross-condition and disease-specific scales, while limiting responder burden through the use of short forms, may address some of these concerns.[5]

Indications for rehabilitation in MS

Situations in which rehabilitation may be utilized to the benefit of MS patients include the following.

- *Education and prevention.* At any stage of the disease, rehabilitation professionals can teach the patient how to minimize the impact of neurologic impairments on the ability to perform daily activities and to fulfill expected roles. This can sometimes be achieved in a single session, a customized home exercise program being most often delivered to the patient at the end of the visit. The goal is to prevent complications and progression of functional limitations, and to empower a patient who often feels frustrated and anxious because of the unpredictable course of the disease. One area of particular interest is the role of exercise, which traditionally was not strongly recommended, or even avoided in MS, out of fear of making symptoms worse or triggering an exacerbation. Results from a few studies have helped understand the role of physical de-conditioning in functional limitations, and the potential benefits of exercise.[45] A controlled study of aerobic exercise in 46 MS patients published by Petajan *et al.* showed improvement of fitness, psychological status

(Profile of Mood States), perceived health status (SIP), and fatigue (Fatigue Severity Scale) in the exercise group compared to the nonexercise group.[43] However, poor adherence to exercise is a concern in MS, and interventions are tested to address this problem.[46] The importance of physical activity and exercise is further emphasized by evidence showing that comorbidities (e.g. cardiovascular, musculoskeletal) have a negative impact on MS-related disability, many of which can be precipitated or worsened by decreased activity and immobility.[47,48]

- *Symptom management.* The management of MS symptoms has become an increasingly complex matter. The necessity to monitor disease activity and manage disease-modifying therapies decreases the time that neurologists can devote to the planning and adjustment of symptomatic therapies. The multiplicity of factors contributing to symptoms, the interaction of consequences from different symptoms, the frequent necessity to combine medications and other interventions, make the rehabilitation approach particularly relevant to this matter, when simple first-line treatments fail to provide adequate relief. For example, a comprehensive fatigue management program should include aerobic exercise and education on energy effectiveness strategies.[49] Another example is spasticity management, where rehabilitation helps achieve optimal outcomes. The effect of most symptomatic medications on function and QOL has not been systematically studied. Dalfampridine was recently approved in the United States, and in the European Union as fampridine, with a specific indication for improving walking in patients with MS. Dalfampridine is an extended-release formulation of 4-aminopyridine (4-AP), a potassium channel blocker shown to facilitate signal conduction along demyelinated axons in vitro. 4-AP has been available as a compounded medication, and safety issues due to compounding errors have been reported.[50] A Phase 2 dose-ranging study of sustained-release 4-AP showed improvement of lower extremity muscle strength and walking speed on the T25FW, with no incremental benefit with doses above 10 mg twice daily, but a dose-dependent increase in the frequency and severity of adverse events.[51] A Phase 3 double-blind, placebo-controlled trial of sustained-release 4-AP[30] showed a significantly higher proportion of responders (subjects who exhibited a sustained improvement in walking speed) in the treatment group compared to the placebo group. The average increase in walking speed was 25.2% in the treatment group and 4.7% in the placebo group (a 20% change has been considered meaningful).[52] No clinical predictors of responder status were found. There was also a significant improvement in lower extremity strength in the treatment group, compared to the placebo group. One can expect a synergy between dalfampridine and gait training, although this combination of interventions has not been formally tested.

- *Focused rehabilitation.* Referral to rehabilitation may be motivated by a specific functional problem. Often, a single rehabilitation professional will be involved, and several sessions will be needed to achieve the desired goal(s). The most frequent example is abnormal limb function (i.e. referral to physical or occupational therapy for difficulty controlling one or both lower or upper extremities). Another example is driver rehabilitation, which can be very helpful when confronted with the difficult decision to deprive a patient of a very important mean of independence because of safety concerns. Treatment often consists of a combination of stretching, strengthening, function-specific training, and the use of assistive/adaptive devices and orthoses. The recommendation, adjustment, and training to the use of most orthotics and assistive devices is most often issued by rehabilitation professionals. Traditional devices such as static and dynamic ankle foot orthoses (AFOs) were found to improve static balance in 14 MS patients, while dynamic balance was challenged, particularly by static AFOs.[53] A more recent study indicated that walking speed did not improve with the use of AFOs.[54] This desire for improved ambulation has led to newer devices that may assist weaker muscles to function more efficiently during the gait cycle. Functional electrical stimulation (FES) of the peroneal nerve has limited evidence in the treatment of foot drop in MS, but recent studies have shown that it improves walking speed and decreases the physiological cost of gait in MS.[55] A recent pilot study demonstrated significant improvement of gait performance at three months and excellent patient satisfaction with a hip flexion assist device (HFAD). In contrast to the ankle dorsiflexor weakness that is treated with an AFO or FES, the HFAD was designed to compensate for the combined weakness of the hip flexor, knee flexor, and ankle dorsiflexor.[56]

- *Reduction or stabilization of chronic activity limitations through comprehensive rehabilitation programs.* Di Fabio *et al.* reported a significant decrease in symptom frequency (MS-Related Symptom Checklist) and level of fatigue at one year in 20 patients receiving weekly outpatient rehabilitation, compared to 26 patients on a waiting list.[40] There was also a slower decline of disability (RIC-FAS) in the treatment group (all patients were diagnosed with progressive MS). In a randomized, single-blind, controlled study of a three-week inpatient rehabilitation program (treatment group; $n = 27$) vs. home exercises (control group; $n = 23$), Solari *et al.* observed that disability (FIM™) improved in the treatment group and worsened in the control group on average.[23] There was also greater improvement of perceived health status (SF-36) in the treatment group. Approximately 20% of patients in each group were diagnosed with relapsing-remitting MS. Freeman *et al.* compared the outcome at six weeks in 32 patients receiving inpatient rehabilitation and 34 patients on a waiting list (all patients had progressive MS). Change in FIM[TM] motor domain scores and London Handicap Scale scores was significantly greater in the treatment group.[21] A one-year uncontrolled longitudinal study in the same institution suggested that improvement of disability, handicap, psychological status, and perceived physical health status, achieved after in-patient rehabilitation on 50 patients with progressive MS, was sustained for at least six months despite worsening of impairments.[22] Another uncontrolled outcomes study in an inpatient setting (n = 28) showed that improvement was most dramatic for ambulation.[57] A more recent study from Australia found improvement in FIM[TM] motor domain scores (but not in MSIS-29 or quality of life scores) in 49 MS patients following an individualized rehabilitation program, compared with 53 wait-list patients.[58]

- *Recovery after acute worsening of disability.* Abrupt loss of function may be secondary to increased disease activity (e.g. exacerbation), or to an intercurrent health event (e.g. infection, surgery). A common conception of rehabilitation, reinforced by the reimbursement guidelines of third-party payors in some countries, favors the concentration of interventions on a relatively short period of time, in response to an acute injury or disease process. Exacerbations or relapses of MS fit into this category, but, for reasons outlined above, rest was recommended in most cases. Some degree of recovery is usually expected after acute worsening, possibly enhanced or accelerated by the use of intravenous methylprednisolone (IVMP),[59] but residual symptoms and functional limitations are frequently reported and observed.[60] The results of a recent randomized controlled trial and an uncontrolled longitudinal study, suggest that multidisciplinary rehabilitation is effective in enhancing functional recovery after exacerbations of MS.[61,62] A randomized single-blind clinical trial of outpatient rehabilitation for six weeks, starting four weeks after IVMP treatment for an MS relapse, showed no significant between-group differences in ISS and SF-36 scores at three months or one year.[63] Although methodological differences between these studies must be taken into consideration, it can be argued that the intensity of rehabilitative interventions may have a significant impact on treatment efficacy after MS exacerbations.

- *Cognitive rehabilitation.* While the indications above referred to physical rehabilitation, there are emerging data supporting the use of cognitive rehabilitation in MS,[64] but there is still a need for further evidence to guide clinical practice.[65]

Implications for clinical practice

An increasing array of interventions are available to improve function and QOL in patients with MS, and many, if not most of them, involve rehabilitation. Many questions remain to be answered about the use of rehabilitation in MS, such

as testing and comparing the efficacy of specific rehabilitation interventions.[66] As is usual in health care, there may not be a single "good answer" to any of these questions for an individual patient. Cultural preferences, the structure of the health care system, availability of services, experience, and beliefs of health care professionals will inevitably and diversely influence the way in which rehabilitation is utilized. It is not possible to present here a catalogue of available interventions and indications. Nevertheless, a few general recommendations can be formulated, based on the information presented above.

- *Intervene early.* Rehabilitation is not a "last resort." For instance, it is important to educate patients early in the course of the disease about the importance of exercising at home to avoid deconditioning, or to stretch daily to reduce the consequences of spasticity. A referral to outpatient rehabilitation helps design an individualized home exercise program.

- *Re-assess periodically.* When a functional or symptomatic problem becomes chronic and/or worsens, a new referral to rehabilitation may be indicated to re-evaluate the situation and to provide new interventions.

- *Define a strategy.* Rehabilitation should be integrated into the plan of care, particularly for symptom management and when the patient reports limitation in his /her ability to carry out daily activities. The patient is more likely to be motivated and compliant with rehabilitative interventions if he / she feels that the prescribing physician is supportive and inquires about outcomes. Single evaluations or short-term interventions by a rehabilitation professional to address a focused problem are often useful, but when the presenting problem is complex, or when rapid and severe loss of function has occurred, more intensive multidisciplinary outpatient or even inpatient rehabilitative interventions are usually indicated.

- *Clarify expectations.* Unrealistic expectations can be as counterproductive as an overly pessimistic attitude. Precise, pragmatic and reasonable goals should be set, with the help of rehabilitation professionals, and feedback on goal achievement should be sought from the patient, as well as by the means of objective assessment.

- *Seek specialized rehabilitation.* Because of the specific challenges faced by MS patients, referral to neurorehabilitation specialists (especially those with experience in MS rehabilitation) is desirable. Even if those specialists are not available in the patient's area, seeking a one-time evaluation in an MS center or neurorehabilitation facility will help in designing an effective and tolerable home exercise program, and recommendations for therapy than can be carried out closer to the patient's home.

Conclusions

There is an increasing body of evidence suggesting that rehabilitative interventions are indeed effective in MS. Increasingly, potent disease-modifying therapies, which do not improve existing symptoms and functional limitations, and unfortunately do not stop all disease activity, have not decreased the need for rehabilitative interventions. Instead, the same principles guiding disease management should be applied to rehabilitation, to allow a more comprehensive approach to the disease and its consequences. Extensive research work is needed to determine or develop appropriate outcomes measures, to gather scientific evidence of the efficacy (and cost-effectiveness) of rehabilitation protocols, to compare different types of interventions, to determine subgroups of patients most likely to benefit from intensive rehabilitation, and to define the best timing of interventions.

References

1. Minaire P. Disease, illness and health: theoretical models of the disablement process. *Bull WHO* 1992;70:373–9.

2. International Classification of Functioning, Disability and Health. Geneva: World Health Organization, 2001.

3. Holper L, Coenen M, Weise A, Stucki G, Cieza A, Kesselring J. Characterization of functioning in multiple sclerosis using the ICF. *J Neurol* 2010;257(1):103–13.

4. Szabo S, The World Health Organization Quality of Life (WHOQOL) assessment instrument. In Spilker B, *Quality of Life and Pharmacoeconomics in Clinical Trials*, 2nd edn Philadelphia: Lippincott-Raven Publishers, 1996.

5. Neuroqol website.

6. Medical Advisory Board of the National Multiple Sclerosis Society, *Rehabilitation: Recommendations for Persons with Multiple Sclerosis*. National Multiple Sclerosis Society 2005: 10 pp.

7. Chard SE. Community neurorehabilitation: a synthesis of current evidence and future research directions. *NeuroRx* 2006;3(4):525–34.

8. Hermens H, Huijgen B, Giacomozzi C, *et al*. Clinical assessment of the HELLODOC tele-rehabilitation service. *Annali Dell'Istituto Superiore di Sanita* 2008.; 44(2):154–63.

9. Cauraugh JH, Summers JJ. Neural plasticity and bilateral movements: a rehabilitation approach for chronic stroke. *Prog Neurobiol* 2005;75(5):309–20.

10. Schaechter JD. Motor rehabilitation and brain plasticity after hemiparetic stroke. *Prog Neurobiol* 2004;73(1):61–72.

11. Kwakkel G, Kollen B, Lindeman E. Understanding the pattern of functional recovery after stroke: facts and theories. *Restor Neurol Neurosci* 2004;22(3–5):281–99.

12. Filippi M, Rocca MA. Disturbed function and plasticity in multiple sclerosis as gleaned from functional magnetic resonance imaging. *Curr Opin Neurol* 2003;16(3):275–82.

13. Beer S, Aschbacher B, Manoglou D, Gamper E, Kool J, Kesselring J. Robot-assisted gait training in multiple sclerosis: a pilot randomized trial. *Mult Scler* 2008;14(2):231–6.

14. Lo AC, Triche EW. Improving gait in multiple sclerosis using robot-assisted, body weight supported treadmill training. *Neurorehab Neural Repair* 2008;22(6):661–71.

15. Carpinella I, Cattaneo D, Abuarqub S, Ferrarin M. Robot-based rehabilitation of the upper limbs in multiple sclerosis: feasibility and preliminary results. *J Rehabil Med* 2009;41(12):966–70.

16. Penner IK, Opwis K, Kappos L. Relation between functional brain imaging, cognitive impairment and cognitive rehabilitation in patients with multiple sclerosis. *J Neurol* 2007;254 Suppl 2:II53–7.

17. Ottenbacher K. Why rehabilitation research does not work (as well as we think it should), *Arch Phys Med Rehabil* 1995;76:123–9.

18. Sharrack B, Hughes R. Clinical scales for multiple sclerosis. *J Neuro Sci* 1996;135:1–9.

19. National Multiple Sclerosis Society.. *M.R.D. Minimal Record Of Disability For Multiple Sclerosis* New York: National Multiple Sclerosis Society, 1985.

20. Willoughby E, Paty D. Scales for rating impairment in multiple sclerosis: a critique. *Neurology* 1988;38:1793–98.

21. Freeman J, Langdon D, Hobart J, Thompson A. The impact of inpatient rehabilitation on progressive multiple sclerosis. *Ann Neurol* 1997;42:236–44.

22. Freeman J, Langdon D, Hobart J, Thompson A. Inpatient rehabilitation in multiple sclerosis: do the benefits carry over in the community? *Neurology* 1999;52:50–6.

23. Solari A, Filippini G, Gasco P, *et al*. Physical rehabilitation has a positive effect on disability in multiple sclerosis patients. *Neurology* 1999;52:57–62.

24. Grasso MG, Pace L, Troisi E, Tonini A, Paolucci S. Prognostic factors in multiple sclerosis rehabilitation. *Eur J Phys Rehabil Med* 2009;45(1):47–51.

25. Solari A, Amato M, Bergamaschi R, *et al*. Accuracy of self-assessment of the minimal record of disability in patients with multiple sclerosis. *Acta Neurol Scand* 1993;87:43–6.

26. Sharrack B, Hughes RA. The Guy's Neurological Disability Scale (GNDS): a new disability measure for multiple sclerosis. *Mult Scler* 1999;5:223–33.

27. Hobart J, Lamping D, Fitzpatrick R, Riazi A, Thompson A. The Multiple Sclerosis Impact Scale (MSIS-29): a new patient-based outcome measure. *Brain* 2001;124:962–73.

28. McGuigan C, Hutchinson M. The multiple sclerosis impact scale (MSIS-29) is a reliable and sensitive measure. *J Neurol Neurosurg Psychiatry* 2004;75:266–9.

29. Fischer J, Rudick R, Cutter G, Reingold S. The Multiple Sclerosis Functional Composite measure (MSFC): an integrated approach to MS clinical outcome assessment. *Mult Scler* 1999;5:244–50.

30. Goodman AD, Brown TR, Krupp LB, *et al*. Sustained-release oral fampridine in multiple sclerosis: a randomised, double-blind, controlled trial. *Lancet* 2009;373(9665):732–8.

31. Créange A, Serre I, Levasseur M, *et al*. Réseau SINDEFI-SEP. Walking capacities in multiple sclerosis measured by global positioning system odometer. *Mult Scler* 2007;13:220–3.

32. Goldman M, Marrie RA, Cohen JA. Evaluation of the six-minute walk in multiple sclerosis subjects and healthy controls. *Mult Scler* 2007;14:383–90.

33. Butland RJ, Pang J, Gross ER, Woodcock AA, Geddes DM. Two-, six-, and 12-minute walking tests in respiratory disease. *Br Med J (Clin Res Ed)*. 1982;284:1607–8.

34. Cattaneo D, Regola A, Meotti M. Validity of six balance disorders scales in persons with multiple sclerosis. *Disabil Rehabil* 2006;28(12):789–95.

35. McConvey J, Bennett SE. Reliability of the Dynamic Gait Index in individuals with multiple sclerosis. *Arch Phys Med Rehabil* 2005 Jan;86(1):130–3.

36. Hauser SL, Dawson DM, Lehrich JR, *et al.* Intensive immunosuppression in progressive multiple sclerosis. A randomized, three-arm study of high-dose intravenous cyclophosphamide, plasma exchange, and ACTH. *N Engl J Med* 1983;308:173–80.

37. Hobart JC, Riazi A, Lamping DL, Fitzpatrick R, Thompson AJ. Measuring the impact of MS on walking ability: the 12-Item MS Walking Scale (MSWS-12). *Neurology* 2003;60:31–6.

38. Granger C, Cotter A, Hamilton B, Fiedler R, Hens M. Functional assessment scales: a study of persons with multiple sclerosis. *Arch Phys Med Rehabil* 1990;71:870–5.

39. Hobart J, Lamping D, Freeman J, *et al.* Evidence-based measurement: which disability scale for neurologic rehabilitation? *Neurology* 2001;57:639–44.

40. Di Fabio R, Soderberg J, Choi T, Hansen C, Schapiro R. Extended outpatient rehabilitation: its influence on symptom frequency, fatigue, and functional status for persons with progressive multiple sclerosis. *Arch Phys Med Rehabil* 1998;79:141–6.

41. Freeman J, Langdon D, Hobart J, Thompson A. Health-related quality of life in people with multiple sclerosis undergoing inpatient rehabilitation. *J Neuro Rehab* 1996;10:185–94.

42. Di Fabio R, Choi T, Soderberg J, Hansen C. Health-related quality of life for patients with multiple sclerosis: influence of rehabilitation. *Phys Ther* 1997;77:1704–16.

43. Petajan J, Gappmaier E, White A, *et al.* Impact of aerobic training on fitness and quality of life in multiple sclerosis. *Ann Neurol* 1996;39:432–441.

44. Freeman J, Hobart J, Thompson A. Does adding MS-specific items to a generic measure (the SF-36) improve measurement? *Neurology* 2001;57:68–74.

45. Ponitchera-Mulcare J. Exercise and multiple sclerosis. *Med Sci Sports Exerc* 1993;25:451–65.

46. McAuley E, Motl RW, Morris KS, *et al.* Enhancing physical activity adherence and well-being in multiple sclerosis: a randomised controlled trial. *Mult Scler* 2007;13(5):652–9.

47. Marrie RA, Rudick R, Horwitz R, *et al.* Vascular comorbidity is associated with more rapid disability progression in multiple sclerosis. *Neurology* 2010;74;1041–7.

48. Dallmeijer AJ, Beckerman H, de Groot V, van de Port IG, Lankhorst GJ, Dekker J. Long-term effect of comorbidity on the course of physical functioning in patients after stroke and with multiple sclerosis. *J Rehabil Med* 2009;41(5):322–6.

49. Multiple Sclerosis Council for Clinical Practice Guidelines. *Fatigue and multiple sclerosis: evidence-based management strategies for fatigue in multiple sclerosis* (Paralyzed Veterans of America, 1998).

50. Burton JM, Bell CM, Walker SE, O'Connor PW. 4-aminopyridine toxicity with unintentional overdose in four patients with multiple sclerosis. *Neurology* 2008;71(22):1833–4.

51. Goodman AD, Cohen JA, Cross A, *et al.* Fampridine-SR in multiple sclerosis: a randomized, double-blind, placebo-controlled, dose-ranging study. *Mult Scler* 2007;13(3):357–68.

52. Schwid SR, Goodman AD, McDermott MP, *et al.* Quantitative functional measures in MS: what is a reliable change? *Neurology* 2002;58:1294–6.

53. Cattaneo D, Marazzini F, Crippa A, Cardini R. Do static or dynamic AFOs improve balance? *Clin Rehabil* 2002;16(8):894–9.

54. Sheffler LR, Hennessey MT, Knutson JS, Naples GG, Chae J. Functional effect of an ankle foot orthosis on gait in multiple sclerosis: a pilot study. *Am J Phys Med Rehabil* 2008;87(1):26–32.

55. Paul L, Rafferty D, Young S, Miller L, Mattison P, McFadyen A. The effect of functional electrical stimulation on the physiological cost of gait in people with multiple sclerosis. *Mult Scler* 2008;14(7):954–61.

56. Sutliff MH, Naft JM, Stough DK, Lee JC, Arrigain SS, Bethoux FA. Efficacy and safety of a hip flexion assist orthosis in ambulatory multiple sclerosis patients. *Arch Phys Med Rehabil* 2008;89(8):1611–17.

57. Greenspun B, Stineman M, Agri R. Multiple sclerosis and rehabilitation outcome. *Arch Phys Med Rehabil* 1987;68:434–437.

58. Khan F. Pallant JF. Brand C. Kilpatrick TJ.. Effectiveness of rehabilitation intervention in persons with multiple sclerosis: a randomised controlled trial. *J Neurol Neurosurg Psychiatry* 2008;79(11):1230–5.

59. Miller DM, Weinstock-Guttman B, Bethoux F, *et al.* A meta-analysis of Methylprednisolone in recovery from multiple sclerosis exacerbations. *Mult Scler* 2000;6:267–73.

60. Bethoux F, Miller D, Kinkel R. Recovery following acute exacerbations of multiple sclerosis: from impairment to quality of life. *Mult Scler* 2000;7:137–42.

61. Craig J, Young CA, Ennis M, Baker G, Boggild M. A randomised controlled trial comparing rehabilitation against standard therapy in multiple sclerosis patients receiving steroid treatment. *J Neurol Neurosurg Psychiatry* 2003;74:1225–30.

62. Liu C, Playford ED, Thompson AJ. Does neurorehabilitation have a role in relapsing remitting multiple sclerosis? *J Neurol* 2003;250(10):1214–18.

63. Bethoux F, Miller DM, Stough D. Efficacy of outpatient rehabilitation after exacerbations of multiple sclerosis. *Arch Phys Med Rehabil* 2005;84:A10.

64. Flavia M, Stampatori C, Zanotti D, Parrinello G, Capra R. Efficacy and specificity of intensive cognitive rehabilitation of attention and executive functions in multiple sclerosis. *J Neurol Sci* 2010;288(1–2):101–5.

65. O'Brien AR, Chiaravalloti N, Goverover Y, Deluca J. Evidenced-based cognitive rehabilitation for persons with multiple sclerosis: a review of the literature. *Arch Phys Med Rehabil* 2008;89(4):761–9.

66. Rasova K, Feys P, Henze T, *et al.* Emerging evidence-based physical rehabilitation for multiple sclerosis – towards an inventory of current content across Europe. *Health Quality of Life Outcomes* 2010;8:76.

Index